Praise for the
American Dietetic Association Complete Food and Nutrition Guide

". . . jam-packed with practical eating and food safety tips."

—USA Today

"This book will appeal to those who want to know a little bit about everything in nutrition but don't have a science background."

—Chris Rosenbloom, PhD, RD, *The Atlanta Journal-Constitution*

"Of the five books closest to my keyboard, this guide is one of the most frequently used. A dynamite resource!"

—Antonia Allegra, CCP, executive director, Symposium for Professional Food Writers; food, wine, travel author

"Bottom line, this is the best consumer nutrition book out. It's user-friendly, and it's complete. From a tidbit to a chapter, if it matters in nutrition, Roberta Duyff has included it. This book is worth its weight in gold."

—Keith Ayoob, EdD, RD, Associate Professor of Pediatrics, Albert Einstein College of Medicine, New York City

". . . this nutrition bible is a good bet. This reputable resource separates fads from facts and answers questions from apples to zucchini, allergies to vegetarian diets."

—Nancy Clark, MS, RD, *Running Network* and *Sweat* magazine

". . . turns a complicated subject into everyday practical information . . . a fun read."

—Claire Lewis, *Today's Health* and *Wellness* magazine

"Sorting out the constantly changing world of nutrition information, diets, and weight loss fads can be tricky, but this book provides all the facts in an easy-to-read format."

—Connie Diekman, MEd, RD, Director of University Nutrition, Washington University

"[A] remarkable reference."

—Graham Kerr, author, culinary expert, TV personality

American Dietetic Association Complete Food and Nutrition Guide

3RD EDITION

Roberta Larson Duyff

MS, RD, FADA, CFCS

WILEY

John Wiley & Sons, Inc.

About the ADA

The American Dietetic Association is the largest group of food and nutrition professionals in the world. As the advocate of the profession, the ADA serves the public by promoting optimal nutrition, health, and well-being.

For more information . . .

Visit the ADA's Web site at *http://www.eatright.org*. The American Dietetic Association's Web site offers nutrition information for consumers and health professionals, and the Find a Dietitian feature to locate a dietetics professional in your area. The ADA's Consumer Nutrition Information line, at (800) 366-1655, also provides referrals to local registered dietitians as well as recorded nutrition messages in English and Spanish.

Illustrations on part and chapter openers and on pages 304, 378, 380, and 398 copyright © 2002 by Jackie Aher.

Published by John Wiley & Sons, Inc., Hoboken, New Jersey
Published simultaneously in Canada

Design and production by Navta Associates, Inc.

For general information about our other products and services, please contact our Customer Care Department within the United States at (800) 762-2974, outside the United States at (317) 572-3993 or fax (317) 572-4002.

Wiley also publishes its books in a variety of electronic formats. Some content that appears in print may not be available in electronic books. For more information about Wiley products, visit our web site at www.wiley.com.

Library of Congress Cataloging-in-Publication Data:

Duyff, Roberta Larson, date.
American Dietetic Association complete food and nutrition guide / Roberta Larson Duyff.—3rd ed.
        p. cm.
    Includes bibliographical references and index.
    ISBN-13 978-0-470-04115-4 (pbk.)
    ISBN-10 0-470-04115-3 (pbk.)
    ISBN-13 978-0-470-04842-9 (cloth)
    ISBN-10 0-470-04842-5 (cloth)
    1. Nutrition—Popular works. I. Title.

RA784.D89 2007
613.2—dc22

                                                                              2006041746

Printed in the United States of America

10 9 8 7 6 5 4 3 2 1

Contents

PART VI   # Resources: More about Healthful Eating

Foreword

Food, nutrition, and physical fitness are the foundation of a healthy lifestyle in today's society. We eat to grow and develop, sustain life, and nourish our bodies, as well as to enjoy food and dining, share meals, and celebrate events. More and more, we equate certain foods and diet patterns with nutritional well-being and realize the complexities of choosing foods wisely. At the same time, however, new information is exploding on the quantity and quality of foods and nutrients needed for optimal health. Some findings may be confusing when one study seems to refute another or one food or nutrient is taken out of context of the total diet. What consumers need is a reliable source based on the best-available scientific evidence. The third edition of the *American Dietetic Association Complete Food and Nutrition Guide* is that source. Updated to reflect new research studies and government recommendations, including the 2005 Dietary Guidelines for Americans and the Dietary Reference Intakes, this comprehensive guide is the foundation of nutrition and physical activity advice for every age and stage of life.

One of the major contributions of this book is its wide and comprehensive scope. Beginning with a framework of food choices and solutions for healthful eating, this guide tackles topics important to today's consumers, including nutrition and fitness standards, the essentials of weight maintenance, being supermarket savvy, eating away from home, diets for chronic disease prevention, food allergies, dietary supplements, and kitchen safety. This guide also examines terms you may have heard, but need to know more about—terms like "discretionary calories," "energy density," "*trans* fatty acids," and "functional foods." As a practical resource, this guide includes fact-filled sidebars, tables, and questionnaires that promote a healthy lifestyle. Recipes, food tips, nutrient charts, and self-help questions keep you informed and motivated. Features like "Your Nutrition Checkup" and "Label Lingo" give this guide a consistent and easy-to-access format. It is a resource that can be consulted again and again.

Scientific evidence will continue to accumulate substantiating the link between diet and a range of chronic diseases, and the *American Dietetic Association Complete Food and Nutrition Guide* will keep you well informed with its extensive list of organizations, Web sites, and resources. Please use and savor this guide for your own health and for those in your care.

Judith A. Gilbride, PhD, RD, FADA
President, American Dietetic Association

Acknowledgments

At every phase in developing the *American Dietetic Association Complete Food and Nutrition Guide*, I've been grateful and indebted to the many professionals, colleagues, and friends—in the fields of nutrition and dietetics; health, family and consumer sciences; food science; culinary arts; education; public policy; and communications—who have shared their knowledge, experience, and expertise throughout my career, and certainly during the development of this book. I'm especially grateful to:

The American Dietetic Association, for the honor of writing this book on behalf of the association's approximately 65,000 members.

Betsy Hornick, editor and registered dietitian, on behalf of ADA Publications, for her nutrition expertise, editorial guidance, and commitment to excellence at every phase in the development of this book in all three editions . . . and for her ongoing friendship.

ADA staff for this third edition: Diana Faulhaber, Publisher, ADA Director of Book Publishing; Krisan Matthews, Editorial Assistant; and Kristen Short, Acquisition Editor, who provided the opportunity to update this consumer-focused, healthy-eating book; and to the ADA staff who previously supported the first and second editions. The ADA Knowledge Center, Sharon Denny, Eleese Cunningham, and Wendy Marcason for their assistance and review to help ensure the scientific accuracy. ADA's Marketing, Communications and Corporate Relations Team for the many promotional efforts for the book.

ADA members—with expertise as either a *registered dietitian* or a *dietetic technician, registered*—and nutrition experts who volunteered countless hours to review manuscripts for content accuracy, clarity, and comprehensiveness:

● To those who provided their unique expertise as reviewers of the second and/or third editions: Keith-Thomas Ayoob, Elizabeth Baily, Leila Beker, Susan Borra, Ann Bouchoux, Felicia Busch, Maureen Callahan, Beverly Clevidence, Sheila Cohen, Mildred Cody, Eleese Cunningham, Sharon Denny, Connie Diekman, Colleen Doyle, Robert Earl, Deborah Fillman, Susan Finn, Lorri Fishman, Julie Fulton, Molly Gee, Shelley Goldberg, Barbara Gollman, Monica Gourovitch, Patricia Harper, Laura Hatch, Dayle Hayes, Beverly Henry, Edith Hogan, Lenore Hodges, Sherri Hoyt, Barbara Ivens, Judith Jarvis, Wendy Reinhardt Kapsak, Lisa Kelly, Cynthia Kupper, Carolyn Margolis, Linda McDonald, Elaine McLaughlin, Julie O'Sullivan Maillet, Reed Mangels, Wendy Marcason, Jacqueline Marcus, Mildred Mattfeldt-Beman, Libby Mills, Farida Mohamedshah, Marlene Most, Beth Ogata, Tammie Otterstein, Anne Piatek, Christine Polisena, Linda Rhodes-Pauly, Christine Rosenbloom, Joan Rothenberg, Diane Quagliani, Allison Sarubin, Lana Shepek, Joanne Slavin, Ceci Snyder, Cathie Squatrito, Patti Steinmuller, Kim Stitzel, Cindi Thomson, Cheryl Toner, and Mary Young

● To those who reviewed the first edition: Susan Borra, Julie Burns, Mary Carey, Suzanne Havala, Dayle Hayes, Marsha Hudnall, Sue Murvich, Nancy Schwartz, Madeleine Sigman-Grant, and Ann Semenske

Sherri Hoyt, colleague and registered dietitian, for her written contributions on food sensitivity, infant and child feeding, and nutrition during pregnancy and breast-feeding for the first edition.

Dietetic students for their careful fact checking: Sehr Jangda, Adrienne Kraemer, Grace Lange, and Kristan Pierce.

Registered dietitians and other food, nutrition, and health professionals in government agencies, food industry, and educational institutions throughout the country, who served as ongoing resources and insightful experts.

Many friends and family who have reviewed the manuscript from their unique consumer and professional perspectives: Ann Hagan Brickman, Linda Carpenter, Julie Duyff, Phil Duyff, Patty Fletcher, Karen Marshall, Patricia McKissack, and Linda Valiga.

Organizations that granted permission for the use of supporting illustrations and graphics.

The fine team of editors, designers, and staff at John Wiley & Sons, including Tom Miller, Christel Winkler, Teryn Kendall, Juliet Grames, and John Simko, who handled the editing and production; the design team at Navta Associates; as well as the John Wiley publishing team for the second edition and the Chronimed Publishing team responsible for its first edition.

Edith Syrjala Eash, Diva Sanjur, and Hazel Spitze, who encouraged my early career as a registered dietitian and as an educator focused on food, nutrition, and health.

Anne Piatek, colleague and culinary dietitian, for encouraging me to write this healthful eating, science-based book for consumers and professionals.

The many readers, media representatives, and colleagues who've called this book their "bible" of nutrition from its first edition, and who've shared ideas for subsequent editions.

My family, especially my mother, Jeane Larson, and my friends, who shared their support, understanding, and encouragement—and my family, who always encouraged the pursuit of life-long learning, commitment to accuracy and a balanced viewpoint, and the joy of educating others.

My husband, Phil, who read every chapter in all three editions for clarity and consumer friendliness . . . and offered the sensitivity and loving support I needed to write this book.

To your health!

Roberta L. Duyff, MS, RD, FADA, CFCS
Author/Food and Nutrition Consultant
Duyff Associates, St. Louis, Mo.

About the Author . . . An award-winning author, national speaker, media writer, and food industry/government consultant, Roberta L. Duyff, MS, RD, FADA, CFCS, promotes the "power of positive nutrition" to consumers of all ages with practical, science-based, great-tasting ways to eat and stay active for health.

Among her books, Roberta has authored three other titles for ADA, including *365 Days of Healthy Eating from the American Dietetic Association*, as well as *Nutrition and Wellness* (a high school text) and several children's healthy eating books. She was the guiding force behind and contributor to the *American Dietetic Association Cooking Healthy Across America* cookbook as Chair of ADA's Food & Culinary Professionals Dietetic Practice Group. She has been recognized with ADA's prestigious Medallion Award for professional excellence, as an ADA Fellow, and with ADA's First Annual President's Lecture.

Unless otherwise noted, the nutrient and calorie data in this book were derived from the U.S. Department of Agriculture, Agricultural Research Service, 2005. *USDA National Nutrient Database for Standard Reference*, Release 18.

Introduction

The *American Dietetic Association Complete Food and Nutrition Guide* has been created for you as a practical, up-to-date resource for healthful eating and active living. From cover to cover, you'll see how smart eating—combined with physical activity—promotes your personal wellness. As important, you'll learn how healthful eating and flavor go hand in hand. And you'll learn how to take steps to customize healthful eating and active living choices—*for you!*

Now in its third edition, this reference for your personal health reflects the most updated, science-based advice for the American public. That includes the 2005 *Dietary Guidelines for Americans*, the fully updated Dietary Reference Intakes, and MyPyramid.

To offer *solutions* for your everyday eating dilemmas, this book is filled with practical advice—whatever your lifestyle or needs. From weight control to heart-healthy eating . . . supermarket shopping to eating out . . . food safety to kitchen nutrition . . . vegetarian eating to sports nutrition, handling food sensitivities, or other food-related health issues, you'll find many tips for ease, convenience, and good taste. Look for today's "hot" food issues, too: healthy weight, phytonutrients, foods with more benefits than from nutrients alone, dietary supplements, and food biotechnology, among others.

As your complete resource on nutrition, you can refer to this book again and again at every age and stage of your life—from choosing the healthiest baby food or feeding a child or teen, to dealing with the unique nutrition needs in a woman's life or the challenges of aging. It's also filled with advice for preventing, slowing, or dealing with heart disease, cancer, diabetes, and other common food-related health problems. This book is meant for you, and for all those you care about . . . perhaps a child, spouse, companion, aging parent, or friend.

For your personal nutrition "checkup," you'll find opportunities to assess your own everyday food choices. Start in chapter 1 with "Looking for 'Healthy Solutions'?" to identify your personal eating challenges. For more information, each question refers you to in-depth answers throughout the book. In fact, in almost every chapter, "Your Nutrition Checkup" gives you a close-up look at your own food decisions.

Whenever nutrition makes the news (print, television, radio, or online), this book can help you judge the headlines and separate sound fact from fad. Its food and nutrition advice comes from the American Dietetic Association, the authority the United States turns to for food and nutrition advice, with more than ninety years of nutrition expertise and research.

With questions posed to nutrition experts—in part through the American Dietetic Association's Knowledge Center—thousands of consumers have helped shape the focus and content of the *American Dietetic Association Complete Food and Nutrition Guide*. We hope the answers to their food and nutrition questions will also answer many of yours. And we hope you'll find practical, positive ways to take simple steps to your own and your family's good health!

Read, enjoy, be active, and eat healthy . . . for life!

Roberta Larson Duyff, MS, RD, FADA, CFCS
Author

PART I

Eat Smart, Live Well

It's about You!

CHAPTER 1

Food Choices: A Fit You!

Your life is filled with choices! Every day you make thousands of choices, many related to food. Some seem trivial. Others are important. A few may even set the course of your life. But as insignificant as a single choice may seem, made over and over, it can have a major impact on your health—and your life!

This book is about choices—those you, your family, and your friends make every day about food, nutrition, and health. Within its pages, you'll find reliable nutrition information and sound advice, based on scientific evidence. It offers you practical ways to make healthful food choices in almost any situation and at every phase of life. And it encourages you to enjoy the pleasures of food. After all, taste is the number one reason most people choose one food over another.

Most important, the practical tips and flexible guidelines on its pages help you choose nutritious, flavorful foods to match your own needs, preferences, and lifestyle—even as your life and family situation change. Eating for health is one of the wisest decisions you'll ever make!

Fitness: Your Overall Health!

What does being fit mean to you? Perhaps being free of disease and other health problems? Or having plenty of energy, a trim or muscular body, or the ability to finish a 10K run or fitness walk? Actually, "fitness" is far broader and more personal. It refers to your own *optimal health and overall well-being*. Fitness, or wellness, is your good health—at its very best.

Being fit defines every aspect of your health—not only your physical health but also your emotional and mental well-being. In fact, they're interconnected. Smart eating and active living are fundamental to all three. When you're fit, you have:

● Energy to do what's important to you and to be more productive

● Stamina and a positive outlook to handle the mental challenges and emotional ups and downs of everyday life, and to deal with stress

● Reduced risk for many health problems, including serious, often life-changing diseases, such as heart disease, cancer, diabetes, and osteoporosis

● The chance to look and feel your best

● Physical strength and endurance to protect yourself in case of an emergency

● A better chance for a higher quality of life, and perhaps a longer one, too

Fit Is Ageless

Fitness at every age and stage in life depends on healthful eating and active living. The sooner you make them your priorities, the better your health.

That, too, is what this book is all about—how to eat for health and stay physically active throughout the cycle of life, and enjoy great-tasting food along the way!

Good nutrition and regular physical activity are two lifestyle habits that promote fitness. But they are certainly not the only ones. To stay fit, make other lifestyle choices for good health, too: get adequate sleep, avoid smoking, manage stress, drink alcoholic beverages only in moderation (if you drink), wear your seat belt, observe good hygiene, get regular medical checkups, obtain adequate health care—to name a few.

Smart Eating: Fuel for Fitness

What does it take to be and to stay fit? You don't need special or costly foods, or fancy exercise equipment or a health club membership. You don't need to give up your favorite foods, or set up a tedious system of eating rules or calorie counting. And you don't need to hit a specific weight on the bathroom scale.

You've heard the term "nutrition" all your life. The food-fitness connection is what it's all about. In a

Make Healthy Choices That Fit Your Lifestyle So You Can Do The Things You Want To Do.

BE REALISTIC
Make small changes over time in what you eat and the level of activity you do. After all, small steps work better than giant leaps.

BE ADVENTUROUS
Expand your tastes to enjoy a variety of foods.

BE FLEXIBLE
Go ahead and balance what you eat and the physical activity you do over several days. No need to worry about just one meal or one day.

BE SENSIBLE
Enjoy all foods, just don't overdo it.

BE ACTIVE
Walk the dog, don't just watch the dog walk.

Source: The Dietary Guidelines Alliance, 2006; © Cattlemen's Beef Board and National Cattlemen's Beef Association.

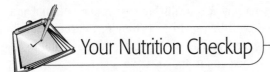

Your Nutrition Checkup

Ready for Healthier Eating?

Where do you fit on this "healthy eating" readiness test? Check one.

☐ *"My food choices are okay as they are."* Okay, but read on to find out why you might consider taking a few steps in the future to eat for better health (and perhaps move more, too).

☐ *"I'll change my eating habits sometime, but I can't make myself do it now."* Good initial thought. Check here for sensible, realistic ways to eat smarter (and move more)—but *now* rather than later. The sooner you start, the greater the benefits.

☐ *"I'm ready to eat smarter, starting now."* Good. Look through these chapters for small steps to healthful eating that you can take. As you achieve them, try a few more. Be active, too.

☐ *"I'm already a 'healthy eater.'"* Great, keep it up! Flip through the book for more practical ways to eat smart. In fact, get adventuresome with your eating. And take time for active living.

☐ *"Healthy eating and active living are second nature to me."* Excellent! Share the practical advice here and your own success with someone else!

nutshell, nutrition is how food nourishes your body. And being well nourished depends on getting enough of the nutrients your body needs—but not too much—and on keeping your weight within a healthy range.

At every stage in life, healthful eating fuels fitness. Well-nourished infants, children, and teens grow, develop, and learn better. Good nutrition helps ensure a healthy pregnancy and successful breast-feeding. Healthful eating and active living help people at any age feel their best, work productively, lower their risks for some diseases—and may even slow aging!

Today, our understanding of nutrition is based on years of scientific study. Interest in food and health actually has a long history and was even recorded by the ancient Greeks. But it wasn't until the nineteenth century that the mysteries of nutrition began to be solved. Since then, scientists have answered many nutrition questions. And research continues as they explore emerging questions about food, nutrients, and phytonutrients, and the roles they play in health.

Today we know that healthful eating along with active living are key to your healthy weight. They're essentials for dramatically lowering the risk for the main causes of disability and death in the United States: heart disease, certain cancers, type 2 diabetes, stroke, and osteoporosis. Good nutrition and regular physical activity also can lower risks for obesity, high blood pressure, and high blood cholesterol—all risk factors for serious disease.

Nutrition advice, with the consensus of today's nutrition experts, is supported by solid scientific evidence. So unlike the ancients, you have a valid basis for choosing food for health. It's up to you to apply nutrition principles and advice for your own well-being.

Smart Eating: Pleasure, Too!

Why do you choose one food over another? Besides the nutrition benefits, food is a source of pleasure, adventure, and great taste! It's no surprise that people entertain and celebrate with food, or look forward to a special dish.

Your own food choices reflect you and what's important to you: your culture, your surroundings, the people around you, your view of yourself, the foods available to you, your emotions, and certainly what you know about food and nutrition. To eat for health, you don't need to give up your food favorites. Simply learn how to fit them in. Good nutrition adds pleasure to eating—especially as you eat a greater variety of vegetables, fruits, whole-grain foods, and other nutrient-rich foods.

Throughout this book, you'll get plenty of guidance to do just that! You'll learn more about nutrition and wellness—and how you can eat foods you like, even try new foods, for eating promotes your personal fitness.

Smart Eating, Active Living: Guidelines for Americans

Healthful eating and active living: they're among your best personal investments! While your genes, age, surroundings, lifestyle, health care, and culture strongly influence your health, what *and* how much you eat and

how much you move are key to your fitness equation.

What's the secret? It's no secret at all, just solid advice. In a nutshell, most people need to eat fewer calories, be more active, and make wiser food choices.

The 2005 Dietary Guidelines for Americans reflect up-to-date scientific knowledge and advice for choosing a nutritious diet, maintaining a healthy weight, getting enough physical activity, and keeping food safe to avoid foodborne illness. By following the guidelines, you may reduce risk factors that lead to many chronic diseases.

Developed by the U.S. Department of Agriculture (USDA) and the U.S. Department of Health and Human Services (USHHS), the Dietary Guidelines present recommendations for all healthy Americans ages two and over. Updated every five years, these 2005 Dietary Guidelines offer the most current, science-based advice, reflecting what we know now. Will the guidelines be updated again? Certainly, as science answers even more food, nutrition, and health questions. Nutrition is, after all, a dynamic science: we're always learning more.

The Dietary Guidelines are based on strong scientific evidence that relates nutrition to promoting health and to lowering chronic disease risks. And they can help you meet the recommendations of the most recent Dietary Reference Intakes, *discussed later in this chapter*. An important premise: most nutrients should come from food! *For the 2005 Dietary Guidelines' key recommendations for the general population, refer to the Appendices.*

The Dietary Guidelines provide the scientific basis that underlies many nutrition initiatives: for example, for setting nutrition policies; for designing nutrition programs for infants and mothers, school food service providers, those receiving food stamps, older adults, and more; for teaching children about nutrition; and for communicating with consumers like you about sound nutrition and active living.

So, if you're not following the Dietary Guidelines' advice already, why not? And why not start now? Let's explore the nine key areas of advice from the 2005 Dietary Guidelines—and consider what they mean for your food and lifestyle choices! *You'll find the Dietary Guidelines' basics in this chapter, with much more about them throughout the book.*

Enough, but Not Too Much!

Adequate Nutrients within Calorie Needs

It's common knowledge: many Americans fall short on their nutrition report card!

Many consume more calories than they need—and too much saturated fat, *trans* fats, cholesterol, added sugars, and salt. On the flip side, both kids and adults often shortchange themselves on calcium, potassium, fiber, magnesium, and vitamin E. Many adults don't consume enough vitamins A (as carotenoids) and C, either. And others, too little vitamin B$_{12}$, folate, vitamin D, and iron.

To improve one's nutrient profile, the Dietary Guidelines advise: (1) eat a variety of nutrient-dense foods and beverages within and among the food groups (including more dark-green vegetables, orange vegetables, legumes, fruits, whole grains, and low-fat milk and milk products) and (2) limit foods with saturated fat, *trans* fats, cholesterol, added sugars, salt, and alcohol. Two tools can help you do that: MyPyramid from USDA and the Dietary Approaches to Stop Hypertension (DASH) eating plan. Both focus on what to eat—and how much.

Why variety? Different food groups—and the nutrients and other substances their foods provide—help keep you healthy in different ways. No one nutrient, food, or food group has all you need, and none works alone. Health benefits come when your overall eating plan is varied and healthful, without excessive calories.

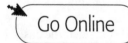 Go Online

Track *Your* Food Choices, Make *Your* "Eat Smart" Plan!

Want a snapshot view of what you eat and how much you move for a day, several days, or even weeks? Judge your meals and snacks and your physical activity online—and see how they match advice from the 2005 Dietary Guidelines. MyPyramid Tracker, an interactive tool available online at USDA's www.MyPyramid.gov, helps you assess your food choices and physical activity level. It also helps you see how well you balance the energy (calories) you consume with how much you use in physical activity.

Healthful eating is about balance, too: balancing the calories you take in with the calories you use. Get the most nutrition from your calories. Choose nutrient-dense foods (foods with substantial amounts of nutrients, yet relatively few calories). And keep calories under control as you follow nutrient and food group advice.

For more about vitamins, minerals, and phytonutrients, refer to chapter 4, with specific nutrient information for infants, children, and teens in chapters 15 and 16, and women and older adults in chapters 17 and 18. Explore MyPyramid in chapter 10 and the DASH eating plan in chapter 22.

"Weight" for Health

Weight Management

Despite known risks, overweight and obesity have become national and global epidemics, and not just for adults. Overweight among children and teens has risen dramatically within the past two decades. Key reasons? In the United States, typical eating and lifestyle patterns provide more calories (energy) than many people need: too many consumed, too few burned in physical activity.

That said, some people don't need to lose weight. Instead they need to strive to keep their healthy weight over the years or gain some if they're underweight.

Are you at your healthy weight? Appearance or fitting into a clothes size are commonly cited reasons to maintain a healthy weight. Yet, even a few pounds of excess weight may be riskier than you think. Research shows that too much body fat increases risks for high blood pressure and unhealthy blood lipid (fats) levels as well as type 2 diabetes, heart disease, stroke, gall bladder disease, breathing problems, gout, osteoarthritis, and certain cancers. Did you know that excess body weight is linked to premature death, too?

No matter what your age, pay attention to your weight. Two measures can help you judge your body fat: body mass index (BMI) and waist size. Abdominal fat has more potential health risk than body fat in other spots. (Strenuous workouts build muscle; extra weight from muscle isn't a problem.) What's your "measure" of fitness? *Check chapter 2 to learn how to find out.*

As an adult, set your goal on achieving or keeping

a weight that's healthy for you. Your calorie needs decrease gradually over time. To combat "weight creep" over time, slowly cut back on your food and beverage calories and move more. If you are over-weight and need to drop a few pounds, aim for slow, steady weight loss. Cut your calories, but keep your nutrient intake adequate—and move! And if you have a health problem or take medication, check with your healthcare provider before starting.

The chance of becoming overweight or obese as adults declines when children and teens keep their healthy weight as they grow. The advice for kids who are mild to moderately overweight: help them slow or prevent continued weight gain so they can grow and develop normally. More active play, fewer sit-down activities (TV, video and computer games), and healthful eating are their best strategies.

At any age, a healthy weight is key to a long, healthy, and productive life. The smart way to a healthy weight range is all about balance: calories from food and drinks balanced with calories used. To eat fewer calories, go easy on added sugars, fats, and alcoholic drinks, and choose sensible portions. Keep physically active, too.

For more about weight management, refer to chapter 2. For specific Dietary Guidelines' advice on healthy weight for children, pregnant and breast-feeding women, and those with chronic disease, check chapters 16, 17, and 22.

Move It!

Physical Activity

Wellness takes more than healthful eating! Regular physical activity promotes health, a sense of well-being, and healthy weight. Yet most Americans don't get enough.

For adults, at least 30 minutes of moderately intense physical activity on most days reduces chronic disease risks. If you move longer or with more vigor, you get even more benefits. Sixty minutes of moderate to vigorous activity on most days helps prevent gradual, unhealthy weight gain that may come with adulthood. Need to lose weight during your adult years? You may need 60 to 90 minutes of moderate activity daily. Children and teens need at least 60 minutes on most, if not all, days of the week. *Refer to "Moderate Activity: What Is It?" in this chapter.*

Get active . . . stay active . . . become more active. Spread out your activity, or do it all at once; either way you get benefits. If you have been inactive, start gradually. Work up to longer, more intense activities.

For overall fitness, fit in a variety of activities:

● *For flexibility*, try stretching, yoga, and dancing.

● *For strength*, try weight-bearing activities (walking, tennis) for bone strength, and resistance exercise, such as carrying groceries or weight lifting, to build muscles.

● *For cardiovascular fitness*, try aerobic activities (running, distance biking) that increase your heart rate and breathing.

Unless you have a health problem, you probably can start moving more now! Talk to your healthcare provider first if you have an ongoing health problem—including heart disease, high blood pressure, diabetes, osteoporosis, arthritis, or obesity—or if you're at high risk for heart disease. Men over age forty and women over age fifty need to check with their doctor, too, if they plan vigorous physical activity, have risk factors for chronic disease, or have health problems. *For Dietary Guidelines' advice on physical activity for pregnant and breast-feeding women and for older adults, refer to chapters 17 and 18.*

Fruits, Veggies, Whole Grains, Milk—Priorities!

Food Groups to Encourage

Eating a variety of nutrient-packed foods every day is basic to good nutrition and health! Today we know

Have You Ever Wondered

. . . if your exercise level is of moderate intensity? Take the "talk-sing" test to find out. If you can talk comfortably as you move, that's moderate activity. If you're too breathless to talk, that activity may be vigorous. If your goal is moderate activity, you might need to slow down. (Remember: Vigorous activity has added benefits.) And if you can sing, that's light-intensity activity; step up your pace! *For another way to target your workout intensity, refer to "Your Physical Activity: How Intense?" in chapter 19.*

MODERATE ACTIVITY: WHAT IS IT?

If some activities use more energy than others, you may wonder . . . just what does "moderate physical activity" really mean? It equates to the energy you need to walk 2 miles in 30 minutes.

Moderate physical activity uses about 3½ to 7 calories a minute, 150 calories a day, or about 1,000 calories a week. For that amount of energy expenditure, you might spend more time on less vigorous activities, such as brisk walking, or spend less time on more vigorous activities, such as running.

COMMON CHORES	DURATION	*Less Vigorous, More Time**	SPORTING ACTIVITIES	DURATION
Washing and waxing a car	45–60 min.	↑	Playing volleyball	45 min.
Washing windows or floors	15–60 min.		Playing touch football	30–45 min.
Gardening	30–45 min.		Walking 1¾ miles (20 min./mile)	35 min
Wheeling self in wheelchair	30–40 min.		Basketball (shooting baskets)	30 min.
Pushing a stroller 1½ miles	30 min.		Bicycling 5 miles	30 min.
Raking leaves	30 min.		Dancing fast (social)	30 min.
Walking 2 miles (15 min./mile)	30 min.		Water aerobics	30 min.
Shoveling snow	15 min.	↓	Swimming laps	20 min.
Stairwalking	15 min.	*More Vigorous, Less Time*	Basketball (playing a game)	15–20 min.
			Jumping rope	15 min.
			Running 1½ miles (15 min./mile)	15–20 min.

* Some activities can be performed at various intensities. The suggested durations correspond to the expected intensity of effort.

Source: Practical Guide to the Identification, Evaluation and Treatment of Overweight and Obesity in Adults, National Institutes of Health, 2001.

much more about health-promoting nutrients found in these nourishing foods.

That means making fruits, vegetables, whole grains, and fat-free and low-fat milk and milk products a personal priority. Eat more of these nutrient-rich foods while you keep your calories under control—and your chances of developing chronic diseases, such as heart disease, stroke, type 2 diabetes, some cancers, and osteoporosis, likely will go down.

Fruits and vegetables . . . Despite their health benefits, many people don't consume enough. Yet, whether they're fresh, frozen, canned, or dried, fruits and vegetables are the major sources of several vitamins and minerals, including vitamins A (as carotenoids) and C, folate, and potassium. And they deliver fiber and other phytonutrients with potential health-promoting qualities.

Exercise Your Options

For more about the benefits of physical activity—and ways to be more physically active—check here:

- *For most healthy people, including those managing their body weight* . . . "Get Physical!" in chapter 2.
- *For children* . . . "Get Up and Move!" in chapter 16.
- *For teens* . . . "Move Your 'Bod'" in chapter 16.
- *For older adults* . . . "Never Too Late for Exercise" in chapter 18.
- *For travelers* . . . "When You're on the Road" in chapter 19.
- *For athletes* . . . "Athlete's Guide: Winning Nutrition" in chapter 19.

Ten Reasons to Make the "Right Moves"

Whether you're involved in sports or simply live an active lifestyle, physical activity pays big dividends. Physical activity is the "right move" for fitness—for almost everyone, not just for athletes. Consider just a few reasons why:

1. *Trimmer body.* If you're physically active, you'll have an easier time maintaining a healthy weight, or losing weight and keeping it off if you're overweight. *For more about physical activity for weight management, refer to chapter 2, "Your Healthy Weight."*

2. *Less risk for health problems.* An active lifestyle—or a sports regimen—can help protect you from many ongoing health problems.

   Studies show that regular physical activity helps lower risk factors. For example, physical activity lowers total and LDL ("bad") cholesterol and triglyceride levels while boosting the HDL ("good") cholesterol level, controls blood pressure, and improves blood sugar levels. Your risks for heart disease, high blood pressure, type 2 diabetes, and certain cancers go down when you fit physical activity into your daily life.

   Active living may also reduce or eliminate the need for medication to lower blood lipids, lower blood pressure, or manage diabetes.

3. *Stronger bones.* Regular, weight-bearing activities—such as walking, running, weight lifting, and cross-country skiing—help make your bones stronger. Even in adulthood, weight-bearing exercise helps maintain your bone strength and reduce your chance of fractures and osteoporosis.

4. *Stronger muscles.* Strength-training activities, such as lifting weights, at least two times a week, keep your body strong for sports and everyday living. When you're strong, it's easier to move, carry, and lift things. When you exercise your muscles, you also give your heart a workout. It's a muscle, too. A strong heart pumps blood and nutrients more easily through your 60,000 miles of blood vessels.

5. *More endurance.* You won't tire as easily when you're physically active. And you may have more stamina during the rest of the day, too.

6. *Better mental outlook.* Active people describe feelings of psychological well-being and self-esteem when they make active living a habit. It's a great way to reinforce that "can do" attitude and positive outlook.

7. *Stress relief and better sleep.* Research shows that physical activity helps your body relax and release emotional tension. That promotes longer, better-quality sleep, and you may fall asleep faster.

8. *Better coordination and flexibility.* Your body moves with greater ease and range of motion when you stay physically active.

9. *Injury protection.* When you're in shape, you more easily can catch yourself if you slip or trip . . . and can move away from impending danger more quickly.

10. *Feel younger longer.* Research suggests that physical activity slows some effects of aging. Active people have more strength and mobility, and fewer limitations.

The nutritional content of fruits and veggies differs, so vary your choices. Choose dark-green, orange, starchy vegetables, legumes (dry beans), and other vegetables several times weekly. How much? If you need 2,000 calories a day, the advice is 2 cups of fruit and 2½ cups of vegetables daily. Adjust the amount slightly if you need more or fewer calories. *Check the Appendices for the right amount for you.*

Whole grains . . . While most people eat enough grain products overall, few consume enough whole grains. The Dietary Guidelines now advise: make at least half your grains whole. What are whole grains?

They're foods made from the entire grain kernel, which includes the fiber-rich bran and germ, and the endosperm. Refined grains contain mostly the endosperm.

Why emphasize whole grains? They're important sources of fiber (typically underconsumed), other phytonutrients, and some key vitamins and minerals. Eating three or more one-ounce equivalents of whole-grain foods daily may lower your chances for some chronic diseases and may help you manage your weight, too.

If at least half of your grains are whole, what about

Source: www.MyPyramid.gov.

the other half? Make them enriched or whole grain, too. Enriched grain products are fortified with certain B vitamins and iron to replace those lost when grains are refined. They're also fortified with folic acid; whole grains may or may not be. *Refer to chapters 5 and 6 for more about whole-grain foods.*

Dairy foods . . . Calcium-rich dairy foods have many health benefits, including bone health. Yet dairy foods often come up short for children, teens, and even adults. The Dietary Guidelines advise: each day consume 3 cups of fat-free or low-fat milk or the equivalent in other milk products, such as low-fat yogurt or low-fat cheese. If you don't or can't drink milk, try lactose-free milk products and/or calcium-fortified foods and beverages.

For more about all five food groups and how to plan healthful meals and snacks, learn about MyPyramid in chapter 10 and the DASH eating plan in chapter 22. Check chapter 16 for specific advice for children and teens.

Know Your Limits

Fats

Fat is a nutrient, essential for your health—and for children's growth. Besides supplying energy, it contains essential fatty acids and carries some fat-soluble vita-

mins (A, D, E, and K) and carotenoids (phytonutrients) into your bloodstream. Fat helps you stay healthy in other ways, too. Yet, it's well known that too much saturated fat, *trans* fats, and cholesterol are linked to a higher risk for unhealthy levels of blood cholesterol and for heart disease. High-fat diets tend to be high in saturated fats and excess calories.

Although many people consume less total fat, saturated fat, and cholesterol than a decade ago, many Americans still consume too much. For health, eating less than 10 percent of your calories from saturated fat and less than 300 milligrams of cholesterol per day are goals to strive for. Keep *trans* fatty acids as low as possible. Limit your total fat intake to 20 to 35 percent of your calories (energy). And get most of your fat from foods such as fish, nuts, and vegetable oils, which contain mostly heart-healthy polyunsaturated and monounsaturated fatty acids. *Dietary Guidelines for fat are somewhat different for children and teens; refer to chapter 16.*

On the flip side, an eating pattern that's too low in fats and oils, with less than 20 percent of calories from fat, isn't healthful either. It's likely low in vitamin E and essential fatty acids. When dietary fat levels dip below 20 percent, blood levels of HDL (good) cholesterol and triglycerides often change in an unhealthy way.

Among the fat-savvy guidelines: learn to choose and prepare lean meat, fish, and poultry; low-fat and fat-free foods, such as milk and milk products; and dry beans. You'll learn how in this book. *For more about fat, saturated fat,* trans *fats, and cholesterol in a healthful eating plan, refer to "Fat Facts," chapter 3.*

Make Your Calories Count!

Carbohydrates

It's true that carbohydrates are important for healthful eating. Two forms of carbohydrates—sugars and starches—are your body's main energy sources. Fiber, a nondigestible carbohydrate, has other health benefits. A high-fiber eating plan can lower your risk for heart disease and help keep your gastrointestinal tract healthy. And a new research area explores the link between fiber and lower risk for type 2 diabetes.

What foods have "carbs"? Fruits, vegetables, grain products, and milk—all nutrient-rich—contain carbohydrates naturally. Fruits and dairy foods, for example, have natural sugars. Grain products, vegetables, and fruits contain starches (complex carbohydrates) that break down into sugars during digestion. In many processed and prepared foods and drinks, sugars are added for flavor and function. To the human body, sugars look and act alike, regardless of their sources.

Yet, it's important to choose your "carbs" wisely! The Dietary Guidelines advise: choose fiber-rich fruits, vegetables, and whole grains often because they're nutrient-rich! Enjoy mostly whole fruit, which has more fiber, rather than fruit juice. Fit in legumes (dry beans and peas) several times weekly. And make at least half your grain choices whole.

Added sugars supply calories, but few nutrients. Notes the *Report of the Dietary Guidelines Advisory Committee on the Dietary Guidelines for Americans 2005*: those who consume a lot of added sugars from food or drinks tend to take in more calories and fewer vitamins and minerals. And there's a likely link between drinking sugary drinks and weight gain. To get enough nutrients and reduce calories, choose and prepare foods and beverages with little added sugars.

How do you know which foods and drinks have added sugars? Check the ingredient list on food labels. Be aware, Nutrition Facts list only amounts of total carbohydrates and total sugars, not added sugars. *Chapter 11 gives label reading tips.*

What about tooth decay? Both sugars and starches contribute to decay. For a healthy smile, brush and floss regularly and consume foods and drinks with sugars or starches less frequently. Drinking fluoridated water helps prevent decay, too; most bottled water isn't fluoridated.

For more about "carbs," refer to chapters 5 and 6.

Check the Nutrition Facts!

Sodium and Potassium

Salt is a combination of two nutrients: sodium and chloride, which help your body regulate fluids and blood pressure. Sodium itself is naturally present in many foods—and so is potassium. So why have Dietary Guidelines's advice for sodium and potassium?

Most Americans consume much more sodium than they need. For many people, the higher their salt intake, the higher their blood pressure. High blood pressure, in turn, increases the risk for heart disease, stroke, heart attacks, and kidney disease. During their lifetime, many Americans will develop high blood pressure. That said, a potassium-rich eating pattern helps counteract the effects of sodium on blood pressure.

Advice for most people: consume less than 2,300 mg (approximately 1 teaspoon of salt) of sodium daily. For those with high blood pressure, African Americans, and middle-aged and older adults, try to limit sodium intake to 1,500 milligrams daily, while consuming 4,700 milligrams of potassium from food. This is wise advice for healthy people, too, who may not know if their blood pressure is sodium-sensitive.

What's the main source of sodium and potassium? Food itself. For sodium, it's mostly from processed food, not the salt shaker. And for potassium, from many fruits and vegetables.

To lower the risk for high blood pressure or delay its onset if you're sodium-sensitive, the general advice is to go easy on salt (and sodium) and consume more potassium. Choose and prepare foods with little salt. Use Nutrition Facts on food labels to find foods with less sodium and more potassium. And consume plenty of potassium-rich foods, such as fruits and vegetables. *For more about salt, sodium, and potassium in a healthful eating plan, refer to chapters 4 and 7.*

Go Easy, If at All

Alcoholic Beverages

Do you enjoy an occasional drink? If so, drink alcoholic beverages only in moderation. That means up to one drink a day for women and two for men. A drink is 12 ounces of beer, 5 ounces of wine, or 1.5 ounces of 80-proof distilled spirits.

On their own, alcoholic beverages offer calories but essentially no nutrients, so they don't nourish your body. In fact, calories from heavy drinking make it difficult to get enough nutrients without overdoing your calorie budget: a potential weight problem. When calories from alcohol replace those from nutritious food and beverages, the risk for poor nutrition goes up—especially for heavy drinkers.

Moderate drinking for middle-aged and older adults (not younger adults) may have some health benefits, perhaps lowering the risk for heart disease.

Generally speaking, more than moderate drinking isn't advised. What are the risks? Too much alcohol impairs judgment, which can lead to accidents and injury, and perhaps to dependency and addiction for some. Excessive drinking is linked to serious health problems, including some liver and pancreatic diseases, damage to the heart and the brain, and, during pregnancy, to a greater likelihood of mental retardation, birth defects, and behavioral and psychosocial problems for the baby.

Can moderate drinking be an issue? Perhaps for some. Heavy drinking is linked to higher chances of accidents and injuries, high blood pressure, stroke, certain cancers, violence, and suicide. During pregnancy moderate drinking may increase the risks for behavioral and developmental problems for the child. And as little as one drink a day may slightly increase a woman's risk for breast cancer.

When should you avoid drinking? Whenever you put yourself and others at risk! Don't drink at all . . . *if* you can't control your drinking, *if* you're a child or teen, *if* you plan to work with equipment that takes attention, skill, or coordination, *if* you plan to drive or operate machinery, *if* you're taking medications that may interact with alcohol, *if* you have certain medical conditions, or *if* you're pregnant, trying to become pregnant, or breast-feeding.

For more about alcoholic beverages and advice for consuming them, refer to "Alcoholic Beverages: In Moderation" in chapter 8.

For Your Health's Sake

Food Safety

Healthful eating is about more than *what* you eat; it's also about *how* you keep food safe from harmful bacteria and viruses (the biggest food safety problem), chemicals, and other contaminants. Foodborne illness strikes millions of Americans each year, causing mild to severe, even life-threatening symptoms. The effects may last a few hours or days, or for weeks, months, or years. Young children, pregnant women, older

adults, and those with weakened immune systems or some chronic diseases are especially vulnerable.

Keeping food safe is up to you, not just the responsibility of farmers, food manufacturers, retailers, and restaurant workers. Many cases of foodborne illness could be avoided if consumers handled food carefully: keep food clean; cook it to safe internal temperatures; separate raw, cooked, and ready-to-eat foods; chill perishable foods promptly; and defrost properly.

Refer to chapter 12 for an in-depth look at foodborne illness and how to keep food safe and healthful. You'll also find specific Dietary Guidelines's advice on food safety for infants, young children, pregnant women, older adults, and those with impaired immunity.

Your Food Choices: The Inside Story

While you enjoy the sensual qualities of food—the mouth-watering appearance, aroma, texture, and flavor—your body relies on the life-sustaining functions that nutrients in food perform. Other food substances, including phytonutrients (or plant substances), appear to offer even more heath benefits beyond nourishment. What's inside your food?

Nutrients—Classified Information

Your body can't make most nutrients from food, or produce energy, without several key nutrients. You need a varied, adequate supply of nutrients from food for your nourishment—and life itself.

Your food choices are digested, or broken down into nutrients, then absorbed into your bloodstream and carried to every cell of your body. Most of the body's work takes place in cells, and food's nutrients are essential to your body's "do list." More than forty nutrients in food, classified into six groups, have specific and unique functions for nourishment. Their work is linked in partnerships for your good health.

Carbohydrates. As your body's main source of energy, or calories, carbohydrates are starches (complex carbohydrates) and sugars. *Chapter 5, "Carbs: Simply Complex," addresses them.*

Fiber, another form of complex carbohydrate, aids

digestion, promotes health, and offers protection from some diseases. Despite its role in health, fiber isn't a nutrient because it is not digested and absorbed into the body. *See chapter 6, "Fiber: Your Body's Broom."*

Fats. Fats supply energy. They support other functions, too, such as nutrient transport, growth, and being part of many body cells. Fats are made of varying combinations of fatty acids. All fatty acids aren't the same. Some are more saturated (harder at room temperature); others, more unsaturated. Fatty acids that your body can't make are considered "essential." *You'll learn about fat and cholesterol (a fatlike substance) in chapter 3.*

Proteins. Proteins are sequenced combinations of amino acids, which build, repair, and maintain all your body tissues. Your body makes nonessential amino acids; others are considered "essential" from food because your body can't make them. Especially when carbohydrates and fats are in short supply, proteins provide energy. If they're broken down and used for energy, amino acids can't be used to maintain body tissue. *For more about amino acids, refer to chapter 20, "The Vegetarian Way."*

Vitamins. Vitamins work like spark plugs, triggering chemical reactions in body cells. Each vitamin regulates different body processes. Because their roles are so specific, one cannot replace another. *To learn more, refer to chapter 4, "Vitamins, Minerals, Phytonutrients: Variety on Your Plate."*

Minerals. Somewhat like vitamins do, minerals spark body processes. They, too, have unique job descriptions. *Refer to chapter 4.*

Water. Water makes up 45 to 75 percent of your body weight—and it's a nutrient, too. It regulates body processes, helps regulate your body temperature, carries nutrients and other body chemicals to your cells, and carries waste products away. *For more about water, see chapter 8, "Fluids: The Power of Water."*

Nutrients: How Much?

Everyone around you needs the same nutrients—just in different amounts. Why differences? For healthy people, age, gender, and body size are among the reasons. Children and teenagers, for example, need more

Feel Better Today, Stay Healthy for Tomorrow

Here's what the Dietary Guidelines advise. *Tip:* MyPyramid offers easy steps to get there!

● *Make smart choices from every food group* . . . in an eating plan that emphasizes fruits, vegetables, whole grains, and fat-free or low-fat milk and milk products, that includes lean meat, poultry, fish, beans, eggs, and nuts, and that's low in saturated fats, *trans* fats, cholesterol, salt (sodium), and added sugars.

● *Find your balance between food and physical activity* . . . by balancing the calories you take in from food with the calories you spend each day.

● *Get the most nutrition out of your calories* . . . by choosing nutrient-rich foods (foods with more nutrients and fewer calories) from each food group every day. Pick fruits, vegetables, whole grains, and fat-free or low-fat milk and milk products more often.

Source: Based on 2005 Dietary Guidelines for Americans.

of some nutrients for growth. Pregnancy and breastfeeding increase the need for some nutrients, too, and for food energy. Because their bodies are typically larger, men often need more of most nutrients than women do.

How much of each nutrient do you need? Dietary Reference Intakes (DRIs), established by the Food and Nutrition Board of the Institute of Medicine, National Academy of Sciences, include daily nutrient recommendations for healthy people in the United States and Canada, based on age and gender. The DRIs include four types of recommendations:

● *Recommended Dietary Allowances (RDAs)* are recommended levels of nutrients that meet the needs of almost all healthy individuals in specific age and gender groups. Consider this advice as your goals.

● *Adequate Intakes (AIs)* are similar in meaning to RDAs. They're used as guidelines for some nutrients that don't have enough scientific evidence to set firm RDAs.

● *Tolerable Upper Intake Levels (ULs)* aren't recommended amounts. In fact, there's no scientific consensus for recommending nutrient levels higher than the RDAs to most healthy people. Instead, ULs represent the maximum intake that probably won't pose risks for health problems for almost all healthy people in a specific age and gender group.

● *Estimated Average Requirement (EAR)* is used to assess groups of people, not individuals.

For carbohydrates, fats, and proteins (all macronutrients), which supply calories (energy), you might also see an *Acceptable Macronutrient Distribution Range (AMDR)*. That range not only reflects what's enough. It's also the amount linked to reduced chronic disease risk. Consuming more than the AMDR may increase the risks for certain chronic diseases and/or for coming up short on essential nutrients.

Groups of experts regularly review the DRIs, using the most current research evidence, and update the dietary recommendations. *A listing of the DRIs appears in the Appendices.*

How do you use the DRIs? For the most part, you don't need to add up the numbers; it takes considerable effort to calculate the nutrients in all your food choices, then make an assessment with DRIs. If you choose to do that, remember, however, that the recommendations—RDAs and AIs—apply to your average nutrient intake over several days, not just one day and certainly not one meal.

More Than Nutrients: Foods' Functional Components

Food contains much more than nutrients! Science is beginning to uncover the benefits of other substances in food: phytonutrients (including fiber), omega fatty acids, conjugated linoleic acid, and pre- and probiotics, to name a few. Described as "functional," these substances do more than nourish you. They appear to promote your health and protect you from health risks related to many major health problems, including heart disease, some cancers, diabetes, and macular degeneration, among others.

At least for now, no DRIs exist for the functional components in food, except for fiber. And scientists don't yet fully understand their roles in health. However, within this book, you'll get a glimpse of emerging knowledge about functional substances in food. You're bound to hear more, as new studies about functional substances in food unfold.

Healthful Eating, Active Living: One Step at a Time!

The sooner you invest in your health, the greater the benefit! If you're ready to eat smarter or move more, use these goal-setting steps to invest in your health and the health of your family, one easy step at a time.

Audit your food choices and lifestyle. Start by keeping track of what you eat or drink, along with how much, when, and why; for example, do you snack when you feel stressed or bored? Use a food log to pinpoint eating behaviors you want to change. *Refer to "Dear Diary . . ." in chapter 2 for tips on keeping a food log, or use MyPyramid Tracker described earlier. Take the personal assessments in "Your Nutrition Checkup" throughout the book.*

Set personal goals. Know what you want—perhaps a healthier weight or lower cholesterol levels. And be realistic. Change doesn't mean giving up a food you like. However, smaller portions, different ways of cooking, or being more physically active give you more "wiggle room" to occasionally enjoy foods with more calories.

Make a plan for change. Divide big goals, such as "I will eat better," into smaller, more specific goals, such as "I will eat more vegetables." List practical steps to achieve your goals. For example:

Goal: Eat more whole-grain foods.

Steps: Make sandwiches and French toast with whole-grain bread. Switch to brown rice. Eat oatmeal or oat flakes for breakfast. Snack on plain popcorn. Add whole barley to vegetable soups.

Be patient. Make gradual changes. Change for the long run takes time, commitment, and encouragement. Most health goals take a lifelong commitment. Stick with your plan, even if success takes time. Remember that small steps toward reaching a goal add up over time!

Monitor your progress. If you get off track, pick up where you left off, and start again. You can do it!

Seek help from a qualified health professional. A registered dietitian can help on your fitness journey.

Reward yourself. Change is hard work that deserves recognition. Pat yourself on the back with a bike ride, a walk with a friend, a new CD, or a new outfit. Feeling good is the best reward!

Reevaluate your plan every month or two. See how changes you made—the simple steps you took—fit with your goals. You may even tackle a new goal!

Looking for "Healthy Solutions"?

Looking for a practical approach to sound nutrition? Check here for sensible, easy solutions to eat for fitness. Some advice is meant for you; other advice may apply to family members or friends.

Do you ...	Yes or no?	For "Healthy Solutions," check here ...
Feel confused by nutrition news and advice?	☐ Yes ☐ No	*Chapter 24, "Well Informed?,"* to decipher today's and tomorrow's news about food and health. (The whole book translates what's known about nutrients, phytonutrients, and health into smart eating.)
Get frustrated trying to control your weight?	☐ Yes ☐ No	*Chapter 2, "Your Healthy Weight,"* to find a way to your healthy weight that works—and sort through diets that don't.
Wonder what to drink when you're thirsty, and even when you're not?	☐ Yes ☐ No	*Chapter 8, "Fluids: The Power of Water,"* to decide what to drink and how much.
Think you need to give up foods you enjoy to eat healthy?	☐ Yes ☐ No	*Chapter 10, "Planning to Eat Smart,"* to see how you can enjoy *any* food and still eat for your good health!
Feel life's just too hectic to eat healthy?	☐ Yes ☐ No	*Chapter 10, "Planning to Eat Smart,"* to find quick, healthful, easy meals and snacks when you're tight on time.
Wonder how to devise a personal, customized plan for healthful eating—one that's just right for you?	☐ Yes ☐ No	*Chapter 10, "Planning to Eat Smart,"* for tips on creating your own individualized food plan—based on your own calorie needs—for what to eat and how much!
Feel overwhelmed by all the food choices in the supermarket?	☐ Yes ☐ No	*Chapter 9, "What's on Today's Table,"* to keep updated on today's "new" foods (functional, health-positioned, organic, ethnic, others), food regulations, and food biotechnology. *Chapter 11, "Savvy Shopping,"* to shop easily for taste, convenience—and good health.
Wonder if the "bug" you caught might be foodborne illness?	☐ Yes ☐ No	*Chapter 12, "The Safe Kitchen,"* for essential ways to keep your food safe for you to eat.

Looking for "Healthy Solutions"? *(continued)*

Do you ...	Yes or No?	For "Healthy Solutions," check here ...
Think healthful cooking takes too much effort?	☐ Yes ☐ No	*Chapter 13, "Kitchen Nutrition: Delicious Decisions,"* for simple ways to healthier food "prep"—for *more* vegetables, fruits, whole grains, fiber, and calcium, *fewer* calories, *less* saturated fats and *trans* fats, salt, and added sugars, and *more.*
Think eating out a lot keeps you from eating right?	☐ Yes ☐ No	*Chapter 14, "Your Food Away from Home,"* to eat out (fast food, ethnic food, sit-down food) your way—and enjoy it, too!
Feel unsure if you're feeding your kids right?	☐ Yes ☐ No	*Chapter 15, "Off to a Healthy Start,"* for baby-feeding basics. *Chapter 16, "Food to Grow On,"* for strategies that work for helping your child or teen learn to eat for their good health—now and in the long run.
Know that women have some special nutrition issues, but not know what they are?	☐ Yes ☐ No	*Chapter 17, "For Women Only,"* for sound eating advice for pregnancy, breast-feeding, menopause, and more.
Want to slow down the aging process?	☐ Yes ☐ No	*Chapter 18, "For Mature Adults: Healthful Eating!"* for smart eating if you're age "fifty plus" or if you're caring for someone that age. (Check this whole book, too.)
Want to "max" your sports performance?	☐ Yes ☐ No	*Chapter 19, "Athlete's Guide: Winning Nutrition,"* for ways to eat for your physical best: before, during, and after a workout.
Feel uncertain about your own (or your teen's) approach to vegetarian eating?	☐ Yes ☐ No	*Chapter 20, "The Vegetarian Way,"* for practical advice, no matter what your approach to vegetarian eating.
Think you have a food allergy or other food sensitivity?	☐ Yes ☐ No	*Chapter 21, "Sensitive about Food,"* to deal with lactose intolerance, a food allergy, or other food sensitivities.
Need help to reduce your risks for—or deal with—specific health problems?	☐ Yes ☐ No	*Chapter 22, "Smart Eating to Prevent and Manage Disease,"* for the healthful eating basics for common health problems—heart disease, diabetes, cancer, and osteoporosis, among others. (This book also is filled with tips!)
Think you need a nutrient or an herbal supplement, but you're not sure what—*and if*?	☐ Yes ☐ No	*Chapter 23, "Dietary Supplement: Use and Abuse,"* to sort through smart advice and misinformation about supplements.

Every "yes" is one more reason to use this book as your healthy eating resource!

PART II

Healthful Eating
The Basics

CHAPTER 2

Your Healthy Weight

We often take it for granted, but good health is one of the most precious gifts of life. A healthy weight—maintained throughout life—helps you achieve good health in many ways: look your best, feel your best, and reduce your risk for many serious and ongoing diseases.

What is a healthy weight? It's the weight that's best for you—not necessarily the lowest weight you think you can be. A healthy weight actually is a range that's statistically related to good health. Being above or below that range increases the risk of health problems, or decreases the likelihood of good health.

The smart approach to your best weight is really no secret—only common sense. A healthful lifestyle, with regular physical activity and an eating pattern chosen for variety, balance, and moderation, makes all the difference. Maintaining a healthy weight throughout life is best for health. Do you need to be "everyday perfect"? No. Just try to manage your weight by eating smart and living actively most of the time.

Body Basics: What's Your Healthy Weight?

The answer isn't as simple as stepping onto a bathroom scale, then comparing your weight to a chart. Your own healthy weight is one that's right for you. It may be quite different from someone else's weight, even if you are the same height, gender, and age.

What makes the difference? Your genetic makeup plays a role because it determines your height and the size and shape of your body frame. A genetic link to body fat also may exist. Of course, genetics isn't the only reason why weight differs from person to person. Your metabolic rate, the rate at which your body burns energy, makes a difference. So does your body composition. Muscle burns more calories than body fat does. Your level of physical activity and what you eat both play an important role, too.

So what's your healthy weight? That depends. Determining your right weight takes several things into account: (1) your body mass index, or your weight in relation to your height; (2) the location and amount of body fat you have; and (3) your overall health and risks for weight-related problems such as diabetes or high blood pressure.

Body Mass Index: Fit or Fat?

Body mass index (BMI) is a number based on body weight in relation to your height that indicates how much your weight affects your risks for weight-related health problems. It doesn't directly measure body fat. For adults, there's no difference in BMI weight ranges for age; health risks appear to be the same, regardless of age. The same chart applies to men and women.

The generous BMI range of healthy weights allows for individual differences. Higher weights within the healthy range typically apply to people with more muscle and a larger frame, such as many men and some women. After all, muscle and bone weigh more than fat. Gaining or losing weight within these ranges isn't necessarily healthful for you.

People with a higher percentage of body fat tend to have a higher BMI than those who have a greater percentage of muscle. Carrying excess body fat puts you at greater risk for health problems such as heart disease, diabetes, certain cancers, and high blood pressure. The higher your BMI, the greater your risk.

What's Your BMI?

Calculate your BMI: (1) Multiply your weight in pounds times 703. (2) Divide that by your height in inches. (3) Divide that by your height in inches again! Or skip the calculations; *check the BMI chart on page 23 or in the Appendices.*

Right for You: Fit at Any Size

Healthy people come in many sizes and shapes: tall or short, stocky or lanky, muscular or not. These differences are a unique part of being human. For this reason, there's no such thing as a "perfect body," or an ideal body weight, shape, or size that everyone should strive for. The most important thing is being healthy, so you can enjoy a healthful life with the body you have.

Likewise, losing weight, or maintaining a healthy weight, is easier for some than others—in spite of their commitment to healthful eating and physical activity. That, too, helps make each of us unique.

Regardless of your size and shape, you can choose a healthful lifestyle—and so live a fuller, more productive life and reduce your risk for health problems:

- Assess your own health habits. Make choices for good health with yourself in mind.
- Be active—no matter what your body size. Start by doing what you can do, anything that gets you moving, even for a few minutes for starters.
- Eat for health with a sensible approach. *See chapter 10.*
- Get regular physical checkups.
- Monitor your "numbers" (blood cholesterol, triglycerides, blood pressure, fasting blood sugar levels). Keep them within a healthy range. *See page 543 for normal levels.*
- Make your goal your personal healthy weight, not some unattainable goal!

Energy in Balance!

There's nothing magical about controlling weight! Dietary Guidelines advise: *To maintain weight in a healthy range, balance calories from foods and beverages with calories expended.* In other words, let calories in equal calories out. Otherwise, you gain or lose weight.

The amount of calories you can consume to match your body's energy (calorie) expenditure is your energy allowance. Think of it as a calorie budget. How do you want to "spend" those calories? If you need to lose or gain, tip the energy balance:

- *For weight loss:* consume fewer calories than you burn each day. Either cut back on calories in, or move more. Better yet, do both!
- *For weight gain:* tip the balance the other way. Take in more calories than your body uses. Still keep moving!

Why focus on energy balance? Your body stores most excess calories consumed as body fat. Just 100 extra calories a day adds up to about 1 pound a month, or a gain of about 10 pounds in a year. Are your calories in balance? To reach energy balance, most people need to move more—and perhaps trim calories in their food choices, too!

If you fit within the healthy range—BMI 18.5 to 24.9—that's good. Take steps to keep it there, especially if your BMI starts to creep up. Be aware: some people fit within the healthy range but still have excess body fat and little muscle.

What if your BMI is above 25? For most people, that's less healthy—unless the extra weight is muscle, not fat. Try to avoid more weight gain. The higher your weight is above the healthy range, the greater your risk for weight-related problems.

What if your BMI falls below "healthy"? That may be okay for you, but also may suggest a health problem. A BMI under 18.5 may indicate increased risk for menstrual irregularity, infertility, and osteoporosis. It also may be an early symptom of a health problem or an eating disorder. Check with your health professional if you lose weight suddenly or unexpectedly.

Use the BMI *only* as a guideline. Age, gender, and ethnicity impact how BMI relates to body fat. For people who have lost muscle mass, including some elderly people, even a BMI within the "healthy" range may not be healthy. Healthy muscular people may have a BMI above the healthy range. Consult your doctor about the BMI that's healthy for you. Your BMI alone doesn't determine whether your weight is healthy. The location and amount of body fat you carry, and your weight-related risk factors, including your family history of health problems, count, too.

Note: This BMI chart is meant for adults, not for growing children or teens. *See the Appendices for the growth charts with body mass index for age percentiles for boys and for girls two to twenty years.* Pediatric charts take individual growth patterns into account.

Body Weight, Body Fat?

Your body composition (how much of your weight is body fat), not necessarily where you fit on any chart, is an important part of evaluating your weight. In fact, the location and amount of body fat may predict your weight-related health risk more than body weight alone. For example, a person's BMI may fit right within the healthy range, but he or she still may carry too much body fat. Conversely, a muscular person may seem to be at increased risk according to charts, but may not be overfat. Why? Muscle weighs more than fat.

How can you determine how much of your weight is body fat (often referred to as percent body fat)? Short of expensive tests such as underwater weighing, getting an exact measure isn't easy, and it's especially hard to figure it out on your own. A health or fitness professional might use a skinfold caliper to measure the fat layer on several parts of your body, such as your arm, midriff, and thigh. New electronic scales and other devices also can measure body fat percentages.

DOES YOUR BMI PUT YOU IN A RISKY ZONE?

BMI—figured at weight in relation to height—indicates how weight may affect your disease risk. As BMI goes up the contribution of weight to disease risk does too. For athletes and those with muscular builds, a higher BMI may overestimate disease risk. BMI ranges shown above are for adults.

Directions: Find your weight on the bottom of the graph. Go straight up from that point until you come to the line that matches your height. Then look to find your weight group.

- BMI 18.5 to 24.9: not a risk factor for weight-related health problems
- BMI 25 to 29.9: some increased risk for weight-related health problems
- BMI 30 or higher: significant increased risk for weight-related health problems

Source: Report of the Dietary Guidelines Advisory Committee on the Dietary Guidelines for Americans, 2000, page 3.

Remember: Your weight on a scale by itself can't tell you if you're carrying too much fat and how your weight is distributed. Most importantly, body weight shouldn't dictate how you feel about yourself.

Here are some other ways to judge how you are doing in terms of body fat and health.

Of Apples and Pears

Stand in front of a full-length mirror, preferably nude. How do you look? Be your own judge. Are you shaped like an apple or a pear? For health, being an "apple" can be riskier than being a "pear."

Where your body stores fat is a clue to your healthy weight. Abdominal or upper body fat (applelike shape) increases the risk for some health problems such as diabetes, high cholesterol levels, early heart disease, and high blood pressure, even when BMI falls within a healthy range. In contrast, excess weight carried in the hips, buttocks, and thighs (pearlike shape) doesn't appear to be as risky for most health problems. However, it may increase your risk for varicose veins and orthopedic problems.

For the most part, being an "apple" or a "pear" is an inherited tendency for those who carry extra weight. In other words, fat distribution is partially influenced by genes. However, smoking and drinking too many alcoholic beverages also seem to increase fat carried in the stomach area; as a result, they increase the risk of weight-related health problems. Conversely, vigorous exercise can help to reduce stomach fat, helping to decrease these health risks.

Waist Whys. Health risks go up as waist size increases. That's especially true if your waist measures more than 35 inches for a woman or more than 40 inches for a man. So a simple tape measure is a tool for assessing abdominal fat. Stand, and measure your waist just above your hipbone. (*Hint:* Relax, breathe out. Don't cinch in the tape measure or pull in your stomach!) *Note:* After menopause many women tend to add weight around the midriff.

What Are Your Health Risks?

Have you ever finished a physical exam feeling that your weight was within a healthy range, only to have

---

RISK OF ASSOCIATED DISEASE ACCORDING TO BMI AND WAIST SIZE

BMI	WAIST LESS THAN OR EQUAL TO 40 IN. (MEN) OR 35 IN. (WOMEN)	WAIST GREATER THAN 40 IN. (MEN) OR 35 IN. (WOMEN)
18.4 or less	–	N/A
18.5–24.9	–	N/A
25.0–29.9	Increased	High
30.0–34.9	High	Very high
35.0–39.9	Very high	Very high
40 or greater	Extremely high	Extremely high

Source: Partnership for Healthy Weight Management (2001).

---

your doctor suggest that you lose—or perhaps gain—a few pounds? For some physical conditions, such as high blood pressure, diabetes, high blood cholesterol, or arthritis, your physician may advise weight loss even though you appear to have a healthy weight. *See "Are You at Risk for Chronic Disease?" on page 25.* The higher your BMI and waist measurement and the more weight-related risk factors you have, the more likely you'll benefit from losing a few pounds.

A doctor may advise some weight gain for other reasons, perhaps to replace weight loss and aid recovery after a prolonged illness or surgery, or to help withstand some medical treatments, perhaps cancer treatment. *For benefits of a healthy weight for women's health, see "Every Age and Stage of Life: Why a Healthy Weight?" in chapter 17.*

Energy Basics: Calorie Math

You can't touch them or see them. Food supplies them, but they're not nutrients. Your body burns them to keep you alive—and moving. What are they? They're calories! To understand how to achieve and maintain a healthy weight, start with calorie basics.

A Measure of Energy

Calories actually are units of energy. Back in science class, you probably learned the technical definition: one calorie is the amount of energy needed to raise the temperature of 1 gram of water by 1 degree Celsius. In the world of nutrition and health, the term "calorie" refers to the amount of energy in food and the amount of energy the body uses.

In food, calories are energy locked inside three groups of nutrients: carbohydrates, fats, and proteins. These nutrients are released from food during digestion, then absorbed into the bloodstream and converted to glucose, or blood sugar.

In your body, the food energy in glucose finally gets released into trillions of body cells, where it's used to power all your body's work—from your heartbeat, to push-ups, to the smile that spreads across your face. Energy from food you don't need right away can be stored as body fat or perhaps as glycogen, a storage form of carbohydrate. If your body doesn't use them, they just "hang around" as stored energy for later use.

Food Power

Read food labels or check a calorie counter. You'll see that most foods supply calories, or energy—some more than others. What accounts for the differences?

Three nutrient groups—carbohydrates, proteins, and fats—and alcohol supply energy, or calories, in food and beverages. Gram for gram, fat and alcohol supply more than either carbohydrate or protein.

Fats provide 9 calories per gram; alcohol, 7 calories per gram; and carbohydrates and proteins, 4 calories per gram. Vitamins, minerals, and water don't provide calories; neither do cholesterol and fiber.

Foods that are watery, watery-crisp (rather than greasy-crisp), or fibrous tend to have fewer calories and more volume than foods that are more fatty or greasy. (Water and fiber are calorie-free.) For example, celery, which has more water and fiber than French fries, also has fewer calories. To turn up the volume on your plate, choose more bulky foods (with more water or fiber) that fill you up with fewer calories. *Check "Eat More Food, but Less Calories!" in chapter 10.*

How Many Calories for You?

Your body's need for energy, or fuel, never stops. Every minute of every day, your body needs a constant supply of energy to stay alive and to function well.

How much? Energy needs vary from person to person. Even your own energy needs change at different ages and stages of life. Your age, basal metabolic rate, body size and composition, physical health, and activity level contribute to how much energy you need.

The Institute of Medicine advises Acceptable Macronutrient Distribution Ranges (AMDR): for adults, calories from carbohydrate (45 to 65 percent), from fat (20 to 35 percent), and from protein (10 to 35 percent). To lose, gain, or maintain your weight, it makes little difference what proportion of nutrients supply your calories. It's your total calories—in and out—that count! *Check chapter 15 for AMDR levels for kids.*

The fewer calories you consume overall, the greater percent of calories needed from protein to meet your protein need.

Powering your body can be compared to fueling your car. Both your car and your body need a source of energy just to keep idling. When you move, your body—like your car—burns more fuel, and uses even

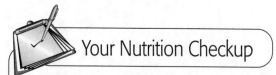

more to go faster and farther. Some bodies—and some cars—are more fuel-efficient than others. That is, they use less energy to do the same amount of work. Age, size, shape, gender, physical condition, and even the type of "fuel" affect fuel efficiency. *"How Does Your Body Use Energy?" on page 26 shows the proportion of energy used for each role in your body.*

Your Basic Energy Needs

Energy for basal metabolism (basic needs) is energy your body burns on "idle." In scientific terms, basal metabolic rate (BMR) is the energy level that keeps involuntary body processes going: pumping your heart, breathing, generating body heat, perspiring, transmitting brain messages, and producing thousands of body chemicals. For most people, basal metabolism represents about 60 percent of their energy needs!

The simple "rule of ten" offers a quick, easy estimate of how much energy your body uses for basal metabolism daily. Figure on 10 calories per pound of body weight for women, and 11 calories per pound for men, to meet routine energy demands. Here's an example:

Consider an active 130-pound female. She would burn about 1,300 calories (130 pounds × 10 calories per pound) per day for basal metabolism and about 2,200 calories total per day. (That's 60 percent of total calories for her basic energy needs.) Now calculate for yourself: about how much energy might your body require for your basic needs?

Why can one person consume more calories day after day and never gain a pound? For another person of the same age, height, and activity level, weight control is a constant challenge. The "rule of ten (or eleven)" doesn't allow for individual differences in basal metabolic rate (BMR). Age, gender, genetics, and body composition and size, among other factors, affect basic energy needs. Although you don't need to know your BMR to achieve and maintain a healthy weight, that may be useful information for some people, perhaps athletes in training. Health or fitness professionals can determine that for you. *Worth noting:* A handheld palm device is available that individuals can use to measure their metabolic rate at rest.

Age Factor. Young people—from infancy through adolescence—need more calories per pound than adults do for growing bone, muscle, and other tissues. During infancy, energy needs are higher per pound of body weight than at any other time in life. And just watch a growing teenager eat; you know that energy needs are high during adolescence! (The "rule of ten" isn't meant for kids—especially not infants.)

By adulthood, food energy (calorie) needs—and BMR—start to decline: 2 percent for each decade. For example, a woman who needs about 2,200 calories per day for her total energy needs at age twenty-five might need 2 percent less, or 2,156 calories per day, at age thirty-five. She may need another 2 percent less by age forty-five, and so on.

Why the decline in BMR? Body composition and hormones change with age. And with less physical activity, muscle mass decreases; body fat takes its place. Because body fat burns less energy than muscle, fewer calories are needed to maintain body weight, and the basal metabolic rate goes down. (As an aside, regular physical activity can help keep your metabolic rate up.)

If you continue to follow your teenage eating habits—and live a less active lifestyle—the extra pounds that creep on with age should come as no surprise! Unused calories get stored as body fat.

Family Matters. Genetic makeup and inherited body build account for some differences in basal metabolic rate—differences you can't change! (Families tend to pass on food habits to one another, too, which also may account for similarities in body weight.)

Body Size, Shape, and Composition. Consider the impact on BMR and energy needs:

● A heavy, full-size car usually burns more fuel per mile than a small, sleek sports car. Likewise, the more you weigh, the more calories you burn. Body size makes a difference. It takes somewhat more effort to move if you weigh 170 pounds compared to 120. That's one reason why men, who often weigh more, use more calories than women.

● A lean, muscular body has a higher metabolic rate than a softly rounded body with more fat tissue. Why? Ounce for ounce, muscle burns more energy than body fat does. So the higher your proportion of muscle to fat, the more calories you need to maintain your weight. A softly rounded body type has a greater tendency to store body fat then a lean, muscular body.

Tip: Stay physically active to maintain your muscle mass—and give your BMR a boost.

● A tall, thin body also has more surface area than a short body, and as a result, more heat loss; the net result—more calories burned (higher BMR) to maintain normal body temperature.

How Does Your Body Use Energy?

If you're like most people, here's how your body uses the energy it "burns" each day:

Basic energy needs (basal metabolism)	60%
Physical activity	30%
Digestion of food and absorption of nutrients	10%
Total energy use for the day	*100%*

Gender Gap. The ratio of muscle to fat differs with gender, accounting for differences in basal metabolic rate. Up to age ten or so, energy needs for boys and girls are about the same, but then puberty triggers change. When boys start developing more muscle, they need more calories; their added height and size demand more energy, too.

By adulthood, men usually have less body fat and 10 to 20 percent more muscle than women of the same age and weight. That's one reason why men's basic energy needs are higher. In contrast, women's bodies naturally keep body fat stores in reserve for pregnancy and breast-feeding when a woman's energy needs go up. *Refer to chapter 17.*

Hot—or Cold? Outside temperature affects internal energy production. On chilly days, your BMR "burns" a little higher to keep you warm during prolonged exposure to cold. Shivering and moving to keep warm use energy, too. And in hot temperatures, your body's air conditioning system burns a bit more energy—for example, as you perspire to cool down.

The Diet Factor. Do you think that skipping meals or following a very-low-calorie eating plan offers a weight-loss edge? Think again. Severe calorie restriction actually can make your body more energy efficient and cause the rate at which your body burns energy from food to slow down! Your body then requires fewer calories to perform the same body processes. This slowdown in metabolic rate is your body's strategy for survival.

Physical Activity: An Energy Burner

Movement of any kind—a blink of your eye, a wave of your hand, or a jog around the block—uses energy. In fact, about 30 percent of your body's energy intake is used to power physical activity! At best, that estimate is imprecise because activity levels differ so much. Very active people need more calories, about 40 percent of their total energy for physical activity.

Common sense says that some physical activities burn more energy than others. The amount of energy used to power physical activity actually depends on three things: the type of activity, its intensity, and how long you do it. Suppose you walk with a friend of the same age and body size. The one who pumps his or her arms and takes an extra lap around the block burns more energy. *The chart "Burning Calories with Activity" on page 28 shows how much energy (calories) get used for common, nonstop activities.*

The Food Connection

Eating itself actually burns calories. Digesting food and absorbing nutrients use about 10 percent of your day's energy expenditure—about 200 calories if you consume 2,000 calories daily. But don't count on these processes to burn up all the energy in anything you eat!

Calorie Myths

Over the years, calorie myths of all kinds have developed. Do these unfounded notions sound familiar?

Have You Ever Wondered

. . . what nutrient-dense foods are? Nutrient-dense, or nutrient-rich, foods such as vegetables, fruit, low-fat milk, and lean meat and poultry have substantial amounts of vitamins and minerals naturally, yet relatively few calories, or food energy. An energy-dense food such as candy and regular soft drinks supplies calories, but relatively few vitamins and minerals. *Refer to chapter 10 to learn more.*

. . . if drinking milk helps you lose weight? Perhaps so. Emerging research suggests that dairy foods (24 ounces per day) as part of a reduced-calorie diet may promote weight loss, more than just cutting calories alone. The potential reasons aren't clear, but any link may be related to the mix of milk's nutrients or perhaps milk's components that appear to boost the body's ability to burn fat and keep muscle. Stay tuned!

. . . if stress promotes weight gain? The role of chronic stress and weight is an area of research. Among the questions: do hormones released with stress increase appetite, and do these hormones promote fat production and deposits, especially in the abdomen? That said, for many people, stress triggers emotional overeating.

. . . what to do when your weight seems to plateau? Be patient. Plateaus are normal with weight loss. Your body requires fewer calories to function as you lose weight. Allow time to readjust. Gradually adding more activity may help nudge you off the weight plateau.

BURNING CALORIES WITH ACTIVITY

CALORIES BURNED PER HOUR, BY BODY WEIGHT			CALORIES BURNED PER HOUR, BY BODY WEIGHT		
ACTIVITY	120 LBS.	170 LBS.	ACTIVITY	120 LBS.	170 LBS.
Aerobic dance	335	500	Racquetball	380	540
Archery	190	270	Reading	70	100
Basketball	330	460	Rowing, stationary	380	540
Bicycling (<10 mph)	220	310	Running, 10 mph	870	1,235
Bowling	165	230	Sitting (watching TV)	55	75
Calisthenics	190	270	Sitting (writing, typing)	100	140
Driving a car	110	155	Skating, roller	380	540
Eating	80	115	Skiing, cross-country	435	615
Food preparation	120	175	Skiing, downhill	325	460
Gardening	220	310	Sleeping	50	70
Golf (walking)	245	345	Soccer	380	540
Hiking	325	460	Swimming, leisure	380	540
Horseback riding	220	310	Tennis	380	540
Housework	135	190	Walking, brisk	205	295
Jogging	380	540	Weight training	165	230
Mowing lawn	245	345			

Calculated from: Ainsworth, BE. *The Compendium of Physical Activities Tracking Guide. Prevention Research Center,* Norman J. Arnold School of Public Health, University of South Carolina, 2002.

Myth: Margarine has fewer calories than butter.

Fact: Either one, regular stick margarine or stick butter, contain about 36 calories per teaspoon. For a spread with fewer calories, try jelly or jam with 16 calories per teaspoon, or whipped butter or lite margarine, about 26 calories per teaspoon.

Myth: A rich, fudgy brownie, before bedtime, is more fattening than the same brownie eaten at lunchtime.

Fact: What you eat, not when, makes the difference. No matter when they're eaten, calories seem to have the same effect in the body. Too many can add up to extra body fat. Timing has no direct effect on how your body uses the calories. However, evidence does suggest that eating regular meals, especially breakfast, helps promote weight loss by reducing fat intake and minimizing impulsive snacking, which can add up to excess calories over the day.

Myth: Potatoes and bread are fattening.

Fact: By themselves, they're not high in calories—88 calories for a medium (4-ounce) potato and 70 calories for an average-size slice of bread. However, high-fat toppings or spreads can add up to excess calories. Consider the calories in one tablespoon: sour cream (about 30 calories), butter or margarine (about 100 calories), and regular mayonnaise (about 100 calories).

Myth: Skip nuts for weight loss.

Fact: A small portion (an ounce or two) of nuts can be okay—and may take the edge off hunger. Enjoy these nutrient-rich foods (with their healthy oils and phytonutrients) from the Meat and Beans Group. And be prudent: ⅓ cup has about 270 calories.

Myth: Excess "carbs," not fats, cause weight gain.

Fact: Excess carbohydrates are no more fattening than excess calories from any source: fats, carbohydrates, and proteins. Despite claims of "low-carb" weight loss regimens, a high-carbohydrate diet doesn't promote body fat storage by enhancing insulin resistance. Excess calories from any source are stored as body fat.

Weighing the Risks

Overweight and obesity are epidemic. According to the National Center for Health Statistics, 30 percent of American adults (60 million people) are obese—and many more are overweight, up significantly over the past two decades! Young people are increasingly overweight, too. An estimated 16 percent of children and teens (over 9 million kids) ages six to nineteen in the United States are considered overweight, triple the number from 1980. (This data was gathered from

Have You Ever Wondered

. . . if my weight problem is really a thyroid problem? Maybe—but before you blame your thyroid, check with your doctor, who may order a test to find out. Hypothyroidism, when the thyroid doesn't produce enough thyroid hormone, is the most common form of thyroid disease; one symptom is weight gain. On the flip side, an overactive thyroid causes hyperthyroidism; one symptom is weight loss. *See chapter 22, page 551, with a "Have You Ever Wondered" question about thyroid disease and high blood cholesterol.*

the National Health and Nutrition Examination Survey for 1999–2002.)

According to the Institute of Medicine, obesity is defined as excess body fat; overweight refers to excess body weight that includes fat, bone, and muscle.

The causes of overweight and obesity? Energy imbalance: more calories consumed than used. Today's inactive lifestyles contribute heavily to weight problems. For example, studies link excessive television viewing to obesity. Today's technology, including computers, video and computer games, and work-saving devices, play a role, too!

The causes underlying energy imbalance and obesity are complex: psychological, social, environmental, physical, and lifestyle. Consider the temptation of food that's so available; big portions from restaurants and vending machines; overscheduled living; and communities designed for driving, not walking or bicycling. The list goes on!

Because it runs in families, genetics may play a role—especially if the conditions are right. For example, people who inherit a sluggish metabolism are more likely to have a weight problem. A child's surroundings and upbringing are factors, too. Families pass on their diet and lifestyle habits. With one obese parent, the chances of being overweight are 40 percent; that doubles when both parents are obese.

What about being too thin? The reasons for being underweight are as complex and unique as being overweight. Genetics may be a factor too. As with obesity, thinness tends to run in families. Some

---

Gaining, or Losing, 1 Pound

One pound of body fat equals about 3,500 calories, so losing 1 pound requires a 3,500-calorie deficit. The opposite is true for weight gain. The following describes how an average person might gain or lose weight.

- To gain 1 pound: *If you added 250 calories* from an extra sandwich, salad, or a bag of chips to your normal eating plan daily—without changing your activity level—how long might it take *to gain 1 pound?*

    3,500 calories = 1 pound of body fat

    3,500 calories ÷ 250 calories per day = *14 days, or 2 weeks*

- To lose 1 pound: *If you burned 100 extra calories* by walking about 30 minutes during your lunch hour 5 days a week—without changing your calorie intake—when would that *pound come off?*

    100 calories per day × 5 days = 500 calories per week

    500 calories per week × 7 weeks = 3,500 total calories burned

    3,500 calories = 1 pound of body fat loss in 7 weeks

people may inherit a speedy metabolism. For many reasons, the brain's appetite center may not signal hunger, so people may feel full even when they're not. Other psychological, physical, economic, social, and lifestyle factors also may get in the way of eating well. *See "Too Thin—a Problem?" later in this chapter.*

Overweight and Obesity: Hazards to Health

Sometime spend an hour or so carrying around a 5-pound bag of flour, a 10-pound bag of potatoes, or a heavy phone book. Tiring? That's the extra burden on your body and heart when you carry extra pounds of body fat. The more excess body fat you have, the greater that burden. Every body system—including the lungs, the heart, and the skeleton—has to work harder just to move.

Many health problems, *noted in the chart "Risky Business" on page 31,* are linked to overweight and obesity. And in 2005, an estimated 112,000 deaths annually were linked to obesity. *Chapter 22 explores the links between overweight and obesity, and cardiovascular health, some cancers, and diabetes.*

Your "Weigh": Figuring Your Energy Needs

How much energy does your body need in a day? For a rough guesstimate, do the following "energy math."

1. *Figure your basic energy needs (BMR).* Multiply your healthy weight (in pounds) by 10 for women and by 11 for men. If you see from your BMI that you're overweight, use the average weight within the healthy weight range for your height in "Does Your BMI Put You in a Risky Zone?" on page 23.

   weight × ____ (either 10 or 11) = ____ calories for basic needs

2. *Figure your energy needs for physical activity.* Check the activity level that matches your lifestyle for most days of the week:

   ____ Sedentary: mainly sitting, driving a car, lying down, sleeping, standing, reading, typing, or other low-intensity activities

   ____ Light activity (for no more than 2 hours daily): light exercise such as light housework, grocery shopping, walking leisurely

   ____ Moderate activity: moderate exercise such as heavy housework, gardening, dancing, or brisk walking (and very little sitting)

   ____ Very active: active physical sports, or in a labor-intensive job such as construction work

   Multiply your basic energy needs by the percent that matches your activity level: sedentary, 20%; light activity, 30%; moderate activity, 40%; or very active, 50%.

   ____ calories for basic needs
   × ____% for activity level
   = ____ calories for physical activity

3. *Figure energy for digestion and absorbing nutrients.* Add your calories for basic needs and calories for physical activity, then multiply the total by 10%.

   (____ calories for basic needs + ____ calories for physical activity) × 10% =

   ____ calories for digestion and absorbing nutrients

4. Add up your total energy needs by adding calories for each purpose.

   + calories for basic needs
   + calories for physical activity
   + calories for digestion and absorbing nutrients
   = ____ calories for your total energy needs

   As an example, consider this 40-year-old female, who works at a desk and walks during her lunch hour. She weighs 125 pounds, which is healthy for her height.

   Basic energy needs: 125 pounds × 10 = 1,250 calories

   Energy for physical activity: 1,250 calories × 0.30 = 375 calories

   Energy for digestion and absorbing nutrients: (1,250 + 375 calories) × 0.10 = 162.5 calories

   Total energy needs: 1,250 calories + 375 calories + 162.5 calories = *1,787.5 calories*

Check the Appendices for the Dietary Reference Intake's Estimated Energy Requirements, as well as MyPyramid's Food Intake Pattern Calorie Levels.

RISKY BUSINESS

**OVERWEIGHT AND OBESITY:
KNOWN RISK FACTORS FOR . . .**

- Diabetes
- Heart disease
- Stroke
- High blood pressure
- Gallbladder disease
- Osteoarthritis (degeneration of the cartilage and bone in joints)
- Sleep apnea and other breathing problems
- Some forms of cancer (uterine, breast, colorectal, kidney, gallbladder, perhaphs others)

OBESITY: ASSOCIATED WITH . . .

- High blood cholesterol
- Complications of pregnancy
- Menstrual irregularities
- Excess body and facial hair
- Stress incontinence (urine leakage cause by weak muscles in the pelvic area)
- Psychological disorders such as depression
- Increased surgical risk

Source: National Institute of Diabetes and Digestive and Kidney Diseases/National Institutes of Health.

Obesity and Kids: A Heavy Burden

America's youth are getting fatter. And inactivity is also on the rise among youth. Effects of childhood overweight and obesity can last a lifetime.

Although obese children don't automatically become obese adults, there's reason for concern. Eating and activity patterns for life often are established during childhood. For these children, the risk for being overweight as teens and adults is higher. According to some studies, those who are overweight as teens have a greater chance for ongoing health problems such as diabetes as adults. What's more, weight problems affect self-image and, as a result, self-esteem. How children feel about themselves can affect almost every aspect of their lives now—and into adulthood.

Weight-loss programs for adults are not meant for children or teens. Young people need enough calories and nutrients for their growth and development. Often increased physical activity, rather than cutting calories, is enough to help overweight children achieve a healthful weight. For them, the goal is to reduce the rate of weight gain as they grow and develop. Before devising a plan to help your child or teenager lose weight, talk to your doctor or registered dietitian (RD).

For more about healthful food choices and lifestyles for children and teens, see chapter 16, "Food to Grow On." There you'll also find guidelines for helping young people reach and maintain a healthy weight.

Obesity can lead to a cycle of inactivity. Often extra body weight makes physical activity more tiring—even for everyday activities such as walking up stairs or through a mall. Inactivity can lead to more weight gain, more muscle loss, and other health problems. Obesity can have an emotional price tag, too, if a negative body image leads to poor self-esteem and social isolation.

Now consider the upside: the health benefits of trimming down. If you need to lose, dropping 5 to 15 percent of your body weight may improve your health and quality of life, and prevent these health problems. For someone who weights 200 pounds, that's a loss of 10 to 30 pounds. Even this small weight shift can help lower the risk factors for many chronic diseases: lower blood pressure, total and LDL blood cholesterol levels, triglyceride levels, and blood sugar. In addition, HDL cholesterol levels may go up. *To learn about total, LDL, and HDL cholesterol and triglycerides, see the "'Fat' Dictionary" in chapter 3.*

Your weight is healthy? Smart eating and active living help you prevent weight gain and stay healthy as you age.

Weight Management: Strategies That Work!

The key to managing your weight throughout your life? A positive "can do" attitude and the right kind of motivation! If you're trying to lose weight to fit into a bathing suit before vacation, or to look good for your

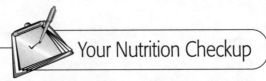

Weight-Loss Readiness Test

Are you ready to lose weight? Your attitude affects your ability to succeed. Take this readiness quiz to see if you're mentally ready before you begin. Mark each statement as "true" or "false." Be honest with yourself! The answers should reflect the way you really think—not how you'd like to be!

1. I have thought a lot about my eating habits and physical activities, and I know what I might change.

2. I know that I need to make permanent, not temporary, changes in my eating and activity patterns.

3. I will feel successful only if I lose a lot of weight.

4. I know that it's best if I lose weight slowly.

5. I'm thinking about losing weight now because I really want to, not because someone else thinks I should.

6. I think losing weight would solve other problems in my life.

7. I am willing and able to increase my regular physical activity.

8. I can lose weight successfully if I have no slipups.

9. I am willing to commit time and effort each week to organize and plan my food and activity choices.

10. Once I lose a few pounds but reach a plateau (I can't seem to lose more), I usually lose the motivation to keep going toward my weight goal.

11. I want to start a weight loss program, even though my life is unusually stressful right now.

NOW SCORE YOURSELF

Look at your answers for items 1, 2, 4, 5, 7, and 9. Score "1" if you answered "true" and "0" if you answered "false." For items 3, 6, 8, 10, and 11, score "0" for each "true" answer and "1" for each false answer.

No one score indicates if you're ready to start losing weight. But the higher your total score, the more likely you'll be successful.

If you scored 8 or higher, you probably have good reasons to lose weight now. And you know some of the steps that can help you succeed.

If you scored 5 to 7 points, you may need to reevaluate your reasons for losing weight and the strategies you'd follow.

If you scored 4 or less, now may not be the right time for you to lose weight. You may be successful initially, but you may not be able to sustain the effort to reach or maintain your weight goal. Reconsider your reasons and approach.

INTERPRET YOUR SCORE

Your answer can clue you in on some stumbling blocks to your weight management success. Any item you scored as "0" suggests a misconception about weight loss, or a problem area for you. So let's look at each item a bit more closely.

1. You can't change what you don't understand, and that includes your eating habits and activity pattern. Keep records for a week to pinpoint when, what, why, and how much you eat—as well as patterns and obstacles to regular physical activity.

2. You may be able to lose weight in the short run with drastic or highly restrictive changes in your eating habits or activity pattern. But they may be hard to live with permanently. Your food and activity plans should be healthful ones you can enjoy and sustain.

3. Many people fantasize about reaching a weight goal that's unrealistically low. If that sounds like you, rethink your meaning of success. A reasonable goal takes body type into consideration—and sets smaller, achievable "mile markers" along the way.

4. If you equate success with fast weight loss, you'll have problems keeping weight off. This "quick fix" attitude can backfire when you face the challenges of weight maintenance. The best and healthiest approach is to lose weight slowly while learning strategies to keep weight off permanently.

5. To be successful, the desire for and commitment to weight loss must come from you—not your best friend or a family member. People who lose weight, then keep it off, take responsibility for their weight goals and choose their own approach.

6. Being overweight may contribute to some social problems, but it's rarely the single cause. While body

image and self-esteem are strongly linked, thinking you can solve all your problems by losing weight isn't realistic. And it may set you up for disappointment.

7. A habit of regular, moderate physical activity is a key factor to successfully losing weight—and keeping it off. For weight control, physical activity doesn't need to be strenuous to be effective. Any moderate physical activity that you enjoy and will do regularly counts.

8. Most people don't expect perfection in their daily lives, yet they often feel they must stick to a weight-loss program perfectly. Perfection at weight loss isn't realistic. Rather than viewing lapses as catastrophes, see them as opportunities to find what triggers your problems and develop strategies for the future.

9. To successfully lose weight, you must take time to assess your problem areas, then develop the approach that's best for you. Success requires planning, commitment, and time.

10. First of all, a plateau in an ongoing weight-loss program is perfectly normal, so don't give up too soon! Before you lose your motivation, think about any past efforts that have failed, then identify strategies that can help you overcome those hurdles.

11. Weight loss itself can be a source of stress, so if you're already under stress, you may find a weight-loss program somewhat difficult to implement right now. Try to resolve other stressors in your life before starting your weight-loss effort.

Source: American Dietetic Association.

---

school reunion, or because your spouse is nagging you to drop a belt size, your commitment and efforts are likely to fizzle out over time. Internal motivators—health, increased energy, self-esteem, feeling in control—increase your chances for lifelong success.

If you're at your healthy weight, these strategies for weight management are meant for you, too. **Caution:** If your weight problem is excessive—too much or too little—or if you have health problems, talk to your doctor before you get started. Children, pregnant women, those with chronic diseases, and people over age sixty-five shouldn't attempt weight loss without advice from their health professional.

Ready? Set . . . Go for It!

Whether your objective is weight loss, weight gain, or weight maintenance, lifelong success depends on some new ways of thinking.

● Make health your weight-management priority. *A potential bonus:* Positive changes in your appearance! Strive for your best weight for health, not necessarily the lowest weight you could be—or what you consider your "ideal" number.

● For weight loss or gain, follow these tactics: (1) healthful eating, (2) regular physical activity, and (3) acceptance of the weight you can achieve through healthful eating and a healthful lifestyle.

● Set realistic, attainable goals—for you! Start with your current weight or lifestyle, not where you want to be. The challenge of trimming 5 pounds at a time may seem more doable than losing 25 or more pounds.

● Focus on a healthful lifestyle—for a lifetime—not on "dieting." Dieting alone is often a short-term tactic without long-term results. The concept of "dieting" carries negative baggage: guilt, "shoulds," and "can't haves." For most people, "dieting" results in failure.

● Focus your strategies: action-oriented and specific. Perhaps you'll walk for 15 minutes each day during your break, or you'll drink low-fat or fat-free milk rather than a milk shake with your fast-food lunch.

● Tailor your strategies to your schedule, your budget, your family situation, and your personal needs, to name a few. Experts have found that two out of three people who were successful at weight control personalized their efforts to fit their lifestyles.

● Think long-term; act gradually. Fasting and starvation-type diets can peel off pounds, but most of the weight that's lost quickly is only water loss, which will come back as fast as it's lost. Grueling exercise regimens may tone the body, but for most people, these tactics aren't realistic ways to live—and are not healthful, either.

Instead of trying quick fixes, plan for a gradual weight shift of $1/2$ to 1 pound a week. That's safe and healthy. With any more weight loss, you may be exercising too much or eating too little.

Weight Cycling—the "Yo-Yo" Problem

Have you gained and lost the same 10, 20, or even 30 pounds over and over again? The cycle of repeatedly losing and regaining weight can make weight management more difficult in the long run. Lost weight that repeatedly comes back may lead to feelings of frustration, failure, and poor self-esteem. According to some studies, weight cycling may even increase the risk for ongoing health problems such as high blood pressure, high cholesterol, and gallbladder disease.

Weight cycling is often an outcome of quick-fix diets, weight-loss gimmicks, and other risky strategies. If repeated "ups and downs" of dieting describe your weight problem, shift your approach to one of lifetime weight management. Break the cycle with long-term approaches rather than short-term results. Make gradual and permanent changes in the way you eat, your activity level, and your lifestyle. It's the only way to be healthy—for life.

If you have weight-cycling history, here's some insight. Most research indicates that weight cycling itself doesn't affect, or lower, your metabolic rate, according to the National Institutes of Health, Weight-Control Information Network. Most people return to their original weight, with the same percentage of lean muscle and fat as before—if their activity level and calorie intake return to the original levels, too. Weight cycling doesn't increase abdominal fat, either. If you adopt a healthier approach to weight loss or maintenance, your past history won't get in the way.

If you need to lose weight, losing about 10 percent of your weight over 6 months likely is safe; that's 20 pounds in 6 months (26 weeks) for someone who weighs 200 pounds. Your extra pounds didn't appear overnight. They don't disappear that way, either!

● Be realistic with your self-talk. Skip the absolutes— "always," "never," and "must" in your tactics. "I'll never eat another French fry." "I must swim twenty laps every other day." Get rid of "shoulds," too. "I should get up early and walk."

● Cut yourself some slack. Nobody's perfect. Allow for occasional slipups in your eating strategies, without feeling guilty.

● Plan to indulge sensibly. By planning for "treats" and "splurges" you may be more successful in the long run.

● Expect success. Reaching life's goals is often a self-fulfilling prophecy. Positive self-talk and an enthusiastic approach to weight management can set you up for success!

Get Physical!

Move it to lose it! Physical activity has been cited as the most powerful tool for weight management. A physically active lifestyle offers many rewards—from heart health to strong bones to stress relief, plus many other benefits. Yet many people don't get enough. *See "Moderate Activity: What Is It?" in chapter 1.*

Think of the impact of the personal computer. Back in the days of the manual typewriter, a typist, on average, burned 15 more calories an hour than someone doing the same work today on a computer. For someone who does word processing for four hours a day, that adds up to 60 calories a day, or 300 calories

Put Action in Your Lifestyle!

Like sound eating habits, regular physical activity is part of a healthful lifestyle. Apply the same principles— variety, balance, and moderation—to both your food choices and your physical activities. Always check with your healthcare provider before beginning any rigorous physical activity program.

● *Variety.* Enjoy many different activities to move different muscles, including your heart: perhaps power walking for your heart and leg muscles, gardening for arm muscles, and sit-ups for abdominal muscles.

● *Balance.* Because different activities have different benefits, balance your physical activity pattern. For overall fitness, choose activities that build cardiovascular endurance (aerobic activities), muscular strength, bone strength, and flexibility.

● *Moderation.* Move enough to keep fit, without overdoing. You don't need a heavy workout. To reduce health risks, at least 30 minutes of moderate physical activity most and preferably all days of the week will do for reducing health risks. To lose or maintain weight, step up to 60 minutes on most days!

over a five-day workweek. When you add up all the energy savings—from escalators and moving side-walks, to cars and motorbikes, to home appliances and electric garage door openers—you can see that inactivity has become a way of life and why weight control has become an everyday challenge. The more you sit, the less energy you need, and the more likely you are to gain weight!

The Active Edge

Study after study shows that people who keep physically active are more successful at losing—and keeping off—extra pounds of body fat. In fact, physical activity appears to be the key to maintaining a healthy weight. Here are eight reasons why. Regular, moderate physical activity:

Twenty Everyday Ways to Get Moving

Do you find it difficult to fit 30 minutes of physical activity into your life every day? It may be easier than you think—even with a busy lifestyle. These everyday activities can count toward your day's total if they're done with moderate intensity—and most take only a little extra time, perhaps 10 minutes at a time.

1. Wake up 30 minutes earlier, and take a brisk walk to start your day. Need someone to get you going? Schedule your walk with your spouse or a neighbor.

2. Forget the drive-through car wash. Wash the car yourself. *Bonus:* You'll save money at the same time.

3. Take stairs instead of the elevator or escalator. Walking up stairs is a great heart exerciser, calorie burner, and muscle builder!

4. Park at the far end of the parking lot for a longer walk. Get off the bus a stop ahead, then walk the rest of the way to your destination. Walk your kids to and from school.

5. Are you a computer user—on and off the job? Give yourself at least 5 minutes off for every hour or two of computer time: walk to the water fountain, or go up and down a few flights of stairs.

6. Walk around your building—outside or inside—during your lunch or coffee break. You'll burn energy rather than being tempted to nibble on a snack.

7. Get a dog, and walk together. No dog? Then borrow a neighbor's dog or push a baby stroller.

8. Play actively with your kids, grandkids, or pets. Some dogs like to play with a Frisbee as much as kids do!

9. Before and after dinner, walk—and talk—with your family. To burn more energy if you have an infant, use a baby carrier on your back rather than pushing a stroller.

10. Do backyard gardening. (*Bonus:* Grow fresh vegetables and herbs if you can.) In the fall, rake leaves.

11. Ride your bike (the kind you pedal) to work or to a friend's home—if it's safe to do. Walk to do nearby errands, such as grocery shopping for small things or going to the post office.

12. While you watch television, do household chores or projects: mop the floor or refinish a piece of furniture. Avoid "couch potato" syndrome.

13. Catch up with your around-the-house work: wash the windows, vacuum or shampoo the carpet, clean the garage or basement, sweep the sidewalk.

14. Use the exercise equipment you already own. Do two things at one time: ride your stationary bicycle while you read the morning paper or a news-magazine. Watch the morning news while you work out on your rowing machine.

15. Push your lawn mower instead of using the power-assisted drive. Skip the snow blower; shovel the snow by hand if you're fit.

16. Make homemade bread. Knead the dough by hand, not with a bread machine or a food processor.

17. Use a rest room at the other end of the building so you get an opportunity to walk.

18. Plan an active family vacation or a weekend outing. Rather than sit on a beach, go canoeing, hiking, or snow skiing.

19. "Walk your talk!" If you like to chat on the phone, move your body while you talk. (Use hand weights while talking on the phone.)

20. Rent an exercise video or DVD rather than a movie. And work out as a leisure-time activity.

● *Burns energy.* The longer, more frequently, and more vigorously you move, the more energy you burn. When you burn more than you consume, your body uses its energy stores, and you lose weight. Just adding thirty minutes of brisk walking to your day makes a difference!

● *Helps you keep muscle and lose body fat.* Without physical activity, you tend to lose lean body tissue along with body fat.

● *Builds lean body mass.* Even when you're not moving, lean body mass requires more energy (calories) to maintain than fat tissue.

● *May suppress appetite a bit.* In fact, people who get regular physical activity often eat less than those who don't.

● *Helps relieve stress.* Remember: Stress may lead to nibbling on more food and consuming more calories than your body needs.

● *Creates a "trimmer" mind-set.* As some people get more physically active, they opt for foods with less fat, fewer calories, and less added sugars. The reason? It just seems to "feel good."

● *"Looks good" on you.* A firm, lean body from physical activity looks trimmer than one that's flabby with more body fat, even at the same weight. Think of your body as a "package" of lean tissue and body fat; muscles take less space than body fat. Although looks aren't the only reason for being physically active, they're a great side effect!

What if you need to *gain* weight? Because the benefits go beyond weight control, everyone needs to get moving. There's no need to cut back on physical activity unless a person's physical activity pattern is excessive—or if a physician advises a slower pace.

Weight control is just one reason to keep physically active. *For other benefits, see "Ten Reasons to Make the 'Right Moves'" in chapter 1.*

Simply Living an Active Lifestyle

To benefit from active living, you don't need to be an exercise fanatic with strenuous daily workouts. Step aerobics at a fitness club, kick boxing, or thirty minutes on an exercise bike every day may not be right for you. That's okay; any kind of moderate, consistent physical activity can do the job. In fact, any activity

you enjoy and stay with can be the right one for you. If it's enjoyable, you're more likely to stick with it.

To get weight loss or maintenance benefits, you need to step up your physical activity, beyond what's advised for lowering chronic disease risk. In Dietary Guidelines' "talk": *To help manage body weight and prevent gradual unhealthy body weight gain in adulthood, engage in approximately 60 minutes of moderate to vigorous activity on most days of the week while not exceeding calorie intake requirements.* For weight loss during adulthood, the Dietary Guidelines advise 60 to 90 minutes daily. You might need to check with your healthcare provider before you start.

Do it all at once, or spread it out: for example, ten minutes of brisk walking during your lunch hour, fifteen minutes of leisure bike riding, and five minutes of sidewalk sweeping at home. If you haven't been physically active, then build up gradually. Get a pedometer to count your steps; work up to 10,000 steps a day. Even a little more physical activity can make a difference.

Remember: *The energy expenditure of physical activity goes up in three ways.* The *longer,* the *more frequent,* and the *more intense* your activity, the more energy you burn. Regardless, choose physical activities that you enjoy and can stick with for the rest of your life.

Even though some weight-loss regimens make "spot-reducing" promises, your body can't get rid of fat in just the problem places. As you exercise and burn more calories than you consume, your body draws energy from all its fat stores, including the problem spots. If you keep on moving, fat will eventually disappear in all the right places.

When You Want to Lose

Use a health-smart approach! The Dietary Guidelines advise: *For those who need to lose weight, aim for slow, steady weight loss by decreasing calorie intake while maintaining an adequate nutrient intake and increasing physical activity.*

The good news: eating for weight control and for good health are one and the same. A simple food plan with physical activity, based on MyPyramid, can accomplish both goals. Use it to tip your energy balance toward weight loss; at the same time, make the calories in your food choices count for good nutrition! *Refer to chapter 10 for a healthful eating plan, created at a calorie level that can help you lose or maintain your healthy weight.*

What's slow, steady weight loss? It's a safe rate of about ½ to 1 pound per week. Experts say that striving for a 250- to 300-calorie deficit per day can help you achieve that. Remember: One pound of body fat contains 3,500 calories worth of stored energy. For weight loss, you need to create a 3,500-calorie deficit for each pound you want to lose: cut back on what you eat, be more physically active—or better yet, do both!

To trim food energy intake, should you count calories? Maybe. But just eating smarter might be enough. Cut back to smaller portions. Eat fewer high-calorie foods. Make your calories count by choosing mostly lean and low-fat foods. Enjoy plenty of fruits and vegetables.

Counting calories to manage weight takes effort. If you choose to do this, start by knowing how many calories you need *and* eat them now. Get a calorie counter that lists calories in many foods, or try a computer program that makes the task easier.

Even when you're trying to lose, not every food you eat needs to be "low cal." Instead your total calorie intake needs to be less than what you use—over several days. If you eat some high-calorie foods, balance them with plenty of lower-calorie foods.

How many calories for weight loss? That depends on you—and how active you are. To get enough nutrients, you need enough nutrient-rich foods, such as vegetables and fruits, from the five food groups. And you need to tip your energy balance toward weight loss—easier if most food choices are lean and low-fat, or low in added sugars. Children and teens especially need adequate calories and nutrients for growth, as well as normal body function and physical activity.

Make calories count with healthful strategies:

● Follow the advice of MyPyramid, at a calorie level targeted for your weight loss. For a ½ to 1 pound a week drop, pick the MyPyramid plan to help you consume up to 250 to 300 calories a day less—without going below 1,600 calories a day (MyPyramid plans are set at twelve calorie levels; *refer to chapter 10.*) If you use an extra 150 calories a day with physical activity, you need to trim only 100 to 150 calories from your day's food choices!

● Watch your portion sizes, and the amount you serve to others. Even calories in low-fat foods can tip your energy balance toward weight gain when portions are bigger than you need.

● When you shop, cook, and eat out, cut back on fat in your food choices. Switching from high- to low-fat foods can make a difference if the calorie content is less. Read Nutrition Facts on food labels to find out.

● Fill up on fruits, vegetables, and whole-grain foods. Being high in fiber and usually low in calories, they can help satisfy you faster. *Bonus:* They may take more time to chew—so you eat less!

● After eating enough nutrient-rich foods spend any extra calories with discretion, perhaps small amounts of foods with more fat and added sugars. If you're physically active, you have more discretionary calo-

Get Portion Savvy

"It's not too big. It's not too small. It's just right!" As a weight management strategy, keep tabs on portion sizes to, in turn, manage the number of calories you consume. Even low-fat foods—for example, pasta, rice, beans, or potatoes—can add up to a hefty calorie count when portions get big.

How portion savvy are you? Without using a measuring cup, try pouring one cup of dry cereal—or scooping a half cup of ice cream—into a bowl. Now check the size with a measuring cup. Chances are, you've overestimated. Most people do. That's why many people quite innocently overdo their calorie intake.

MyPyramid gives guidelines for healthful eating in household measures. Use measuring cups and spoons, and perhaps a kitchen scale to compare your helpings with MyPyramid recommendations or the serving sizes listed on the Nutrition Facts of food labels.

Need specific strategies to be more portion savvy? Check here for "how-tos":

● Size up your servings—see chapter 10.

● Be aware of portion distortion—see chapter 10.

● Control restaurant portions—see chapter 14.

Check It Out!

Ready to start a weight control plan? To make sure the approach is healthful and effective, ask yourself a few questions before you begin. Does the program include:

- A variety of foods from all the food groups of MyPyramid—and the right amount (enough, not too much)? (See chapter 10.)
- Appealing foods you will enjoy eating for the rest of your life, not just a few weeks or months?
- Foods that are available at the supermarket where you usually shop?
- The chance to eat your favorite foods—in fact, any foods?
- Eating strategies that fit your lifestyle and budget?
- Enough regular physical activity? (See page 35.)

If you *cannot* answer "yes" to all these questions, chances are this weight-loss program won't bring long-term success because you may not stick to it. Success is possible only when you make healthful, permanent changes in your eating and physical activity habits.

ries to spend! *See chapter 10 to learn about discretionary calories.*

● Learn how to eat what you like! No one food can make you fat. You'll more likely stick to your eating plan if you don't deprive yourself. Just eat small amounts of higher-calorie food. *For tips on taming food cravings, see "Eat What You Crave!" later in this chapter.*

● Use the Nutrition Facts on food labels to compare calories and nutrients in different foods. The amount for one standard serving is on the label. A serving isn't necessarily the whole package! Check the front of the label, too, where you may find nutrition claims for foods with fewer calories. What do the label terms mean? *Check "Label Lingo: Calories" on page 39.*

● Go easy on wine, beer, spirits, and other alcoholic drinks: no more than one drink a day for women and two for men. Alcohol supplies calories—7 calories per gram. A 12-ounce beer contains about 150 calories, a 5-ounce glass of white wine, and 1½ ounces of spirits have about 100 calories. Downing a six-pack of beer on a hot summer day can add up to a whopping 900 calories, and splitting a 1-liter bottle of wine

can supply 325 calories or more; excessive amounts aren't healthful, either. Drinking alcoholic beverages also can stimulate your appetite so you may eat more.

● Snack smart. It's easy to think about meals yet forget about snacks. Choose snacks wisely by the calories and nutrients they supply. Practice the art of calorie balancing so you can enjoy some higher-fat snacks, such as chocolate bars, nuts, ice cream, or chips. Just eat them less often, in small amounts. Balance them with lower-calorie, lower-fat snacks—pretzels, raisins, yogurt, fruit, or raw vegetables—next time.

● Ask a registered dietitian for more guidance on choosing healthful foods for weight loss.

Slimming Habits

Look at your eating habits. Do you snack on high-calorie foods at work because everyone else does? Do you eat fast so you can get on quickly with your day? Are you a stand-up diner?

● Rethink your old ways of eating—and identify those habits that promote weight gain. Consider what, when, why, where, and how you eat. Then, if you need to, make some changes.

● Plan meals and snacks ahead. Haphazard eating often becomes high-calorie eating. Pack low-calorie snacks, such as raw vegetables, to eat at work when others snack on candy, doughnuts, or chips.

● Shop on a full stomach to help avoid the temptation to buy extra goodies or to nibble on free

Need specific calorie-cutting strategies? Check here for "how-tos":

- Take control of calories in alcoholic drinks—see chapter 8.
- Snack smart for fewer calories—see chapter 10.
- Get "calorie-wise" as you shop—see chapter 11.
- Cut calories by trimming fat and added sugars in food "prep"—see chapter 13.
- Eat out with calorie savvy—see chapter 14.

Label Lingo

Calories

Nutrition Facts on the food label list the calories in a single serving. In addition, "calorie lingo" on the package can alert you to lower-calorie food products as you search supermarket displays.

LABEL TERM	MEANS
Calorie-free	Less than 5 calories
Low-calorie	40 calories or less
Reduced or fewer calories	At least 25% fewer calories*
Light or lite	One-third fewer calories or 50% less fat*; if more than half the calories are from fat, fat content must be reduced by 50% or more
Low-calorie meals	120 calories or less per 100 grams
Light meal	"Low-fat" or "low-calorie" meal

*As compared with a standard serving size of the traditional food

samples. Write out your shopping list when you're not hungry.

● Stick to a regular eating schedule. (There's no hard-and-fast rule about eating three meals a day.) Studies show that missed meals can lead to impulsive snacking and overeating and may lower the rate at which your body burns energy. Eat breakfast!

● Eat from plates, not from packages. When you nibble chips or crackers from a package or snack on ice cream from the carton, you don't know how much you've eaten. It may be more, much more, than you think!

● Serve preportioned sensible amounts of foods on the dinner plate. You'll likely eat less. Use smaller bowls and dinner plates so small portions look like more. *See "Get Portion Savvy" earlier in this chapter for more on portion control.*

● Eat slowly. Savor the flavor of each bite. After all, it takes about twenty minutes for your stomach to signal your brain that you're full—which curbs your urge for a second helping. Slow down by putting down your fork between bites. Eat with chopsticks if they slow you down. Sip, rather than gulp, beverages. Swallow before refilling your fork.

● Eat when you're hungry; stop when you're full. Learn body signals for fullness and real hunger. Forget the "clean-plate club." You don't need to eat everything on your plate if you're satisfied.

● Sit down to eat, rather than nibble while you do other things. Focus on your food. That way you know that you've eaten.

● Make eating the only event—and enjoy it. Eating unconsciously while you watch television, read, talk on the phone, or drive may lead to eating more than you think.

LOW-"CAL" AND LOW-FAT: NOT THE SAME!

Read the label! Compare the calories. Being fat-free doesn't make a food calorie-free. A fat-free or reduced-fat product may have as many (even more) calories per serving than regular products. Many people eat larger quantities of fat-free or low-fat foods, believing they are healthier.

Fig cookie (1)	
Fat-free	48 calories
Regular	56 calories
Vanilla frozen yogurt (1/2 cup)	
Nonfat	110 calories
Regular	117 calories
Caramel topping (2 tablespoons)	
Fat-free	105 calories
Homemade with butter	102 calories
Peanut butter (2 tablespoons)	
Reduced-fat	166 calories
Regular	188 calories
Cereal bar (1.3 ounce)	
Low-fat	133 calories
Regular	140 calories

Source: U.S. Department of Agriculture, Agricultural Research Service, 2005. *USDA National Nutrient Database for Standard Reference*, Release 18, and food industry Web sites, as appropriate.

● Choose foods that take more time to eat. For example, peeling and eating an orange takes longer than drinking a glass of orange juice.

● Stop eating when you leave the table. Avoid the urge to nibble on leftovers as you clean up.

● When you get the urge to nibble (especially if you're not hungry), do something else. Jog, call a friend, walk the dog, or step out into your garden.

● Be aware of the influence of others. You don't need to eat cake, muffins, or bagels in the break room just because your officemate brought it to work.

Eating Triggers

You have all the best intentions. Then something triggers your desire to eat—even though you're not hungry. Instead of looking inside the refrigera-

Dear Diary . . .

Help yourself to weight control by keeping tabs on what you eat. Research shows that people who keep a food and activity diary are often more successful at weight management than those who don't.

There's nothing complicated about keeping a record. Use a notebook, or buy a day-to-day food and activity diary for handwritten records. If you carry your laptop computer everywhere, keep your records there. Or get a hand-held palm monitoring device with software to log the data and carry with you.

For the record, keep track of the amounts and kinds of foods and beverages you eat. To get a handle on any eating "triggers," write your mood and rate your hunger level each time you eat. Put down the time and place, too. List the amount of time you spend in physical activity, along with what you do. Keep your food and activity record for at least a week or two. Then review it for a close look at your eating and physical activity habits.

Most people can spot problem areas easily. Keeping records offers one way to identify areas you might need to change. It also can help you focus on your weight goals—and think twice before indulging in a high-fat snack when you're not hungry.

For an online food and physical activity tracker, check www.MyPyramid.gov.

Emotional Overeating: Take Control!

To relax, quell anger, or overcome depression or loneliness, mood-triggered eating may feel good—at first. But eating to cope with emotions can lead to more negative feelings (guilt, lack of personal control, and poor self-esteem) and perhaps to a cycle of mood-triggered eating. Any excessive calorie intake can promote weight gain. Just as important, using food to satisfy emotions may distract you from handling serious issues in your life.

On the plus side, learning to control mood-triggered eating promotes feelings of personal power and self-esteem!

Learn to deal with emotions in a positive, appropriate way. Address the real problems. Resolve your moods with positive self-talk or a brief change of scenery. Compared with nibbling, physical activity—perhaps a brisk walk, a bike ride, or a tennis game—often does the trick. Regular physical activity is a great stress buster!

tor or diving into a bowl of snacks, get in touch with the emotions and situations that trigger your eating. Learn to differentiate between physical hunger and other, emotionally driven hungers. Find an appropriate diversion. Limit temptations whenever possible.

● Do you eat when you're bored or stressed? Find some other options. Make a list of fun activities: enjoy your garden, play with the dog, go shopping, call a friend, surf the Internet, or play with your kids. Post your list on the refrigerator. When you're bored or upset, pick one of these activities instead of eating. *See "Emotional Overeating: Take Control!" above.*

● Be aware of social situations that trigger eating—such as parties, entertaining friends, dating, talking around the coffeepot at work, and happy-hour business meetings. Create your ways to avoid overeating.

● Remember: Out of sight, out of mind. If the sight of candy, chips, and other high-calorie foods lures you, store them in an inconvenient place. Better yet, don't keep them around. Instead stock up on fruit, raw vegetables, and other foods with fewer calories.

● Accomplished something special? Reward yourself, but not with food. Treat yourself to a massage or a day spa. Buy something new to wear or read, or something to entertain you. Go to a play, concert, or sports event.

● Watch out for seasonal triggers: perhaps nibbling while watching fall and winter sports on television, "cooling off" in hot weather with a few beers or an extra-large soft drink, or eating and entertaining during the holidays. Or eat smaller portions or different foods if only eating will do. If you're not sure what triggers your eating, keep a food diary for a week or two. *"Dear Diary . . ." on page 40 offers some help.*

Party "Tid-bites"

Just because you're trying to eat healthfully doesn't mean you need to avoid celebrations or accept a few extra party pounds. Any foods—even traditional holiday fare—can fit into a healthful eating plan for the calorie-conscious. The secret is moderation and balance.

Kitchen Nutrition

Celebration Meals Go Lean!

Celebration menus—or almost any meal—may be modified to lower the calories and the fat content. Often the differences go almost unnoticed. Compare this traditional menu with its leaner version. *Then see chapter 13 for tips on trimming calories and fat in food preparation.*

ORIGINAL MENU	LEANER MENU
3½ oz. roasted turkey with skin	3½ oz. skinless, roasted turkey
½ cup stuffing	½ cup wild rice pilaf
½ cup broccoli with 2 tbsp. hollandaise sauce	½ cup broccoli with lemon juice
½ cup cranberry relish	¼ cup cranberry relish
1 medium crescent roll	1 whole-grain roll
1 slice pecan pie	1 slice pumpkin pie
Total calories: 1,140	*Total calories:* 735
Total fat: 50 g	*Total fat:* 20 g

Whether a stand-up event or a sit-down dinner, these party tips can help you hold the line:

● Be realistic. Trying to lose weight during the holidays may be a self-defeating goal. Instead strive to maintain your weight.

● Balance party eating with other meals. Eat small, lower-calorie meals during the day so you can enjoy celebration foods, too—without overdoing your energy intake for the day.

● Take the edge off your hunger before a party. Eat a small, low-fat snack such as fruit or whole-grain toast. Feeling hungry can sabotage even the strongest willpower!

● When you arrive at a party, avoid rushing to the food. Greet people you know—conversation is calorie-free! Get a beverage, and settle into the festivities before eating. You may eat less.

● Ask for sparkling water and a lime twist rather than wine, champagne, or a mixed drink. Sparkling water doesn't supply calories.

● Move your socializing away from the buffet table. When conversations take your attention away from food, unconscious nibbling becomes too easy.

● Make just one trip to the party buffet. And be selective. Choose only the foods you really want to eat, and keep portions small. Often just a taste satisfies a craving or curiosity.

● Opt for lower-calorie party foods. Perhaps enjoy raw vegetables with a small dollop of dip, just enough to coat the end of the vegetable. Try boiled shrimp or scallops with cocktail sauce or lemon. Go easy on fried appetizers and cheese cubes.

● If you're bringing a dish, make it healthfully delicious—and low-calorie, too. That way, you'll know there's something with fewer calories you can munch on. Perhaps bring raw vegetables with a yogurt or cottage cheese dip, or bring a platter of juicy, fresh fruit.

● Enjoying a sit-down dinner party? Make your first helping small—especially if your host or hostess expects you to take seconds. The total amount may be about the same as your normal-size portions.

● Forget the all-or-nothing mind-set. Depriving yourself of special holiday foods, or feeling guilty

Noodlin' over "Carb" Headlines?

Can "carbs" make you fat—as some headlines suggest? The Dietary Guidelines for Americans and MyPyramid recommend an eating pattern with starches (complex carbohydrates) from foods such as whole-grain breads, cereals, rice, pasta, fruits, vegetables, and legumes (dry beans).

Limited research notes that carbohydrate-rich foods may cause weight gain in "insulin-resistant" people. For these individuals, it's speculated, the body reacts to sugars and starches by overproducing insulin—and so causing too much carbohydrate to be stored as fat. However, most of us don't gain weight on a high-carbohydrate diet, unless it provides excess calories. The real culprits for weight are inactivity, high-fat eating, and uncontrolled portion sizes from any source of food, including bread, pasta, and other grain products. *See "Insulin Resistance Syndrome, or 'Metabolic Syndrome'" in chapter 22.*

when you do enjoy them, isn't a healthful eating strategy. And deprivation and guilt certainly are not part of the holiday spirit!

● When you're entertaining, make over your menus with fewer calories and fat. Your guests probably won't detect the difference. Be sensitive to any guests with weight goals in mind, too. *For a dinner makeover, see "Kitchen Nutrition: Celebration Meals Go Lean!" earlier in this chapter.*

● Have fun! Sharing food at many celebrations and enjoying a traditional holiday meal and party foods with family and friends doesn't need to destroy healthful food habits you nurtured all year.

● Balance "party calories" with more physical activity.

Motivation Boosters

With weight control as part of your lifestyle, healthful eating and physical activity become second nature. When you need a boost to stay on track, try this!

● Make lifestyle changes with a friend or a family member! A partner increases the enjoyment factor of physical activity and healthful eating.

● Enlist support. Family and friends can help you

keep on track. Those who have the support of family members, particularly a spouse, more likely manage their weight successfully. Watch out for those who attempt to sabotage your efforts. If it's right for you, join a support group.

● Track your progress—daily or weekly, whichever way helps keep you on track. Be aware that weight fluctuates from day to day due to fluid loss and retention. If daily weighing is confusing or discouraging, know that once a week is enough.

● Do try to track your steps to keep your body moving. Get a pedometer. Are you stepping 10,000 steps a day?

● Give it time. For women, weight gain from water retention may be a normal part of a monthly menstrual cycle. Usually that passes in a few days.

● Celebrate any success. Weight loss doesn't need to be "all-or-nothing." If you carry around excess pounds, even small changes can make a difference in your health and reduce your disease risk.

● Enjoy how good your healthy weight feels. Reward yourself with a new garment, a bouquet of flowers, a new CD, or a special outing. Still, there's no greater motivation or reward than knowing you're in control and caring for yourself and improving your health!

Too Thin—a Problem?

Maybe. Being too thin can be a health risk, especially if underweight results from undereating. An eating pattern with too few calories may not supply enough nutrients to keep the body running normally. Children who undereat may not get enough nutrients or energy for growth and development either. A lack of food energy may cause fatigue, irritability, and lack of concentration. And those with a poor diet may have trouble warding off infections.

For normal-weight people, a layer of body fat just under the skin helps protect the body from cold. But very thin people have only a very thin fat layer, so they lack insulation to keep them warm. That becomes an increasing problem for the thin, frail elderly, especially if they don't have adequate heating in their homes.

If you lose weight suddenly and don't know the

<table>
<tr><td></td></tr>
</table>

Have You Ever Wondered

... why it seemed easy to lose weight in your teens and twenties ... and why it's so hard now? There could be several reasons why it seems harder as an adult—a less active lifestyle, different eating habits, or changes in your body. Metabolism slows during each decade of your adult years.

Being inactive complicates the picture if you lose muscle mass and put on extra body fat, too. Fat tissue requires fewer calories to maintain than muscle does. The remedy? Move more. Physical activity burns fat and can build muscle, making weight loss easier. Increased physical activity can boost the rate at which your body uses energy for your basic energy needs.

... if your stomach shrinks when you eat less? No, your body doesn't work that way. Although your stomach can expand to accommodate a large intake of food, it doesn't stretch out indefinitely. As food passes to your intestines, the stomach goes back to its normal size. When you cut back on calories, your stomach keeps its normal size, even if your appetite isn't as big.

... if every person's body has a unique set point, or a preset weight, that it tries to return to? That's a theory with no conclusive evidence. Even if a set point exists, it's probably a range that can be set a little lower with more physical activity and food choices with fewer calories and fat. Or for someone who's too thin, eating a few extra calories may help adjust the set point a bit higher.

cause, talk to your doctor. This may be an early symptom of other health problems.

When You Want to Gain

There's plenty written about weight loss. However, some people need to gain weight. Weight gain can be as hard as weight loss!

The obvious approach for weight gain is this—consume more energy than your body burns. For every pound of body weight you gain, you need to consume 3,500 calories more than your body burns. As with weight loss, do so in a healthful way. *Note:* The suggestions indicated here are not meant for people with eating disorders, whose weight problems are complex and often life-threatening.

● Follow MyPyramid guidelines—and eat more food-group foods. MyPyramid has twelve plans for healthy eating, each at a different calorie level. To make your calories count for good nutrition, pick a plan with more calories than you eat now. You may have room for "extra" discretionary calories from foods with more fat or added sugars. *Refer to chapter 10 for more about MyPyramid and how to fit extras in, without overdoing it.*

● Even though higher-fat foods deliver more calories, be fat savvy. Keep your overall eating plan moderate in total fat and low in saturated fat and *trans* fats. Choose healthy fats. *See chapter 3.*

● Choose some foods with concentrated calories. That way you won't need to increase the volume of food too much. Try dried fruits. Fortify soups, casseroles, and fluid milk with dry milk powder. Enjoy some higher-calorie condiments, such as a dollop of sour cream on a baked potato. Garnish salads with olives, avocados, nuts, and cheese, which have more calories.

● Eat more frequently—five to six small meals a day—if your appetite is small. Eating two or three large meals during the day may be too much to handle at one time.

● Drink fluids thirty minutes before and after meals—not with meals. By limiting beverages at mealtime, you'll have more room for food.

● Focus on nutrient-rich foods and beverages. Don't fill up on low- and no-calorie foods or drinks, such as diet sodas or diet candies. Rather than coffee, tea, and water, drink juice, milk, and shakes.

● Enjoy a snack before bedtime.

● Stimulate your appetite if you just don't feel like eating. *See the following section, "No Appetite?"*

● Use the Nutrition Facts on food labels to choose nutrient-rich foods, which also supply more calories. *See chapter 11 for more on label reading.*

● Try adding a commercial liquid meal replacement, or make a shake or smoothie if you can't get enough calories from your regular meals and snacks.

● Ask a registered dietitian for more guidance on choosing healthful foods for weight gain. *See chapter 24, "Well-Informed?" for tips on finding a qualified nutrition expert in your area.*

● Stay physically active—good for muscle building and feeling energetic. It also may help stimulate your appetite!

Source: Adapted from Gail Farmer, *Pass the Calories, Please!* (Chicago: The American Dietetic Association, 1994). Used with permission.

No Appetite?

People lose their appetite for all kinds of reasons: illness, pain, fatigue, depression, stress, medication, disease, or a combination of these.

If that happens, the appetite control center of your brain might be affected, signaling that you're not hungry even when you should be. You may lose your appetite and tolerance for food when you're sick—even though you need nourishment to get well. Or emotional stress may affect your desire for and ability to handle food.

Cope with a loss of appetite. Eat by the clock rather than by hunger. It may be easier to consume all the calories you need. Take advantage of the "up" times. When you feel well and your appetite is good, eat and enjoy! To stimulate your appetite:

● Add some pizzazz to your foods! Colorful foods, appealing texture, and an appetizing aroma are helpful aids to increasing food intake.

● Drink a glass of beer or wine before meals. This often gives your appetite a jump start. But check with your doctor first.

● Eat meals with friends. The pleasure of being with others may be an appetite booster.

● Fill the house with enticing food aromas such as freshly baked bread, cake, or cookies.

● Keep favorite foods on hand. You may eat more when food is readily available.

● Make mealtimes pleasant. A relaxed and attractive setting with soft music or flowers on the table may perk up your appetite.

● Try eating your meal away from the dining room table, such as picnic style in the living room or at a candlelit table in front of the fireplace. Sometimes a change of place helps.

● Plan for longer mealtimes. Don't schedule activities close to meals.

● Walk before meals. A short walk often helps stimulate an appetite.

● Stay away from unpleasant or unsettling topics of conversation at mealtimes, especially if stress is a problem for you.

Source: Adapted from Gail Farmer, *Pass the Calories, Please!* (Chicago: The American Dietetic Association, 1994). Used with permission.

Disordered Eating: Problems, Signs, and Help

An estimated eight million Americans suffer from disordered eating, according to the National Association of Anorexia Nervosa and Associated Disorders (ANAD). Between 5 and 20 percent will die from medical complications as a result. Eating disorders—anorexia nervosa, bulimia, and binge eating disorder—are actually distorted eating habits often related to emotional problems. Anorexia typically results in low body weight; it's linked to menstrual irregularity, osteoporosis in women, and greater risk of early death in women and men. Bulimia may or may not be linked to low body weight. And binge eating disorder, probably the most common eating disorder, typically results in overweight and often in repeated weight gain and loss. All require qualified medical attention.

Anorexia and Bulimia: What Are They?

Anorexia nervosa is sometimes called the "starvation sickness." Obsessed with food, weight, and thinness, people suffering from anorexia deny their hunger and refuse to eat—even after extreme weight loss. As they consume too few calories for their basic needs, their bodies slowly waste away. By starving themselves, people with anorexia don't get the nutrients they need for normal bodily functions.

Bulimia nervosa is marked by binge eating and purging (self-induced vomiting). The person gorges, usually on high-calorie foods, and then intentionally vomits or uses laxatives or diuretics. The consequences are serious: dehydration, organ damage, internal bleeding from the stress of vomiting, tooth decay from acids in vomit, and in some cases, death. Many people with these eating disorders alternate between anorexia and bulimia. Reports indicate that 60 percent of people who have dieted extensively or starved themselves resort to bingeing, then purging to keep weight off.

Disordered eating is more than the "big three." Also getting attention: night eating syndrome (not just eating at night) and orthorexia nervosa, a popular name for compulsive attitudes and behavior about healthful eating. Compulsive exercising is a related concern.

When does an eating disorder start? Generally it begins with an ordinary weight-loss diet, begun just before or after a major life change or trauma. However, there's no clear understanding of the exact causes.

We do know, however, that eating disorders are more than food problems. The person's whole life—schoolwork or career, family life, overall health—gets wrapped up in the eating issues.

Who's at Risk for Anorexia and Bulimia?

People of almost any age and either gender may develop an eating disorder. However, some groups of people are more at risk than others.

- Females clearly are the most susceptible. In fact, approximately 90 to 95 percent of all people with anorexia or bulimia are women.

- Adolescents are at particular risk. Estimates indicate that as many as 1 of every 100 teenage girls in the United States will develop anorexia according to ANAD.

- Athletes such as dancers and gymnasts, who must control their weight, are susceptible.

- Eating disorders are being increasingly identified in males, as well as in adults and even in children as young as eight, nine, and ten years old.

Anorexia and Bulimia: The Warning Signs

Eating disorders produce warning signs. If you or someone you know shows any combination of these symptoms, be concerned!

People with anorexia may:

- Eat tiny portions, refuse to eat, and deny they are hungry.

Three Things to Know about Disordered Eating

Experts aren't certain about the exact causes of disordered eating. But they do agree on these key points:

1. **Food itself is not the primary problem.** Instead, eating patterns are symptoms of serious distress.

2. **Early detection is crucial.** The sooner the person gets help, the better the chance for permanent recovery.

3. **Help is available.** Team treatment, including medical and dental care, psychotherapy, nutrition education, and family counseling, provides the best results.

- Show abnormal weight loss—as much as 15 percent or more of body weight—or a large weight loss in a short time.

- Act hyperactive, depressed, moody, or insecure.

- Have an intense fear of being fat.

- See themselves as fat, wanting to lose more weight, even when they are very thin.

- Exercise excessively and compulsively.

- Suffer from constipation or irregular menstrual periods.

- Develop fine, downy hair on their arms and face.

- Complain of nausea or bloating after eating normal amounts of food.

- Binge-eat, then purge, perhaps by vomiting or using laxatives or diuretics.

People with bulimia may:

- Eat mainly in private.

- Disappear after eating—often to the bathroom.

- Show great fluctuations in weight, and may be of normal weight or be overweight.

- Feel out of control when eating.

- Eat enormous meals but not gain weight.

- Feel ashamed and depressed after gorging.

● Have swollen parotid glands. The parotid glands, near the ears, are one type of salivary glands.

● Experience irregular menstrual periods.

● Binge-eat, then purge.

● Abuse alcohol or drugs.

● Become dependent on laxatives, diuretics, emetics, or diet pills to lose weight. Emetics such as syrup of ipecac induce vomiting.

● Develop dental problems caused by acid from vomiting. Acids eat away at tooth enamel.

Binge Eating Disorder: A More Common Problem

Binge eating disorder (BED), different from occasional overindulging, is the uncontrollable eating of large amounts of food in a short time. Unlike bulimia, a person with BED usually doesn't purge, fast, abuse diuretics or laxatives, or overexercise. Estimates suggest that 2 percent of Americans (as many as 4 million) have this disorder—many are obese or overweight.

The concerns are physical, psychological, and social. Large amounts of food eaten by binge eaters are typically high in fats and added sugars, and may lack sufficient vitamins and minerals. With the likelihood of overweight and obesity comes an increased risk for serious health problems, including diabetes, heart disease, high blood pressure, gallbladder disease, and some cancers. Binge eating often results in depression, embarrassment, and social isolation; those with the disorder are often upset by both the problem and their inability to control their eating.

Although the cause of BED isn't clear, there's a link to depression and other negative emotions. Among the areas of research: the effect of brain chemicals and metabolism, and whether depression is a cause or a result of binge eating disorder.

Who's at Risk for Binge Eating Disorder?

Although many people with BED are overweight or obese (often severely obese), even normal-weight people have this disorder. More women than men deal with BED, but it's the most common eating disorder among men.

BED: The Warning Signs

Being overstuffed after an exceptional meal isn't necessarily a warning sign. Instead, people with binge eating disorder typically have several characteristics:

● Feel out of control when eating.

● Eat unusually large amounts of food.

● Eat very fast.

● Eat until they feel uncomfortable.

● Eat a lot, even when they aren't hungry.

● Feel embarrassed about the amount of food they eat, so eat alone.

● Feel disgusted, depressed, or guilty about overeating.

What to Do

If you suspect a friend or a family member has anorexia, bulimia, or binge eating disorder, don't wait until a severe weight problem or a serious medical problem proves you are right. There's plenty you can do before that happens:

● *Act to get help.* Speak to the person about your concern. Enlist assistance from family and friends. Talk to medical professionals, a social worker, or the school nurse or counselor if the person is a student. Call your local mental health association. A registered dietitian also can give you an expert perspective on eating disorders. *See chapter 24, "Well Informed?" to locate a registered dietitian in your area.*

As an aside: People with disordered eating may encourage disordered eating among others; today that problem has spread through the use of Web sites with private chat rooms.

For people with BED, a weight-loss diet alone may not be successful. Losing weight and keeping it off may be harder (for physical and emotional reasons) than for people without an eating disorder. Normal-weight people with binge eating disorder shouldn't be on a weight-loss diet.

The best treatment for disordered eating combines medical, psychological, and nutrition counseling. Participation in self-help groups for the patient, as well as group counseling for family members, are important parts of treatment.

● *Expect resistance.* A person with anorexia usually doesn't believe that he or she needs assistance or is in any danger. Someone with bulimia or BED may acknowledge the problem but still refuse to seek help. But the faster he or she gets help, the greater the chances for recovery.

● *Prepare for long-term treatment.* Recovery may take several months to several years. Symptoms and attitudes related to eating disorders rarely disappear quickly. Treatment includes helping people achieve an appropriate weight. Family support groups are particularly effective in helping relatives of people with disordered eating survive the long ordeal.

For more guidance, see "More Weighty Problems for Children—Fear of Weight Gain" and "Mainly for Girls . . . Pressure to Be Thin" in chapter 16.

"Diets" That Don't Work!

Every year Americans spend billions of dollars on the weight-loss industry—often for diet plans, diet books, services, and gimmicks that don't work! The lure of quick, easy weight loss is hard to resist, especially for those unwilling to make a commitment to lifelong behavioral change. Although the diets are ineffective in the long run, weight-loss hopefuls willingly give the next craze a chance. The result? Perhaps temporary results. But overall, wasted money, weight regained, a feeling of failure, and perhaps damage to health.

The next craze is often a past craze that's simply resurfaced with a new name, a new twist, yet still no sound science to back up the claims. Fad diets typically rely on nonscientific, unproved claims, personal stories, testimonials, or poorly controlled studies. Not surprisingly, many people feel confusion and diet fatigue as they sort through contradictory popular approaches to weight loss. Sound familiar? For those who try one fad diet after another, weight cycling becomes a common, frustrating problem. *See "Weight Cycling—The 'Yo-Yo' Problem" earlier in this chapter.*

"Magical, One-Food" Diets

The "grapefruit diet," the "all-you-can-eat fruit diet," the "rice diet," "the cabbage soup diet," "the no dairy foods diet"! There's a weight-loss diet for almost every taste.

The facts are . . . Often touted to help melt fat away, no single-food or single-food-group diet has any special ability to do that. These diets don't work for several reasons. They lack variety. They don't provide adequate amounts of all the nutrients and protective phytonutrients the body needs for health, especially when some foods are off-limits. With unlimited quantities of "magical foods," the dieter runs the risk of overeating the foods featured on the so-called diet plan. Any weight loss—and lower calorie intake—comes from eliminating entire groups of other foods, not to any single food or food group.

The bottom line is that no super food can reverse weight gain resulting from inactivity and overeating. Eliminating a food or food category doesn't work either. Also, because these diets don't teach new eating habits, people usually don't stick with them!

Low-"Carb," High-Protein Diets

Recent headlines and best-selling books promote low-carb and high-protein eating as a great solution to weight loss and fitness. Carbohydrates—starches and/or sugars—are often falsely accused as the culprits for weight gain. In fact, these diet plans aren't new. They've been around with different names for years.

QUICK CHECK: DOES THIS DIET WORK?

Popular diets may not work—at least not in the long run—if they promote:

● Foods and approaches with "miracle" fat- or weight-loss qualities.

● Odd amounts of foods or rigid food combining.

● Overemphasis on any one food or type of food.

● Quick weight loss.

● A food or product you must buy for success.

● Little, if any physical activity.

The facts are . . . Simply because these diets are lower in calories, they may promote loss—if you stick with them. Here's what happens. By consuming fewer "carbs," your body burns stored carbohydrates and releases water, thus water weight. If your "carb" intake is very low, your body also burns some fat, creating ketone bodies, which suppress appetite. If your total calorie intake (from any "energy nutrients") is low enough, you lose weight and muscle tissue.

A high-protein diet doesn't build muscle and burn fat, as some people think. Only regular physical activity and training build muscle strength and burn calories stored in body fat.

Because these weight loss plans are common today, research is under way looking at low to moderate carbohydrate diets for weight loss. They may be appropriate for some people, perhaps those with insulin resistance. Stay tuned. *See "Insulin Resistance Syndrome, or Metabolic Syndrome" in chapter 22.* A moderate-carbohydrate diet with more protein may help some people lose body fat while maintaining muscle as they lose weight.

For most people, a low-carbohydrate, high-protein eating approach for weight loss raises concerns:

● These diets do promote rapid weight loss—at first. Their diuretic effect promotes loss of water weight, not body fat, however. The psychological lift offers a false sense of success that's quickly gone when water weight returns.

● Depending on the foods consumed, a high-protein, low-"carb" diet may be high in total fat, saturated fat, and cholesterol. Inconsistent with sound nutrition advice, this weight loss regimen over time can increase the risk for heart disease and perhaps some forms of cancer.

● A diet that restricts many starchy foods is often low in fiber. The possible result? Constipation and other gastrointestinal disorders. A low-fiber diet isn't consistent with guidelines for health.

● A condition called ketosis (increased blood ketones from incomplete fat breakdown) can result with these regimens. Ketosis suppresses hunger and thus contributes to lower calorie intake. Some popular diets claim that ketosis hastens weight loss. In truth, muscle also breaks down

due to a lack of carbohydrate for energy. In addition, ketosis can cause weakness, nausea, dehydration, light-headedness, and irritability. It can be fatal to people with diabetes, and during pregnancy may cause birth defects or fetal death.

High-Fiber, Low-Calorie Diets

The flip side of the high-protein craze may be the high-fiber approach to dieting. It's true that most of us need more fiber to promote good health. Depending on your age and gender, 25 to 38 grams of fiber a day are advised for adults. *See chapter 6 for specific recommendations.* Too much—perhaps resulting from fiber supplements—may be too much of a good thing!

The facts are . . . As a food component, fiber isn't absorbed, so it doesn't contribute calories. That's why high-fiber foods such as whole grains, vegetables, legumes, and fruits—usually lower in calories—are included in weight-loss diets. These diets are quite filling, so you might eat less overall.

Very-high-fiber diets may come up short on protein foods. And they can cause constipation and dehydration if extra fluids aren't consumed.

Bulk fillers, which are high in fiber, aren't advised. They reduce hunger by first absorbing liquid, then swelling up in the stomach. These products can be harmful when they obstruct the digestive tract. *See "Supplement Watch: About Fiber Pills and Powders . . ." in chapter 6.*

Eating enough fiber-rich foods, as part of a healthful weight-loss plan, is a smarter idea!

Very-Low-Calorie Liquid Diets

Very-low-calorie liquid formulas have been developed for short-term use under a doctor's supervision. To help some obese people, they may aid short-term weight loss—if there's also a commitment to new eating and active living habits. Used as a liquid diet without other foods, they're very low in calories, providing just 400 to 800 calories a day.

These formulas were changed after deaths were attributed to their use. Newer formulas have more vitamins, minerals, and high-quality protein.

The facts are . . . Without medical supervision and nutrition education, liquid diets don't teach new ways

Eat What You Crave!

If the sight of certain foods puts your mind into a tailspin, you may need to readjust your approach to eating. An overly restrictive diet may "feed" a food craving—and set you up to overindulge!

The jury is still out on the true cause of food cravings. It may be physiological, psychological, or both. We don't yet know if food cravings are linked to a need to resupply the body with nutrients it lacks, or if cravings are reinforced by positive emotional and social links to certain foods.

Studies suggest that avoiding certain foods altogether often makes them irresistible. The result? Giving in to a food craving, and perhaps overeating. Then guilt creeps in, and people try to resist those foods once again, only to overindulge and feel guilty again.

What's a better approach? Eat a small portion of any food you enjoy—even if it's higher in fat or calories. Even when you're trying to shed pounds, you can enjoy some high-calorie foods as long as your eating plan is healthful, and you eat fewer calories overall than your body uses. As another option, try to satisfy your palate with a low-fat, low-calorie version.

of eating. Since people usually don't stay with them, there's usually no long-term weight loss. They also may result in fatigue, constipation, nausea, diarrhea, or hair loss. For people with some health problems, such as insulin-dependent diabetes or kidney disease, a very-low-calorie liquid diet can be harmful.

Fasting

As a tactic, does fasting jump-start weight loss?

The facts are . . . As with very-low-calorie diets, fasting deprives the body of energy and nutrients needed for normal functions. Any rapid weight loss is mostly water and muscle loss. Fasting also may cause fatigue and dizziness, with less energy for physical activity. And it feeds the cycle of "yo-yo" dieting.

As an aside, there's a misconception that fasting "cleans out" the system, removing toxic wastes. To the contrary, body chemicals called ketones build up in the body when carbohydrates aren't available for energy. Ketosis puts a burden on the kidneys; as noted, ketones that accumulate can be harmful to health.

Gimmicks, Gadgets, and Other "Miracles"

Promoters advertise "easy ways to weight loss"—weight-loss patches, electric muscle stimulators, spirulina (a species of blue-green algae), starch and fat blockers, creams that melt fat away, and many others. *Chapter 23 addresses some weight-loss supplements.*

The facts are . . . All these products have been offered for sale and purport to promote weight loss. Yet none proves effective. Some even may be harmful. And they're all a waste of money!

The popular press often advertises massages and other therapies for losing "cellulite," dimpled fat on thighs and hips. Cellulite is simply normal body fat under the skin that looks lumpy when the fat layer gets thick, allowing connective, fibrous-looking tissue that holds fat in place to show. The lumpy look can lessen or disappear with normal weight loss.

You've probably seen weight-loss programs that sweat off extra weight. Sweating in a sauna—or wearing a rubber belt or nylon clothes that make you perspire during exercise—may cause weight loss. However, the pounds that disappear are water loss, not body fat. When you drink or eat, weight returns.

Instead of helping to achieve a healthful weight goal, "sweating off" pounds may damage health through dehydration. *See chapter 8, "Fluids: The Power of Water," for more about the need for water.*

When You Need Help . . .

If you have weight problems of any kind or more questions about controlling your own weight, it's okay to

Have You Ever Wondered

. . . if meal replacements are effective for weight loss? Research has shown that meal replacements (such as liquid drinks, meal bars, and portion-controlled meals) can be an effective weight management aid for some people. They can offer convenience, ease, and portion and calorie control, and perhaps reduce sensory stimulation from food itself. Like any food, they should be nutrient dense.

seek outside advice and help. But be wary. Not every weight-loss "professional" is qualified to give the help you need. Steer clear of weight-loss programs and products that offer claims for quick fixes. They often promise far more than they can deliver.

First and foremost, choose a program that suits your personality and lifestyle. In addition, find a program with a maintenance plan that includes physical activity, and counseling that focuses on realistic behavioral changes. In the end, you supply your own motivation, but the plan must promote your good health. Above all, choose a sound plan you can live with.

If you need help finding a weight-control program, talk with a registered dietitian, who is trained to help you figure out what kind of weight-management system will fit your lifestyle. *For more help in finding a qualified nutrition professional and for reliable information about nutrition and health, see chapter 24.*

If you become ill after using a weight-loss product or service, contact the U.S. Food and Drug Administration at 1-800-332-1088.

Questions to Ask . . . about Diet Programs

Millions of Americans participate in organized weight-loss programs each year. Today the Internet even provides this service. Many of these programs are run by qualified medical and nutrition experts who can effectively help their clients lose weight and keep it off permanently. However, others make overblown claims and tout products that are ineffective and costly, and their staff may not have appropriate credentials. Before you sign on the dotted line, ask:

Need more strategies for sensible, effective weight management? Check here for "how tos":

- Help your child or teen keep a healthy weight—see chapter 16.
- Encourage your kids to move more and sit less—see chapter 16.
- Stay physically active in your later years—see chapter 18.
- Gain, maintain, or lose weight as an older adult—see chapter 18.

Have You Ever Wondered ❓

. . . if the glycemic index is useful for a weight-loss diet? Probably not. The glycemic index (GI) measures how individual foods affect blood sugar levels. But it's not easily applied to real-world eating. And there's insufficient research at this time showing how the glycemic index of a food in a meal affects weight loss or gain. *For more about GI, refer to chapter 5.*

. . . if getting more sleep helps with weight loss? Maybe. Scientists are investigating if sleep affects hormones that regulate hunger, feeling full, or metabolic rate. Research also is looking at the links between sleep and heart disease, diabetes, and immunity. Snooze enough, and stay tuned!

. . . why clothes look different on a mannequin than on you? Store mannequins don't represent average U.S. women. Mannequins are typically 6 feet tall, with a 34-inch bust, 23-inch waist, and 34-inch hips!

- What is the approach? What are the program goals?
- What are the health risks?
- How will you assess my health status before recommending the program? Many programs recommend a medical checkup before starting.
- Will the program include instruction, guidance, and skill building to help me learn to eat in a more healthful way for the long term? How?
- Will the program include guidance on physical activity for a lifetime? How?
- What data can you show me that prove your program works? What has been written about the program's success besides individual testimonials?
- Do customers keep off the weight after they leave the diet program? Ask for results over two to five years. The Federal Trade Commission requires weight-loss companies to back up their claims.
- What are the costs for membership, weekly fees, food, supplements, maintenance, and counseling? What's the payment schedule? Are any costs covered under health insurance? Do you give refunds if I drop out?
- Will you monitor my success at three- to six-month intervals, then modify the program if needed?

● Do you have a maintenance program? Is it part of the package, or does it cost extra?

● What kind of professional support is provided? What are the credentials and experiences of these professionals? (Detailed information should be available on request.)

● What are the program's requirements? Are there special menus or foods, counseling visits, or exercise plans?

For more guidance on evaluating a weight-control plan, see "Check It Out!" earlier in this chapter.

Have You Ever Wondered

. . . if food combining can help you lose weight? Forget this claim! It's just wishful thinking. No scientific evidence suggests that combining certain foods or eating them in careful sequence aids weight loss, or causes food to turn to body fat or produce toxins.

. . . if over-the-counter diet pills help with weight loss? Over-the-counter diet pills, or appetite suppressants, work by curbing appetite, but usually just for a few weeks. Some have unpleasant side effects, and some can be addictive, with potential damage to the heart and the nervous system. They may be prescribed to help a person start a lifelong program for weight management, but they're not a substitute for healthful eating habits over the long term. They should never be taken for very long—and only under a doctor's supervision.

. . . if obesity can be controlled with medication? For some people, medication may be prescribed—under a doctor's care—as part of an obesity treatment program. Such medication isn't effective for everyone, and can have potential side effects. The U.S. Food and Drug Administration (FDA) has approved two kinds for long-term use. Sibutramine is an appetite suppressant that seems to work with natural hormones (norepinephrine and serotonin) in the brain; however, it may increase blood pressure and induce an abnormally rapid heartbeat. Over-the-counter Orlistat reduces the absorption of dietary fat; however, it may reduce the absorption of some fat-soluble vitamins, too. The FDA has approved two others for short-term use: phentermine and diethyl-propion, which both work as appetite suppressants. Rimonabant, which also suppresses appetite, is awaiting FDA approval. Each has possible side effects and should be taken under a doctor's supervision Research continues on medications to manage obesity.

. . . if surgery and liposuction are options for weight loss? Not for most people. Gastric bypass surgery, done by shortening the small intestine or by making the stom-ach smaller, does promote weight loss. However, because the side effects can be harmful with lifelong implications, doctors generally advise surgery only as a final resort for people who are at least 100 pounds over-weight when other approaches haven't worked. Another approach, called adjustable gastric banding, can alter stomach capacity and emptying time. Lipo-suction, the surgical removal of fat tissue from various body areas, is often only a short-term solution. If eating and exercise habits remain the same, it's likely that weight will be regained.

. . . if you should join a support group to lose weight? Perhaps, but that's an individual matter. Weight-loss organizations and support groups often educate participants as they offer psychological support. And many, but not all, are coordinated by qualified nutrition experts. The section *"Questions to Ask . . . about Diet Programs"* can help you judge. For some people, peer support offers motivation, especially if they pay to attend the program. There's a downside, however. Without a weight maintenance program, many people gain weight again when they're no longer in the group.

. . . if "cyberdieting" works? Logging on to the Internet may offer support for weight loss. Some people like the anonymity; others like personalized help with feedback at home. Some research suggests that well-designed, interactive programs are effective—at least in the short term. The challenge is finding a site that offers sound guidance and privacy of personal data, rather than one that's mostly in business to sell products. There's another potential problem. Face-to-face weight-loss counseling with a registered dietitian addresses other issues—related health problems, personal lifestyles, and food preferences, among others—that may affect your weight-loss success; cyberdieting may not. *See "Nutrition in Cyberspace" in chapter 24.*

CHAPTER 3

Fat Facts

For more than two decades, fats have been in the limelight! With the health advice of today's experts, we're advised to moderate the total fat and lower the saturated fats, *trans* fats, and cholesterol in our food choices. Certainly media continues to report new research linking various types of fats and cholesterol to health outcomes. Culinary experts provide flavorful ways to use sensible amounts of fat in food prep. And the food industry has launched many fat-modified products: "reduced fat," "0 grams *trans* fat," and "with omega-3s." Not surprisingly, many consumers hear the message and consider the "fat facts" as they buy and prepare food.

While other nutrition-related concerns have emerged, attention to fat likely will be around for some time. Evidence indicates that a diet high in saturated fats, *trans* fats, and cholesterol increases risks for unhealthy levels of blood cholesterol, and therefore cardiovascular disease. High-fat eating (more than 35 percent calories from fat) is likely high in saturated fat, and risky for heart health. Managing excess calories is also harder with high-fat eating. There may be a link to some cancers, too. As science reveals more, it's also becoming clear that the links between the different types of fat and health are more complex than once thought.

Aging baby boomers are being forced to face the "fat facts of life." And people of all ages recognize that cutting back to a moderate fat intake—and eating less "sat fats," *trans* fats, and cholesterol and replacing some with healthy oils—will promote good health in the long run.

Many Americans already have cut down on their total fat intake to moderate levels. Yet there's still room to improve, to make healthier food and fat choices, and to consume less saturated and *trans* fats.

Fats Matter

Suppose your doctor said, "You need to get your serum cholesterol level down. Your triglycerides are borderline high. And cut the fat, especially the saturated fat, in your diet." Just what would this mean to you? And what would you do? To understand the role of fats in food, health, and chronic disease, we need to start with the basics.

Fat: A Nutrient for Health

With all the attention on fat, you may be surprised to learn that fats have fundamental health functions and positive benefits. Fat is a nutrient necessary for your health. In moderate amounts, fats perform a full workload of body functions. You actually can't live without them! That's why a fat-free diet isn't a healthful goal. There's more to healthful eating than simply cutting back on fats. In fact, the type of fat you eat may be just as important as the total amount of fat in your diet. Evidence suggests that the various types of fats in foods have different effects on health; some fats may even offer health-protective benefits. So just how does fat help keep you healthy?

Fats: Essential Work

Fats work as partners in your body with other nutrients. Just as sugar dissolves in water, some vitamins dissolve in fat. That's how vitamins A, D, E, and K, as

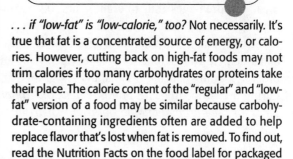

HOW MUCH OMEGA-3?

	OMEGA-3S (GRAMS)	TOTAL FAT (GRAMS)
Fatty fish, about 3 ounces, cooked		
Atlantic herring	1.8	9.8
Anchovy, canned in oil, drained	1.8	8.3
Atlantic salmon, farmed	1.8	10.5
Chinook salmon	1.7	11.4
Atlantic mackerel	1.1	15.1
Rainbow trout, farmed	1.0	6.1
Less fatty fish, about 3 ounces, cooked		
Tuna, white, canned in water, drained	0.7	2.5
Halibut, Atlantic and Pacific	0.5	2.5
Flounder	0.5	1.3
Shrimp	0.3	1.0
Tuna, light, canned in water, drained	0.2	0.7
Catfish, farmed	0.2	6.8
Codfish, Atlantic	0.1	0.7

PLANT-BASED FOODS	ALA (CONVERTS TO OMEGA-3S (GRAMS)*	TOTAL FAT (GRAMS)
Ground flaxseed, 2 tbsp.	3.2	6
Walnuts, 1 oz. (14 halves)	2.6	18.5
Canola oil, 1 tbsp.	1.3	14
Soy nuts, ¼ cup	0.7	11

*About 35 percent of ALA is converted to omega-3s.

Source: U.S. Department of Agriculture, Agricultural Research Service, 2005. *USDA National Nutrient Database for Standard Reference*, Release 18.

Figures have been rounded.

well as carotenoids, are carried in food and into your bloodstream. Without fats, these fat-soluble vitamins cannot fully nourish your body.

Certain fats are considered essential, specifically two fatty acids—linoleic acid and alpha-linolenic acid (ALA)—which your body can't make. (Fatty acids are the building blocks of fat.) For children to grow normally and for adults and children to maintain healthy skin, food choices must supply linoleic acid. For children, alpha-linolenic acid is important, too. Alpha-linolenic acid converts to omega-3 fatty acids, which keep your brain and nervous system functioning normally. You may know some omega-3s by their nicknames: EPA (eicosapentaenoic acid) and DHA (docosahexaenoic acid). Linoleic acid is an omega-6 fatty acid. *See "Functional Nutrition: Eat Your Omega-3s and -6s" on page 56.*

Both linoleic acid and alpha-linolenic acid are widely available in food: for example, linoleic acid from vegetable oils and poultry fat, and alpha-linolenic acid (converts to omega-3s) from soy oil, nuts, and seeds. If your food choices are varied, getting enough of these fatty acids is easy. EPA and DHA are naturally part of some foods, especially fatty fish and fish oils.

Have You Ever Wondered

. . . if "low-fat" is "low-calorie," too? Not necessarily. It's true that fat is a concentrated source of energy, or calories. However, cutting back on high-fat foods may not trim calories if too many carbohydrates or proteins take their place. The calorie content of the "regular" and "low-fat" version of a food may be similar because carbohydrate-containing ingredients often are added to help replace flavor that's lost when fat is removed. To find out, read the Nutrition Facts on the food label for packaged foods. Even if the calories are less, go easy on your amount of low-fat or fat-free foods. Eating a whole box of fat-free cookies isn't a "low-calorie" experience! (*See page 39.*)

. . . if a reduced-fat food is always "low-fat"? Not necessarily. It just may have less fat (at least 25 percent less) than its full-fat counterpart. Check the Nutrition Facts on food labels to find out. *See "Label Lingo" later in this chapter to know what the terms mean.*

How much omega-3s? The recommended amount isn't much; it adds up to 10 to 15 calories a day. The Institute of Medicine has set a daily Adequate Intake level: children ages four to eight years, 0.9 grams; boys ages nine to thirteen, 1.2 grams; girls ages nine to thirteen years, 1 gram; males ages fourteen years and older, 1.6 grams; females ages fourteen years and older 1.1 grams; during pregnancy, 1.4 grams, and during breast-feeding, 1.3 grams. *Check the Appendices for the Acceptable Macronutrient Distribution Range.*

A "Power Source"

Like carbohydrates and proteins, fats supply energy, or calories, to power your physical activity and the many body processes that keep you alive. (Remember: A calorie is a unit of energy.) Fats are a concentrated energy source, supplying 9 calories per gram. To compare, carbohydrates and proteins provide just 4 calories per gram. Although your body uses fat for energy, it's not the body's preferred fuel source. And often fat isn't used for energy.

If you consume more energy from fat than your body needs, your body saves the extra in your body's fatty tissues, mostly in fat cells. Body fat also is known as adipose tissue. When you need an extra energy supply, your body can draw on this stored fat. Other body cells and blood plasma have some fat, too.

Fat for Satiety

A little fat in food adds more than flavor. It also helps satisfy hunger by making you feel full. Why? Because fats take longer to leave your stomach than carbohydrates or proteins do. If you eat a very-low-fat meal, you may feel hungry again within an hour or two.

Body Fat: Its Role

You need a certain amount of body fat: to cushion and position your body organs, to protect your bones from injury, and as a fat layer under your skin, which offers insulation, helping you stay warm on a cold day. The soft fat pads on your buttocks and the palms of your hands protect your bones from bumps, bangs, and jolts. Fat that's stored around your organs isn't accessed for energy.

Why Foods Contain Fat

Fat offers sensory qualities that make food taste good. As an ingredient, fat carries flavor. It also gives a smooth, creamy texture to foods such as ice cream and peanut butter. When foods such as a brownie seem to melt in your mouth, that's just what's happening—the fat is melting! From meat to baked foods, fat makes many foods moist and tender, or brown and crispy.

Can you cut the fat in a recipe? To a certain extent, yes. The recipe may work if you use less. But eliminating fat altogether may not give the result you expect.

In baked foods. Fat tenderizes; adds moisture; holds in air so baked foods are light; and affects shape, for example, in cookies. With too little fat, baked goods might be tough or dry, or may not rise properly.

In sauces. Fat keeps sauces from curdling and forms part of an emulsion. An emulsion is a mixture of two substances, such as fat and water, that stay together instead of separating, as they normally would.

Your "Fat Tooth"

Have a craving for rich chocolates or desserts? Your "fat tooth," not your "sweet tooth," may account for that urge. In this world of high-fat foods, a preference for them may be culturally conditioned. Research suggests that happens early, when infants and young children learn through experience that fat is associated with satiety (reduction of hunger).

A smooth, creamy milk shake; a flaky, tender pastry; and a juicy steak: the appeal of high-fat foods may come from qualities that fat imparts. Or perhaps the appeal stems from on-again, off-again dieting. Some studies say that dieting may amplify a fat craving, or more likely, the craving for sweetened fat like that found in many rich desserts.

No matter what the reason for a "fat tooth," you can overcome, or manage, your preference for fatty foods:

- Fool your tastebuds. Get a smooth, creamy consistency with low-fat and fat-free ingredients: low-fat yogurt in savory dips; thick, pureed fruit as a dessert sauce; and creamy buttermilk as a milk shake base.
- Indulge a "fat tooth." Share a rich dessert to cut your fat grams and calories in half.
- Gradually shift to lower-fat foods.

In other cooked foods. Fat helps conduct heat as food cooks—for example, when food is sautéed (cooked quickly in a small amount of fat) or fried.

In cooked meat, poultry, and fish. Fat seals in moisture as foods are basted, or brushed with liquid during cooking. Sometimes the surface gets dry if it isn't basted.

For foods cooked in a pan. Fat lubricates the pan so food won't stick.

In all kinds of food. Fat helps carry flavor and nutrients, provides texture (mouth feel), and adds satiety.

Sorting the Fats

The dictionary of fat terms seems endless and often confusing. In fact, there's no one kind of fat. Some terms describe fats in the body; others apply to fats in food; and some to both. Just what do all these terms really mean?

"Fat" Dictionary

Lipid. Scientific term that refers to all fats, cholesterol, and other fatlike substances; lipids do not dissolve in water.

Lipoproteins. Protein-coated packages that carry lipids, including cholesterol, in the bloodstream. Without the protein coating, lipids cannot travel through the bloodstream.

Cholesterol. Waxy, fatlike substance found in foods of animal origin and in every body cell. It's essential for cell building.

Blood (serum) cholesterol. Cholesterol that travels in the bloodstream. The body manufactures most of its blood cholesterol; some is also absorbed from foods you eat.

Dietary cholesterol. Cholesterol in food, found only in foods of animal origin, and never from plant sources, even if they contain fat.

HDL ("good") blood cholesterol. Cholesterol carried by high-density lipoproteins (HDLs). HDLs carry cholesterol and other blood lipids away from body cells to the liver so they can be broken down and excreted. HDLs—with a higher ratio of protein to cholesterol—are made in the liver in response to physical activity and some foods. Food doesn't have them.

LDL ("bad") blood cholesterol. Cholesterol carried by low-density lipoproteins (LDLs). LDLs circulate to body cells, carrying cholesterol and other lipids, where they may be used. LDL cholesterol may form deposits on artery and other blood vessel walls. LDLs—with a higher ratio of cholesterol to protein—are also manufactured in the liver. They are only in the body, not in food.

Fats. Group of compounds made of glycerol and fatty acids. Fats are one of three macronutrient groups that supply energy; the others are carbohydrates and proteins. Fats can be stored in the body.

Adipose tissue. Scientific term for body fat.

Dietary fat. Fats in food.

Triglycerides. Scientific name for the common form of fat found both in the body and in foods. Most body fat is stored in the form of triglycerides; triglycerides also circulate in the blood. Triglycerides, made of three fatty acids and glycerol, act like saturated fat: they trigger the liver to make more cholesterol so levels of total and LDL cholesterol rise.

Fatty acids. Basic units of fat molecules arranged as chains of carbon, hydrogen, and oxygen. Fats are mixtures of about sixteen different fatty acids, categorized by their structure. Each has its own unique physiological effect in your body. The terms "fats" and "fatty acids" are often used interchangeably.

Monounsaturated fatty acids (MUFAs). Fatty acids missing one hydrogen pair on their chemical chain. They trigger less total or LDL cholesterol, and more HDL cholesterol, production. Canola, nut, and olive oils are high in monounsaturated fatty acids.

Polyunsaturated fatty acids (PUFAs). Fatty acids missing two or more hydrogen pairs on their chemical chains. They also trigger lower total blood cholesterol, as well as lower LDL and HDL cholesterol, production. Corn, safflower, soybean, sesame, and sunflower oils are high in polyunsaturated fatty acids. Fatty acids in seafood are mainly polyunsaturated, too.

Saturated fatty acids. Fatty acids that have all the hydrogen they can hold on their chemical chains. They trigger the liver to make more total and LDL cholesterol. In food, they come mainly

Functional Nutrition: Eat Your Omega-3s and -6s

No doubt about it: seafood can be good for your health. Overall, it has less total fat and less saturated fat than meat and poultry. For this reason, eating fish regularly may help lower your blood cholesterol levels. Moreover, seafood supplies several vitamins and minerals. Recently there's been interest in the functional food benefits provided by the omega-3 fatty acid content of fish.

Omega-3 fatty acids—polyunsaturated fatty acids of a somewhat different structure—are found mostly in seafood, especially higher-fat, cold-water varieties such as mackerel, albacore tuna, salmon, sardines, Atlantic herring, swordfish, and lake trout. Flaxseed oil, soybean oil, and canola oil, as well as walnuts, supply omega-3s, too, in the form of alpha-linolenic acid, which converts to omega-3s. And some eggs have more omega-3s if the chicken feed supplied it.

Research suggests that omega-3s may help thin blood and prevent blood platelets from clotting and sticking to artery walls. That, in turn, may help lower the risk for blocked blood vessels and heart attacks and strokes. Omega-3s may help prevent arteries from hardening, lower levels of triglycerides, and modestly reduce blood pressure levels.

Even if scientific evidence eventually completely understands the link, omega-3 fatty acids by themselves aren't a magic remedy for heart disease—and you can't simply add them to your meals and snacks to get the potential benefits. Combined with eating less saturated fat in an overall healthful diet, they may have a protective effect. Researchers are exploring other links between omega-3 fatty acids and health: eye health, rheumatoid arthritis, and immunity. Stay tuned!

To enjoy nutritional and omega-3s' benefits from some seafood, make fish a regular part of your eating style; try to eat fatty fish twice weekly (8 ounces total per week). And try using foods with omega-3s in place of foods with more saturated fats.

Although fish oil supplements contain omega-3 fatty acids, they're not advised as a substitute for fish—or as a dietary supplement for most people. Popping a fish oil capsule won't undo the effects of an otherwise unhealthful diet. Instead, enjoy fish for its nutritional benefits, flavor—and variety in your eating style. The American Heart Association advises a fish oil capsule for some people with elevated triglycerides—and under a physician's care.

What about omega-6s (polyunsaturated fatty acids in vegetable oils)? They, too, may help reduce cardiovascular disease risk by helping to lower total and LDL-cholesterol blood levels; however, they also may lower HDL levels.

Another fatty acid—conjugated linoleic acid (CLA)—may offer functional benefits, too. CLAs are found in dairy foods and some meat products (beef, lamb). Research is exploring a potential link to decreased risk for certain cancers and a role in improved body composition. Little human research has yet been done.

---

from animal-based foods such as meat, poultry, butter, whole milk, and whole milk products, and from coconut, palm, and palm kernel oils.

Oil. Fat in liquid form.

Omega-3 fatty acids. Fatty acids (EPA and DHA) that are highly polyunsaturated. They may help reduce blood clotting in the arteries and protect from hardening of the arteries. Mostly they come from seafood, especially fatty fish such as albacore tuna, mackerel, and salmon, and in the form of alpha-linoleic acid in walnuts, and soy, canola, and flaxseed oils.

Omega-6 (linoleic) fatty acids. Another group of polyunsaturated fatty acids. They, too, may help promote heart health by lowering total and LDL cholesterol. Vegetable oils—soybean, corn, safflower—are good sources.

Trans *fatty acids.* One type of fatty acid, formed during the process of partial hydrogenation. Although they're found naturally in some foods, most *trans* fatty acids in the diet come from partially hydrogenated fats. In the body, man-made *trans* fats act like saturated fats and tend to raise blood cholesterol levels.

Hydrogenated fats. Unsaturated fats that are processed to make them more saturated, and stable and solid at room temperature—for example, in many packaged foods (such as crackers and cookies) and stick margarine. Hydrogen is added to their chemical makeup and makes them firmer and more saturated while

FATS AND OILS: HOW DO THEY COMPARE?

DIETARY FAT	Saturated Fat	Monounsaturated Fat	Alpha-Linolenic Acid (an Omega-3 Fatty Acid)	Linoleic Acid (an Omega-6 Fatty Acid)
Canola oil	7	61	11	21
Safflower oil	8	77	1	14
Flaxseed oil	9	16	57	18
Sunflower oil	12	16	1	71
Corn oil	13	29	1	57
Olive oil	15	75	1	9
Soybean oil	15	23	8	54
Peanut oil	19	48	*	33
Cottonseed oil	27	19	*	54
Lard	43	47	1	9
Palm oil	51	39	*	10
Butterfat	68	28	1	3
Coconut oil	91	7		2

Fatty acid content normalized to 100 percent

*Trace

SOURCE: POS PILOT PLANT CORPORATION; www.canolainfo.org.

extending their shelf life. The extent of hydrogenation determines whether there's a little or a lot of *trans* fats.

Fats: Not Created Equal

Whether solid or liquid, the fats that we consume are broken down into fatty acids and glycerol in the body. In turn, the body uses them to form other lipids, which are used for a variety of bodily functions. When fat is stored in your body, it's in the form of a triglyceride.

In scientific terms, fatty acids are chains of carbon, hydrogen, and oxygen. They may be saturated or unsaturated. The term "saturation" refers to how many hydrogen atoms link to each carbon in the chain.

- When carbon atoms have as many hydrogens attached as possible on the chain, a fatty acid is *saturated*.

- When hydrogen atoms are missing, the fatty acid is *unsaturated*. A polyunsaturated fatty acid has two or more missing hydrogen pairs; a monounsaturated fatty acid is missing one hydrogen pair on its chemical chain.

Now what makes margarine different from vegetable oil? The fatty acid content. All foods with fats have a mixture of fatty acids: saturated, polyunsaturated, and monounsaturated. The proportion and differences in fatty acid content account for their varying characteristics—for example, liquid oil as compared with firm margarine. Their degree of saturation also has a significant role in how fatty acids from food affect health.

- Fats made mostly of saturated fatty acids usually are solid at room temperature. Animal-based foods and tropical vegetable oils (coconut, palm kernel, and palm) contain mainly saturated fatty acids. In general, harder and more stable fats are more saturated. They include butter, stick margarine, shortening, and the fat in cheese and meat.

- By contrast, fats that contain mostly polyunsaturated fatty acids usually are liquid at room temperature. Safflower, sunflower, corn, and soybean oils contain the highest amounts of polyunsaturated fats.

- Foods with mostly monounsaturated fatty acids are liquid at room temperature. They're found in more significant amounts in some vegetable oils, such as canola, olive, and peanut oils.

Besides fats and oils, the proportion of fatty acids varies in other fat-containing foods. For example, seafood and meat both have saturated and unsaturated fatty acids. However, seafood has a higher proportion

AT A GLANCE: HOW DIETARY FAT AFFECTS BLOOD LIPIDS

TYPE OF FATTY ACIDS	EFFECTS ON BLOOD LIPIDS
Saturated	↑ total cholesterol, ↑ LDL cholesterol
Polyunsaturated	↓ total cholesterol, ↓ LDL cholesterol, ↓ HDL cholesterol*
Monounsaturated	↓ total cholesterol, ↓ LDL cholesterol, may ↑ HDL cholesterol*
Omega-3	↓ triglycerides, ↓ total cholesterol*
Trans	↑ total cholesterol, ↑ LDL cholesterol, may ↓ HDL cholesterol

*Unsaturated fatty acids may have a beneficial effect if they replace saturated fats, but not if they're simply added, making the diet higher in fat.

of polyunsaturated fatty acids; meat, more saturated fatty acids.

About Trans Fats

Processing can change the structure of fat, making it more saturated. The process is called partial hydrogenation because missing hydrogen is added to fatty acid chains in their chemical makeup. As a result, oils become semisolid and more stable at room temperature. Usually hydrogenation is partial, making fat 5 to 60 percent saturated. The result: *trans* fatty acids.

The term "trans" simply describes the chemical makeup of a fatty acid. Beef, pork, lamb, butter, and milk naturally have small amounts of *trans* fatty acids. Naturally occurring *trans* fatty acids have different, potentially beneficial, health effects, from man-made *trans* fats. They don't have the same cholesterol-raising effects.

All margarines are made from vegetable oil. In stick margarine, the fatty acids are more hydrogenated, with a higher proportion of saturated fatty acids and *trans* fats, making it more firm than soft margarine sold in tubs or as "squeeze" margarine. Tub and squeeze margarines contain more water, and may have air whipped in so they may be lower in fat and calories. Butter-margarine blends may be even firmer than stick margarine; saturated fatty acids in butter help keep the product firm.

Why hydrogenate the oil? This process gives desirable qualities to food. For example, because hydrogenated fats are more stable, they extend the shelf life of foods such as crackers and margarine so they don't develop a rancid flavor and odor as quickly. Hydrogenating the oil in peanut butter gives a creamy consistency; oil stays mixed in and doesn't rise to the top. Stick margarine and shortening remain firm at room temperature when their oil is partially hydrogenated. In the fast-food industry, many foods are fried with these fats. The food industry is developing ways of hydrogenating fat without forming man-made *trans* fats.

Why the concern about *trans* fats? *Trans* fatty acids act like saturated fats, raising LDL blood cholesterol levels and potentially decreasing HDL cholesterol. That, in turn, may increase the risk for fatty deposits on blood vessel walls and heart attacks. *Trans* fatty acids supply about 2 to 3 percent of total calories

Have You Ever Wondered ❓

. . . what trans-free spreads are? They're usually margarine-type products processed with little or no *trans* fatty acids. Their formulas differ and may contain fat replacers. Look for *trans* fat amounts on food labels.

. . . if melting a fat such as butter, stick margarine, or lard makes it less saturated? While unsaturated fats are liquid at room temperature, simply heating and melting doesn't change saturated fatty acids to unsaturated fatty acids. As soon as lard, margarine, or butter is cooled to room temperature, it's solid again.

. . . what stearic acid is? It's another saturated fat, found in animal products and some plant foods, under scientific study. Research suggests that its effect may be neutral, neither raising nor lowering blood cholesterol levels. For now, there's not enough evidence to offer advice—but enough to suggest that even saturated fats work in different ways. One third of the saturated fat in beef is stearic acid.

. . . what shortening really is? It's simply another term that refers to fat. Solid at room temperature, shortening is vegetable oil (often partially hydrogenated soybean or cottonseed oil, palm oil, or coconut oil) sometimes combined with animal fat. Their being high in "*trans* fats" and perhaps "sat fats," go easy on shortening or foods made with shortening.

for American adults; saturated fat intake is 4 to 5 times higher. Still, it's wise to be prudent, especially if you have high cholesterol levels already. You don't need *trans* fats for normal health. As the Dietary Guidelines advise: *Keep* trans *fatty acid consumption as low as possible.* And at the same time, consume a healthful eating plan; you can't eliminate *trans* fats completely.

How can you cut back on *trans* fats? Check food labels and go easy on foods with "partially hydrogenated vegetable oil" as one of the first ingredients: stick margarine, vegetable shortening, and many prepared foods, cakes, cookies, crackers, snack foods, and commercially fried foods, including fried fast foods. Look for *trans* fat amounts on food labels. Because of rounding, a product with partially hydrogenated oil may say "0 *trans* fats" on the label; up to 0.5 grams of *trans* fats are considered zero.

As food products are being reformulated, *trans* fat content is dropping. Newer fats such as rice bran oil may be used instead.

Fat: More Than Meets the Eye!

Visible or not, almost all foods contain fat in varying amounts. Some are very high in fat; others have just trace amounts.

The fat content of some foods is obvious: for example, in butter, oil, and margarine. Even in certain cuts of meat and poultry with the skin on, fat is easy to see—and easy to trim off.

In most foods, however, clues to a food's fat content appear on food labels. The Nutrition Facts panel tells how much per label serving. Salad dressings, many baked foods, chips, crackers, chocolate, nuts, avocados, sauces, meat, poultry, fish, cheese, dairy products, and egg yolks, for example, all contain varying amounts of fat. Obviously, fried foods contain more fat than those that are baked or steamed.

Which foods typically supply the most fat?

● On average, most fat in the American diet comes directly from fats and oils, as well as salad dressings, candy, gravies, and sauces.

● Animal-based foods provide varying amounts of fat, as well as saturated fat. With lean and fat-modified products on the market, check the Nutrition Facts on food labels to know how much and which types.

● With only a few exceptions (avocados and olives), fruits and vegetables don't supply much fat naturally. That's true for most grain products, too—unless it's added during food preparation or processing. French fries, fried okra, croissants, and hush puppies are all higher-fat choices.

About Fat Replacers . . .

Today's supermarkets sell options! Foods made with fat replacers can help you consume less fat if they really replace full-fat products in your food choices. These foods have much of the taste, texture, and appearance of their higher-fat counterparts. Besides being lower in fat, they're usually, but not always, lower in saturated fat, cholesterol, and calories as well.

Fat gives unique characteristics to food, so when fat is removed from a "recipe," perhaps to make a low-fat cookie, many characteristics of the food change, too. Fat replacers often give these foods a familiar texture, appearance, and taste.

Food manufacturers use different types of fat replacers: carbohydrate-, protein-, and fat-based. Most contribute calories, although less than fat does. Because no fat replacer acts exactly like fat, most reduced-fat and fat-free products contain a mixture. From a food safety standpoint, scientific research and review by the U.S. Food and Drug Administration (FDA) recognize fat replacers as safe.

Carbohydrate-Based Fat Replacers

Modified starches, dextrins, cellulose, gums, and other carbohydrate ingredients work by combining with water to provide texture, appearance, and mouth feel that are similar to fat. Fat-free salad dressings, for example, contain carbohydrate-based substitutes. The calories in carbohydrate-based replacers range from almost nothing to 4 calories per gram. The difference is that some, such as modified starches and dextrins, are digested; others, such as cellulose and other fibers,

Have You Ever Wondered

. . . if olive oil has fewer calories and less fat than butter? Because liquid oils are concentrated, and solid fats may contain a small amount of other ingredients besides fat, oils generally contain slightly more fat and calories than equal amounts of solid fat. Per tablespoon, olive oil contains about 14 grams of fat and 120 calories compared to butter, with about 12 grams of fat and 100 calories. The main difference is the types of fatty acids. Olive oil has a higher proportion of healthier monounsaturated fatty acids; butter is more saturated.

. . . which has more saturated fat: butter or margarine? Although stick margarine has more *trans* fats than butter, it still has less saturated fat. Another way to compare is to look at the total of saturated fats plus *trans* fats. One tablespoon of butter has about 7 grams of saturated plus about 0.5 grams *trans* fats; the same amount of some stick margarine has about 2 grams of saturated fat plus about 3 grams of *trans* fats. Total fat is comparable.

Primer: Fat, Saturated Fat, and Cholesterol in Food

	Total Fat (g)	Saturated Fatty Acids (g)	Cholesterol (mg)	Calories
Breads, Cereals, Rice, Pasta				
Bread, 1 slice				
White (from refined wheat)	1	Trace	Trace	70
Whole-wheat	1	Trace	0	65
Egg bagel, ½ small (3-in. diameter)	1	Trace	9	100
Biscuit, 1 small, 2½-in. diameter	6	1	0	130
Roll, dinner, 1 (1 oz.)	2	0.5	0	85
Croissant, 1 medium	12	7	38	230
Blueberry muffin, 1 small	4	1	20	185
Pancake, 1 (4-in. diameter)	4	1	22	90
Waffle, 1 (4-in. square)	3.5	0.5	5	100
Doughnut, yeast, 1 (3¾-in. diameter)	14	3.5	4	245
Danish pastry, 1 (4¼-in. diameter)	13	3.5	81	265
Oatmeal, cooked, ½ cup	1	Trace	0	65
Shredded wheat, 1 large biscuit	0.5	Trace	0	85
Granola, ⅓ cup	10	2	0	220
Rice, white, cooked, ½ cup	Trace	Trace	0	120
Fried rice (with egg and vegetables), ½ cup	6	1	21	120
Cookie, 1 medium				
Oatmeal (2⅝-in. diameter)	3	0.5	5	65
Chocolate chip (2¼-in. diameter)	4.5	1	5	85
Cake, chocolate, frosted (2-in. square)	10.5	3	27	235
Milk, Yogurt, Cheese				
Milk, 1 cup				
Whole	8	4.5	24	150
2% reduced-fat	5	3	20	120
1% low-fat	2.5	1.5	12	100
Fat-free	Trace	Trace	5	85
Yogurt, 1 cup				
Nonfat plain	Trace	Trace	5	135
Low-fat plain	4	2.5	15	155
Low-fat fruit flavored	3	2	14	240
Cottage cheese, ½ cup				
Creamed	5	3	17	115
1% low-fat	1	1	5	80
Cheese, 1 oz.				
Natural Cheddar	9.5	6	30	115
Low-fat Cheddar	2	1	6	50
Mozzarella, part fat-free	6	3.5	15	85
Process American	7	4.5	18	95
Vanilla ice cream, ½ cup	8	5	32	145
Vanilla reduced-fat ice cream, ½ cup	4	2	21	125
Frozen yogurt, ½ cup	3	2	11	110

	Total Fat (g)	Saturated Fatty Acids (g)	Cholesterol (mg)	Calories
Vegetables				
Potatoes				
Boiled, ½ cup	Trace	Trace	0	70
Potato salad, ½ cup	10	2	85	180
French fries, 10 strips	5	1	0	200
Au gratin, ½ cup	9	6	28	160
Chips, 1 oz.	11	3	0	155
Cabbage, ½ cup				
Cooked	Trace	Trace	0	15
Creamy coleslaw	7	1	5	100
Celery and carrot sticks, 8	Trace	0	0	10
Stir-fried vegetables, ½ cup	Trace	Trace	0	45
Meats, Poultry, Fish, Beans, Eggs, and Nuts				
Beef				
Lean cut (eye of round), roasted, 3 oz.				
Lean and fat	13	5	61	210
Lean only	4	1.5	46	145
Fattier cut (chuck blade), braised, 3 oz.				
Lean and fat	29	12	88	355
Lean only	11	4.5	90	215
Ground, cooked, 3 oz. patty				
Regular	15	6	70	230
Lean (80%)	13.5	5	73	210
Extra lean (95%)	5	2	65	140
Pork center loin, roasted, 3 oz.				
Lean and fat	11.5	4	68	200
Lean	8	3	67	170
Beef liver, braised, 3 oz.	4.5	1.5	337	160
Chicken, light and dark meat, roasted, 3 oz.				
With skin	12	3	74	200
Without skin	6	2	75	160
Halibut fillets, baked, 3 oz.	2.5	Trace	35	120
Salmon, Atlantic, farmed, cooked, 3 oz.	10.5	2	54	175
Tuna, canned, 3 oz.				
In oil	7	1	26	160
In water	2.5	Trace	36	110
Crabs, canned, 3 oz.	1.5	Trace	85	90
Shrimp, steamed or boiled, 8 large	0.5	Trace	86	180
Frankfurters, 2 (3 oz.)	27	10	80	300
Dry beans, cooked, ½ cup	Trace	Trace	0	110
Peanut butter, 2 tbsp.	16	3	0	190
Sunflower seeds, 2 tbsp.	8	1	0	95
Egg, large, cooked, 1	5.5	2	212	80
Yolk	4.5	2	210	55
White	Trace	0	0	15

PRIMER: FAT, SATURATED FAT, AND CHOLESTEROL IN FOOD *(continued)*

	TOTAL FAT (G)	SATURATED FATTY ACIDS (G)	CHOLESTEROL (MG)	CALORIES
Fruits				
Apple, 1 medium (2¾-in. diameter)	Trace	Trace	0	70
Avocado, ½ medium	15	2	0	160
Banana, 1 medium (7 to 8 in. long)	0.5	Trace	0	105
Olives, 5 large				
Green	3.5	Trace	0	30
Ripe	2.5	Trace	0	25
Orange, 1 medium (2½-in. diameter)	Trace	Trace	0	60
Peach, 1 medium (2½-in. diameter)	Trace	Trace	0	40
Strawberries, 5 medium	Trace	Trace	0	20
Mixed fruit cup with cream dressing, ½ cup	3	2	9	80
Fats, Oils, Sweets				
Butter, 1 tbsp.	11.5	7	31	100
Butter-margarine blend, 1 tbsp.	11.5	4	12	100
Margarine, 1 tbsp.				
Soft	11.5	2	0	100
Stick	11.5	2	0	100
Liquid (squeezable)	11.5	2	0	100
Light	5.5	1	0	50
Vegetable oil (corn), 1 tbsp.	14	2	0	120
Hydrogenated vegetable shortening, 1 tbsp.	13	3	0	115
Salad dressing, 1 tbsp.				
Mayonnaise (regular)	11	2	5	100
Mayonnaise, reduced-calorie	5	1	5	50
Mayonnaise-type	5	1	4	60
Mayonnaise-type, reduced-calorie	3	0.5	4	40
Italian	5.5	1	0	55
Italian, reduced-fat	1	Trace	1	10
Cream, 1 tbsp.				
Sour	2.5	1.5	5	25
Light (table)	3	2	10	30
Nondairy, frozen	1	Trace	0	20
Cream cheese, 1 tbsp.	5	3	16	50
Pie, apple, ⅛ of 9-inch	19.5	5	0	410
Cheesecake, 1/12 of 9-inch	25	10	86	405
Sherbet, ½ cup	1.5	1	0	110
Milk chocolate bar, 1 oz.	8.5	4	7	150

Source: U.S. Department of Agriculture, Agricultural Research Service, 2005. *USDA National Nutrient Database for Standard Reference*, Release 18.

aren't digested, so they provide no energy. Most of these fat replacers can withstand some heat; however, they can't be used for frying.

Pureed prunes (dried plums) and applesauce sometimes are used as fat replacers in baked foods. They're an easy fat substitute you can try yourself. Pureed prunes and applesauce add bulk, flavor, and nutrition.

Protein-Based Fat Replacers

Made with protein from egg whites or fat-free milk, these fat replacers provide a creamy sensation and improve appearance and texture when fat is removed. Low-fat cheese made with a protein-based substitute gives an appearance and texture that come close to full-fat cheese. Most protein-based replacers aren't used in foods prepared at high temperatures. That's because the protein coagulates, and they no longer function in ways similar to fat.

Protein-based replacers contribute 1 to 4 calories per gram, compared with 9 calories per fat gram. What accounts for the calorie range? These replacers may be blended with ingredients such as cellulose that can't be digested. Protein-based replacers also provide small amounts of amino acids.

Fat-Based Replacers

These are made with fats that have been chemically altered. They provide few or no calories as compared to fat because the body is unable to fully absorb the fatty acids. They may be used in baked foods, some fried foods, cake mixes, frosting, and dairy foods.

Olestra is a calorie-free fat replacer made from vegetable oils and sugar. It contributes no calories because it passes through the body without being digested and absorbed. Olestra provides the characteristics of fat in cooking, especially for frying and snack foods. Olean is the brand name for olestra that you'll see on food labels. Because olestra isn't digested, some vitamins carried by fat aren't fully

absorbed. For this reason, fat-soluble vitamins are added to foods made with olestra. For some people, consuming foods with olestra may be linked to digestive discomfort.

Salatrim is another fat-based replacer used in baked goods, dairy products, and confection-type products. It provides calories, but only 5 calories per gram (as compared to 9 calories per gram in fat) because it is only partially absorbed in the body.

What Foods Contain Fat Replacers?

If you scan the supermarket shelves you see low-fat or fat-free versions of full-fat foods: margarine, salad dressing, mayonnaise, cheese, sour cream, ice cream, cookies, baked foods, and candy, to name a few. They're made by replacing some or all of the fat with fat replacers.

FAT REPLACERS: ONE WAY TO LOWER FAT AND CALORIES

Fat-modified foods can make a difference in the calories and fat of a meal. Foods with fat replacers may have more carbohydrates; that's why the percent of fat reduction may be higher than the percent of calorie reduction.

	CALORIES	FAT (GRAMS)
Regular Lunch		
2 slices bread	130	2
1 oz. American cheese	95	7
2 oz. bologna	175	14
1 tbsp. mayonnaise	100	11
Banana	105	0
2 chocolate chip cookies (30 g)	160	9
Total	765	43
Lunch with Fat-Modified Foods		
2 slices bread	130	2
l oz. reduced-fat cheese product	60	3
2 oz. fat-free bologna	45	0
1 tbsp. low-fat mayonnaise/dressing	50	5
Banana	105	0
2 reduced-fat chocolate chip cookies (30 g)	140	5
Total	530	15

Source: Adapted from International Food Information Council Foundation, ific.org and *USDA National Nutrient Database for Standard Reference*, Release 18.

To some degree, fat replacers supply calories, so the energy contributed by fat-modified foods may or may not be less than the original food. For the calories and fat per serving, check the Nutrition Facts panel on the food label. And go easy. Less fat is no license to overeat!

The bottom line: Fat replacers can be a safe and effective option for making meals and snacks appealing—and at the same time, control the fat and energy in your food choices.

Cholesterol: Different from Fat

To clear up a common misperception, cholesterol is a fatlike substance, but it's not a fat itself. Cholesterol has a different structure from fat and performs different functions in the human body. Some functions promote health; some don't. Because fat and cholesterol often appear together in foods of animal origin, and because their roles in health are so intertwined, they're easily mixed up.

Like fat, cholesterol often gets a "bad rap," yet it's part of every body cell and of some hormones, including sex hormones such as estrogen. As part of a body chemical called bile, it helps the body digest and absorb fat, too. With the help of sunlight, a form of cholesterol in your skin can change to vitamin D, a nutrient essential for bone building. However, too much cholesterol in the bloodstream is linked to heart disease.

Have You Ever Wondered?

... what a label stating "98% fat-free" means? You might think this means that only 2% of the total calories come from fat. Actually, the percent is referring to weight and not calories. So "98% fat-free" means that 2% of the weight of the total serving comes from fat. By law, when manufacturers use a "% fat-free" on a label, the amount of total fat must be below 3 grams of fat per serving. This amount is quite low, but may be more than you'd think when reading the "% fat-free" claim.

Functional Nutrition: Stanol- and Sterol-Based Ingredients

New cholesterol-lowering spreads contain unique, functional ingredients: plant stanol esters or plant sterol esters. Stanols and sterols are naturally present in small amounts in vegetables and plant oils. In fact, the average person consumes about 250 milligrams of plant stanols and sterols daily from many plant-based foods, not enough to lower blood cholesterol.

Naturally occurring plant stanols and sterols, however, can be modified and added to fat-containing foods. For example, butterlike spreads with plant sterol or stanol esters are promoted for their ability to lower LDL blood cholesterol by up to 14 percent; they don't affect HDLs. For a significant cholesterol-lowering effect, the health claim states that you need to consume two servings of a spread that contains plant stanol or sterol esters daily—with meals—as part of an eating plan that's low in saturated fat and cholesterol. Read the package label for the serving size.

These spreads offer cholesterol-lowering benefits to anyone. Research shows that people with elevated cholesterol levels benefit most. In fact, the 2001 National Cholesterol Education Program of the National Institutes of Health recommends the addition of 2 grams per day of stanols or sterols as part of the dietary management for high blood cholesterol levels. People on statin drug therapy can use these spreads for additional cholesterol-lowering as part of their healthful eating.

Two spreads—Take Control and Benecol—contain these unique dietary ingredients. Use them in food preparation, not only as a spread. Benecol regular spread (with plant stanol esters) can be used in cooking and baking without changing the flavor of food. Use it like any other margarine, substituting it equally for the fat, oil, or shortening in a recipe. A spread that contains plant sterols (Take Control) isn't recommended for baking or frying; use it in foods that aren't cooked.

The health claim for stanols and sterols can apply to spreads, salad dressings, snack bars, and soft-gel dietary supplements made with stanol and sterol esters. In the future, a broader array of foods may be approved as well.

Have You Ever Wondered

. . . if using olive oil and canola oil in your food prep is healthful? Sure—if you substitute and take saturated fats away, too. Both oils are high in monounsaturated fatty acids and low in saturated fatty acids. Monounsaturated fatty acids may help lower blood cholesterol levels more than polyunsaturated fatty acids do. However, simply adding olive or canola oil to an already high-fat diet is not the point. These oils are still 100 percent fat, with about 120 calories per tablespoon.

. . . what's the source of canola oil? The canola plant, developed from its close relation to the rapeseed plant, using traditional methods of plant breeding. Extracted from canola seeds, canola oil is very low in saturated fat, yet a great source of mono- and polyunsaturated fats.

Canola oil differs from rapeseed oil (consumed in Europe and Asia) in a significant way. To clarify a misperception, canola oil is extremely low in erucic acid. While erucic acid hasn't been shown to affect human health, it's been linked to cardiac abnormalities in experimental animals. The U.S. Food and Drug Administration deems canola oil safe in food.

. . . if cholesterol supplies calories? Often confused with fat, cholesterol isn't a source of energy, or calories. Unlike fats, carbohydrates, and proteins, cholesterol isn't broken down, so the body cannot derive any energy from it.

. . . what tropical oils are? And how they stack up for nutrition? Tropical oils (coconut, palm, palm kernel) come from the fruit or nuts of the tropical plants they're named for. In processed foods they impart qualities similar to partially hydrogenated oils. There's debate, however, about their impact on blood cholesterol levels. While tropical oils contain saturated fats, palm oil too has quite a bit of polyunsaturated fat; coconut oil contains a fatty acid, called lauric acid, with possible health benefits. Until more is known, limit foods made with tropical oils.

Blood vs. Dietary Cholesterol

Confused about cholesterol? You're not alone! Actually, the term itself refers to two different types. Blood, or serum, cholesterol circulates in the bloodstream. Dietary cholesterol comes from food.

While many factors affect blood cholesterol levels, the cholesterol that circulates in your body comes from two sources:

● *Your body produces cholesterol*—enough for your needs. Your liver makes most of it, but every body cell can make cholesterol, too. In fact, when the body makes too much, the risk for heart disease goes up. Unlike adults, infants and young children's bodies don't produce enough cholesterol, so for children under age two, it's important that their food choices supply cholesterol.

● *Cholesterol also comes from foods and beverages of animal origin:* eggs, meat, poultry, fish, and dairy foods. Animals produce cholesterol, but plants don't. A diet high in cholesterol is one factor that elevates blood cholesterol levels for some people. That's why the Dietary Guidelines advise: *Consume less than 300 milligrams of cholesterol a day*. Dietary cholesterol doesn't automatically become blood cholesterol. Saturated fat and *trans* fats in your food choices have a more significant effect on blood cholesterol levels than dietary cholesterol alone does.

The "Good" and the "Bad"

Have you ever wondered what the terms "good" cholesterol and "bad" cholesterol really mean? They refer to cholesterol carried in your blood by two types of lipoproteins, and not to cholesterol in food.

Because cholesterol doesn't mix with water, it can't be carried alone in your bloodstream. Instead, it's combined in "packages" with fats and proteins. These packages, called lipoproteins, carry cholesterol both to and from your body cells.

The nicknames "good" and "bad" cholesterol relate to risk factors for heart disease. High levels of HDL, or "good," cholesterol are linked to *lower* heart disease risk; high levels of LDL, or "bad," cholesterol, to *higher* heart disease risk. Think "high" for health and "low" for less healthy. Total blood cholesterol consists of both HDL and LDL cholesterol.

Although HDL and LDL cholesterol aren't found in food, your food choices do influence LDL levels. If you lower the saturated fat, *trans* fat, and cholesterol in your diet, you'll likely bring down LDL blood cholesterol levels. And if you're physically active, you'll likely lower your LDL cholesterol and keep your HDL blood cholesterol higher. What you eat and how active you are are just two of many factors that affect LDL, HDL, and total blood cholesterol levels. *Refer to "HDLs and LDLs: The Ups and the Downs" on page 546.*

Cholesterol: In What Foods?

What foods contain cholesterol? Only foods of animal origin. Egg yolks and organ meats are especially high in cholesterol. And in varying amounts, meat, poultry, seafood, dairy products, and animal fats such as butter or lard all supply cholesterol, too. Cholesterol is not found in vegetable oils, margarine, or egg whites, or in plant-based foods such as grains, fruits, vegetables, beans, and peas.

As mentioned before, cholesterol and saturated fatty acids often occur together in animal-based foods. That's why they sometimes get confused. Sirloin steak, butter, and Cheddar cheese, for example, all contain both saturated fatty acids and cholesterol. On the other hand, shellfish and organ meats are high in cholesterol, yet they're low in saturated fatty acids.

In foods of animal origin, both lean and fatty tissues contain cholesterol. That's why some low-fat foods, such as squid and shrimp, can be relatively high in cholesterol. The sauce or butter they're dipped in can boost their cholesterol content, too.

Even though some plant-based foods (margarine, vegetable oil, nuts, and seeds) are high in fat or saturated fat, they have no cholesterol, even margarines made with *trans* fats.

So why do some vegetable dishes and grain-based baked goods contain cholesterol? It's the added ingre-

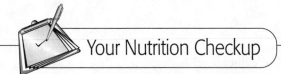

Your Nutrition Checkup

Fat and Cholesterol Audit

What's the fat and cholesterol quotient of your eating style? For each section, check one box in each column that matches your usual food choices over the course of a day or several days. Choosing from every column is okay. That's part of making trade-offs! Remember: Your overall fat intake over time is what counts—not each individual choice.

COLUMN 1 (3 POINTS)	COLUMN 2 (2 POINTS)	COLUMN 3 (1 POINT)
☐ Reasonable portions, equivalent to 5 to 7 oz., of meat, poultry, or fish per day (or less if you also eat protein-rich beans, eggs, and nuts)	☐ Some reasonable portions and some bigger portions, equivalent to somewhat more than 7 oz., of meat, poultry, or fish per day	☐ Big portions of meat, poultry, and fish, equivalent to much more than 7 oz. per day
☐ Low-fat and fat-free milk dairy products	☐ Both low-fat and whole-milk dairy products, and some higher-fat products, such as cheese	☐ Whole-milk dairy products and higher-fat products, such as cheese
☐ Variety of lean meat, skinless poultry, and fish	☐ Some lean and some higher-fat meat and poultry	☐ High-fat meat, such as juicy steak or high-fat sausage, or poultry with skin on

COLUMN 1 (3 POINTS)	COLUMN 2 (2 POINTS)	COLUMN 3 (1 POINT)
☐ Broiled, grilled, or roasted foods such as meat, poultry, and fish, and steamed, boiled, or baked vegetables	☐ Some broiled, grilled, or roasted foods, and others that are fried	☐ Mostly fried or sautéed meat, poultry, fish, and vegetables
☐ Little or no gravy or creamy, high-fat sauces	☐ Some gravy or high-fat sauces	☐ Plenty of gravy and/or high-fat sauces
☐ Low-fat salad dressing or small amount (1 tbsp. per serving) of regular salad dressing	☐ Some regular salad dressing	☐ Liberal use of regular salad dressing
☐ Fruit, frozen yogurt, and other low-fat desserts, and low-fat or *trans*-free snacks	☐ Some low-fat desserts and snacks, and some with more fat, such as regular ice cream, cake, cookies, and regular chips	☐ Plenty of high-fat desserts and snacks
☐ Small amounts of stick margarine, butter, or high-fat spread or toppings on breads or vegetables—and healthy oils	☐ Mostly just small amounts of stick margarine, butter, or other high-fat spreads or toppings on breads or vegetables	☐ Liberal amounts of stick margarine, butter, or other high-fat spreads or toppings on bread or vegetables
☐ Bagels, bread, tortillas, and other low-fat breads	☐ Some low-fat breads and some higher-fat breads such as croissants, muffins, and doughnuts	☐ Mostly higher-fat breads
☐ An egg yolk or less a day	☐ Usually an egg yolk or less a day, but sometimes more	☐ 2 or 3 egg yolk breakfasts, almost daily
Column 1 subtotal _____	*Column 2 subtotal* _____	*Column 3 subtotal* _____

Now for the totals . . .

Your score: _____. Each box is worth 3, 2, or 1 point(s).

If you scored . . .

20 to 30 points—You're savvy about the fat in your food choices.

16 to 19 points—You've got the idea. Yet you still have room to trim fat, especially saturated fat and *trans* fat and cholesterol, in your food choices a bit more. Read on!

10 to 15 points—For your good health, you're wise to rethink your overall eating style for less total fat, saturated fat, *trans* fat, and cholesterol. Read on for simple, practical tips!

dients: egg yolks, cheese, milk, meat, poultry, butter, or lard. Some common examples are refried beans made with lard, greens cooked with bacon, and muffins made with butter and egg yolks. The amount of cholesterol per serving varies with the recipe.

When shopping, if you spot a food that's labeled "no cholesterol" or "cholesterol-free," it cannot have any more than 2 grams of saturated fat. However, you'll want to read the rest of the food label to find out about the total fat content; it could still be high in fat.

Too Much of a Good Thing?

Today, many Americans think about the amount of fat in their diets. Rightly so. Our total fat and cholesterol intake have dropped. That may account partly for a slight, recent decline in death rates from heart disease. Yet many still exceed the amounts advised by health experts for total fat, and especially for saturated fats and *trans* fats.

High-fat eating, especially high saturated fat and excessive *trans* fats, is linked to higher blood cholesterol levels and so a greater chance for heart disease. There's more reason for caution: eating a high-fat diet also increases the risk for obesity, and a diet high in saturated fat, for colon and prostate cancers.

Weight control is a good reason to go easy on fat since high-fat foods are often high in calories, too. Whether they're saturated or unsaturated, calories from fat are all alike. Every fat gram supplies 9 calories, or more than twice the amount provided by 1 gram of carbohydrate or protein. And excess calories, whether from fats, carbohydrates, or proteins, are stored in the body as fat. Remember: The total amount of calories eaten, not just the calories from fat, is the issue in weight management. *Check "Primer: Fat, Saturated Fat, and Cholesterol in Food" earlier in this chapter to compare the calories in higher-fat foods.*

For more about the effects of fat, saturated fat, trans fat, and cholesterol on heart disease and cancer, see "Your Healthy Heart" and "Cancer Connection" in chapter 22.

Fat and Cholesterol: Know Your Limits

How much fat is enough? That depends. The Dietary Reference Intakes recommend a range, not a single amount. Age is factored into the recommendations. And specific amounts depend on how many calories you consume overall. For adults, the 2005 Dietary Guidelines advise:

● *Keep your total fat intake between 20 and 35 percent of your calories from fat, with most fats coming from sources of polyunsaturated and monounsaturated fatty acids, such as fish, nuts, and vegetable oils.*

● *Consume less than 10 percent of your calories from saturated fatty acids, less than 300 mg per day of cholesterol, and keep* trans *fatty acids as low as possible.*

The Dietary Guideline for fat for children and teens is discussed in chapter 16.

Why Healthy Oils?

You know you need fat for health, energy, and for kids, growth. Most of it should be polyunsaturated or monounsaturated, the kinds you find in oils, such as canola, corn, olive, and soybean oils.

All fats are made of saturated, polyunsaturated, and monounsaturated fatty acids, but the proportions differ; see *"Fats and Oils: How Do They Compare?" earlier in this chapter.* Their differences determine how they affect your health.

Polyunsaturated fats contain essential fatty acids, necessary for health. That's why MyPyramid has a category for oil; *refer to chapter 10 to learn more.* Besides their essential fatty acids, oils are the major source of vitamin E for most Americans. Another reason to consume healthy oils in place of solid fats: neither monounsaturated nor polyunsaturated fats raise LDL ("bad") cholesterol levels in the blood.

That said, oils do provide calories: 120 calories per tablespoon, about the same as solid fats. You need to limit how much you consume to stay within your calorie budget; *see chapter 10.*

What if you eat less than 20 percent of your calories from fat and oils? You might come up short on vitamin E, a fat-soluble vitamin with antioxidant powers that may be cardioprotective. Another possibility: missing out on essential fatty acids, which only food provides.

Of the other 65 to 80 percent of calories, 45 to 65 percent should come from carbohydrates, mostly starches (complex carbohydrates) from foods such as bread, cereal, rice, pasta, vegetables, and fruit; the remainder, from protein.

To clear up any confusion, advice for fat intake applies to your total diet, *not* to a single food or a single meal. And the percent of calories you consume from fat—over several days—impacts your health. So don't worry or feel guilty if you occasionally eat more. Just make it up by eating less on other days.

In real numbers, how much is 20 to 35 percent calories from total fat—and less than 10 percent calories from "sat fat"? The specific amount depends on your energy needs. And that depends on your age, gender, body size, and activity level. You can check the bottom of the Nutrition Facts panel on many food labels.

What's Your Limit on Fat and Saturated Fat?

IF YOU CONSUME THIS AMOUNT OF CALORIES A DAY . . .	KEEP YOUR DAILY TOTAL FAT INTAKE WITHIN THIS RANGE* . . .	LIMIT YOUR DAY'S SATURATED FAT INTAKE* TO . . .
1,600	36 to 62 g	less than 18 g
2,000	44 to 78 g	less than 20 g
2,200	49 to 86 g	less than 24 g
2,500	56 to 97 g	less than 25 g
2,800	62 to 109 g	less than 31 g

*Reflects 20 to 35 percent calories from total fat and less than 10 percent of calories from saturated fat, which are the adult recommendations.
Source: Institute of Medicine; *Dietary Reference Intakes for Macronutrients,* National Academies Press, 2002.

For a 2,000- and a 2,500-calorie diet, it shows how many fat grams equal less than 30 percent of calories from fat. Guidelines for saturated fat from the American Heart Association are lower; *see chapter 22.*

To guesstimate your calorie need, see "Your 'Weigh': Figuring Your Energy Needs" in chapter 2.

Trim Fat in Your Eating Style

Do you consume too many calories from fat? Too much saturated or *trans* fat? From a health standpoint, you'd probably benefit by cutting back!

The advice of the Dietary Guidelines: *When selecting and preparing meat, poultry, dry beans, and milk or milk products, make choices that are lean, low-fat, or fat-free. Limit intake of fats and oils high in saturated and/or trans fatty acids, and choose products low in such fats and oil.*

Cutting back on fat or switching to healthier fats doesn't need to be a huge change. Even small changes add up. Often eating a smaller portion of a high-fat dessert, switching to lean meat and low-fat or nonfat dairy products, and eating broiled rather than fried foods are enough to make a daily difference.

Keep in mind that you can reduce fat, including saturated fat and *trans* fat, from your food choices in many ways. To start, try a few strategies listed here.

For Less Total Fat . . .

● Know where fat comes from. You can't cut back unless you know the sources of fat. *See "Primer: Fat, Saturated Fat, and Cholesterol in Food" earlier in this chapter.*

Check the Nutrition Facts on food labels for how much fat, including saturated fat, *trans* fat, and cholesterol a single label serving contains. *To learn how to best use the Nutrition Facts panel, see "Get All the Facts!" in chapter 11.*

● Look for nutrient content claims on the label, perhaps "low-fat" or "lean." As you shop, use these clues to help guide your food purchases. *To learn what these claims mean, see "Label Lingo: Fats and Cholesterol" later in this chapter.*

● Choose lean meat (beef, veal, and/or pork) and skinless poultry. Loin and round cuts of meat have less fat. Trim visible fat from meat and poultry, too. Lean meat isn't fat-free; it just has less fat.

Lean meat contains cholesterol in both the fat and in lean muscle tissue. Trimming the fat and buying lean cuts reduce the cholesterol in meat but won't make it cholesterol-free.

● Make your meals "fishy." Enjoy seafood several times a week, prepared a low-fat way. Go for fish, preferably fattier fish such as salmon, twice a week, to get the potential omega-3 benefits.

● Eat plenty of fruits and vegetables. Besides being low in fat they fill you up and help curb your appetite for higher-fat foods. Soluble fiber in some fruits, vegetables, and grain products also has a cholesterol-lowering effect. *To think about the variety of tasty fruits and vegetables in today's supermarkets, see "Garden of Eatin': Less Common Vegetables" and "Fresh Ideas: Uncommon Fruit" in chapter 9.*

● Go for grains, including whole grains! Choose lower-fat grain products—pasta, rice, breakfast cereal, bagels, tortillas, pita, and other lower-fat breads. Go easy on doughnuts, sweet rolls, higher-fat muffins, cakes, and cookies. Consume more of your food energy from carbohydrate-rich foods and less from fat!

● Choose mostly low-fat or fat-free dairy products.

The bone-building nutrients in low-fat and whole-milk products are about the same.

● Moderate fats overall. That includes vegetable oils, butter, margarine, lard, cream cheese, and bacon used in cooking, as well as high-fat salad dressings, sauces, and many candies. Add flavor with herbs and seasonings rather than high-fat sauces.

● Consider today's fat-modified foods on supermarket shelves: for example, fat-free salad dressing, low-fat snacks, *trans*-free spreads, and eggs with omega-3s. Remember: Many lower-fat processed foods have the same or more total calories than their traditional counterparts. Read the Nutrition Facts on the food label to compare.

● Watch your "snack fats." Smart snacks fill in missing nutrient gaps, help control hunger, and can provide an energy boost between meals. But some popular snack foods are higher in fat, perhaps saturated fat and *trans* fat, than you may realize.

● Defat your cooking style without losing flavor. For example, broil, bake, boil, steam, stir-fry, or microwave foods, rather than fry.

● Add flavor with herbs and spices instead of high-fat flavorings or sauces. Rub mixtures of seasonings on tender cuts of meat before cooking for wonderful blends of flavors. Use low-fat or fat-free marinades to tenderize and add flavor to lean cuts of meat.

● When you can, substitute foods and ingredients high in unsaturated fatty acids for those high in saturated fatty acids. *The chart "Easy Substitutions to Cut Fat and/or Cholesterol" in chapter 13 offers a list of easy ways.*

● Watch your portion sizes. The amount of fat and cholesterol in your food choices depends on both what you eat and how much. Extra-large portions of higher-fat foods provide extra-large amounts of fat.

● Make beans the "main event" at meals occasionally. Meals with cooked dry beans as the main protein source have several cholesterol-lowering qualities. *Usually* bean dishes are lower in total fat, saturated fat, and cholesterol—yet higher in starches (complex carbohydrates) and fiber—than dishes made with meat or cheese.

● Order "lean" when you order out. In a fast-food or

CHECK OUT THE DIFFERENCE: SNACKS WITH MORE AND WITH LESS FAT!

SNACKS	TOTAL FAT (GRAMS)	CALORIES
Apple (1 medium)	0	70
Spiced applesauce (½ cup)	0	100
Apple pie (⅛ of 9-in.)	20	410
Banana (1)	0	105
Milk chocolate bar (1½ oz.)	13	235
Broccoli, raw (½ cup)	0	15
Chocolate chip cookie 2¼-in. (1)	4	80
Carrot (1 medium)	0	25
Carrot cake (1/12 of 9-in.)	11	240
Orange (1 medium)	0	60
Corn chips (1 oz.)	8	150
Strawberries (½ cup)	0	25
French fries (10)	5	200
Salsa (¼ cup)	0	20
Sour cream dip (¼ cup)	12	125
Saltines (10 crackers, or 1 oz.)	4	130
Potato chips (1 oz.)	11	155
Frozen yogurt (½ cup)	3	110
Ice cream, regular (½ cup)	8	145
Angel food cake (1/12 of cake)	0	130
Pound cake (1/16 of loaf cake)	13	230
Gingersnaps (4) (1 oz.)	3	120
Butter cookies 2-in. (6) (1 oz.)	6	135
Bagel 3½-in. (1)		
With 2 tbsp. jam	1	295
With 2 tbsp. part skim ricotta cheese	4	225
With 2 tbsp. cream cheese	11	285
Doughnut (1 glazed/sugared)	10	190

table-service restaurant, look for menu clues that suggest less fat, such as "grilled" or "broiled." Ask questions about how food is prepared. And go easy on foods that are fried, breaded, or prepared with rich sauces or gravy.

Yogurt Cheese

Create your own "fat replacer": yogurt cheese as a thick spread, creamy dip, or baked potato topper. It's low in fat, yet high in calcium.

Line a strainer with a paper coffee filter, or use a strainer specially meant for making yogurt cheese. Place it over a deep bowl. Spoon gelatin-free yogurt (plain or flavored) in the strainer; cover. (Check the label to see if it contains gelatin.) Refrigerate. Drain the liquid whey for 2 to 24 hours, depending on the firmness you want. Drained for 24 hours, 32 ounces of yogurt yields about 1½ cups of yogurt cheese.

Add flavor with apricot preserves and chopped nuts; crumbled blue cheese and grated apple or pear; salmon and chopped green onion; or herb blend.

Source: St. Louis District Dairy Council.

For Less Saturated Fat and Trans Fat . . .

● Limit solid fats such as butter, stick margarine, lard, and partially hydrogenated shortenings; when you can, use vegetable oils instead. Liquid vegetable oils have less saturated and *trans* fatty acids and more unsaturated fatty acids than fats that are firm at room temperature. Go easy on animal fats, too, since they're more saturated. For example, choose soft tub or squeeze (liquid) margarine in place of stick margarine or butter. And try polyunsaturated or monounsaturated oil in recipes calling for melted shortening or butter. *Check "Lean Tips . . . for Baked Goods" in chapter 13 for substitutions with vegetable oil in baked goods.*

● Cut back on total fat. You'll likely reduce saturated fats—and *trans* fats, too. *Tip:* Less "sat fat" gives leeway for plant-based foods with unsaturated fat.

● Check the Nutrition Facts for the saturated fat and *trans* fat in one label serving; choose foods with less. Check the ingredient list, too. If any of these ingredi-

FUNCTIONAL NUTRITION: A QUICK LOOK AT FATTY ACIDS, STANOLS, AND STEROLS

DIFFERENT TYPES OF FATTY ACIDS, STANOLS, AND STEROLS	WHAT THEY APPEAR TO DO	WHERE THEY'RE FOUND (SOME FOOD SOURCES)
MUFAs	● May reduce risk of coronary heart disease (CHD)	● Tree nuts
PUFAs: omega-3 fatty acids—ALA	● May contribute to maintenance of mental and visual function	● Walnuts, flaxseed
PUFAs: omega-3 fatty acids—DHA/EPA	● May reduce the risk of CHD ● May help maintain mental and visual function	● Salmon, tuna, marine and other fish oils
PUFAs: conjugated linoleic acid	● May help maintain desirable body composition and healthy immune function	● Beef, lamb, some cheese
Free Stanols/Sterols*	● May reduce risk of CHD	● Corn, soy, wheat, wood oils, fortified foods and drinks
Stanol/Sterol Esters*	● May reduce risk of CHD	● Fortified table spreads, stanol ester dietary supplements

* The U.S. Food and Drug Administration has approved a health claim for this food component.
Source: Adapted from the International Food Information Council Foundation, 2004.

ents is among the first several listed, the food is likely higher in saturated fat: butter, partially hydrogenated vegetable oil, coconut oil, palm oil, palm kernel oil, cocoa butter, meat fat, lard, egg yolks, whole milk solids, cream, or cheese.

For Less Cholesterol . . .

● Go easy on egg yolks, including eggs in prepared foods such as bread, cakes, and pancakes. The yolk has all the cholesterol—about 215 milligrams from a large egg. *Tip:* Substitute two whites for one whole egg in baked goods, or use an egg substitute.

● Go easy on organ meats such as liver. Even though they're nutritious, they're high in cholesterol.

● Look for lean meat, fish, poultry, and low-fat dairy foods. You'll trim away some cholesterol along with fat.

● Check labels to find low-cholesterol or cholesterol-

Need more lean and low-fat strategies for healthful eating? Check here for "how-tos":

● Shop for foods with less fat and cholesterol—see chapter 11.

● Trim fat in your kitchen without giving up flavor—see chapter 13.

● Cut back on fat in restaurant orders—and enjoy food, too—see chapter 14.

● Enjoy a vegetarian approach to lower-fat eating—see chapter 20.

● Handle fats, "sat fats," and *trans* fats and cholesterol to manage heart disease and other chronic diseases—see chapter 22.

Have You Ever Wondered

. . . if coconut milk is high in fat? One cup of canned coconut milk (made by combining grated coconut meat and coconut water) contains 445 calories and 48 fat grams (of which 43 fat grams are saturated). Coconut water, or liquid, drained from a fresh coconut—without any grated coconut meat—has just 46 calories and less than 1 fat gram per cup. Just ¼ cup of dried, sweetened coconut has 87 calories and 6 fat grams. Look for canned coconut milk with less fat.

. . . if salmon is lower in fat than chicken? Salmon has about 185 calories and 9 fat grams per 3-ounce cooked portion compared with 190 calories and 9 fat grams in the same portion of roasted, light-meat chicken with the skin on. Skinless, this same portion of chicken contains about 150 calories and 3 fat grams. The potential benefits of salmon: more omega-3 fatty acids.

. . . if air-popped popcorn is always low in fat? Not always. If you buy it ready-made, check the Nutrition Facts for total fat, saturated fat, and *trans* fat content. Although the package may say "air-popped," oil may be added after popping as a flavoring. For microwave popcorn, check the label to see if oil is added—and how much and what kind. And what about the bucket of popcorn you buy in malls or movie theaters? It's usually loaded with fat; satisfy your appetite with the small-size order.

. . . if ghee is a good substitute for butter? Commonly used in the cuisine of India, ghee is clarified butter. It's been heated, then strained to remove milk solids so the fat is slightly concentrated—with more fat and calories per teaspoon. Why clarify butter? Without the milk solids, it can be heated to a higher temperature without burning.

. . . how the fat in feta cheese compares with that in other cheeses? It's somewhat lower—but not much. An ounce of feta cheese has 6 grams of fat, which includes 4 grams of saturated fat. By comparison, 1 ounce of Cheddar cheese has 9 total fat grams, including 6 grams of saturated fat. With their intense flavors, small amounts of strong cheeses such as feta, Parmesan, and blue cheese go a long way in delivering flavor.

free foods. *See "Label Lingo: Fats and Cholesterol" below.*

Choose Healthy Oils

● Use vegetable oils—canola, corn, cottonseed, olive, safflower, soybean, sunflower—in place of stick margarine or butter. Mayonnaise, certain salad dressings, and soft (tub or squeeze) margarine with no *trans* fats are mainly oils, too.

● Fit nuts, olives, avocados, and fatty fish into a healthful eating plan. These foods have healthy oils, too!

Label Lingo
Fats and Cholesterol

Check food labels for clues about fat and cholesterol. You may find nutrient content claims.

LABEL TERM ...	MEANS ...	LABEL TERM ..	MEANS ...
For Fat Content ...		Reduced or less saturated fat	At least 25% less saturated fat*
Fat-free	Less than 0.5 gram fat per serving	*For Cholesterol Content ...*	
Low-fat	3 grams or less of fat per serving	Cholesterol-free	Less than 2 milligrams cholesterol and 2 grams or less of saturated fat per serving
Reduced or less fat	At least 25% less fat* per serving	Low cholesterol	20 milligrams or less cholesterol and 2 grams or less of saturated fat per serving
Light	1/3 fewer calories or 50% less fat* per serving	Reduced or less cholesterol	At least 25% less cholesterol* and 2 grams or less of saturated fat per serving
____ % fat-free	The food meets the definition of "low-fat" or "fat-free" if stated as 100% fat-free		
Light meal	"Low-fat" (at least 50% less fat per serving*) or "low-calorie" meal (at least 1/3 fewer calories per serving*)	*For Fat, Saturated Fat, and Cholesterol Content ...*	
		Lean†	Less than 10 grams total fat, 4.5 grams or less saturated fat, and 95 milligrams cholesterol per 3-ounce serving and per 100 grams
Low-fat meal	3 grams or less fat per 100 grams, and 30 percent or less calories from fat	Extra lean†	Less than 5 grams total fat, 2 grams saturated fat, and 95 milligrams cholesterol per 3-ounce serving and per 100 grams
For Saturated Fat Content ...			
Saturated-fat-free	Less than 0.5 gram saturated fat and less than 0.5 gram *trans* fatty acids per serving		
Low saturated fat	1 gram or less saturated fat per serving and no more than 15% of calories from saturated fat		

*Compared with a standard serving size of traditional food

†On packaged seafood or game meat, cooked meat, or cooked poultry

Note: Although not a nutrient content claim per se, look for packages that say "0 g *trans* fat" or "no *trans* fat."

CHAPTER 4

Vitamins, Minerals, and Phytonutrients

Variety on Your Plate!

Vitamins, minerals, and phytonutrients: your body needs them—*perhaps more of them*—for your good health. That's positive nutrition! Just how much do you need for optimal health? What foods are your best sources? And how do these food substances keep you fit?

Although headlines may seem confounding, there's plenty that's well known about the roles of vitamins, minerals, and phytonutrients (plant substances) in health. Over the past century, research has unlocked puzzles related to widespread deficiencies. Today's nutrition breakthroughs focus less on cures and more on the roles of nutrients, phytonutrients, and other food components in health promotion and in protection from cancer, heart disease, and osteoporosis, among other health concerns.

● *Today,* more than forty nutrients, including vitamins and minerals, have been identified. Their functions, the amount you need at different stages of life, and their food sources are better understood. Today's vitamin and mineral research is extending well beyond their well-known, important roles in health, noted in this chapter.

● *Today,* we know more about the balance of vitamins and minerals—and the variety of foods—that allow the body to absorb and use them most efficiently. We're discovering what's enough, but not too much, for our unique, individual needs.

● *Today,* science is exploring a new frontier: food components, including phytonutrients, that offer health benefits beyond basic nourishment.

The bottom line? A variety of food—with plenty of vitamins, minerals, and phytonutrients—is part of your ticket to good health!

Vitamins and Minerals: Team Players!

Vitamins and minerals are key to every process that takes place in your body. They don't work alone, but instead in close partnership with other nutrients to make every body process happen normally: from helping carbohydrates, fats, and proteins produce energy, to assisting with protein synthesis (the creation of new proteins), to building your healthy bones, to helping you think about the words on this page.

● Vitamins are complex substances that regulate body processes. Often they act as coenzymes, or partners, with enzymes, the proteins that cause reactions to take place in your body.

● Minerals are part of many cells, including (but not only) the hard parts: bone, teeth, and nails. Minerals also are part of enzymes and may trigger your body's enzymatic reactions.

Compared with carbohydrates, proteins, and fats, your body needs vitamins and minerals in only small amounts, so they're called *micro*nutrients. Don't let these small amounts fool you, however. Vitamins and minerals don't supply energy directly. But they do regulate many processes that produce energy—and do a whole lot more!

Read on to explore the many vitamins and minerals we know most about: their varied, yet integrated roles in health, recommended intakes, and food sources. *The Appendices give specific recommendations—Dietary Reference Intakes (DRIs)—for vitamins and minerals.* Within this chapter, you'll learn about the vitamins and minerals that the Dietary Guidelines regard with concern for Americans: for adults, calcium, potassium, magnesium, vitamins A, C, and E; for children and teens, calcium, potassium, magnesium, and vitamin E; and for some others, vitamin B_{12}, D, and E, folate, and iron.

Vitamins: The Basics

Vitamins belong in two groups: water-soluble and fat-soluble. Their category describes how they are carried in food and transported in your body.

As their name implies, water-soluble vitamins (B-complex vitamins and vitamin C) dissolve in water. They're carried in your bloodstream. For the most part,

---

Alphabet Soup: What Are DRIs?

Dietary Reference Intakes (DRIs). Daily nutrient recommendations—expressed as RDAs or AIs—based on age and gender; set at levels to decrease the risk of chronic disease.

Recommended Dietary Allowances (RDAs). Recommended daily levels of nutrients to meet the needs of almost all healthy individuals in a specific age and gender group; used when there's scientific consensus for a firm nutrient recommendation.

Adequate Intakes (AIs). Similar to RDAs, and used for nutrients that lack sufficient scientific evidence to determine a firm RDA.

Tolerable Upper Intake Level (UL). Not a recommendation; maximum intake that most likely won't pose risks for health problems for almost all healthy people in that age and gender group.

Source: Institute of Medicine, National Academy of Sciences.

Daily Values (DVs) for nutrients aren't DRIs, although they are based on RDA values from the past. DVs are used for food labeling.

Click Here!

How do your favorite foods stack up for vitamins and minerals? Other nutrients? Calories? All these facts are within your easy reach; just check the Nutrition Facts on a food package. *For the nutrient database from the U.S. Department of Agriculture, click onto www.ars.usda.gov/foodsearch for the "What's in the Foods You Eat—Search Tool." Or use USDA's www.nal.usda.gov/fnic/foodcomp/search/.*

---

water-soluble vitamins aren't stored in your body—at least not in significant amounts. Instead, your body uses what it needs, then excretes the extra through urine. Since they aren't stored, you need a regular supply of water-soluble vitamins from your food choices.

How much do you need? Enough, but not too much. Even though you excrete excess amounts of water-soluble vitamins, moderation is the best approach. For example, taking large doses of vitamin C from a dietary supplement may create extra work for your kidneys, causing kidney stones, as well as diarrhea. Likewise, too much niacin, vitamin B_6, folate, or pantothenic acid also may be harmful.

Fat-soluble vitamins (vitamins A, D, E, and K) dissolve in fat. That's how they're carried into your bloodstream and throughout your body—attached to substances within your body made with lipids, or fat. That's one reason why you need moderate amounts of fat in your overall food choices.

Your body can store fat-soluble vitamins in body fat, so consuming excessive amounts of any fat-soluble vitamins for too long can be harmful. Vitamins A and D, for example, can build up to harmful levels. High intakes of vitamins E and K usually aren't linked to unhealthy symptoms.

Read on to find out how vitamins keep you healthy: their functions, effects of getting too little or too much, Dietary Reference Intakes (DRIs), and their food sources. *Note:* On the following pages, the amounts of vitamins in food have been rounded.

Fat-Soluble Vitamins

Vitamin A (and Carotenoids)

See also "Carotenoids: 'Color' Your Food Healthy" in this chapter.

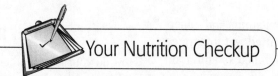

Your Nutrition Checkup

How Do Your Fruits and Veggies Stack Up?

Fruits and vegetables are among your body's best sources of many (but not all) vitamins and minerals—and phytonutrients, including fiber. Fruits and vegetables are rich sources of carotenoids (which form vitamin A), vitamin C, folate, and potassium; *for examples, see the chart "Produce Package" in the Appendices.* And even though they're filling, most are naturally low in calories and fat.

That's why the Dietary Guidelines for Americans advise:

● *Consume enough!* That adds up to 2 cups of fruit and 2½ cups of vegetables a day, if you eat 2,000 calories a day, with somewhat more or less, depending on your energy needs.

● *Vary your veggies.* Choose from all these subgroups, several times a week: darkgreen vegetables, orange vegetables, legumes (dry beans), starchy vegetables, other vegetables.

● *Focus on fruits.* Eat a variety—whether fresh, frozen, canned, or dried. Choose whole fruit, rather than juice, most of the time.

Now take a moment to consider what and how much you ate yesterday. Then keep track of what you eat and drink today.

HOW MUCH?

	VEGETABLES	FRUITS
At breakfast?	_____	_____
At lunch?	_____	_____
For snacks?	_____	_____
At dinner?	_____	_____
For dessert?	_____	_____
Subtotals	_____	_____

½ cup fruit or vegetables equates to:

● ½ cup raw or cooked vegetables

● ½ cup cooked dry beans

● 1 cup fresh leafy greens

● ½ cup fruit or vegetable juice

● ½ cup cut-up or canned fruit

● 1 small orange, peach, or banana; ½ grapefruit; or ½ small apple

● ¼ cup dried fruit

Now repeat this exercise for two more days . . . and keep track. Answer "yes" or "no." Did you consume . . . ?

	Day 1	Day 2	Day 3
About 2½ cups vegetables?	_____	_____	_____
About 2 cups of fruit?	_____	_____	_____
A colorful variety?	_____	_____	_____
More whole fruit than juice?	_____	_____	_____

If most of your answers are "yes," you get the nutrient benefits of plenty of fruits and vegetables. If you mostly answered "no," *check out the ideas in chapters 10 and 13 for fitting in more fruits and vegetables.*

What it does:

● Promotes normal vision, and helps your eyes see normally in the dark, helping adjust to the lower level of light.

● Promotes the growth and health of cells and tissues throughout your body; important for reproduction and development of the embryo.

● Protects you from infections by keeping skin and

On the Label

Without looking, do you know which vitamins and minerals appear on food labels? The four required on the Nutrition Facts need your special attention: vitamins A and C, calcium, and iron. Consume enough of these nutrients to reduce your risk for some common health problems. Other nutrients may appear on the label: some voluntarily, others required if these nutrients are added.

Be aware: Daily Values (DVs) for nutrients, used with food labeling, may differ from today's DRIs. DVs for nutrients are based on previous RDAs. *See "% Daily Values: What Are They Based On?" in the Appendices.*

Nutrition Facts

Serving Size 1 cup (228g)
Servings Per Container 2

Amount Per Serving	
Calories 260	Calories from Fat 120

	% Daily Value*
Total Fat 13g	**20%**
Saturated Fat 5g	**25%**
Trans Fat 2g	
Cholesterol 30mg	**10%**
Sodium 660mg	**28%**
Total Carbohydrate 31g	**10%**
Dietary Fiber 0g	**0%**
Sugars 5g	
Protein 5g	

Vitamin A 4%	•	Vitamin C 2%	
Calcium 15%	•	Iron 4%	

* Percent Daily Values are based on a 2,000 calorie diet. Your Daily Values may be higher or lower depending on your calorie needs:

	Calories:	2,000	2,500
Total Fat	Less than	65g	80g
Sat Fat	Less than	20g	25g
Cholesterol	Less than	300mg	300mg
Sodium	Less than	2,400mg	2,400mg
Total Carbohydrate		300g	375g
Dietary Fiber		25g	30g

Calories per gram:
Fat 9 • Carbohydrate 4 • Protein 4

tissues in your mouth, stomach, intestines, and respiratory, genital, and urinary tracts healthy.

● Helps regulate immune system.

● Works as an antioxidant in the form of carotenoids, and may reduce your risk for certain cancers and other diseases of aging.

Carotenoids (which form vitamin A) are thought to have other health benefits; *these potential health benefits are addressed later in this chapter.*

If you don't get enough: Night blindness; other eye problems; dry, scaly skin; problems with reproduction; diminished immunity, and poor growth are symptoms of a significant deficiency. The deficiency disease from too little vitamin A is called xerophthalmia.

If you consume excess amounts: Because it's stored in your body, large intakes of vitamin A, taken over time, can be quite harmful: headaches, dry and scaly skin, liver damage, bone and joint pain, vomiting or appetite loss, abnormal bone growth, nerve damage, and birth defects. These symptoms more likely result from high intakes of vitamin A from dietary supplements. Beta carotene from fruits and vegetables is okay! Converting carotenoids to vitamin A decreases once the body stores enough vitamin A. High carotenoid intake may turn skin yellow, but that's not considered harmful.

The Tolerable Upper Intake Level is 2,800 micrograms of Retinal Activity Equivalent (RAE) daily for ages fourteen to eighteen, and 3,000 micrograms daily during adulthood. (Retinol, beta carotene, and other provitamin A carotenoids determine RAE.)

How much you need: From age fourteen on, the RDA is 900 micrograms RAE (3,000 IU) of vitamin A for males and 700 micrograms RAE (2,333 IU) for females. During pregnancy, the recommendation is 770 micrograms per day, and during breast-feeding, 1,200 micrograms RAE daily.

Note: The 2001 RDAs measure vitamin A in Retinol Activity Equivalents (RAEs), reflecting retinol and carotenoid units. You might see vitamin A expressed in other ways: International Units (IU)—used for food labels and dietary supplements, or as Retinol Equivalents (RE)—used in the 1989 RDAs and many nutrient databases.

Convert Retinol Equivalents to Retinol Activity Equivalents. For vitamin A derived from:

● Animal-based foods or supplements 1 RE = 1 RAE

● Plant-based foods 1 RE divided by 2 = 1 RAE

Where it's mostly found:

● In animal sources of foods, vitamin A, in the form of retinol, is completely made (or preformed). Vitamin A comes from liver, fish oil, eggs, milk fortified with vitamin A, and other vitamin A-fortified foods.

● Carotenoids, such as alpha carotene and beta carotene, come from foods of plant origin. Certain carotenoids are modified to form vitamin A (referred to as "provitamin A carotenoids") in your body. Carotenoids are found in red, yellow, orange, and many dark-green leafy vegetables. Plant sources of carotenoids are especially important to those who eat few animal-based foods.

Do you get most or all of your beta carotene (which turns to vitamin A) from fruits and vegetables? If so, you may need to eat more of them! According to the 2001 DRI report from the Institute of Medicine, the conversion of carotenoids to vitamin A was overestimated in the past. In fact, it takes twice the amount of carotene-rich foods to meet the body's vitamin A needs as once thought.

Vitamin D

See "Vitamin D: The Sunshine Vitamin," chapter 18.
What it does:

- Promotes absorption of calcium and phosphorus; regulates how much calcium remains in blood.
- Helps deposit these minerals in bones and teeth.

- Helps regulate cell growth.
- Plays a role in immunity.

If you don't get enough: In your older years, you may have greater loss of bone mass (osteoporosis), and your risk of softening of the bones (osteomalacia) increases. Children with a significant vitamin D deficiency may develop rickets, or defective bone growth. Fortifying milk with vitamin D had virtually wiped out rickets in the United States. Rickets is reemerging as a concern, however, possibly related to regularly consuming juice or soft drinks in place of milk. That's happening even though some juices are vitamin D fortified.

Vitamin A and Carotenoids: Good Picks

Besides supplying essential carotenoids, enjoy carotene-rich fruit or vegetables daily for the antioxidant power, too!
Vitamin A content is given below in two ways: in approximate Retinol Equivalents (currently used in many nutrient databases) and in approximate Retinol Activity Equivalents (used with 2001 RDAs for vitamin A).

Food	Retinol Equivalents (RE)* (approximate)	Retinol Activity Equivalents (RAE)* (approximate)	Food	Retinol Equivalents (RE)* (approximate)	Retinol Activity Equivalents (RAE)* (approximate)
Beef liver, cooked (3 oz.)	8,025	8,025	Milk, fat-free (1 cup)	150	150
Sweet potato, mashed (½ cup)	2,580	1,290	Tomato, medium, raw (1)	105	50
Carrot (1 medium)	1,030	515	Mango, medium (½)	80	40
Collards, frozen, boiled (½ cup)	980	490	Egg, large (1)	70	70
Kale, boiled (½ cup)	890	445	Milk, whole (1 cup)	70	70
Turnip greens, cooked (½ cup)	550	275	Broccoli, raw (½ cup)	30	15
Cantaloupe (½ cup)	300	150	Green bell pepper, raw (½ cup)	30	15
Spinach, raw (1 cup)	280	140	Orange, medium (1)	30	15
Romaine lettuce (1 cup)	270	135			
Red bell pepper, raw (½ cup)	235	115			
Apricot (3)	200	100			
Papaya, medium (½)	170	85			

Many fortified foods, including breakfast cereals, supply vitamin A, too. Read the Nutrition Facts on food labels to see how much.

*The % Daily Values—used on food labels and many dietary supplements—are based in International Units (IUs) for vitamin A (not REs or RAEs).

If you consume excess amounts: Because it's stored in your body, too much vitamin D can be toxic, possibly leading to kidney stones or damage, weak muscles and bones, excessive bleeding, and other problems. An overdose usually comes from dietary supplements, not food—and not from overexposure to sunlight. For that reason, an upper limit, or Tolerable Upper Intake Level (UL), of 2,000 International Units (IU), or 50 micrograms, per day for people ages one and over was set.

How much you need: From birth through age fifty, Adequate Intake (AI) has been set at 5 micrograms cholecalciferol (which is the form of vitamin D in an animal-based food) or 200 International Units (IU) daily, with no increased need during pregnancy or breast-feeding. One microgram cholecalciferol = 40 IU vitamin D. To maintain healthy bones, advice for vitamin D goes up to 10 micrograms, or 400 IU, daily for adults over age fifty. Over seventy years, advice increases to 15 micrograms, or 600 IU, per day.

Vitamin D from plant-based foods is in a different form.

The Dietary Guidelines offer specific advice: *for older adults, people with dark skin, and people exposed to insufficient ultraviolet band radiation (i.e., sunlight), consume extra vitamin D from vitamin D-fortified foods and/or supplements.*

Where it's mostly found: Known as the "sunshine vitamin," your body can make vitamin D after sunlight, or ultraviolet light, hits your skin, even on cloudy days. That's no excuse for overexposure to sun from sunbathing. Ten to 15 minutes of sunlight without sunscreen on your hands, arms, and face (or arms and legs) twice weekly usually is enough. Darker skin needs more sun exposure; lighter skin, less. **Caution:** Routinely protect your skin *after those 10 to 15 minutes* with sunscreen having an SPF of 15 or more!

Some fatty fish naturally supply vitamin D— another reason to enjoy salmon and tuna. As a public health strategy, most milk is vitamin D fortified, with 100 IU of vitamin D in an 8-ounce serving. Today's supermarkets also carry vitamin-D fortified yogurt, cheese, juices, soy drinks, breakfast cereals, breads, and cereal bars, as well as eggs from hens raised on vitamin D-fortified feed.

Vitamin-Rich Cures

Nutrition history is full of fascinating stories of nutrient-deficiency diseases that confounded doctors of the past.

- The scourge of *scurvy,* which plagued seafarers several hundred years ago, was finally cured by stocking ships with lemons, oranges, and limes; hence, British sailors were called "limeys." Scurvy is caused by a deficiency of vitamin C, a nutrient that citrus fruits provide in abundance.

- *Night blindness,* often caused by a deficiency of vitamin A, was known in ancient Egypt. The recommended cure of the day: eating ox or rooster livers. Today it's well known that liver contains more vitamin A than many other foods.

- Giving children cod liver oil to prevent *rickets* was practiced in the nineteenth century. But not until 1922, when vitamin D was discovered, did scientists know what substance in cod liver oil gave protection.

- *Beriberi,* a deficiency of thiamin, was noted in Asia as polished, or white, rice became more popular than unrefined, or brown, rice. The cure was discovered accidentally when chickens with symptoms of beriberi ate the part of rice that was discarded after polishing. It contained the vitamin-rich germ. Today the process of enrichment adds thiamin and other B vitamins back to polished rice; today rice is fortified with folic acid, too.

FOOD	VITAMIN D (INTERNATIONAL UNITS)
Salmon with bones, canned (3 oz.)	190–535
Milk, most types (1 cup)	100
Orange juice, vitamin D fortified (1 cup)	50
Cornflakes (1 cup)	20

Vitamin E

See also "Vitamin E: One Main Mission" in this chapter.

What it does:

- Works as an antioxidant, preventing the oxidation of LDL cholesterol, and perhaps lowering the risk for heart disease and stroke. Its antioxidant activity also may help reduce the risk of other health problems, such as some types of cancer.

● As an antioxidant, protects essential fatty acids and vitamin A. *See "Antioxidant Vitamins: A Closer Look" later in this chapter.*

If you don't get enough: Many Americans consume enough vitamin E, yet it's still a nutrient of concern, according to the Dietary Guidelines, 2005. Two more exceptions are premature, very-low-birthweight infants and people with poor fat absorption, cystic fibrosis, or some other chronic health problems. In these cases, the nervous system can be affected. Because vegetable oils are good sources of vitamin E, people who cut back on total fat may not get enough. Vitamin E-fortified cereal may be a good choice.

If you consume excess amounts: Eating plenty of vitamin E-rich foods doesn't appear problematic. However, taking large doses of vitamin E as a supplement hasn't been shown conclusively to have benefits—and isn't recommended. Too much may increase the risk of bleeding, may impair vitamin K action, and may increase the effect of anticoagulant medication.

That's why a Tolerable Upper Intake Level (UL) has been set: 800 milligrams daily for teens ages fourteen to eighteen; 1,000 milligrams of alpha-tocopherol daily for adults ages nineteen and over. If you take a supplement, 1,000 milligrams equal about 1,500 IU of natural vitamin E or 1,100 IU of dl-alpha-tocopherol synthetic vitamin E.

How much you need: The RDA guideline for males and females age fourteen and over is 15 milligrams of alpha-tocopherol each day. Children need less, depending on their age. During pregnancy, women still need 15 milligrams daily; during breast-feeding the recommendation goes up to 19 milligrams daily.

Note: Vitamin E is a group of substances called tocopherols with different potencies. Alpha-tocopherol is its most potent form. On food and supplement labels, the amount is given in International Units (IU) of alpha-tocopherol, not in milligrams.

To make the conversion, 15 milligrams of alpha-tocopherol (the RDA for adults) equal:

● About 22 IU of d-alpha-tocopherol ("natural" vitamin E in some supplements)

● About 33 IU of dl-alpha-tocopherol (a synthetic form in fortified foods and some supplements)

The "natural" form of vitamin E is more fully used than the synthetic form. That's why there's a difference in the conversion factor.

Where it's mostly found: The best sources of vitamin E are vegetable oils—for example, soybean, corn, cottonseed, and safflower. That includes margarine, salad dressing, and other foods made from oil. Nuts (especially almonds and hazelnuts), seeds (especially sunflower seeds), and wheat germ—all high in oil—are good sources, too, as are some fortified breakfast cereals. Green, leafy vegetables provide smaller amounts.

FOOD	VITAMIN E (MG ALPHA-TOCOPHEROL)
Sunflower seeds (1 oz.)	11
Almonds (1 oz. or 24 nuts)	7
Wheat germ (¼ cup)	5
Hazelnuts (1 oz.)	4
Soy beverage (1 cup)	3
Peanut butter (2 tbsp.)	3
Corn oil (1 tbsp.)	3
Spinach, cooked (½ cup)	2
Turnip greens, cooked (½ cup)	1

Vitamin K

What it does:

● Makes proteins that cause your blood to coagulate, or clot, when you bleed. That way, bleeding stops.

● Helps your body make some other body proteins for your blood, bones, and kidneys.

If you don't get enough: Blood doesn't coagulate normally. Except for rare health problems, a deficiency of vitamin K is very unlikely. Prolonged use of antibiotics could be a problem since they destroy some bacteria in your intestines that produce vitamin K.

If you consume excess amounts: No symptoms have been observed, but moderation is still the best approach. People taking blood-thinning drugs, or anticoagulants, need to eat foods with vitamin K in moderation. Too much can make blood clot faster. No Tolerable Upper Intake Level (UL) is established.

How much you need: The Adequate Intake (AI) advises 75 micrograms daily for teens ages fourteen to eighteen. During adulthood the intake goes up: 120 micrograms daily for men and 90 micrograms daily for women. Neither pregnancy nor breast-feeding increases the recommendation. To make sure infants have enough, newborns typically receive a shot of vitamin K.

Where it's mostly found: Like vitamin D, your body can produce vitamin K on its own—this time from certain bacteria in your intestines.

The best food sources are green, leafy vegetables such as spinach and broccoli. However, a variety of foods provide smaller amounts, including some fruits, vegetables, and nuts.

FOOD	VITAMIN K (MCG)
Spinach, raw (1 cup)	145
Broccoli, raw (½ cup)	45
Black-eyed peas, cooked (½ cup)	20
Canola oil (1 tbsp.)	17
Blueberries (½ cup)	15
Pine nuts (1 oz.)	15
Pistachios (1 oz.)	5
Raspberries (½ cup)	5

Water-Soluble Vitamins

Thiamin (vitamin B₁)

What it does:

- Helps produce energy from carbohydrates in all the cells of your body.

If you don't get enough: Because most people consume many grain products, a thiamin deficiency is rare in the United States today, with one exception: chronic alcoholics. Symptoms include fatigue, weak muscles, and nerve damage. Before refined grains were enriched with thiamin, a deficiency was common, sometimes resulting in a disease called beriberi, which affects mainly the cardiovascular and nervous systems.

If you consume excess amounts: Your body excretes any excess amount you may consume. Contrary to popular claims, extra amounts have no energy-boosting effect.

How much you need: The RDA for thiamin is tied to your energy needs: 1.2 milligrams daily for males age fourteen through adulthood. For females, the recommendation is 1.0 milligram daily from ages fourteen through eighteen and 1.1 milligrams daily from age nineteen on. During pregnancy and breast-feeding, the amount recommended goes up to 1.4 milligrams daily.

Where it's mostly found: Whole-grain and enriched grain products such as bread, rice, pasta, tortillas, and fortified cereals provide much of the thiamin we eat. Enrichment adds back nutrients, including many B vitamins, lost when grains are refined. Pork, liver, and other organ meats provide significant amounts, too.

FOOD	THIAMIN (MG)
Pork, lean, broiled (3 oz.)	1.0
Beef liver, braised (3 oz.)	0.2
Enriched flour tortilla (1)	0.2
Enriched rice, cooked (½ cup)	0.2
Whole-grain bread (1 slice)	0.1

Riboflavin (vitamin B₂)

What it does:

● Helps produce energy in all cells of your body.

● Helps change the amino acid called tryptophan in your food into niacin. (Protein is made of many different amino acids.)

If you don't get enough: Except for people who are severely malnourished, a deficiency isn't likely. Deficiency symptoms include eye disorders (including cataracts); dry and flaky skin; and a sore, red tongue. Contrary to popular myth, riboflavin deficiency doesn't cause hair loss.

If you consume excess amounts: No reports suggest problems from consuming too much.

How much you need: Like thiamin, the RDA for riboflavin is tied to your energy needs. Adult men need 1.3 milligrams daily and adult women need 1.1 milligrams daily. During pregnancy, the recommendation is 1.4 milligrams; during breast-feeding, the amount goes up to 1.6 milligrams daily.

Where it's mostly found: Milk and other dairy foods are major sources of riboflavin. Some organ meats—liver, kidney, and heart—are excellent sources. Enriched bread and other grain products; eggs; meat; green, leafy vegetables; and nuts supply smaller amounts. Because ultraviolet light, such as sunlight, destroys riboflavin, most milk is packed in opaque plastic or cardboard containers, not clear glass.

FOOD	RIBOFLAVIN (MG)
Beef liver, braised (3 oz.)	3.5
Yogurt, fat-free with dry milk solids (1 cup)	0.4
Milk, fat-free (1 cup)	0.4
Spinach, cooked (½ cup)	0.2
Egg, large (1)	0.2
Enriched corn tortilla (1)	0.1
Whole-grain bread (1 slice)	0.1

Niacin

What it does:

● Helps your body use sugars and fatty acids.

● Helps enzymes function normally in your body.

● Helps produce energy in all body cells.

If you don't get enough: For people who consume adequate amounts of protein-rich foods, a niacin deficiency isn't likely. Pellagra is caused by a significant niacin deficiency. Symptoms include diarrhea, mental disorientation, and skin problems.

If you consume excess amounts: Consuming excessive amounts, not likely from food, may cause flushed skin, rashes, or liver damage. The Tolerable Upper Intake Level (UL) is 35 milligrams daily for adults, and 30 milligrams daily for teens ages fourteen to eighteen. Self-prescribing large doses of niacin to lower blood cholesterol may lead to adverse effects—and may not give cholesterol-lowering benefits. If your doctor prescribes niacin, take it in the recommended dosage.

How much you need: Niacin recommendations are given in NE, or niacin equivalents. That's because it comes from two sources: niacin itself and from the amino acid called tryptophan, part of which converts to niacin.

Like thiamin and riboflavin, the recommendation is tied to energy needs. The advice for adult males is 16 milligrams NE daily, and for adult females, 14 milligrams NE daily. During pregnancy, 18 milligrams NE is advised; during breast-feeding, 17 milligrams NE daily.

Where it's mostly found: Foods high in protein are typically good sources of niacin: poultry, fish, beef, peanut butter, and legumes. Niacin is also added to many enriched and fortified grain products.

FOOD	NIACIN (MG NE)
Turkey breast, roasted, without skin (3 oz.)	6.0
Peanut butter (2 tbsp.)	4.0
Codfish, cooked (3 oz.)	2.0
Enriched flour tortilla (1)	1.5
Enriched spaghetti, cooked (½ cup)	1.0
Black-eyed peas, frozen, cooked (½ cup)	0.5
Lima beans, boiled (½ cup)	0.5
Yogurt, fat-free with dry milk solids (1 cup)	0.5

Pyridoxine (vitamin B₆)

What it does:

● Helps your body make nonessential amino acids, or protein components, which are then used to make body cells.

● Helps turn the amino acid called tryptophan into two important body substances: niacin and serotonin (a messenger in your brain).

● Helps produce other body chemicals, including insulin, hemoglobin, and antibodies that fight infection.

If you don't get enough: A deficiency can cause mental convulsions among infants; depression; nausea; or greasy, flaky skin. For infants, breast milk and properly prepared infant formulas contain enough.

If you consume excess amounts: Large doses, over time, can cause nerve damage. The Tolerable Upper Intake Level (UL) is 100 milligrams daily for adults; 80 milligrams daily for teens, fourteen to eighteen.

How much you need: The RDA is 1.3 milligrams daily for adult males and females through age fifty. After age fifty, the RDA increases to 1.7 milligrams daily for males and 1.5 milligrams for females. The amount increases to 1.9 milligrams daily during pregnancy and 2.0 milligrams daily during breast-feeding.

Where it's mostly found: Chicken, fish, pork, liver, and kidney are the best sources. Whole grains, nuts, and legumes also supply reasonable amounts.

FOOD	PYRIDOXINE (MG)
Chicken, light meat, skinless, roasted (3 oz.)	0.5
Pork, loin, roasted (3 oz.)	0.4
Peanut butter (2 tbsp.)	0.2
Black beans, boiled (½ cup)	0.1
Whole-wheat spaghetti, cooked (½ cup)	0.1
Almonds (1 oz. or 24 almonds)	<0.1

Folate (folic acid or folacin)

What it does:

● Plays an essential role in making new body cells by helping to produce DNA and RNA, the cell's master plan for cell reproduction.

Have You Ever Wondered ?

. . . about the difference between the terms "enriched" and "fortified"? Both terms indicate that nutrients—usually vitamins or minerals—were added to make a food more nutritious. *Enriched* means adding back nutrients that were lost during food processing. For example, B vitamins, lost when wheat is processed, are added back to refined white flour. *Fortified* means adding nutrients that weren't present originally. For example, milk is fortified with vitamin D, a nutrient that helps your body absorb milk's calcium and phosphorus. According to a recent law, most enriched grain products are now fortified with folic acid to reduce the incidence of certain birth defects.

. . . if microwave cooking destroys vitamins? Even if you cook foods properly, some water-soluble vitamins, such as B vitamins and vitamin C, can be destroyed. For several reasons, more vitamins are retained with microwave cooking than with most other methods: very short cooking time, covered cooking, and little or no cooking water.

● Works with vitamin B_{12} to form hemoglobin in red blood cells.

● May help protect against heart disease.

● Helps lower the risk of delivering a baby with neural tube defects such as spina bifida.

● Helps control plasma homocysteine levels, linked to increased cardiovascular disease risk.

If you don't get enough: A deficiency affects normal cell division and protein synthesis, especially impairing growth. Anemia, caused by malformed blood cells that can't carry as much oxygen, may result from a folate deficiency.

Pregnant women who don't get enough folate, especially during the first trimester, have a greater risk of delivering a baby with neural tube defects such as spina bifida. To reduce the risk the Dietary Guidelines advise: *for women of childbearing age who may become pregnant and those in the first trimester of pregnancy, consume adequate synthetic folic acid daily from fortified foods or supplements in addition to food forms of folate from a varied diet.*

If you consume excess amounts: Consuming too much can mask a vitamin B_{12} deficiency and may interfere with certain medications and offers no known benefits. For adults, the Tolerable Upper Intake Level (UL) is 1,000 micrograms daily of folic acid, the form of folate in fortified foods and supplements. For teens ages fourteen to eighteen, it's 800 micrograms daily.

How much you need: For folate, the RDA for males from age fourteen through adulthood is 400 micrograms daily. Folate can come from foods with naturally occurring folate, as well as from foods fortified with folic acid and from supplements.

Women capable of becoming pregnant (fourteen to fifty years) should get 400 micrograms of folic acid daily from fortified foods, vitamin supplements, or a combination, in addition to the folate found naturally in foods. Pregnancy increases the recommended amount to 600 micrograms daily; during breast-feeding, 500 micrograms are advised.

Where it's mostly found: Orange juice, lentils, dried beans, spinach, broccoli, peanuts, and avocados are among the good sources of naturally occurring folate. Enriched grain products—such as most breads, flour,

crackers, rice, macaroni, and noodles—must be fortified with folic acid, a form of folate. Some breakfast cereals are fully fortified at 400 micrograms per serving—100 percent of the daily recommendation for many people. Unenriched grain products, such as some imported pastas, may not be fortified with folic acid. Check the Nutrition Facts on the label of grain products to see if folic acid has been added and how much. Many whole-grain breads and other whole-grain products are not fortified with folic acid, but check the label.

FOOD	FOLATE (MCG)
Breakfast cereals, fortified with folic acid (¾–1 cup)	100–400
Spinach, boiled (½ cup)	130
Navy beans, boiled (½ cup)	125
Orange juice (1 cup)	110
Wheat germ (¼ cup)	100
Avocado (½)	80
Pasta, fortified with folic acid, cooked (½ cup)	50
Rice, fortified with folic acid, cooked (½ cup)	45
Peanuts, dry roasted (1 oz.)	40
Bread, fortified with folic acid (1 slice)	30
Romaine lettuce, shredded (½ cup)	30

Vitamin B_{12} (cobalamin)

See "Vitamin B_{12}: A Challenge for Vegans" in chapter 20.

What it does:

● Works with folate to make red blood cells.

● Serves as a vital part of many body chemicals and so occurs in every body cell.

● Helps your body use fatty acids and some amino acids.

If you don't get enough: A deficiency may result in anemia, fatigue, nerve damage, a smooth tongue, or very sensitive skin. A deficiency of vitamin B_{12} can be masked—and even progress—if extra folic acid is taken to treat or prevent anemia.

For either genetic or medical reasons, some people develop a deficiency—pernicious anemia—because they can't absorb vitamin B_{12}. They're missing a body chemical called intrinsic factor that comes from their stomach lining. This problem can be medically treated with injections of vitamin B_{12}.

Strict vegetarians, who eat no animal products, and the infants of vegan mothers are at risk for developing a vitamin B_{12} deficiency. This could cause severe anemia and irreversible nerve damage. The elderly also are at risk. Including foods fortified with vitamin B_{12} or dietary supplements can prevent vitamin B_{12} deficiency. The Dietary Guidelines advise: *for people over age fifty, consume vitamin B_{12} in its crystalline form (e.g., fortified foods or supplements).*

If you consume excess amounts: No symptoms are known, but taking extra vitamin B_{12} to boost energy has no basis in science.

How much you need: The RDA is 2.4 micrograms daily for adults. The recommendation increases to 2.6 micrograms daily during pregnancy and 2.8 micrograms daily during breast-feeding.

Where it's mostly found: Vitamin B_{12} comes from animal products—meat, fish, poultry, eggs, milk, and other dairy foods. Some fortified foods may contain it.

Food	Vitamin B_{12} (mcg)
Salmon, cooked (3 oz.)	3.0
Beef tenderloin lean, broiled (3 oz.)	2.3
Yogurt, fat-free (1 cup)	1.5
Shrimp, cooked (3 oz.)	1.3
Milk (1 cup)	1.3
Egg, large (1)	0.7
Chicken, light meat, skinless, roasted (3 oz.)	0.3

Biotin

What it does:

● Helps your body produce energy in your cells.

● Helps metabolize (or use) proteins, fats, and carbohydrates from food.

If you don't get enough: That's rarely a problem for healthy people who eat a healthful diet because the body also produces biotin from intestinal bacteria. In rare cases of deficiency, these symptoms may appear: heart abnormalities, appetite loss, fatigue, depression, or dry skin.

If you consume excess amounts: There are no reported effects of consuming excess amounts.

How much you need: The Adequate Intake (AI) for biotin is 30 micrograms daily for adult males and females, including during pregnancy. The AI increases to 35 micrograms daily during breast-feeding.

Where it's mostly found: Biotin is found in a wide variety of foods. Eggs, liver, yeast breads, and cereals are among the best sources.

Food	Biotin (mcg)
Egg, large (1)	11
Wheat germ (¼ cup)	5
Peanuts (½ cup)	5
Cottage cheese (½ cup)	5
Whole-grain bread (1 slice)	2

Pantothenic Acid

What it does:

● Helps your body cells produce energy.

● Helps metabolize (or use) proteins, fats, and carbohydrates from food.

If you don't get enough: That's rarely a problem for healthy people who eat a healthful diet.

If you consume excess amounts: The only apparent effects are occasional diarrhea and water retention.

How much you need: The Adequate Intake (AI) for pantothenic acid is 5 milligrams daily for teens ages fourteen to eighteen and for adults. During pregnancy and breast-feeding, the AI increases to 6 and 7 milligrams, respectively.

Where it's mostly found: Pantothenic acid is widely available in food. Meat, poultry, fish, whole-grain cereals, and legumes are among the better sources. Milk, vegetables, and fruits also contain varying amounts.

FOOD	PANTOTHENIC ACID (MG)
Yogurt, fat-free (1 cup)	1.5
Salmon, cooked (3 oz.)	1.3
Sweet potato, mashed, cooked (½ cup)	1.0
Milk, fat-free (1 cup)	0.9
Chicken, light meat, skinless, roasted (3 oz.)	0.8
Corn, boiled (½ cup)	0.7
Egg, large (1)	0.7
Ham, lean (3 oz.)	0.5
Whole-wheat macaroni, cooked (½ cup)	0.3
Kidney beans, cooked (½ cup)	0.2

Choline

What it does: Choline, a vitaminlike substance, plays a role in many body processes.

- Promotes the transport of fats and helps make substances that form cell membranes.

- Helps make acetylcholine, which is a neurotransmitter in your body needed for many functions, including muscle control and memory storage.

- Plays a role in liver function and reproductive health.

If you don't get enough: No clear cases of deficiencies in humans have been identified, but choline status may depend on consuming enough folate. Since scientific data are insufficient, it's not known if choline is essential in the diet; if so, how much is needed; and the effects of a deficiency.

If you consume excess amounts: The Tolerable Upper Intake Level (UL) for adults is 3.5 grams of choline daily; for teens ages fourteen to eighteen, 3.0 grams daily.

How much you need: There is no RDA for choline. However, Adequate Intake (AI) levels were set in 1998: 550 milligrams daily for males ages fourteen and older; 400 milligrams daily for girls ages fourteen to eighteen; and 425 milligrams daily for women. During pregnancy and breast-feeding, the AI increases to 450 milligrams and 550 milligrams, respectively.

Where it's mostly found: Choline, a natural food component, is widely distributed in food. Meat, liver, eggs, soybeans, and peanuts are especially good sources. Since the U.S. Food and Drug Administration has authorized nutrient content claims on food labels for choline, you may find new choline-fortified products.

FOOD	CHOLINE (MG)
Beef liver (3 oz.)	425
Egg, large (1)	255
Beef, extra-lean (3 oz.)	85
Pistachios (1 oz.)	70
Milk, fat-free (1 cup)	15

Vitamin C (ascorbic acid)

See "Vitamin C: More Jobs than You Think!" later in this chapter.

What it does:

- Helps produce collagen, a connective tissue that holds muscles, bones, and other tissues together.

- Helps keep capillary walls and blood vessels firm, and so protects you from bruising.

- Helps your body absorb iron and folate from plant sources of food.

- Helps keep your gums healthy.

- Helps heal any cuts and wounds.

- Protects you from infection by stimulating the formation of antibodies and so boosting immunity.

- Works as an antioxidant to inhibit damage to body cells.

Have You Ever Wondered

. . . if bleeding gums mean you're not getting enough vitamin C? It's not likely unless you have a severe deficiency. Most cases of bleeding gums come from poor oral hygiene. Brushing and flossing regularly help keep your gums healthy. *For more about healthy gums, see chapter 22.*

Vitamin C: More than Citrus

Citrus fruits—oranges, grapefruits, tangerines—are well-known sources of vitamin C. Yet many other fruits and vegetables are excellent sources, too.

Food	Vitamin C (mg)
Red bell pepper (½ cup)	140
Guava, medium (1)	125
Papaya, medium (½)	95
Orange juice, from frozen concentrate (¾ cup)	75
Orange, medium (1)	70
Green bell pepper (½ cup)	60
Broccoli, boiled (½ cup)	50
Strawberries (½ cup)	50
Kohlrabi, boiled (½ cup)	45
Grapefruit, white (½)	40
Tomato juice (¾ cup)	35
Cantaloupe (½ cup)	30
Mango, medium (½)	30
Tangerine, medium (1)	25
Cabbage, red, raw (½ cup)	25
Collard greens, frozen, boiled (½ cup)	25
Potato, medium, baked with skin (1)	20
Tomato, medium, raw (1)	15
Spinach, raw (1 cup)	10

Some fruit drinks, bottled waters, and other processed foods are fortified with vitamin C. Check the Nutrition Facts on the label for the amount per serving. And remember, if you rely only on fortified foods as your vitamin C source, you may miss out on other nutrients and compounds present in foods with naturally occurring vitamin C.

If you don't get enough: Eventually, a severe deficiency of vitamin C leads to scurvy, a disease that causes loose teeth, excessive bleeding, and swollen gums. Wounds may not heal properly either. Because vitamin C-rich foods are widely available, scurvy is rare in the United States today.

If you consume an excess amount: Because vitamin C is water-soluble, your body excretes the excess; high levels of vitamin C in urine can mask the results of tests for diabetes. Very large doses may cause kidney stones and/or diarrhea, and for those with iron overload (hemochromatosis), excessive vitamin C (which enhances iron absorption) can make the problem worse. But the effects of taking large amounts for a long time isn't known. A Tolerable Upper Intake Level (UL) for vitamin C has been set: 2,000 milligrams daily for adults; 1,800 milligrams daily for teens ages fourteen to eighteen.

How much you need: The RDA for females and males ages fourteen to eighteen is 65 milligrams and 75 milligrams of vitamin C daily, respectively. Adult males need 90 milligrams daily; adult females, 75 milligrams of vitamin C daily for everyday needs (about the amount in ¾ cup of orange juice). Women need somewhat more during pregnancy (80 to 85 milligrams) and breast-feeding (115 to 120 milligrams).

For people who smoke, the RDA for vitamin C is *increased* by 35 milligrams daily to help counteract the oxidative damage from nicotine.

Where it's mostly found: Vitamin C mainly comes from plant sources of food. All citrus fruits, including oranges, grapefruits, and tangerines, are good sources. And many other fruits and vegetables, including berries, melons, peppers, many dark green, leafy vegetables, potatoes, and tomatoes supply significant amounts, too. *See "Vitamin C: More Than Citrus" on this page for a list of good sources and amounts.*

Antioxidant Vitamins: A Closer Look

You've probably read the headlines "Antioxidants Promote Health!" or "Antioxidants Prevent Aging." A quick trip through the supermarket shows that many food manufacturers are fortifying food with beta carotene (which forms vitamin A in the body), vitamin C, and vitamin E, as well as selenium (a mineral).

Just what are antioxidants? They're a handful of vitamins, minerals, carotenoids, and polyphenols present in a variety of foods that significantly slow or prevent the oxidative (damage from oxygen) process and so prevent or repair damage to your body cells. They may also improve immune function and perhaps lower risk for infection and cancer. What makes them unique? What foods supply them naturally? How might they work in your body? And how may antioxidants promote health and reduce chronic disease risk? Since antioxidants research is new, there's no conclusive evidence yet on their role in health. However, *"Rounding Up Free Radicals" later in this chapter explains how antioxidants appear to work.*

Carotenoids: "Color" Your Food Healthy

Imagine a beautiful autumn day. Leaves of red, orange, and yellow rustle in the branches overhead. The colors of the season belong to carotenoids, or plant pigments that generally are red, orange, and deep yellow.

The array of colors in fruits and vegetables also comes from carotenoids. The clues to their presence are obvious in the vibrant palette of produce in your supermarket. It's no surprise that apricots, cantaloupes, mangoes, carrots, red and yellow peppers, and sweet potatoes, for example, all contain carotene. Broccoli, kale, romaine lettuce, and spinach have carotene, too—even though they're dark green! The orange-yellow color of their carotene gets hidden by the chlorophyll in the leaves. *"Vitamin A and Carotenoids: Good Picks" earlier in this chapter lists good food sources and amounts.*

Beta carotene is the carotenoid most familiar to us. Actually, the plant world has more than six hundred known carotenoids. Of those, only a few have been analyzed in fruits and vegetables: alpha carotene, beta carotene, beta cryptoxanthin, gamma carotene, lycopene, lutein, and zeaxanthin; even then, the data are limited.

Beta carotene and other carotenoids perform as precursors to vitamin A; *also see "Vitamins: The*

Have You Ever Wondered

. . . if beta carotene supplements offer protection for smokers? No research supports any benefit. More importantly, a large study of smokers indicated that beta carotene supplements may be harmful to smokers. Smokers who used supplemental beta carotene had a higher incidence of lung cancer than those who didn't. For nonsmokers, it's still unknown whether higher intakes of beta carotene offer benefits. Unless your doctor prescribes it, don't consume large amounts of supplemental beta carotene or other carotenoids.

Basics" in this chapter. Carotenoids also play a functional role in health—many antioxidants potentially offer protection from some diseases and degenerative changes that accompany aging.

For foods high in beta carotene and other carotenoids, try to choose red, orange, deep-yellow, and some dark-green leafy vegetables every day. Color is a clue, not an assurance, that fruits and vegetables are good sources of beta carotene. For example, despite their color, neither corn nor snow peas have much beta carotene—but they do supply other nutrients.

No Dietary Reference Intakes (no RDA, AI, or UL) specifically for carotenoids have been established yet except as precursors to vitamin A. Be cautious; consuming too much of them from dietary supplements may have an adverse effect. *See "Vitamin/Mineral Supplements: Benefits and Risks" in chapter 23.*

Vitamin C: More Jobs Than You Think!

Over the years, vitamin C, also known as ascorbic acid, developed celebrity status with claims that it can prevent or cure the common cold. Although those claims have been overblown, an adequate intake of vitamin C does play an important role in fighting infection. For colds, extra vitamin C may have a mild antihistamine effect, perhaps shortening the duration of a cold and making the symptoms more mild. However, scientific evidence doesn't justify taking large doses of vitamin C regularly to boost immunity. For those who choose to take vitamin C for colds, research suggests that the placebo effect may be responsible for more benefits than taking extra vitamin C.

Here's what we do know: vitamin C is a water-soluble vitamin with many functions in health. Among them, vitamin C helps form the connective tissue that holds the many parts of your body together. It keeps capillaries healthy so you don't bruise easily, and your gums healthy so they don't bleed.

Vitamin C works in partnership with iron, too, helping the body to absorb iron from plant sources of food. *See "Iron in Foods: Heme vs. Nonheme" later in this chapter.* In fact, an adequate daily supply of vitamin C in your food choices can increase the absorption of nonheme iron (mostly from plant sources) by as much as two to four times. For those who get most of their iron from plant sources of food, including vegetarians, vitamin C is of special importance.

Of newer interest, as an antioxidant, vitamin C may protect your body in much the same way that beta carotene and vitamin E do. However, vitamin C attacks free radicals in body fluids, not in fat tissue. Preliminary research is exploring a link to reduced risk of cataracts and cancer protection; no evidence exists to advise consuming more than the RDA for vitamin C.

Because vitamin C isn't stored in the body, you're wise to consume a vitamin C-rich food daily. *"Vitamin C: More than Citrus" earlier in this chapter lists several good sources.* If you habitually consume a vitamin C-rich fruit or juice with breakfast, you probably consume enough.

Vitamin E: One Main Mission

For years, vitamin E has been surrounded by pseudo-scientific myths. It's been misguidedly acclaimed as a cure for almost all that ails you: for example, improving sexual prowess, curing infertility, preventing aging, curing heart disease and cancer, and improving athletic performance, to name just a few. The benefits of vitamin E don't extend this far, but it does appear to play a broad role in promoting your health.

The main role of vitamin E—a fat-soluble vitamin—appears to be as an antioxidant. It may help prevent the oxidation of LDL, or "bad," cholesterol, which contributes to plaque buildup in the arteries; although the jury's still out, that may help reduce the risk for heart disease and stroke. Vitamin E also may help protect from cell damage that can lead ultimately to health problems such as cancer. Vitamin E appears to work with other antioxidants such as vitamin C and selenium.

Vitamin E is actually a group of substances called tocopherols, all with different potencies. For this reason they're often measured as milligrams of alpha-tocopherol equivalents.

Where do you get vitamin E? Vitamin E is found most abundantly in vegetable oils, salad dressings, margarine, and other processed foods made with vegetable oils. For those looking for nutrient-rich sources of vitamin E, which deliver many nutrients besides fat, vitamin E is also in many fortified breakfast cereals, wheat germ, whole-grain products, seeds, nuts (especially hazelnuts and almonds), and peanut butter. In addition, vitamin E is added to processed foods as a preservative. *Note:* Heating vegetable oils to high temperatures, as in frying, destroys vitamin E.

In vegetable oils, nuts, and seeds, vitamin E protects their unsaturated fats from oxidation. Typically, foods high in unsaturated fats also are good sources of vitamin E.

Rounding Up Free Radicals

Just how do antioxidant vitamins work? First let's learn more about oxygen. To produce energy, every cell in your body needs a constant supply of oxygen. For this reason, oxygen is basic to life.

There's another side to the oxygen story. When body cells burn oxygen, they form free radicals, or oxygen by-products; a free radical is an unstable molecule with a missing electron. Free radicals can damage body cells and tissues, as well as the DNA, your body's master plan for reproducing cells. Environmental factors such as cigarette smoke and ultraviolet light also cause free radicals to form in your body.

Damage caused by oxidation is quite familiar: for example, the quick browning on a cut apple or pear, and rancidity in oils. However, if you dip your apple or pear in orange juice, which has vitamin C, it stays white. And if vitamin E is added as a preservative to vegetable oil, it doesn't turn rancid as fast.

In your body, the process is similar. Free radicals cause oxidation, or cell damage, as they "steal" an

Label Lingo

Vitamins and Minerals

The lingo on the front of many food packages describes the amount of vitamins or minerals found in a single serving. For specific amounts of the nutrients described, check the Nutrition Facts on the label.

High, Rich in, Excellent source of means 20% or more of the Daily Value.*

Good source, Contains, Provides means 10 to 19% of the Daily Value.*

More, Enriched, Fortified, Added means 10% or more of the Daily Value.*

*As compared with a standard serving size of the traditional food

electron from body cells to become stable. Over time, that may lead to cell dysfunction and contribute to the onset of health problems such as cancer, artery and heart disease, cataracts, age-related macular degeneration, diabetes, Alzheimer's disease, and some deterioration that goes with aging. Antioxidants in your body counteract the action of free radicals.

Three antioxidant vitamins appear to neutralize free radicals: beta carotene and other carotenoids, vitamin C, and vitamin E. Some enzymes that have trace minerals—selenium, copper, zinc, and manganese—and some phytonutrients act as antioxidants, too. As scavengers, antioxidant vitamins mop up free radicals by donating an electron of their own. The result? Antioxidants may control free radicals or convert them to harmless waste products that get eliminated before they do damage. Antioxidants even may help undo some damage already done to body cells.

Each antioxidant has its own biological job description. Being water-soluble, vitamin C removes free radicals from fluids inside and outside of body cells. Beta carotene and vitamin E, because they're fat-soluble, are present in lipids and fat tissues in your body. Antioxidants seem to complement each other. Because they work together, an excess or a deficiency of one may inhibit the benefits of other antioxidants.

Scientific evidence can't promise that antioxidant nutrients provide a "safety shield" from chronic diseases. Their role and potential interactions in reducing the risks are among the many unknowns. And we don't know the potentially adverse affects of ongoing, high intakes of these nutrients from supplements, either. Still, a varied diet—that follows MyPyramid—with plenty of antioxidant-containing fruits, vegetables, and whole grains is smart eating!

A "Garden" of Antioxidants

Where should your antioxidant vitamins come from? An eating style with plenty of fruits and vegetables is undisputed as the wisest approach to good health.

Fruits and Vegetables: A Look at Their Antioxidant Potential

A food's health-promoting benefits likely come from many antioxidants, not just a single antioxidant nutrient or food substance. With this in mind, a scientific scoring method—the ORAC (oxygen radical absorbency capacity) score—has been created to estimate the overall antioxidant potential of fruits and vegetables. The higher the ORAC score, the greater the antioxidant potential.

FRUIT (RAW)	ORAC UNITS	VEGETABLES (RAW)	ORAC UNITS
Dried plums (prunes) (4)	1,939	Kale (1 cup)	1,186
Blueberries (½ cup)	1,740	Beets (½ cup)	571
Blackberries (½ cup)	1,466	Red bell peppers (½ cup)	533
Strawberries (½ cup)	1,170	Brussels sprouts (½ cup)	431
Raisins (¼ cup)	1,026	Corn (½ cup)	420
Raspberries (½ cup)	756	Spinach (1 cup)	378
Oranges (½ cup sections)	675	Onions (½ cup)	360
Plums (1)	626	Broccoli florets (½ cup)	320
Red grapes (½ cup)	591	Eggplant (½ cup)	320
Cherries (½ cup)	516	Alfalfa sprouts (½ cup)	149

Sources: USDA Agricultural Research Service, *Food and Nutrition Research Briefs* (April 1999). Calculated to serving sizes, J. Walsh, "The Growing Allure of Antioxidants," *Environmental Nutrition* (January 2000).

Remember: The ORAC score offers a scientific method for looking at food in a new way. No guidelines exist to suggest how many ORAC units you need. *Be aware:* A high ORAC value doesn't mean a food performs better as an antioxidant source; the bioavailability of these antioxidants isn't known, either.

Eating plenty of whole-grain foods, as well as nuts, containing vitamin E provides them, too.

Many foods on supermarket shelves are fortified with antioxidant vitamins: C, E, and beta carotene. While these foods may not supply enough antioxidant vitamins for their possible protective benefits, they're often good sources. For carotenoids and vitamin C, fruits and vegetables still are the best sources, as they contain other phytonutrients that may help prevent health problems such as some cancers and heart disease.

Antioxidants in Supplements

Even if a little is good, a lot may not be better. So far no research proves that taking beta carotene, vitamins C or E, or other antioxidant supplements prevents disease.

To date, scientists haven't pinpointed which antioxidants offer specific benefits, how much would be enough—or how many years you'd need to take them. They don't know enough about side effects from taking supplemental antioxidants over long periods of time. Moreover, the mix of antioxidants in food, not just one or two from supplements, may offer positive and powerful antioxidant action.

Other antioxidant issues need research, too. For one, high doses from antioxidant supplements may be harmful, perhaps by working as pro-oxidants that promote, rather than neutralize, oxidation. Second, not all free radicals are harmful. Some offer protection by attacking harmful bacteria or cancer cells in the body. Very high intakes of antioxidants may destroy or hinder these protective free radicals.

Until more is known, continue to enjoy the wide variety of fruits, vegetables, whole-grain products, and nuts and seeds, with their many naturally occurring antioxidants. And avoid high doses from supplement sources. *For more about dietary supplements, see chapter 23.*

Minerals—Not "Heavy Metal"

The term "minerals" may conjure up thoughts of rocks. But to your body, minerals are another group of essential nutrients, needed to both regulate body processes and give your body structure.

Have You Ever Wondered

. . . how tortillas made with corn could have calcium? Made in the traditional Mexican way, corn tortillas can supply significant amounts of calcium, especially to people who eat them as the main bread in their everyday diet. Corn itself doesn't have calcium. But to prepare corn for tortillas, it's first soaked in slaked lime to remove the hard coating on corn kernels. Not from citrus fruit, this lime is instead calcium hydroxide, which is safe to eat when used this way in food processing.

. . . how frozen yogurt compares nutritionally to regular yogurt? Regular yogurt—plain or fruit-flavored—supplies considerably more calcium than frozen yogurt. The nutrient content of frozen yogurt is variable but more similar to low-fat ice cream than to regular yogurt. No federal standards exist for frozen yogurt. Read the label to learn the nutrient and calorie content.

As an aside, some regular and frozen yogurts contain "active live cultures" with possible health benefits; see *"Prebiotics and Probiotics: What Are They?" later in this chapter.* For frozen yogurt, very low temperatures slow the action of any live cultures. To find yogurt that contains these cultures, look for the seal from the National Yogurt Association.

Like vitamins, minerals help trigger, or regulate, a myriad of processes that continually take place in your body, so they are essential to your life. For example, they regulate fluid balance, muscle contractions, and nerve impulses.

Even though they make up only a small percentage—about 4 percent—of your weight, minerals also help give your body structure. They not only give structure to bones and teeth, but muscles, blood, and other body tissues all contain minerals, too.

Unlike vitamins, minerals are inorganic. Minerals can't be destroyed by heat or other food-handling processes. In fact, if you've ever completely burned food, perhaps while cooking over a fire, the little bit of ash left over is its mineral content.

Think of minerals in two categories—major minerals and trace minerals—depending on how much you need. Regardless of amount, they're all essential.

● *Major minerals:* Major minerals are needed in greater amounts than trace minerals are—more than

250 milligrams are recommended daily for each one. Calcium, phosphorus, and magnesium fit in this category, along with three electrolytes—sodium, chloride, and potassium.

Electrolytes, grouped together because their work is interrelated, regulate body fluids in and out of every cell. Electrolytes also transmit nerve, or electrical, impulses. *To learn more, see "Sodium and Potassium: You Need Some!" in chapter 7.*

● *Trace minerals:* Your body needs just small amounts—fewer than 20 milligrams daily—for each of the trace minerals, or trace elements: chromium, copper, fluoride, iodine, iron, manganese, molybdenum, selenium, and zinc. Recommended Dietary Allowances have been set for only some: copper, iodine, iron, molybdenum, selenium, and zinc. Others are presented in DRI Charts as Adequate Intake Levels (AIs).

Nutrition experts have reviewed research on other trace elements: arsenic, boron, nickel, silicon, and vanadium. They don't appear to have a role in human health. However, Tolerable Upper Intake Levels (UL) have been set for some: boron (20 milligrams a day), nickel (1.0 milligram a day), and vanadium (1.8 milligrams a day) for adult levels.

All minerals are absorbed in your intestines, then transported and stored in your body in different ways. Some pass directly into your bloodstream, where they're carried to cells; any excess passes out of the body through urine. Others attach to proteins and become part of your body structure; because they're stored, excess amounts can be harmful if the levels consumed are too high for too long.

Note: On the following pages, the amounts of minerals in foods have been rounded.

Major Minerals

Calcium

See "Calcium: A Closer Look" later in this chapter.

What it does:

● Builds bones, in both length and strength, becoming part of bone tissue.

● Helps your bones remain strong by slowing the rate of bone loss as you age.

● Helps your muscles contract and your heart beat.

● Plays a role in normal nerve function.

● Helps your blood clot if you're bleeding.

If you don't get enough: For children, not getting enough calcium may interfere with growth; a severe deficiency may keep children from reaching their potential adult height. Even a mild deficiency over a lifetime can affect bone density and bone loss, increasing the risk for osteoporosis, or brittle bone disease. *See "Bone Up on Calcium" later in this chapter.*

If you consume excess amounts: Unless the doses are very large (more than 2,500 milligrams daily), adverse effects for adults are unlikely. Very large doses over a prolonged time may cause kidney stones and poor kidney function, and may affect the absorption of other minerals such as iron, magnesium, and zinc. Regular consumption of milk and milk products won't result in excessive amounts of calcium. The Tolerable Upper Intake Level (UL) from the Dietary Reference Intakes is set at 2,500 milligrams daily from age one through adulthood.

How much you need: For ages nine through eighteen, the Adequate Intake (AI) is 1,300 milligrams daily. As an adult through age fifty, the AI is 1,000 milligrams of calcium daily. After that, the recommendation goes back up, to 1,200 milligrams of calcium daily for both men and women to help maintain bone mass. Calcium recommendations for women who are pregnant or breast-feeding are the same as for other women in their respective age group.

To reduce the risks of osteoporosis, many nutrition experts believe that even more calcium is better for your bones. The National Osteoporosis Foundation advises at least 1,200 milligrams of calcium daily, and vitamin D each day, along with regular physical activity (weight-bearing, resistance training).

Where it's mostly found: Milk and other dairy foods such as yogurt and most cheeses are the best sources of calcium. In addition, some dark-green leafy vegetables (kale, broccoli, bok choy), fish with edible bones, calcium-fortified soy beverage, and tofu made with calcium sulfate also supply significant amounts. There's also juice, bottled water, and bread that may be calcium fortified. *See "Counting Up Calcium" later in this chapter for a list of good sources and amounts.*

Phosphorus

What it does:

- Helps generate energy in every cell of your body.
- Acts as the main regulator of energy metabolism in your body's organs.
- Is a major component of bones and teeth, second only to calcium.
- Serves as part of DNA and RNA, which are your body's master plan for cell growth and repair.

If you don't get enough: A deficiency is quite rare, except for small, premature babies who consume only breast milk, or for people who take an antacid with aluminum hydroxide for a long time. In those rare cases, the symptoms include bone loss, weakness, loss of appetite, and pain.

If you consume excess amounts: An excess amount may lower the level of calcium in the blood—a problem if calcium intake is low. As a result, bone loss may increase. Besides that, consuming too much phosphorus doesn't appear to be a problem in the United States. The Tolerable Upper Intake Level (UL) for phosphorus is 4,000 milligrams a day for people ages nine through seventy; after age seventy, it's 3,000 milligrams of phosphorus daily. For pregnancy, the level drops slightly, to 3,500 milligrams of phosphorus daily.

How much you need: The RDA for phosphorus is 1,250 milligrams daily for ages nine through eighteen, then decreases to 700 milligrams daily for adults of all ages. Scientific evidence shows that people need less than previously thought.

Where it's mostly found: Almost all foods contain phosphorus. Protein-rich foods—milk, meat, poultry, fish, and eggs—contain the most. Legumes (dry beans) and nuts are good sources as well. Even bread and other baked foods have some. You'll also find phosphorus in colas and pepper-type soft drinks.

FOOD	PHOSPHORUS (MG)
Milk, fat-free (1 cup)	245
Perch, cooked (3 oz.)	220
Lean ground beef, cooked (3 oz.)	195
Cheddar cheese (1 oz.)	145
Kidney beans, cooked (½ cup)	125
Tofu (½ cup)	120
Peanut butter (2 tbsp.)	115
Egg, large (1)	95
Cola (12 oz.)	40

Magnesium

What it does:

- Serves as an important part of more than three hundred body enzymes. Enzymes are body chemicals that regulate all kinds of bodily functions, including producing energy, making body protein, and muscle contractions.
- Helps maintain body cells in nerves and muscles, and signals muscles to relax and contract.
- Serves as a component of bones.

If you don't get enough: A deficiency is rare except in diseases where the body doesn't absorb magnesium properly. Then symptoms might include irregular heartbeat, nausea, weakness, and/or mental derangement.

If you consume an excess amount: Consuming too much magnesium from food probably won't do any harm—unless it can't be excreted properly due to kidney disease. The Tolerable Upper Intake Level is 350 milligrams a day; this amount is less than the RDA because it represents only the amount of magnesium in supplements or drugs.

How much you need: The RDA for teenage boys is 410 milligrams of magnesium daily to age eighteen; for teenage girls, 360 milligrams daily. The RDA for adult males is 400 milligrams daily through age thirty, then 420 milligrams daily after that. For females, the recommendation is 310 milligrams daily through age thirty, then 320 milligrams daily after age thirty. Neither pregnancy nor breast-feeding increases the need for magnesium.

Where it's mostly found: Magnesium is found in varying amounts in all kinds of foods. The best sources are legumes, nuts, and whole grains. Green vegetables are good sources, too.

FOOD	MAGNESIUM (MG)
Spinach, boiled (½ cup)	80
Peanut butter (2 tbsp.)	50
Black-eyed peas, boiled (½ cup)	45

FOOD	MAGNESIUM (MG)
Pecans, dried (1 oz.)	40
Lima beans, boiled (½ cup)	40
Whole-wheat bread (1 slice)	25
Parsnips, boiled (½ cup)	25
Whole-wheat spaghetti, cooked (½ cup)	20

Major Minerals: Electrolytes

Chloride

What it does:

- Helps regulate fluids in and out of body cells.
- As a component of stomach acid, helps with the digestion of your food and the absorption of nutrients.
- Helps transmit nerve impulses, or signals.

If you don't get enough: Because salt is such a common part of the diet, a deficiency of chloride isn't likely. If deficient, however, symptoms are similar to sodium deficiency.

If you consume excess amounts: For people who are sensitive, along with sodium, there may be a link to high blood pressure, but more study is needed. The Tolerable Upper Intake Level (UL) is 3,400 milligrams daily for kids ages nine to thirteen; after that, the UL is 3,600 milligrams daily for teens and adults.

How much you need: The Adequate Intake for all aged nine to fifty (including during pregnancy and breast-feeding) is 2,300 milligrams a day. For ages fifty-one to seventy years, it goes down to 2,000 milligrams a day; after age seventy, it's 1,800 milligrams daily.

Where it's mostly found: Salt is sodium plus chloride. Salt and salty foods are the main chloride sources: ¼ teaspoon of salt has 750 milligrams of chloride.

Potassium

See chapter 7, "Sodium and Potassium: A Salty Subject."

What it does:

- Helps regulate fluids and mineral balance in and out of body cells.
- Helps maintain your normal blood pressure by blunting sodium's effects on blood pressure.
- Helps transmit nerve impulses, or signals.
- Helps your muscles contract.

If you don't get enough: For healthy people, a potassium deficiency is rare. When vomiting, diarrhea, or laxative use goes on for too long, the body may lose excess amounts. Kidney problems also may cause severe loss. Deficiency symptoms include muscle cramps, weakness, appetite loss, nausea, and fatigue. You may need a potassium supplement if you're on medication for high blood pressure. Talk to your doctor.

If you consume excess amounts: Harmful effects from consuming too much from food are rare because excess amounts usually are excreted. If an excess can't be excreted, it can cause heart problems and possible sudden death. People with kidney problems may not be able to get rid of excess potassium and may be advised to limit potassium-containing foods and to avoid using potassium chloride as a salt substitute. There is no Tolerable Upper Intake Level for potassium.

How much you need: The Adequate Intake (AI) level for potassium is 4,500 milligrams daily for those ages nine to thirteen. From ages fourteen on up, the AI is 4,700 milligrams daily, including pregnancy. For breast-feeding women, the AI is 5,100 milligrams. People on some diuretics or heart disease medicines should get less than the AI; check with your doctor.

Where it's mostly found: Potassium is found in a wide range of foods, especially fruits, many vegetables, legumes, dairy foods, meat, poultry, fish and nuts. Less processed foods tend to have more potassium.

FOOD	POTASSIUM (MG)
Banana, medium (1)	420
Milk, fat-free (1 cup)	380
Kidney beans, cooked (½ cup)	360
Haddock, cooked (3 oz.)	340
Potato, baked, with skin (2 oz.)	330
Tomato, medium (1)	290
Orange, medium (1)	235

Turkey, light and dark meat, roasted, skinless (3 oz.)	225
Almonds (1 oz. or 24 almonds)	210
Spinach, raw (1 cup)	170
Okra, boiled (½ cup)	110

FOOD	SODIUM (MG)
Beef bologna (1 oz.)	310
Cheddar cheese (1 oz.)	175
Whole-wheat bread (1 slice)	150
Milk, fat-free (1 cup)	105

Sodium

See chapter 7, "Sodium and Potassium: A Salty Subject."

What it does:

● Helps regulate the movement of body fluids in and out of your body cells.

● Helps muscles, including your heart, relax.

● Helps transmit nerve impulses, or signals.

● Helps regulate your blood pressure.

If you don't get enough: Unless you have prolonged diarrhea or vomiting, or have kidney problems, a sodium deficiency isn't likely. If it happens, symptoms might include nausea, dizziness, and muscle cramps.

If you consume an excess amount: For healthy people, excess sodium is excreted, but some kidney diseases interfere with sodium excretion, causing fluid retention and swelling. For people with sodium sensitivity, a high-sodium diet can increase blood pressure.

The Tolerable Upper Intake Level (UL) is 2,200 milligrams daily for kids ages nine to thirteen; after that, the UL is 2,300 milligrams daily for teens and adults, including pregnant or breast-feeding women. This advice is set for people who don't have high blood pressure; the UL may be too high for those who already have it.

How much you need: The Adequate Intake (AI) for males and females ages nine to fifty is 1,500 milligrams a day. The level stays the same during pregnancy and breast-feeding. For ages fifty to seventy, it goes down to 1,300 milligrams a day; after age seventy, it's 1,200 milligrams daily.

Where it's mostly found: Processed foods account for about 77 percent of the sodium in food. The rest comes from table salt and the small amount that occurs naturally in food. As a point of reference, ¼ teaspoon of salt contains about 500 milligrams of sodium.

The Nutrition Facts on food labels tell how much sodium comes from a single label serving of food. *See "Get All the Facts!" in chapter 11 on food labeling.*

Trace Minerals

Chromium

What it does:

● Works with insulin to help your body use glucose, or blood sugar. *See "Sugar: What Is It?" in chapter 5 to learn more about glucose.*

If you don't get enough: Because chromium works closely with insulin, a deficiency can look like diabetes. *See "Diabetes: A Growing Health Concern" in chapter 22 for more about diabetes.*

If you consume excess amounts: Consuming harmful amounts from dietary sources is highly unlikely.

How much you need: A level of Adequate Intake (AI) has been set for chromium: 35 micrograms per day for males ages fourteen to fifty, and 30 micrograms per day from age fifty-one on. For females, 24 micrograms daily from ages fourteen to eighteen; 25 micrograms daily from ages nineteen through fifty; and 20 micrograms daily from age fifty-one on. During pregnancy, the AI level is 5 micrograms daily higher; during breast-feeding, an additional 20 micrograms.

Where it's mostly found: Meat, eggs, whole-grain products, and cheese are all good sources.

FOOD	CHROMIUM (MCG)
Cheese, American (1 oz.)	48
Liver, braised (3 oz.)	42
Shredded wheat (1 oz.)	33
Peas (½ cup)	30
Egg, large (1)	26

Copper

What it does:

- Helps your body make hemoglobin, needed to carry oxygen in red blood cells.
- Serves as a part of many body enzymes.
- Helps your body develop connective tissue, myelin, and melanin.
- Helps your body produce energy in the cells.

If you don't get enough: A deficiency rarely comes from a lack of copper, but instead from genetic problems. Another cause: excess zinc from supplement sources can hinder copper absorption.

If you consume excess amounts: Harmful effects of copper from dietary sources are extremely rare in the United States. The Tolerable Upper Intake Level (UL) is 8,000 micrograms daily for teens ages fourteen to eighteen, and 10,000 micrograms daily for adults.

How much you need: The RDA for copper is set at 890 micrograms per day for teens ages fourteen to eighteen, and 900 micrograms daily for adults. During pregnancy the level is 1,000 micrograms daily; during breast-feeding it's 1,300 micrograms daily.

Where it's mostly found: Organ meats, especially liver; seafood; nuts; and seeds are the best sources. Cooking in copper pots increases the copper in food.

FOOD	COPPER (MCG)
Beef liver, braised (3 oz.)	12,140
Clams, cooked (3 oz.)	590
Sunflower seeds, dry roasted (1 oz.)	520
Peanuts, dry roasted (1 oz.)	190
Mushrooms, canned (½ cup)	180

Fluoride

See "The Fluoride Connection" in chapter 8.

What it does:

- Helps harden tooth enamel and so helps protect your teeth from decay.
- May offer some protection from osteoporosis, or brittle bone disease, by helping to strengthen bones.

If you don't get enough: Tooth enamel may be weak.

If you consume excess amounts: With excessive fluoride, teeth become mottled, or marked with brown stains, although teeth are healthy in every other way. Be aware that these stains may have other causes as well. The Tolerable Upper Intake Level (UL) is 2.2 milligrams of fluoride daily for children ages four through eight; from age nine through adulthood, the UL is 10 milligrams of fluoride daily.

How much you need: An Adequate Intake (AI) for fluoride has been set. AI levels for children are as follows: ages four to eight, 1 milligram of fluoride daily, and ages nine to thirteen, 2 milligrams of fluoride daily. For teens the AI is set at 3 milligrams of fluoride daily. For adults, the guideline is 4 milligrams of fluoride daily for males and 3 milligrams daily for females. There are no increased needs during pregnancy or breast-feeding. A fluoride supplement may be prescribed by a dentist or doctor for some infants and children. *See "Vitamin and Mineral Supplements for Breast-Fed Babies" in chapter 15.*

Where it's mostly found: Fluoride is not widely available in food. Two significant sources are tea, especially if it's made with fluoridated water, and fish with edible bones, such as canned salmon.

The main means for obtaining fluoride is drinking and cooking with fluoridated (fluoride added) water. Many municipal water supplies are fluoridated; however, most bottled waters are not. Some types of cooking utensils, such as Teflon with its fluoride-containing polymer, also can increase the fluoride content of food. The fluoride content in food varies and is affected by the environment in which the food originated.

Iodine

What it does:

- Serves as part of thyroid hormones such as thyroxin, which regulate the rate at which your body uses energy.

If you don't get enough: With an iodine deficiency, the body can't make enough thyroxin. As a result, the rate at which the body burns energy slows down, and weight gain may become a problem. Goiter, an enlarged thyroid gland, is the deficiency disease often caused by a lack of iodine. With the use of iodized salt, goiter rarely is caused by an iodine deficiency.

If you consume excess amounts: Goiter also can be induced when people consume high levels of iodine—but not at levels consumed in the United States. Too much also can result in irregular heartbeat and confusion. The Tolerable Upper Intake Level (UL) is 900 micrograms daily for teens ages fourteen to eighteen, and 1,100 micrograms daily during adulthood.

How much you need: The RDA for iodine is 150 micrograms daily for adults. During pregnancy, the recommendation goes up to 220 micrograms; during breast-feeding, 290 micrograms daily.

Where it's mostly found: Iodine is found naturally in saltwater fish. Foods grown near coastal areas also contain iodine, but many people don't have access to these foods. For this reason, salt is iodized, assuring an adequate amount of iodine in the food supply, even if you consume only modest amounts of salt. One-half teaspoon of iodized salt provides almost enough iodine to reach the RDA for a day.

FOOD	IODINE (MCG)
Cod, cooked (3 oz.)	99
Table salt, iodized (¼ tsp.)	98
Potato, cooked (1 medium)	54
Turkey breast, baked (3 oz.)	34
Navy beans, cooked (½ cup)	31

Iron

See "Iron: A Closer Look" later in this chapter.

What it does:

- Serves as an essential part of hemoglobin, which carries oxygen in your blood from your lungs to every body cell, and other enzymes.
- Helps in brain development.
- Supports a healthy immune system.

If you don't get enough: Although there may be other causes, an iron deficiency can lead to anemia, along with fatigue and infections. Among women with regular menstrual loss, iron deficiency is more common. In fact, in the United States, iron deficiency is the most common nutrient deficiency.

If you consume excess amounts: Iron can build up to dangerous levels for people with a genetic problem called hemochromatosis, whereby the body absorbs and stores too much iron. That excess can cause an enlarged liver, bronze skin pigmentation, and diabetes, as well as pancreatic, liver, cardiac, and other organ damage. Ten times more common in men, symptoms of hemochromatosis usually begin to appear in adulthood, often in the thirties.

Taking adult iron supplements can be dangerous for children. Children should get immediate medical attention if they take an overdose of iron supplements. The Tolerable Upper Intake Level (UL) is 45 milligrams of iron per day for ages fourteen and over.

How much you need: The RDA for teen males ages fourteen to eighteen is 11 milligrams of iron daily; for adult men it's 8 milligrams daily. For teen females to age eighteen, 15 milligrams of iron daily; for females ages nineteen to fifty, 18 milligrams are recommended daily. From age fifty-one on, women need about 8 milligrams of iron daily.

During pregnancy the recommendation goes up to 27 milligrams daily; during breast-feeding, the RDA is 10 milligrams daily for females age eighteen and younger and 9 milligrams daily for females ages nineteen and over.

Where it's mostly found: Iron comes from foods of both animal (heme iron) and plant (nonheme) sources. It's much better absorbed from heme iron and when

Have You Ever Wondered

... about sulfate—since it's considered an electrolyte? Inorganic sulfate is a nutrient with electrolyte properties. The Dietary Reference Intakes (DRIs) identify sulfate, but don't show an Adequate Intake (AI) level. Food, water, and the metabolic breakdown of amino acids in the body provide enough. Dried fruit and fruit juice, wine, beer, soy flour, bread, and meat supply sulfate. No Tolerable Upper Intake Level (UL) exists, either. The odor and off-flavor usually limit how much people consume. That said, when the water supply has a high level of sulfate, diarrhea may result.

vitamin C is consumed with nonheme iron at the same meal. *See "Counting Up Iron" later in this chapter for a list of good sources and amounts.*

Manganese

What it does:

- Serves as part of many enzymes.
- Helps in bone formation.
- Helps in the metabolism of energy from carbohydrates, fats, and proteins.

If you don't get enough: The chances of not getting enough are very low since manganese is so widely distributed in the food supply.

If you consume excess amounts: Consuming harmful levels from food is very rare, too. The Tolerable Upper Intake Level (UL) is set at 9 milligrams daily for teens ages fourteen to eighteen, and at 11 milligrams daily during adulthood.

How much you need: There is no RDA for manganese. However, the AI is set at 2.2 milligrams and 1.6 milligrams daily for males and females ages fourteen to eighteen, respectively. For adults the AI is 2.3 milligrams daily for males and 1.8 milligrams daily for females. During pregnancy (teens and adults), the AI is 2.0 milligrams daily; during breast-feeding, 2.6 milligrams daily.

Where it's mostly found: Whole-grain products are the best sources of manganese, along with some fruits and vegetables. Tea also is a good source.

FOOD	MANGANESE (MG)
Pineapple, raw (½ cup)	1.2
Whole-wheat spaghetti, cooked (½ cup)	1
Tea, instant powder (1 tsp.)	0.9
Whole-wheat bread (1 slice)	0.7
Lentils, boiled (½ cup)	0.5
Kale, boiled (½ cup)	0.3
Strawberries (½ cup)	0.3

Molybdenum

What it does:

- Works with riboflavin to incorporate the iron stored in the body into hemoglobin for making red blood cells.
- Is part of many body enzymes.

If you don't get enough: With a normal diet, there's no need to worry about a deficiency. A deficiency of the enzymes made with molybdenum affects the nervous system, and in extreme cases may result in death.

If you consume excess amounts: Too much may have reproductive effects, but harmful levels are quite uncommon. The Tolerable Upper Intake Level (UL) is 1,700 micrograms daily during the years fourteen to eighteen, and 2,000 micrograms daily during adulthood.

How much you need: The RDA for molybdenum is 43 micrograms daily during the years fourteen to eighteen, and 45 micrograms daily during adulthood. During pregnancy and breast-feeding, the RDA level goes up to 50 micrograms daily for teen and adult women.

Where it's mostly found: Molybdenum is found mostly in milk, legumes, liver, breads, and grain products. The amount consumed in a typical eating pattern appears adequate. Little is known about the actual amounts in foods.

Selenium

What it does:

- Works as an antioxidant with vitamin E, to protect cells from damage that may lead to heart disease, and perhaps cancer and other health problems.
- Aids cell growth.
- Boosts immune function.

If you don't get enough: The general signs of a deficiency in humans aren't clear, but it may affect the heart muscle.

If you consume excess amounts: A normal diet with a variety of foods generally provides moderate levels of selenium. Very high levels from dietary supplements can be quite harmful. The Tolerable Upper Intake Level (UL) is set at 400 micrograms daily for people ages fourteen and over.

How much you need: The RDA is 55 micrograms daily for people ages fourteen and over. During pregnancy the recommendation remains the same, 55 micrograms daily; during breast-feeding it goes up to 70 micrograms daily.

Where it's mostly found: The richest sources are seafood, liver, and kidney, as well as other meats. Grain products and seeds contain selenium, but the amount depends on the selenium content of the soil in which they're grown. Fruits and vegetables generally don't have much.

FOOD	SELENIUM (MCG)
Chicken, light meat, skinless (3 oz.)	24
Egg, large (1)	16
Brown rice, cooked (½ cup)	10
Whole-wheat bread (1 slice)	10
Peanuts (¼ cup)	3

Zinc

What it does:

● Promotes cell reproduction and tissue growth and repair. Adequate zinc intake is essential for growth.

● Associated with more than two hundred enzymes.

● Helps your body use carbohydrates, proteins, and fats.

If you don't get enough: A deficiency during childhood can impair growth, and during pregnancy can cause birth defects. Other symptoms include appetite loss, skin changes, and reduced resistance to infections.

If you consume excess amounts: Too much zinc from dietary supplements can have harmful side effects, including impaired copper absorption. The Tolerable Upper Intake Level (UL) for zinc is 34 milligrams daily for teens ages fourteen to eighteen, and 40 milligrams daily for adults.

How much you need: The RDA for males is 11 milligrams daily for ages fourteen on. For females it's 9 milligrams daily for teens ages fourteen to eighteen, and 8 milligrams daily during adulthood. During pregnancy the recommendation increases to 13 milligrams daily for teens, and 11 milligrams daily for adults; during breast-feeding, 14 milligrams and 12 milligrams daily, respectively.

Where it's mostly found: Good sources of zinc include foods of animal origin, including meat, seafood, and liver. Eggs and milk supply zinc in smaller amounts.

Whole-grain products, wheat germ, black-eyed peas, and fermented soybean paste (miso) also contain zinc, but in a form that's less available to the body.

FOOD	ZINC (MG)
Beef, ground lean (3 oz.)	5.5
Wheat germ (¼ cup)	4.7
Crab, canned (3 oz.)	3.5
Wheat bran (½ cup)	2
Sunflower seeds (1 oz.)	1.5
Black-eyed peas, frozen, boiled (½ cup)	1
Almonds (1 oz.)	1
Milk, fat-free (1 cup)	1
Tofu, raw (½ cup)	1
Peanut butter (2 tbsp.)	0.9
Tuna, canned, packed in water (3 oz.)	0.7
Egg, large (1)	0.6
Whole-wheat bread (1 slice)	0.5

Calcium: A Closer Look

The human body contains more calcium than any other mineral. For an average 130-pound adult, about 1,200 grams—almost 3 pounds—of the body is calcium. Your body composition, of course, depends on the size of your body frame; the density of your bones; and, if you're older, how much bone you've lost through aging.

Of that amount, about 99 percent of your body's calcium is in your bones. The remaining 1 percent is in your other body fluids and cells. Calcium is as important to you as an adult as it was during your childhood. The reasons really aren't that different.

Bone Up on Calcium

Most of us mentally connect the growing years with the need for calcium. That's true, but "boning up" is actually a lifelong process—starting at the moment of conception. During the childhood and teen years, bones grow long and wide. In fact, 40 percent or more of the body's bone mass is formed during adolescence. By age twenty or so, that phase of bone building is complete. But the period of building toward peak bone mass continues until the early thirties. Bones become stronger and more dense as more calcium becomes part of the bone matrix.

Your bones are in a constant state of change. Because bones are living tissue, calcium gets deposited and withdrawn daily from your skeleton, much like money in a bank, in a process called remodeling. As small amounts are withdrawn, they're used for other body functions; at the same time, calcium is deposited in bones. To keep your bones strong and to

reduce bone loss, you need to make regular calcium deposits to replace the losses—and even build up a little "savings account" of calcium for when your food choices come up short.

Calcium doesn't work alone. It works in partnership with other nutrients, including phosphorus and vitamin D. Vitamin D helps absorb and deposit calcium in bones and teeth, making them stronger. Phosphorus also is an important part of bone structure. There's another way the body can absorb calcium

Your Nutrition Checkup

Yesterday . . . Did You Consume Enough Calcium?

Food	No. of Servings	Calcium Quality Points	Score	Food	No. of Servings	Calcium Quality Points	Score
8 oz. milk (any type)	_____	× 3 =	_____	1 cup cooked greens (mustard, dandelion, beet)	_____	1	_____
8 oz. yogurt	_____	3					
3½ oz. sardines	_____	3	_____	1 cup cooked soybeans	_____	1	_____
½ cup ricotta cheese	_____	3		1 cup cooked acorn squash or butternut squash	_____	1	_____
10 oz. milkshake	_____	3					
2 slices processed cheese	_____	3	_____	1 cup tofu (treated with calcium sulfate)	_____	1	_____
8 oz. calcium-fortified orange juice*	_____	3		1 packet instant oatmeal	_____	1	_____
8 oz. calcium-fortified soy beverage**	_____	3		1 English muffin	_____	1	_____
1 oz. hard cheese	_____	2		½ cup softserve vanilla ice milk	_____	1	_____
⅓ cup grated cheese	_____	2					
1 cup black-eyed peas	_____	2	_____	½ cup chocolate, vanilla, tapioca, or rice pudding	_____	1	_____
2 tbsp. blackstrap molasses	_____	2	_____	1 slice medium cheese pizza	_____	1	_____
3 oz. canned salmon with bones	_____	2	_____	1 medium cheeseburger	_____	1	_____
1 cup frozen yogurt	_____	2		*Total calcium score*			_____
1 cup cottage cheese	_____	1				× 100	
1 cup baked beans	_____	1		Approximate milligrams of calcium			_____
1 cup cooked broccoli, kale, or bok choy	_____	1	_____				

*Fortified at about 500 milligrams calcium per 8 ounces

**See page 265 for calcium equivalencies for calcium-fortified soy beverages without vitamin D; however, that mechanism requires even more calcium intake!

If you don't consume enough calcium—or if your body doesn't adequately absorb it (perhaps because you're short on vitamin D)—your body may withdraw more calcium from bones than you deposit. You need calcium, for example, for muscle contraction and your heartbeat, too. This process gradually depletes bone, leaving a void where calcium otherwise would be deposited, eventually making bones more porous and fragile. *See "Which Bone Is Healthy?" in chapter 22 to compare healthy and osteoporotic bone.*

After age thirty or so, bones slowly lose minerals that give them strength. That's a natural part of aging. Whatever calcium a woman has "banked" in her skeleton will be the amount in her bones when she enters menopause. Even then, consuming enough calcium can help women retain their bone density and lower the risk for osteoporosis later.

During the childbearing years, the hormone estrogen appears to protect bones, keeping them strong. But with the onset of menopause, bone loss speeds up for women as estrogen levels go down. If women achieve their peak bone mass as younger adults, their risk for osteoporosis, or brittle bone disease, later in life is reduced. Their bones are strong enough before menopause to offer protection.

For older adults (ages fifty-one and over), calcium remains important for bone health as well as for protection from high blood pressure and cancer. It's not too late to get the benefits from consuming more calcium, even if you're starting now.

An adequate calcium intake is one important factor in building healthy bones. Adequate exercise is another. Regular, weight-bearing physical activities such as walking, strength-training, dancing, kick-boxing, and tennis stimulate bone formation. These types of activities trigger nerve impulses that, in turn, activate body chemicals to deposit calcium in bones.

Women—and men, too: You can build bone until about age thirty. After that, you can only slow the bone loss that comes with aging. Follow these tips:

- Consume adequate amounts of calcium and vitamin D—at every age and stage of life!

- Be careful with weight loss; eating plans that

severely restrict food often restrict calcium. If you're concerned about calories or fat, choose fat-free or low-fat milk for bone building.

- Participate regularly—at least three times weekly—in weight-bearing activities.

- Avoid smoking and an excessive intake of alcoholic drinks; both interfere with bone health.

For more about calcium during the bone-building adolescent years, see "Calcium: A Growing Issue" in chapter 16. For other factors that relate to osteoporosis, see "Osteoporosis: Reduce the Risks" in chapter 22.

Have You Ever Wondered

... if calcium supplements or calcium-fortified foods can substitute for dairy foods? For most people, fortified foods and supplements are meant to supplement, not replace, foods with naturally occurring calcium.

Although they may fill the calcium gap, supplements and calcium-fortified foods (such as in some juice, cereal, pasta, and rice) don't supply all the other health-promoting nutrients and food substances found in dairy foods. Besides calcium, Milk Group foods are key sources of protein, vitamins A, B$_2$ (riboflavin), B$_{12}$, and D (if fortified) and the minerals phosphorus, potassium, magnesium, and zinc. Beyond that, dairy foods offer substances with potential functional benefits: conjugated linoleic acid (CLA), sphingolipid, and butyric acid, which may help protect you from some cancers and other health conditions. *For more about CLA, see "Functional Nutrition: Eat Your Omega-3s and -6s" in chapter 3. See page 265 for more about calcium-fortified soy beverages.*

You can overdo calcium if you regularly consume calcium-fortified juice and/or calcium-fortified breakfast cereal—and take a calcium supplement as "insurance." What's the downside? Too much calcium, most likely from fortified foods and supplements, may limit the absorption of iron and zinc, two minerals that often come up short for many Americans.

... if eggs count as a calcium-rich dairy food? Although they're typically sold in the dairy case, eggs aren't a dairy food! Since you don't eat the shell (your body can't use that form of calcium), eggs supply very little calcium.

More than Bone Health!

Looking for ways to stay healthy? Bone-building benefits are just one reason to make calcium a smart-eating priority! Like other nutrients, calcium is well known for "multitasking."

Daily "Chores." Although used in just a small amount, calcium helps your muscles contract, your heart beat, your blood clot, and your nervous system send messages. These functions are vital to your health.

More Protection. Calcium appears to play an important role in promoting health and protecting you from several health risks that begin to appear in midlife.

● Calcium helps your blood pressure. The good news: research shows that a low-fat diet with low-fat

---

Counting Up Calcium

Dairy foods supply about 72 percent of all the calcium available in the U.S. food supply. Some dark-green leafy vegetables and fish with edible bones provide significant amounts. Many processed foods such as soy beverage, tofu, orange juice, and breakfast cereal may be fortified with calcium.

Green, leafy vegetables and grain products supply some calcium. However, some vegetables such as spinach contain oxalates; grains may contain phytates. Both bind with some minerals, including calcium, magnesium, and iron, partially blocking their absorption. Caffeine slightly interferes with calcium absorption.

Food	Calcium (mg)	Food	Calcium (mg)
Yogurt, plain, nonfat (1 cup)	490	Okra (½ cup)	90
Yogurt, plain, low-fat (1 cup)	450	Cottage cheese (½ cup)	75
Tofu, regular (processed with calcium*) (½ cup)	435	Parmesan cheese (1 tbsp.)	65
Yogurt, fruit (1 cup)	370	Tofu, raw (processed without calcium*) (½ cup)	60
Milk, fat-free (1 cup)	305	Milk chocolate bar (1 oz.)	55
Chocolate milk, 1% (1 cup)	290	Dried figs (3)	50
Milk, 2% (1 cup)	285	Mustard greens, boiled (½ cup)	50
Milk, whole (1 cup)	275	Orange (1)	50
Chocolate milk, 2% (1 cup)	270	Kale, boiled (½ cup)	45
Swiss cheese, low-fat (1 oz.)	270	Anchovies with edible bones (5)	45
Calcium-fortified orange juice (¾ cup)	260	Tortillas (made from slaked lime-processed corn*)	45
Calcium-fortified soy beverage (8 oz.)	250–350	Pinto beans, boiled (½ cup)	40
Cheese pizza[†] (⅛ of 15-in. pizza)	220	Rutabaga, boiled (½ cup)	40
Mozzarella cheese, part skim (1 oz.)	210	Chinese cabbage, raw (½ cup)	35
Cheddar cheese (1 oz.)	205	Broccoli (½ cup)	30
Salmon, canned with edible bones (3 oz.)	205	Cream cheese (2 tbsp.)	25
Blackstrap molasses (1 tbsp.)	170	Tuna, canned (3 oz.)	10
Pudding (½ cup)	160	Lettuce greens (1/2 cup)	10
Macaroni and cheese[†] (½ cup)	150		
Sardines with edible bones (1 oz.)	110		
Turnip greens, boiled (½ cup)	100		
Frozen yogurt (½ cup)	90		
Ice cream (½ cup)	90		
Tempeh (½ cup)	90		

*Read the labels.

[†]The amount of calcium may vary, depending on the ingredients.

Source: U.S. Department of Agriculture, Agricultural Research Service, 2005. *USDA National Nutrient Database for Standard Reference,* Release 18.

dairy foods, fruits, and vegetables may help reduce your risk for hypertension (high blood pressure). Already hypertensive? Consuming adequate calcium may help bring your blood pressure level down. *Read about the DASH (Dietary Approaches to Stop Hypertension) eating plan and calcium link in chapter 22.*

● Are you at risk for colon cancer, perhaps with a history of polyps? Although the research isn't conclusive, calcium-rich or low-fat dairy foods appear to offer protection from abnormal cell growth in the colon—more protection than calcium supplements offer.

● Although research has just begun, calcium or dairy foods may reduce the risk of other health problems: kidney stones, premenstrual syndrome, polycystic ovary syndrome, breast cancer, lead toxicity, and obesity. Stay tuned—and consume enough calcium!

Calcium: When You Need More . . .

As an extra safeguard, many doctors also recommend calcium supplements, especially for menopausal and postmenopausal women to help slow bone loss that comes with hormonal changes. Many women simply don't consume enough calcium.

If you're advised to take calcium supplements, use them to fill the calcium gap—not to substitute for calcium-rich foods. *See "Calcium Supplements: A Bone Builder" in chapter 23 for ways to get the most benefit.*

Calci-Yumm: How to Eat More!

Need more calcium in your food choices? Give your meal and snack choices a calcium boost.

● Make it a habit! Eat 3 cups or an equivalent of foods from the Milk Group each day. Include 8 ounces of fruit yogurt with breakfast and a refreshing cup of milk for lunch or dinner. Three cups of milk, regardless of whether it's whole, fat-free, or flavored, supply about 900 milligrams of calcium.

● Reach for milk—during your "coffee break." If there's no place to buy a carton of milk, bring it from home. Refrigerate milk for a day at work in a small water bottle. Some experts say that just choosing milk at snacktime could make a big impact toward reducing the risk for osteoporosis.

● Give other dairy drinks a try: buttermilk, drinkable yogurt, kefir, even goat milk. In fact, 8 ounces of buttermilk delivers 235 milligrams of calcium, for just 200 calories and 2 fat grams.

● For the "new taste" of milk, try flavored milk—blueberry, banana, peanut butter—or yogurt-fruit drinks. Or make your own fruity drinks by blending milk or yogurt with fruit and ice in a blender.

● Enjoy snacks as calcium sources: frozen yogurt, cheese with crackers, plain yogurt, pudding, milk, or calcium-fortified juice. *For a calcium-rich, low-fat dip or cracker spread, see "Kitchen Nutrition: Yogurt Cheese" in chapter 3.*

● At a coffee bar, order latte (steamed milk with espresso coffee) or cappuccino. Lower the calories by asking for fat-free milk. For more flavor, sprinkle on cinnamon or nutmeg. Does caffeine interfere with calcium absorption? The effect is very small and easily offset by consuming the amount of steamed milk typically added to latte or cappuccino.

● Lighten up with milk. Add milk to your coffee or tea (milk tea), rather than drinking it black. Milk has more calcium than powdered nondairy creamer.

● Choose vegetables and fruits with more calcium: dark-green leafy greens such as kale and mustard, collard, and turnip greens; broccoli, dried beans, and bok choy are good sources. Other nondairy options include dried figs and calcium-fortified fruit juices.

● Drink calcium-fortified soy beverage (from the carton or blended in smoothies), and use it in cooking, especially if you choose to avoid milk.

● Say "cheese" when you make or order sandwiches.

● Choose canned fish with edible bones: salmon, sardines, and anchovies. Mix salmon in salads, casseroles, pasta dishes, salmon cakes, and other mixed dishes.

● Add tofu (soybean curd) made with calcium to salads, casseroles, chili, stir-fries, smoothies, and other dishes.

● Boost the calcium in your food preparation. Make soups, chowders, and hot cereal with milk. Top salads, soups, and stews with shredded cheese. Mix dry milk powder into meat loaf and casseroles. Make vegetable dips with plain yogurt, calcium-fortified tofu, or cottage cheese. Add bok choy, broccoli, or kale to soups, casseroles, and other mixed dishes. *For more*

Kitchen Nutrition: Milk Plus

You say you're not a milk drinker? Just whisk one or two ingredients, such as those below, with one cup of milk—cold or hot, fat-free or whole—and give it a refreshing new flavor! (And enjoy the added benefits of 300 milligrams of calcium from a cup of milk.)

- ½ cup of fresh or frozen pureed berries: strawberries, raspberries, blackberries, or blueberries
- 2 tablespoons of fruit juice concentrate or 1 pureed peach and ½ teaspoon of flavor extract
- ¼ teaspoon of almond, anise, hazelnut, maple, or vanilla extract. Or try a flavored oil, perhaps cinnamon or peppermint: use 2 drops of flavored oil in place of ¼ teaspoon of extract.
- ½ cup of cranberry juice cocktail and a small scoop of low-fat vanilla ice cream or frozen yogurt
- 1 tablespoon of creamy peanut butter and 2 tablespoons of chocolate syrup

ways to add calcium-rich foods in food preparation, see "Calcium Boosters" in chapter 13.

● Look for calcium-rich foods in the grocery store. Check the Nutrition Facts on food labels, listing the calcium in a single label serving. The amount is given as the % Daily Value, which approximates the percentage of your day's calcium need supplied by one label serving of that food.

● Try high-calcium milk. If milk is fortified with extra calcium, you'll find the amount per serving (perhaps 500 milligrams in one cup of milk) listed in the Nutrition Facts on the label.

Descriptions on food labels help you identify non-dairy foods that are good calcium sources. Look for "calcium-rich," "good source of calcium," and "more calcium." *See "Label Lingo: Vitamins and Minerals" earlier in this chapter for what these descriptions mean.*

Note: If you frequently have gas, cramping, and bloating after consuming milk and milk products, you may be lactose-intolerant. *For ways to include calcium-rich foods in your meals and snacks, see "Lactose Intolerance: A Matter of Degree" in chapter 21.*

Iron: A Closer Look

Iron: it's a mineral widely available in food. You need small amounts to keep healthy. Yet, iron deficiency is a common nutrition problem around the world. Iron deficiency often leads to anemia and its symptoms: fatigue, weakness, and poor health, all interfering with a person's physical ability to perform at full potential.

Iron: Its Mission

Although iron has many biological functions, its main job is to carry oxygen in the hemoglobin of red blood cells. In fact, about two-thirds of your body's iron is in hemoglobin. Hemoglobin takes oxygen to your body cells, where it's used to produce energy. Iron in red blood cells also helps take away carbon dioxide, a by-product of energy production. Red blood cells have a "life span" of about four months. After that, some of their iron gets recycled; either it's stored or used immediately to make new red blood cells. This recycling action helps protect you from iron deficiency.

What happens when you don't consume enough iron—or when the iron stored in your body gets too low? Red blood cells can't carry as much oxygen, likely making you feel tired, perhaps weak, and less able to perform at your peak efficiency. These are among the symptoms of anemia. However, anemia has several causes—not just iron deficiency. *See "Anemia: More Than One Cause" in chapter 22.*

As part of its job description, iron also helps protect you from infections as part of an enzyme in your immune system. Iron helps change beta carotene to vitamin A, helps produce collagen (which holds tissues of your body together), and helps make body proteins (amino acids), among its other tasks.

How much iron do you need to consume? Your body is highly adaptive, absorbing more iron when its iron stores are low, and less when they're higher. Regardless, the Recommended Dietary Allowances (RDA) are set to meet the needs of the broad population.

Iron needs are highest during periods of rapid growth: childhood, adolescence, childbearing years for women, and pregnancy. Prior to menopause, women need enough iron to replace losses from menstrual flow. Iron needs also go up to support increases of blood volume during pregnancy. Not surprisingly, iron-deficiency anemia is most common among people at these ages and stages of life, too, when the dietary need for iron is highest. In fact, it's hard to get enough without taking an iron supplement.

The Dietary Guidelines advise: *For women of childbearing age or who may become pregnant, eat foods high in heme iron and/or consume iron-rich plant foods or iron-fortified foods with an enhancer of iron absorption, such as vitamin C-rich foods.*

With menopause, iron needs drop. That's the time to *stop* taking an iron supplement, especially for women at risk for hemochromatosis, a genetic disorder that results in high levels of stored iron in the body. Iron-rich foods can supply as much as most postmenopausal women need. *See the earlier discussion of iron in this chapter for a brief explanation of hemochromatosis.*

Iron in Foods: Heme vs. Nonheme

If iron is abundant, why don't many of us "pump enough iron" from food? Iron comes from a wide variety of foods—of both animal and plant origin. Most of the iron from meat, poultry, and fish is heme iron. That name comes from the way it's carried in food—as part of the hemoglobin and myoglobin (similar to hemoglobin in humans) in animal tissue. Foods of plant origin contain only nonheme iron. And egg yolks have mostly nonheme iron.

The deep-red color of animal muscle comes from hemoglobin. The darker the color, the higher the content of heme iron. For example, beef liver, which is redder than roast beef, has more iron. And dark turkey meat has more heme iron than the light meat.

COUNTING UP IRON

This chart shows the amount of total iron in food. But remember, iron from most animal sources (heme iron) usually is better absorbed than iron from plant sources of food (nonheme iron).

To help reduce iron-deficiency anemia, many foods on today's supermarket shelves are enriched or fortified with iron: iron-enriched flour (also used in baked goods and pasta) and iron-fortified breakfast cereals.

FOOD	IRON (MG)	FOOD	IRON (MG)
Sources of Mostly Heme Iron		*Sources of Nonheme Iron (continued)*	
Beef liver, braised (3 oz.)	5.6	Enriched rice, cooked (½ cup)	1.4
Lean sirloin, broiled (3 oz.)	2.9	Pretzels (1 oz.)	1.2
Lean ground beef, broiled (3 oz.)	2.5	Dried plums (prunes) (5)	1.0
Skinless chicken, roasted dark meat (3 oz.)	1.1	Whole-wheat bread (1 slice)	0.9
Skinless chicken, roasted white meat (3 oz.)	0.9	White bread made with enriched refined flour (1 slice)	0.9
Pork, lean, roasted (3 oz.)	0.9	Egg, large (1)	0.9
Salmon, canned with bone (3 oz.)	0.7	Raisins, seedless (¼ cup)	0.8
Sources of Nonheme Iron		Green beans, cooked (½ cup)	0.6
Fortified breakfast cereal (1 cup)*	4.5–18	Peanut butter, (2 tbsp.)	0.6
Pumpkin seed kernels (1 oz.)	4.2	Apricots, dried (3)	0.6
Soybean nuts (½ cup)	3.4	Grapes (½ cup)	0.3
Blackstrap molasses (1 tbsp.)	3.2	Zucchini, cooked (½ cup)	0.3
Spinach, boiled (½ cup)	3.2	Cranberry juice cocktail (¾ cup)	0.2
Wheat bran (½ cup)	3.0	Unenriched rice, cooked (½ cup)	0.2
Red kidney beans, cooked (½ cup)	2.6	Egg white, large (1)	<0.1
Prune juice (¾ cup)	2.3		
Lima beans, cooked (½ cup)	2.2		

*The amount varies. Read the Nutrition Facts on food labels.

Source: U.S. Department of Agriculture, Agricultural Research Service, 2005. *USDA National Nutrient Database for Standard Reference,* Release 18.

What makes this difference nutritionally significant? First, consider that iron in food isn't absorbed efficiently. Much of the iron you consume never gets absorbed into your bloodstream. (Fortunately, the RDAs take this fact into account.) The amount of iron your body absorbs depends on several factors: among them, how much iron you consume and in what form (heme or nonheme); other nutrients in the meal or snack that can enhance or hinder its absorption; and how much iron your body has stored already. In fact, the bioavailability of iron in a mixed U.S. diet (animal- and plant-based foods) is about 18 percent; in a vegetarian diet, about 10 percent.

Heme iron is absorbed into your body more readily than nonheme iron. Depending on how much you already have stored, 15 to 35 percent of heme iron gets absorbed. That's good news.

Nonheme iron is a different story. Only 2 to 20 percent of nonheme iron gets absorbed. Even though

Have You Ever Wondered

. . . if spinach will make you strong, as the famous cartoon character Popeye believed? It's true that spinach contains iron. But another food component in spinach, called oxalic acid, binds with iron, impairing its absorption, so it's not the best source. Only physical activity, not iron or any other nutrient, builds muscle strength.

. . . if cooking in an iron skillet improves the iron content of food? It does. Before the days of aluminum and stainless steel cookware, great-great-grandma unknowingly supplemented her family's diet with iron from her iron pots and pans. If you have cast iron cookware, you can get the benefits, too. Foods with acids such as tomato juice, citrus juice, and vinegar help dissolve small amounts of iron from the pot into the cooking liquids—especially good for foods that simmer for a while.

. . . if you need more iron if you seem tired all the time? Maybe—or maybe you need more sleep, less stress, or perhaps more physical activity to increase your stamina! Fatigue is a symptom of anemia, however. Check with your physician for a blood test. *See "Anemia: 'Tired Blood'" in chapter 22 for more about anemia and blood testing.*

Iron: The Power of Partnership

To help your body absorb more iron, pair foods like these at your meals and snacks. Meat, poultry, fish (all three with heme iron), and vitamin C-rich foods help release more nonheme iron from foods of plant origin and egg yolks.

ABSORPTION ENHANCERS	NONHEME IRON SOURCES
Sirloin strips	With spinach salad
Barbecued beef	With refried beans and tortillas
Ground beef	With a whole-grain roll
Pork	With bean soup
Chicken	With brown rice
Ham	With scrambled eggs
Grapefruit	With bran cereal
Strawberries	With oatmeal
Red bell pepper	With whole-grain pasta
Papaya	With whole-wheat toast
Orange	With a peanut butter sandwich on whole-wheat bread

Source: Adapted from National Cattlemen's Beef Association, *Iron in Human Nutrition* (Chicago, 1998).

foods with nonheme iron often contain more iron than those with heme iron, you may get less than you think. You can enhance your body's ability to absorb nonheme iron. Consuming vitamin C and foods such as meat with heme iron aids nonheme iron absorption.

On the reverse side, some phytonutrients—oxalic acid in spinach and chocolate; phytic acid in wheat bran and legumes; tannins in coffee and tea; and polyphenols in coffee—seem to inhibit nonheme iron absorption. But again, consuming vitamin C or iron from meat, fish, and poultry at the same time helps overcome these "inhibitors."

These quick nutrition tips can help your body better absorb iron (nonheme) from foods of plant origin and from egg yolks:

● Enjoy a vitamin C-rich food—such as an orange, cantaloupe, green pepper, or broccoli—right along with it; for example, you get more iron from a peanut butter sandwich on whole-wheat bread if you eat it with a glass of orange juice. This is especially important for vegetarians, who get most of their iron from plant sources. Add a little meat, poultry, or fish (with heme iron) to foods of plant origin and egg yolks; for example, include some ground beef in a pot of chili, or sliced lean ham in an egg omelette. The presence of heme iron boosts the absorption of nonheme iron.

● Drink coffee or tea between meals—not with meals.

● Cook in an iron skillet.

For more combinations, see "Iron: The Power of Partnership" on page 106.

Need more strategies to boost your vitamin and mineral quotient? Check here for "how-tos":

● Explore new-to-you fruits, vegetables, and grain products—see chapter 9.

● Plan a day's food choices that deliver enough vitamins and minerals and plenty of phytonutrients—see chapter 10.

● Scout for nutrient-rich, phytonutrient-rich foods when you shop—see chapter 11.

● Lock vitamins in and boost calcium, too, when you prepare food—see chapter 13.

● Enjoy the flavors and get the benefits of fruits and vegetables—see chapters 13 and 14.

● Use nutrient supplements wisely—see chapter 23.

Phytonutrients—a "Crop" for Good Health

Besides nutrients, plant-based foods (legumes, vegetables, fruits, whole grains, nuts, seeds, and teas as well as herbs and spices) have another "crop" of naturally occurring compounds with potential health benefits. Collectively they're called phytonutrients, or phytochemicals, meaning plant chemicals. "Phyto" means plant. Think *fight* for "phytos," since they appear to promote health by sparking body processes that fight, or reduce the risk for the development of some diseases.

Why have phytonutrients captured our attention?

Because of their potential for health promotion! Today consumers are more interested in positive nutrition and self-care: adding (not avoiding) foods that may enhance health, boost immunity, slow aging, and prevent or slow the chance for chronic disease. Sound like you? Research on phytonutrients is the new frontier in nutrition, as exciting today as vitamin discoveries were a hundred years ago!

Phytonutrients: What Role in Health?

As public interest in phytonutrients soars, science is exploring their benefits. In fact, consumer and media interest often is ahead of scientific evidence. Functional benefits are those that extend beyond basic nutritional effects. In fact, the benefits are all about what you can eat, *not* what you can't!

Phytonutrients are bioactive compounds in food that promote your health by helping to slow the aging process or reducing the risk for many diseases. Since the early 1980s, research has intensified in investigating how phytonutrients protect against some cancers, heart disease, stroke, high blood pressure, cataracts, osteoporosis, urinary tract infections, and other chronic health conditions.

These are among the ways that phytonutrients might work: serve as antioxidants, enhance immunity,

Functional Nutrition: More to Learn!

Phytonutrients aren't the only food substances with functional benefits. Check here to learn more:

● *"Prebiotics and Probiotics: What Are They?"* in this chapter.

● *"Eat Your Omega-3s and -6s"* in chapter 3.

● *"Stanol- and Sterol-Based Ingredients"* in chapter 3.

● *"Sugar Alcohols: Sugar Replacers,"* about sugar alcohols, in chapter 5.

● *"Fiber: Your Body's Broom,"* chapter 6.

● *"Teatime: Health Benefits?"* in chapter 8.

● *"Functional Foods: A New Wave"* in chapter 9.

● *"A Toast to Heart Health"* in chapter 22.

● *"Functional Foods: What Does Research Say?"* in the Appendices.

enhance communication among body cells, cause cancer cells to die, detoxify carcinogens, and repair damage to DNA that's caused by smoking and other toxins. Yet the benefits and actions of phytonutrients are still uncertain. Do they work independently, together, with nutrients and fiber, or do their actions add up?

"Phytos": In a Class of Their Own

Neither vitamins nor minerals, phytonutrients are substances that plants produce naturally to protect themselves against viruses, bacteria, and fungi, as well as insects, drought, and even the sun. Beyond that, they provide the color, aroma, texture, and flavor that give food so much sensual appeal. Of the thousands of phytonutrients, more than two thousand are plant pigments that put a rainbow of colors on your plate! *See "Paint Your Plate with Color!" in chapter 13.*

Like nutrients, phytonutrients are grouped according to their biochemical characteristics and probable protective functions. Only a few hundred have yet

Boosting Phytonutrient Benefits

Research suggests that what you do in the kitchen can make a difference in food's phytonutrients benefits.

- Cooking or food processing may enhance the body's ability to use (bioavailability) some phytonutrients. Carotenoids (including lycopene) are one example. In addition, dietary fat may enhance the absorption of carotenoids; dietary fiber impedes it.
- Heat damages anthocyanins, which are flavonoids. On the flip side, the anthocyanin content may increase in fresh fruit if it's stored for a few days.
- Flaxseed needs to be crushed or ground to get the benefits.
- For the most benefit from tea's polyphenols, brew each cup fresh (preferably in water that's not hard) and drink it soon. Three to five minutes of brewing for one tea bag brings out 80 percent of the catechins, which are flavonoids.
- Chop garlic for about fifteen minutes before heating to allow allyl sulfides to fully develop.

Functional Nutrition Prebiotics and Probiotics: What Are They?

As other functional components of foods, prebiotics and probiotics may promote healthy bacteria, or microflora, in your intestines—and perhaps improve your health. *Prebiotics* stimulate or help activate bacteria growth; *probiotics* are the live cultures, or bacteria, themselves. *Syn*biotic combines both.

- *Prebiotics* are nondigestible substances such as oligosaccharides, inulin, and polydextrose (indigestible carbohydrate) in food that promote the growth of normal, healthful bacteria that are already in your colon. Other substances in food, such as dietary fiber, starch, and sugar alcohols, may work as prebiotics, too.

- *Probiotics* are active cultures, such as some strains of lactic acid bacteria, or foods that contain them, that help reintroduce or change bacteria in the intestine. *Lactobacilli* and *Bifidobacteria* in yogurt with live cultures and other fermented dairy food and some nondairy foods have probiotic cultures.

Research suggests that probiotic cultures may help keep your immune system healthy and help maintain the "good" bacteria in your intestine. Probiotics also may help reduce the risk of some health problems—for example, shorten the duration of diarrhea, reduce the symptoms of lactose intolerance, decrease the risk of some cancers, help prevent some allergy symptoms, and reduce symptoms of irritable bowel disease, among others.

been studied. What we know today is merely the "appetizer."

Research has revealed a few things. Most fruits and vegetables contain phytonutrients. Different plant-based foods supply different kinds and amounts; some have a remarkable variety. An orange, for example, has more than 170 different phytonutrients! In any fruit or vegetable, these substances appear to work together with nutrients and fiber for your good health.

Check the Appendices, "Functional Foods: What Does Research Say? to learn more.

For phytonutrients, food databases are limited, with only a few key carotenoids and phytoestrogens. A USDA database for flavonoids is being developed.

FUNCTIONAL NUTRITION: A QUICK LOOK AT KEY PHYTONUTRIENTS

A HANDFUL OF PHYTONUTRIENTS*	WHAT THEY APPEAR TO DO	WHERE THEY'RE FOUND (SOME FOOD SOURCES)
Carotenoids		
Beta carotene	● As an antioxidant, neutralizes free radicals that may damage cells ● Bolsters antioxidant defenses in cells	● *Yellow-orange fruits and vegetables* such as apricots, cantaloupes, papayas, carrots, pumpkins, sweet potatoes, winter squash ● *Green vegetables* such as broccoli, spinach, kale
Lutein	● May contribute to maintaining healthy vision	● *Green vegetables* such as kale, spinach, collard greens, Swiss chard, Romaine lettuce, broccoli, Brussels sprouts ● Kiwifruit ● Egg yolks
Lycopene	● May reduce risk of prostate cancer	● *Most red fruits and vegetables* such as tomatoes, processed tomato products, pink grapefruit, guava, watermelon (The red pigment in red peppers is from keto carotenoids, not lycopene.)
Zeaxanthin	● May contribute to maintaining healthy vision	● Corn, spinach, winter squash, green vegetables, citrus fruits (Eggs have a small amount of zeaxanthin, too.)
Flavonoids		
Anthocyanidins	● As an antioxidant, neutralizes free radicals that may damage cells ● May contribute to maintaining brain function ● May contribute to maintenance of healthy immune function	● Blueberries, blackberries, cranberries, cherries, strawberries, kiwifruit, plums, red grapes, red cabbage, eggplant (skin)
Flavanols: catechins, epicatechins, procyanidins	● May contribute to maintaining heart health	● Apples, chocolate, cocoa, grapes, tea (black, oolong, or green), wine
Flavanones: hesperetin, naringenin	● Neutralizes free radicals that may damage cells ● Bolsters antioxidant defenses in cells	● Citrus fruit
Flavonols (quercetin)	● Neutralize free radicals that may damage cells ● Bolster antioxidant defenses in cells	● Apples, broccoli, onions, tea

A Handful of Phytonutrients*	What They Appear to Do	Where They're Found (some food sources)
Flavonoids *(continued)*		
Proanthocyanidins	● May contribute to maintaining urinary tract health and heart health	● Apples, cinnamon, cocoa, cranberries, grapes, peanuts, strawberries, wine
Resveratrol	● Bolsters antioxidant defenses in cells ● May contribute to maintaining heart health	● Red grapes, red grape juice, red wine, peanuts
Isothiocyanates		
Sulphoraphane	● As an antioxidant, neutralizes free radicals that may damage cells ● May aid in detoxification of undesirable compounds ● Bolsters antioxidant defenses in cells	● Cruciferous vegetables, such as bok choy, broccoli, broccoli sprouts, cabbage, cauliflower, collard greens, kale, turnips, turnip greens
Phenols		
Caffeic acid, ferulic acid	● May bolster cellular antioxidant defenses ● May contribute to maintaining healthy vision and heart health	● Fruits, including apples, citrus, pears, some vegetables
Ellagic acid	● Neutralize free radicals that may damage cells ● Bolster antioxidant defenses in cells	● Berries, red grapes, kiwifruit
Polyols		
Sugar alcohols: lactitol, mannitol, sorbitol, xylitol	● May reduce risk of dental caries	● Some chewing gums ● Other food applications
Phytoestrogens		
Isoflavones: daidzein, genestein	● May reduce menopause symptoms, such as hot flashes ● May contribute to maintenance of bone health ● May contribute to healthy brain function and immune function	● Soybeans, soy-based foods
Lignans	● May contribute to heart health and healthy immune function	● Flaxseed (not flaxseed oil unless hull remains), rye, wheat bran, oatmeal, barley, vegetables
Phytic acid	● May contribute to maintaining normal blood sugar levels and maintaining heart health ● Neutralizes free radicals that may damage cells ● Bolsters antioxidant defenses in cells	● Cereal grains, nuts, seeds

A Handful of Phytonutrients*	What They Appear to Do	Where They're Found (some food sources)
Prebiotics and Probiotics		
Inulin, fructo-oligosaccharides, polydextrose	● May improve gastrointestinal health ● May improve calcium absorption	● Whole grains, onions, some fruits, garlic, honey, leeks, fortified foods and beverages
Lactobacilli, bifidobacteria	● May improve gastrointestinal health and systemic immunity	● Yogurt, other dairy and non-dairy applications
Soy Protein		
Soy protein	● May reduce risk for coronary heart disease (CHD)	● Soybeans, soy-based foods
Sulfides/Thiols		
Allyl methyl trisulfide, diallyl sulfide	● May help maintain heart health ● May help maintain a healthy immune system ● May aid in detoxification of undesirable compounds	● Chives, garlic, onions, leeks, scallions
Dithiolthiones	● Contributes to maintenance of healthy immune function	● Cruciferous vegetables

Source: Adapted from: International Food Information Council Foundation, 2004.

Other phytonutrients are addressed elsewhere: fiber in chapter 6 and stanols and sterols in chapter 3. Animal-based foods also contain some functional substances, e.g., some fatty acids; see chapter 3.

No Dietary Reference Intakes exist for them yet.

Bottom line: Already there's overwhelming evidence for the health benefits of plant-based foods: fruits, vegetables, legumes (including soy), nuts, seeds, and grains, especially whole grains. Research shows that you *lower the odds* for some cancers, heart disease, and other health problems by *eating more* fruits, vegetables, and grains.

Count on a variety of foods to reap the benefits of the many phytonutrients from all kinds of plant-based foods. Supplements with just one or a few phytonutrients haven't been shown to be effective.

CHAPTER 5

Carbs
Simply Complex

Carbohydrates get attention today, with a fresh new mind-set! When you think of "carbs," what comes to mind: hearty whole-grain bread . . . piping hot basmati rice . . . tender fettuccini . . . freshly popped popcorn . . . naturally sweet sweet potatoes . . . crunchy celery . . . summer-fresh corn on the cob . . . juicy peaches or sweet mangos . . . a fresh banana . . . savory baked beans . . . ice-cold milk . . . delicious fruit smoothies?

All these nourishing foods can put carbohydrates, an important nutrient category, on your plate!

"Carbs": The Basics

Sugars, starches, and fiber: they all belong to a unique macronutrient category called carbohydrates. As energy nutrients, sugars and starches are your body's main fuel source.

"Carbs": What Are They?

All carbohydrates are made of the same three elements: carbon, hydrogen, and oxygen. The name "carbohydrate" comes from its chemical makeup. "Carbo-" means carbon; "-hydrate" means water, or H_2O. To make different types of carbohydrates, these elements first are arranged in single units. Sugars are made of just one or two units; they're considered "simple." Made of many sugar units, starches and fiber are more complex.

Carbohydrate's "Short Form"

Were you born with a "sweet tooth"? Probably, yes. Studies show that newborns respond to the sweet tastes of sugars quicker than to other tastes: bitter, sour, or salty. Sweetness adds to the pleasure of eating!

When people hear the word "sugar," table sugar often comes to mind. Yet that's just one of several sugars referred to as simple carbohydrates. Some sugars occur in foods naturally. Others are added. Regardless, your body can't tell the difference.

In scientific language, sugars are either monosaccharides with one sugar unit or disaccharides with two sugar units. ("Mono-" means one, "di-" means two, and "-saccharide" means sugar.) Monosaccharides are fructose, galactose, and glucose. When two join together chemically, they become disaccharides:

sucrose = glucose + fructose

lactose = glucose + galactose

maltose = glucose + glucose

Sucrose is just another name for table sugar; this same sugar is found naturally in many fruits and some vegetables and grains, too. Lactose is the naturally occurring sugar in milk, while fructose is the sugar in fruit and in honey. And maltose is formed when starch breaks down to simple sugars.

Starches and Fiber: Made of Many Sugars

Starches and fiber have something in common. They're polysaccharides. "Poly-" means many. If you concluded that they're composed of many sugar units, you're absolutely right! They're just longer chains of sugars. Starch comes from plant-based foods, such as rice, pasta, potatoes, beans, and grain products.

You may wonder—if starch is made of sugars, why doesn't it taste sweet? Molecule size makes the difference. Starch molecules are bigger. Unlike smaller sugars, starch molecules are too big to fit on the receptors of your taste buds, so they don't taste sweet. But keep a starchy cracker in your mouth for a while. Once digestive enzymes in saliva break down its starch into sugar, the cracker starts to taste sweet. The sugar molecules are small enough to taste. Get a cracker; try it!

Another polysaccharide, called glycogen, is the form of carbohydrate that your body stores. Stored glycogen is important to athletes doing endurance sports. *For more about energy for sports, refer to "Energy to Burn" in chapter 19.*

From Complex to Simple . . .

From complex to simple! In a nutshell, that's what happens when starches are digested. Before they can be absorbed from your digestive tract into your bloodstream, they're broken down to the simplest sugars: glucose, galactose, and fructose. Then, in your bloodstream, single sugars move into your body cells, where they're converted to energy. Except for fiber, carbohydrates—sugars and starches—break down to single sugars during digestion. Your body doesn't distinguish their food source.

Being single sugars already, monosaccharides, such as the fructose in fruits, can be absorbed as they are. That's not true for disaccharides: sucrose, lactose, and maltose. Digestive enzymes break them down, too. Some people don't produce enough of an enzyme called lactase; they have trouble digesting lactose, or milk sugar. *Refer to chapter 21, "Lactose Intolerance: A Matter of Degree."*

Only fiber, another polysaccharide, remains somewhat intact in the body. Many animals can digest fiber. However, human digestive enzymes can't break down fiber into units that are small enough for absorption. So fiber can't be an energy source. That very quality makes fiber uniquely qualified to promote your health in other ways. *Refer to chapter 6, "Fiber: Your Body's Broom."*

Carbohydrates: Your "Power" Source

Carbohydrates are your body's main energy source, powering everything from jogging, to breathing, to thinking, and even to digesting food. Actually, glucose is the main form of carbohydrate used for energy. Because it circulates in your bloodstream, it's often called blood sugar. It's carried to every body cell, each with its own "powerhouse" for producing energy.

Carbohydrates, absorbed from your digestive tract, cause blood sugar (glucose) levels to rise. Insulin helps glucose enter cells, where it's used for energy.

Your body doesn't turn all of its blood sugar to energy at the same time. As blood sugar levels rise above normal, insulin (a hormone from your pancreas) signals your liver, muscles, and other cells to store the extra. Some gets stored in the muscles and liver as glycogen, a storage form of carbohydrate. Some glucose also may be converted to body fat—if you consume more calories than you need.

When blood sugar levels drop below normal, another hormone called glucagon triggers the conversion of glycogen to glucose. That's how blood sugar levels stay within normal range between meals. Once glucose is back in your bloodstream, it's again ready to fuel your body cells.

Your body also derives energy from fat and protein, but "carbs" should be your main energy source. Protein should be saved for what only protein can do: build and repair body tissues. If your energy intake is less than what your body needs and if your limited glycogen stores are spent, body proteins are broken down for energy. In a low-"carb," high-fat diet, fat becomes an energy source; in the process, potentially harmful ketones can build up in blood—not healthful either.

From sugar or starch, 1 gram of carbohydrate fuels your body with the same amount of energy: 4 calories per gram. By comparison, protein also supplies 4 calories per gram; fat supplies 9 calories per gram. For health's sake, make nutrient-rich, starchy foods your body's main energy source. Usually these same foods are loaded with vitamins, minerals, and perhaps fiber, too. *An added bonus:* Many starchy foods are low in fat.

How Much Carbohydrate?

For total carbohydrates, including starch and sugars, the Institute of Medicine (IOM) recommends a

... if honey or brown sugar is more nutritious than white sugar? That's a common misperception. Honey is several sugars (fructose, glucose, sucrose, and others), formed from nectar by bees. Ounce for ounce, the nutrients in honey and white (or table) sugar are nearly the same. Why a difference? A teaspoon of honey weighs slightly more than a teaspoon of white sugar, so it has slightly more calories and carbohydrate: a teaspoon of white sugar has about 15 calories and 4 grams of carbohydrate; a teaspoon of honey, about 21 calories and 4.5 grams of "carbs."

Honey is sweeter than white sugar, so you need less to sweeten foods. Brown sugar is merely sugar crystals, flavored with molasses. Nutritionwise, it too has about 15 calories and 4 grams of carbohydrate per teaspoon—about the same amounts as white sugar. No sugars contain vitamins, minerals, or fiber.

... what refined sugar is? Refined sugar is most simply described as sugar, separated either from the stalk of sugarcane or from the root of a sugar beet. The sugar-containing juice of the plant is extracted, then processed into dried sugar crystals. It's sold as granulated or white sugar. Molasses is the thick syrup that's left after sugar beets or cane is processed for table sugar.

... what raw sugar really is? Raw sugar comes from processing cane sugar. It's a coarse, granulated solid sugar left when clarified sugarcane juice evaporates. Because of its impurities, you can't buy 100 percent raw sugar. But you can buy turbinado sugar. Light-tan, turbinado sugar is raw sugar, refined in a centrifuge under sanitary conditions. Nutritionally speaking, its calorie and carbohydrate content are the same as refined, or table sugar. So-called natural sugars (raw sugar, date sugar, honey, maple syrup) aren't nutritionally better than other sugars.

minimum level for normal brain function and a range for overall healthy eating.

The Adequate Intake level (AI) is based on the lowest amount of glucose (blood sugar) needed daily for normal brain function. For people ages one year or over, that's a minimum of 130 grams of carbohydrate, which equals 520 calories, or 25 percent of the calories in a 2,000-calorie daily diet. The minimum needed

for brain function is more than the amount recommended in the early stages of some weight loss regimens! The AI for pregnancy is 175 grams; for breast-feeding, 210 grams.

An eating plan that simply meets the AI for carbohydrates is likely inadequate for other nutrients and fiber, and may be high in fat. For that reason, the IOM set Acceptable Macronutrient Distribution Ranges (AMDR) for energy nutrients. For carbohydrates, that's a range of 45 to 65 percent (for children, teens, and adults) of total daily calories, adding up to 225 to 325 grams of carbohydrates daily in a 2,000-calorie-a-day eating plan. The actual amount you need depends on your total calorie need; *see chapter 2*. For added sugars only, the advice is not more than 25 percent of

Fructose: A Sweeter Message

Is fructose any more healthful than sucrose, or table sugar? Surprisingly, the answer is no. All sugars nourish your body in the same way. Fructose and sucrose are just different sugars; both are simple carbohydrates. In fact, your body eventually breaks down sucrose into fructose and glucose.

Fructose is found naturally in fruit. But it's also added to certain foods, either as crystalline fructose or as high-fructose corn syrup (HFCS). Crystalline fructose is made from cornstarch, and looks and tastes much like sucrose. HFCS is a combination of fructose and dextrose, a sugar that comes from corn. Currently it's one of the most commonly consumed sweeteners in the United States. Like any sugar, crystalline fructose and HFCS supply 4 calories per gram.

Where does high-fructose corn syrup (HFCS) fit within the obesity epidemic? It's a source of extra calories, often from beverages such as soft drinks. Despite recent theories, there is *not* enough scientific evidence to say that HFCS changes metabolism, or that it increases body fat or boosts appetite. To help trim calories, ease up on added sugars of all kinds, including HFCS from nondiet snacks drinks.

You might find crystalline fructose on the ingredient list of baked foods, frozen foods, beverages, and tabletop sweeteners. HFCS is used in nondiet soft drinks, fruit drinks, salad dressings, pickle products, ketchup, baked foods, tabletop syrups, fruits, candies, gums, and desserts.

Just a Spoonful of Sugar . . .

1 teaspoon honey	21 calories
1 teaspoon jelly	16 calories
1 teaspoon brown sugar	16 calories
1 teaspoon table sugar	15 calories
1 teaspoon maple syrup	17 calories
1 teaspoon corn syrup, light or dark	19 calories

total calories, or 125 grams of carbohydrates from added sugars. Added sugars do not include naturally occurring sugars. The IOM advice for fiber is separate—and *discussed in chapter 6.*

Why limit added sugars? For one, they just contribute calories. Many foods high in added sugars supply energy but few other nutrients, and may replace more nutritious foods, along with the vitamins and minerals they provide. To compare, many starchy vegetables, legumes (dry beans), and grain products have less fat, but more vitamins, minerals, and fiber. Second, added sugars—like starches and naturally occurring sugars—can promote tooth decay, especially with frequent snacking.

When you're really active, you may need more calories. If your overall eating plan is healthful, added sugars can supply some of that extra energy as discretionary calories.

Carbohydrates and Health

At different periods over the decades, carbohydrates have been given a bad rap. Unfair, since they're among the six categories of nutrients essential to your health!

"Carbs" Count!

Carbohydrates: they're important since glucose is the only form of energy your brain can use! Besides being the main power source for your brain and muscles, carbohydrates spare protein for building and repairing body cells.

Chosen wisely, carbohydrate-rich foods—whole and enriched grain foods, fruits, vegetables, beans—deliver more than energy. Much attention has been given to their role in lowering the risk for heart disease, stroke, high blood pressure, and some cancers. Many "carb"-containing foods also provide important vitamins, minerals, and phytonutrients. And fiber-rich foods deliver a host of benefits; *see chapter 6.* That's why the Dietary Guidelines advise: *Choose fiber-rich fruits, vegetables, and whole grains often.*

Nutrient-dense carbohydrate-containing foods may help with weight regulation, especially when combined with regular physical activity. Among the research areas: (1) carbohydrate-containing foods, especially those rich in fiber, may aid satiety so people eat less, (2) a high-"carb" diet may have fewer calories for the same amount of food than a high-fat diet does; and (3) excess carbohydrate doesn't change as efficiently to body fat as calories from other sources. Stay tuned!

Your Smile: Carbohydrates and Oral Health

Imagine the wide smile that comes with those popular words: "Look, Mom, no cavities!" Today, more than 50 percent of America's children have cavity-free teeth. And the number has been climbing. Good dental care, along with the widespread presence of fluoride toothpaste, fluoride rinses, sealants, and fluoridated water, is making smiles healthier than ever.

Have You Ever Wondered

. . . if presweetened cereals are more cavity-promoting than unsweetened cereals? There's really no difference. Carbohydrates in both starches and sugars "nourish" bacteria that promote decay. Whether or not they're presweetened, their cavity factor depends on how long cereals stick between teeth or in the crevices in molars. Cavity-causing potential doesn't depend on the amount of carbohydrates.

Although not a dental health issue, presweetened cereals often have more calories per serving—but perhaps no more than the same amount of unsweetened cereal with a spoonful of sugar sprinkled on, too. Breakfast cereal, including presweetened cereal, contributes only 5 percent of the sugar in kids' diets, according to NHANES 2001-02 data.

Hot Topic: Glycemic Index

Glycemic index rates carbohydrate-containing foods on how they affect the body's blood sugar (glucose) levels after eating them. A food's glycemic index (GI) is ranked against a glucose solution, set at the top level of 100. Foods with a higher glycemic index produce a greater increase in blood glucose levels than low GI foods.

That said, figuring the body's response sounds simpler than it really is. So be wary of products marketed using glycemic index. Glycemic index is calculated for a specific amount of food, usually 50 grams of total carbohydrate minus the fiber. Many factors affect glycemic index for a single food, including its ripeness, its variety, how it's prepared or processed, the type of sugar and starch, how much fat and fiber it contains, and how long it takes to digest.

In general, nonstarchy vegetables, most fruits, legumes (dry beans), and milk tend to have a low glycemic index. For example, ½ cup of kidney beans has a glycemic index of 52; a medium apple, 38. White bread (from refined flour), crackers, and cornflakes are high-GI foods. The glycemic index of a medium baked potato (no skin) is 85, considered high. Yet this rule of thumb doesn't always hold true. Foods like watermelon and carrots also have a high glycemic index.

To clarify two common misperceptions: (1) The GI doesn't measure how fast blood glucose levels rise. Regardless of the carbohydrate source, blood glucose levels peak at about the same time. (2) The body's insulin response to a specific food isn't directly related to its GI value or its carbohydrate content.

The glycemic index of a single food isn't reliable for helping most healthy consumers make food choices. Why? First, the food is usually eaten with other foods; glycemic index doesn't measure what happens with mixed foods. A high-GI food eaten with a low-GI food may give a moderate GI response. Second, the amount eaten may be more or less than the amount for calculating glycemic response; to address that issue, glycemic loads for standard portions have been determined. And third, the GI of a food can vary from one person to another. A person's individual response may vary from day to day, too.

That said, glycemic index is being used in research related to type 2 diabetes, heart disease, and obesity—with potential for more use in the future. Currently no evidence shows that eliminating foods with a higher glycemic index, such as baked potatoes or cornflakes, promotes weight loss or helps with appetite control. And these foods may offer nutrient and phytonutrient benefits.

For people with diabetes, glycemic index can be useful as one tool to manage blood sugar levels, along with blood glucose monitoring and monitoring total grams of carbohydrate. That should be guided by a registered dietitian or other health professional. *Refer to "Diabetes: A Growing Health Concern" in chapter 22.*

The Dietary Guidelines advise: *Reduce the incidence of dental caries by practicing good oral hygiene and consuming sugar- and starch-containing foods and beverages less frequently.*

Just what causes cavities—and how can you protect your teeth? For years, we've connected tooth decay to eating sugary foods. But whether or not you get cavities depends on many factors—and certainly not diet alone! Heredity, as well as the makeup and flow of saliva, are factors. Although part of the equation, sugar itself isn't the culprit as once thought.

Plaque Attack!

The cavity-producing process starts when bacteria in your mouth mix with carbohydrates—both sugars and starches—to make acids. Bacteria are found in dental plaque, an invisible film that forms in your mouth and clings to the surfaces of your teeth and along your gum line.

Acids, produced by oral bacteria, can eat away tooth enamel, causing tooth decay, also known as dental caries. Every time you eat sugars and starches, acids begin to bathe your teeth. The cavity-producing action continues for 20 minutes or more after you eat something starchy or sugary.

These two "equations" offer a quick summary of the action that takes place in your mouth when bacteria in plaque mix with carbohydrate in food:

plaque + carbohydrate = acid
acid + tooth enamel = potential tooth decay

A Sticky Issue

Hard candy offers no more threat to your teeth than pasta does. Surprised? Any food that contains carbohydrate—pasta, bread, rice, chips, fruit, even milk, as well as cake, cookies, and candy—can "feed" the bacteria in plaque.

Table sugar, or sucrose, isn't the only sugar that plays a role in oral health, either. Any sugar—whether it's added or naturally occurring—has the potential to promote cavities. Fructose in fruit and lactose in milk, for example, also cause bacteria to produce plaque acids. So too, fruit juice–sweetened cookies have the same cavity potential as cookies made with table sugar.

Among young children, baby-bottle tooth decay is caused when teeth or gums are exposed to milk, breast milk, formula, fruit juice, or another sweet drink for extended periods of time. This happens most often when babies fall asleep sucking on a bottle or fall asleep frequently while breast-feeding. *For more on baby-bottle tooth decay, refer to chapter 15, "Caring for Baby Teeth."*

Do some foods promote cavities more than others? There's no definitive list that ranks the cavity-forming potential of food. However, two factors that make a difference include how often you eat (or how often carbohydrate comes in contact with your teeth) and how long it stays on your teeth.

Frequency. The more often you eat carbohydrate foods, especially between meals, the more likely acid attacks teeth. Sucking hard candy or cough drops, nibbling chips, or slowly sipping a sweetened drink nourishes bacteria and bathes teeth with plaque acids for a while. The action continues for 20 minutes or longer after you finish each candy, nibble each chip, or drink each sip of regular soft drink or juice.

Type of Food. Because some foods stick to your teeth, plaque acids continue their action long after you stop eating or drinking. The word "sticky" may conjure up thoughts of caramels. Yet caramels dissolve and leave your mouth faster than bread or chips that stick between your teeth or in the pits of your molars. It may take hours for the food particles to finally leave

---

Keep Teeth and Gums Healthy

- Follow MyPyramid advice (*see chapter 10*) for healthful eating. An adequate supply of nutrients from all five food groups promotes healthy teeth and gums.

- Go easy on between-meal snacks. When you do snack, try to eat the snack at one time rather than over a longer period.

- Brush twice a day. Floss or use an interdental cleaner between your teeth daily. Use a fluoride mouth rinse. Before age six a fluoride rinse, which should not be swallowed, isn't advised; after that, use it only with your dentist's advice. For some people, an interdental cleaner, made of soft rubber, can help clean the food particles and plaque between teeth; ask your dentist if it's right for you.

- Be aware that brushing too often may be abrasive to your tooth enamel.

- Use a fluoride toothpaste with the American Dental Association Seal of Acceptance. The optimal amount of fluoride from toothpaste comes from brushing twice a day, not any more often.

- Teach children over age two years to brush with just a pea-size amount of fluoride toothpaste and to spit out, not swallow, toothpaste to reduce the chances of mottled teeth (dark spots) from too much fluoride. For kids under age two, talk to your doctor about fluoride toothpaste.

- Have regular dental checkups, which include a thorough cleaning.

- Talk to your dentist about sealants, which protect against decay in the pits and fissures of your teeth. (They're not just for kids.)

- For infants, avoid the urge to pacify your baby with a bottle of juice, formula, or milk. If you choose to use a bottle as a pacifier, fill it with water only.

- For children, talk to your dentist, doctor, or pediatric nurse about what amount of fluoride your child should have. If you live in a community that doesn't have an optimal amount of fluoride in the water, supplements may be recommended.

your mouth. The faster food dissolves and leaves your mouth, the less chance it has to produce plaque acid. For example, sticky dried fruit, granola bars, and raisins may stay on your teeth longer than a soft drink or a hot fudge sundae does.

Will a box of raisins or a bunch of grapes be more cavity-promoting than a single raisin or single grape? Eaten at one time, portion size makes no difference. Any amount of carbohydrate gets the decay process going. It's the frequency of snacking that seems to have a bigger impact on cavity formation than snack size.

Brushing and flossing after eating removes the "decay duo": plaque and food particles. Swishing water around your mouth after meals and snacks may help rinse away food particles and sugars but won't remove plaque bacteria.

"Carbs"—Not the Only Link to Oral Health

Carbohydrates aren't the only nutrition factor linked to oral health. Some nutrients make teeth stronger. And some are even described as "anti-cavity" foods.

For children, an overall nutritious diet promotes healthy teeth, making them stronger and more resistant to cavities. Several nutrients are especially important, including calcium, phosphorus, and vitamin D. These nutrients also build the jawbone, which helps keep teeth in place. For adults, calcium intake has little effect on keeping teeth healthy. But these same nutrients help keep your jawbone strong.

Tooth loss, common among the elderly, may be linked to periodontal, or gum, disease. Constant infection causes the bone structure of the jaw to gradually deteriorate. *Refer to "Keep Smiling: Prevent Gum Disease" in chapter 22.*

Before fluoridation of water was common, tooth decay was much more prevalent. Now, adding fluoride—to drinking water, toothpaste, and mouth rinses—is one of the most effective ways to prevent cavities. Fluoride makes the structure of teeth stronger by helping to add minerals back to microscopic cavities on the surface of tooth enamel. With the popularity of bottled water, which generally isn't fluoridated, many Americans may not get enough fluoride for oral health. *Refer to chapter 8, "The Fluoride Connection."*

Get your juices flowing! Your body produces up to

Snack for a Healthy Smile

Keep your smile healthy! For everyone, especially children, smart snacking can lead to good oral health.

● Overcome the urge to snack frequently. Bacteria in plaque produce acids that can damage teeth for 20 minutes or more after each exposure to carbohydrates.

● Choose snacks wisely for a well-balanced eating plan. Eat raw vegetables, fruits (such as apples), plain yogurt, cheese, milk, and popcorn.

● Even though sugars from hard candy, cough drops, and lollipops may leave your mouth faster than snacks that stick between your teeth, go easy on sugary snacks that dissolve slowly in your mouth. Sucking on foods prolongs the time that sugar bathes your teeth. Slowly sipping a sweetened beverage or soft drink has the same effect.

● Brush as soon as you can after snacking. This removes plaque and so stops the cavity-producing action of bacteria. Or at least rinse your mouth with water to get rid of food particles.

---

one quart of saliva a day—especially if you drink enough fluids. That's good news because saliva helps protect your teeth from decay. By clearing carbohydrates from your mouth faster, saliva helps to reduce the time that plaque acids can form. Minerals in saliva—calcium, phosphorus, and fluoride—may have a protective effect, too.

Smile, and say cheese! Some aged cheeses—for example, sharp Cheddar, Monterey Jack, and Swiss—may offer modest cavity protection. By increasing saliva flow, they lower acid levels. Both milk and cheese contain nutrients, including calcium, phosphorus, and protein, which may help protect tooth enamel.

"Carb" Myths

Other than their role in tooth decay, carbohydrates don't directly relate to most health problems—unless you consume too many! Yet "carb" myths are widespread. Here's the scoop on some common misconceptions about "carbs."

Makes You Fat?

No. Eating too many calories, not just starches and sugars, causes your body to produce extra pounds of body fat. That includes too many calories from any source—carbohydrates, fats, or proteins. Actually, excess calories from fats turn into body fat first, before extra calories from carbohydrates do. Sugar itself isn't the villain, either. Instead, being overweight results from a complex interaction, including genetics, environment, inactivity, and overall food choices.

Contrary to some popular diet gurus, sugar won't cause your body to make or store fat. It's true that insulin levels rise when "carbs" are absorbed. That's normal. Insulin regulates energy storage, allowing your body to move blood glucose elsewhere, perhaps to your cells for energy or to your muscles or liver for storage. Once accomplished, insulin and glucose levels drop to normal if you're healthy. Glucose is converted to body fat only if you consume more calories than your body needs.

That said, neither sugar itself nor a carbohydrate-rich diet causes an insulin reaction that results in weight gain—although some popular diet book gurus may say so. Consuming carbohydrate-rich foods doesn't cause insulin resistance; excessive calories do. People who are overweight and sedentary may have symptoms of insulin resistance, a condition often diminished with moderate physical activity and weight loss.

Do people with weight problems consume more sugars than normal-weight individuals? And do they have a "sweeter tooth"? No evidence says so. In fact, they may eat less sugar—but perhaps more fat and likely more calories. For those who are calorie conscious, some sweet flavors may help to make a low-calorie diet more appealing. So, just because many people like sweet tastes doesn't mean that eating sugary foods will lead to overindulgence. Eating sweets won't stimulate the appetite for more!

To keep your weight healthy, you're wise to control all calories, including those from starches and sugars, in your food choices. Sugary foods, for example, sweet, rich desserts and snacks, can supply more calories than you need. Those extra calories may come from fats, as well as carbohydrates. A "fat tooth," rather than a "sweet tooth," may be the reason some people overindulge. To maintain your weight ("no

gain, no loss") you've got to balance the calories you eat with those you burn. Use MyPyramid as your guide, and stay physically active.

Linked to Hyperactivity?

Following an afternoon of sweet snacks, friends, and active play, kids may be "all wired up." But don't blame the candy, cupcakes, or sweet drink for a "sugar high." Sugar has been wrongly accused as a cause of hyperactivity or attention deficit-hyperactive disorder (ADHD). Even though no scientific evidence supports any link between the intake of sugars and hyperactivity, many parents and other caregivers seem reluctant to put this notion aside.

Causes of nervous, aggressive, and impulsive behavior and a short attention span aren't understood completely. But experts advise adults to take stock of a child's overall environment. The excitement of a party or a special event, such as trick-or-treating or a visit to Santa—not the sweet snacks that go with the fun—may account for unruly behavior. To the contrary, some studies suggest that sugars may have a calming effect. There's not enough research yet, but a body chemical called serotonin produced in and released from the brain may be a factor.

Causes Diabetes?

Again, the answer is "no." Sugars—and other carbohydrates—don't cause diabetes. Even though the scientific community debunked the sugar myth about twenty-five years ago, the misperception persists.

In diabetes, the body can't use sugar normally. The causes are complex and still not fully known. Genetics certainly play a role, but illness, being overweight, or simply getting older also may trigger diabetes. Being overweight seems to be a key factor in the growing diabetes epidemic, including type 2 diabetes among kids.

While food choices don't cause diabetes, diet is part of the strategy for managing diabetes—along with physical activity and perhaps medication. To control blood sugar levels, people with diabetes manage the overall carbohydrates, proteins, fats, and alcoholic drinks in their meals and snacks.

In the past, people with diabetes were warned to

avoid or strictly limit sugar in their food choices. But today, experts recognize that added sugars, naturally occurring sugars, and starches have similar effects on blood sugar levels. For people with diabetes, the amount of carbohydrate, not the source, is the issue. In fact, blood sugar levels after a meal or snack are linked to many factors, including how the food is prepared, the meal size, how much fat was eaten, the other foods in the whole meal or snack, the absorption rate of the sugars (digested from sugars and starches)—and certainly a person's health status.

According to current advice from the American Diabetes Association, moderate amounts of sugar, in fact all carbohydrates, can be part of a well-balanced diabetic diet. For people with diabetes, a registered dietitian or certified diabetes educator can help plan and monitor their diet. *For more on diabetes, as well as insulin resistance, refer to chapter 22, "Diabetes: A Growing Health Concern."*

Triggers Hypoglycemia?

It's highly unlikely. Yet many people explain away anxiety, headaches, and chronic fatigue as hypoglycemia caused by eating foods with sugar. Often self-diagnosed, hypoglycemic disorders are actually quite rare.

Hypoglycemia, or low blood sugar, is actually a condition, not a disease. Between meals, blood sugar levels naturally drop—but they remain fairly constant, between 60 and 110 milligrams per deciliter (mg/dL). A signal for hypoglycemia is when levels drop below about 40 mg/dL. When blood sugars fall below normal levels, there's not enough glucose immediately available for cells to produce energy. That can cause several symptoms, including sweating, rapid heartbeat, trembling, and hunger.

Among people with diabetes, hypoglycemia is caused by taking too much insulin, by exercising too much, or by not eating enough. In most other cases, low blood sugar is linked to other serious medical problems, such as liver disease or a tumor of the pancreas.

In rare cases, a disorder called reactive hypoglycemia occurs. As a rebound effect, the body secretes too much insulin after eating a large meal. The result is a drop in blood sugar well below normal, and symptoms such as shakiness, sweating, rapid heartbeat, and trembling may occur—but not until about two to four hours after eating. These symptoms are not to be confused with extreme hunger, which is characterized by gradually increased stomach rumbling, headache, and feelings of weakness—usually occurring six to eight hours after a meal.

If you think you're among those rare cases and that you have symptoms of reactive hypoglycemia, pay

Have You Ever Wondered

. . . if a "sugar-free" food is also "calorie free"? Not necessarily, so don't let the term confuse you. A sugar-free food may not contain sugar, but may contain calories from other carbohydrates, fats, and proteins. To find the calories and total sugars in one label serving of any packaged food, read the Nutrition Facts.

. . . if "low carb" is "low calorie"? No again. If protein replaces carbohydrates, the calories per label serving may not change. If you're out to manage your weight, you can't count "carbs" and ignore the calories. Read the Nutrition Facts!

. . . if "carbs" affect your mood? No consistent research supports this. Studies have investigated the link between stress and serotonin, a body brain chemical. Serotonin breaks down to help relieve stress. Although carbohydrates may help replenish the body's serotonin, no conclusive research suggests a calming effect. Does a bowl of ice cream or mug of hot chocolate give you a feeling of comfort or calm? Perhaps. It's really a link to pleasant memories.

. . . what goes in when food manufacturers take "carbs" out? Traditional products may use higher-protein ingredients in place of some carbohydrates, for example, soy flour, soy protein, or wheat protein in place of wheat flour. Or, as in candy, ice cream, and other sweets, sugar alcohols may replace some sugars. To go "low carb," high-fiber fillers also may replace whole grains; however, that means missing out on grain's nutrient and phytonutrient benefits.

attention to how you feel two to four hours after eating. Then talk to your physician about a medical checkup and testing your blood glucose level while you're experiencing symptoms.

Also be cautious of so-called health clinics that diagnose "sugar-induced hypoglycemia" and offer treatment with costly remedies.

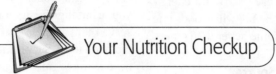

Your Nutrition Checkup

Sweet and Nutrient-Rich, Too?

Here's your chance to check your "sweet" choices. Are they packed with nutrients, too? Or do they provide mostly calories, added sugars, and few nutrients? Check the space that describes what choices you make!

Do You . . . ?	ALWAYS	MOSTLY	SOMETIMES	NEVER
Reach for fruit as a snack, rather than candy or cookies?	___	___	___	___
Drink 100% juice—or milk—with lunch or dinner, rather than soft drinks?	___	___	___	___
Top your cereal with fruit instead of—or along with—sugar?	___	___	___	___
Sweeten waffles, pancakes, or French toast with fruit, rather than just syrup?	___	___	___	___
Top ice cream with fruit, not just chocolate or caramel syrup?	___	___	___	___
Make water or milk your snack drink choice?	___	___	___	___
Choose fruit for dessert, not a rich, high-calorie dessert?	___	___	___	___
Go for the smaller rather than the bigger slice of pie or cake?	___	___	___	___
Snack on two or three cookies with milk, rather than simply down five or six cookies, or the whole package?	___	___	___	___
Make hot cocoa with milk, not just water?	___	___	___	___

Now rate your choices.

Total the points in each column. For each answer, give yourself:

4 points for "always"
3 points for "mostly"
2 points for "sometimes"
1 point for "never"

If you scored . . .

30 or above. Your "sweet" choices are mostly high in nutrients, too. In fact, enjoy a bit of sugar now and then, to add pleasure to eating.

20 to 29. If your overall diet is balanced and you're not overspending your calorie budget, your preference for sweets is probably okay.

10 to 19. Your "sweet tooth" may be crowding out nutritious foods. Check them out and consider some sweet options such as fruit, with fewer or no added sugars. You'll find great ideas for nutrient-rich "carb" foods in this chapter!

Carbohydrates in Food

We casually refer to a vast array of foods as "carbs," when we really mean carb-containing foods. And "good carbs" and "bad carbs"? Misnomers, too, that typically refer to nutrient-dense (rich) and energy-dense foods with carbohydrates. So, what foods contain carbohydrates—and are some better than others?

Starches and Sugars: Their Sources

Most carbohydrates come from plant-based foods. Through photosynthesis, plants transform the sun's energy into carbohydrates as food for their own growth. As a result, carbohydrates—sugars and starches—naturally form in fruits and vegetables, including legumes (dry beans), grain products, nuts, and seeds. As an aside, all these foods are rich in other nutrients, too.

Plants have the unique ability to change their car-bohydrates. As fruit matures, its carbohydrate shifts from starch to sugars, making fruit much sweeter and more appealing. By contrast, many vegetables—among them peas, carrots, and corn—are sweetest when they're young. As they mature, their sugars change to starches. What's the "chef's" lesson? If you're buying "fresh," look for young vegetables—and serve them at their peak. In other words, don't store them too long. Serve fruits when they're ripe; you may need to allow ripening time after you buy them.

Milk, too, derives some of its pleasing flavor from lactose, its own naturally occurring sugar. Milk isn't perceived as a sweet beverage, however. Lactose is only one-sixth as sweet as sucrose.

In one form or another sugars are added to many prepared foods for function, flavor, or both. *See "Added Sugars: What Foods?" on this page.* Soft drinks, candy, other sweet snacks, desserts, and sweet baked goods are obvious sources; added sugars end up in many other processed and prepared foods. Check the ingredient lists on their labels to identify them. Naturally occurring sugars are not included in the ingredient list.

One more source of added sugars: potentially your own kitchen. In one form or another, you're likely adding sugar to food, too, with your food prep: white and brown sugar, corn syrup, molasses, and honey, as well as jam, jelly, and syrup – and the ingredients you may use, processed with added sugars.

Sugars: Their Roles in Food

Eighty-five years ago, homemakers baked with sugars and honey, prepared jellies and jams with sugars, and flavored homemade baked beans with molasses or sorghum molasses. Today sugars are added to food during commercial food processing, as more and more households depend on convenience foods, rather than home cooking and baking.

The sweetness of sugars is the attribute that gets attention. Yet sugars contribute far more than flavor. That's why they're added to many processed and prepared foods. From the standpoint of kitchen chemistry, sugars work as multipurpose ingredients, fulfilling functions that you may not even think about:

In yeast breads . . . sugars are "food" for yeast, allowing the dough to rise. Yeast doesn't consume all the

---

Added Sugars: What Foods?

Do you eat a lot of these foods? If so, you may need to cut back. They contribute more than 5 percent of the added sugars in the typical American diet, in descending order:

	PERCENT* OF ADDED SUGARS INTAKE
● Soft drinks (not diet or sugar free)	33
● Sugars and candy	16
● Cakes, cookies, pies	13
● Fruit drinks (fruitades and fruit punch)	10
● Dairy desserts and milk products (ice cream, sweetened yogurt, sweetened milk)	9
● Other grains (cinnamon toast, honey-nut waffles)	6

(*Percentage is rounded.)

Source: Guthrie, *Journal of the American Dietetic Association,* 2000.
Printed in: Dietary Guidelines for Americans, 2005.

sugar, however. The rest adds flavor and contributes to the aroma and delicate-brown color of the crust.

In cakes . . . sugars contribute to the bulk, tenderness, smooth crumb texture, and lightly browned surface. In cakes that have air whipped in, such as angel food cake and sponge cake, sugars help hold the form.

In cookies . . . as sugars and shortening are creamed together, sugars help bring air into the dough. Sugars also contribute to the light-brown color, crisp texture, and even to the "cracked" surface of sugar cookies and gingersnaps.

In canned jams, jellies, and preserves . . . sugars help inhibit the growth of molds and yeast by tying up the water that these microorganisms need to multiply. For this reason, sugars act as preservatives.

In candy . . . sugar contributes to the texture, for example, the smoothness of hard candy and the creaminess of fudge. And as it cooks, turning from white to yellow to brown, sugar develops a unique, tasty flavor.

In all kinds of food . . . sugar adds to the flavor, aroma, texture, color, and body of food. Sometimes, just a small amount of sugar is added to a recipe to bring out the flavors of other ingredients, such as in tomato-based sauce or salad dressing.

What happens if you cut back on sugar in recipes? That depends. In some recipes, there's little difference—except for taste. In others, you'll notice a difference in volume, texture, color, and aroma. And in jams, jellies, and preserves, mold will grow quickly, even if they're refrigerated.

"Carbs" on the Food Label

Hunting for the carbohydrate content of food? Check the food label. Clues come from the ingredient list, the Nutrition Facts, and nutrient content claims.

If you're curious about a food's "recipe"—and how much added sugars and fiber it has—check the ingredient list. If sugar appears as the first or second ingredient, or if several sugars are listed, the food likely has a lot of added sugars.

Even if you don't see the word "sugar" on the ingredient list, it may have added sugars. Terms ending in "-ose" mean sugars. Words such as "maltose," "dextrin," and "corn syrup" are sugars, too, often made of several types of sugars. Among the many sugars that may appear (besides those ending in "–ose":

brown sugar	honey
cane sugar	high-fructose corn syrup (HFCS)
confectioner's sugar	invert sugar
corn sweeteners	malt syrup
corn syrup	maple syrup
crystallized cane sugar	molasses
dextrin	raw sugar
evaporated cane juice	syrup
fruit juice concentrate	turbinado sugar

You can also check the USDA Database for Added Sugars Content of Selected Foods, 2006: www.nal.usda.gov/fnic/foodcomp/Data/add_sug/addsug01.pdf.

For "carb" amounts check the Nutrition Facts. Almost all food labels carry a Nutrition Facts panel with the amount of calories, total carbohydrate, sugars, and fiber in a standard label serving. As defined by FDA for the Nutrition Fact panel:

● *Total Carbohydrate* includes starches, naturally occurring and added sugars, sugar alcohols, and fiber, as well as organic acids and preservatives (which don't weigh much).

● *Sugars* are the sum of all naturally occurring and added sugars, and they contribute to the total carbohydrate amount. You'll find sugars in all kinds of foods, including those without added sugars—such as milk, fruit, and grain products. On the label, added sugars are included in sugars; they're not listed separately in the Nutrition Facts.

● *Dietary Fiber*, also part of total carbohydrates, is listed. By checking the label, you'll see that whole-grain foods usually have more fiber than those made from refined grains. *Refer to chapter 6 for more on fiber in whole grains and spotting fiber-rich foods.*

● *Sugar alcohols* might be included on a separate line, too. *Read about them later in this chapter.*

Know the meaning of nutrient content claims. You may find words such as "sugar free" or "no sugar added" on flavored yogurt, canned fruit, breakfast cereal, or other foods. If these claims catch your

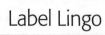

Label Lingo

Sugars and Calories

Although the FDA hasn't approved nutrient content claims for total carbohydrates, you may find claims related to calories and sugar. Look for these terms as you walk the supermarket aisles:

LABEL TERM . . .	MEANS . . .
Calorie free	less than 5 calories per serving
Sugar free	less than 0.5 gram sugars per serving
Reduced sugar or less sugar	at least 25% less* sugar or sugars per serving
No added sugars, without added sugar, no sugar	no sugars added during processing or packing, including ingredients that contain sugar such as juice or dry fruit

*As compared with a standard serving size of the traditional food

attention, check the Nutrition Facts for specifics. *Refer to "Label Lingo: Sugars and Calories" in this chapter.*

What do terms like "net carbs," "low carb," or "net impact carbs" on labels mean—*and not mean*? Often they're "defined" as consumer confusion! Although currently allowed, these terms aren't regulated by the FDA, at least not now. Their meaning is unclear, varying among food manufacturers and weight-loss plans. "Net carbs" may be total carbohydrates minus fiber, *or* minus fiber and sugar alcohols. The idea is: they aren't counted because fiber isn't absorbed and sugar alcohols aren't completely absorbed. This issue is under scientific debate. Until regulated, the FDA recommends that labels explain the term and its calculation. For diabetes management, talk to your registered dietitian or certified diabetes educator about how foods labeled with these terms fit in your food plan.

Refer to chapter 11, Supermarket Smarts, to learn about health and structure-function claims on food labels, related to carbohydrate-containing foods.

"Carbs": Choose by the Company They Keep!

Vegetables, fruits, legumes (dry beans), grain products, and milk: all these nutrient-rich foods supply carbohydrates! Get most of the "carbs" you need from these foods that also supply a host of vitamins, minerals, fiber, and other phytonutrients. *Refer to chapter 10 to learn how to fit these foods in.* Go easy on energy-dense options, or those that deliver more calories (and added sugars) and fewer nutrients.

Starchy Foods: Healthful and Easy!

Plenty of starchy foods deliver great nutrition. Consider this to make the best choices.

● Read labels. Choose starchy foods that deliver plenty of other nutrients.

● Partner! Serve grain foods with other nutrient-rich foods: for example, brown rice with vegetable stir-fry, whole-wheat pita stuffed with a garden salad, or baked potato topped with chili beans.

● Fit variety in: starchy vegetables (for example, potatoes, sweet potatoes, squash, beans), other veggies, and grain products, including whole grains. Follow the guidance of MyPyramid for amounts; *see chapter 10.*

● Pick grain products with fewer fats and added sugars: for example, bagels in place of donuts, crackers without *trans* fats rather than chips, baked potatoes rather than fries.

● Substitute whole-grain products for those made with refined flour, for more nutritional benefits from "carb-rich" foods! Make half your grain choices whole grain.

● Be sensible about portions. It's easy to serve up 3 cups of pasta when half that amount may be plenty!

Sugars: In Healthful Eating

Naturally occurring or added, sugars are part of healthful eating. By adding taste, aroma, texture, color, and body to all kinds of foods, sugars make many foods more appealing.

That said, be mindful of the amount, especially of added sugars. The more foods with large amounts of added sugars consumed, the harder it is to get enough nutrients without weight gain—especially true if your energy needs are low.

The Dietary Guidelines advise: *Choose and prepare foods and beverages with little added sugars or calorie sweeteners, such as the amounts suggested in MyPyramid and the DASH eating plan. Refer to chapters 10 and 22.*

● Enjoy the sweet flavor of fruit and fruit juice—and reap the nutritional benefits! Fruit gets its sweet flavor from fructose. At the same time, it supplies beta carotene (which forms vitamin A), vitamin C, or both—and folate, potassium, and fiber, as well as other nutrients and phytonutrients. Some fruits aren't sweet, but are instead sour or bitter. Cranberries and limes are two examples; sugars may be added to make these nutritious fruits or their juices more enjoyable.

● Drink water often. Enjoy milk, too. Soft drinks—sugar- or calorie-free—shouldn't replace calcium-rich beverages you need for healthy bones.

Fruit Snacks: Sweet & Nutritious

Next time you have a craving for a sweet snack, reach for fruit! Besides satisfying a taste for sweets, fruit is packed with nutrients.

Fruit Pops. For a nutritious "fruit pop," freeze pureed fruit (mango, papaya, or apricot) or juice in ice cube trays or paper cups with wooden sticks.

Frozen Bananas. Push a wooden stick into half of a peeled banana. Roll in yogurt or a light coating of chocolate syrup, then in crunchy cornflakes. Wrap; freeze.

Fruit-Mix. Mix up a zipper-top bag of dried fruits of your choice: apple slices, apricots, blueberries, cherries, cranberries, pear slices, and raisins, among others. (*Hint:* Brush your teeth—or rinse your mouth with water—after nibbling because dried fruit sticks to teeth!)

Frozen Chips. Slice bananas into thin rounds. Spread them flat on a baking pan; cover. Freeze and serve frozen as a fun snack. (*Hint:* The same technique works for seedless grapes or berries.)

Frugurt. Top a rainbow of cut-up fruit with low-fat yogurt. (*Hint:* It looks pretty in a clear glass or plastic cup.)

● Go easy on foods with mostly sugars, but few other nutrients: candy, some soft drinks and fruit drinks, jelly, jams, and syrup. Make sugar trade-offs to fit some in. Balance sugary foods, such as cake or pastries, with those having less sugars, such as bread or crackers. That way you can enjoy them within your calorie budget for the day. *Check chapter 10 for more about your discretionary calorie budget.*

● Read labels on all kinds of processed and prepared foods. Some have little or no added sugars, such as some canned and frozen fruit. Others may be sweetened with an intense sweetener (with few calories), such as in candy, beverages, yogurt, and some baked foods.

● Go easy on added sugars in your food preparation. *For tips, refer to "Sugar Savers" in chapter 13.*

● Use a light touch with your sugar spoon. Sweeten coffee or tea with just a bit of sugar. For a hint of "sweet" without the calories, try a touch of cinnamon. The same goes for sugar sprinkled on cereal or French toast. Use just a bit. Or sweeten with fresh fruit instead.

● Go "50-50"—and cut calories in half. Or eat small portions. Perhaps eat a miniature-size candy, not a large candy bar, or share a sugary dessert or snack with a friend. Then eat it slowly to get the most enjoyment.

● Try intense sweeteners to add flavor—yet few calories. *For tips, refer to "Cooking with Intense Sweeteners."*

How do foods with added sugars (sugars you add in food prep or added sugars in prepared foods) fit in? Certainly they're part of healthful eating. Besides their very real culinary functions, they may add appeal to nutritious foods you otherwise would avoid. The health issues are: (1) how much—and whether you have enough extra, or discretionary calories, to spend on foods with added sugars, and (2) whether high-sugar, low-nutrient foods crowd out more nutritious options. One example is when soft drinks, rather than milk or fruit juice, frequently accompany a meal. *Refer to chapter 10 to learn how to fit added sugars into your healthful eating plan.*

Sugar Alcohols: Sugar Replacers

Polyols, or sugar alcohols, are another category of nutritive sweeteners. Why nutritive? Like sugars, they provide energy, or calories. Usually they replace sugar on an equal basis. Why the term "sugar alcohol"? To clarify, "sugar" and "alcohol" refer only to their chemical structure. Sugar alcohols don't contain ethanol, as alcoholic beverages do. They also may be referred to as "sugar replacers" or "reduced-calorie sweeteners."

Sugar alcohols are naturally present in many foods you already enjoy, including berries, other fruits, and vegetables. In fact, they're carbohydrates. They're also a category of commercial ingredients, derived from sucrose, glucose, and starch: for example, sorbitol, mannitol, and hydrogenated starch hydrolysates.

Sweet, Fewer Calories

Because sugar alcohols are carbohydrates, they supply energy, but fewer calories per gram than sugar does: anywhere from 1.5 to 3 calories per gram. Sugars provide 4 calories per gram. To compare, sorbitol has 2.6 calories per gram; mannitol, 1.6 calories per gram. As an energy source, however, they're absorbed slowly and incompletely, and require little or no insulin for metabolism. That's why foods made with polyols may offer alternatives for people with diabetes.

Their sweetness varies, from 25 percent to 100 percent as sweet as sugar. Sorbitol and mannitol, for example, may be half as sweet as table sugar; however, xylitol is just as sweet. Often they're combined with intense sweeteners, such as aspartame or saccharin, for a sweeter flavor.

Sugar alcohols aren't cavity-promoting either. Why? They aren't converted to acids by oral bacteria that produce cavities, so they offer a functional food benefit. In fact, the FDA has approved the health claim for gum, candies, beverages, and snack foods with sugar alcohols, noting that sugar alcohols in these foods do not promote tooth decay. For some people, sorbitol and mannitol may produce abdominal gas or discomfort or may have a laxative effect when consumed in excess. You might see this label statement: "excess consumption may have a laxative effect." Eat foods with these sweeteners in moderation or perhaps with other foods if your tolerance is lower.

What about their safety? The FDA regulates their use. The following sugar alcohols are on the GRAS list (generally recognized as safe) or are approved as additives: erythritol, hydrogenated starch hydrolysates (HSH), isomalt, lactitol, maltitol, mannitol, sorbitol, and xylitol. *See chapter 4 for a brief discussion of prebiotics, "Prebiotics and Probiotics: What Are They?"*

Kitchen Nutrition

Sweet Seasons

Bring out the flavors of foods with seasonings that offer the perception of sweetness: allspice, cardamom, cinnamon, ginger, mace, nutmeg, and citrus juices.

- Add ginger to a fruit glaze. Blend frozen raspberries with a pinch of ginger and a small amount of fruit juice concentrate or sweetener. Toss the glaze with fresh berries or sliced fruit.

- Add a "sweet" spice of your choice to dry coffee grounds before brewing.

- Add zest and sweet flavor to oatmeal and other cooked breakfast cereals with allspice, mace, or nutmeg. In place of water, cook it in fruit juice (or milk for more calcium and phosphorus)! Toss with dried fruits, such as cranberries or apricots. Or top with fresh fruit.

- For a hint of sweet flavor in rice, cook with cardamom, cinnamon, or ginger. You might substitute juice for part of the cooking liquid. Perhaps toss in raisins or other dried fruits, too!

- Add a touch of sweetness to cooked vegetables: for example, carrots with a hint of ginger, mashed sweet potatoes with cinnamon, and spinach with a sprinkle of nutmeg.

- Squeeze citrus juice—lemon, lime, or orange—over fresh fruit to enhance the flavor. *Calorie-saving tip:* You save about 45 calories with a "squeeze" of juice rather than one tablespoon of sugar.

- Create "syrup" for pancakes or waffles. In a blender, puree sliced peaches, berries, or apples with a little fruit juice, honey, and a pinch of cinnamon.

Pairing Sugars and Chocolate!

A love for chocolate can be traced through the centuries. Known as a food of the gods, chocolate was highly prized in the Americas in pre-Columbian times. Native Americans from what is now Mexico served chocolate to European explorers as early as the 1500s.

By itself, chocolate has a bitter taste. But sugar, transported from plantations in the American and Caribbean colonies, made chocolate tasty to the European palate. By the mid-1600s, the popularity of chocolate, sweetened with sugar, had spread throughout Europe. In 1847, milk chocolate was created, and it quickly became popular around the world.

As an ingredient with a distinctive flavor, chocolate can fit within a healthful eating plan. It may add a flavor spark that makes nutritious foods, such as milk, more appealing. Chocolate, a plant-based ingredient, also contains a category of phytonutrients called polyphenols, which may offer some health benefits. *Refer to chapter 4 on phytonutrients.* Research is exploring links to heart health; chocolate appears to have significant antioxidant potential.

The chocolate challenge? Sugary, chocolate-flavored foods are typically high calorie, often low in nutrients. And they may crowd out more nutritious foods—for example, if a chocolate bar replaces fruit in your lunch bag—or when you can't control a chocolate urge. Much of the chocolate we consume is found in confectionery and baked products that are fat laden, too.

Now let's melt away a few chocolate myths:

- *Myth: Chocolate causes acne.* That misconception has captured the attention of teens for years. However, hormonal changes during adolescence are the usual cause of acne, not chocolate.

- *Myth: Carob bars are more healthful than chocolate bars.* Actually a carob bar has the same amount of calories and fat as a similar-size chocolate bar. Carob, a common substitute for chocolate, comes from the seeds of the carob tree, which are different from cocoa beans.

- *Myth: Chocolate has a lot of caffeine.* Chocolate supplies caffeine, but the amount is quite small. Eight ounces of chocolate milk have about 5 milligrams of caffeine, compared with 3 milligrams in 5 ounces of decaffeinated coffee. In contrast, 5 ounces of regular-brew coffee contains 115 milligrams of caffeine.

- *Myth: Some people are "chocoholics."* Not true—although some people do have a stronger preference for chocolate than others, perhaps because of its taste, aroma, and texture. While popping chocolate candies may become a high-calorie habit with a pleasurable sensation, eating chocolate itself can't become truly addictive. Research is exploring any potential role of chocolate to brain neurotransmitters that regulate serotonin and dopamine, often referred to as "feel good" body substances.

Sugar Alcohols in Foods

Besides adding sweetness to some sugar-free foods, sugar alcohols add texture and bulk to a wide range of foods: baked goods, ice cream, fruit spreads, and candies. They also help foods stay moist, prevent browning when food is heated, and give a cooling effect to the taste of food. Baked foods made with sugar alcohols won't have a crisp brown surface unless the color comes from another ingredient. Sugar alcohols also are used in chewing gum, toothpaste, and mouthwash.

With weight management and diabetes as key health issues, more sugar-alcohol-containing foods appear on supermarket shelves these days. How can you spot them on a food label? The ingredient list may give the specific name, perhaps sorbitol. If a nutrition content claim is made, perhaps "sugar free," the sugar alcohol content must appear with the Nutrition Facts separately, under carbohydrates, as grams of "sugar alcohols" or of the specific polyol. The label may also say that the food has fewer calories per gram than other similar foods with nutritive sweeteners.

Anyone can enjoy foods made with sugar alcohols. But since they're lower in calories than sugars, sugar alcohols have potential advantages for people managing diabetes or weight. That said, for diabetes management, sugar alcohols aren't "free foods." They aren't calorie free; instead, 2 grams of sugar alcohols are generally counted as 1 gram of carbohydrate. If

Have You Ever Wondered ?

...if chocolate milk is okay for kids? Like unflavored milk, chocolate and other flavored milk supplies calcium, phosphorus, protein, riboflavin, and vitamin D. Flavored milk contains more calories from added sugars; the sugars are no more cavity-promoting than any other carbohydrate.

... whether the FDA has guidelines for sugar replacers? The FDA has set "acceptable daily intakes" (ADIs) for sugar replacers (sugar alcohols and intense sweeteners), used as food additives. The ADI for each, set at a very conservative level, is how much can be consumed daily over a lifetime without posing a risk.

you're managing diabetes, have a registered dietitian or certified diabetes educator help you fit foods with sugar alcohols into a healthful eating plan.

Intense Sweeteners: Flavor without Calories

"Low in calories" and "sugar free"! For many weight-conscious people and those with diabetes, these are sweet messages.

When it comes to sweetness, sugar is "top of mind." Yet intense sweeteners can deliver sweet taste with just a fraction of the calories, and they're many times sweeter than the same amount of sugar. With intense sweeteners, you need only a very small amount. *Refer to "Sweet Comparisons."*

Intense sweeteners also are known by other names: non-nutritive sweeteners, very-low-calorie sweeteners, or alternative sweeteners. They contribute little if any energy, so the term "non-nutritive" is appropriate. In comparison, nutritive sweeteners, such as sugars and sugar alcohols, supply your body with energy in the form of calories.

Intense sweeteners can fit into healthful eating for just about anyone. Alone or blended with other sweeteners, they provide sweetness in foods such as yogurt and pudding, without adding calories or compromising nutrients. The intense sweeteners used today won't promote tooth decay since they aren't carbohydrates.

Sweet Options

Perhaps no ingredient has been scrutinized by researchers as much as intense sweeteners. Before being used in food—or as a tabletop sweetener—they're first tested extensively to meet the guidelines and safety standards of the FDA. That includes assigning Acceptable Daily Intakes (ADIs).

Currently in the United States, six intense sweeteners have been approved: acesulfame potassium, aspartame, neotame, saccharin, sucralose, and tagalose. But watch for news about others. Approval from the FDA is being sought for alitame and cyclamate. If you travel abroad, you may hear of stevioside or thaumatin, too.

Acesulfame Potassium

Acesulfame potassium (or acesulfame K) entered the food world in 1967. Approved for use in the United States in 1988, acesulfame potassium is marketed under the brand name Sunette.

A white, odorless, crystalline sweetener, this intense sweetener provides no calories. Like saccharin, acesulfame potassium can't be broken down by the body, and it's eliminated in the urine unchanged. Again, no calories, and a potential benefit for people with diabetes.

Acesulfame potassium is 200 times sweeter than table sugar, adding its sweet taste to candies, baked goods, desserts, noncarbonated drinks, dairy products, sauces, alcoholic drinks, and tabletop sweeteners, such as Sweet One and Swiss Sweet. By itself in some foods, a high concentration of acesulfame potassium may leave a slight aftertaste. So it's often combined with other sweeteners, both traditional and intense.

Cooking tip: Because acesulfame potassium is heat stable, you can use it in cooked and baked foods. Like saccharin, it gives no bulk, or volume, as sugar does, so it may not work in some recipes. *Refer to "Cooking with Intense Sweeteners."*

Aspartame

Aspartame is also about 200 times sweeter than table sugar. Discovered in 1965 and approved by the FDA in 1981, aspartame was first marketed as NutraSweet and sold as the tabletop sweetener Equal. Aspartame is now available in a variety of tabletop sweeteners.

Aspartame isn't sugar. Instead it's a combination of two amino acids—aspartic acid and the methyl ester of phenylalanine. While amino acids are the building blocks of protein, aspartic acid and phenylalanine are joined in a way that's perceived as sweet in your mouth. These same two amino acids are also found naturally in common foods such as meat, fat-free milk, fruit, and vegetables. When digested, your body treats them like any other amino acid in food.

Like other protein, aspartame actually has 4 calories per gram. However, so little is used that the calorie impact on the diet is negligible.

Because aspartame contains phenylalanine, people with phenylketonuria (PKU) need to be cautious about consuming foods and beverages with it. On food labels, look for "aspartame" in the ingredient list, as well as this statement: "Phenylketonurics: Contains Phenylalanine." PKU is a rare genetic disorder that doesn't allow the body to metabolize phenylalanine properly. It afflicts about one in 15,000 people in the United States. In the United States, all infants are screened for PKU at birth. *Refer to chapter 21, "Sensitive about Food."*

Because it's not heat stable, aspartame is used mostly in foods that don't require cooking or baking. Most aspartame consumed in the United States is in soft drinks. Among other commercial uses are puddings, gelatins, frozen desserts, yogurt, hot cocoa mix, powdered soft drinks, teas, breath mints, chewing gum, and tabletop sweeteners, such as Equal and SweetMate.

Cooking tip: When aspartame is heated for a long time, it may lose its sweetness. When you prepare food with a tabletop sweetener containing aspartame, add it toward the end of cooking. Or sprinkle it on a cooked or baked product after removing it from the heat.

Saccharin

Discovered in 1879, saccharin has been used as a noncaloric sweetener for about 100 years. It's produced from a naturally occurring substance in grapes. Today, saccharin is used in soft drinks and in tabletop sweeteners, such as Sweet 'N Low and Sweet 10. The benefits? Calorie free, not cavity-promoting, not metabolized by humans, and safe.

Being 300 to 500 times sweeter than table sugar, a small amount of saccharin adds a lot of flavor—without adding calories. Just 20 milligrams of saccharin gives the same sweetness as one teaspoon (4,000 milligrams, or 4 grams) of table sugar. Because the body can't break it down, saccharin doesn't provide energy. Instead it's eliminated in urine.

What about its bitter aftertaste? It's usually blended with other sweeteners to make the flavor pleasing.

After decades of research, saccharin was removed from the government's list of potential carcinogens and, since the 1970s, has had interim approval. Scientific consensus in the government's 2000 Report on Carcinogens deemed that cancer data on rats was not relevant to human physiology. In the past, a few studies hinted that saccharin—in very large amounts

Sweet Comparisons

Many ingredients have a sweet flavor, some much more than others. For intense sweeteners, such as saccharin, a little bit goes a long way!

SWEETENER	COMPARING THE SWEETNESS TO SUCROSE (WHITE OR TABLE SUGAR)
Hydrogenated starch hydrolysates	0.25 to 0.5
Lacititol	0.3 to 0.4
Isomalt	0.45 to .65
Sorbitol	0.5 to 0.7
Mannitol	0. 5 to 0.7
Sucrose	1.0
Xylitol	1.0
High-fructose corn syrup (HFCS)	1.5
Fructose (crystalline)	1.5
Cyclamate*	30
Aspartame	200
Acesulfame K	200
Saccharin	300–500
Sucralose	600
Alitame*	2,000
Neotame	8,000

*Not yet approved for use in food or beverages in the United States

(equivalent to 750 cans of soft drinks or 10,000 saccharin tablets daily)—may cause cancer in laboratory
rats. No human studies have ever confirmed the findings. A warning label related to risk in lab animals
still appears—until the FDA or Congress removes it.
As with any food or food substance, keep moderation
in mind.

Cooking tip: Saccharin keeps its sweet flavor when
heated, so it can be used in cooked and baked foods.
Because it doesn't have the bulk that sugar has, it may
not work in some recipes. *Refer to "Cooking with
Intense Sweeteners."*

Sucralose

Of the low-calorie sweeteners, sucralose is the only
one that's made from sugar. It's actually 600 times
sweeter. Discovered in 1976 and approved in 1998 for
U.S. use, sucralose is marketed as Splenda.

Unlike sugar, the body doesn't recognize sucralose
as a carbohydrate. As a result, it doesn't promote tooth
decay and supplies no calories, either. Sucralose can't
be digested, absorbed, or metabolized for energy, so
it doesn't affect blood glucose levels or insulin production, either. Instead it passes through the body
unchanged—a benefit for people with diabetes. As a
non-nutritive powder, it's used in beverages, processed
foods, chewing gum, and tabletop sweeteners.

Cooking tip: Sucralose offers the sweet sugar
flavor, without the calories, and performs like sugar
in cooking and baking. However, it doesn't give bulk
to baked goods. It's highly heat stable, even for a prolonged time. And it keeps its flavor in foods, even
when stored for a long time. Like sugar, it dissolves
easily in water. Use sucralose as a sweetener in food
preparation and beverages.

Tagatose and Neotame

Two others have been recently approved: tagatose
(2001) and neotame (2002). Tagatose is a low-calorie
sweetener (1.5 calories per gram) derived from lactose, which is found in some dairy foods. It may be
used as a food and beverage ingredient; check the
ingredient list to find out. Neotame is a noncaloric
sweetener that's 8,000 times sweeter than sucrose,
used in food and beverages.

Intense Sweeteners: For Whom?

In the 1970s the Baby Boom generation became intent
on slimness; in the 1980s, on fitness; then, in the 1990s
and now in this century, diabetes and overweight have
become bigger issues, too. The growing use of intense
sweeteners has paralleled these health interests and
concerns.

From a health perspective, almost anyone can consume foods and beverages flavored with intense sweeteners. It's a matter of personal choice.

Watching your weight? You can't lose weight just by
using sugar substitutes! But, because they're usually
lower in calories, foods sweetened with intense sweeteners can help you keep trim—if you control calories
in your whole eating plan. Calorie control—from a

Have You Ever Wondered

. . . why intense sweeteners don't cause tooth decay?
As sweeteners, aspartame, acesulfame potassium, saccharin, or sucralose won't promote cavities because they
aren't broken down by bacteria in plaque. Since they
don't "feed" bacteria, no acids form. Sugarless gum, flavored with an intense sweetener, may actually promote
dental health. First, it doesn't have any carbohydrate.
Second, gum chewing increases saliva flow, which actually helps neutralize plaque acids.

. . . if aspartame is safe? Aspartame, approved as safe
by the FDA, has been intensely studied for its safety to
humans. Yet unreputable unidentified scares appear on
the Internet. No scientific evidence shows links between
aspartame and health problems, including attention
deficit disorder and seizures among children.

. . . what's stevia? It's an herb that's sweeter than sugar,
but calorie free. It hasn't been approved by the FDA
as a sweetener, but it's sold as a supplement. Like
other supplements, talk to a health professional before
using it.

*. . . if foods with intense sweeteners increase your
appetite and so promote weight gain?* No research evidence shows that these sweeteners stimulate appetite.
That said, they can be an aid to weight management,
by adding flavor in an overall approach to healthful eating and active living.

variety of foods—is one part of the weight management formula; regular physical activity is the other.

For people with diabetes: Intense sweeteners can satisfy a taste for sweets without affecting insulin or blood sugar levels. They also can help with weight control.

During pregnancy and breast-feeding: Eating a variety of foods with enough calories and nutrients is the real issue. In moderation, foods with intense sweeteners can satisfy a desire for a sweet flavor, without adding excess calories. That leaves room for nutritious foods.

For children: Intense sweeteners are safe, but not intended for infants and young children. Kids need ample calories for rapid growth and active play. Foods and beverages sweetened with intense sweeteners are okay occasionally—if children eat enough from a variety of nutrient-rich foods.

Cooking with Intense Sweeteners

With their sugarlike flavor, intense sweeteners can be used in many recipes you already enjoy, perhaps to reduce calories. For example, sweetening an apple cobbler with saccharin rather than brown sugar might save 67 calories per serving (if a recipe to serve four calls for ½ cup of brown sugar).

If you use intense sweeteners, be prepared to adjust your recipe or food preparation technique. Remember: Their unique cooking qualities differ from sugar. And they have limitations in baked goods.

● Check the food label on sweetener packages for usage. You'll see the sugar equivalents. Since some intense sweeteners have ingredients added to give them bulk, the substitution equivalents may vary.

● Know that recipes prepared with an intense sweetener may not turn out exactly like the same recipe made with sugar—especially if they don't have a bulking agent added. That's especially true of baked foods. Sugar has many functions other than sweetness. Check label directions for advice on using specific intense sweeteners.

● If intense sweeteners are new to you, experiment. Add just a little sweetener until you get the sweetness you want. Adding too much can ruin the flavor.

Need more carb-smart strategies for healthful eating? Check here for "how-tos":

● Get the scoop on fiber, another "carb"—chapter 6.

● Shop to make "carb foods" count—chapter 11.

● Sweeten food in your kitchen, and cook for health, too—chapter 13.

● Enjoy sweet flavors in restaurant foods—and eat smart, too—chapter 14.

● Manage "carbs" if you're an athlete—chapter 19.

● Handle carbohydrates on a diabetic eating plan—chapter 22.

● Use any intense sweetener in recipes that don't require heat, such as cold beverages, salads, chilled soups, frozen desserts, or fruit sauces. Be aware, however, that intense sweeteners don't add bulk or volume as sugar does.

● Use saccharin, acesulfame potassium, and sucralose-based sweeteners in all kinds of recipes—uncooked, cooked, and baked—according to package directions. They retain their sweetness when heated.

● Add aspartame-based sweeteners close to the end of the cooking or baking process. Prolonged and high heat breaks down aspartame, causing a loss of sweetness. But don't worry if it does get heated. Although you may lose flavor, aspartame is still safe to consume.

● Expect a lower volume and less browning when cooking and baking with intense sweeteners instead of sugar. Sugar adds bulk. Intense sweeteners with a bulking agent help bring up the volume. Or go "50–50" by substituting saccharin- or acesulfame potassium-based sweeteners for half the sugar, according to package directions. The volume still won't be as high as with 100 percent sugar.

Need more guidance? Contact the manufacturers of intense sweeteners. They can provide tips and recipes for using their products to sweeten your palate.

CHAPTER 6

Fiber
Your Body's Broom

Your ancestors probably consumed more fiber than you do!

Before the days of advanced milling technology, gristmills ground wheat, corn, and other grains into meal or flour. Using the power of a moving river, grain was milled between two coarse stones. Then it was sifted to remove the inedible chaff, or husk, leaving all the edible parts of the grain. The bran and the germ that contain fiber and many essential nutrients remained. Whole grains were the only grains people knew. In some parts of the world, that's still true today; in fact, some people still pound their grain by hand to make flour.

As technology improved, the bran and the germ were separated and removed, leaving refined white flour. With this new process came new status. White bread with its softer texture and high-class appeal became more desirable than coarser, darker bread. But it was more expensive and only available to those who could afford it. For the same reasons, white rice became more desirable than brown rice. Simply put, refined was "in"!

With this switch to refined grains, however, people became short-changed on many nutrients—including fiber—without knowing it. In the 1940s, recognizing the health consequences, manufacturers began enriching many grain products. Now, some nutrients lost during processing—thiamin, riboflavin, niacin, and iron—are added back. In some, fiber is added back, too. Since the late 1990s, enriched grain products have also been fortified with folic acid.

Only within the past thirty-five or so years have health experts recognized that fiber offers more than bulk to food. It's loaded with health benefits. Today whole-grain products, along with other fiber-rich foods—vegetables, fruits, and legumes—are "in" again. And today's experts advise: make at least half your grains whole!

Just what is fiber? How does it promote your health?

Fiber: It's Very Important!

We talk about fiber as a single component of food, but it's not that simple. Actually, dietary fiber is a general term, referring to certain complex carbohydrates and lignin that your body cannot digest or absorb into your bloodstream. Instead of being used for energy like other carbohydrates, fiber is eliminated.

Fiber is considered to be a phytonutrient, a component of food that promotes your good health in many other ways.

Fiber: Just What Is It?

Plants—and foods of plant origin—count on fiber for their shape. It's fiber that gives celery its rigid stalk and gives spinach the strong stems that hold up its leaves. That same structure "bulks up" the contents inside your digestive tract.

Like starch, most fibers are made of many sugar units, so they're actually polysaccharides. But unlike starch, fiber's chains of sugars can't be digested in the

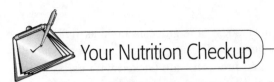

Your Nutrition Checkup

What's Your Fiber Factor— in Your Food Choices?

That's up to you—and what you choose to eat. If you had a choice, which would you pick for your meals or snacks?

1 medium unpeeled apple	or	½ cup applesauce
1 slice whole-wheat bread	or	1 slice white bread toast (from refined flour)
3½-oz. cooked meat patty	or	½ cup baked beans
⅓ cup bran flakes	or	⅓ cup corn flakes
1 carrot stick	or	1 bread stick
½ cup white rice	or	½ cup brown rice
½ cup strawberries	or	½ cup grapes
½ cup spinach	or	½ cup peas
½ cup peanuts	or	1 oz. cheese
2 figs	or	2 dried plums (prunes)
2 tbsp. bean dip (hummus)	or	2 tbsp. sour cream
¾ cup orange juice	or	1 orange
1 baked potato with skin	or	½ cup mashed potatoes (no skin)
1 tbsp. wheat germ	or	1 tbsp. wheat bran

Now check your answers . . .

For each pair, these foods contain more fiber: unpeeled apple, whole-wheat bread, baked beans, bran flakes, carrot stick, brown rice, strawberries, peas, peanuts, figs, bean dip (hummus), orange, baked potato with skin, and wheat bran.

To compare the specific amounts of fiber in these food pairs, see the chart "How Much Fiber?" later in this chapter. Give yourself 5 points each time you picked the higher-fiber choice; 70 points is the highest score you can get. The higher your score, the more fiber in your diet—if these foods truly would be your "picks" for the day!

human body into simple sugars. *For more about carbohydrates, see chapter 5.*

In dairy cows, bacteria in digestive juices break down fiber in their grassy meals, providing energy to produce milk. However, human digestive enzymes cannot break fiber into units that are small enough for absorption. That's why fiber isn't converted to energy, or calories, in your body. That very quality gives fiber its own unique roles in health. (Technically, your body can digest very small amounts of some fibers. But the amount is much too small to count.)

Not well studied, some nondigestible carbohydrates also come from animal-based foods. This type of fiber may have benefits to human health, too.

Not All Fibers Are Alike!

Soluble and insoluble: different types of fiber with different missions! What makes them unique? Soluble fiber dissolves in water, and insoluble fiber doesn't. These differing qualities allow them to keep you healthy in different ways although some major health benefits are attributed to both. With the mixture of foods people eat, about two-thirds to three-quarters of their fiber intake is likely soluble.

Insoluble Fiber: Aid to Digestion

Insoluble fiber: you know it as "roughage." This group of fibers—cellulose, hemicellulose, and lignin—gives structure to plant cell walls. Wheat bran, for example, is high in insoluble fiber.

Although they don't dissolve, insoluble fibers do hold on to water. And they move waste through the intestinal tract without being broken down themselves, earning fiber its title as "nature's broom." By adding bulk and softness to stools, insoluble fibers promote regularity and help prevent constipation. By moving waste through the colon, insoluble fibers increase the rate at which wastes are removed. This reduces the time that potentially harmful substances in waste come in contact with the intestinal lining.

Soluble Fiber: Protective Benefits

Soft, liquid foods may have fiber, too. Surprised? Instead of giving a coarse texture to food, soluble fibers, such as those in oat bran, dissolve to become gummy or viscous. They're often used in low-fat and

What Is a Whole Grain?

A whole grain is the entire edible part of any grain: wheat, corn, oats, and rice, among others. In the life cycle of plants, it's the seed from which other plants grow. Nutrients in these seeds supply the first nourishment for the plant . . . before the roots are formed. The whole grain, or seed, contains three parts: endosperm, bran, and germ.

The *bran* makes up the outer layers of the grain. It supplies antioxidants, B vitamins, trace minerals, and dietary fiber.

The *endosperm,* which is the inner part of the grain, has most of the proteins and carbohydrates, and just small amounts of vitamins and minerals. White flour is ground from the endosperm.

The *germ* is small but very important. It sprouts, generating a new plant. It has B vitamins, vitamin E, trace minerals, antioxidants, and essential fats.

It's clear why whole-grain products have more fiber; the bran and the germ supply most of the fiber. When milled to produce white flour, only the grain's endosperm remains. Most of the fibrous bran and the germ are removed—along with important nutrients and phytonutrients, including fiber.

Most foods with significant amounts of fiber—such as legumes (dry beans), whole-wheat bread, strawberries, and broccoli—are packed with carbohydrates (complex or simple) and other essential nutrients. For example, many fruits and vegetables contribute antioxidant vitamins (beta carotene and vitamin C), which may help protect against some cancers. Whole grains contain antioxidant nutrients (such as vitamin E and selenium), iron, magnesium, zinc, and B vitamins. And legumes supply protein as well as B vitamins and iron. Foods with more fiber often have less fat, too.

Most fiber-rich foods are loaded with phytonutrients that offer a wide range of health-promoting benefits. Consider this: besides fiber, whole-grain foods supply lignan, which may block estrogen activity in cells and perhaps reduce the risk of breast, ovarian, colon, and prostate cancers. Whole grains also supply phytic acid, which, by binding to minerals, may prevent free radicals from forming and perhaps reduce cancer risk. *See "Functional Nutrition: A Quick Look at Key Phytonutrients" in chapter 4, indicating those in fruits, vegetables, and grain products, and "Functional Nutrition: A Quick Look at Fiber" on page 135.*

nonfat food to add texture and consistency. Fibers called gums, mucilages, and pectin are all soluble.

If you've ever made jam or jelly, you're probably familiar with pectin. Pectin gives them their thick, gel-like consistency. In your body, pectin plays a different role, binding to fatty substances and promoting their excretion as waste. This quality seems to help lower blood cholesterol levels. Soluble fibers also help regulate the body's use of sugars.

Fiber's "Benefit Package": A Closer Look

Unlike many nutrients, life doesn't depend on fiber—but your overall health may! Fiber's "benefit package" not only promotes health, it also may help reduce the risk for some chronic diseases. The Dietary Guidelines for Americans encourage: *Choose fiber-rich fruits, vegetables, and whole grains often.*

Fiber: Bundled with Nutrients and Phytonutrients

Fiber isn't a "lonely" component of food. And fiber's benefits in food can't be easily separated from the contributions of other nutrients and plant substances.

Which Bread Is Whole Grain?

Being brown doesn't make bread whole wheat! Terms such as "7 grain" or "multigrain" are no assurance, either. Whole-grain breads usually are browner than breads made with refined white flour. However, the rich brown color may come from coloring, often listed on the label as "caramel coloring." What's more, a different grain variety called "white wheat" is used to make some whole-wheat flour. So today, some whole-wheat bread looks white. Traditionally a red wheat variety was usually used!

Finding whole-grain bread takes label skills. Any bread labeled "whole wheat" must be made with 100 percent whole-wheat flour. "Wheat bread" may contain both white refined and whole-wheat flours; proportions vary. The ingredient list gives a general idea; the flour listed first is in the greater amount. Find loaves made mostly with whole-wheat or other whole-grain flour.

Other whole-grain label clues: (1) a whole-grain health claim, which requires the product to contain 51 percent or more whole-grain ingredients by weight and (2) the Whole Grains Council's voluntary Whole Grain Stamp. *Refer to chapter 11 on labeling.* Whole-grain breads may or may not be high in fiber.

Avoiding the Trio: Constipation, Hemorrhoids, Diverticulosis

You already read about the benefits of insoluble fiber—the kind in wheat bran. It holds onto water, helping to soften and add bulk to waste in the intestines. This action helps stools pass through the intestinal tract more quickly with normal frequency and ease. As a result, fiber helps prevent constipation and the discomfort that goes with it.

When soft stools easily pass out of the body, there's no need for strained bowel movements. As a result, hemorrhoids—a painful swelling of the vein near the anus—are less likely to form. Softer, bulkier stools put less pressure on the colon walls and so reduce the chance of hemorrhoids, too. With diverticulosis, tiny sacs form when the intestinal wall, especially in the colon, gets weak. These sacs may become infected and quite painful, a problem called diverticulitis.

For more about dealing with these health conditions, see "Gastrointestinal Conditions" in chapter 22.

Cancer Connection?

Eating plenty of fiber-rich foods over the years may help prevent certain cancers. About thirty-five years ago scientists noted that some cancers were more common in Western countries where people ate less fiber. Today, research studies show strong evidence linking fiber-rich foods (vegetables, fruits, and whole grains) to cancer prevention, although their protective role is complex.

The link between a high-fiber diet and lowered risk for some cancers or polyps hasn't been clearly established, although they seem associated. Despite the inconsistency in studies, most scientific research points to consuming more fiber-rich foods.

A high-fiber diet may help reduce cancer risk in several ways: (1) by speeding the time it takes for waste to pass through the digestive tract,

(2) by forming a bulkier, heavier stool, and (3) by controlling the intestinal pH balance (the level of acidity or alkalinity). Slow movement of food waste through the digestive tract allows more time for potentially harmful substances to come in contact with intestinal walls. Bulkier stools help dilute the concentration of potential carcinogens. And insoluble fibers help keep the pH at a level that reduces the ability of intestinal microbes to produce carcinogens.

Is it fiber that protects? Or is it something else? It's difficult to know. Many fiber-rich foods supply plenty of nutrients, including antioxidant nutrients and phytonutrients. The anticancer power of fiber-rich foods may come from the interaction or the additive benefits of their many substances. In addition, a high-saturated-fat diet is associated with the risk for colon cancer. Since a high-fiber diet is usually lower in fat, it may be another reason why cancer risk seems to go down among people who eat more fiber.

FUNCTIONAL NUTRITION: A QUICK LOOK AT FIBER

DIFFERENT TYPES OF DIETARY FIBER	WHAT THEY APPEAR TO DO	WHERE THEY'RE FOUND (SOME FOOD SOURCES)
Insoluble fiber	● May contribute to maintenance of a healthy digestive tract	● Wheat bran
Beta glucan*	● May reduce the risk of coronary heart disease (CHD)	● Oat bran, rolled oats, oat flout
Soluble fiber*	● May reduce risk of CHD	● Psyllium seed husk
Whole grains*	● May reduce the risk of CHD and cancer; may contribute to maintenance of healthy blood glucose levels	● Cereal grains

*The U.S. Food and Drug Administration has approved a health claim for this food component.

Source: Adapted from International Food Information Council Foundation (2004).

Have You Ever Wondered ?

. . . which one to buy: wheat germ or wheat bran? They're two different parts of the grain, so their benefits differ. The germ is the nutrient-rich inner part, and the bran is the outer coating. From a nutritional standpoint, 1 ounce (⅓ cup) of wheat bran has a lot more fiber, about 13 grams, than the 4.4 grams of fiber in 1 ounce (¼ cup) of wheat germ. Wheat germ has more protein, and more of some vitamins and minerals.

. . . what psyllium is? (When you pronounce it, the "p" is silent.) Psyllium—high in soluble fiber—is a seed husk used in some bulk-forming natural laxatives; it also has potential cholesterol-lowering qualities. Some supplements have it. Its source is plantago, a plant that grows in India and the Mediterranean. Although some people may be allergic to psyllium, in moderate amounts it's safe for most people.

"Waistline Watchers"

Fiber-rich foods may help your body keep trim! Often they're lower in calories, fat, and added sugars, and they're less energy dense. Because they take longer to chew, fiber-rich foods may help slow your eating down, so you may eat less. With their added bulk, they help you feel full sooner, so you eat less. Fiber itself can't be fattening or provide calories—it isn't digested.

To make a fiber-rich diet work for your waistline, remember to keep your calorie intake low at the same time. (An active lifestyle is important, too.)

Help for People with Diabetes

For people with diabetes, fiber, especially soluble fiber, may perform another important function—helping to control the rise of blood sugar levels after eating. For some people with diabetes, fiber's role in blood sugar control may help reduce the need for insulin, or medication. Incorporating fiber-rich foods, including those with soluble fiber such as legumes (dry beans) and oats, into an overall healthful eating plan to manage diabetes is wise.

The reason why soluble fibers may help lower blood sugar levels isn't fully understood. Perhaps it's because fiber makes the stomach contents more viscous (more sticky and gummy) and so prolongs its emptying time.

Because carbohydrates break down more slowly, sugar is released and absorbed more slowly, too. That in turn slows the rise of blood glucose levels. *To learn more about blood sugar and its role in diabetes, see "What Is Diabetes?" in chapter 22.*

If you have diabetes and want to consume more fiber to help control blood sugars, talk to a registered dietitian or certified diabetes educator.

Fiber—Heart Healthy, Too!

Another potential benefit: Some soluble fibers (mostly beta glucan and pectin) may help lower the level of total blood cholesterol, mainly by lowering LDL cholesterol, or "bad" cholesterol. In the small intestine, soluble fiber acts like a sponge, binding cholesterol-rich bile acids. As a result, they can't be reabsorbed, but instead pass through the intestine as waste. As a result, the body absorbs less dietary cholesterol, and the liver pulls more cholesterol from the blood to replace the lost bile acids. That may make blood cholesterol levels drop.

Years of research show that soluble fibers in beans, psyllium, oats, flaxseed, and oat bran seem to help lower blood cholesterol levels in some people. In fact, there's enough sound research for the U.S. Food and Drug Administration to allow foods to carry health claims linking oats, psyllium, and whole grains with heart health. *See "Health Claims on the Label" in chapter 11 for more about health claims.* Those same high-fiber diets were lower in fat, too. What's more, these foods have other substances besides fiber that may affect the way the body uses lipids (fats). Yet another benefit: fiber-rich foods may displace fattier foods in meals and snacks.

The benefits of fiber-rich foods for heart health are truly complex. Until more is known about lowering blood cholesterol levels, continue to consume fiber-rich foods of all kinds; limit your intake of saturated fats and *trans* fats, while consuming healthful fats in moderation; maintain a healthy weight; and live a physically active lifestyle. Another area of research: a potential link between higher fiber intake and reduced blood pressure.

Tip: You need to consume a lot of soluble fiber for heart-healthy benefits. Research suggests that it takes 3 grams a day for a cholesterol-lowering effect. Here are some equivalents: 1½ cups of cooked oatmeal, *or* 1½ cups of some ready-to-eat oat bran cereals, *or* ¾ cup of uncooked oatmeal (added to meat loaf, salmon cakes, muffin batter, or as a topping for yogurt or fruit).

For more about blood cholesterol levels, see "Prevention: Cholesterol Countdown" on page 546.

Intestinal Gas: Part of Fiber's "Action"

Intestinal gas is a common complaint—and a normal side effect—of eating a high-fiber diet. If your eating plan has been typically low in fiber, minimize the discomfort that comes with "bulking up." Increase your fiber intake slowly over several months. Drink enough water, too, to help reduce the effects of intestinal gas and prevent impacted stools.

People especially complain—and sometimes joke—about beans and vegetables in the cabbage family: "They give me gas!" Gas forms in the intestines because humans lack the right enzymes to digest certain carbohydrates, leaving people feeling gassy and bloated. Other foods or ingredients reported to cause gas for some include milk, wheat germ, onions, carrots, celery, bananas, raisins, dried apricots, prune juice, and sorbitol. Sorbitol, which is slowly digested, is actually a sugar alcohol, not a sugar.

To help tame the gas caused by beans:

Label Lingo

Fiber

Although the Nutrition Facts panel on a food label gives the specific amount of fiber in foods, "fiber lingo" on the label may offer a quick description. Look for these terms as you walk the supermarket aisles:

LABEL TERM ...	MEANS ...
High fiber	5 g or more per serving
Good source	2.5 to 4.9 g per serving
More or added fiber	At least 2.5 g more* per serving

*As compared with a standard serving size of the traditional food

● When preparing dry beans, soak them overnight, then discard the soaking water. Some gas-producing carbohydrates get absorbed in the soaking water. For cooking the beans, use fresh water.

● Allow enough time to cook dry beans thoroughly. That makes them easier to digest.

● If bean dishes or other foods cause gas, take smaller helpings.

● "Degas" canned beans by draining off the liquid, then rinsing the beans. That also reduces the sodium.

If you need more relief from intestinal gas, several nonprescription products may help. Products containing charcoal, which are taken at the end of a meal, help absorb gas in the intestines. They can interfere with the absorption of medications, however, and are not recommended for children. Products with a food enzyme called alpha-galactosidase help convert gas-producing carbohydrates to more easily digestible sugars. They're sold in the form of tablets or drops taken before a meal. Products with simethicone help relieve gas symptoms but do not prevent them. This substance works by breaking large pockets of gas in the intestines into smaller bubbles.

Be aware that other gas-reducing or gas-preventing products are sold, some with questionable claims. You're wise to check with your doctor before using any gas-reduction products.

Fiber: How Much Is Enough?

If you're like most Americans, your day's meals and snacks come up short on fiber, supplying only about half (about 14 grams) the amount your body needs.

How much total fiber do you need? That depends on your age and gender. For men up to age fifty years, the Institute of Medicine advises an Adequate Intake (AI) of 38 grams daily; for women that age, it's 25 grams daily. During pregnancy and breast-feeding, the advice is slightly higher. If you're age fifty-one years or more, the AI is less: 30 grams of total fiber daily for men; 21 grams for women. *Chapter 16 gives fiber recommendations for children and teens.*

Although fiber comes from foods of plant origin, you don't need to eat huge amounts of whole-grain products, legumes, vegetables, and fruits to meet your

Defining Fiber!

If you read about fiber, you'll likely see a slew of terms: dietary fiber, functional fiber, total fiber, and a few more. What's the difference? What do they mean?

What we understand about fiber is in flux—with more to learn more about measuring food's fiber content and its many physiological effects. This includes fiber's ability to bind cholesterol, how it speeds intestinal transit time to protect against cancer and constipation, and how its fermentation benefits digestive health. These issues impact how we talk about fiber.

The Institute of Medicine's (IOM) Dietary Reference Intakes use "total fiber," defined as dietary fiber plus functional fiber. In this book, "dietary fiber" is the fiber that's naturally present in plant-based foods. Also with health benefits, "functional fiber" is manufactured from plant or animal products. For example, inulin and FOS (fructooligosaccharides or frucan) work as prebiotics; methylcellulose is a bulking agent.

For labeling "dietary fiber" is used, yet its definition differs around the world. As more is learned, fiber's definitions will be clarified. In the future clearer terms will likely be used rather than the terms "soluble fiber" and "insoluble fiber," too; after all, most foods have both types of fiber. Nutrition truly is an evolving science!

fiber goal. By following the advice of MyPyramid, your everyday food choices can supply all you need if you eat more fruits and vegetables, and make at least half your grain food choices whole. *Check the chart "How Much Fiber?" later in this chapter to "guesstimate" your fiber intake.* You'll see that most of the grain products, fruits, and vegetables you eat have only 1 to 3 grams of fiber per standard serving.

However, when it comes to fiber, you can overdo a good thing! Too much fiber can move food through the digestive tract faster than some nutrients can be absorbed. By eating more than 50 to 60 grams of fiber a day, your body may lower the absorption of vitamins and minerals, among them zinc, iron, magnesium, and calcium. An excessive amount of fiber may cause gas, diarrhea, and bloating. By filling up with too many high-fiber foods or supplements, you may not have an appetite for other nutrient-rich foods. As an aside, since fiber makes food bulky, most people feel full before they eat too much.

How might you get too much fiber? By eating a lot of bran, very-high-fiber cereals, or perhaps using a fiber supplement in an eating plan that already has plenty of vegetables, fruits, and whole grains!

For Fiber—Variety!

As laboratory procedures have improved, consumers now know the "dietary fiber" content of food, which reflects both soluble and insoluble fiber. Today you'll find dietary fiber listed on the Nutrition Facts on the labels of most packaged food products.

Foods for Fiber

Do you like to nibble on popcorn? It's a whole-grain snack that helps boost fiber in your diet. Again, dietary fiber comes only from plant sources of food: fruits, vegetables, legumes, grains, nuts, and seeds. Plant-based foods actually contain a "mixed bag" of dietary fibers, having some of both types: soluble and insoluble. Good sources of soluble fiber may supply some insoluble fiber, too, and vice versa. For example, fruits and vegetables have both pectin (soluble) and cellulose (insoluble). However, fruit usually has more pectin; vegetables, more cellulose. Both oatmeal and beans have some of both: soluble and insoluble fiber.

Have You Ever Wondered

. . . if "whole grain" is "high fiber"? And if "high fiber" is "whole grain"? In either case, not necessarily. First, the amount of fiber differs naturally in different types of grain, depending on their proportion of bran, germ, and endosperm. Other ingredients and moisture in whole-grain foods also affect fiber content. Second, high-fiber foods, such as bran cereals, may have more fiber even though they aren't whole grain. For fiber content, read the label's Nutrition Facts; if a label serving has 20 percent or more Daily Value, it's "high fiber." As another clue, check for a whole-grain labeling claim, *described in chapter 11.*

. . . if cornmeal is whole grain? Yes—but only if it's made with the whole corn kernel. Cornmeal that's labeled "degerminated" or "degermed" has been refined; it's not whole grain.

Have You Ever Wondered

. . . what grains are whole grain? Buckwheat, brown rice, bulgur, whole kernel corn (hominy), millet, popcorn, quinoa, sorghum, triticale, whole oats and oatmeal, wheat berries, whole barley (not pearl barley), whole rye, and whole wheat are more common whole grains in the United States. Cracked wheat is whole berry wheat, too—just broken into coarse, medium, or fine particles.

. . . what graham flour is? It's a whole-wheat flour that's a little coarser than regular whole-wheat flour. Try it!

(Beta glucan is the soluble fiber in oats and barley.)

These foods provide significant amounts of insoluble and soluble fibers. Their texture is a clue.

● *Insoluble fibers:* whole-wheat products; wheat, oat, and corn bran; flaxseeds; and many vegetables (such as cauliflower, green beans, and potatoes), including the skins of fruits and root vegetables, and beans. In fact, their tough, chewy texture comes from insoluble fibers.

● *Soluble fibers:* dried beans and peas, oats, barley, flaxseeds, and many fruits and vegetables (such as apples, oranges, and carrots). When cooked, their soft, mushy texture comes from their soluble fibers. Psyllium seed husks also supply soluble fiber.

For the record: Any nondigestible carbohydrate in animal-based foods is not currently defined as "dietary fiber" on food labels. But stay tuned in the future for possible changes in fiber labeling on food.

From grain to grain, brans aren't all alike. The bran layers in different grains—wheat, rice, corn, oats, and others—have varying types and different amounts of fiber. Wheat bran, for example, has a higher concentration of fiber than most other bran, and its bran is mainly insoluble. To compare, oat bran contains mainly soluble fiber.

The fiber content of vegetables and fruits varies; some are better sources than others. A heaping bowl of fresh lettuce greens may seem loaded with fiber. However, one cup of lettuce contains just about 1 gram of fiber; instead, it's mostly water. In contrast, ½ cup of a three-bean salad (mainly legumes) supplies more than 3 fiber grams.

Food preparation or processing also may affect the fiber content of foods. Just as a sponge changes in its ability to hold water when it's chopped into very fine pieces, so properties of fiber may change a bit when the structure is altered by food processing or preparation. Fiber content drops, too, when the fiber-rich part of a food is removed. *See "Which Apple for Fiber?" to compare the fiber content in different forms of an apple, including juice.*

When it comes to making food choices, don't get hung up on which fiber is which—just consume enough overall. Enjoy a variety of plant-based foods: vegetables (including legumes), fruits, whole-grain foods, and nuts. Minimally processed foods are generally better fiber sources.

Have You Ever Wondered

. . . if soybeans are a good fiber source, what about tofu? Half a cup of soybeans has more than 5 grams of fiber. That's great! But when soybeans are processed to make tofu, fibrous substances are strained out, and what's left is high in soy protein. Half a cup of tofu has only less than 1 gram of fiber.

. . . what's the difference between a lignin and a lignan? The terms often get confused. Classified as an insoluble fiber, lignin actually isn't a carbohydrate but a complex molecule that's a woody part of the stems and seeds of fruits and vegetables and the bran in cereals. Its properties may help prevent cancers. Lignans are phytonutrients found in whole grains and flaxseeds; research is examining their roles as phytoestrogens and anticancer agents.

. . . if oat bran has "magic" that defies heart disease? Since the early 1980s research has shown that soluble fiber in oat bran has a blood cholesterol-lowering effect. That's why it's been added to breakfast cereals, muffins, and other foods. Its soluble fiber may be just one of the heart-healthy benefits of foods made with oat bran. Regardless, no single food, not even oat bran, offers ultimate protection. Your overall eating plan, including oat bran and other high-fiber foods, along with less fat (especially saturated fat), offers the benefits!

Which Apple for Fiber?

Apple juice, applesauce, a whole apple—which has the most fiber? An apple of any variety with the peel on has more fiber than an apple without the peel. And as food changes form, its fiber content may change, too.

1 whole medium apple with peel	3.3 grams fiber
1 whole medium apple without peel	1.7 grams fiber
½ cup applesauce	1.5 grams fiber
¾ cup apple juice	0.2 gram fiber

Need a Fiber Boost?

Try to eat 4½ cups of fruit and vegetables daily if you eat 2,000 calories daily, and slightly more if you need more calories. And make at least half your grain choices whole: equal to 3 ounces of whole-grain foods or more each day. Consume legumes often (about 3 cups a week). With that you can meet your fiber goal!

If you boost your fiber intake, do so gradually! Give the bacteria in your stomach and intestines time to adjust. If you add more fiber to your diet too quickly— or consume too much on a regular basis—you may end up with gas, diarrhea, cramps, and bloating.

Drink plenty of water and other fluids, too, when you eat extra fiber. Remember that fiber acts like a large sponge in your colon. It holds water as it keeps waste moving along. That's how it helps prevent constipation and related intestinal problems. For fiber to do its job, you need to consume enough fluids. *How much fluid a day? Refer to chapter 8.*

Caution: Before You Boost Fiber in Meals and Snacks . . .

For young children: Eating a lot of high-fiber foods may fill young children up too quickly. That may take away their appetite for other nutritious foods with nutrients their bodies need for proper growth. Excessive amounts of fiber also may interfere with their body's absorption of vitamins and minerals.

For elderly people and people who have had gastrointestinal surgery: If you're older than sixty-five or have had surgery on some part of your stomach, intestines, colon, or rectum, check with your doctor before adding fiber to your meals and snacks. You may feel the effects of added fiber more than others.

Supplement Watch: About Fiber Pills and Powders . . .

Should you take a fiber supplement—or not? Depending on the supplement, adding a fiber pill or powder to the foods you already eat may not make much difference to your health, although it may help relieve constipation. Fiber-rich foods can supply more fiber than many fiber pills do. Also, supplements with fiber may inhibit the absorption of some minerals—a problem for people whose diets are nutrient-deficient. If you decide to take fiber supplements for "regularity," your body might come to rely on them.

In contrast, fiber-rich foods—whole-grain foods, fruits, legumes, and vegetables—provide the added benefits associated with a high-fiber diet: little or no fat, especially saturated fat, and a good supply of other nutrients. Fiber pills and powders don't add benefits.

Can fiber supplements help you lose weight and keep weight off? No scientific evidence supports this claim. You can't trick your appetite in the long run. Rather than fiber pills and powders, choose a low-fat, high-fiber diet with plenty of fruits, vegetables, whole-grain foods, and beans to get the fullness feeling. Research doesn't show a link between fiber supplements and reduced cancer risk, either.

Ten Great Ways to "Fiber Up"!

Are you ready to eat more fiber? These ten tips can put your day's food choices within range.

1. Eat a variety of foods. You'll benefit from a mix of fibers—both soluble and insoluble.

Need more strategies for fitting fiber in? Check here for "how-tos":

- Shop for whole-grain and fiber-rich foods—see chapter 11.

- Boost the fiber factor in your food preparation—see chapter 13.

HOW MUCH FIBER?

	SERVING SIZE*	CALORIES	DIETARY FIBER (G) TOTAL
Fruits			
Apple	1 medium	75	3.3
Applesauce	½ cup	95	1.5
Apple juice	¾ cup	85	0.2
Banana	1 medium	105	3.1
Blueberries	½ cup	40	1.7
Cantaloupe	½ cup	30	0.8
Cherries	10	45	1.4
Dates (dried)	5	115	3.3
Figs (dried)	3	65	2.5
Fruit cocktail	½ cup	55	1.2
Grapefruit	½ medium	50	2.0
Grapes	½ cup	55	0.7
Grape juice	¾ cup	115	0.2
Kiwifruit	1 medium	45	2.3
Orange	1 medium	60	3.1
Orange juice	¾ cup	80	0.4
Prunes (dried plums)	5	100	3.0
Peach	1 medium	40	1.5
Pineapple	½ cup	40	1.1
Pear	1 medium	95	5.1
Raisins	¼ cup	125	1.5
Raspberries	½ cup	30	4.0
Strawberries	½ cup	25	1.7
Watermelon	½ cup	25	0.3
Vegetables, cooked			
Asparagus	½ cup	20	1.8
Broccoli	½ cup	25	2.6
Brussels sprouts	½ cup	35	3.2
Corn	½ cup	90	2.2
Green beans	½ cup	20	2.0
Peas	½ cup	65	4.4
Potato (mashed)	½ cup	120	1.6
Potato (baked, plain, with skin)	1 medium	160	3.8
Spinach	½ cup	20	2.2
Sweet potato (baked, plain)	1 medium	105	3.8
Zucchini	½ cup	15	1.3
Vegetables, raw			
Carrot	1 medium	25	1.7
Celery	1 medium stalk	5	0.6
Cucumber (sliced)	½ cup	10	0.3
Lettuce (romaine)	1 cup	10	1.0
Mushrooms (sliced)	½ cup	10	0.3
Spinach	1 cup	5	0.7
Tomato	1 medium	20	1.5
Legumes, cooked			
Baked beans (vegetarian)	½ cup	120	5.2
Garbanzo beans (chickpeas)	½ cup	135	6.2
Kidney beans	½ cup	110	6.5
Lentils	½ cup	115	7.8
Navy beans	½ cup	125	9.6
Soybeans	½ cup	150	5.2

HOW MUCH FIBER? *(continued)*

	SERVING SIZE*	CALORIES	DIETARY FIBER (G) TOTAL
Breads, grains, pasta			
Bagel	½ (3½-in. diameter)	90	0.8
Barley, cooked	½ cup	95	3.0
Bread, whole wheat	1 slice	70	1.9
Bread, pumpernickel	1 slice	65	1.7
Bread sticks	2 (4½-in.) sticks	40	0.3
Bread, French	1 slice, small	90	1.0
Bread, white	1 slice	65	0.6
Bun (hamburger or hot dog)	½	60	0.5
Pasta (cooked)	½ cup	110	1.3
Pita	½ (6½-in. diameter)	80	0.7
Rice, brown (cooked)	½ cup	110	1.8
Rice, white (cooked)	½ cup	120	0.3
Breakfast cereals			
100% bran	1 oz.	85	8.3
Bran flakes	1 oz.	95	5.3
Corn flakes	1 oz.	100	1.3
Granola	1 oz.	140	2.4
Oatmeal (cooked)	½ cup	75	2.0
Puffed rice	1 oz.	115	0.5
Raisin bran	1 oz.	90	3.4
Whole grain oats cereal	1 oz.	105	2.9
Snacks			
Corn chips	1 oz.	140	1.5
Hummus dip	2 tbsp.	45	1.5
Peanuts (dry roasted)	¼ cup	215	2.9
Popcorn (air-popped, plain)	3 cups	95	3.5
Pretzels	1 oz.	110	0.8
Sunflower seeds	¼ cup	185	3.6
Walnuts	¼ cup	190	2.0
Added ingredients			
Flaxseeds, ground	1 tbsp.	35	1.9
Gums	0.1 oz.	5	2.8
Oat bran	1 tbsp.	15	0.9
Psyllium	1 tbsp.	5	6.0
Rice bran	1 tbsp.	25	1.5
Seaweed	1 tbsp.	1	0.1
Wheat bran	1 tbsp.	10	1.6
Wheat germ	1 tbsp.	25	0.9

*The serving sizes are standardized amounts often used in dietary guidance or for comparing similar foods.

Source: U.S. Department of Agriculture, Agricultural Research Service, 2005. *USDA National Nutrient Database for Standard Reference*, Release 18.

2. Check the food label. Nutrition Facts on food labels can help you find foods with more fiber. Look for words such as "high in fiber" or "more fiber" on labels, too. *See "Label Lingo: Fiber" earlier in this chapter to see what these claims mean.* Spot fiber-rich ingredients on the ingredient list. Look for "bran," "whole grain," or "whole-wheat flour," too.

3. Remember breakfast—a good time for fiber-rich foods. Besides bran cereal or another fiber-rich breakfast cereal, enjoy oatmeal, whole-bran muffins, whole-wheat waffles, or fiber-rich breakfast/cereal bars. Check food labels for a cereal with 5 or more grams of fiber per serving. Top with fruit for a little more fiber.

4. Switch to whole grains—in bread, cereals, buns,

bagels, crackers, and pasta, to name a few—at least some of the time. Make at least half of your Grains Group choices whole grain! For breads, that includes cornbread from whole, ground cornmeal; cracked wheat bread; oatmeal bread; pumpernickel bread; rye bread; and the perennial favorite, whole-wheat bread. Eat breads made with bran, too, such as bran muffins.

5. Give brown rice a try sometimes, or mix half brown and half white rice.

6. Plan to eat legumes (dry beans) several times a week. They're among the best fiber sources around. And they add flavor and texture to dishes.

7. Fit in fruits and veggies: about 4½ cups total a day, if you eat 2,000 calories a day. You might plan cooked vegetables and a salad for dinner, whole fruit and carrot sticks for lunch. How about a fruit or veggie snack?

8. Enjoy fruits and vegetables with the edible skin on. With the skin, a medium potato has 3.8 grams of fiber. Skinless, it has less—2.3 grams. Also enjoy the flavor and crunch of edible seeds—for example, in all kinds of berries, kiwifruit, and figs. They, too, supply fiber.

9. Choose whole fruit more often than juice. Fiber comes mainly from the peel and pulp; usually both are removed when juice is made. Juice usually has almost no fiber.

10. "Fiberize" your cooking style. Substitute higher-fiber ingredients in recipes, such as using part whole-wheat flour in baked food. And fortify mixed dishes with high-fiber ingredients, perhaps bran or oatmeal added to meat loaf or ground flaxseeds added to baked goods.

Refer to "Cooking Grain by Grain" in chapter 13.

Legumes: A Nutritious Fiber Source

All over the world, people eat and enjoy beans, peas, and other legumes! Legumes come from plants whose seed pods split on two sides when they're ripe.

Because they're a nutritious, flavorful, and inexpensive protein source and because they're easy to grow and store, legumes have been a staple for thousands of years. Today we recognize another benefit. Besides their versatility, legumes are among the

world's best fiber sources! No matter what the variety or form (fresh, frozen, canned, or dried), legumes are loaded with proteins, starches (complex carbohydrates), and fiber, along with B vitamins (including folate), iron, other vitamins and minerals, and phytonutrients.

In MyPyramid, legumes fit into the Meat and Beans Group and the Vegetable Group, but not both at the same time. Choose one. Like meat, they're good protein sources. One-quarter cup of cooked legumes (beans or lentils) counts as 1 ounce of meat; 5 to 7 ounces are recommended daily. One-half cup of cooked legumes count as ½ cup of vegetables.

Cooking a Pot o' Beans

If you're short on time, go for canned, frozen, or fresh beans. If not, try the traditional way, by soaking dry beans first. *Tip:* Dry legumes need soaking; lentils or split peas don't.

To soak beans, do this:

● *Leisurely method.* Reduce cooking time by up to half by soaking beans for at least four hours or overnight in a pot filled with room-temperature water. Choose a pot that's big enough; beans expand!

● *Quick method.* Time short? Then bring water to a boil, and let beans soak in hot water for one to four hours, depending on the variety of beans.

To reduce the gas you might experience, rinse beans, discard the soaking water and any debris, and cook in fresh water. Not to worry—the beans, not the soaking water, retain most of the essential nutrients.

To cook, cover beans with fresh water: about 6 cups of fresh water for each pound of dry beans. Add seasonings to the cooking water. Salt toughens beans by taking out the moisture; and acid foods, such as tomatoes or vinegar, slow their softening. Wait until the end of the cooking time to add these ingredients.

Cover the pot partially. To keep legumes from foaming as they cook, add a little cooking oil (¼ teaspoon) to the water. Simmer beans until they're cooked. *See the chart "Bean Bag" in this chapter for simmering times.* Add cooked beans or peas to your favorite dish.

BEAN BAG

Beans of all kinds are sold as dried, canned, frozen, and fresh. Each type has a distinctive appearance and flavor, varying cooking times, and somewhat different uses. Use of a variety bag that includes several types of beans is an easy way to taste the flavors of many types of different beans.

On average, 1 pound of dry beans equals about 2¼ cups of dry beans, or 5 to 6 cups of cooked beans. The yield for lentils is less; for 2¼ cups of dry lentils, figure about 3½ to 4 cups cooked. One can (15½ ounces) of drained, canned beans or lentils equals about 1⅔ cups cooked. As an aside, rinsing canned beans reduces the sodium content by 23 to 45 percent.

BEANS AND PEAS	SIZE AND COLOR	FLAVOR	SIMMERING TIME (HOURS)*	COMMON USES†
Adzuki or azuki bean	Small, red, shiny	Slightly sweet	½ to 1	Salads, poultry stuffing, casseroles, soups
Black bean	Small, black, shiny, kidney-shaped	Slightly sweet	1½ to 2	Stew, soup, Brazilian *feijoada*, Cuban rice and beans
Black-eyed pea or cowpea	Small, cream-colored, ovals with black spots	Vegetablelike, full-flavored	1 to 1½	Southern dishes with ham or rice, bean cakes, curries, *Hoppin' John*
Cannellini or white kidney bean	Elongated, slender, creamy white	Mild	2	Soups, stews, salads, casseroles, Italian side dishes, *pasta e fagioli*
Chickpea, or garbanzo bean	Golden, hard, pea-shaped	Nutty	2¼ to 4	Casseroles, cooked with couscous, soups, stews, *hummus, caldo gallego*
Fava or broad bean	Broad, large, oval, light brown	Nutty	1½ to 2	Stews, side dishes
Flageolet or green haricot bean	Small to medium, pale green	Nutty	1½ to 2	Mixed bean salads, vegetable side dish
Great northern	Large, white	Mild	1 to 1½	Soups, casseroles, mixed bean dishes
Lentils‡	Yellow, green, or orange	Earthy	¾	Soup, *pease pudding, dhal,* curry dishes
Lima bean	Large or small, creamy white or pale green, kidney-shaped	Like chestnuts	1½	Casseroles, soups, salads, *succotash*
Mung bean	Small, olive green	Earthy	1	Soups, casseroles, purees, Asian and Indian dishes, "sprouted" for salads
Navy bean	Small, oval, white	Mild	1 to 1½	*Boston baked beans*
Pigeon pea	Small, round, slightly flat, beige, brown flecks	Mild	¾ to 1	Caribbean peas and rice
Pinto bean	Orange-pink, with rust-colored flecks, oval	Earthy, full-flavored	1 to 1½	*Mexican rice and beans, refried beans,* stew
Red kidney bean	Dark, red-brown, kidney-shaped	Full-flavored, "meaty"	1½ to 2	Stew, mixed bean salad, Cajun bean dishes, *chili con carne*
Soybean	Small, yellow or black	Full-flavored	3½ to 4	Side dish, soups, used to make tofu (bean curd), "sprouted" for salads

*Simmering time for dry beans.

†Traditional and ethnic dishes, italicized throughout the chart, commonly use the type of bean indicated.

‡Lentils don't require soaking, only shorter cooking times.

CHAPTER 7

Sodium and Potassium
A Salty Subject

From your doctor, the media, and government experts, you've heard the messages: "Check food labels for sodium," "Cook with less salt," "Put away the salt shaker." These are today's headlines. Yet salt has made news for centuries!

Throughout recorded history, salt has played an important economic and political role—and has always been part of the world's food supply. Until the past two hundred years, salt was used heavily for preserving foods: meat, fish, vegetables, and even fruit. Cheese, too, was salted more than it is today. Especially in Mediterranean regions, cooks used herbs and spices to mask strong, salty flavors from preservation. Nations that controlled the salt trade also controlled distribution and preservation of food, especially in times of shortage.

The ancient Greeks valued salt so highly that they used it for currency. Salt was even traded for slaves, hence the phrase "He's not worth his salt." Originally Roman soldiers were given a handful of salt every day. Later they received money to buy their own salt, which was referred to as *salarium argentum;* that means "salt money." The word "salary" in English is derived from this Latin term.

Because of its value, salt historically has been used symbolically, too. To the ancient Romans, salt given to a newborn symbolized the giving of wisdom. In Europe, a pinch of salt tossed three times over the left shoulder helped fend off evil. Even today, we reflect our doubts with the comment "Take it with a grain of salt."

Until the late 1700s, salty flavors were common due to their use in food preservation. In the nineteenth century, tastes began to change, and people preferred less salty foods. Concurrently, other food preservation methods got started: canning, freezing, and refrigeration. By the twentieth century, commercially available canning, freezing, and refrigeration combined with the transportation system enabled people to have a variety of foods at any time of year. Today most salt is used for industrial purposes rather than in the food supply.

In ancient times, salt's ability to preserve food helped provide a varied supply of nutrients to the population. Any other link to health or to ongoing health problems, such as high blood pressure, was unknown. As science advanced, we've learned that the blood pressure of some people may be sensitive to salt, or to the sodium it's made from. And now we recognize that the blood pressure link to nutrition may be more complex, with potassium, magnesium, and calcium also playing a role.

Did you know . . .

. . . 1 teaspoon of salt contains about 2,300 milligrams of sodium?

. . . most sodium that Americans consume comes from processed or prepared food, not from the salt shaker at the kitchen table?

. . . a preference for salty foods is acquired?

. . . you can cut back on salt in your food choices without giving up flavor?

Sodium, Potassium, and Your Health

Salt . . . or sodium? Although we often refer to them in the same breath, salt and sodium aren't the same thing. Table salt is actually the common name for "sodium chloride." It's 40 percent sodium and 60 percent chloride. And potassium? Like sodium and chloride, it's an essential mineral, too.

Sodium and Potassium: You Need Them!

The link between sodium and high blood pressure is well publicized, yet few people know the flip side of the sodium story—why sodium is essential to health.

Sodium is a mineral that occurs naturally in food. Some of the most basic work your body does depends on sodium: maintaining proper fluid balance—controlling the movement of fluids in and out of your cells; regulating your blood pressure; transmitting nerve impulses; and helping your muscles, including your heart muscle, relax.

Sodium, along with other minerals such as chloride and potassium, are collectively called electrolytes. They get their name because they transmit electrical current in your body. You can compare them to electrically charged particles, or ions, in flashlight batteries.

If you lick your upper lip after sweating a lot, you know that body fluids have salt. You can taste it! Sodium, chloride, and potassium dissolve in body fluids, where they become separate ions. With their electrical charge, they transmit nerve impulses throughout your body. And they send messages from your brain to your muscles, causing them to relax or to contract.

Have you ever sprinkled salt on a sliced eggplant or potato, then watched the liquid come to its outer surface? Salt drew fluid out of the plant cells. That same reaction happens with electrolytes in your body. They control the balance of fluids in and out of cells. Sodium and chloride mostly work outside your body cells, and potassium works mainly inside. Together they regulate the balance of fluids.

Fluid balance—moving fluid in and out of cells—has important health implications. Among them, electrolytes help move nutrients into cells and help take

wastes away. Both nutrients and wastes are carried in body fluids.

For more about these minerals, see "Major Minerals: Electrolytes" in chapter 4.

Sodium: Keeping the Balance

Your kidneys regulate the sodium level in your body. If you're healthy, your body doesn't retain excess sodium—even when you consume more than you need. And excess amounts don't get stored.

Instead your body rids itself of the extra. Excess sodium passes out through urine and, to a much lesser extent, through perspiration. If, for example, you eat foods high in sodium, you may urinate more. Then you probably feel thirsty because you lost fluids, too.

Is extra sodium always removed? No. When kidneys don't work properly, perhaps due to kidney disease, extra sodium isn't excreted. This causes swelling, often in the face, legs, and feet. In medical terms, this swelling is called edema.

Can you have a sodium deficiency? Yes, but this doesn't happen under normal circumstances. However, if a person vomits or has diarrhea for a prolonged period, or if he or she has a kidney problem, sodium levels might get too low. Unless sweating is profuse and extended over a long time and the person drinks a lot of water, sodium levels will remain normal if healthy. Your body conserves sodium when your intake is low, but it is less effective with potassium. Make up for it with more potassium-rich foods.

Links to Blood Pressure

High blood pressure, or hypertension, is a major risk factor for heart disease, stroke, kidney failure, and other conditions. It affects about 65 million Americans ages six years and over—and about one-third of adults. Many don't know it. Are you at risk? These are some factors linked to high blood pressure: family history of high blood pressure, overweight, excessive alcohol intake, advancing age, and smoking.

Why is attention given to sodium? There's a direct, progressive link between increased high blood pressure and sodium intake. For many people, high-sodium intake is one dietary factor linked to high blood pressure or perhaps its early prehypertension stage. Likewise, reducing sodium intake may help to lower blood pressure if it's high.

Regarding blood pressure, there are other nutrition angles to consider. Three other minerals may be just as important in regulating blood pressure: potassium from fruits and vegetables; calcium from dairy foods and some vegetables; and magnesium from whole grains, legumes, nuts, and green vegetables.

Although the scientific reasons aren't yet fully understood, foods high in potassium may help protect against high blood pressure. Potassium appears to blunt the effect of sodium on blood pressure.

In fact, the DASH (Dietary Approaches to Stop Hypertension) plan—an eating plan that's low in fat, with low-fat and fat-free dairy foods and plenty of vegetables and fruits—may help lower blood pressure, even among people within the "normal" range. *See chapter 22 for normal blood pressure ranges.* The reason is unclear; it may be that the DASH approach to eating is high in potassium, calcium, and magnesium.

For some people, even 2,300 milligrams (the upper daily recommended level) for sodium may be too much. In the DASH-Sodium study supported by the National Heart, Lung, and Blood Institute of the National Institutes of Health, people who followed

---

Potassium: Another Reason for Fruits and Veggies!

Fruits and vegetables are among the best sources of potassium, a mineral that helps normalize blood pressure. Here are some fruits and vegetables that are good potassium sources:

Apricot	Potato
Banana	Prunes (dried plums)
Broccoli	Raisins
Cantaloupe	Spinach
Carrot	Sweet potato
Dates	Swiss chard
Mushrooms	Watermelon
Orange	Winter squash
Parsnip	

Other good potassium sources: Dry beans, lentils, peas, almonds, and peanuts. Milk and yogurt supply calcium and potassium, perhaps protecting against high blood pressure.

Note: Potassium chloride, as a salt substitute, isn't recommended. Unless used under medical supervision, it can be harmful to health.

Have You Ever Wondered

... how you know if you're sodium-sensitive? There's no way yet to predict who may have blood pressure that's sodium-sensitive. Your best clue? Check your family history. If you have a blood relative who controls blood pressure with antihypertensive or diuretic drugs, or a low-sodium diet, that's one hint. Often the condition is inherited. (Diuretics help the body get rid of excess fluids and so help control high blood pressure.) African Americans and older adults are among those at higher risk.

... if a high-salt diet is okay if you're not salt-sensitive? Moderation is always a better rule of thumb for anything you eat, so it's wise to be sensible. Choose and prepare foods with little salt, and hedge your bets with the DASH approach to eating: dairy foods, plenty of fruit and vegetables, whole-grain foods and low-fat foods. The body excretes more calcium in urine when salt intake is high. To help lower calcium loss, cut back on salt.

---

the DASH plan diet and lowered their sodium intake to 1,500 milligrams daily had even better blood-pressure-lowering results—especially if they had hypertension. *To learn more, see "Blood Pressure: Under Control?" and specifically "DASH to Health" in chapter 22.*

Consider following the DASH plan whether or not you have high blood pressure. If you have it or some other health condition, your doctor might recommend less sodium than you consume now. Consult your doctor for the right sodium level for you, and a registered dietitian (RD) to help you follow this advice.

Research suggests another benefit of cutting back on salt: possibly less calcium loss from bone, and as a result, reduced risk of osteoporosis and bone fractures.

Sodium and Potassium: How Much Is Enough?

To keep your body running normally, you need sodium. But you likely consume more than enough. On average most adults consume about 3,200 milligrams of sodium daily. There's no known advantage to consuming this much. Those at risk for or with high blood pressure are better off with less.

How much then? The Institute of Medicine's Daily Reference Intakes recommend a maximum for sodium intake: for the general public the Tolerable Upper Intake Level is 2,300 milligrams of sodium daily, and somewhat less for children ages thirteen and under. That's about the amount in 1 teaspoon of salt.

The Dietary Guidelines say *less than* 2,300 milligrams is better. In fact, for most healthy people ages nine to fifty, the Adequate Intake (AI) of 1,500 milligrams of sodium daily is enough. The AI is somewhat less for adults over age fifty and children eight years and under. Getting enough other nutrients, including potassium, isn't easy, however, in an eating plan at 1,500 milligrams of sodium daily.

When you sweat after strenuous physical activity, do you need extra salt—from the salt shaker, a salt tablet, or a sports drink? Probably not. Food eaten after exertion normally replenishes sodium lost in sweat. That said, sodium's AI level doesn't apply to highly active people, such as those doing endurance sports.

What's the potassium recommendation? For ages fourteen on up, the AI is 4,700 milligrams daily.

Note: For people with hypertension, African Americans, and middle-aged and older adults, the Dietary Guidelines advise: *Aim to consume no more than 1,500 milligrams of sodium per day, and meet the potassium recommendation (4,700 milligrams per day) with food.*

Advice . . . Even for Healthy People

As part of the healthful eating message, the Dietary Guidelines for Americans advise: *Choose and prepare foods with little salt.* It's the best way to cut back on sodium. *At the same time, consume potassium-rich foods, such as fruits and vegetables.*

Why is this advice given to healthy people? For one, there's no way to tell if your blood pressure is sodium-sensitive. You may—or may not—develop high blood pressure from consuming too much sodium. So stick to the recommendation. Second, consuming less sodium or little salt certainly isn't harmful to healthy adults. Even if you don't have high blood pressure now, cutting back may offer protection, just in case.

Sodium in Your Food Choices

Salt and sodium—are they just in food for flavor? Or do they have other roles, too? It's easier to spot foods with salt or sodium if you know what they do.

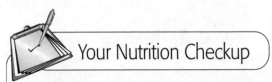

Your Nutrition Checkup

Sodium: A Healthful "Shake"

You know the guideline for healthful eating: *Choose and prepare foods with little salt.* How have you addressed this "salty issue"? Check off the tips that apply to your approach to eating. *Do you . . .*

☐ Shake a little salt on your food only *after* you taste it?

☐ Enjoy plenty of fresh vegetables?

☐ Keep the salt shaker in the cabinet, not on the table or kitchen counter where it's easier to use?

☐ Skip the salt in cooking water—for pasta, rice, and vegetables?

☐ Season food mostly with herbs and spices?

☐ Read Nutrition Facts on food labels to check the amount of sodium in food and buy foods with less?

☐ Consider the salt or sodium in restaurant food or fast food if you eat out regularly?

☐ Enjoy processed meats such as corned beef, ham, bacon, bologna, salami, hot dogs, and pastrami only occasionally?

☐ Buy brands of prepared foods and snack foods that have reduced sodium or salt or no added salt?

☐ Go easy on condiments such as mustard, ketchup, soy sauce, and tartar sauce, or use brands with less sodium?

☐ Balance your food choices: if you enjoy some foods with more sodium, also eat others with less?

How many boxes did you check?

If you said yes to . . .

Nine to eleven items: you're likely consuming moderate amounts of sodium and salt. Read on for more ideas.

Six to eight items: you're controlling the sodium and salt in your food choices but may be able to "shake the sodium habit" even more. Read on.

Five or fewer items: it's time to read on and try the tips in this chapter to consume a healthful amount of salt and potassium.

Salt and Sodium: More Than Flavor

Why are salt and other sodium-containing ingredients added in food preparation and processing? Flavor probably comes to mind first. Just a few grains of salt can bring out food's natural flavors—even in sweet foods. However, sodium-containing ingredients play a broader role in the food supply.

● Before the days of refrigeration, people relied on salt to *preserve* many foods. Salt and sodium-containing ingredients preserve food by inhibiting the growth of bacteria, yeast, and molds—and so prevent food spoilage and foodborne illness.

Even today, many cured foods use salt or an ingredient made with sodium (such as sodium nitrate) as a preservative. For example, ham, sausage, corned beef, and Canadian bacon are cured meats. Another way to preserve vegetables is to soak them in brine, or a solution of water and salt. Eat pickles? Cucumbers and okra are pickled in brine.

● In many foods, salt *affects the texture*. For example, yeast breads with salt have a finer texture; salt-free yeast breads tend to be coarser.

● In some foods, such as cheese, bread dough, and sauerkraut, salt *controls the speed of fermentation*. Fermentation changes the chemistry of food, and as a result its appearance and flavor.

● In whipping egg whites or cream, a pinch of salt *increases and stabilizes the volume*.

● In processed meats, including sausage, salt and sodium-containing ingredients *help hold meat together*.

Have You Ever Wondered

. . . if rinsing canned beans reduces the sodium content? If you rinse canned vegetables, including beans, in a strainer under cool running water, you can reduce their sodium content by 23 to 45 percent. The rest remains. You also rinse away some nutrients, such as some B vitamins, that leach from vegetables into the canning liquid.

. . . if celery has a lot of sodium? Many people think so. But a celery stalk has just 35 milligrams of sodium.

Where Does Sodium Come From?

Many people think their taste buds offer all the clues they need to the sodium content of food. However, you can't always judge food's sodium content by its taste! Many foods with sodium don't have a salty flavor.

A shake here and a shake there—the amount of salt we sprinkle on food can add up quickly. The same is true for sodium-containing condiments such as soy sauce, mustard, and tartar sauce. However, only about 11 percent of the sodium in the food most people eat comes from the salt shaker or from sodium added during cooking or at the table.

Prepared foods are the main sources of sodium in the average American diet: about 77 percent. Because salt and sodium-containing ingredients serve several functions in the food supply, it's not surprising that processed foods contain varying levels of sodium. For example, two cookies or crackers may have 25 to 270 milligrams of sodium. A frozen dinner might vary from 550 to 1,300 milligrams of sodium. And two

Ingredients with Sodium	What They Do
Baking soda (sodium bicarbonate)	Leavening agent
Baking powder	Leavening agent
Brine (salt and water)	Preservative
Disodium phosphate	Emulsifier, stabilizer
Monosodium glutamate (MSG)	Flavor enhancer
NaCl (salt or sodium chloride)	Flavor enhancer, preservative
Sodium benzoate	Preservative
Sodium caseinate	Thickener, binder
Sodium citrate	Acid controller, stabilizer
Sodium erythorbate	Antioxidant
Sodium nitrate/nitrite	Preservative
Sodium propionate	Preservative, mold inhibitor
Sodium sulfite	Preservative for dried fruits
Soy sauce	Flavor enhancer
Teriyaki sauce	Flavor enhancer

Salty Terms

When a recipe calls for salt, which one will you use? Most recipes call for table salt. How does table salt compare with other types of salt for nutrition and culinary uses?

● *Iodized salt:* table salt with iodine added. The human body needs just small amounts of iodine. By adding it to salt, people get enough iodine—even when they go easy on salt. An important nutrient, iodine helps prevent goiter, which is a thyroid gland condition.

● *Kosher salt:* coarse grain salt that adds a crunchy texture to some dishes and some drinks, such as margaritas. Kosher salt is also used to prepare meat by religious Jews. "Kosher salt" may have anticaking additives.

  Tip: ¼ teaspoon of kosher salt has somewhat less sodium than ¼ teaspoon of table salt. That's because kosher salt has a coarser grain, so less fits in the spoon. For the same saltiness in a cooked dish, you need the same amount by *weight*—and that has the same amount of sodium, kosher or not.

● *Lite salt:* salt that is "50–50": half sodium chloride (regular salt) and half potassium chloride. It has less sodium than table salt, but it's not sodium-free.

● *Pickling salt:* fine-grained salt used to make brines for sauerkraut or pickles. Unlike table salt, it has no iodine or anticaking additives. Additives would make the brine cloudy or would settle to the bottom.

● *Popcorn salt:* very finely granulated salt that sticks well to popcorn, fries, and chips

● *Rock salt:* large, chunky crystals of salt used in a crank-style ice cream maker or as a "bed" for serving foods such as clams or oysters. Not commonly used in recipes, rock salt contains some harmless impurities.

● *Salt substitute:* made of potassium chloride and contains no sodium. It may be recommended by a healthcare provider for people on a sodium-restricted diet.

● *Sea salt:* salt—either fine-grained or in larger crystals—produced by evaporation of seawater—for example, Black Sea, French (fleur de sel), Celtic, or Hawaiian sea salt. It has trace amounts of other minerals that may offer a somewhat different flavor. Still, it's sodium chloride. Even though sea salt is often promoted as a healthful alternative to ordinary table salt, the sodium content is comparable; the small amount of other minerals offers no known health advantages. As with other salts, use sea salt judiciously. If the grain is coarse, it may have less sodium per teaspoon, but not by weight.

  Tip: With canning, trace minerals in sea salt may discolor food.

● *Seasoned salt:* salt with herbs and other flavorings added, such as celery salt, garlic salt, onion salt, or other seasoned salts. Seasoned salt has less sodium than table salt but more than herbs alone.

  Tip: For less sodium in cooking, use just herbs—for example, celery seed, garlic powder, or onion flakes. Check the ingredient list for salt.

● *Table salt:* fine, granulated salt commonly used in cooking and in salt shakers. An anticaking additive—calcium silicate—helps table salt flow freely and not get lumpy.

---

slices of bacon may deliver 500 to 800 milligrams of sodium. Even "reduced-sodium" foods may be higher in sodium than you think!

For clues to the sodium in processed foods, check the label for sodium-containing ingredients. If an ingredient has *Na, salt, soda,* or *sodium* in its name, that's a clue for sodium. ("Na" is the scientific symbol for sodium.) Foods described as "broth," "cured," "corned," "pickled," or "smoked" usually contain sodium, too; cured ham often contains about 350 milligrams of sodium per ounce. *Page 149 shows just a few ingredients with sodium.*

Because sodium occurs naturally, too, even unprocessed foods may contain sodium. But the amounts (about 12 percent of our overall sodium intake) aren't high enough for concern.

How do you know if a food has a lot of sodium, or a little? Check the amount of sodium in one label serving of a food, using the label's Nutrition Facts. If one serving contains 5 percent or less of the Daily Value (DV) for sodium, that's low. If it contains 20 percent or more DV, that's a lot. Remember: Two servings double the sodium. *For tips on using food labels, see "Today's Food Labels" in chapter 11.*

Which food groups have the most sodium? The sodium content of foods varies—even in very similar

Need more strategies to shake the salt habit? Check here for "how-tos":

- Shop for foods with less sodium—see chapter 11.
- Fit in more fruits and veggies (and more potassium)—see chapter 13.
- Cut salt in your cooking—see chapter 13.
- Give food a flavor burst with herbs and spices, not salt—see chapter 13.
- Order restaurant foods with less sodium—see chapter 14.
- Follow the DASH eating plan—see chapter 22.

foods. The difference comes from the way foods are prepared and processed. Foods in every group of MyPyramid may contain sodium.

Flavor . . . with Little Salt and Less Sodium

Do you like the taste of salty snacks? Does food seem to taste better after a few shakes of the salt shaker? Most people eat what they like. According to consumer research, taste ranks first in making food choices. Good news: you can enjoy plenty of flavorful foods prepared with *less* salt and sodium.

"Salty"—an Acquired Taste

A preference for strong, salty tastes is acquired, probably starting in childhood. It's the saltiness that people like, not the sodium. In fact, chloride in salt may have more to do with flavor than sodium does.

Except for the sensory experience, the body adjusts easily to eating less salt. Interestingly, when people gradually cut back and learn to go with less salt in their food choices, the desire for salty tastes declines, too. Over time, the less salt they consume, the less they want.

For taste perception, no other foods truly substitute for the taste of salt. Even salt substitutes, suggested for some people, don't give the same taste sensation. They may taste somewhat bitter or sharp.

About Salt Substitutes

Are salt substitutes good for moderating sodium in food choices? That depends. Salt substitutes aren't appropriate—and may not be healthful—for everyone.

MSG–Another Flavor Enhancer

You probably know about monosodium glutamate, or more simply, MSG. Common in many types of ethnic cooking, MSG is a flavor enhancer. It blends well with salty or sour flavors . . . and brings out the flavor of many prepared foods, such as "heat 'n' eat" meals, sauces, and canned soups.

Besides accenting the natural flavor of foods, MSG adds a unique taste of its own. Called "umami," its taste is described as "meaty" or "brothlike." Studies show "umami" actually elicits a fifth taste sensation, distinctive in cheese, meat, and tomatoes. Sweet, sour, salty, and bitter are the other four taste sensations. *For more about taste, see "'Flavor' the Difference" in chapter 13.*

As its name implies, monosodium glutamate contains sodium and glutamate or glutamic acid. Glutamic acid is an amino acid found naturally in your body and in high-protein foods. Meat, fish, dairy foods, and some vegetables contain glutamic acid.

Over the years, consumers have asked about the safety of MSG. The U.S. Food and Drug Administration considers MSG "generally recognized as safe" (GRAS) for consumption. Other GRAS substances include commonplace food "additives" such as sugar, salt, and baking soda. *See "Testing, Testing" in chapter 9 for more about the GRAS list. Also see "Have You Ever Wondered . . . if You Can Be Sensitive to MSG?" in chapter 21.*

MSG has nutrition-related benefits that may go unrecognized. Since a little goes a long way, MSG provides a bigger "bang" for the "shake." With only a third as much sodium as a comparable amount of salt, it may be an option for controlling sodium intake.

Adding MSG to foods such as soups and stews may make eating more enjoyable for older adults. As we grow older, our sense of smell may weaken and our taste buds decrease in number. As a result, foods lose some of their "taste appeal." The decline in smell and taste often causes seniors to lose interest in eating, putting them at nutritional risk. Adding MSG to certain foods can perk up the flavor! *See "Aging with 'Taste'" for more about taste and older adults in chapter 18.*

Many salt substitutes contain potassium in place of all or some of the sodium. For some people, potassium consumed in excess can be harmful. For example, those with kidney problems may not be able to rid their bodies of excess levels of potassium. If you're under medical care—especially for a kidney problem—check with your doctor before using salt substitutes.

Rather than salt substitutes (potassium chloride), try herb-spice blends as a flavorful alternative to salt—or lemon or lime juice. Today's supermarkets carry a variety of salt-free seasoning blends. Remember to read the ingredient list and the Nutrition Facts on the label. Some herb-spice blends are neither salt- nor sodium-free. As an alternative, make your own; *see "Kitchen Nutrition: Salt-Free Herb Blends" on page 153. For more about the sensations of taste and flavor, see "'Flavor' the Difference" in chapter 13.*

Taming Your Taste Buds

Enjoying what you eat is a top priority! Fortunately, healthful foods don't need to taste bland. And you don't need to give up your favorite high-sodium foods—just eat them in moderation. Here's how:

● Cut back on high-sodium foods gradually if you're accustomed to salty tastes. Because a preference for a salty taste is learned, it takes time to unlearn it, too—and to appreciate new flavor combinations.

● Taste food before salting it. Maybe it tastes great just as it is! Keep the salt shaker in the kitchen cabinet, not on the stove or the table. Use it as needed—not just as a habit.

● Enjoy plenty of fruits and vegetables. Most contain only small amounts of sodium (unless added in processing), and they're rich in potassium. Eat them as low-sodium snacks!

● Choose foods within a food group that have less sodium, such as fresh meats, poultry, fish, dry and fresh legumes, unsalted nuts, eggs, milk, and yogurt. Plain rice, pasta, and oatmeal don't have much sodium, either. Their sodium content goes up only if high-sodium ingredients are added during prep.

● Season with herbs, spices, herbed vinegars, herb rubs, and fruit juices instead of salt. *"A Pinch of Flavor: How to Cook with Herbs and Spices" in chapter 13 offers many ways to use herbs and spices. Or prepare the easy blends on page 153 to keep on hand.*

● Prepare food with little salt or fewer high-sodium ingredients. For example, skip the salt in cooking water for pasta, rice, cereals, and vegetables. Salt toughens many vegetables, especially beans, as they're cooked. Salt draws water out of the plant cells. *For*

Look at the Differences

To eat less salt and sodium, fresh foods are an ideal choice. You can enjoy processed and prepared foods, too.

Some processed foods have more sodium than others: cured and processed meats; many canned foods such as legumes, vegetables, and fish; cheese; condiments; boxed convenience foods such as pasta mixes or rice side dishes; and salted snack foods. For many, you can find lower-sodium versions. Read Nutrition Facts on food labels to compare similar products.

FOOD	SODIUM (MG)
2 oz. canned tuna	215
2 oz. low-sodium canned tuna	135
1 medium dill pickle	835
1 medium low-sodium dill pickle	10
3 oz. ham	1,110
3 oz. reduced-sodium ham	825
3 oz. lean pork loin	55
3 cups regular microwave popcorn	265
3 cups air-popped popcorn	<5
3 cups salt-free microwave popcorn	0
1 oz. salted peanuts	160–230
1 oz. lightly salted peanuts	50
1 cup boxed convenience rice	1,600
1 cup plain brown or white rice seasoned with herbs	5
1 cup vegetable beef soup	860
1 cup reduced-sodium vegetable beef soup	50
½ cup canned green beans	175
½ cup canned no-salt-added green beans	<5
½ cup frozen green beans	5
½ cup fresh green beans	<5
1 cup chicken broth	490–1,480
1 cup low-sodium chicken broth	70

more ways, see chapter 13 on "Kitchen Nutrition: Delicious Decisions."

● Balance: if you eat high-sodium foods occasionally, balance them by eating foods with less sodium. How much salt and sodium you consume over several days is what counts.

● To buy processed and prepared foods with less sodium and salt, read Nutrition Facts on food labels. You'll find the sodium content in milligrams and the % Daily Value for sodium in a single label serving. The Daily Value is based on 2,400 milligrams of sodium for the day.

● Scan the nutrient content claims on the front of food labels as you walk the supermarket aisles. From soup, canned fish, vegetables, and vegetable juice to crack-ers, popcorn, and snack foods, you'll find a variety of food products described as "unsalted," "no salt added," "reduced sodium," "sodium-free," or "low in sodium." *To learn what these words mean, see "Label Lingo: Salt and Sodium" later in this chapter.*

● Buy foods with less sodium. Try reduced-sodium products, which may offer more flavor than low-sodium products. They're still lower in sodium than the traditional versions.

● Whether you eat in a sit-down or a fast-food restaurant, be sodium-conscious if you eat out regularly. *See "Eating Out" on page 154 for simple ways to cut back.*

● Try lightly salted or unsalted nuts, popcorn, pretzels, and crackers if an urge for a salty flavor strikes.

Kitchen Nutrition

Salt-Free Herb Blends

Enhance the flavor of food with salt-free herb and spice combinations. To make ½ cup, combine the ingredients in a jar. Cover tightly and shake. Keep in a cool, dark, dry place. Then rub or sprinkle them on food for flavor. *(Tip:* They make great hospitality gifts!)

Chinese five-spice . . . for chicken, fish, or pork.

Blend ¼ cup of ground ginger, 2 tablespoons of ground cinnamon, 1 tablespoon each of ground all-spice and anise seeds, and 2 teaspoons of ground cloves.

Mixed herb blend . . . for salads, pasta salads, steamed vegetables, vegetable soup, or fish.

Blend ¼ cup of dried parsley flakes, 2 tablespoons of dried tarragon, and 1 tablespoon each of dried oregano, dill weed, and celery flakes.

Curry blend . . . for rice, lentil, and vegetable dishes, and chicken.

Blend 2 tablespoons each of turmeric and ground coriander, 1 tablespoon of ground cumin, 2 tea-spoons each of ground cardamom, ground ginger, and black pepper, and 1 teaspoon each of pow-dered cloves, cinnamon, and ground nutmeg.

Italian blend . . . for tomato-based soups and pasta dishes, chicken, pizza, focaccia, and herbed bread.

Blend 2 tablespoons each of dried basil and dried marjoram, 1 tablespoon each of garlic powder and dried oregano, and 2 teaspoons each of thyme, crushed dried rosemary, and crushed red pepper.

Mexican chile blend . . . for chili with beans, enchiladas, tacos, fajitas, chicken, pork, and beef.

Blend ¼ cup of chile powder, 1 tablespoon each of ground cumin and onion powder, 1 teaspoon each of dried oregano, garlic powder, and ground red pepper, and ½ teaspoon of cinnamon.

Greek blend . . . for seafood, poultry, and herbed bread.

Blend 3 tablespoons each of garlic powder and dried lemon peel, 2 tablespoons of dried oregano, and 1 teaspoon of black pepper.

Easy dip blend . . . for mixing with cottage cheese, yogurt cheese *(see "Kitchen Nutrition: Yogurt Cheese" in chapter 3),* or low-fat sour cream; also nice on chicken and fish.

Blend ¼ cup of dried dill weed and 1 tablespoon each of dried chives, garlic powder, dried lemon peel, and dried chervil.

Eating Out

Unlike foods you buy at the supermarket, you usually don't know the sodium content of items on a restaurant menu. Yet, if you eat out a lot, the sodium from restaurant meals and snacks could be significant. To eat less salt from foods you order out:

● Move the salt shaker to another table, or taste before you shake. Ask for a lemon wedge, or bring your own herb blend to enhance the food's flavor.

● Recognize menu terms that may indicate a high sodium content: pickled, smoked, au jus, soy sauce, or in broth.

● Nibble on raw veggies rather than salty snacks.

● Go easy on condiments such as mustard, catsup, pickles, and tartar sauce for burgers, hot dogs, and sandwiches. Enjoy lettuce, onions, and tomatoes. Remember that bacon tends to be high in sodium.

● Ask the server to have your food prepared without added salt; ask for sauces and salad dressings on the side since they're often high in sodium. For a salad, use a twist of lemon, a splash of vinegar, or a light drizzle of dressing.

● Keep your order simple. Order broiled or grilled meat—without salty seasonings—rather than entrées cooked in sauces. Often special sauces and toppings add sodium.

See chapter 14 for more on eating out.

Label Lingo

Salt and Sodium

Does the term "sodium" or "salt" appear on the front of the food label? If so, here's what the descriptions mean. For the specific sodium content in a standard serving, check the Nutrition Facts.

LABEL TERM	MEANS
Sodium-free	Less than 5 milligrams of sodium per serving
Very low sodium	35 milligrams or less of sodium per serving
Low sodium	140 milligrams or less of sodium per serving
Reduced or less sodium	At least 25% less sodium*
Light in sodium	50% less sodium*; restricted to foods with more than 40 calories per serving or more than 3 grams of fat per serving
Salt-free	Less than 5 milligrams of sodium per serving
Low-sodium meat	140 milligrams or less of sodium per 100 grams (3½ ounces)
Unsalted or butter, no added salt	No salt added during processing; does not necessarily mean sodium-free

*As compared with a standard serving size of the traditional food

CHAPTER 8

Fluids

The Power of Water

Water? Unless your throat feels parched and sweat drips from your brow, you probably give little thought to water. Yet this clear, refreshing fluid is one of your body's most essential nutrients.

You've probably heard that water is vital to health—and to life itself. While you may survive for six weeks without food, you cannot live longer than a week or so without water. In fact, losing more than 10 percent of your body weight from dehydration, or water loss, causes extreme weakness and potential heat stroke. And a 20 percent loss is life-threatening. Water truly is the beverage of life!

A Fluid Asset

Water is the most abundant substance in the human body as well as the most common substance on earth. Like the oxygen you breathe, you can't live without it.

On average, body weight is 45 to 75 percent water—or for many, about 10 to 12 gallons of water. The specific percentage varies from person to person, relating to body composition, age, and gender, among other factors.

Compared with body fat, lean tissue holds much more water, so the leaner you are, the higher proportion of water in your body. Males, with more muscle, carry a higher percentage of water in their bodies than females do. And younger individuals usually have more than older adults. Water accounts for about 75 percent of a newborn's weight, while the amount dwindles in the elderly to about 50 percent.

Body tissues of all types contain water—some more than others. The fact that blood contains water is certainly no surprise; your blood is about 83 percent water. Lean muscle tissue is about 73 percent water; body fat, about 25 percent. Even though bones seem hard, they, too, contain water, about 22 percent by weight.

Water: An Essential Nutrient

What does water do in your body? Far more than satisfy your thirst! Thirst is actually more like a warning light that's flashing on the dashboard of your car. This physical sensation signals to you that your body needs more fluid to perform its many functions. To satisfy thirst, you drink fluids.

Water itself is a simple substance, containing just one part oxygen and two parts hydrogen. It supplies no calories. Yet every body cell, tissue, and organ, and almost every life-sustaining body process, needs water to function. In fact, water is the nutrient your body needs in the greatest amount.

Whether inside or surrounding your cells, nearly every function of the human body takes place in a watery medium. Water regulates your body temperature, keeping it constant at about 98.6° F. Many body processes produce heat, including any physical activity. Through perspiration, heat escapes from your body as water evaporates on your skin.

Water transports nutrients and oxygen to your body cells and carries waste products away. It moistens body tissues such as those in your mouth, eyes, and nose. Water is the main part of every body fluid, including blood, gastric (stomach) juice, saliva, amniotic fluid (for a developing fetus), and urine. By softening stools, water helps prevent constipation. It helps lubricate joints and cushion organs and tissues.

To keep your body functioning normally and to avoid dehydration, your body needs an ongoing water supply. During a strenuous workout, losing water weight is common, especially on a hot, humid day. Losing just one or two pounds of your body's water weight can trigger a feeling of thirst. With a little more fluid loss, the body loses strength and endurance; even mild dehydration can interfere with physical performance. With even more water loss and prolonged exposure to high temperatures, a person may suffer from heat exhaustion or risk heat stroke. With a 20 percent drop in water weight, a person can barely survive.

Of all the nutrients in your diet, water is most abundant. Drinking water and other beverages are the main sources. But you "eat" quite a bit of water in solid foods, too—perhaps more than you think. Juicy fruits and vegetables such as celery, lettuce, tomatoes, and watermelons contain more than 90 percent water. Even dry foods, such as bread, supply some water. *Check the chart "Food: A Water Source" on page 157.*

Your body has still another water source. About 15 percent of your body's total water supply forms in your body cells when energy is produced from carbohydrates, proteins, and fats. Along with energy, water is an end product of your body's metabolism.

Fluids: How Much Is Enough?

The average adult loses about 2½ quarts or more (about 10 or more cups) of water daily through perspiration (even when sitting), urination, bowel movements, and even breathing. During hot, humid weather or strenuous physical activity, fluid loss may be much higher. Unlike some other nutrients, the human body doesn't store extra water for those times when you need more. To avoid dehydration and to keep your body working normally, replace the fluids lost through normal bodily functions.

Dehydration: Look for Body Signals!

The effects of dehydration, or loss of body water, are progressive: thirst, then fatigue, next weakness, followed by delirium, and finally death. Although you need to pay attention to the signals of water loss, all these steps won't happen in a single day.

PERCENT LOSS OF BODY WATER BY TOTAL BODY WEIGHT	PROGRESSIVE EFFECTS OF DEHYDRATION (PARTIAL LIST)
0 to 1	Thirst
2 to 5	Dry mouth, flushed skin, fatigue, headache, impaired physical performance
6	Increased body temperature, breathing rate, pulse rate
8	Dizziness, increased weakness, labored breathing with exercise
10	Muscle spasms, swollen tongue, delirium, wakefulness
11	Poor blood circulation, failing kidney function

How much water do you need each day? The Dietary Reference Intakes from the Institute of Medicine (IOM) advise an Adequate Intake (AI) level of 3.7 liters (125 ounces) of total water daily for males ages nineteen and over; for females nineteen and over, it's 2.7 liters (91 ounces) daily. (A liter is about 1 quart or about 4 cups.) Teens and children need somewhat less; *refer to the Appendices for recommended amounts.* The AI is set for generally healthy people living in temperate climates. The IOM notes that people can be properly hydrated at higher or lower levels of water intake, too.

These amounts may seem like a lot, but "total water" comes from many sources—from drinking water, other beverages, and water in solid foods. Body weight is one factor affecting fluid need. Additional factors that may cause a need for more water include climate, level of physical activity, diet, and other physical differences. For example:

- When you're exposed to extreme temperatures—very hot or very cold—your body uses more water to maintain its normal temperature.

- With strenuous work or exercise, your body loses water through perspiration. Drink before physical activity. And drink early and often during exercise. As a good practical guide, check the color of your urine (*see below*). *For signs that you need to drink more, see "Dehydration Alert!" in chapter 19.*

- When you're exposed to heated or recirculated air for a long time, water evaporates from your skin. Dry, recirculated air on planes promotes dehydration.

- Pregnancy and breast-feeding increase the amount of fluid a woman's body needs. The AI level advised for pregnancy is 3 liters daily; for breast-feeding, 3.8 liters daily.

- Being sick makes a difference. Fever, diarrhea, and vomiting cause increased water loss. Follow the advice of your healthcare provider; drink plenty of water and other fluids to prevent dehydration.

- On a high-fiber diet, your body needs extra water to process more roughage and prevent constipation.

In healthy people, water intake and water loss balance out. If you consume more than you need, your kidneys simply eliminate the excess, about 24 ounces of fluid an hour! You probably won't overdo on water. When you don't consume enough, your body may trigger a sensation of thirst.

Thirst signals the need for fluids, but it isn't a foolproof mechanism, especially for elderly people, children, and during illness, hot weather, or strenuous physical activity. Waiting until you feel thirsty to drink may be too long. By then, two or more cups of body fluids may be gone—even when you're healthy. *For more on fluids for older adults, see chapter 18.*

To see if you're drinking enough fluid, check your urine. A small volume of dark-colored urine indicates that you aren't consuming enough fluid. Besides feeling thirsty, this is your signal to drink more. Pale or almost colorless urine means you're drinking enough.

As another option, weigh yourself before and after strenuous physical activity. For every pound of weight you lose, replace it with two cups of fluid.

Caution: If you always seem thirsty or urinate too

Food: A Water Source

It's not easy to calculate just how much water you consume each day. While drinks supply a good portion of your water needs, solid food also provides a surprising amount.

FOOD	PERCENT WATER BY WEIGHT
Lettuce	95
Watermelon	91
Broccoli	89
Grapefruit	89
Milk	89
Orange juice	88
Carrot	88
Apple	86
Yogurt	85
Potato, baked with skin	75
Tuna, canned, drained	74
Rice, cooked	70
Kidney beans, boiled	67
Chicken, roasted, no skin	65
Pasta, cooked	62
Whole-wheat bread	38
Cheddar cheese	37
Honey	17
Butter or margarine	16
Raisins	15
Pecans, dried	4
Vegetable oil	0

Source: U.S. Department of Agriculture, Agricultural Research Service, 2005. *USDA National Nutrient Database for Standard Reference,* Release 18.

much, talk to your healthcare provider. This may be a sign of diabetes. On the other hand, water retention, for reasons other than premenstrual syndrome, may suggest a kidney or a liver problem.

While rare, water toxicity can happen if someone drinks too much water. The effect can be life-threatening. Since it's so unlikely, a Tolerable Upper Intake Level for water wasn't set.

Water: In Balance

To maintain your body's fluid balance, you need to replace the amount of water you lose each day. If you lose a little more, such as through perspiration, you'll need to drink more fluids to balance out.

Your body loses water daily through . . .

Urine	2 to 4 cups
Perspiration (lose through skin)	2 to 8 cups
Breath (expired air)	1 to 1 ½ cups
Feces	⅔ cup

You replace water in your body daily through . . .

Water and other fluids	9 to 12 ½ cups* (depending on gender)
Solid foods	2 ⅓ to 3 cups (depending on gender)
Water from metabolism	1 to 1 ½ cups

*Based on estimated minimum losses and production of water in healthy sedentary adults. If you consumer a little more than your body needs, your body will excrete any extra.

Calculated from "Table: Estimation of Minimum Daily Water Losses and Production,: *Dietary References Intakes for Water, Potassium, Sodium, Chloride, and Sulfate*, 2004.

Drinking for Health

To keep your body well hydrated, consume enough water. Follow your thirst, and drink beverages with meals. Because milk, juice, and some other beverages are mostly water, they count toward your daily water intake. So does water from solid foods, although you can't really measure it. On average, moisture in food provides about 20 percent of your water intake. Surprised?

Caffeinated beverages—coffee, tea, and some soft drinks—contribute to your day's total water intake, as noncaffeinated drinks do. While a high intake of caffeine may have a diuretic effect, the effect likely won't last long. Diuretic effect means water loss through increased urination. Any diuretic effect from alcoholic drinks appears to be short term, too; the effect may change during the day and may depend on how much water you drink before meals.

To increase your water intake . . .

● Take water breaks during the day instead of coffee breaks. If you're a subconscious "sipper," keep a cup of water on your desk.

● When you buy a vending machine or convenience store drink, reach for bottled water.

● "Water down" your meals and snacks. Complement food with more water, milk, or juice. Occasionally, start your meals with soup.

● When you walk by a water fountain, drink!

● Refresh yourself at snack time with juice, milk, or sparkling water.

● Drink sparkling water at social gatherings.

● Before, during, and after any physical activity, drink water, especially in hot weather. Consume ½ to 2 cups of water every fifteen to twenty minutes while you exercise. Don't wait until you feel thirsty! *For more on fluids during exercise, see chapter 19.*

● Keep a bottle of water with you as you commute, while you work, as you run errands. Travel with a supply of bottled water, too, even for day outings. Airline travel promotes dehydration. *For tips on drinking fluids in flight, see page 364.*

Hydration for the Seasons

From the bone-chilling days of winter to the hot, sultry days of summer, your body needs water to maintain its normal temperature.

In hot, humid weather your body perspires, increasing water loss. Cool, refreshing drinks may help cool your overheated body. *An interesting side note:* Your body has a harder time cooling down in hot, humid weather than in hot, dry weather. That's because perspiration doesn't evaporate from your skin to cool you down. Instead your skin feels sticky and hot.

Dehydration may seem like just a summer issue. But keeping your body well hydrated during winter is just as important. When the weather turns chilly, most people head indoors. There heated air evaporates the moisture on your skin. Although you may not feel thirsty, you still need to replace water loss. Even in the cold outdoors, you may perspire . . . perhaps from the physical exertion of shoveling snow, skating or skiing, or from being bundled up with many layers of clothing.

The Fluoride Connection

For children and adults, fluoride, a mineral, helps harden developing tooth enamel and so protects teeth from decay. It's also important for bone health. Many municipal water systems contain a natural supply of fluoride. But in areas where fluoride levels are low, the water system may be fluoridated to levels recommended by the U.S. Public Health Service. The optimum fluoride level is 0.7 to 1.2 parts fluoride per million parts water.

Fluoride is not only ingested through the water supply. In areas where water isn't fluoridated, dentists may prescribe fluoride supplements for children. If you're not sure about fluoride in your municipal water system, check with your local water department or public health department. If you have your own well, have it tested for fluoride.

"Topical" fluoride—applied directly to teeth with fluoride toothpaste, oral rinses, gels, foams, and treatments from a dental office—also helps strengthen tooth enamel. To reduce the chance for developing brown spots (*see below*) on permanent teeth, children shouldn't swallow fluoride toothpaste or rinses.

Consuming too much fluoride can cause the teeth to be mottled, or marked with brown spots, even though they're healthy in other ways. That most likely happens with excessive supplement doses. The Tolerable Upper Intake Level for fluoride is 2.2 milligrams daily for children ages four through eight; from age nine through adulthood, it's 10 milligrams of fluoride daily.

People who drink mostly bottled water may not consume enough decay-preventative fluoride. Remember: Tap water is often fluoridated. The fluoride content of bottled water varies. Check the label. It's hard to know how much it has since the U.S. FDA only requires fluoride labeling on bottled water if it's added in processing.

For more about healthy teeth, see "Your Smile: Sugar and Oral Health" in chapter 5 and "Caring for Baby Teeth" in chapter 15.

What's to Drink?

Just plain water: It's the most available fluid around and often your best choice! Juice and milk make good beverage options, too, since they supply other nutrients besides water. For example, juice offers vitamins A or C, or both, and milk is calcium-rich. Other beverage choices—coffee, tea, soft drinks, and alcoholic drinks—don't offer the nutrient benefits of milk, fortified soy beverage, or juice.

Why drink water? For starters, water has no calories. If you're trying to avoid extra calories, that's a definite advantage. In other beverages, such as regular soft drinks and alcoholic beverages, calories really can add up. Water is also low in sodium and has no fat or cholesterol. Watching your caffeine intake? Unlike many coffees, teas, and some soft drinks, you won't find caffeine in water either.

Tap Water or Bottled Water?

Tap water or bottled water: Which should you drink? Both are regulated stringently by the government—tap water by the Environmental Protection Agency (EPA) and bottled water by the U.S. Food and Drug Administration (FDA). Especially when it comes from large municipal water systems, tap water is just as safe for drinking as bottled water.

Right from the Tap

Just turn on your faucet! Most drinking water in the United States comes right from the tap. Most of us take this for granted, but in many parts of the world, drinkable tap water is a luxury. If you live in an urban area, your tap water probably comes from a surface water source: river, lake, or reservoir, fed by a watershed, or land area. In a rural area, you likely drink groundwater that's pumped from an aquifer, an underground, natural reservoir. Either way, water must be treated with chemicals and filtered to ensure its quality and safety.

Treated: For Safety's Sake. No matter what the original source, water isn't naturally pure. Impurities dissolve or absorb in water as it flows through rivers and streams, filters through soil and rocks, and collects in lakes and reservoirs.

To make tap water safe from public health problems, the EPA has established standards for contaminants that may occur in drinking water. Standards are set at a low enough level to protect most people, including children. Treatment protects you from microbes such as bacteria and viruses, inorganic contaminants such as chemicals, and lead, arsenic, and other minerals.

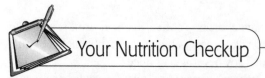

Your Nutrition Checkup

"Wet" Your Appetite?

Now that you've read about the value of water to your health, just how much fluid do you drink during a typical day?

If yesterday was typical for you, write down what you drank and about how much. Include beverages consumed with meals and snacks. Remember to include water you drank from a water fountain, tap, or dispenser on the refrigerator.

WATER	OTHER BEVERAGES	HOW MUCH?
Morning		
_____	_____	_____
_____	_____	_____
_____	_____	_____
_____	_____	_____
Afternoon		
_____	_____	_____
_____	_____	_____
_____	_____	_____
_____	_____	_____
Evening		
_____	_____	_____
_____	_____	_____
_____	_____	_____
_____	_____	_____

About how many cups of fluids did you drink? _____

For good health, consume enough fluids: about 9 cups or more for women, and about 12½ cups or more for men. That adds up to about 80 percent of the AI for water. Drink more if you've been physically active or if it's a hot day. The rest of the water you consume (about 20 percent) comes from the food you eat. If you came up short, read on for ways you might drink a little more!

Tip: Alcoholic beverages don't provide a complete fluid-replacement benefit because of their mild diuretic effect.

To find out about a public water supply, ask for the annual report, or Consumer Confidence Report, from your community water supplier. It indicates the water source, the presence or level of contaminants, and what you can do to protect your drinking water.

Water may be disinfected chemically, or by a physical process such as ultraviolet light. Chlorination is a tried-and-true method for effectively treating water and keeping you safe from most immediate microbial reactions such as diarrhea and vomiting, and from outbreaks of cholera, hepatitis, and other microbial diseases.

There's been some question about a by-product called trihalomethane (THM), created when chlorine reacts with organic matter in water. The very low amount of THM created in the process of making water safe to drink isn't enough to create a cancer risk. From a public health standpoint, protecting people from disease outbreaks far outweighs the insignificant effect of THM.

If you want to know the THM level of your water, check your municipal water quality report; home testing is unreliable. The THM standard from the EPA is an average (per quarter of the year) of 80 parts per billion (ppb) as of January 2002. Home water filters can reduce these compounds in your drinking water if you choose to use one.

Water quality is continually assessed for safety. For example, in a few spots in the nation, low levels of arsenic in drinking water (from natural and commercial sources), consumed over time, were identified as a potential cancer risk. For that reason, new standards for arsenic in drinking water were adopted in 2006. The arsenic level in water must be at a maximum level of 10 parts per billion (ppb). *For more information, check http://www.epa.gov/safewater/arsenic.html—EPA's Web address.*

Hard or Soft? Surprisingly, water itself may not be the only nutrient in drinking water. Unless distilled, or demineralized, drinking water may contain minerals in varying amounts, such as fluoride, calcium, sodium, iron, and magnesium. The water source and how it's processed determine the actual composition of drinking water. Water from underground wells, springs, and aquifers may contain high mineral concentrations. As water from rain and snow seeps through rocks, gravel, and sand, it picks up minerals along the way. That's how some underground water becomes naturally fluoridated. *"The Fluoride Connection" earlier in this chapter describes the link between fluoridated water and oral health.*

Water may be described as "hard" or "soft" depending on its mineral content. Hard water contains more calcium and magnesium, while soft water has more sodium. With one exception there's essentially no difference in flavor between hard and soft water. Small amounts of iron give a metallic taste to hard water—but not enough to make it a significant source of dietary iron.

Where water is naturally hard, some consumers choose to use a water softener, which adds sodium and removes other minerals. The reason? The decision to soften water isn't a nutrition issue; instead, softening water can make soap work more efficiently, extend the life of a water heater, and avoid residue buildup in pipes. The amount of softening (salt added) depends on the hardness of the water. For well water that must be fully softened, the amount of sodium per cup of water is about 39 milligrams. Usually well water doesn't need to be fully softened; however, the average softened municipal water may contain about 22 milligrams of sodium per cup. Again, your own water supply may not be softened. For most people, the amount of sodium in softened water isn't significant.

If you have your own water softener, you might soften only hot water typically used for washing, not

Have You Ever Wondered

. . . where to get your water tested? Whether you're checking for lead, trihalomethanes, or other contaminants, or having a private well tested, skip home testing kits. They're unreliable. Instead, contact the EPA or your local public health department.

. . . what you can do to help keep drinking water safe? Find out how to dispose of toxic trash such as household cleaners and batteries with lead or mercury. Your town may have a special collection site. Take used motor oil to a recycling center; don't discard it in your trash or storm sewer. Don't put any chemicals in places that seep into groundwater, such as septic systems, drainage wells, or dry wells.

Water: In Case of Emergencies

Disaster can hit anyone, anywhere! To ensure a safe water supply for your family, disaster experts advise these precautions.

● Store a week's supply of bottled water for everyone in your family. Figure about 1 gallon of water per person per day.

● Store containers of water in a cool, dry place away from direct sunlight.

● Label bottles of water with the date. Replace them every six months to ensure freshness.

cooking or drinking. If you're sodium-sensitive, you won't have extra sodium in cold drinking water.

What about Bottled Water?

Do you carry a bottle of water? In recent years, consumption of bottled water has soared. The bottled-water industry began in the late 1950s, and by 2005 total annual sales for Americans was about 7.5 billion gallons. Except for soft drinks, people living in the United States drink more bottled water than any other beverage! With today's consumer demand, soft-drink companies have added bottled water to their line. The most common types include mineral water, purified water, sparkling water, spring water, and well water . . . plain or lightly flavored.

Since both tap and bottled water are safe, why drink bottled water? According to consumer research, some people prefer the taste. Bottled water usually doesn't contain chlorine, which can give water a slight flavor. It's convenient: portable for the office, a picnic, a drive, or a workout, and often easy to buy. Many people drink bottled water for what it doesn't contain: calories, caffeine, or alcohol.

About Bottled Water. Bottled water that's sold state to state is regulated by the FDA to assure its quality, safety, and accurate labeling. Terms on labels for bottled water, such as "spring water" or "mineral water," are defined legally. If bottled water comes from a municipal water supply, the label must state that fact, unless it's been processed to be purified water. By regulation, bottled water can't contain sweeteners or additives—besides flavors, extracts, or essences from food or spices (less than 1 percent by weight). And it must be calorie- and sugar-free.

Instead of chlorine, bottled water usually is disinfected in other ways, including filtration; reverse osmosis; ultraviolet (UV) light; or ozone, a highly reactive form of oxygen. *See "Have You Ever Wondered?" later in this chapter for a brief background on water filtration systems.* Depending on the method, bottled water may or may not be 100 percent pathogen-free. If you're at risk with suppressed immune function, talk to your healthcare provider to find bottled water that's pathogen-free.

Ever see "NSF-certified" or "IBWA Bottler Member" on bottled water labels? IBWA stands for International Bottled Water Association. These label statements indicate that a voluntary inspection, using standards set by the National Sanitation Foundation, was conducted with the water source and the finished product checked against FDA regulations. Safe water may not have a label since the inspection is voluntary. If you see "FDA-Approved" or "EPA-Certified," beware; neither agency conducts these inspections.

On bottled waters marketed for infants, you might see the term "sterile." That means the water meets the FDA's standards for commercial sterilization, so it's safe from bacteria. If not, the label must state that the product isn't sterile and should be used to prepare infant formula only as directed by a doctor or according to infant formula preparation instructions. For safety, follow that guideline. Look for fluoridated bottled water if your child or infant consumes only bottled water.

Consumer Tips for Bottled Water. If you like it, buy it. But know that you may pay 240 to more than 10,000 times as much per gallon for bottled water that's no more healthful than most United States' tap water.

From a nutritional standpoint, there's no significant difference, except that bottled water likely doesn't have as much fluoride. In large municipal water systems, either bottled or tap water is safe and healthful. In fact, some bottled water *is* tap water, reprocessed to change its taste and composition.

Some bottled waters may be a good beverage choice for those at high risk; *see "Drinking Water: For Special Health Needs" on page 163.* In places

Label Lingo

Bottled Waters

Today's supermarket shelves offer bottled waters—some flavored, others plain. But what do the terms on the label mean? According to the FDA:

- *Artesian water* is a certain type of well water, collected without mechanical pumping. The well must tap a confined aquifer that has water standing much higher than the rock, gravel, or sand. An aquifer is an underground layer of rock or sand with water.

- *Well water* is collected from an underground aquifer, too, but with a mechanical pump.

- *Drinking water* is bottled water from an approved source. It must meet state and federal standards and go through minimal filtration and disinfection.

- *Mineral water* contains minerals at a standard level, no less than 250 parts per million (ppm) of total dissolved solids, or minerals. These minerals must be naturally present, not added. If the level is less than 500 ppm, it will be labeled "low mineral content"; if higher than 1,500 ppm, "high mineral content."

- *Purified water* has been processed to remove minerals and other solids. The process may be distillation, deionization, reverse osmosis, or another suitable process. *Tip:* "Purified" doesn't mean that purified water is any more "pure" or better for you than tap water.

- *Distilled water,* which is one type of purified water, has been evaporated to steam, then recondensed to remove minerals.

- *Sparkling water* is water with a "fizz." Either carbon dioxide is added, or water is naturally carbonated. If carbon dioxide is added, it can't have any more than its naturally carbonated level. It can be labeled as natural sparkling water only if there's no added carbonation. Seltzer, tonic water, and club soda are considered soft drinks, not sparkling water, and may contain sugar and calories.

- *Spring water* comes from an underground source and naturally flows to the surface. It must be collected at the spring or through a bored hole that taps an underground source of the spring. If it's collected by an external (not natural force), it must have the same composition and physical qualities (perhaps carbonated) as the naturally flowing spring water.

where the lead or nitrate content of water is a concern, bottled water may be a good alternative, particularly for pregnant women or families with children. Bottled water doesn't contain lead.

Some cooks prefer bottled or filtered water for cooking. It usually doesn't contain chlorine, which may slightly alter the flavor of soups and stews. In homes with lead pipes or lead solder, bottled water may be a good alternative in soups, stews, and other long-cooking dishes. During extended cooking times, any lead in tap water may become more concentrated.

Consider this: most bottled water isn't chlorinated. So if you sip from the bottle for several days, it's subject to bacterial contamination. Drink it right away; wash the bottle with soapy water if you plan to reuse it.

Safe Enough to Drink

For any nation, water safety is a top public health priority. In the United States, infectious disease spread by untreated water has been almost nonexistent, except during natural disasters such as floods, earthquakes, or accidental contamination of wells or municipal water. Any of these incidents can devastate a community's drinking water supply, so you're wise to know what to do in a water emergency.

When the safety of your water supply is in doubt, don't drink it! Instead, take steps to make it safe from bacteria that spread infectious disease.

● Report your concern to your water company or local public health department. They may test the water or refer you to a qualified private laboratory.

● If you rely on a private well or spring, have it tested annually by a certified water testing laboratory for coliform bacteria, nitrate, and perhaps other contaminants such as radon, pesticides, or industrial wastes. Do it more often if your sample exceeds the standard. People who draw their water from a private water source are responsible for the safety of their own water supply. *For tips on how to protect a private water supply, http://www.epa.gov/safewater/ is the EPA's Web site.*

● Purify contaminated drinking water by boiling tap water for at least one minute, then pouring the boiled water into a sterile container. At high altitudes, perhaps if you're camping, boil water longer. Why? At high altitudes water boils at a lower temperature, which may be less effective at killing bacteria.

● Use iodine or chlorine tablets to disinfect your water supply, strictly following directions on the package. These products are generally available in camping stores. Campers, hikers, and others who rely on water supplied by lakes and streams in wilderness areas might use water filtration and purification devices as well as iodine or chlorine tablets.

● Contact the EPA's Safe Drinking Water Hotline or Web site; your state certification officer for referral to a certified water testing lab; or your local health department. *See "Resources You Can Use" at the back of this book.*

In some countries, contaminated water is an ongoing problem, spreading diarrhea and even life-threatening diseases such as cholera and hepatitis. For

---

Drinking Water: For Special Health Needs

Some people are more vulnerable to microbial contaminants such as *Cryptosporidium* (or "crypto"), which isn't destroyed by chlorination. More often found in surface water than ground water, "crypto" may cause nausea, diarrhea, or stomach cramps when healthy people ingest it. For people who are more vulnerable, the symptoms may be more severe and perhaps life-threatening. That includes people with HIV/AIDS or other immune system disorders (such as lupus or Crohn's disease), organ transplants, the elderly, children, and those undergoing chemotherapy.

In 2001, new EPA standards put more controls on disinfecting procedures for microbial contaminants, including "crypto," for surface water. However, at-risk people should still talk to their healthcare provider and take careful precautions.

Boiling tap water and pasteurizing bottled water destroy "crypto." Filters with an "absolute 1-micron" rating are relatively effective; see *"Have You Ever Wondered? . . . if you need a water filter"* in this chapter. Bottled waters—processed by distillation or reverse osmosis, or commercially filtered with an NSF International Standard 53 filter before bottling—are safe. Not all bottled waters are handled in this way.

globe-trotters, water is a common source of travelers' diarrhea. *See "What's Safe to Drink?" in chapter 14 for guidance on safe drinking water for travelers.* For added safety in less-developed areas, you might travel with a supply of iodine or chlorine tablets.

Get the Lead Out (and the Nitrates and Nitrites, Too)!

With the spread of infectious disease from drinking water under control, concern in the United States has shifted to certain compounds in water. Lead is a major issue.

Excessive lead in drinking and cooking water poses a serious health risk. Over time, too much lead consumed in food and beverages can build up in the body, potentially damaging the brain, nervous system, kidneys, and red blood cells. Infants, children, and unborn babies are more vulnerable to lead poisoning.

If the water supply is monitored, where does lead come from? Often, lead can come from plumbing inside the home or from service lines. In the past,

many houses and multifamily dwellings were constructed with water pipes, fittings, or fixtures made of lead. Additionally, lead service lines in older communities may connect a house with the municipal water system. According to 1996 amendments to the U.S. Safe Drinking Water Act, all pipe, fittings, and fixtures introduced into commerce must be lead-free.

If you are concerned, check your pipes and water supply. Even copper pipes might use lead solder in the joints; brass faucets and fittings may contain lead, too. To have your water tested, contact your local public health department or water utility company. They may have a free testing kit, or may refer you to a government-certified laboratory that tests water safety.

If the lead problem in your water supply is severe, you might install a water filtering device or use bottled water for drinking and cooking. If less severe, follow these guidelines to help ensure the safety of your water:

● Avoid drinking water that has been in lead plumbing for six hours or more.

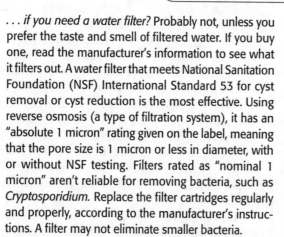

Have You Ever Wondered

. . . if you need a water filter? Probably not, unless you prefer the taste and smell of filtered water. If you buy one, read the manufacturer's information to see what it filters out. A water filter that meets National Sanitation Foundation (NSF) International Standard 53 for cyst removal or cyst reduction is the most effective. Using reverse osmosis (a type of filtration system), it has an "absolute 1 micron" rating given on the label, meaning that the pore size is 1 micron or less in diameter, with or without NSF testing. Filters rated as "nominal 1 micron" aren't reliable for removing bacteria, such as *Cryptosporidium.* Replace the filter cartridges regularly and properly, according to the manufacturer's instructions. A filter may not eliminate smaller bacteria.

. . . if seltzer and club soda are the same as bottled water? No. Still safe to drink, neither is required to meet the quality standards of bottled water. Some seltzer and club soda products contain sugar and sodium, whereas bottled water, by definition, cannot.

. . . what flavored waters really are? Flavored waters

may have just a hint of flavor, derived from a natural fruit essence. Check the label carefully, though, because some clear beverages also contain sugar, other sweeteners, and artificial flavors. If they do, they're soft drinks or "water beverages," not bottled water. Being clear doesn't mean that a beverage is simply water!

. . . if oxygen-enhanced drinks offer unique benefits such as a boost in athletic performance? No. It's just marketing hype.

First, consider "oxygen-enhanced" water. Under pressure, only a tiny amount (about the amount in one breath) of oxygen can be forced into water. It quickly bubbles out as soon as you open the bottle.

Even if some "extra oxygen" in water made it to your mouth, your digestive tract would get it, not your lungs. Your lungs, not your intestines, process oxygen that's captured by the heme (iron) portion of blood. Fortunately, there's enough oxygen in the environment to sustain life. To most efficiently use the oxygen you do breathe in, get regular aerobic activity.

• For drinking and cooking water, let the cold water faucet run for sixty seconds or more to clear water that has been in the pipes and faucet. This helps flush out water with the heaviest lead concentration.

• For cooking and baby formula preparation, use cold water from your tap or bottled water. Hot water dissolves lead from the pipes more quickly than cold water does. Boiling water doesn't get rid of the lead!

• To minimize lead in drinking and cooking water, install a water-softening system only on your hot-water faucet. Then for drinking and cooking use the hard water from your cold-water faucet. It won't pick up as much lead as soft water from your hot-water faucet. Use soft water for washing.

• Use bottled water for cooking and drinking.

As a precaution: The American Academy of Pediatrics and the Centers for Disease Control and Prevention (CDC) advise lead screening for infants and toddlers at ages one and two. If you have a young child between six months and three years old, talk to your doctor about possible sources of lead in your home or child care setting. *As a reminder about lead poisoning and kids, refer to chapter 16.* When children test above 10 micrograms per deciliter, sources of lead in the child's environment should be identified and corrected, according to the CDC.

Another alert: If your water supplier alerts you to nitrate or nitrite levels that exceed EPA standards *and* if you have a child under six months of age, talk to your healthcare provider. Ingesting that water could cause "blue baby syndrome," which can be life-threatening without immediate medical attention. The symptoms are a bluish skin tone and shortness of breath.

Find a different and safe water source for preparing baby formula. Nitrates are inorganic and can't be destroyed as bacteria can be. As with lead, boiling water just concentrates nitrates and so increases the risk.

Water may become unsafe to drink for other reasons. Be aware of water alerts during natural disasters. Sanitize your refrigerator's icemaker and water disperser regularly, according to appliance guidelines. *For more about food and water safety, refer to chapter 12.*

Juicy Story: Fruit Juice, Juice Drink, Fruit Drink . . . or Just Plain Water?

When you're thirsty, a refreshing, fruity beverage often hits the spot. Which will you reach for: fruit juice, juice drink, fruit drink, or water? All replace fluid. When you're choosing a "thirst quencher," go easy on juice or juice drinks since their calories can add up; drink more water. For a flavorful refresher, dilute juice with water. As an aside, the Dietary Guidelines advise that most Fruit Group amounts come from whole fruit rather than juice for more fiber.

Depending on the fruits and perhaps the vegetables they're made from, juices and juice drinks supply varying amounts of vitamins A and C. When it comes to terminology, only 100 percent juice can be called "juice." If juice is diluted (<100 percent juice), the product label must identify it with a different name: "juice drink," "juice beverage," or "juice cocktail"; these terms can be used interchangeably. Or it may be called "diluted ____ juice"—for example, diluted apple juice. A "fruit drink" is simply flavored

Did You Stop to Think

. . . that with so many bottled drinks on the market today, you must be a label reader? Serving sizes aren't always the same. A single bottle may have two or more label servings, for at least twice the calories. And many water beverages, teas, and coffee drinks are high in added sugars.

. . . that a large, regular soda (32 ounces) adds up to about 400 calories? Drinking one drink that size three times a week adds up to 1,200 calories per week, or about 60,000 calories over a fifty-week work year. A pound of body fat is about 3,500 calories. Do the math! That adds up to several pounds of added body fat if you don't make other changes in your food or lifestyle habits!

. . . that "slow sipping" a regular soft drink, sweetened ice tea, or juice drink bathes your teeth in cavity-promoting sugars? And the effect continues for twenty or more minutes after your last sip!

. . . that 8 ounces of milk provide a quarter to almost a third of your day's calcium recommendation? Great for bones! A 12-ounce can of diet soda instead provides "zero" calcium.

water (with no juice), perhaps fortified with vitamin C or other nutrients, phytonutrients, or herbs.

Does 100 percent juice have more vitamin C than a juice drink? Not necessarily. The percentage of juice is just part of the nutrition story. Some 100 percent fruit juices contain less than 100 percent of the Daily Value (DV) for vitamin C, while some juice drinks are fortified to supply at least 100 percent in a single label serving:

¾ CUP	% DAILY VALUE OF VITAMIN C
Orange juice	100
Fortified juice (such as cranberry)	100
Apple juice (unfortified)	3
Grape juice (unfortified)	0

To learn how to use Nutrition Facts on fruit juice and juice drink labels, see "Today's Food Labels" in chapter 11; you'll also find advice on refrigerated juice safety.

All juice products contain water and sugar. Fruit juice contains naturally occurring fructose, or fruit sugar, whereas juice drinks have added sugars such as high-fructose corn syrup as well as some fructose. Scientific evidence shows that your body can't distinguish between naturally occurring and added sugars, so regardless of whether a juice or juice drink is naturally sweet or sweetened, its sugars are used by your body in the same way. *See chapter 5, "Carbs: Simply Complex!"* Depending on the amount of sugars added, there may be a difference in the amount of calories per label serving between fruit drinks and fruit juices.

On the label, 100 percent juices, such as orange juice, won't list sugar and water as separate ingredients. They're naturally present in juice. Sometimes tart juices, such as cranberry, are blended with other juices, water, and sweeteners to make them more pleasing. Some juice drinks are flavorful blends, such as cranberry-mango or tangerine-grapefruit. A nutritional difference between fruit juices and fruit drinks is that fruit juices often contain more of other important nutrients and phytonutrients, such as folate in orange juice or antioxidants in blueberry juice.

Does fruit come to mind first when you think of

juice? Give vegetable juice, such as tomato juice or a vegetable juice mixture, a try, too.

For guidelines on fruit juice for infants and children from the American Academy of Pediatrics, see chapters 15 and 16.

Juicing Fruits and Vegetables

Some juice-machine promoters may lead you to believe that juicing makes fruits and vegetables healthier. Of course, their juices are healthful, offering most of the vitamins, minerals, and phytonutrients found in the whole fruit or vegetables. However, juices typically have less fiber; it gets left behind in the pulp. And in spite of the "cure-all" claims, simply changing the form of food by juicing can't deliver added benefits. Enjoy juice as one way to get the benefits of fruits and vegetables—but don't expect miracles!

Milk, Cocoa, and Flavored Milks: Calcium-Rich Choices

Like all beverages, milk supplies that essential nutrient water: about 89 percent by weight. And as one of the best calcium sources in the American diet, milk offers a lot more.

Along with water, milk supplies many essential nutrients; here's what just 1 cup (8 ounces) supplies. Do a little math to see what the recommended three cups of milk (or the equivalent) daily from the Milk Group provide.

NUTRIENTS IN 8 OUNCES	% DAILY VALUE
Calcium (305 mg.)	30
Vitamin D (100 IU)	25
Vitamin A (500 IU)	10
Protein (8 g.)	16
Potassium (380 mg.)	11
Riboflavin (0.4 mg.)	26
Vitamin B_{12} (1.3 mcg.)	22
Phosphorus (245 mg.)	25
Niacin and niacin equivalents (2 NE)	10

Among the various types of milk—whole, 2 percent reduced-fat, 1 percent low-fat, and fat-free—the fat content varies, along with the calorie content. However, the contributions of other nutrients, including water, are about the same.

Flavored milk, perhaps fruit- or chocolate-flavored, can be a healthful option. For chocolate milk, the difference is an additional 60 calories per 8-ounce serving from the added sweetener, and chocolate or cocoa. Whether it's flavored or unflavored, milk supplies the same amounts of calcium, phosphorus, protein, riboflavin, and vitamin D. *To compare the calories and nutrients in various milk, see "Milk: A Good Calcium Source" in chapter 10.*

The fact that many kids like flavored milk has prompted the question: do the sugar and caffeine in chocolate milk cause hyperactivity? No scientific evidence suggests a link between sugar and hyperactivity, mood swings, or academic performance. The amount of caffeine in the chocolate or cocoa is very small. Some soft drinks provide much more caffeine. *See the chart "Caffeine: What Sources, How Much?" later in this chapter.*

Among other dairy options: drinkable yogurt, smoothies, and hot cocoa made with milk rather than water. They, too, deliver calcium; read the label's ingredient list and the Nutrition Facts to compare the calories and other nutrients. Drinkable yogurt and yogurt drinks may have active live cultures with probiotic benefits; check the label to find out.

Drinks: With or without Caffeine?

Caffeine, a mild stimulant, has been part of the human diet for centuries. As far back as five thousand years ago, records suggest that the Chinese were brewing tea. About twenty-five hundred years ago, highly valued coffee beans were used in Africa as currency. And in the Americas, the Aztecs enjoyed chocolate drinks. Today, caffeine-containing foods and beverages are a growing part of our food pattern. Does coffee in the morning go with your "wakeup" routine?

A naturally occurring substance in plants, caffeine is found in leaves, seeds, and fruits of more than sixty plants, among them coffee and cocoa beans, tea leaves, and kola nuts. We consume these products as coffee, chocolate, tea, and cola drinks. Caffeine also is used in more than a thousand over-the-counter drugs as well as in prescription drugs, and as a subtle flavoring.

Coffee remains the chief source of caffeine in the United States. That includes drinks made with coffee, such as latte, mocha, and cappuccino. The amount of caffeine depends on the type of coffee, the amount, the brewing method, and whether it's caffeinated.

Soft drinks and teas are the main sources of caffeine for children and teens. Among soft drinks, cola isn't the only beverage with caffeine; some citrus-flavored beverages contain caffeine as well.

Caffeine acts as a mild stimulant to the central nervous system. That's why some people drink coffee: to keep alert and prevent fatigue. Does caffeine improve physical performance? *See chapter 19.*

Caffeine: A Health Connection?

Over the years many studies have explored the connection between caffeine and health. No scientific evidence has been found to link caffeine intake to any health risks, including cancer (pancreatic, breast, or other types), fibrocystic breast disease (benign fibrous lumps), cardiovascular disease, blood cholesterol levels, ulcers, inflammatory bowel disease, infertility, birth defects, or osteoporosis.

Concerned about your blood pressure? Caffeine doesn't cause hypertension or a lasting increase in blood pressure. However, it may cause a temporary

Have You Ever Wondered

. . . if sports drinks are good fluid replacers? The optimal drink for many sports is water! Sports drinks are meant to replace fluids, supply calories for energy, and replace sodium and potassium lost through perspiration. Most athletes don't need a sports drink unless they've exercised for an hour or more. Even then, the body mainly needs fluids. If you're more likely to drink a sports drink than water during physical activity, then by all means do. Just be aware that these drinks contain added sugars, so they also supply calories. As a regular beverage choice, remember that their calories can add up: often 50 to 100 calories per cup. *For more information on fluids and sports, see "Thirst for Success!" in chapter 19.*

rise that lasts only a few hours and adds up to less than the rise from climbing stairs.

Caffeine may have a mild diuretic effect, increasing water loss through urination. However, the fluid in the beverage usually cancels any loss. The diuretic effect depends on the amount of caffeine. Caffeinated drinks won't cause dehydration or electrolyte imbalance, either. If you have trouble with diarrhea, avoiding caffeine might be advised.

While caffeine can increase slightly the amount of calcium lost through urine and feces, it's the amount of calcium in about 1 tablespoon of milk that's lost for each cup of regular coffee. To help counter this effect and boost the calcium benefit, enjoy coffee drinks made with plenty of milk. A 12-ounce caffe latte, made with fat-free milk and no added syrups or whipped cream, has about 400 milligrams of calcium and 110 calories. Moderate amounts of caffeine don't appear to raise the risk for osteoporosis. By the way, you don't need to use whole milk to get a foam on cappuccino. Low-fat or fat-free milk and soy beverage also will do the trick.

Chic coffee drinks? Shots of caramel, chocolate, fruit syrups, or cream can load coffee bar beverages (lattes, mochas, cappuccinos, or other drinks) with plenty of added sugars, total fat, saturated fat, and calories. The larger the size, the more calories they rack up! If you can customize your coffee drink, make it healthier. Ask for the smallest size. Request fat-free milk (no or less whipped cream) or soy beverage, and perhaps sugar-free syrup or a dusting of cocoa powder or cinnamon. Bottled coffee drinks may not have as much calcium as you think—and perhaps more added sugars and calories; read the Nutrition Facts.

Although many think coffee can help "sober up" someone who drinks too much alcohol, caffeine won't counteract the effects of alcoholic drinks. Neither will a cold shower or a long walk. Only time can make someone sober.

In varying degrees, excessive caffeine intake may cause "coffee jitters," anxiety, or insomnia. Caffeine also may speed heart rate temporarily. These physical effects don't last long since caffeine doesn't accumulate in the body. Within three to four hours, most is excreted in healthy people; for smokers, it's slightly faster. Some people are more caffeine sensitive than others.

Caffeine: What Sources, How Much?

The amount of caffeine in foods or beverages depends on several factors: type of product, its preparation method, and portion size. Caffeine occurs naturally in some products, such as coffee and chocolate, and is added as a flavoring agent in some others, such as soft drinks.

	CAFFEINE (MG)	
BEVERAGE	TYPICAL	RANGE
Coffee* (8-oz. serving)		
Brewed, drip method	85	60–120
Brewed, perculator	75	60–85
Decaffeinated	3	2–4
Espresso coffee (1-oz. serving)	40	30–50
Tea (8-oz. serving)		
Brewed	40	20–90
Instant	28	24–31
Iced	25	9–50
Some soft drinks (8 oz.)	24	20–40
"Energy" drinks (8 oz.)	80	0–80
Cocoa beverage (8 oz.)	6	3–32
Chocolate milk beverage (8 oz.)	5	2–7
Milk chocolate (1 oz.)	6	1–15
Dark chocolate, semisweet (1 oz.)	20	5-35
Baker's chocolate (1 oz.)	26	26
Chocolate-flavored syrup (1 oz.)	4	4

*For the coffee and tea products, the range varies due to brewing method, plant variety, brand of product, etc.
Source: U.S. Food and Drug Administration and National Soft Drink Association.

"Excessive" caffeine intake is individual. Caffeine sensitivity depends on the amount and frequency of caffeine intake, body weight, physical condition, and overall anxiety level, among other factors. Tolerance to caffeine develops over time. A regular coffee drinker may not notice the effects as quickly as someone who drinks an occasional cup. For most healthy adults, moderate amounts of caffeine—200 to 300 milligrams a day, from about two to three cups of coffee—pose no physical problems. For kids, use common sense. No evidence shows that caffeine in levels normally found in food and beverages are harmful or that kids are any more sensitive to caffeine than adults. That said, some kids do consume a lot of caffeine from soft drinks.

Can you become addicted to caffeine? No, but caffeinated drinks may become a habit. If you drink them regularly, then suddenly stop, you may have short-term symptoms—drowsiness, headache, perhaps less concentration—that disappear in a day or two.

According to the National Institutes of Health, caffeine affects children and adults in the same way. No studies show that caffeine causes attention deficit disorder or affects growth in children.

● *If you're pregnant or nursing* . . . up to 300 milligrams of caffeine (about two to three 8 oz. cups of brewed coffee) doesn't appear to have adverse affects, and it doesn't affect fertility. Although most physicians agree on its safety, sensitivity to caffeine may increase during pregnancy. In breast milk, caffeine can pass to the baby, but the very small quantity in usual amounts isn't enough to affect the infant. During breast-feeding, limit caffeine drinks, advises the American Academy of Pediatrics; you don't need to avoid them.

● *If you have a medical problem* . . . ask your physician to guide you on caffeine consumption, particularly if you suffer from gastritis, ulcers, or high blood pressure, or if you're taking beta-blockers. People with stomach problems may be wise to steer clear of both caffeinated beverages and their decaffeinated counterparts. Substances in both stimulate the flow of stomach acids, potentially irritating the stomach lining.

● *If you're older* . . . your sensitivity to caffeine may increase with age.

● *At any age* . . . pay attention to how caffeine affects you, especially if coffee, tea, or soft drinks take the place of more nutritious foods or beverages.

For most people who choose caffeinated beverages, two to three cups of coffee (or that amount of caffeine) are likely reasonable. If you decide to reduce your caffeine intake, it's easy. Here's how:

● Cut back gradually—if you've been ingesting a lot of caffeine—to get your body accustomed to consuming less. A gradual cutback helps avoid any temporary headaches or drowsiness.

● Try to mix half-regular and half-decaffeinated coffee.

● Drink decaffeinated coffee, which has almost no caffeine at all. Some bottled coffee drinks also are decaffeinated; check the label.

● Brew tea for a shorter time. A one-minute brew may contain just half the caffeine that a three-minute brew contains.

● Drink decaffeinated tea or caffeine-free herbal tea.

● Keep a cup of water handy to sip. If you drink coffee, tea, or soft drinks mindlessly, you may be drinking more caffeine than you realize.

● Read soft drink labels; many soft drinks consumed in the United States contain caffeine. If you drink soft drinks, look for decaffeinated drinks or those without caffeine. Color doesn't indicate the presence of caffeine; both clear and caramel-colored soft drinks may have caffeine. Caffeine is listed in the ingredient list if it is present in the product.

● Read medication labels carefully, or check with your pharmacist. One dose of an over-the-counter pain relief capsule can contain as much caffeine as one or two cups of coffee.

● For those with insomnia, avoid coffee or other caffeine sources in the evening.

Take Time for Tea

Tea: next to water, it's the most common beverage choice throughout the world. Whether it's black, green, or oolong tea, tea comes from the same plant, called *Camellia sinensis.* Differences in color and flavor depend on processing.

● For *black tea,* the most popular type in the United States, tea leaves are exposed to air. The natural biochemical process turns them a deep red-brown color and imparts a unique, rich flavor. Many flavored specialty teas start with black tea. As an aside, orange pekoe isn't made with orange flavor; instead "pekoe" or "orange pekoe" refers to the grade and size of the tea leaves.

● For *green tea,* typically served in Chinese and Japanese restaurants, the tea leaves are not processed as much. Instead, they're just heated or steamed quickly to keep their green color and delicate flavor.

● *Oolong tea* is an "in-between" tea: between black and green tea.

Teatime: Health Benefits?

Whether black or green or oolong, tea appears to have potential health benefits, perhaps derived from its flavonoids. Flavonoids and other polyphenols, which are phytonutrients, work as antioxidants that may help protect body cells from damage done by free radicals. Using the oxygen radical absorbency capacity (ORAC) score, which ranks the antioxidant potential of plant-based foods, tea ranks as high as or higher than many fruits and vegetables. *To learn more about antioxidants, the ORAC score, and phytonutrients, see chapter 4.*

Can tea drinking help keep you healthy? Maybe, but the research linking tea consumption and disease prevention is too new for certainty. And there's not enough evidence yet to offer specific advice about tea drinking. Some promising areas of study suggest that tea or tea's flavonoids may reduce risk of gastric, esophageal, and skin cancers and may offer protection from heart disease and stroke—if you consume enough (four to six cups a day). Some studies are investigating whether tea plays a role in relaxation or mental performance.

Tea may supply fluoride, which helps strengthen tooth enamel, if it's made with fluoridated water. Tea also may help fight cavities by reducing plaque formation and hindering cavity-forming bacteria. You still need to brush and floss!

For now, enjoy tea; brew it for at least three minutes to bring out most of the flavonoids. Then stay tuned for science-based advice.

Creative Ways to Enjoy Tea

● Try bottled teas as a portable beverage choice. Many bottled or canned ice tea drinks have as much added sugars as a regular soda; read the label to check the calories. Look for those flavored with noncaloric sweeteners.

● Watching calories? Enjoy tea without added sugar or honey. For a touch of flavor in unsweetened tea, just add a slice of lemon or lime, fresh ginger, or fresh mint leaves.

● Add citrus juice for flavor and smart nutrition! Tea's flavonoids partly inhibit the absorption of nonheme iron (iron from legumes, grain products, and eggs). A squeeze of vitamin C-rich lemon, orange, or lime juice in your tea can counteract some of the action.

● For more calcium, enjoy "milk tea": hot or cold tea added to milk. Some believe that adding milk to tea lowers tea's antioxidant power. However, no scientific evidence proves that milk binds to and inactivates polyphenols. If you enjoy milk in your tea, certainly add some!

● Experiment with culinary uses of dried tea leaves: as a flavor rub for a roast, for tea-marinated meat, or in homemade sorbet.

● Use tea—perhaps a flavored variety—in place of water in dough or batter for breads, cookies, cakes, and brownies.

Pour a "Herbal"?

Have a sip of apple-cinnamon tea, mint tea, or ginger tea. Interest in herbal teas has been rising for those seeking an alternative to caffeinated beverages—and for those hoping for other health benefits.

To clear up a misconception: many branded herbal teas are really tea leaves with added herbs and perhaps fruit juice, honey, sweeteners, or flavor extracts; they have caffeine unless the label indicates "decaf." The ingredient list will include "tea." And some herbal teas on the market aren't tea at all. Instead, they're infusions made with herbs, flowers, roots, spices, or various other parts of many plants. The more correct term for them is "tisane," which means tealike substance.

When it comes to health benefits, herbal teas haven't been studied, so not much is known. Some research suggests that their polyphenols, one type of phytonutrient, may bind iron before it can be absorbed. Most major branded herbal teas are considered safe to drink. Still, you're wise to consume only common varieties sold by major manufacturers.

Some herbal teas interfere with over-the-counter or prescription medications. Talk to your doctor or pharmacist before drinking them when you're on medication.

Because of their potential harmful effects, be careful about using herbs to make "teas"—comfrey, lobelia, woodruff, tonka beans, melilot, sassafras root, and many others may be harmful in large amounts. For example, comfrey may cause liver damage. Woodruff, an anticoagulant, may cause bleeding. Lobelia may cause breathing problems. Even chamomile may cause an allergic reaction.

For more on herbal teas and remedies, see "For Herbal and Other Botanical Supplements . . ." in chapter 23.

Soft Drinks: Okay?

Flavored, carbonated drinks have been around for about two hundred years. And their popularity continues to grow—overtaking more nutritious beverages among some age groups.

The term "soft drink" originally was coined to distinguish these beverages from "hard" liquor. Yet a hundred years ago, consumers asked for "pop," named for the sound made by popping open the bottle cap. Today, "soft drink"—or "soda" in some parts of the United States—refers to a beverage made with carbonated water and usually flavoring ingredients.

What's in a soft drink? Whether they're regular or diet varieties, soft drinks contain water: about 90 percent for regular soft drinks and about 99 percent for diet soft drinks. Carbon dioxide, added just before sealing the bottle or can, gives the fizz. Regular soft drinks are sweetened with sugar, perhaps high-fructose corn syrup and/or sugar; diet drinks, with saccharin, aspartame, and other alternative sweeteners. *See chapter 5 for more about sugar and alternative sweeteners.* Additional flavor comes from artificial and natural flavors. Acids such as citric acid and phosphoric acid give a tart taste and act as preservatives. Coloring may be added. Some caffeine may be added to enhance the flavor, while other ingredients may add consistency.

As soft drink consumption goes up, the nutritional concerns do, too:

● Soft drinks can take the place of more nutritious beverages such as calcium-rich milk. Except for water and for carbohydrates in the form of sugars, soft drinks don't supply significant amounts of nutrients. A 12-ounce can of regular cola, for example, supplies water and about 150 calories (from almost 10 teaspoons of sugar), but little else. A 20-ounce bottle or cup has 250 calories! A diet soft drink is a source of water and has almost no calories.

● Added sugars, especially in drinks, are linked to higher calorie intake. That, in turn, may contribute to the growing problem of overweight and obesity. Consuming less added sugars, especially from drinks, may help prevent weight gain and may aid weight loss.

● Soft drinks fortified with antioxidants have hit the market, too. Be wary. For the potential benefits, fruits, vegetables, and whole-grain foods are much more effective sources. *See "Antioxidant Vitamins: A Closer Look" in chapter 4.*

Functional Beverages

Improve your memory? Lift your mood? Relieve tension? Fight fat? Give you energy? A growing market of functional beverages—juice, tea, soft drinks, flavored water, isotonic drinks, enhanced with herbs, phytonutrients, and other functional ingredients—are marketed with promises to improve health. Do they offer benefits?

Most functional beverages aren't likely to offer benefits to most healthy people. Among the issues: Claims that aren't proven; *for what we know and don't know about the ingredients (gingko, kava, ginseng, and St. John's wort, among many others), see "Dietary Supplements: What Are They?" in chapter 23.* The amount of the added ingredient is neither standardized nor identified on the label. And their safety—optimal doses, interactions, and long-term consequences—isn't known.

Will "energy drinks" really give you more energy? High caffeine and "carbs" are the so-called power behind their marketing hype. It's not the ideal drink for athletes, or for "grab-and-go energy." Extra caffeine may give a boost at first, but with too much caffeine, performance may suffer; *see chapter 19 for more about beverages for athletic performance.* The concentrated sugar content can slow the body's absorption of water, so energy drinks aren't the best fluid replacers. And as a mixer in alcoholic drinks, the stimulating effect of caffeine may mask the effects of too much alcohol—a potential danger. Energy drinks sold as nutritional supplements, with the potentially dangerous stimulant ephedrine, were banned by FDA in 2004 although there have been legal challenges to this ruling.

Functional drinks won't counter dysfunctional eating or living. The best approach for health and for feeling energetic? Healthful eating, regular physical activity, enough rest—and learning to deal with stress. The best fitness drink with moderate exercise: water!

Drink Smart—and Get Your Zzzzzzzs!

Do you wake up with a sleep deficit? Do you regularly have trouble sleeping? Adequate rest, along with good nutrition and regular physical activity, are part of any formula for fitness. Consider these tips for the "rest" of your life:

- If you're caffeine-sensitive, avoid caffeinated drinks six to eight hours before sleeptime. For meals and snacks later in the day, opt for milk, juice, water, or decaffeinated drinks.

- Don't expect a glass of wine or other alcoholic beverage to help you sleep well. A drink might help you feel drowsy at first, but even if you sip a drink two or three hours before bedtime, your sleep might be light instead of the deep, most restful kind of sleep pattern.

   An added note: Promote rest through regular physical activity. Being active actually helps your body relax and sleep soundly. Just refrain from exercise too close to bedtime. Exercise speeds up your metabolism for a while, perhaps keeping you "pumped up" and unable to sleep right away.

As your best guideline, enjoy soft drinks in moderation—as long as you consume the nutrients you need from other sources and don't overdo on calories in your overall diet. Remember: Regular soft drinks deliver calories, but little else.

Alcoholic Beverages: In Moderation

No one's sure who first invented beer, wine, or spirits, but historians do know that societies have enjoyed these beverages throughout recorded history.

Today, moderate amounts still add pleasure to eating. For some, a single drink may be relaxing—perhaps in the company of another. For older adults and people with some chronic illnesses, a drink before a meal may enhance appetite. And evidence suggests that moderate drinking may lower the risk for heart disease among some people; healthful eating and active living are part of the equation, too.

The key to potential benefits is sensibility: moderation and understanding alcohol equivalency.

- *Moderation:* up to one drink a day for women and up to two drinks daily for men

- *Equivalency of one drink:* 12 fluid ounces of regular beer (150 calories), *or* 5 ounces of fluid wine (100 calories), *or* 1.5 fluid ounces of 80-proof distilled spirits (100 calories). Each contains the same amount of alcohol—approximately 14 grams (or 0.6 fluid ounces) of pure ethanol. Distilled spirits include bourbon, brandy, gin, rum, vodka, whisky, and liqueurs.

The Dietary Guidelines advises: *Those who choose to drink alcoholic beverages should do so sensibly and in moderation.* The guidelines continue, giving specific precautions, among them: never drink if it puts you or others at risk!

Alcoholic Beverages: The Health Effects

For most adults, one alcohol-containing drink or two a day offers little risk for problems related to drinking. Are there any benefits? What are the risks?

Unlike nutrients, most alcohol isn't broken down through digestion. Its "pathway" to body cells moves much faster, including directly through the stomach lining and wall of the small intestine. With no food in the stomach to slow it down, absorption into the blood-

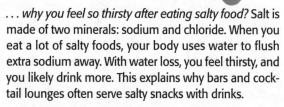

Have You Ever Wondered

. . . why you feel so thirsty after eating salty food? Salt is made of two minerals: sodium and chloride. When you eat a lot of salty foods, your body uses water to flush extra sodium away. With water loss, you feel thirsty, and you likely drink more. This explains why bars and cocktail lounges often serve salty snacks with drinks.

. . . if a few cold beers on a hot day are as good as water to replace fluids? Not really. Alcohol is a mild diuretic, which increases urine output and so promotes dehydration—not the best fluid replacement when you're sweating! If you enjoy a beer, drink water, too.

. . . what's rooibos tea? Pronounced ROY-boss, rooibos isn't a tea at all, but instead a herbal brew. First popularized in South Africa, this red brew in nutty, flowery, and fruity flavors is purported to have antioxidant benefits. Research doesn't back up the advertised claims. Like other herbals, be cautious.

stream is even faster (within about twenty minutes). From the bloodstream, it goes to every cell of the body, to some degree depressing cell activity.

Although some people drink to be the "life of the party," alcohol actually is a depressant, not a stimulant. The initial "lift" that may come with drinking is short-lived. By dulling various brain centers, alcohol may reduce concentration, coordination, and response time; cause drowsiness and interfere with normal sleep patterns; and result in slurred speech and blurred vision. Because they have a short-term diuretic effect, some people may feel thirsty after drinking a lot—perhaps the morning after.

The alcohol concentration in blood depends on the amount of alcohol consumed over a period of time as well as body composition, body size, metabolism, and medications. A healthy liver detoxifies much of the alcohol consumed—at a rate of about $\frac{1}{2}$ ounce per hour. The higher the blood alcohol concentration level, the longer it takes. For two regular-size drinks consumed during a sixty-minute "happy hour," the body needs two to three hours to break it down.

A single alcoholic drink affects women more than men, due in part to differences in body size and metabolism. Alcohol is carried in the body's fluids, not in body fat. Because women have a smaller volume of water in their bodies than men do, the same amount of alcohol is more concentrated in the bloodstream and so potentially has a greater effect. The enzyme that helps metabolize alcohol in the body is also less active in women. As a result, women are at greater risk for problems related to alcoholism.

Caution: *The Risks.* The Dietary Guidelines for Americans notes risks related to alcoholic beverage consumption. The hazards of heavy drinking are well known and include an increased risk for several health problems, including high blood pressure, liver cirrhosis, and several forms of cancer, as well as motor vehicle accidents, other injuries, violence, and death. During pregnancy, drinking increases the chances for birth defects. For women, moderate drinking may slightly increase the risk for breast cancer.

Heavy drinkers may have social and psychological problems: for example, altered judgment and a potential dependency. Excessive drinking also can lead to brain and heart damage, cirrhosis of the liver, and an inflamed pancreas.

Potential Benefits? Moderate drinking may offer health benefits: lower risk for heart disease, mostly for middle-age and older adults. The benefits appear to come from moderation of any alcoholic beverage: wine, beer, or distilled spirits.

An alcoholic drink before a meal may stimulate the appetite and make a meal more appealing. Talk to your healthcare provider if you have a health problem linked to appetite loss. That said, the potential benefits aren't reason enough to start drinking or to drink more frequently.

Watch the Calories, Mind Your Nutrients!

Alcohol is actually a fermentation product of carbohydrates: both sugars and starches. In beverages or food, it supplies energy, or calories. Alcohol provides 7 calories for every gram, compared with 4 calories

Red Wine: Heart-Healthy?

Does red wine protect against heart disease? There's no conclusive answer. Research suggests that a moderate amount of alcoholic beverages—red wine as well as white wine, beer, and distilled spirits—may help lower the risk for heart disease. Possibly a small amount may help increase HDL blood cholesterol, or "good" cholesterol, and it may prevent LDL, or "bad" cholesterol, from forming. However, factors other than ethanol (alcohol) also may play a role.

Phytonutrients such as resveratrol and tannins in wine may offer heart-healthy benefits. Resveratrol, a flavonoid in the skins and seeds of grapes, has estrogenlike qualities that may help increase HDLs or increase the oxidation, or breakdown, of LDLs. (Grape skins are needed to make red wine.) Also speculated, resveratrol may boost the body's natural clot-dissolving enzyme; when blood platelets clot, they decrease blood flow, which can lead to a heart attack or a stroke. Tannins also may inhibit platelet clotting.

Scientists don't know enough to offer definitive advice, so if you don't drink, protecting your heart isn't a reason to start. If you do, a drink a day of any alcoholic beverage may offer a benefit. Remember: Other lifestyle habits—such as healthful eating, regular exercise, not smoking, and keeping a healthy weight—offer the most protection against heart disease! See "A Toast to Heart Health" in chapter 22.

per gram of carbohydrate and protein, and 9 calories per gram of fat. A 1½-ounce jigger or "shot" of vodka, for example, may be on average 40 percent alcohol, or up to 0.6 ounce of alcohol. That equals about 14 grams and contributes about 100 calories. The additional calories in beer, wine, or liqueurs come from carbohydrates.

The alcohol content of a single drink depends on the type of alcoholic beverage and the serving size. "Special" alcoholic drinks advertised on restaurant table tents usually contain more alcohol because they're bigger. The calorie content also is determined by the amount of alcohol and, for mixed drinks, the other ingredients in the drink. *See the chart "Alcohol and Calories: How Much?" later in this chapter for alcohol and calories in standard-size servings.*

Does drinking lead to weight gain? Probably not for moderate drinkers. In fact, a few scientific studies suggest that the body uses energy (calories) from alcohol differently than energy from other sources.

For some people who drink to excess, however, a "beer belly" is aptly named. Calories from alcoholic beverages can add up, contributing to excess overall body weight. For example, a six-pack of beer, consumed on a hot summer day, supplies 900 calories. To burn off those calories, a person would need to jog without a break for about two hours. A 5-ounce glass of dry wine before dinner supplies 100 calories, or 700 calories if consumed every day of the week. Within five weeks that adds up to a pound of body fat. (A pound of body fat equals 3,500 calories.) The mixers added to drinks make the calories add up even more, yet often add few nutrients; for example, the soft drink in a rum-and-cola drink, coconut cream in a pina colada, and sugar in a daiquiri or hot buttered rum.

Although it supplies calories, alcohol isn't a nutrient. On the contrary, because alcohol may interfere with nutrient absorption, heavy drinkers may not benefit from all the vitamins and minerals they consume. Unless juice or milk beverages are mixers, alcoholic beverages themselves supply few if any nutrients.

Moderate drinking isn't associated with poor nutrition. However, alcoholic beverages shouldn't take the place of nutritious foods and beverages—for example, when a glass of wine with dinner takes the place of calcium-rich milk. By limiting your intake of beer, wine, and spirits, there's room in your eating plan for more nutritious foods and drinks. For the casual or moderate drinker, this may not be much of a problem; malnutrition is a significant concern for very heavy drinkers.

Drinking: For Some Not Advised

The Dietary Guidelines for Americans advise: *For those who drink alcoholic beverages, do so sensibly and in moderation.* However, some people are wise to avoid alcoholic drinks entirely. Besides the risks mentioned earlier, avoid drinking . . .

. . . if you're a teenager or a child. Young people should not drink. That includes new fortified fruit-flavored wines and hard (alcoholic) ciders. Since the risk of alcohol dependence goes up when drinking starts at an early age, kids who drink can set themselves up for the same health-related risks that adults have. For inexperienced teenage drivers, alcohol and driving is a very risky combination. Besides, buying alcoholic beverages is illegal in the United States for anyone under age twenty-one.

Label Lingo

Alcoholic Beverages

You'll find this warning statement on the label of beverages containing alcohol. On wine and beer labels, you may also find information on sulfite content. *See "For the Sulfite-Sensitive . . ." in chapter 21.* (*Tip:* If you're sulfite-sensitive, distilled spirits and sake, a type of rice wine, don't contain sulfites.)

GOVERNMENT WARNING:

(1) ACCORDING TO THE SURGEON GENERAL, WOMEN SHOULD NOT DRINK ALCOHOLIC BEVERAGES DURING PREGNANCY BECAUSE OF THE RISK OF BIRTH DEFECTS. (2) CONSUMPTION OF ALCOHOLIC BEVERAGES IMPAIRS YOUR ABILITY TO DRIVE A CAR OR OPERATE MACHINERY, AND MAY CAUSE HEALTH PROBLEMS.

CONTAINS SULFITES found in most wines to protect flavor and color.

. . . *if you can't moderate your drinking.* As part of a lifelong commitment, recovering alcoholics and problem drinkers should abstain from any alcoholic drink. Because of the genetic link to alcoholism, people with alcoholism in their family are wise to moderate their intake of alcoholic beverages, too—or avoid them.

. . . *if your work requires attention, skill, or coordination.* Alcohol affects productivity, which can affect your work output and your personal safety. Even with moderate drinking—a glass of wine or beer—alcohol stays in your blood for about one hour, and two glasses, for two hours or more.

. . . *if you plan to drive or handle potentially dangerous equipment.* Even low levels of blood alcohol from a single drink can make you more accident-prone for an hour or so. If you plan to drink, designate another driver from the start who won't be drinking!

. . . *if you're pregnant or trying to get pregnant.* In the United States, drinking during pregnancy is the leading known cause of birth defects. Fetal alcohol syndrome is characterized by mental retardation, and by behavioral and psychosocial problems. While there's not enough proof that an occasional drink is harmful, even moderate drinking may have behavioral and mental consequences. No safe level has been established for a woman any time during pregnancy, including the first few weeks. Too often, women drink before they even know they're pregnant, potentially compromising their baby for life. *See "Pregnancy and Alcoholic Beverages Don't Mix!" in chapter 17 for more on fetal alcohol syndrome.* Heavy drinking may not be wise for dad, either. According to research, excessive alcohol may decrease sperm count and potency and so affect fertility.

. . . *if you're breast-feeding.* The level of alcohol in your breast milk will mirror that of your blood alcohol content if you consume alcoholic drinks. And even low to moderate drinking may adversely affect a baby's feeding and behavior.

. . . *if you have certain medical conditions,* such as liver disease. Talk with your doctor.

. . . *if you're on medication, even over-the-counter kinds.* Alcohol may interact with certain medicines, making them either less effective or more potent. The medication itself may raise blood alcohol levels or increase its adverse affects on the brain. The result: a single drink will impair judgment, coordination, and skill faster. Check warnings on over-the-counter medications. Talk with your doctor, pharmacist, or healthcare provider about your prescribed and over-the-counter medications. *See "Food and Medicine" in chapter 22.*

. . . *if you suffer from allergies.* Sulfites in wine may trigger histamine production and allergy symptoms.

Have You Ever Wondered

. . . if a little "nip" of brandy will help fight a cold? On the contrary, if you have a cold or a chronic health problem that lowers your immunity, you're wise to abstain. Alcohol can impair the body's ability to fight infectious bacteria and may interfere with medication.

. . . if an alcoholic drink will warm you up in cold weather? No. Alcohol tends to increase the body's heat loss, making people more susceptible to cold. If you're ice fishing, cross-country skiing, or watching outside winter sports, an alcoholic drink won't keep you warm.

. . . what the term "80 Proof" means on a bottle of liquor? The term "Proof" indicates the amount of alcohol. The proof is twice the alcohol content. If a label on a bottle of liquor states "80 Proof," this means that the liquor contains 40 percent alcohol. The proof will vary depending on the type of liquor.

. . . if a nightcap will help you sleep? It may put you to sleep, but not help you stay asleep—with the deep, restful sleep you need. A drink with dinner probably won't affect your sleep habits.

. . . how much alcohol burns off or evaporates in cooking? That depends on the cooking time, temperature, and the amount of distilled spirits, wine, or beer used. Added to uncooked foods, the alcohol content doesn't change. However, added to boiling liquid at the end of cooking, about 85 percent of the alcohol may be retained, compared to only about 5 percent if the dish was braised for 2½ hours. A flamed (flambé) dish may retain about 75 percent of its alcohol content.

. . . how cooking wine compares to regular table wine? Cooking wine is usually high in sodium. From a flavor standpoint, regular wine may be better.

Substitutions for Alcoholic Ingredients

Baby back ribs, chicken, or seafood tenderized in a beer marinade, a touch of distilled spirits to enhance the flavor of cooking juices, light biscuits or bread made with beer, chicken braised in wine. Wine, beer, and distilled spirits can add to the flavor, tenderness, and texture of your culinary creations.

If you choose to avoid wine, beer, or distilled spirits, it's easy to make a quick, flavorful substitution. To equal the amount of liquid from the alcoholic ingredient, you may need to add water, broth, or apple or white grape juice. (*Note:* Extracts may have small amounts of alcohol.)

IN A RECIPE THAT CALLS FOR . . .	USE THIS INSTEAD . . .
¼ cup or more white wine	Equal amount of: *In any dish:* white grape juice, apple juice, nonalcoholic wine* *In salad dressings:* lemon juice *In marinades:* vinegar *For savory dishes:* chicken, vegetable, or clam broth (Use ⅞ cup broth plus 2 tbsp. lemon juice or vinegar.) (*Add 1 tbsp. vinegar to balance sweetness.)
¼ cup or more red wine	Equal amount of: *In any dish:* red grape juice, cranberry juice, nonalcoholic wine* *In salad dressings:* lemon juice *In marinades:* vinegar *For savory dishes:* tomato juice, fruit-flavored vinegar, or beef, chicken, or vegetable broth (*Add 1 tbsp. vinegar to balance sweetness.)
¼ cup or more port wine, rum, brandy, sweet sherry	Equal amount of apple or apple juice plus 1 tsp. vanilla extract
¼ cup or more beer	*For soups, stews, and other cooked dishes:* Equal amount of nonalcoholic beer, apple cider, or broth
2 tbsp. almond-flavored liqueur, such as Amaretto	¼ to ½ tsp. almond extract
2 tbsp. bourbon	1 to 2 tsp. vanilla extract
2 tbsp. coffee liqueur, such as Kahlua	2 tbsp. double-strength espresso *or* 2 tbsp. instant coffee, made with 4 to 6 times the usual amount in a cup of coffee
2 tbsp. orange-flavored liqueur, such as Grand Marnier	2 tbsp. orange juice concentrate *or* 2 tbsp. orange juice plus a little orange rind
2 tbsp. chocolate/coffee-flavored liqueur	½ to 1 tsp. chocolate extract plus ½ to 1 tsp. instant coffee in 2 tbsp. water
1 tbsp. dry vermouth	1 tbsp. apple cider
2 tbsp. dry sherry or bourbon	2 tbsp. orange or pineapple juice *or* 1 to 2 tsp. vanilla extract
2 tbsp. rum or brandy	½ to 1 tsp. vanilla, rum, or brandy extract *or* 2 tbsp. orange or pineapple juice

Taking Control: Drinking Responsibly!

If you choose to drink alcoholic beverages, always do so responsibly. Here's how you can go easy . . .

● Start with a nonalcoholic beverage. Satisfy your thirst first. Then enjoy your alcoholic beverage more slowly.

● Don't drink on an empty stomach. Eating a little food helps slow the absorption of alcohol.

● Decide ahead to limit drinks, preferably no more than one per day if you're a female or two per day if you're a male. If you choose to drink more, pace yourself. On average, the body can detoxify only one standard-size drink (about ½ ounce of alcohol) per hour. The rest continues to circulate until it's finally broken down.

● To slow your drinking pace, put your drink down. Socialize instead.

● If you have one alcoholic drink, make the next one nonalcoholic. When you do this, you consume less alcohol and give your body a chance to process the alcohol you've consumed already.

● Measure liquor for mixed drinks with a jigger. Use a 1-ounce jigger, not the 1½-ounce size. You'll likely use less with a jigger than if you pour from the bottle right into the glass.

● Make an alcoholic drink last longer; you'll less likely order another. Learn to sip, not gulp; perhaps use a straw for mixed drinks. Dilute drinks with water, ice, club soda, or juice to increase the volume. *Tip:* Frozen drinks often take longer to sip.

● If you feel thirsty, drink bottled water or a soft drink instead of another alcoholic beverage. Remember: Alcohol actually has a diuretic effect.

● Prefer a wine cooler? Instead of commercial drinks, mix your own using less wine. For mixers, try sparkling water or fruit juice.

● Lighten up! Order low-alcohol beer, light wine, or a light distilled spirit instead. Each has less alcohol. Or try nonalcoholic beer.

● At the table, have a glass of water by your plate, too. You'll probably drink less alcoholic drinks.

● Skip the last round before the bar closes! And,

Super Sippers

Hot-weather thirst quenchers:

● For a subtle citrus flavor in ice water, add slices of lemon, lime, or orange. Or add fruited or floral ice cubes: freeze fruit juice or edible flowers in your ice cube trays. *To learn about edible flowers, see "Please Don't Eat the Daffodils" in chapter 13.*

● Combine one 6-ounce can of grapefruit juice or cranberry-mango cocktail concentrate with two 12-ounce bottles of chilled club soda. Serve with a sprig of fresh mint. Serves four.

● Make a fruit smoothie. In a blender, puree berries, sliced kiwifruit, mango, or pineapple chunks, and frozen limeade concentrate. Perhaps add a little fresh mint. For convenience, try canned and frozen fruit for smoothies!

● Create your own shakes. In a blender, puree melon chunks or peach slices with buttermilk, crushed ice, and a touch of ginger or cinnamon until smooth.

● Use silken tofu as a great nondairy alternative in a creamy shake. Add a little juice and frozen fruit; puree until smooth.

Cold-weather belly warmers:

● Simmer cranberry-apple juice with cinnamon, cloves, allspice, and orange peel for about twenty minutes. Strain. Stir in fat-free dry milk powder and vanilla extract. Heat through.

● Add anise seeds, ground cinnamon, and ground cloves to ground coffee. Prepare hot coffee using the spiced ground coffee. Lighten with warm milk.

● Scoop praline or chocolate-swirl frozen yogurt into a mug. Pour hot cocoa or coffee over the top. Stir with a cinnamon stick.

as a host, don't feel a need to refresh your guests' drinks.

● Order a "virgin" cocktail: nonalcoholic mixers without the liquor. Mix in juice, carbonated water, or a soft drink instead. Remember the garnish! *See "Kitchen Nutrition: Super Sippers" for more ideas.*

● Bring bottled water or soft drinks to a picnic or a sports event to be sure you have a nonalcoholic option.

Alcohol and Calories: How Much?

Although their calorie content differs, these standard-size drinks each supply about the same amount of alcohol—about 14 grams of pure ethanol. (*Note:* Alcoholic drinks are not 100 percent alcohol; that's why the volume differs.)

ALCOHOLIC DRINK	CALORIES
Beer, regular, 12 oz.	150
Beer, light, 12 oz.	100
Wine, dry, 5 oz.	100
Wine cooler, 12 oz.	180
Distilled spirits (80-proof), 1½ oz.*	100
Cordial or liqueur, 1½ oz.*	160 (varies widely)

*An added mixer, such as a soft drink, adds more calories.

Beer and Wine: What's in a Name?

Today these products appear on supermarket shelves. But just what do the descriptions mean, and how much alcohol do they contain?

Near beer: Malt beverage that has an alcohol content below 0.5 percent by volume. It also can be labeled a "malt beverage," a "cereal beverage," or when the label says "contains less than 0.5 percent alcohol by volume" as "nonalcoholic."

Low-alcohol or reduced-alcohol beer: Malt beverage with less than 2.5 percent alcohol by volume.

Alcohol-free malt beverage: Malt beverage that contains no alcohol.

Flavored malt beverage: Malt beverage (beer, lager, ale, porter, stout) flavored after fermentation, perhaps with juice, fruit, or juice concentrate—for example berry-, lemon-, or orange-flavored beer.

Aperitif wine: Wine with an alcohol content of 15 to 24 percent by volume, made from grape wine and added brandy, or alcohol flavored with herbs or other natural aromatic flavorings.

Fortified wine: Wine that has brandy or distilled spirits added to it. Dessert wine has 14 to 24 percent alcohol by volume, more than table wine.

Table wine: Wine that has 7 to 14 percent alcohol by volume. Light wine, red wine, and sweet table wine are all types of table wine.

Low-alcohol wine: Wine, or fermented fruit beverage, that is less than 7 percent alcohol by volume. Low-alcohol wine isn't necessarily lower in calories; it may have more sugars than other wine.

Wine cooler: Diluted wine product (diluted with fruit juice, water, and/or added sugars) with an alcohol content of less than 7 percent by volume. Read the label's Nutrition Facts for calorie content per serving. Wine coolers may have more alcohol and calories than you think since a serving is usually bigger: often 12 ounces, rather than a 5-fluid-ounce glass of table wine.

Sources: Bureau of Alcohol, Tobacco, and Firearms (2001); U.S. Food and Drug Administration (personal communication, 2001).

As an aside, most beers contain 5.0 to 5.5 percent alcohol by volume. In the United States and Europe, a pale beer (usually a lager), rather than a dark beer, may be referred to as a light beer. The alcohol content is about the same as in regular beer, but the calories are somewhat less. An alcoholic beverage with more than 24 percent alcohol by volume is defined (and taxed) as a distilled spirit.

Need more strategies to boost your fluid intake? Check here for "how-tos":

- Buy the type of milk, including soy beverage, that matches your needs—see chapter 11.

- Scout for nutrient-rich drinks when you eat out—see chapter 14.

- Get enough fluids when you're physically active—see chapter 19.

- Know how to fit milk in if you're lactose intolerant—see chapter 21.

PART III

Smart Eating
The Consumer Marketplace

CHAPTER 9

What's on Today's Table?

From all the foods available for today's table, why do consumers—why do you—choose one food over another? Consumer research says taste is the top reason—followed by nutrition, food safety, price, and convenience!

In the past decade or two there's been a real "change of plate" on the family table. As a consumer, perhaps you've noticed a shift with even more health- or flavor-focused food products, or in your own shopping and cooking patterns, lifestyles, and attitudes about food and health. You may be eating smarter to promote health. Like many others, you may be more adventuresome with food and want more flavor. Or in spite of ever better kitchens and cooking equipment, convenience and speed may be more important to you than before.

The diversity of foods in today's marketplace reflects the diversity of today's consumers. Rather than selling just to the mass market, food producers know the value of "different strokes for different folks." As a result, a variety of foods are produced and marketed to match unique needs: age, gender, health, lifestyle, ethnic or religious background, preferences, and economic resources, among others.

Food: What's "in Store" for You?

Frozen skillet meals, bagged salad mixes, or marinated ready-to-cook beef roast for *convenience* . . . almond milk, ostrich tenderloin, blue potatoes, or doughnut-shaped peaches for *something new* . . . hummus, guava juice, or pad Thai for *ethnic adventure* . . . multigrain cereal with flaxseed, or juice with added antioxidants for their *health benefits*. You'll find these foods alongside your traditional favorites in today's supermarkets.

When it comes to food choices, consumers in the United States seem to have more variety of food to choose from every year—and more ways to eat for health. A single supermarket stocks, on average, about fifty thousand different items, including nonfood items. In a typical year, about ten thousand new food products may be introduced in the marketplace. Yet only about 2 percent make it past the consumer cut.

When you eat away from home, you may notice that some fast-food menus are offering more variety, along with more whole-grain, fruit, and vegetable choices, and more grilled, broiled, steamed, and stir-fried, not just fried, food anymore. Many supermarkets sell fully prepared meals. Traditional restaurant menus and recipes for at-home cooking reflect an interest in healthful eating, ethnic cuisine, flavor, local ingredients, and a blending (or fusion) of ingredients and cooking styles.

More choices mean more decisions and more for you to know about your food supply.

Healthy Eating Sells!

Packaging promotes foods' health benefits: "lowers cholesterol," "promotes immunity," "build strong bones." Nutrition Facts on labels display the calories, nutrient, cholesterol, and fiber content per serving. Signs in many produce departments remind you to eat plenty of colorful fruits and vegetables daily. You can hardly walk through a supermarket without being exposed to healthful eating messages!

Functional Foods: A New Wave

"Functional foods" describes foods and beverages with health benefits beyond (and in addition to) basic nutrition. These foods or beverages may enhance your health, protect you from certain diseases, or do both. With functional nutrition, what you *do* eat, not what you *don't* eat, makes the difference!

Currently no legal definition for a "functional food" exists. Technically, all foods, in one way or another, are functional and provide health benefits. Among the big sellers are health bars and products made with soy. Traditional foods such as tomatoes, oranges, oatmeal, yogurt, and tuna also have functional messages to share. That said, it's a market that's rapidly growing!

Why the interest? Attention to personal health is on the rise, and many people—perhaps even you— want control over their health, especially as health-care costs go up. An aging population seeks avenues for health protection. Rapid advances in science provide a growing body of credible evidence for functional nutrition, and agricultural and food science technology can produce foods that offer potential functional benefits. In addition, changes in food regulation that began in the mid-1990s allow labels to include health claims and structure/function claims.

What makes foods functional? Food components that do more than nourish you! Consider a few examples:

- Many fruits, vegetables, and grain products have phytonutrients, or plant substances (carotenoids, flavonoids, isoflavones, or indoles, to name a few), that may reduce the risk for certain diseases including prostate cancer, heart disease, and macular degeneration. Phytonutrients that give health benefits also deliver flavor and color.

- Strong scientific evidence supports the belief that oats help lower cholesterol levels.

- Prebiotics/probiotics such as fructo-oligosaccharides in shallots and lactobacillus in some dairy foods may improve the balance of "good" intestinal bacteria.

- Fatty fish have fatty acids known as "omega-3s," which may lower your risk for heart disease and improve your mental performance.

- Dairy foods and some meat (beef, lamb) have another fatty acid, conjugated linoleic acid (CLA), which may help lower your risk for cancer.

- Calcium-rich foods such as dairy foods may help protect you from high blood pressure and colon cancer and may play a role in weight control.

- Soy protein in many soy-based foods may help lower your cholesterol levels.

In most foods, functional benefits probably come from several—perhaps many—food components. The heart-healthy benefits of oats come not only from its soluble fiber (beta glucan) but also from its antioxidants, amino acids, and natural plant sterols. Cancer protection from legumes may come from fiber as well as isoflavones, saponins, and protease inhibitors.

For more examples, refer to chapters 3, 4, and 6.

Different types. "Tried and true" or "innovative and new," functional foods belong in several categories:

- *Unmodified whole foods* such as oats, carrots, tomatoes, grapes, blueberries, nuts, beans, salmon, and yogurt with live, active cultures, to name a few!

- *Modified foods,* including those fortified or enriched with nutrients, or enhanced with phytonutrients or botanicals, such as high-fiber cereals, calcium-fortified orange juice, vegetable juice with added lutein, flour with added folic acid, and beverages with more vitamin E, even cereals with herbal additives.

- *New foods created for functional and other benefits* such as shakes and snack foods with soy protein, omega-3 and flaxseed food bars, and spreads with plant stanol or sterol esters that help lower blood cholesterol.

- *Foods produced through biotechnology* for functional benefits such as tomatoes with more lycopene, or rice with added beta carotene and iron. *See "Food Biotechnology: Nutrition Opportunity!" later in this chapter.*

Fitting functional foods in. Credible research shows that functional foods certainly play a role in wellness (*see Appendices*) when combined with balanced food choices and plenty of physical activity. However, they're not "magic bullets" for health. Functional foods can't make up for poor eating habits or an unhealthy lifestyle.

Functional benefits of food—their bioactive components and their physiological action—are full of unknowns. To get their known benefits, as well as those that science may reveal in the future:

● Eat a *variety* of foods with potentially healthful benefits, on a *regular basis,* and in *adequate amounts.* To be effective, you need enough regularly over a period of time.

● Choose from all five food groups and the healthful oils of MyPyramid. Foods in each group

Functional Nutrition: What's in a Name?

With the advent of functional foods, new terms have entered our vocabulary. Although not legally defined, here's what they generally mean and how they differ.

● *Functional foods:* foods that provide health benefits beyond basic nutrition

● *Phytonutrients:* substances in plant-based foods with physiologically active components that have functional food benefits; also called phytochemicals

● *Prebiotics:* nondigestible food substance that may stimulate the growth and activity of health-promoting, or "good," bacteria in the intestine

● *Probiotics:* live bacteria that may promote health by improving the balance of "good" bacteria in the intestine

● *Synbiotics:* products with both prebiotic and probiotic substances that work together to keep the balance of "good" bacteria in the intestine

● *Zoonutrients:* a term sometimes used for substances, such as omega-3 fatty acids, with physiologically active components, in animal-based foods; also called zoochemicals.

For more about phytonutrients, prebiotics and probiotics, and substances in animal-based foods that promote health, see chapter 4.

—plant- and animal-based foods—offer bioactive, potentially beneficial substances.

● For the functional benefits, enjoy food first, rather than supplements. Food has many more functional components that likely work best when eaten together, as nature provided.

● Choose wisely. Foods fortified for functional benefits may not be the best choice, especially if they didn't have many nutrients or perhaps had a lot of calories to start with.

● Use claims on food labels to find foods that match your needs. *To understand what functional claims mean—and don't mean—see "Health Claims on the Label" and "Structure/Function Claims on the Label" in chapter 11.*

● Enjoy foods with functional benefits as part of your fat strategy for better health, not in place of appropriate medical care or medications. Tell your healthcare provider what you're doing.

● Be savvy when you read about foods promoted with functional benefits. Junk science abounds! Nutrition research that's either misinterpreted or oversimplified often makes headlines. *To help you sort through the information maze, see chapter 24, "Well Informed?"*

Nutrient-Modified Foods: "The Haves and the Have-Nots"

Shop for foods positioned for nutrition-conscious consumers. For example, you'll find "good source of calcium," "more fiber," and "fat-free" foods. In many cases these foods are modified versions of traditional foods—often produced with less fat, saturated fat, *trans* fat, cholesterol, sugar, or sodium, or with more fiber or certain vitamins or minerals. Fat-free taco chips and fat-free refried beans, high-fiber cereal, and reduced-sodium soup are some examples.

To create these foods, the food industry adjusts the ingredients. By modifying the nutrient content, the qualities of food often change. For example, to cut back on fat, some foods may contain more carbohydrates, such as starch or added sugar. Conversely, to lower "carbs," fat may be bumped up. These modifications may change the flavor and the mouth feel of foods you're accustomed to. Formulating foods with less salt often makes them less flavorful, too—unless other flavor-intense ingredients, such as herbs or spices, are added.

How can you fit today's nutrient-modified foods into a healthful eating plan?

● Remember the big picture. Enjoy them in an overall way of eating that's varied, moderate, and balanced. For example, being "fat-free" doesn't mean calorie-free. And "calcium added" juice doesn't make it a substitute for all the nutrients in milk, although the juice may be a calcium-rich source for strict vegetarians or those with lactose intolerance.

● Check the Nutrition Facts on food labels for foods with nutrient content claims. For example, cutting back on fat won't necessarily make a food low in calories. *See "Get All the Facts!" in chapter 11.*

● Count nutrient-modified foods in your eating plan just as you'd count their traditional counterparts. Either way, 1½ ounces of fat-free or of regular Cheddar cheese count as an 8-ounce equivalent from the Milk Group of MyPyramid. *See "MyPyramid: Your Healthful Eating Guide" in chapter 10.*

● Look for products with flavor-boosting spices, herbs, and other ingredients—for example, reduced-fat or low-fat sausages with herbs. Extra seasonings boost flavor in products with less fat or sodium.

Flavor Sells: The Multicultural Palate

With global communications, travel, and food imports, our "world of food" is more connected than ever, offering more ethnic and regional foods. But not that long ago, bagels, pita bread, pastas of every shape, and tortillas were considered trendy, ethnic foods—and salsa was a new flavor experience! Today these foods and many other ethnic foods are now supermarket mainstream.

What sparks interest in and availability of ethnic and regional foods? Perhaps a sense of curiosity and adventure as well as a desire to learn—and the search for nutritious, flavorful alternatives. Celebrity chefs entertain by preparing ethnic foods, even taking us via media to global markets and kitchens. Travel, cooking classes, Web sites, magazines, newspapers, cook-

books, and restaurants expose us to unique flavors: ingredients, seasonings, and dishes. Supermarkets stock their shelves with ethnic and regionally inspired foods, partly to meet the demand from diverse populations, partly to match flavor trends.

As a result, consumers have more food variety, food combinations, and ways to eat for flavor, health, and pleasure. Many ethnic and regional cuisines offer health benefits, especially those that focus on grains, vegetables, legumes, and fruits. *For many nutritious, good-tasting dishes in ethnic cuisines, see "Vegetarian Dishes in the Global Kitchen" in chapter 20.*

Our Edible Heritage

"Ethnic food" isn't new. Throughout history, the foods of one culture have traveled to another, infusing cuisines with more variety and new flavors. Those foods also became new sources of nutrients and food energy.

The quest for flavor—exotic Eastern spices—launched the Age of Discovery and the exploration of the New World. Among the discoveries: a vast array of foods! Among other foods, the Americas contributed tomatoes to Italy, potatoes to Ireland, peanuts (or groundnuts) to West Africa, and hot chiles to Thailand. And foods unknown to the Americas five hundred years ago came from all parts of the Old World—for example, chickens, pigs, beef, wheat, oats, barley, okra, Asian rice, peaches, pears, watermelons, citrus fruits, bananas, and lettuce.

American cuisine has strong roots in its native foods: corn, legumes, pumpkins, peanuts, potatoes, tomatoes, peppers, pineapples, squash, wild rice, and turkey, among many others. Each immigrant wave has contributed its own ethnic cuisine. In time, many ethnic foods were adapted and became "typically American"— for example, pizza, tacos, and chop suey. "Food immigration" continues as new waves of immigrants—mostly Latin Americans, Asians, Eastern Europeans, and Middle Easterners—influence American cuisine today.

Regional specialties develop as people adapt their cooking style to foods that are available. And many foods once eaten as regional specialties become nationally popular—for example, sweet potato pie, cooked collard greens, and black-eyed peas and rice from the South, created by African American cooks; crab cakes and clam chowder on the Atlantic coast; tamales, bean burritos, and cactus salad from the Southwest; and smoked salmon and berry cobblers from the Pacific Northwest.

A Fusion of Flavor

The blending of cuisines, sometimes called "fusion cuisine," is one of today's hot culinary phenomena. It combines the ingredients or cooking techniques of two or more cultures not geographically close together. The result: new cuisines, such as Thai-French, Southwest-Asian, Cuban-French, and unique dishes such as Moroccan couscous topped with Chinese stir-fried vegetables. Even fast-food menus reflect the trend, with Mexican pizza, chili in a pita pocket, or a Thai wrap tucked in a tortilla.

The fusion of ingredients and flavors isn't new. It's been going on for centuries as people gradually adapted their cuisines to the available food supply—sometimes by choice, often by necessity. Interestingly, about 50 percent of foods eaten in the world today originated in the Americas.

Today, fusion cooking brings an explosion of new dishes to the American table. In many cases, new "fused" dishes uniquely combine grain products, fruits, and vegetables. Their combinations may offer nutritional benefits for you. *For ways to "fuse" ingredients in your meals and snacks, see "Ethnic Table: For Variety, Health, and Eating Pleasure!" later in this chapter.*

Simply adding seasonings from an ethnic cuisine also creates fusion: perhaps a touch of curry powder from India blended in pumpkin soup . . . or basil and garlic, borrowed from Italian cooking, added to beef stew. *For more about seasoning combinations, see "Flavor Profile!" in chapter 13.*

What's New Is What's Old, Too

What's new on the table is also what's old. Grandma's meat loaf, mashed potatoes, soup, and biscuits are "dressed" with today's seasonings, such as sun-dried tomatoes, garlic, wasabi, lemongrass, and fresh herbs. Often sold in farmers' markets, heirloom vegetables and fruits—with their unique flavors, colors, shapes, and scents—add more variety to the table. "Heirlooms" are open-pollinated (grown from seed) cultivars grown for at least fifty years. Examples? Flavorful, pinkish-red Brandywine tomatoes (Amish); purple-striped Cherokee Trail of Tears pole beans (Native American); and sweet, lime-green Jenny Lind melons.

Culture on Your Plate

Moroccan or Lebanese, Nuevo Latino or Thai, Indian or Ethiopian, ethnic fare has captured consumer interest. Many people want to go beyond "ethnic" basics—Italian, Chinese, and Mexican—and explore regional ethnic foods: Tuscan, Liguria Roman, Calabrian, and Lazio (Italian); Sichuan, Peking, and Cantonese (Chinese); and Yucatán, Oaxacan, and Michoacan (Mexican). If you're among those who want to go beyond the basics . . .

● Try an ethnic or a regional restaurant; do "tastings" at community ethnic festivals. Order food that's new to you. *For restaurant tips, see "Eating Out Ethnic Style" in chapter 14.* Ethnic foods and other new food combinations often get introduced first in restaurants! If you're cautious, try an appetizer portion.

Take Your Taste Buds to the Mediterranean

There's no single cuisine for regions that border the Mediterranean Sea. The dishes of Greece, southern Italy, Spain, southern France, Tunisia, Lebanon, and Morocco, for example, are all distinctive. Yet they typically contain plenty of grain products, vegetables, legumes, nuts, and fruits; less meat and poultry; more fish; and (except in Muslim areas) moderate amounts of wine. Their fat is mostly monounsaturated (from olive oil). And yogurt and cheese offer other sources of animal protein.

Traditional Mediterranean eating may have several health benefits—especially for reducing risks of heart disease, and perhaps for some cancers. Studies show that the death rate from heart disease and the incidence of cancer are lower among many Mediterranean populations. And the incidence of these health problems has gone up among people who no longer eat in their traditional way. The reasons for this are not yet clear to scientists.

In general, the total fat intake of the Mediterranean diet isn't lower than the typical American diet. It's just shifted to more monounsaturated fat. Other dietary factors, not fully understood, may offer some protection.

Before you switch your eating style, be aware that the benefits of the Mediterranean lifestyle may go well beyond food. Traditionally, the people studied in the region were also more physically active. Body weight and genetics are factors, too. And the overall lifestyle was more relaxed.

● Shop from the ethnic food section of your supermarket. Or in an ethnic food store, shop and ask for advice on food preparation—perhaps from other customers!

● Get an ethnic cookbook; check one out from a library. Try a dish with more grains, vegetables, beans, or fruits—perhaps Mediterranean tabouli (bulgur salad) or cucumber-yogurt dip, Japanese sukiyaki (stir-fried meat and vegetables) with udon noodles, Brazilian black bean soup, or vegetarian curries from India. Check food TV, and culinary magazines and Web sites.

Your Nutrition Checkup

Food Neophobia: Do You Have It?

Enjoying more variety of fruits, vegetables, and grain products puts more nutrients and phytonutrients on your plate! Measure your sense of food adventure.

1. How would you describe your willingness to try new foods?

I don't experiment.	1
I'll try if offered.	2
I'm a willing adventurer.	3

2. When was the last time you bought an unfamiliar vegetable or fruit at the store?

Last year or longer	1
Last month	2
Last week	3

3. When a new food product hits the market . . .

I'm rarely aware of it.	1
I give it a try after it's been on the market a while.	2
I try it right away—if it matches my needs.	3

4. I try to eat a wide variety of foods.

Never	1
Sometimes	2
Almost always	3

5. I look for new ways to prepare familiar foods . . . perhaps from cookbooks, magazines, newspapers, TV, Web sites or from friends.

Never	1
Sometimes	2
All the time	3

6. The variety of foods becoming available due to today's agriculture . . .

Doesn't interest me	1
Mildly interests me	2
Intrigues me	3

7. When was the last time you ate at an ethnic restaurant (other than Italian, Chinese, or Mexican)?

Last year or longer	1
Within the past six months	2
Within the past month	3

8. If preparing an Italian meal, I would make . . .

Spaghetti noodles	1
Spaghetti noodles or some other type of pasta (e.g., whole wheat)	2
Any type of pasta, polenta, or risotto	3

How did you fare? Add up your points.

NOW SCORE YOURSELF

20 to 24: You're probably a "foodie" who enjoys food adventure and flavor. Being a food adventurer adds variety—along with more than forty different nutrients and hundreds of phytonutrients—for your good health.

13 to 19: You're open to experiencing new foods . . . a healthy attitude toward eating! Be aware that the same food may taste different to different people, perhaps because they have a different number of taste buds. That may be why some people like spicy-hot flavors and others don't.

8 to 12: You're more comfortable with your "tried and true." But does your cautious approach mean missing out on a variety of nutritious foods? Don't be surprised if you don't like a food the first time you taste it. The more often you try a food, the more familiar it gets—and often, the more you like it!

Read on for new foods to add to your plate.

● Learn "hands on" about ethnic ingredients, food prep, and flavors. Take a cooking class; take a culinary vacation.

● Be adventuresome with food when you travel, rather than head for familiar fast-food fare.

● Learn from a friend: someone who prepares his or her own family's ethnic dishes.

What's "New"?

Supermarket shelves and restaurant menus feature a broad array of foods that weren't easily available a few short years ago—all offering more ways you can eat for health, flavor, convenience, "on the go" lifestyles, and enjoyment! Today's food manufacturers and packaging provides you with:

● *More convenience.* You'll find more prepackaged foods—precooked meat and poultry, meal kits, speed scratch meals, and take-out—to help you serve a nutritious "home served" meal in record time.

● *More variety of fruits and vegetables.* With more health-consciousness, produce departments—even the canned and frozen aisles—stock a greater variety of fruits and vegetables year-round, including "exotics" and varietals. For example, an apple isn't just an apple anymore; it may be a Granny Smith, a Rome Beauty, or a Gala! Specialty produce also comes in different colors and miniatures: *red* carrots, okra, and corn; *purple* asparagus, artichokes, Brussels sprouts, kohlrabi, wax beans, and yams; *white* eggplant and sweet potato; *yellow* beets; *golden* kiwifruit; and *miniature* avocados, eggplant, squash, corn, bananas, and kiwifruit.

● *More variety of grains.* Interest in breads has shifted to more coarse-textured, denser, whole-grain breads. Breakfast cereals are made with more whole grains—and not just corn, oats, or wheat. And whole grains of all kinds are also used in salads, soups, and mixed dishes. Eating more whole grains and whole-grain foods is easier with so many new whole-grain products to select from.

● *More "fresh."* Even in mixes, you'll find more fresh foods—fresh salad mixes, stew and stir-fry mixes, vegetable snacks, and herbs. Mixes for breadmaking machines let you bake bread without effort. Fresh

pasta is sold in refrigerated displays. And the fresh seafood department is commonplace. Fresh foods aren't necessarily more nutritious. *See "Fresh vs. Processed: Either Way to Health" later in this chapter.*

● *More function and personal customization. See "Functional Foods: A New Wave" earlier in this chapter.*

● *More vegetarian entrées.* With growing interest in vegetarian eating, you'll find more meatless, prepared entrées, such as bean burritos or vegetarian lasagna. There's a greater variety of pasta, vegetables, and legumes (dry, canned, and fresh) for home-cooked vegetarian meals, too. Enjoy legumes—perhaps in vegetarian entrées—several times a week.

● *More specialty foods.* With growing food sophistication, more gourmet and unique foods are available, too. Being "gourmet" doesn't make food any better. Read the Nutrition Facts on the food label.

● *More flavor.* The influence of ethnic cuisine, herbs, and other flavor ingredients has put more flavors in canned, frozen, and packaged foods; recipes; and restaurant foods. Consider the availability of hot sauces!

● *More indulgence.* There's a flip side to the growing array of foods marketed for health. There are now more indulgence foods: richer, higher-fat frozen desserts, bigger portions, and more high-calorie snack foods, among others. If you choose these foods, fit them into a smart strategy without overdoing on calories.

Look for new foods in stores. Of the eighty thousand known edible plants, only about three hundred are cultivated for food! Only twelve are major food staples.

Garden of Eatin': Less Common Vegetables

Looking for new ways to enjoy a colorful variety of fruits and vegetables? Starting here, identify all the vegetables that you've never tried before. Then make a point of buying and trying one or two of them the next time you're in a supermarket or restaurant—and get their nutrient and phytonutrient benefits.

● *Arugula (ah-ROO-gu-lah)* is a green, leafy vegetable with a distinctive flavor. It's used raw in mixed garden salads, or cooked and tossed with pasta or risotto.

Ethnic Table: For Variety, Health, and Eating Pleasure!

Look for this multicultural array of foods in your supermarket aisles. Then enjoy these quick-to-fix dishes at home.

	Cuisine*	Serving/Preparation Ideas	Nutrient Contribution
Grain Group			
Whole-wheat couscous (tiny, round pasta)	Moroccan	Serve hot with tomato sauce and Parmesan cheese, or serve cold as a salad with raisins, mandarin oranges, and spices.	Starches, B vitamins, fiber
Kasha (buckwheat kernels)	East European	Serve as a hot side dish with chicken or beef. Mix with pasta shapes.	Starches, B vitamins, fiber
Pozole (soup made with fermented corn kernels)	Mexican	Serve warm with diced onion, shredded cabbage, and a lime wedge.	Starches, fiber
Wonton wrappers (thin wheat dough used to wrap spring rolls)	Chinese, Vietnamese	Wrap thin strips of cooked lean barbecued pork or chicken, and shredded cabbage and carrots inside, then steam.	Starches, B vitamins
Vegetable Group			
Jicama	Mexican	Slice in thin strips and dip into salsa or reduced-fat or fat-free ranch dressing. Use to replace water chestnuts in stir-fry dishes.	Negligible
Collard greens	African American/Southern	Boil greens with chopped, smoked turkey, vinegar, and seasonings.	Beta carotene, fiber
Tomatillos	Mexican	Dice, and boil with jalapeño peppers for salsa. Dice, and combine with onions for an omelette.	Vitamin C, beta carotene, potassium, fiber
Shiitake mushrooms	Japanese	Add raw to salads and sandwiches, or toss in stir-fry dishes.	Negligible
Fruit Group			
Lychee	Chinese	Serve on top of frozen yogurt.	Vitamin C, potassium
Kumquat	Chinese	Pack a few for snacking, or slice for fruit salad.	Vitamin C, beta carotene, folate
Papaya	Mexican, Central American	Blend with pineapple for tropical juices, dice and add to salsas, or simmer in a chutney recipe.	Vitamin C, beta carotene, potassium
Plantain	Puerto Rican, Central American	Cube, and add to stews and soups.	Potassium, starches
Mango	Caribbean	Slice for fruit salads, or simmer in a chutney recipe.	Vitamin C, beta carotene, potassium

	CUISINE*	SERVING/PREPARATION IDEAS	NUTRIENT CONTRIBUTION
Meat and Beans Group			
Squid	Mediterranean, Asian	Slice in rings, and broil. Serve with marinara sauce. Or cook in stir-fry dishes.	Protein, iron, B vitamins
Veal, lamb	Mediterranean	Marinate in Italian vinaigrette, then grill.	Protein, iron, B vitamins
Hummus (mashed chick-peas)	Middle Eastern	Serve as a dip for raw veg-etables or pita triangles.	Protein, B vitamins, fiber
Chorizo (sausage)	Mexican	Slice in bite-size pieces, add to omelettes or stews.	Protein, iron, B vitamins
Tofu	Japanese, Chinese	Slice for stir-fry dishes, or dice for salads or soups.	Protein, calcium
Black beans	Latin American	Use in place of red beans in chili or soup, mash for homemade refried beans, or mix with rice.	Protein, B vitamins, fiber
Milk Group			
Plain yogurt	Middle Eastern	Top falafel sandwiches (chickpea- and vegetable-stuffed pita). Blend with mint as a dip or dressing for cucumbers.	Protein, calcium, riboflavin
Goat milk	Middle Eastern, African (some areas)	Drink goat milk plain. Make a thick drink by mixing with juice. Use it in place of cow milk in baking.	Protein, calcium, riboflavin
Ricotta cheese	Italian	Use in lasagna, or stuffed jumbo pasta shells.	Protein, calcium, riboflavin
Queso blanco (white cheese)**	Mexican	Shred, and melt over enchi-ladas and quesadillas.	Protein, calcium, riboflavin

*These foods may be used in the dishes of many global cuisines.
**To reduce the risk of foodborne illness, look for queso blanco made from pasteurized milk.
Refer to chapter 14 for common food-group foods in Italian, Mexican, and Chinese cuisines.
Source: American Dietetic Association.

● *Bok choy (BAHK choy) (or pak choi)* is a Chinese cabbage. It doesn't form a head, but instead has several white, bunched stems with thick green leaves. It can be eaten raw or cooked, and is used often in stir-fry dishes.

● *Breadfruit* looks like a green, bumpy melon (brown when ripe) on the outside, and is creamy white on the inside. Like other starchy vegetables, it's peeled, then baked, boiled, fried, grilled, or cooked with stew and soup. Its flavor is somewhat sweet, yet mild. Some Caribbean dishes are made with breadfruit.

● *Broccoli raab,* with 6- to 9-inch stalks and small broccolilike buds, is strong and bitter. Use it raw in salads, cooked as a side dish, or in mixed dishes.

● *Cactus pads (nopales, or noh-PAH-lays),* which are cactus leaves, are used in a variety of Mexican and Southwest dishes. Their thorns are removed before cooking them. Then they're usually sliced, then sim-mered or cooked in a microwave oven. You also can buy canned nopales.

● *Cassava (kah-SAH-vah) (manioc, or MA-nee-ahk; yuca, or YOO-kah, root),* a starchy root vegetable, has a thick, brown peel, but inside it's white or yellow like a potato. It's often cooked in dishes similar to the way potatoes are used.

● *Celeriac (seh-LER-ee-ak),* a member of the celery family, is enjoyed for its root, not its stalks. It has a fibrous, brown, bumpy peel . . . and a sweet, celery flavor inside. Once peeled, enjoy it raw, perhaps in salads, or cooked—boiled, steamed, or fried. Use it in soups or stews, perhaps in place of celery.

● *Chard,* actually a white-rooted beet, is grown for its leaves, and creamy-white or red stalks. With its mild yet distinctive flavor, it's used much like spinach.

● *Chayote (cheye-OH-tay)* is a pale-green, pear-shaped vegetable with a mild flavor. Baked, boiled, braised, or stuffed, it complements the flavors of other ingredients in mixed dishes. Use it like squash.

● *Chicory (curly endive)* has a frizzy green leaf in a loose head of greens. Its bitter flavor adds a nice touch to salads—in small amounts.

● *Daikon (DEYE-kuhn)* is a Japanese radish that looks like a smooth, white parsnip. It has a stronger, more bitter flavor than a red radish. Often it's used to make sushi (fish rolled with rice in seaweed) and in vegetable carvings.

● *Dasheen (dah-SHEEN)* is a large, round root vegetable with a coarse, brown peel that's similar to taro. Usually prepared either boiled or baked, dasheen is starchy, somewhat like a potato.

● *Escarole (EHS-kah-role)* is a somewhat bitter salad green. Sometimes its green leaves have a reddish tinge. Unlike iceberg lettuce, it forms a loose head.

● *Fennel* looks like a squat bunch of celery with feathery leaves. Its flavor is distinctive, like a sweet, delicate anise. The bulb and stalks are often braised, steamed, sautéed, or used in soups. The feathery leaves may be used in salads, as an herb, or as a garnish.

● *Jerusalem artichoke*—native to North America—has nothing in common with a globe artichoke, except for its name. Like a potato, it's a tuber, grown under the ground. But it is knobby and irregularly shaped, with a sweet flavor and a light-brown or purplish-red peel. It's often cooked in its peel; a little lemon juice in the cooking water keeps peeled Jerusalem artichokes from browning. Use them in dishes that call for potatoes, or eat them raw.

● *Jicama (HEE-kah-mah),* another root vegetable, is crisp and slightly sweet. It's often peeled, sliced, and eaten raw, perhaps in salads. Or it's cooked in stews and stir-fried dishes.

● *Kale,* a leafy vegetable in the cabbage family, doesn't form a head. It has a curly, purple-tinged, green leaf. Use it in salads and in ways that you would cook spinach.

● *Kelp* is brown seaweed, often used in Japanese cooking and wrapped around sushi.

● *Kohlrabi (KOLE-rah-bee),* a member of the cabbage family, looks and tastes somewhat like a turnip. It's light green in color. It can be used in recipes that call for turnips, or sliced and used in stir-fry dishes, or peeled and eaten raw or in salads.

● *Leeks* are onions and look like a bigger, sturdier, flat-leaved version of green onions. Both the bulbs and the leaves are eaten. Bulbs usually are sliced and steamed in soups or baked in casseroles. The leaves are often used in salads. They need to be cleaned well to remove soil that gets between the leaves.

● *Lotus root,* which is the root of the water lily, often is peeled, sliced, then cooked—stir-fried, steamed, or braised, with mixed Chinese dishes. It has the texture of a potato and a flavor more similar to fresh coconut.

● *Plantain* actually belongs to the banana family, but it's longer and thicker, starchier, and less sweet. For that reason it's eaten as a vegetable—always cooked. It can be eaten at any of its three stages: green, yellow, or black, but it's sweetest when it's black. Plantains are cooked in or out of the peel. They may be baked, boiled, or fried, and often are mixed in stews.

● *Radicchio (rah-DEE-chee-oh)* is a small, purplish head of leaves with white ribs. It's somewhat bitter, and adds a nice touch to salads, pasta, and stir-fry dishes.

● *Rutabaga (ROO-tuh-bay-guh)* is a root vegetable, with a turniplike flavor and appearance. Use it in recipes that call for turnips—stews, soups, and casseroles.

● *Salsify,* a white root vegetable tasting like delicate oysters, usually is eaten as a plain vegetable or perhaps in soups.

● *Seaphire* is a halophyte, or saltwater crop. With an asparagus-grass look, seaphire is crisp, crunchy, and salty. Since it's high in sodium, enjoy it in small amounts as a flavoring in salads, stir-fries, and vegetable dishes, especially if you're sodium-sensitive. Three ounces have 1,350 milligrams of sodium.

● *Seaweed,* used most often in Asian dishes and some Irish, Welsh, and Scottish dishes, includes many types.

Kelp may be the most commonly used in the United States. Many Japanese dishes use nori (NOH-ree).

● *Squash* includes many varieties for cooked dishes: acorn, buttermilk, crockneck, delicata, golden nugget, hubbard, kabocha, mini pumpkin, spaghetti (as an alternative to pasta), sunburst, and turban.

● *Taro (TAIR-oh)* is a rough, brown or purplish tuber vegetable that looks much like a yam, although some varieties look different. It has edible leaves, which are called callaloo in the Caribbean. Taro is peeled and usually boiled, baked, or fried, much like potatoes. Hawaiian poi is made from taro.

● *Tomatillo (tohm-ah-TEE-oh),* a member of the tomato family, has a paperlike husk. Under the husk it looks like a small green tomato. It's often used in food like a green tomato, although the flavor is more citruslike. It is often used in Southwest and Mexican dishes, including salsa and salads.

Fresh Ideas: Uncommon Fruit

Rather than reaching for fruit you know already, try something new! Many fruits aren't well known in the United States because they grow in tropical or sub-tropical areas. Fortunately, today's transportation systems are increasing the variety of fruits available from near and far—at all times of the year. Look for these or other unusual fruits in the produce department of your store, in the canned food aisle of your supermarket, or in Asian and Hispanic food stores.

Red bananas, amnazano bananas, apple bananas, plantains—not just yellow bananas! To help make fruit an adventure, try different varietals of common fruits, too—perhaps apples, bananas, oranges, plums, and pears—for their unique flavors, textures, and perhaps cooking qualities.

● *African horned melon,* also known as Kiwano, is unique in appearance: spiked, oblong shape, golden-orange color, with juicy green fruit inside that tastes like cucumber, banana, and lime.

● *Asian pear* looks like a yellow apple—and has a similar firm, crunchy texture. It's sweet and juicy and nice to eat as a whole fruit or mixed in salads.

● *Atemoya (a-teh-MOH-ee-yah)* is a cross between two fruits: cherimoya and sweetsop. With a green skin,

it has a petal-like look. Inside, the cream-colored, custardlike pulp is studded with large black seeds and offers a mango-vanilla flavor.

● *Blood orange* is a tart, yet sweet orange with flesh that's either bright red or white with red streaks.

● *Cherimoya (chair-ih-MOY-ah) (custard apple)* has a custardlike consistency and flavor. On the outside it looks like a little green pineapple without leaves. The inside has little black seeds. It tastes like a mixture of fruit flavors: strawberry, banana, pineapple, and mango. It's best to eat it as whole fruit; just cut it in half, remove the seeds, and scoop out the fruit.

● *Cape gooseberries* are juicy and bittersweet beneath their "Chinese lantern" skin. They're tasty with meat, other savory dishes, and desserts.

● *Feijoa (fay-YOH-ah, or fay-JOH-ah)* looks like a kiwifruit without fuzz. Inside its cream-colored flesh is sweet, fragrant, and pearl-like. To eat it, remove the skin, which may be bitter, cut it in half, and scoop out the fruit. It's a great recipe substitute for apples or bananas.

● *Guava (GWAH-vah) (guayaba, or gwey-AH-bah)* is a sweet, fragrant fruit that's about the size of a lemon. Its peel varies in color from yellow to purple, and the fruit inside may be yellow, pink, or red. Eat guavas as whole fruit, or in sauces, salads, juices, frozen desserts, and jams.

● *Kumquat (KUHM-kwaht),* in the citrus family, looks like a small, olive-shaped orange. Because the peel is very thin, a kumquat is eaten with the peel on—either uncooked or cooked with meat, poultry, or fish. Slice it as a garnish or for salads.

● *Longan (LONG-uhn)* is a small, round, cherry-sized fruit with a thick, nonedible brown shell. Inside, the white, juicy fruit, which surrounds a large black seed, is fragrant and sweet.

● *Loquat (LOH-kwaht),* a small, pear-shaped fruit, is light orange in color on the inside and the outside. Somewhat tart, it has a pit, which must be removed. Loquats are eaten whole, and often prepared in salads or in cooked poultry dishes.

● *Lychee (LEE-chee) (litchi),* a fruit that's just 1 or 2 inches in diameter and has a pink to red shell. Inside, the fruit is white and sweet with a consistency like a grape. Its seed isn't edible. Lychees make a nice snack or a dessert just as they are.

● *Mango,* a sweet-tart and juicy fruit, ranges in size and shape. It can be about 6 ounces to 5 pounds, and it may be round or long. Its inedible peel is orange when ripe, with orange fruit inside and a large seed. The best way to eat a mango is to either peel back the skin and eat it with a spoon . . . or remove both peel and seed and cut into pieces. Mangoes are eaten in fruit salads, smoothies, and desserts and may be prepared with cooked meat, poultry, rice, or grain dishes.

● *Mangosteen (MAN-goh-steen),* small in size, has an inedible leathery brown skin. Inside, the soft, white, juicy fruit divides into segments. Buy this fruit canned; it's rarely available fresh.

● *Papaya (pah-PEYE-ah) (pawpaw)* may weigh from 1 to 20 pounds in an elongated, oval shape. Its inedible peel is yellow or orange, with an orange fruit inside and many black seeds. It has a tart, sweet flavor that is delicious as is or mixed in salads.

● *Passion fruit (granadilla, or gra-nah-DEE-yah)* is a small, spherical fruit with a leathery peel, which may appear shriveled. It has a perfumelike, sweet-tart flavor. The color varies from light yellow to reddish-purple. It may be eaten as a whole fruit or added to salads, sauces, desserts, or beverages.

● *Pepino (puh-PEE-noh),* ranging in size from a plum to a papaya, is a fragrant fruit with a smooth, golden skin that's streaked with purple. Inside, the yellow flesh is juicy sweet. Enjoy a peeled pepino whole, or cut it for salads or garnishes.

● *Persimmon (puhr-SIHM-uhn)* looks somewhat like an orange-red tomato with a pointy end. If it's ripe, it's sweet. If not, a persimmon is mouth-puckering, bitter, and sour. It may be eaten as whole fruit or used in desserts and baked foods.

● *Pomegranate (PAH-meh-gran-uht)* is unlike any other fruit. It has a red, leatherlike peel; inside, membranes hold clusters of small, edible seeds with juicy red fruit around the seeds. The flavor is both tart and sweet. Pomegranate seeds are often used in salads and in many cooked dishes.

● *Pomelo (pom-EH-loh),* a huge citrus fruit, can be as big as a watermelon! But it's more commonly the size of a cantaloupe. In many ways it looks and tastes like a grapefruit, but the sections are not as juicy.

● *Prickly pear (cactus pear),* which is yellow-green to deep yellow, is the fruit of the cactus plant. It has a sweet, mild flavor. It should be peeled and seeded before eating. It may have small hairs or needles in the peel that can be uncomfortable if they get into your skin. The fruit itself is eaten fresh or used in salads, sauces, and other dishes.

● *Sapodilla (sah-poh-DEE-yah)* is a small, egg-shaped fruit that has a rough, brown peel. Only the creamy pulp inside is edible—when it's ripe. The flavor is mild, much like vanilla custard.

● *Starfruit (carambola, or kar-am-BOH-lah),* with its unique shape, forms stars when the fruit is sliced. The flavor varies from sweet to tart. It can be eaten as fresh fruit, in salads, or as a garnish.

● *Tamarillo (tam-uh-RIH-yoh),* with its tough but thin peel, is about the size and shape of a small egg. Because it's so tart, it is often sweetened with sugar. Often it is used in baked or cooked foods.

● *Ugli (UH-glee)* fruit is a cross between a tangerine and a grapefruit. It's sectioned on the inside but looks like a small grapefruit on the outside.

● *Zapote (zah-POH-tay) (white sapote)* is a sweet, yellowish fruit about the size of an orange.

Have You Ever Wondered

. . . if couscous is a grain? Actually, it's not. Instead, couscous is a form of pasta. Traditionally, couscous (made from ground millet) has been the pasta of northern Africa. In the United States it's made from ground semolina wheat and often used in salads, mixed with fruit, and used in other grain dishes. Because it's made from wheat, it's a good source of B vitamins. Look for whole-wheat couscous, too.

. . . what Quorn is? It's a mycoprotein, or a plant-based protein derived from the mushroom family. Sold in Europe for nearly two decades and now in the United States, this meat alternative is marketed as burgers, sausages, cold cuts, and other meat substitutes. Quorn supplies protein and fiber, with less fat and saturated fat than meat.

Today's Grains

Looking for a creative, even exotic, way to eat more grains? Most of today's "new" grains are really as old as the hills. Although unfamiliar to many in the United States, some are staple foods that nourish millions of people around the world.

Today's grains are full of health benefits. Many whole grains are good fiber sources that help to protect against heart disease, but also constipation, diabetes, and diverticular disease, along with other phytonutrients; they also supply B vitamins (including folate), vitamin E, and trace minerals such as copper and zinc. Refined grains are enriched with vitamins and minerals. What's more, all grains are rich in starches (complex carbohydrates) and low in fat. The fat they supply is mostly unsaturated—a heart health benefit. Seeds such as amaranth and wild rice are high in protein and often are used as grain substitutes.

● *Amaranth (AM-ah-ranth),* a seed rather than a true grain, is a protein-rich food. The seeds may be used as a cereal grain.

● *Arborio (ar-BOH-ree-oh)* rice, a plump medium- or long-grain rice, absorbs a lot of liquid. The result is a creamy-textured rice. Often it's used to make Italian risotto, a rice-based dish; the rice usually is cooked in broth.

● *Barley,* sold pearled (polished) and hulled, makes a hearty addition to stews, soups, salads, and casseroles. In its hulled form it's a whole-grain with more nutrients. Look for barley grits, flakes, and flour, which is hulless, but still uses the whole-grain kernel.

● *Basmati (bahz-MAH-tee)* rice, a long-grained aromatic rice, has a distinctive nutlike, fruity flavor. It's often used in Asian and Middle Eastern recipes—and in salads—because it's light and fluffy. Basmati rice may be polished or brown (whole-grain) rice.

● *Brown rice* is the whole grain of rice with only the inedible outer husk removed. Unlike refined white rice, brown rice still contains the bran, germ, and endosperm parts of the grain. *For more about whole grains and their nutrient content, see "What Is a Whole Grain?" in chapter 6.* Any variety of rice—long-, medium-, or short-grain—can be brown rice.

● *Buckwheat,* considered a whole grain, often is pre-pared like rice. The crushed, hulled kernels, called buckwheat groats, most commonly are used in dishes of Russian origin, such as kasha.

● *Bulgur,* whole-wheat kernels that have been parboiled, dried, and crushed, has a variety of textures—from coarse to fine. It has a soft but chewy texture that's nice in many grain-based dishes such as pilaf and tabouli. Try adding it to bread dough, too. Bulgur isn't quite the same as cracked wheat.

● *Glutinous rice,* either black or white, is very sticky because it's high in starch, making it easier to pick up with chopsticks. The grain is either short- or medium-grain. This is the type of rice typically served in Japanese and Chinese restaurants.

● *Hominy (HAH-mih-nee)* is the dried corn kernel with the hull removed. It's usually soaked in liquid to soften, then cooked, often in stews, casseroles, or other mixed dishes. *Note:* Although we eat corn as a vegetable, it's really a whole grain.

● *Jasmine (JAZ-mihn) rice,* another aromatic rice, is used in many Asian dishes. But it's equally nice whenever a subtle "sweet" side dish is called for, perhaps with pork or fruit-glazed poultry. A polished rice, it's often sold in specialty stores.

● *Kamut (kah-MOOT),* a high-protein wheat, has a nutty flavor. Its contribution of other nutrients is higher than traditional wheat as well.

● *Millet,* a small, round, yellow grain, is a staple whole grain in many parts of the world, including Europe, Asia, and northern Africa. It's less commonly used as food in the United States. Mild in flavor, millet cooks fast. It's used for mixed dishes such as pilaf or casseroles; for cooked cereal; and, when ground into flour, for bread such as roti from India.

● *Pearl barley* is an ancient, hardy grain used throughout the world. Pearl barley, with the bran removed, is the more polished and most common form of barley; the vitamins and minerals lost in processing are added back. Whole-grain barley is sold, too. Barley typically is served in soups.

● *Quinoa (KEEN-wah),* a whole grain native to South America, cooks much like rice but faster. Nutritionally it stands out because it's higher in protein than other grains, and it's a good source of iron and magnesium. The grain itself is small, ivory in color, and bead-shaped. With its bland flavor, quinoa can be used in soups, salads, and casseroles, and in any dishes that call for rice.

● *Sorghum (or milo)*, a gluten-free whole grain, can be eaten as a cooked cereal or used as a flour for baked foods.

● *Texmati rice* (sometimes called popcorn rice), from Texas, is a cross between American long-grain rice and basmati rice. Less fragrant than basmati rice, it's a good all-purpose aromatic rice.

● *Triticale (trih-tih-KAY-lee)* is a modern whole grain, developed as a hybrid of both rye and wheat. The result: a nutty-flavored grain with more protein and less gluten than wheat alone. Cooked as a whole berry (not as flour), it is used in hearty grain-based salads, casseroles, and other grain dishes. Look for flaked and cracked varieties, too, which can be added to bread dough.

● *Waxy rice*, or sweet rice or sticky rice (opaque white or deep, dark purple) is moist and very sticky when cooked. The purple variety has a subtle fruity flavor.

● *Wehani rice*, a basmati rice, is sold with the bran intact. When cooked it looks like wild rice.

● *Wheat berries* are whole grains that haven't been processed. They're often cooked and used in grain-based dishes. Cracked wheat isn't bulgur but instead is wheat berries that have been crushed. Also look for rye berries in specialty stores.

● *Wild rice* isn't a grain, but the seed of a water grass. With its nutlike flavor, it's often used in place of grains, or perhaps mixed with them. As a seed it's higher in protein and a good fiber source.

To learn how to prepare these grains, see "Cooking Grain by Grain" in chapter 13. For a list of whole grains, see page 139.

Ensuring Your Food Supply

The United States' food supply offers a safe, plentiful variety of food—anywhere, at any time of year. Compared with other nations, eating in the United States costs less: about 10 percent of our income, compared with 14 percent in Europe, 21 percent in Japan, and 48 percent in China! Even though food

---

Need more strategies to enjoy the food variety from today's marketplace? Check here for "how-tos":

● Use label claims to get clued in to foods' nutrient benefits—see chapter 11.

● Know how to fit all kinds of foods—including less common fruits, veggies, and grain products—into your eat-smart plan—see chapter 10.

● Add more food variety, perhaps functional ingredients, in your food "prep"—see chapter 13.

● Be more adventurous with food when you eat out—see chapter 14.

---

safety remains a consumer concern, strict regulations safeguard the U.S. food supply and minimize potential health risks.

Modern methods of agriculture, food processing, biotechnology, and transportation systems work together to put food on your table. The average U.S. farmer feeds you plus 127 other people here and in other nations; just 75 years ago, 1 farmer fed only 20 people. Still, hunger is a serious problem in the United States and certainly throughout the world.

Processing—Making Food Available

Throughout much of recorded history, people have processed foods to make them edible and to preserve them for times of scarcity. In Europe and other parts of the world eight thousand years ago, foods were smoked and dried. In the Middle East, cheesemaking developed forty-five hundred years ago as a way to store milk. And about twenty-five hundred years ago, Egyptians and Europeans mastered skills needed to salt foods for preservation.

Modern processing methods began in the 1800s with canning, giving perishable food a longer shelf life. People finally could eat a variety of fruits and vegetables year-round. During the nineteenth century, pasteurization—a process of heating milk or other liquids to kill disease-causing bacteria—was developed.

Have You Ever Wondered ?

. . . why boxed fluid milk is sold on the grocery shelf, not the dairy case? Aseptic packaging, a relatively new food processing and packaging method in the United States, allows fluid milk to be stored on the shelf at room temperature for up to a year without preservatives. Sterilization is the key to preventing spoilage. Food is first heated quickly (three to fifteen seconds) to ultrahigh temperatures to kill bacteria. Then it's packaged in a sterilized container, such as a box, within a sterile surrounding. This process of flash heating minimizes loss of nutrients, texture, color, and flavor—and extends shelf life. Besides milk, look for many other grocery items sold in aseptic packaging—for example, soup, tofu, liquid eggs, tomatoes, soy beverages, juice and juice drinks, syrup, nondairy creamers, and wine. In the future, you'll find even more!

Today foods are still pasteurized, or perhaps ultrapasteurized at higher temperatures, to keep food safe and flavorful and extend shelf life. Early-twentieth-century technology launched frozen foods. Later, lightweight, freeze-dried foods were developed for the space program; today backpackers and cyclists use them. Processing makes it easy to have foods, such as olive oil, that may not be grown, harvested, or produced where you live. In reality, most of our food supply is processed for the benefits of consumer safety and food variety.

What are today's newer contributions to food processing? Many relate to health—for example, adding substances for their nutrient benefits or functional qualities . . . using fat replacers and intense sweeteners to cut back on fat and added sugars . . . and irradiating food for improved food safety. And many add flavor, too.

Fresh vs. Processed: Either Way to Health

The flavor of fresh produce in season is hard to beat: freshly picked, handled properly, and eaten right away! For convenience, their canned and frozen counterparts offer another option. Research shows that canned and frozen ingredients are comparable in nutrition to cooked fresh counterparts.

The moment you pick a fruit or a vegetable, or catch a fish, or milk a cow, food starts to change texture, taste, perhaps color, and nutrient content. That's why food producers usually process food as fast as possible, while nutrient content and overall quality are at their peak. Immediate processing helps lock these qualities into food. In canneries on board some fishing vessels, seafood is processed as it's brought in. Tomatoes are canned just yards away from the fields. The same is true for commercially frozen foods.

As long as processed foods are handled properly—from the food manufacturer to the supermarket to your home—there's little nutrient loss. Freezing, drying, and canning retain the nutritional quality of foods.

A processing method called fortification increases the nutritional value of food by adding nutrients, such as vitamins or minerals, not present naturally or replacing nutrients removed. Milk, for example, is fortified with vitamin D, which helps the body handle calcium for bone-building; grain products are fortified with folic acid to reduce risk for birth detects. The nutritional quality of fresh fruit and vegetables depends on their care after harvest. Handled or cooked improperly or stored too long, they may not be quite as nutritious as their canned or frozen counterparts.

Whether food is fresh or processed, it's up to you to minimize nutrient loss in your kitchen. Store, prepare, and handle all foods with care. *See "Food 'Prep': The Nutrition-Flavor Connection" in chapter 13.*

Irradiated Foods: Safe to Eat?

Like canning and freezing, irradiation is a food processing method that enhances an already safe food supply. It extends the freshness of food, helping to retain its quality and safety longer.

Since it uses no heat, yet destroys disease-causing bacteria, irradiation is sometimes called "cold pasteurization." Poultry and beef can be irradiated to ensure pathogens that are especially harmful to children, the elderly, and people with weak immune systems are destroyed. That includes *Escherichia coli O157:H7, Salmonella,* and *Campylobacter.* Irradiation also slows ripening and retards sprouting—for example, in potatoes.

Irradiation destroys bacteria, mold, fungi, and insects by passing food through a field of radiant energy, much like sunlight passes through a window or like microwaves pass through food. It leaves no residue. A small number of new compounds are formed when food is irradiated, just as new compounds are formed when food is exposed to heat. These changes are the same as those caused by cooking, steaming, roasting, pasteurization, freezing, and other food preparation.

Irradiated foods generally retain their nutrient value. Like freezing, canning, drying, and pasteurization, irradiation results in minimal nutrient loss. The amount lost is often too insignificant to measure. Irradiation can't take the place of good food handling practices—nor improve the quality of food. As a consumer, you still need to store, prepare, and cook food in clean, safe ways to avoid foodborne illness.

Besides food safety, what are some other advantages of irradiation? Agricultural losses caused by insects, parasites, or spoilage can be cut dramatically. Foods that stay fresh longer can mean less food waste in your kitchen. Like other processing methods, irradiation is regulated and approved by the U.S. Food and Drug Administration (FDA).

By law, whole foods that have been irradiated must be labeled on the package. Look for the international Radura symbol *(to the right)* and the phrase "Treated by Irradiation" or "Treated with Radiation." Irradiated ingredients in prepared, deli, or restaurant foods usually aren't labeled.

As a way to control foodborne illness, irradiation—studied for safety by the FDA for forty years—was approved in 1997 by the FDA for fresh and frozen meats, including beef, pork, lamb, and poultry. The process protects these foods from contamination by *Escherichia coli O157:H7* and *Salmonella,* but doesn't compromise the nutritional quality of meat. *For more about foodborne illness, see chapter 12.* Irradiation also is used for vegetables, fruit, wheat flour, and spices. Research continues to evaluate irradiation as part of the overall system of ensuring food safety.

Additives: Safe at the Plate

Do you consider that most peanut butters don't separate? That products made from prepared baking mixes

Uncanny Safety, Nutrition Inside

Quick and convenient: more than fifteen hundred varieties of canned foods appear on today's supermarket shelves: traditional fare, along with a variety of nutritionally positioned products—for example, sodium-free, low-fat, no-added-sugar, and others. Some benefits:

- *Long shelf life.* Canned fruits and vegetables are preservative-free; the canning process (high temperatures and sterile containers) destroys organisms that would cause spoilage. Canned food remains safe as long as the container remains intact. Although most canned foods are coded with "use by" dates, you're wise to rotate them. Change your supply of canned products at least every other year.

- *Nutritious.* Canned foods—and dishes made with canned ingredients—are as nutritious as cooked fresh, according to research, and perhaps more so, if fresh aren't handled properly. Lycopene in canned tomatoes is more bioavailable than in uncooked fresh tomatoes.

- *Convenient, portable, quick.* They're ready to eat. Canned soups, stews, and vegetables only need heating since they're already cooked in the can.

- *Tamper resistance.* Cans are very tamper-resistant. Any opening is clearly evident. Rust spots on the outer surface or dents don't affect the contents of the can as long as the can doesn't bulge or leak.

- *Food safety.* Food is heated to destroy bacteria and then sealed in cans within hours of harvesting. Washing, peeling, and other steps in the canning process remove almost any pesticide residues left on unprocessed foods. For maximum flavor and nutritional value from canned foods, use the product immediately after opening it. Handle any leftover as a perishable food—stored in the refrigerator in a clean, sealed container to retain taste and nutritional quality.

rise in the oven? That ice cream is smooth and creamy? And that breakfast cereal has been fortified with many vitamins you need for health? Probably not. Most likely you take many desirable qualities of food for granted. Even if you do, you may not attribute these qualities to food additives. Food additives are any substances added to food for purposes such as these.

Adding substances to food for preservation, flavor,

or appearance is a centuries-old practice. Before refrigeration, salt preserved meat, fish, and poultry; vegetables were pickled in vinegar; and sugar was added to cut fruit to prevent spoilage. Ancient Egyptians used food colorings, and Romans used sulfites to help preserve wine. The spice trade among Asia, the Middle East, and Europe flourished because the public demanded the flavors that spices added to food.

Today more than three thousand substances are used as food additives. Direct additives are added for specific functions. Many are common household ingredients: sugar, salt, and corn syrup. Very small amounts of other substances—called indirect additives—also may pass into food during packaging, storage, or other handling. One example is the small amount of packaging material that may come from the food container. Both direct and indirect additives are subject to government review and safety regulations.

What do they do? Additives help foods retain their original qualities, which might otherwise change through temperature changes, storage, oxidation, and contact with microbes. The benefits include nutritional value, freshness and safety, convenience, affordability, color, and flavor appeal. Many additives offer qualities that you've probably come to expect. All additives are listed by name in the ingredient lists on food labels.

Have You Ever Wondered

... if cereal fortified with 100% Daily Value for nutrients is always your best choice? It's certainly one choice. But you may not need "100%" if you're already getting enough variety and balance in your day's food choices. Breakfast cereals fortified at a lower level may offer enough nutrition for you.

... how "natural" and "artificial" additives differ? So-called natural ingredients come from natural sources, such as soybeans or corn to make lecithin for product consistency, or beets to make food coloring. Others are man-made because they can be produced with greater purity, consistent quality, and perhaps more economically. For example, vitamin C made in a lab or from fruit is the same. Whatever their source, additives must follow the same standards for safety.

For Better Nutrition

Vitamins, minerals, or fiber are added to almost every category of processed foods to maintain or to improve their nutrition and health-promoting qualities. Until the past seventy-five years or so, nutritional deficiency diseases such as goiter, rickets, scurvy, and pellagra were relatively common. Adding nutrients to food has almost eliminated most nutrient deficiencies. Today nutrients are added to help protect against other health problems, too. Added nutrients contribute to nutrient density—an important approach toward optimal nutrition.

● *Enrichment:* replacing nutrients that are lost in processing. "Enriched" means that nutrients are added back to foods. If the grain's "refined," bread, flour, and rice are enriched with B vitamins and iron.

● *Fortification:* adding nutrients and food substances not present before processing: for example, iodine in salt, vitamins A and D in milk and some soy beverages, folic acid in most products made with refined grains, calcium in some fruit juices, and fiber in breakfast cereal and other foods. Fortification adds nutrients often lacking in a typical eating pattern; for example, fortifying salt with iodine in the United States has eliminated goiter. Today fortification also enhances food's functional qualities.

What nutrients and food substances are added? Check the food label. Any added nutrient shows up in two places: (1) in the ingredient list, and (2) on the Nutrition Facts panel, telling the total amount or contribution (% Daily Value) of that nutrient in a single label serving. *See "Get All the Facts!" in chapter 11.*

For Freshness and Safety ...

Air, bacteria, fungi, mold, and yeast promote food spoilage. Some additives, called preservatives, slow spoilage and help maintain food's appeal and wholesome qualities. You've likely heard of antioxidants. Some preservatives work as antioxidants, protecting food from chemical changes caused by contact with oxygen. Others are antimicrobials that inhibit the growth of mold, bacteria, and yeast. Some foods contain both.

● *Tocopherols (vitamin E), BHA, and BHT* help delay or prevent vegetable oils and salad dressings from rancidity. Working as antioxidants, they help protect naturally present nutrients in foods: essential fatty acids (linoleic and linolenic acids) and fat-soluble vitamins (A, D, E, and K). Studies verify the safety of BHA and BHT as GRAS ("generally recognized as safe") substances.

● *Citric acid,* a natural component of citrus fruits, works as an antioxidant, helping food keep its color. Coating sliced apples with lemon juice does the same thing—keeping the apple from turning brown. Ascorbic acid (vitamin C) does this, too.

● *Sulfites* help prevent color and flavor changes in dried fruits and vegetables. They're used to inhibit bacterial growth in wine and other fermented products. Some baked foods, snack foods, and condiments also may contain sulfites. Most people have no adverse reactions to sulfites. But packaged and processed foods containing sulfites are labeled for the small percentage of the population who are sulfite-sensitive. *For more on sulfites, see "For the Sulfite-Sensitive . . ." in chapter 21.*

● *Calcium propionate,* produced naturally in Swiss cheese, is a preservative that keeps bread and other baked foods from getting moldy too quickly.

● *Sodium nitrite,* used as a preservative in processed meats such as ham, hot dogs, and lunch meat, keeps the meat safe from botulism bacteria. It also adds to the flavor and pink color. *For more on botulism, see "Bacteria: Hard Hitters" in chapter 12.*

What foods have additives for freshness?

● *Antimicrobials* (to prevent spoilage from mold, bacteria, and yeast) . . . in baked foods, beverages, bread, cheese, cured meats, fruit juice, fruit products, margarine, pie filling, table syrup, and wine, among others.

● *Antioxidants* (to prevent rancidity or discoloration) . . . in baked goods, cereals, fats, oils, processed foods, salad dressings, and high-fat foods such as chips and doughnuts, among others.

For Food Preparation or Processing . . .

From helping bread rise . . . to keeping chocolate suspended in chocolate milk . . . to keeping seasoning blends from clumping, food additives fulfill a wide variety of tasks in food production. Without them,

food manufacturers couldn't achieve many food qualities or appeal that consumers want.

● *Anticaking agents* keep seasonings, baking powder, confectioners' sugar, table salt, and other powdered or granular products flowing freely. Because they keep food from absorbing moisture, it won't lump together. Calcium silicate and silicon dioxide are two anticaking agents.

● *Emulsifiers* are mixers that keep ingredients and flavorings blended by holding fat on one end and water on the other end of their chemical structure. For example, they're used to keep the oil, vinegar, and seasonings in salad dressings from separating. In peanut butter, emulsifiers keep the peanuts and the oil from separating. Even in baked foods, they help keep the dough uniform. Some emulsifiers come from food itself: for example, lecithin (from soybeans, milk, and egg yolks), alginates (salts from algae), and mono- and diglycerides (from vegetables and beef tallow).

● *Humectants* such as glycerine or sorbitol, help foods keep their moisture and soft texture. Shredded coconut stays moist and marshmallows stay soft because a humectant is added.

● *Leavening agents* help create the light texture of waffles, bread, muffins, and other baked goods. Baking soda (sodium bicarbonate) and baking powder (sodium bicarbonate and acid salts), as well as yeast, produce carbon dioxide that makes dough rise. Without them, the texture would be compact and heavy.

● *Maturing and bleaching agents* improve the baking qualities of foods made with wheat flour and improve the appearance of certain cheeses. When the yellow pigment of wheat flour is bleached, the dough becomes more elastic and the baking results, better. The white curd in some cheeses, such as gorgonzola and blue cheese, is the result of adding a bleaching agent to milk.

● *pH control agents* influence the texture, taste, and safety of foods by adjusting their acidity or alkalinity. Adding acids (acidulants) such as lactic acid or citric acid gives a tart taste to frozen desserts and beverages; they also inhibit the growth of bacteria in low-acid processed foods such as beets, and help prevent discoloration and rancidity. Alkalizers neutralize acids in foods such as chocolate so the flavor is milder.

● *Thickeners and stabilizers* give food a uniform texture. In ice cream they keep the texture smooth without forming ice crystals. In chocolate milk they allow the chocolate particles to stay in suspension. With stabilizers, oils that add flavor to food also stay in food. Proteins and carbohydrates in food—such as gelatin from animal bones, carrageenan from seaweed, and pectin from fruit—commonly are used as thickeners and stabilizers.

What foods have additives to aid food processing or preparation?

● *Anticaking agents* (to prevent lumping) . . . in baking powder, powdered foods, and salt, among others.

● *Emulsifiers* (to distribute particles evenly) . . . in baked foods, bread, breakfast cereal, chocolate, chocolate milk, cocoa, frozen desserts, margarine, mayonnaise, nut butter, pie and pudding mixes, and salad dressings, among others.

● *Humectants* (to retain moisture) . . . in candy, shredded coconut, gum, and marshmallows, among others.

● *Leaveners* (to help food rise) . . . in baked goods such as bread, cake, freezer waffles, and muffins, among others.

● *Maturing and bleaching agents* (to improve baking quality) . . . in bread, cereal, some cheese, flour, and instant potatoes, among others.

● *pH control agents* (to control pH levels) . . . in baked goods, candy, chocolate, gelatin desserts, processed cheese, salad dressings, sauces, soft drinks, and vegetable oils, among others.

● *Stabilizers, thickeners, and texturizers* (for smooth, thick, uniform texture) . . . in baked goods, beverages, candy, cream cheese, frozen desserts, jam, jelly, pie filling, pudding, salad dressings, sauces, and soups, among others.

For Flavor and Appeal . . .

Some additives add adventure to eating. They may add color, provide flavor or enhance it, or sweeten food.

● *Colorings* won't affect the nutrients, safety, or taste of food, but they make a nutritional contribution when they make food look more appealing to eat. Cheese and margarine often get their yellow coloring from annatto, which comes from the tropical annatto tree. Ice cream and many baked foods also are among the many foods with added coloring.

Food colors may be added to food for many reasons: to offset any color that's lost from being exposed to light, air, temperature extremes, moisture, and storage; to correct natural color variations; to enhance natural colors; and to give color to fun or colorless foods.

Both natural and synthetic colors are used in food.

No Surprises

Additives in food are no secret to consumers. Just by reading the ingredient lists on food labels, you can identify specific additives in any food. Note the "contains" statement for food allergen labeling.

Emulsifier
to keep ingredients blended

Flavoring
to add sweetness

INGREDIENTS: CRUST: WHEAT FLOUR WITH MALTED BARLEY FLOUR, WATER, PARTIALLY HYDROGENATED VEGETABLE OIL (SOYBEAN AND/OR COTTONSEED OIL) WITH SOY LECITHIN, ARTIFICIAL FLAVOR AND ARTIFICIAL COLOR (BETA CAROTENE), SOYBEAN OIL, YEAST, HIGH FRUCTOSE CORN SYRUP, SALT, CALCIUM PROPIONATE ADDED TO RETARD SPOILAGE OF CRUST, L-CYSTEINE MONOHYDROCHLORIDE; **SAUCE:** TOMATO PUREE (WATER, TOMATO PASTE), WATER GREEN PEPPERS, SALT, LACTOSE AND FLAVORING, SPICES, FOOD STARCH - MODIFIED, SUGAR, CORN OIL, XANTHAN GUM, GARLIC POWDER, **TOPPING:** LOW MOISTURE PART SKIM MOZZARELLA CHEESE (PASTEURIZED MILK, CHEESE CULTURES, SALT, ENZYMES). **CONTAINS WHEAT, MILK, SOY.**

Preservative
to retard spoilage

Thickener
to give a
uniform texture

Nine certified colors, such as Yellow #5 and Red #2, are approved in the United States. They offer intense and uniform color, without undesirable flavor. More and more natural pigments from vegetables, minerals, and animal sources are being used to color food; they're exempt from certification but still meet regulations for safety and purity. For example, look for foods colored with annatto extract, beet juice, paprika, carrot oil, beta carotene, grape skin extract, or saffron. Only one food coloring is known to cause allergic reactions, in rare cases: Yellow #5. *See "Coloring . . . by Any Other Name!" in chapter 21 for more about it.*

● *Flavorings,* which may be natural or synthetic, make up about seventeen hundred of the additives approved for use in food. They include spices, herbs, essential oils and their extracts, fruit juices, caffeine, and other seasonings. To make artificial flavorings, food scientists carefully study the makeup of natural flavors, then approximate the complexity of the natural flavor. Natural flavors come from food itself after a minimum amount of processing. They're often taken from one food and added to another. The chemical structure of natural and artificial flavors is similar, although artificial flavors may not have all the complex elements that give a distinctive natural taste.

● *Flavor enhancers* don't add flavor of their own. Instead, they heighten natural flavors already present in food. A well-known flavor enhancer is monosodium glutamate (MSG). MSG comes from a common amino acid, which is a protein called glutamic acid. MSG comes mostly from vegetable proteins. *For more about MSG, see "MSG—Another Flavor Enhancer" in chapter 7.*

● *Sweeteners* are flavorings, but they're grouped separately from the others. Some, such as sucrose (table sugar), fructose, dextrose, and mannitol, are nutritive, which means they produce energy in your body. Besides adding a sweet flavor, these sugars add mouth feel and work as browning agents in food. And they may be used as a preservative. Intense, or non-nutritive, sweeteners such as saccharin and aspartame don't contribute calories, or food energy. *For more about sugars and other sweeteners, see chapter 5, "Carbs: Simply Complex."*

What foods have additives to increase food appeal?

● *Colorings* . . . in baked goods, candy, cheese, gelatin mixes, ice cream, jam, jelly, margarine, pie, and pudding fillings, among others.

● *Flavorings* . . . in baked goods, candy, gelatin, pie filling, pudding, salad dressing mix, sauces, and soft drinks, among others.

● *Flavor enhancers* . . . in canned vegetables, gravy, processed meats, sauce mixes, and soups, among others.

● *Sweeteners* . . . in baked foods, canned and frozen fruit, frozen desserts, fruit yogurt, fruit juice drinks, gelatin mixes, jam, jelly, pudding mixes, and soft drinks, among others.

As a reference for specific additives, see "A Close-Up Look at Additives" in the Appendices.

Testing, Testing

Did you know that new additives must pass rigid safety tests before they can be used? During the past eighty years, the use of food additives has allowed a more varied and plentiful food supply. And beginning in 1938, government regulations have

Have You Ever Wondered

. . . if food additives are okay for everyone? Except for those few with specific allergies who may react, food additives are "safe at the plate." In fact, a primary use of additives is protecting food quality and safety. For someone with a sensitivity to an additive, the reaction should be similar whether the additive is natural or synthetic. The chemical makeup is quite similar. *For specifics about rare cases of allergic responses, see "Sensitive to Additives? Maybe, Maybe Not" in chapter 21.*

. . . if people with gluten intolerance should avoid certain additives? Yes; they need to read food labels carefully to avoid additives with gluten. See *"Gluten Intolerance: Often a Lifelong Condition" in chapter 21.*

. . . what's Culinology? It's a term coined for bringing food science and culinary arts together to create appealing food for the consumer table.

helped guide and ensure the safety of their use in food.

Today food additives are regulated more tightly than at any other time in history—with safety as the primary goal. In 1958 the federal government passed the Food Additives Amendment, which gave the U.S. Food and Drug Administration (FDA) responsibility for approving additives used in food. The FDA sets safety standards, determining whether a substance is safe for its intended use. If it's found to be safe, the FDA decides what types of foods the additive may be used in, in what amounts, and how it must be indicated on a food label.

Federal food laws distinguish among additives: those generally recognized as safe (GRAS), prior-approved additives, regulated additives, and color additives.

Generally recognized as safe (GRAS). In 1959 the FDA established a list of about seven hundred additives that were exempt from the regulatory process. This list—called the GRAS list—recognized that many additives had an extensive history or existing scientific evidence of their safe use in food. Additives that appear on the list include salt, sugar, spices, vitamins, and monosodium glutamate.

From time to time, GRAS ingredients are reevaluated by the FDA and the U.S. Department of Agriculture (USDA), and perhaps removed from the list or reclassified. That occurred in 1986 for sulfites because research showed that some people are sensitive to sulfites. *For more about sulfite sensitivity, see "For the Sulfite-Sensitive" in chapter 21.*

Prior-approved substances. Before the 1958 Food Additives Amendment, some additives—such as nitrites used to preserve processed meat—had been approved by the FDA or the USDA. If used as originally approved, these substances didn't need to go through the approval process again; the government already had judged them safe.

As with the GRAS list, prior-approved substances are continually monitored. Current scientific evidence of their link to health is reviewed, recognizing that the statutes of prior-approved substances can be changed.

Regulated additives. Any additive not considered as GRAS or prior-approved must be approved before it can be marketed and used in food. The evaluation addresses: the substance's composition and qualities,

the amount typically consumed, the immediate and long-term effects, and safety factors. These are the regulatory steps:

- First, the additive manufacturer must prove that the additive is effective—that the additive does what it is supposed to do, and that it can be detected and measured when put into a food.

- Second, the manufacturer must prove that large amounts of the food additive, when given to two kinds of test animals over an extended time, won't cause cancer, birth defects, or other problems. Results of human studies may be submitted.

- The FDA reviews the results, then invites public response to the manufacturer's petition.

- If approval is given, the FDA establishes regulations for the types of food in which the additive can be used, the maximum amount, and how the substance must be described on the label. The level approved is much lower than the amount that may have any expected adverse effect.

When the food industry proposes an additive for use in meat or poultry products, another approval also is required—this time from the U.S. Department of Agriculture's Food Safety and Inspection Service (FSIS), which applies different standards that consider the unique characteristics of meat and poultry. For example, the FSIS doesn't allow the use of sorbic acid, which is an approved additive, in meat salads because it could mask spoilage.

Color additives. In 1960 the federal government passed another law—the Color Additives Amendments, which required that dyes used in foods, drugs, cosmetics, and medical devices needed testing, similar to tests for regulated food additives.

Safety Check

Approval of additives, including those on the GRAS and prior-sanctioned lists, doesn't guarantee that they'll be used in food forever, nor does it infer absolute certainty of zero risk. However, based on the best available science, FDA approval reflects reasonable certainty of no harm to consumers when the additive is used as proposed. The FDA continues to review all categories of food additives, and it judges them by the latest scientific standards and consumer consumption of that additive. Based on new evidence, approval is either maintained or withdrawn.

As another safety check, the Food Additives Amendment also has a section called the Delaney Clause, which states that no additive known to cause cancer in animals or humans can be put in food in any amount. One artificial sweetener called cyclamate was removed from the GRAS list for that reason. Tests showed that large amounts were linked to cancer in test animals. The safety of cyclamate is currently being reevaluated; it is approved for use in some other countries.

To monitor and investigate complaints of adverse reactions to additives, the FDA also maintains the computerized Adverse Reaction Monitoring System (ARMS), which records updated safety data. Incidences of allergic reactions to food and color additives and to dietary supplements, reported by individuals or their doctors, are recorded, too. These reports help determine whether further investigation is warranted—and if action is required to maintain public health. *For more about adverse reactions to food additives, see "Sensitive to Additives? Maybe, Maybe Not" in chapter 21.*

Good Manufacturing Practices (GMP) regulations also limit the amount of additive use: only as much needed for the desired result.

Additives—Your Choice

With such an array of foods available, consumers have considerable choice about food additives. If you have a history of food-related allergies, you may need to limit or avoid foods with ingredients, including additives, that you're sensitive to. Learn to read the ingredient lists on labels. *See "A Word about Ingredients..." in chapter 11. If you have a food reaction and think it may be additive-related, talk to your doctor.*

Pesticides: Carefully Controlled

The vast array of safe, nutritious foods available in your supermarket throughout the year doesn't happen by chance. Successful growers carefully manage their croplands and orchards to control about eighty thousand plant diseases, thirty thousand weed species, a thousand species of nematodes, and more than ten thousand insect species! In the United States alone, about $20 billion of crops (10 percent of our production) are lost yearly with these problems. If you've ever

struggled with mildew, insects, weeds, and rodents in your own garden, just multiply the problem!

To produce high-quality produce with adequate yields, most farmers use some pesticides—either in the field or the grove, or just after harvest—to prevent mold or insect damage during transport or storage.

Without prudent use of pesticides, many farmers couldn't control crop damage from disease, insects, molds and fungi, weeds, and other pests. And their crop yields would be much lower. In spite of pesticide use, U.S. farmers annually lose a significant amount of crops because of damage from pests. That number would be far higher without careful use of pesticides.

About Pesticides . . .

Pesticides include a broad range of chemicals that protect crops. They're applied by dusting, fogging, spraying, or injecting them into the soil:

- *Herbicides* control weeds.
- *Fungicides* control mold, mildew, and fungi that cause plant disease, and inhibit molds that may be harmful to consumers.
- *Insecticides* control harmful insects, often those that damage crops or carry plant disease.
- *Rodenticides* control rodents in the field.
- *Disinfectants* act against bacteria and other disease-carrying microorganisms.

When people think of pesticides, synthetic chemicals often come to mind. However, naturally occurring chemicals in the environment, such as copper, nicotine, and sulfur, and some bacteria also are used to control pests. And many plants protect themselves by producing their own pesticides in low levels.

IPM—Best of Both Worlds

What does sex have to do with pest control? Interestingly, sex scents, called pheromones, can confuse pest mating patterns, allowing farmers to use less pesticides. It's part of a biological system of pest control.

IPM stands for integrated pest management—a contemporary farming approach that uses pesticides, biological control, and biotechnology to reduce crop damage. As farmers work in partnership with nature, they apply pesticides on crops selectively, ultimately using less.

IPM incorporates a variety of strategies—not just limited pesticide use—into pest management.

● Crop rotation—for example, switching from soybeans to corn—helps limit pest buildup because insects lose their natural food source.

● Farmers may use living organisms to help control pest diseases, or use pest predators (when "good" bugs eat "bad" bugs).

● Growers may choose plant varieties that are more resistant to pests. Traditional plant breeding and genetic engineering can help crops develop their own natural resistance. *See "Food Biotechnology: Nutrition Opportunity" later in this chapter.*

● Computers can help growers forecast disease and weather conditions. The more they know, the more prudent they can be with pesticides.

Safety: Whose Job?

Safety starts with growers; most are prudent with pesticides for many reasons. One is cost. Pesticides are expensive, so farmers use them judiciously to remain profitable. Second, successful growers project toward the future. By using too much pesticide with one year's crop, they may cause crop damage in the future. Some pesticide residues remain in the soil. Third, today's farmers are more aware than ever of the environment (wildlife, groundwater, soil quality)—their livelihood depends on it. Most farmers are trained in the responsible, legal use of agricultural chemicals; some pesticides must be applied only by people certified or licensed to do so.

Pesticide manufacturers bear responsibility for the effects of pesticide use among consumers, farm workers, and the environment. If research indicates that pesticide use would not meet standards for toxicology, crop residues, or environmental impact, the Environmental Protection Agency (EPA) can stop or change its use. Several government agencies regulate and monitor pesticide safety in food:

● The *EPA* regulates the manufacture, labeling, and use of pesticides—and sets maximum levels, or tolerances, for pesticide residues. Before a pesticide can be used on crops, it must be thoroughly tested to assure that it's safe for the environment and for human health. If approved, the EPA may limit its use—amount, frequency, or crop—and require that these limitations be listed on the product label. Growers who misuse pesticides, even mistakenly, risk having their crop seized or destroyed. And the grower may be charged with a civil or a criminal lawsuit.

Regulations established in 1996 under the Food Quality Protection Act set even stricter safety standards. Among other measures, this law further protects children and infants from pesticide risk, requires testing and information about any estrogenlike effects of pesticide residues, and considers exposure of pesticides to drinking water.

● The *U.S. Food and Drug Administration (FDA)* monitors pesticide residues in most foods (not meat, poultry, and eggs)—both raw and processed—and enforces the tolerance levels set by the EPA. If residues exceed these levels, the food can be seized or destroyed, and a lawsuit may be filed. Any pesticide residues that remain on raw foods are usually removed during washing or peeling.

● Like the FDA, the USDA's *Food Safety and Inspection Service (FSIS)* monitors pesticide residues and enforces tolerance levels for meat, poultry, and eggs.

● Several states, including California, that grow many fruits and vegetables have their own regulations, too.

Tolerances, or maximum levels, for pesticide residues are set in parts per million, parts per billion, and parts per trillion. For example, 1 part per million would mean 1 gram of residue is the maximum allowed in 1 million grams of food. That equates to 1 cherry in about 20,000 1-pound cans.

Tolerances for pesticide residues are legal limits. In most foods, levels are well below that. Tolerances are a hundred to a thousand times lower than the amount that might pose a health risk, so there's a very wide margin of safety. FDA testing has shown that foods rarely exceed limits, and many samples are below the tolerance level or show no residues at all. To pass through U.S. customs, imported foods must meet the same stringent standards set for foods grown domestically.

Benefits vs. Risks

The presence of low levels of pesticide residues doesn't signal a risk. Tolerances are legal limits, not medical limits—set far below what is considered safe for the most sensitive part of the population, including infants and children.

In fact, the use of pesticides may reduce other risks related to food. For example, fungicides help control aflatoxin B2, a naturally occurring toxin in grains and peanuts. Most important, the prudent use of pesticides helps ensure a wide variety of fruits and vegetables, which supply important vitamins, minerals, dietary fiber, and other phytonutrients for human health.

What You Can Do . . .

Any pesticide residues in foods you buy are present at minimal levels. It's safe to say that they probably won't pose any risk to your health. You can add more to your safety net by the way you handle food in your kitchen . . . or by the way you grow fruits and vegetables in your own garden:

● Choose produce carefully. Avoid fruits and vegetables with cuts, insect holes, mold, or decay.

● Wash fresh fruits (including melons) and vegetables with water to remove residues on the surface and in the crevices. For foods such as carrots, squash, apples, and pears, use a vegetable brush to clean them even more—if you eat the fiber-rich skin. Rinse well. Avoid soap, unless it's especially meant for produce, because it leaves its own residues. As an option, use a produce wash formulated to remove soil, wax, and pesticides. Rinse well after using a produce wash.

● Remove outer leaves of lettuce, cabbage, and other leafy vegetables.

● Although you could peel some fruits and vegetables, recognize what you'd be giving up—the nutrients and the fiber that the peel contains.

● Eat a variety of foods. Not only do you get the nutritional benefits of food variety, but you also minimize pesticide risks. Different crops require different pesticides, so variety limits exposure to any one type.

Have You Ever Wondered ❓

. . . what BST refers to? BST, or bovine somatotropin (also called bovine growth hormone, or BGH), is a naturally occurring protein in all cow milk and meat. When given as a supplement in small, controlled doses it helps improve cows' efficiency in producing milk. Even without supplementation, BST naturally occurs in cow milk, in small quantities. It has no effect on humans. Like other proteins, it's broken down during digestion. With BST supplementation, a cow's milk production goes up, but the normal level of BST in milk itself doesn't change; the cow uses it up itself. In addition, there's no change in the flavor or nutritional qualities of milk produced from supplemented cows. As always, milk remains an excellent source of calcium, protein, vitamins, and other nutrients.

In 1990, the National Institutes of Health reinforced that BST is safe for humans. In 1993 the U.S. FDA approved BST supplementation based on its safety for humans, cows, and the environment. And regulatory agencies around the world have authorized milk and meat from cows receiving BST as safe for people of all ages.

. . . if wax on fruits and vegetables is safe to eat? Yes.

There's no need to peel waxed produce. Just wash it with water—*no* soap. You might use a brush to remove any dirt, bacteria, and pesticide residues. The thin, waxy coating on foods such as cucumbers and apples is applied after picking to replace natural wax and to help produce stay fresh and edible; a little fungicide often mixed with the wax helps control mold and rot. Wax helps by retaining moisture, protecting the food from bruising, and preventing spoilage. By long-standing federal law, waxed produce must be labeled.

. . . if you should avoid any specific fruit or vegetable to reduce your exposure to pesticides? No. For any crop, pesticide use varies with the time of year, the soil conditions, the climate, and the presence of pests. There's no way you can tell the difference. The best guideline: wash produce thoroughly, remove outer leaves on leafy greens—then enjoy the nutritional benefits that all fruits and vegetables provide.

. . . if food grown in soil that's depleted of minerals or nitrogen is less nutritious? When soil lacks minerals or nitrogen, plants don't grow properly and may not produce their potential yield. If soil can grow crops, the food produced is nutritious.

- If you're a home gardener, minimize your use of pesticides, and follow the directions for their safe use, storage, and disposal. Contact your county extension service if you need guidance. *See "Resources You Can Use" in this book to help locate your local extension service.*

- Wash and sanitize your refrigerator drawers frequently.

- Remember: Being "organic" doesn't guarantee safety. Clean organic produce well.

Organically Produced

If you've scanned the shopping aisles you know: organic foods, once available mostly from health food stores, now sell in mainstream supermarkets. Organic farming is expanding fast—not only with fruits, vegetables, and grains, but also eggs, dairy foods, meat, poultry, packaged foods, oils, baby foods, and even wine and beer! Just what are organic foods? And how do they compare with their conventionally produced counterparts?

The term "organic" is a misnomer. All foods come from living organisms—plant and animal. Because they all contain carbon, they're all organic. Foods referred to as "organic" are really "organically grown" or "organically produced"—with little or no synthetic fertilizers or pesticides and no antibiotics or hormones.

Perspective: Organically Produced Foods

Organic farming offers choice: an alternative to conventional agriculture and an alternative for you at point of purchase. Sold fresh, frozen, and canned, organic products have grown in quality, availability, and popularity! And they're often a good option.

Pesticide-free? Maybe and maybe not. Organic farmers may use insects and crop rotation to control pests that damage crops. Certain insects, for example, are natural predators for other insects that cause crop damage. Or farmers may use chemicals found naturally in the environment, such as sulfur, nicotine, copper, or pyrethrins, as pesticides. When these methods don't work, organic farmers can use other substances (biological, botanical, or synthetic) from a list approved by the National Organic Program of the U.S.

Department of Agriculture. To compare, pesticide levels with conventional farming are set low, so they're not harmful to health; *see "Pesticides: Carefully Controlled" earlier in this chapter.*

With organic farming, manure, compost, and other organic wastes fertilize crops; there are some allowed synthetic fertilizers. The soil is also managed with crop rotation, tillage, and cover crops. Organic fertilizers are effective, yet plants can't distinguish them from synthetic fertilizers. Both types of fertilizer break down in the soil to nurture growing plants.

The criteria for organically raised livestock and poultry and for animals raised for milk and eggs are equally stringent. From the last third of gestation, or for poultry, the second day of life, animals are fed only 100 percent organic feed, and they must have outdoor access and be humanely treated. Although vitamin and mineral supplements are allowed, hormones for growth and antibiotics are not. Any animal treated with medication can't be sold as organic.

Despite common perception, no conclusive scientific evidence shows that organically produced foods are healthier or safer. Both approaches—organic and conventional farming—supply nutritionally comparable foods. Climate and soil conditions, genetic differences, maturity at harvest, and the way food is handled—not the type of fertilizer—affect the nutrient content of raw foods.

How do taste and appearance compare? Studies show no significant flavor difference between organically grown and conventionally grown foods. Instead, taste differences appear to come from the food varietal, its growing conditions, and its maturity at harvest time. Most of today's organic foods compare very favorably in appearance with conventionally grown foods.

Organically produced foods often cost more. That's usually due to higher production costs (more labor, more management intensive, more crop losses, and smaller farms or yields). In the future, costs may go down as organic farmers develop more cost-efficient techniques and farming systems and get larger yields.

On a large-scale basis, today's organic farming alone can't produce enough food for the world's exploding population. However, more large food companies now offer organic options. The marketplace does offer many choices if you prefer organically produced food.

Have You Ever Wondered

. . . how sustainable agriculture fits within food production? Sustainable agriculture is a way to allocate resources for the needs of the current generation, without compromising the future. Many strategies to achieve this goal are local, for example, encouraging local food production and supporting local farmers' markets. Others may be practiced by farmers anywhere around the globe, such as conserving natural resources, following ecologically sound farming practices, and working as communities to promote agriculture and the environment.

To be successful, the ability to feed the world's growing population and to support local economies with minimal environmental impact will require a multifaceted approach to food production, which includes local sustainable agriculture. *For ways to support local growers through farmers' markets, see chapter 11. Refer to "The 'Eco' Kitchen" in chapter 12 for ways to conserve resources as you handle food.*

. . . what are hydroponically grown foods? They're foods from plants raised in water, not soil; "hydro" means water. The hydroponic solution—which varies by crop and environmental conditions—supplies roots with elements found in soil and fertilizer. With hydroponic farming, high-quality food can be produced almost anywhere: a desert, outer space, and areas with poor soil. Nutritionally, hydroponically grown foods are comparable to those grown in soil; undamaged by weather, they may look better.

A few more terms in modern agriculture: aeroponics is a way of growing plants by spraying the roots with nutrient solution; aquaculture is raising fish in a controlled environment.

. . . if hormones used in beef production affect humans? The FDA and the FSIS work together to provide consumers with a safe food product by ensuring the proper use of hormones in cattle. In very small amounts, certain hormones have been approved by the FDA to improve the feed efficiency or weight gain of beef cattle and sheep. For naturally occurring hormones used in production, the amounts of hormone in meat must fit within the same range as for untreated animals. With the use of synthetic hormones, producers must show that any hormones in meat after treatment remain below a level that's too low to affect humans.

If you prefer meat from untreated animals, you have choices. Beef products may be labeled "no hormones administered"—if sufficient evidence is provided by the producer to the FSIS showing that hormones were not used to raise the animals. What about pork or chicken? Federal regulations prohibit the use of added hormones in raising hogs or poultry.

Coming to Terms

The National Organic Program ensures that the production, processing, and certification of organic foods match a comprehensive standard. If you prefer organic foods, now you can be confident about what you buy.

Under the Organic Foods Production Act, federal regulations require consistent and uniform standards. Organic farming or processing operations that take in more than $5,000 gross must be certified. Even smaller, uncertified organic operations must abide by the standards and may label their products. Certification allows organic labeling, with terms that have a consistent meaning: "100 percent organic," "organic," and "made with organic ingredients." The "USDA Organic" seal may appear on any foods that contain at least 70 percent organic ingredients. In organic food production, food irradiation (to destroy foodborne bacteria), sewage sludge, and genetic engineering can't be used. A product with less than 70 percent organic ingredients can list only specific organically produced ingredients on the ingredient list. *For more about organic labeling, see chapter 11.*

Food Biotechnology: Nutrition Opportunity!

In the twenty-first century your shopping cart will be filled with an array of new products: foods that taste fresher and more flavorful, more health-promoting varieties of foods, and a greater variety of produce all year long. Today's food biotechnology has already put these foods on your table: canola, corn, soybean, and cottonseed oils. Varieties of potatoes, squash, tomatoes, papaya, and others have been developed, too.

Modern biotechnology is simply applying plant

science and genetics to improving food production—and food itself. Simply put, it's applied science.

"Traditional" biotechnology began perhaps ten thousand years ago, as farmers raised animals and grew plants to produce food with desirable traits: higher yields, new food varieties, better taste, faster ripening, and more resistance to drought. Five thousand years ago in Peru, potatoes were grown selectively. In ancient Egypt—forty-five hundred years ago—domesticated geese were fed to make them bigger and tastier. About twenty-three hundred years ago, Greeks grafted trees, a technique that led to orchards and a more abundant fruit supply. In fact, products as commonplace as grapefruit and wine came from traditional biotechnology or traditional breeding and selection.

Over the years, farmers have replanted seeds or cross-pollinated from their best crops. And they've bred new livestock from their best animals. For example, within the past few decades, hogs have been bred to be leaner, in turn producing lean cuts of pork for today's consumers.

With traditional breeding, farmers changed the genetic makeup of plants and animals by selecting those with desirable traits. They then raised and selected again and again until a new, more desirable breed or food variety was established. Even in the "old days," this breeding resulted in genetic change.

Traditional cross-breeding takes time. Often it's unpredictable. Each time one plant pollinates another, or one animal inseminates another, thousands of genes cross together. Along the way, less desirable traits—and the genes that cause them—may pass with desir-able ones. Several generations of breeding, perhaps ten to twelve years, may go by before desirable traits get established and less desirable qualities are bred away.

Modern biotechnology offers a faster and more precise way to establish new traits in both plants and animals—and so provide improved foods that are safe, nutritious, healthful, abundant, and tasty.

Food Biotechnology Today: What's It All About?

In a nutshell, modern biotechnology refers to using living organisms—plants, animals, and bacteria—to develop new products, not just for food, but also for medical treatment, waste management, and alternative fuels, among others.

Today's food biotechnology started about thirty-five years ago, as scientists learned more about DNA (deoxyribonucleic acid), genes, and the genetic code in living things, and applied this knowledge to plant and animal breeding practices. In fact, the latest advances in food biotechnology have spawned a new vocabulary. Popular media may use "genetically modified foods," or "GM foods," to refer to these foods. Other terms, such as "genetic engineering," "gene splicing," "cell culture," and "recombinant DNA," refer to some methods of modern biotechnology. Recombinant DNA is the process of inserting genes from one organism into the genetic code, or DNA, of another. That's how a trait is transferred.

To understand how modern food biotechnology works, think about writing a book on a computer. With a click of your keyboard, you can copy a single quote from one document to another, without merging the two, or you can highlight or delete a single phrase. Likewise, agricultural scientists can pinpoint specific genes that carry traits they want, such as disease resistance, better nutrient quality, or flavor. Then they can transfer a single gene from one plant or from an unrelated species, such as a bacterium, to another. Or they can extract a certain gene, leaving undesirable traits behind. The latest advances in food biotechnology are

Source: American Dietetic Association.

more efficient, more predictable, and less time-consuming than traditional breeding.

The Benefits Package

Food biotechnology offers an approach for protecting the environment while producing a high-quality, abundant, healthful, and inexpensive food supply.

Healthier crops, higher yields. Crops produced using biotechnology can thrive with less environmental impact. For the farmers, that means lower production costs; for the environment, more protection.

For example, some cotton and corn varieties have been enhanced through biotechnology to contain *Bacillus thuringiensis* (*Bt*), a common soil bacterium that lets corn protect itself from certain insects that eat and destroy plants. That lowers the use of insecticides. "Bt" itself isn't new, however. Organic farmers have sprayed it on their crops for more than forty years.

Enhanced farming is developing other crops to resist plant viruses and other diseases, or to require less insecticide or more environmentally friendly herbicides (glyphosphate). Newly developed soybeans, as well as some corn, canola, cotton, and potatoes, flourish with less insecticides.

Weather-resistant crops. Crops are being genetically improved to withstand severe weather, reducing crop loss for farmers and extending the growing season and region to make more fresh fruits, vegetables, and grains available year round.

Fresher foods, better flavor. By transferring desirable genetic traits, fruits and vegetables with different ripening qualities can be shipped longer and farther, without spoilage or damage: bananas, pineapples, and strawberries for example, that resist mold. This means fresher, better-tasting produce such as sweeter peppers, or potatoes with fewer dark spots, year round.

Healthier foods. Modern food biotechnology may help to promote public health, providing fruits, vegetables, and grains with more nutritious benefits: more proteins, vitamins, and minerals, or less fat and saturated fat. In the future, fruits and vegetables such as sweet potatoes with higher levels of antioxidants (vitamins C and E, and beta carotene) may help reduce heart disease and cancer risk.

Already some vegetable oils have a better fatty acid profile—less saturated fat and *trans* fat and more monounsaturated fat—for heart health. Food biotechnology also has enhanced soybeans, canola, and other oil seeds so they have less saturated fat and more oleic acid, an unsaturated fatty acid that is a benefit to heart health. Enhanced flaxseeds could bring more omega-3 benefits to vegetable-based cooking oils.

For those with food allergies, biotechnology is seeking ways to reduce the allergens in wheat, peanuts, and other crops.

In parts of the world, nutrient-enhanced crops may help address problems of malnutrition. For example, "golden rice" with beta carotene (vitamin A) and iron may address two health problems: blindness among children caused by a lack of vitamin A, and low iron intakes, which is harmful to many children and women. Protein-rich potatoes and cassava (a staple in Africa) could address malnutrition.

Safer foods. With food biotechnology, foodborne bacteria and viruses may be easier to detect, so the risk of foodborne illness may decline.

Medical uses. Products of food biotechnology might treat health problems: bananas grown to include vaccines to deliver to developing nations. Other nonfood applications of biotechnology may result someday in new vaccines and medications to treat heart disease, cancer, and diabetes, among others, and the ability to produce human insulin to help treat diabetes.

Efficient food production. Foods can be grown in a better way to produce higher yields, reducing costs and efforts for farmers.

Food biotechnology also can use simple organisms to produce the same food components found in nature. One example is an additive called rennin. In fact, 70 percent of cheese produced in the United States is made with an enzyme available through biotechnology. Traditionally, rennet—an enzyme extracted from the lining of calves' stomachs—was used to form curds and whey from milk, a first step in making cheese. Through the use of food biotechnology, scientists have transferred the calf gene into "friendly" bacteria, where it produces the same enzyme. This enzyme is more active and more pure than rennet—and consistently available to food manufacturers.

New food varieties. Food biotechnology can extend

Today's Meat

Through breeding, feeding, and management at the farm, hogs and beef cattle are leaner than ever. In addition, processing methods help create leaner meat. The reason? The need to provide products for consumers with high nutrient content, yet lower levels of total fat and saturated fat. For example, pork cuts sold in the supermarket today have an average of 43 percent less fat than they did in 1983, and compared with the 1970s, beef has 27 percent less trimmable fat.

One reason for leaner hogs is genetics. Some of the eight major hog breeds in the United States carry genes that produce leaner, meatier hogs. With selective breeding, hog producers have changed the fat and muscle composition of hogs, gradually producing leaner animals over the past few decades.

As with humans, a hog's food and "lifestyle" affect its body composition. With a scientifically balanced diet matched to its age, current weight, and nutrient needs, a hog is fed what it needs without excess.

The next step in producing lean meat is with the meat packers or processors. They usually trim the fat surrounding cuts of meat to $\frac{1}{8}$ to $\frac{1}{16}$ inch, rather than $\frac{1}{2}$ to $\frac{1}{4}$ inch, as in the past. For example, with beef, many cuts have no outside fat at all. Financial incentives may be offered by the packer to the farmer for producing lean animals. Even processed meat is produced with less fat and cholesterol than before, yet it's still tender, moist, and flavorful. Look for lean ground beef and low-fat pork sausages: just 5 fat grams and 6 fat grams, respectively, per 3-ounce serving. That's about 50 percent less than for regular meat.

Finally, it's up to you to keep lean meat lean and flavorful . . . by using low-fat cooking methods and avoiding high-fat sauces, and by cooking to a safe internal temperature, without overcooking. *For more about preparing meat, see chapter 13. For tips on buying lean meat, see chapter 11.*

to advances in traditional cross-breeding, allowing for new food varieties: for example, broccoflower (green cauliflower); single-serving, seedless melons; mini avocadoes; blood oranges; baby pineapples; donut peaches; and red sweet corn. By understanding the plant genome, traditional breeding can also develop food varieties with better flavor, other agronomic qualities, and a better nutrient profile. And it can help scientists understand the thousands of edible plant species yet unexplored that may contribute to modern agriculture.

More food grown on less land. Food biotechnology can help farmers produce enough food to meet the world's rapidly growing population—expected to double in less than fifty years. Within just the next twenty years, the world will need 40 percent more rice, wheat, corn, and other grains!

Weather-resistant crops can turn regions with poor climate or soil conditions into productive agricultural land. Higher-yielding crops can feed more people, using less farmland.

Protection for the environment. With enhanced farming, greater crop yields can reduce the need to clear forests for farmland. Better weed control with herbicide-tolerant crops allows farmers to use no-till or other forms of conservation tillage that lead to less erosion of valuable topsoil because the soil isn't turned over as much and there is less run-off. Crops with traits that repel pests require fewer insecticides. As a result, fewer residues pass into water supplies. With "environmentally friendly" animal feed, less unwanted phosphorus passes into manure, then on to the water supply.

As another nonfood application, biotechnology may provide cost-effective options for renewable, non-polluting sources of fuel—for example, from corn. These fuel sources can reduce dependence on nonrenewable energy sources such as petroleum.

Now about Food Safety. . .

With any new technology, consumer safety is one of the first questions. The U.S. Food and Drug Administration subjects products of food biotechnology to the same stringent standards of labeling and safety as all foods sold in the United States.

Most foods enhanced through biotechnology don't differ in composition, nutritional quality, or safety from those that are conventionally produced—unless that's the trait specifically desired. And like other foods in the U.S. marketplace, any foods produced through biotechnology are rigorously tested and strictly regulated.

Who's responsible for safety? Several federal agencies and some state agencies regulate and ensure the safety of foods produced through biotechnology: the

Food and Drug Administration (FDA), the Environmental Protection Agency (EPA), and the U.S. Department of Agriculture (USDA). The FDA's key role is assuring the safety of the product as a food for humans or as animal feed. The EPA regulates the safety of pest control properties of crops, including the impacts on the environment and food supply. The USDA assesses the safety of crops growing in the field.

Seed manufacturers conduct thorough research and demonstrate proof of testing for every crop brought to market—for example, showing proper nutrient levels, status of allergens or natural toxins, how the improved crop functions as food or animal feed, scientific procedures for product development, environmental effects, and the history of safe use. For substances that differ significantly from existing foods and ingredients, special testing is required. In fact, products are tested at many stages of development before they reach consumers.

With new technology come change and controversy. However, evaluation procedures used by manufacturers and regulators to ensure safety for consumers are endorsed internationally by the Food and Agriculture Organization (FAO) of the United Nations and the World Health Organization (WHO). In the United States, the National Academy of Sciences, the American Medical Association, Society of Technology, and the American Dietetic Association among others support the safety of the foods produced by biotechnology.

Biotechnology Labeling: When You Need to Know

Most foods produced through biotechnology do not seem different from foods you enjoy already. They taste good, look fresh, and are available throughout the year. In addition, most of these foods do not need a special food label because they have been proven to be the same as other foods.

Foods developed through biotechnology are subject to the same FDA labeling regulations and carry the same food labels, including allergen labeling, as any other foods. Additional labeling is required on biotech food and foods with ingredients derived from biotechnology under some circumstances:

. . . if a known allergen is introduced into the food. Allergic reactions come from proteins in foods, and genes direct the production of proteins. So if a gene is taken from a food known to cause allergic reactions (such as peanuts), then transferred to another food (such as potatoes or corn), the new food must be labeled as potentially containing that particular allergen. No foods introduced to the food supply to date contain proteins from known allergenic foods. (*Note:* Through biotechnology, research is under way to remove known allergens from food—for example, to develop allergen-free or allergen-reduced peanuts.)

. . . if the nutritional content of the food changes. Foods that are enhanced to change their nutritional content must be labeled. Perhaps rice with more protein or an orange with more vitamin C.

. . . if the food composition changes substantially. Perhaps it would be labeled with a new varietal name; or maybe, like broccoflower, a new identity.

According to federal regulation, manufacturers may voluntarily label their foods as produced with or without the use of ingredients enhanced or produced

Natural Toxins

Plants have built-in mechanisms for pest control: fungi, insects, and animal predators. Unlike animals, plants can't flee when they sense danger, so they produce natural compounds—actually, low levels of pesticides—to protect against these invading organisms.

The level of natural toxins in food may be many times higher than any level of synthetic pesticide residue, according to the National Academy of Sciences. And according to FDA estimates, Americans ingest ten thousand times (by weight) more natural pesticides than synthetic ones—with no apparent health risk.

Natural toxins are found in foods you eat every day—for example, oxalates in rhubarb, solanine in green potatoes, nitrates in broccoli, and cyanide in lima beans. At high levels, some might cause illness or may be carcinogenic (cancer-causing). However, in the amounts normally eaten in a varied diet, none has been shown to pose a cancer risk.

Through advances in biotechnology, scientists now can identify genes that produce natural toxins, then either remove them or suppress their action, to provide a health benefit.

through biotechnology. The phrases "derived through biotechnology" or "bioengineered" have been suggested by the FDA for labeling. A recent American Medical Association report indicates no scientific justification for labeling most foods.

Growing Possibilities . . .

Food biotechnology, which holds great promise for feeding the world, is developing in the global marketplace, not just in the United States. Gradually you might find these foods in your supermarket:

● Tomatoes with more lycopene, an antioxidant that protects against prostate cancer

● Low-fat potato chips or French fries, made from higher-starch potatoes that absorb less fat

● Vegetables and fruits with higher levels of antioxidants (vitamins C and E, and beta carotene) to help reduce risks for some health problems such as cancer and heart disease

● Rice with higher-quality protein (more amino acids) produced with genes from pea plants

● Vegetable oils—canola, corn, soybean, and others—with more stearate (a form of stearic acid, a saturated fat that doesn't appear to affect blood cholesterol levels) for use in margarine and spreads

● Garlic with more allicin, a phytonutrient that may help lower cholesterol levels

● Peanuts with less of the naturally occurring protein that causes allergic reactions

● Strawberries with more ellagic acid, a cancer-fighting phytonutrient

● Drought-resistant corn and rice for growing in regions with extreme heat and drought

● Fruits that can deliver vaccines in regions of the world without adequate refrigeration to store vaccines

● Folate-rich grains

● As an ingredient, high linolenic acid soybean oil that is more stable, so less *trans* fats are formed during processing

Have You Ever Wondered?

. . . what nutrigenomics is—and what it may mean for you? Decoding the human genome, a remarkable feat completed within this new millennium, will offer a personalized way to approach health and nutrition decisions. Nutrigenomics is the study of genes and their link to nutrition. It's how nutrients and other food components interact with a person's genetic makeup, regulating particular genes to increase or decrease the risk for certain diseases.

Nutrigenomics offers a huge opportunity to customize what people eat for their unique genetic makeup. The goal: the potential to slow and even prevent all kinds of diseases—some directly nutrition-related, such as celiac disease, diabetes, obesity, cancer, and heart disease, others not, such as sickle cell disease, cystic fibrosis, and Alzheimer's disease—for those at risk. Understanding functional foods and nutrigenomics goes hand in hand, as science reveals the unique ways that foods' many substances work and interact within body cells.

That said, a great deal of research is needed before gene-based nutrition advice becomes a reality. But the first steps are being taken, already within our lifetime!

. . . if antibiotics used in agriculture affect human health? Antibiotics have been used in animal agriculture for many years to prevent or cure diseases in animals. The FDA and the FSIS work together to provide safe food by ensuring the proper use of animal antibiotics in agriculture. The FDA regulates and monitors the use of animal antibiotics to ensure that any residues are minimal and at very safe levels. Currently, questions have been posed about the possibility of "antibiotic resistance" in humans if animal antibiotics are used in cattle production; definitive research is needed to determine any effect from the use of animal antibiotics on human health. (Penicillin, important to human health, is not used with cattle.) Meat and poultry may be labeled "no antibiotics added" or "raised without antibiotics" if there's enough substantiated proof to the FSIS that animals were raised without them.

CHAPTER 10

Planning to Eat Smart

Food, glorious food! We've explored how nutrients function in human health. But it's the wide array of food, not nutrients, that entices most people to eat. The aromas, flavors, textures, and appearance of all kinds of food stimulate your appetite, satisfy your tastebuds, and give you the contented feeling that goes with a wonderful meal or a tasty snack.

These wise and flavorful decisions deliver much more, of course. The choices you make about food each day, along with physical activity, affect your health and how you feel today, tomorrow, and in the future.

You're ready to harness the power of healthy eating. But how? The Dietary Guidelines—*summed up in chapter 1*—describe "a healthy diet" this way:

● Emphasizes fruits, vegetables, whole grains, and fat-free or low-fat milk and milk products

● Includes lean meats, poultry, fish, beans, eggs, and nuts

● Is low in saturated fats, *trans* fats, cholesterol, salt (sodium), and added sugars

● Is handled and prepared to keep food safe.

Making healthful food choices has its own challenges: often lack of time, too much effort needed, and limited "know how." Sound familiar? The goal is to satisfy your hunger, appetite, and desire for certain foods, while ensuring that your meals and snacks have the food variety, balance, and moderation that help to maintain, and even improve, your health. The solution? Quick, simple, and convenient ways to eat smart for a healthier *you*, especially when you're short on time and energy.

MyPyramid: An Eating Guide for a Healthier You!

Looking for a sensible strategy for smart eating—meant for you? No matter what you like to eat or your eating style, MyPyramid is just that! It's a plan from the U.S. Department of Agriculture, designed to help you choose the foods and amounts that are right for you, to balance with your daily physical activity. Meant for healthy people ages two on up, it helps you—and your family—put sound nutrition advice, based on the latest science, into action. Think of it as your practical, everyday strategy for making the Dietary Guidelines for Americans and other nutrition standards work in your life.

Best of all, MyPyramid has enough flexibility to fit in foods that match your lifestyle, your food preferences, and your personal nutrition and health needs. It truly is . . . all about you!

MyPyramid Power

For healthful eating, MyPyramid symbolizes that one size doesn't fit all. Instead it's personal, meant for healthful eating and physical activity—your way, each day. In a nutshell, MyPyramid says:

● *Be active.* The person climbing up the steps reminds you to fit physical activity into every day.

● *Vary your choices.* The six bands stand for the five food groups plus an area for oils. For health, consume a variety among and within these groups to get the array of nutrients you need. No one food or food group supplies all the nutrients, fiber, and other substances your body needs. (Besides, variety adds flavor, interest, and pleasure to eating!)

● *Think in proportions.* The food-group bands differ in width, reminding you to eat more of some types of foods than others. These widths are just estimates—not specifically the amount that's right for you. Because you're unique, your pattern is unique, too.

● *Make moderation your mind-set*—and your everyday eating habit. For each food group, the wider base stands for foods with little or no solid fats or added sugars; eat them more often. The narrower top stands for foods with more added sugars and solid fats; go easy! The more active you are, the more of these foods you can consume. Another great reason to live an active lifestyle!

● *Customize.* You have many options for healthful eating and active living. Use the Web site—www.MyPyramid.com—to choose the kinds and amounts of food just right for you.

● *Improve gradually.* Take small steps to healthier eating and active living. Small steps add up to big benefits!

MyPyramid—for You

MyPyramid is meant for any healthy person, ages two on up—unless he or she is on a special diet to manage a health problem. Refer to:

● MyPyramid for Kids—chapter 16.

● MyPyramid for Vegetarians—chapter 20.

● DASH Eating Plan as another approach to eat for health—chapter 22.

A Food Group Plan—For You

With MyPyramid you can: (1) make smart choices from every food group, (2) find your balance between food and physical activity, and (3) get the most nutrition out of your calories. Where do you start? First know roughly how many calories you need in a day. Then plan your day's food and beverage choices to match. *Refer to "Your Nutrition CheckUp" in this chapter to do that!*

For ease MyPyramid provides twelve food-group plans, each created for a different calorie level, from 1,600 to 3,200 calories. How much *you* need from each food group and oils depends on how many calories *you* need overall. The more energy (calories) your body uses, the more calories you need. Your energy needs depend on your age, gender, height and weight, and level of physical activity. MyPyramid's daily advice shows how you can get enough

Source: www.MyPyramid.gov.

MyPyramid: In a Nutshell

Food Group*	Food Group Strategies Steps for making smart food group choices appear throughout this book.	How Much? For a 2,000-calorie diet, you need this amount every day**
Grains Make half your grains whole.	● Eat at least 3 ounces of whole grains: cereals, breads, crackers, rice, or pasta. ● 1 ounce is about 1 slice of bread, *or* about 1 cup of breakfast cereal, *or* ½ cup of cooked rice, cereal, or pasta.	6 ounce equivalents
Vegetables Vary your veggies.	● Eat more dark-green veggies like broccoli, spinach, and other dark leafy greens. ● Eat more orange vegetables like carrots and sweet potatoes. ● Eat more dry beans and peas like pinto beans, kidney beans, and lentils.	2½ cups
Fruit Focus on fruits.	● Eat a variety of fruit. ● Choose fresh, frozen, canned, or dried fruit. ● Go easy on fruit juices.	2 cups
Milk Get your calcium-rich foods.	● Go low-fat or fat-free when you choose milk, yogurt, and other milk products. ● If you don't or can't consume milk, choose lactose-free products or other calcium sources such as calcium-fortified food and beverage.	3 cups (For kids aged 2 to 8, it's 2 cups.)
Meat and Beans Go lean with protein.	● Choose low-fat or lean meats and poultry. ● Bake it, broil it, or grill it. ● Vary your protein routine —choose more fish, beans, peas, nuts, and seeds.	5½ ounces

MyPyramid.gov
STEPS TO A HEALTHIER YOU

Find your balance between food and physical activity.
● Be sure to stay within your daily calorie needs.
● Be physically active for at least 30 minutes most days of the week.
● About 60 minutes a day of physical activity may be needed to prevent weight gain.
● For sustaining weight loss, at least 60 to 90 minutes a day of physical activity may be required.
● Children and teenagers should be physically active for 60 minutes every day, or most days.

Know the limits on fats, sugars, and salt (sodium).
● Make most of your fat sources from fish, nuts, and vegetable oils.
● Limit solid fats like butter, margarine, shortening, and lard, as well as foods that contain these.
● Check the Nutrition Facts label to keep saturated fats, *trans* fats, and sodium low.
● Choose foods and beverages low in added sugars. Added sugars contribute calories with few, if any, nutrients.

Source: www.MyPyramid.gov.

*Some foods don't fit into any group. These "extras" may be mainly fat or added sugar—limit your intake of these.

**For the amounts that are right for you, check "MyPyramid: Food Intake Patterns" in the Appendices, or go to www.MyPyramid.gov.

nutrients within a calorie budget. *Refer to "MyPyramid: Food Intake Patterns" in the Appendices to plan for your calorie level* or go to www.MyPyramid.gov.

For the five food groups and oils, recommendations are given in cups and ounces, not in servings and serving sizes. Your entire day's choices are what count, not how many food-group servings you eat during a meal or snack.

"MyPyramid: In a Nutshell" shows how you might spread out your food choices if you need 2,000 calories a day.

Right-Sizing Your Portions

So, how does your plate of pasta fit within your eating plan? The large muffin from the bakery? The refreshing 20-ounce fruit smoothie? To follow MyPyramid guidance and keep your calories in balance for maintaining your healthy weight, become portion savvy. Learn to estimate your food and drink portions (in cups and ounces) and to judge how much you eat overall on a typical day.

What's the right amount? Try to make the overall amounts from the food groups and oils for the day add up to about what you need within your calorie goal. If your only lunchtime veggie is a few carrot sticks, eat a bigger dinner salad and perhaps fill your dinner plate with more vegetables.

Not sure about how much you eat (size of your helpings)? Take out the measuring cups and a kitchen scale. Serve your amount of food on a plate. Then measure or weigh them. Surprised? Your amount may be bigger or smaller than you think! To get the right-size helpings for you:

● Get to know visual clues for portions. *See "Your Guide to Amounts" on the next page.*

● Use smaller dishes, bowls, mugs, and cups. A meal served on a lunch plate rather than a dinner plate looks like more!

● Let veggies, fruit, and grain products fill most of your plate. Meat, chicken, or fish don't need to take the biggest plate space.

● Eat from a plate, not a package, so you know how much you eat. Put the opened package out of sight to resist temptation.

● Repackage big packages into several smaller containers—enough to use one at a time. Or buy portion-controlled "singles."

● Whether you feed yourself or serve others, start with small helpings. Put the rest out of sight. Then eat slowly, paying attention to hunger and fullness cues. Go for seconds only if you're still truly hungry.

For more ways to overcome over-sizing, refer to the tips in chapters 11 and 14.

The Nutrition Facts panel on a food label, meant for nutrient and calorie information and comparisons, offers serving sizes. Use them to gauge your portions. *"Get All the Facts!" in chapter 11 explains serving sizes on food labels.*

MyPyramid amounts are meant to guide your food choices so you think about how much you need and how much you eat. You don't need to get out the tape measure for each piece of fruit or vegetable! Skip undo attention to precision!

Extra Calories: Spend Wisely within Your Budget!

You need calories for two key reasons: some to keep your body functioning and some to power your physical activity. Together those calories add up to your total calorie budget. *For calorie basics, refer to chapter 2.*

Calorie "essentials" are the minimum amount to meet your nutrient needs. Following MyPyramid advice—by choosing lean, low-fat, and fat-free forms of foods and by eating the recommended amount of oils—supplies that amount. The leftover is discretionary calories that reflect the extra energy (calories) you can eat to match your energy expenditure. Call them "your choice" calories!

Make food choices to get your nutrients, then decide how to spend the extra calories! If you made good nutrition "buys" from the food groups (nutrient rich and relatively low in energy density), you may have calories left in your calorie budget. The best nutrition "buys" are generally the most nutrient-rich. You can spend your "extra" discretionary calories on luxuries like solid fats (higher in saturated fats), added sugars, and alcoholic drinks, or on more foods from any food group. *For more about nutrient density and energy density, check later in this chapter.*

YOUR GUIDE TO AMOUNTS

How do 3 ounces of meat look? How about ½ cup green beans, 1 cup cooked pasta, or 1½ ounces cheese? To *guess-timate*, use visual clues to compare food amounts to everyday objects.

For vegetables, fruit, dried fruit, beans, rice, pasta, cereal, yogurt, shredded cheese:
  ¼ cup = 1 large egg
  ½ cup = 1 small computer mouse
  1 cup = 1 3-inch diameter baseball

For milk and juice:
  1 cup = 8-ounce carton
  ½ cup = 4-ounce carton

For meat, poultry, or fish:
  2 to 3 ounces = 1 standard-size deck of cards

For nut butter, nuts, seeds, oils, salad dressing, and spreads:
  2 tablespoons = 1 roll 35mm film
  1 tablespoon (1 ounce) = 1 nine-volt battery

For cheese:
  1½ ounces = 2 nine-volt batteries

For bread:
  1–ounce slice = 1 computer disk

For a potato:
  1 small = 1 small computer mouse
  1 medium = 1 baseball

For an apple:
  1 3-inch diameter = 1 baseball

For French fries:
  ½ cup (10) = 1 standard-size deck of cards

How It Works. Assume your calorie budget is 2,000 calories per day. Of these calories, you need to spend at least 1,750 calories on foods that deliver essential nutrients. You'd spend that many calories if you chose wisely from the food groups. You now have 250 discretionary calories yet to spend. Now think about your meals and snacks: how will you spend them? You can:

● Eat more nutrient-rich foods from any food group—more than what you need to match your healthful eating plan.

● *Or* eat some higher-calorie versions of food-group foods, with a little more solid fats or added sugars. A few examples: whole milk, cheese, sausage, biscuits, sweetened cereal, or sweetened yogurt.

● *Or* flavor your meals with some added fats or sweeteners, perhaps with sauces, salad dressings, sugar, syrup, or butter—or more healthy oils.

● *Or* enjoy a small portion of candy, soft drinks, wine, beer, or other calorie-dense foods.

Whatever option you choose, go easy. Many people take in more "extra" calories than they need to maintain their weight, consuming more fats, added sugars, and alcoholic drinks than their discretionary calorie allowance—perhaps even before lunch! Your discretionary calorie allowance probably isn't very big. Before you know it, those calories can get spent in higher-calorie choices, such as higher-fat meats, cheese, whole milk, or sweetened baked foods. Typically people have just 100 to 300 extra calories to spend, especially if they don't move much.

Good news: the more you get your body moving, the more "extra" calories you have to spend. Physical activity is *the* best way to get more discretionary calories to spend! Notice that MyPyramid also offers advice about physical activity, *addressed in other chapters*.

Save Calories, Spend Elsewhere. Are some of your favorite foods higher in calories—perhaps in fat and added sugars, too? You don't need to give them up, but just figure out how to fit them in. It's your food choices and calories over the course of the day or several days that count. For example, save calories so you may have room to spend discretionary calories elsewhere.

● Enjoy a baked potato (without a high-fat topping) for supper rather than French fries, so you may fit a small dish of ice cream in your calorie budget.

● Top homemade pizza with reduced-fat, rather than regular mozzarella, so you may enjoy a cookie later as a snack. Top French toast with sliced fresh peaches, rather than syrup, which is mostly added sugars.

● Enjoy fruit canned in natural juices as a snack, rather than fruit packed in syrup, to save on calories for jam or honey on your dinner biscuit.

Portion Distortion: A 20-Year Shift!

Today's portions seem to say "Eat until you feel stuffed, not just until you're satisfied." With this attitude, it's easy to see how adults and kids might lose their ability to regulate how much they eat, as they listen *less* to their hunger and fullness cues. Larger restaurant portions and dinnerware have changed our perceptions of portion sizes. And many Americans typically underestimate how much they eat by 50 percent!

That's problematic, of course, since overeating leads to excess calories. Besides leading to overweight, diet-related health risks may go up as mega portions "over deliver" total fat, including saturated fats and *trans* fats, cholesterol, sodium, and added sugars, too.

CALORIES IN PORTIONS . . .

Food	20 Years Ago	Today
Bagel	140 calories (3-inch diameter)	350 calories (6-inch diameter)
Fast food cheeseburger	333 calories	590 calories
Spaghetti and meatballs	500 calories (1 cup spaghetti with sauce and 3 small meatballs)	1,025 calories (2 cups spaghetti and 3 large meatballs)
Bottle of soda	85 calories (6½ ounces)	250 calories (20 ounces)
Fast food French fries	210 calories (2.4 ounces)	610 (6.9 ounces)
Turkey sandwich	320 calories	820 calories (10-inch sub)

Source: Dietary Guidelines for Americans, 2005, and National Heart, Lung, and Blood Institute.

To make "calorie budgeting" easier, read the Nutrition Facts on food labels. Check the label's serving size and the calories per label serving.

Remember: Your goal isn't to eliminate foods, but to moderate and balance your day's meal and snack choices to make MyPyramid work for you!

Inside MyPyramid

Local foods, ethnic foods, your favorite foods, restaurant foods, snack foods, foods you grow yourself, supermarket foods—all kinds of food fit within MyPyramid! Foods are grouped together because their nutrient content is similar. Foods within each food group and the oils category promote health in comparable ways. In fact, foods from each group supply your body with some, but not all, nutrients and phytonutrients needed for energy, health, and, for kids, growth.

Let's take a look inside MyPyramid, and check out some tips and ideas to start you toward more healthful eating and to make your calories count for good nutrition. That's a nutrition-rich approach! *Then check chapters that follow, filled with MyPyramid pointers for food shopping (chapter 11), food prep (chapter 13), and eating out (chapter 14).*

Grains Group: Make at Least Half Your Grains Whole!

What's a grain product? It's any food made from wheat, rice, oats, cornmeal, barley, or another cereal grain. Bread, pasta, oatmeal, breakfast cereals, tortillas, and grits are among the many foods in the Grains Group. *You'll find more ideas in "Today's Grains" in chapter 9.*

Whatever grain product comes to mind, it's made with whole grains, refined grains, or perhaps both. Whole grains are the whole grain kernel, with the bran, germ, and endosperm intact. *Refer to the list of whole grains, including whole-wheat flour, oatmeal, whole cornmeal, and brown rice, in chapter 5.* When refined grains are milled for a finer texture or longer shelf life, the bran and the germ are removed, taking dietary fiber, iron, and many B vitamins along with

HOW MANY DISCRETIONARY CALORIES DO YOU HAVE TO SPEND?

"Extra" discretionary calories are estimated by age and gender. If you're more physically active, you can eat a little more. Discretionary calories are part of your total estimated calorie needs, *not* in addition to them.

	NOT PHYSICALLY ACTIVE . . .*		PHYSICALLY ACTIVE . . . **	
	Estimated total calorie need	Estimated discretionary calorie allowance	Estimated total calorie need	Estimated discretionary calorie allowance
Females 31 to 50 years	1,800	195	2,000 to 2,200	265 to 290
Males 31 to 50 years	2,200	290	2,400 to 3,000	360 to 510

*<30 minutes of moderate physical activity on most days
**30 minutes (lower calorie level) to at least 60 minutes (higher calorie level) of moderate physical activity on most days
Source: www.MyPyramid.gov.

For other age groups, refer to "How Many Discretionary Calories Can You Have?" in the Appendices.

them. White refined flour, degermed cornmeal, most white bread, and white rice are refined grain products.

Most refined grain products are enriched, meaning nutrients (thiamin, riboflavin, niacin, and iron) lost in processing are added back. Fiber isn't added back to enriched grains. Most refined grain products and some whole grains are also fortified with folic acid. The ingredient list on grain products is your way to find out if a grain product is enriched, fortified, or both; *see chapter 11.*

Why Eat Grain Products?

Grain products, especially whole grains, offer a bundle of health and body maintenance benefits from their many nutrients and phytonutrients.

Key nutrients: Grain products deliver starches (complex carbohydrates), several B vitamins (thiamin, riboflavin, niacin, and folate), minerals (iron, magnesium, and selenium), and dietary fiber from whole-grain foods.

Important health benefits: Grain's carbohydrates are your body's main energy source, and their B vitamins help your cells produce that energy. Their folic acid from fortified grains, consumed before and during pregnancy, helps protect against some birth defects. And whole grains, as part of healthful eating, help reduce the risk of some chronic diseases, including heart disease, diabetes, and cancer, and help prevent constipation. To help you manage your weight, make at least half your grain choices whole.

Grain Products: How Much?

Hit your "carb" goal with nutrient-rich foods! Just how much do you need from the Grains Group? Specific advice for you depends on your age, gender, height and weight, and your level of physical activity. If you need 2,000 calories a day, the recommended daily amount adds up to 6 ounces of grain products. *Check "MyPyramid: Food Intake Patterns" in the Appendices for the amount that matches your calorie level.*

At least half of your daily grain choices should be whole grain. Most Americans consume enough grains, but few as whole grains. Look for "whole" before the grain name on the ingredient list.

One Ounce of Grain Equals: In general, an ounce is 1 slice of bread, or 1 cup of ready-to-eat cereal, or ½ cup of cooked rice, pasta, or cereal. Specifically, here's what an ounce means:

- 1 regular (1 ounce) whole-grain or enriched bread slice, or 1 small slice French bread, or 4 snack-size slices rye
- 1 (1-ounce) bagel
- ½ English muffin
- 1 small (2-inch diameter) biscuit, 1 small (2½-inch diameter) muffin
- 5 whole-wheat crackers, or 2 rye crispbreads, or 7 square or round crackers
- 1 ounce ready-to-eat cereal (1 cup flakes or rounds, or 1¼ cup puffed)
- ½ cup (made from 1 ounce dry) cooked oatmeal
- ½ cup cooked barley, bulgur, millet, quinoa, or other whole grains
- ½ cup cooked (made from 1 ounce dry) rice or pasta
- 1 (6-inch) corn or flour tortilla
- 3 cups popped popcorn
- 1 (4½-inch diameter) pancake, or 2 small (3-inch diameter) pancakes

MyPyramid Pointers

Choose grain products by the company they keep! Make at least half your choices whole grain for their fiber and other benefits. Go easy on those made with more fat, cholesterol, and added sugars, such as croissants, pastries, doughnuts, hush puppies, fried rice, and regular tortilla chips.

- Make pasta, rice, or other grain foods, especially their whole-grain versions, center stage at your meal or snack. Add flavor and nutrition with vegetables, small amounts of seafood, lean beef, or skinless poultry, or fresh herbs.

- Boost your whole-grain choices: whole-grain or oat bread for sandwiches, oat cereal for breakfast, brown rice as a stir-fry side dish, whole barley in soup, or bulgur in salads and casseroles.

- Opt for bagels, bread sticks, English muffins, Italian bread, hamburger buns, pita bread, or corn and flour tortillas—especially their whole-grain counterparts. Ease up on croissants, doughnuts, and sweet rolls.

Eat More Food, but Less Calories!

"More food, less calories" may sound great if you love to eat! In fact, fiber-rich, watery foods deliver more volume to your plate for fewer calories. So fit them into your food-group choices. Ounce per ounce, foods with more fat and with less fiber and water are more energy dense, with more calories per ounce. Energy-dense foods add up to a lot less food for the same calories than those low in energy density.

To compare, 1 cup of sliced raw carrots has 50 calories, and so does just 0.33 ounce of chips. (Even a small snack bag of chips is at least 1 ounce, or 150 calories.) And the carrots give you more nutrients and fiber, take longer to eat, and can leave you feeling satisfied with fewer calories. Other foods high in volume but low in energy density include broth-based soups, fruits and vegetables, fat-free and low-fat milk and yogurt, and beans. *Refer to "Food: A Water Source" in chapter 8 for the percentage of water in common foods.*

- Be aware that many grain products are a mix of whole-grain and refined-grain ingredients. They don't count as a *full* whole-grain portion.

- Try less common Grains Group foods, perhaps quinoa, buckwheat, millet, amaranth, or couscous. Enjoy grain-based salads, perhaps pasta salad, rice pilaf salad, or tabouli (made with bulgur). Or enjoy risotto (made with arborio rice) or polenta (made with cornmeal). *Refer to "Today's Grains" in chapter 9.*

- Try these snack options: air-popped popcorn, graham crackers, matzos, pretzels, rice cakes, saltines, bread sticks, zweiback, baked tortilla chips, and whole-grain crackers. Many taste great with vegetable dips or fruit spreads.

- For sweet desserts from the Grains Group, consider angel food cake, gingersnaps, and oatmeal cookies more often than frosted cake, brownies, and pie. Count the "extra" calories as "discretionary."

- Check the ingredient list on food labels to find foods made with whole grains, and to find grain products fortified with folic acid and other nutrients. *Check chapter 6 for ways to identify whole-grain foods.*

- Use whole-grain bread for sandwiches, toast, and more. It's hard to make at least half your grains whole if you don't.

Have You Ever Wondered

...where potato chips and corn chips fit in MyPyramid? Potato chips fit within the Vegetable Group; corn chips, within the Grains Group. Yet they supply more fat and more calories (more energy density) than other foods in those groups. Eat these foods with discretion; try baked varieties, which have fewer calories and less fat. Count their calories as part of your discretionary calories that you can spend.

...if potatoes can substitute for bread since they're both high in starches? Potatoes are among the starchy vegetables in the Vegetable Group. Breadfruit, cassava, corn, green peas, hominy, lima beans, rutabaga, taro, and yautia are some others. Although high in starches, vegetables have different nutrients and phytonutrients than foods in the Grains Group. Potatoes, for example, supply vitamin C and potassium; Grains Group foods supply some B vitamins and iron.

Vegetable Group: Vary Your Veggies!

Raw or cooked . . . fresh, frozen, or canned . . . whole, cut-up, or mashed . . . dried or dehydrated . . . or juiced. No matter how you enjoy them, a colorful, bountiful array of vegetables fits within this food group. The more variety and color you eat, the better! *Check chapter 9, "Garden of Eatin': Less Common Vegetables," for more ideas.*

Why Eat Vegetables?

More than a colorful garnish on your plate or crisp texture in a sandwich, vegetables are loaded with different nutrients and phytonutrients. Eat plenty of them to promote your overall health.

Key nutrients. Vegetables are important sources of many nutrients, including carbohydrates, vitamins A, C, and E, folate, potassium, and dietary fiber. Unless you add sauces and other seasonings, most vegetables are naturally low in fat and calories. None have cholesterol.

Different vegetables supply different nutrients. That's why you need variety! Dark-green leafy vegetables are great sources of beta carotene (forms vitamin A), as well as vitamin C, folate, calcium, magnesium, and potassium. Deep-orange vegetables, such as sweet potatoes and carrots, supply beta carotene. Others, such as Brussels sprouts, bell pepper, and tomato, have more vitamin C. Many are rich in folate. Besides their complex carbohydrates, starchy vegetables supply niacin, vitamin B_6, zinc, and potassium. Legumes (dry beans) provide protein, as well as thiamin, folate, iron, magnesium, phosphorus, zinc, potassium, and fiber. *To learn about their phytonutrients, refer to chapter 4, "Phytonutrients—A 'Crop' for Good Health," and "'Paint' Your Plate with Color" in chapter 12.*

Important health benefits: Vegetables deliver a host of benefits. The vitamin C they contain not only helps to heal wounds and keep teeth and gums healthy, but also aids iron absorption. Their vitamin A keeps eyes and skin healthy and helps to protect against infections. Their vitamin E works as an antioxidant. Their folate helps form red blood cells, and helps prevent against some birth defects. Their potassium helps maintain healthy blood pressure. And their fiber has many roles: lowering total blood cholesterol and heart disease risk, aiding digestion, reducing constipation and diverticulosis, and possibly filling you up with fewer calories.

Vegetables: How Much?

Veggies: how much? That depends on your age, gender, height and weight, and your level of physical activity. For 2,000 calories a day, the advice adds up to 2½ cups of vegetables a day. Most people come up short. *Check "MyPyramid: Food Intake Patterns" in the Appendices for the amount that matches your calorie level.*

To get the nutrient variety that different vegetables provide, MyPyramid provides weekly advice, too, from the vegetable subgroups. If you need 2,000 calories a day, strive for:

- Dark-green vegetables   3 cups per week
- Orange vegetables   2 cups per week
- Dry beans and peas   3 cups per week
- Starchy vegetables   3 cups per week
- Other vegetables   6½ cups per week

VARY YOUR VEGGIES! TRY SOMETHING NEW!

Vegetables fit into five subgroups, depending on their nutrient content.

Dark-green vegetables
bok choy
broccoli
collard greens
dark-green leafy lettuce
kale
mesclun (young salad green mix)
mustard greens
romaine lettuce
spinach
turnip greens
watercress

Orange vegetables
acorn squash
butternut squash
carrots
hubbard squash
pumpkin
sweet potatoes

Dry beans and peas
black beans
black-eyed peas
garbanzo beans (chickpeas)
kidney beans
lentils
lima beans (mature)
navy beans
pinto beans
soybeans
split peas
tofu (bean curd made from soybeans)
white beans

Starchy vegetables
corn
green peas
lima beans (green)
potatoes

Other vegetables
artichokes
asparagus
bean sprouts
beets
Brussels sprouts
cabbage
cauliflower
celery
cucumbers
eggplant
green beans
green or red peppers
iceberg (head) lettuce
mushrooms
okra
onions
parsnips
tomatoes
tomato juice
vegetable juice
turnips
wax beans
zucchini

For advice based on age and gender, see "Vegetable Variety: Your Weekly Goal, Too!" on page 242.

One Cup of Vegetables Equals: For most vegetables, here's a simple rule of thumb—one cup is either: 1 cup of raw or cooked vegetables or vegetable juice, or 2 cups of raw leafy greens. To extend the list, here's what counts as one cup:

● 2 cups raw lettuce, spinach, watercress, or other leafy greens

● 1 cup chopped, mashed, or sliced nonleafy vegetables

● 1 cup tofu in ½-inch cubes

● 1 cup vegetable juice

● 1 cup (12) baby carrots

● 1 cup cooked legumes (beans, peas, or lentils)

● 1 large (3-inch-diameter) bell pepper

● 1 large (3-inch-diameter) tomato

● 1 medium (2½- to 3-inch-diameter) baked or boiled potato

● 3 spears (5 inches long) broccoli

● 2 stalks (11- to 12-inch) celery

● 2 medium carrots

● 1 large ear (8 to 9 inches) corn

● 20 medium (2½- to 4-inch) French fries

MyPyramid Pointers

Vary the types and colors: dark-green leafy, deep-yellow vegetables, red, orange, white! Because vegetables supply different amounts and types of nutrients, phytonutrients, and fiber, variety makes good health sense. Ease up on ever-popular French fries and fried onion rings, or salads with heavy dressing; their preparation and/or toppings increase the calorie and fat content.

● Try different greens in salads: arugula, beet greens, bibb lettuce, chicory, fennel greens, kale, leaf lettuce, romaine, spinach, and watercress. Keep edible peels on potatoes, cucumber, and summer squash.

● Enjoy vegetables you've always eaten—just more of them! Or broaden your vegetable repertoire. Besides green beans and broccoli, try okra, snow peas, or Brussels sprouts. Roast parsnips and beets with your carrots and potatoes. Shred fresh spinach for slaw. Need more ideas? *Besides the ideas in this chapter and in chapter 9*, a walk through the produce department and grocery aisles may spark your creativity!

● Add more vegetables to everyday meals. "Fortify" pizza or pasta dishes with steamed, sliced vegetables: zucchini, carrots, broccoli, and bell peppers. Add tomato or cucumber slices and spinach to sandwiches. Top baked potatoes with vegetable salsa or stir-fried veggies. Add spinach to hot soup. *For more ideas, refer to "Fruits and Vegetables: Fitting More In!" in chapter 13.*

● Snack on veggies. Keep cleaned, raw veggies in the fridge, ready for a quick nibble. Tuck a can of 100 percent vegetable juice in your lunch or snack bag.

● As a sandwich side, enjoy broccoli florets, baby carrots, or pepper strips.

● Enjoy more beans (legumes). Legumes have a "split personality." Count them in either the Vegetable Group or the Meat and Beans Group. Keep in mind that the same bowl of beans can't count for both.

Fruit Group: Focus on Fruits!

What's in the fruit bowl? You'll find all of America's favorites: apples, oranges, and bananas, as well as berries and melons. And you'll find some we may eat less often: cherries, mangoes, nectarines, pineapple, and kiwifruit. For more variety, fill your fruit bowl with less common fruits, too, such as lychees, loquats,

Have You Ever Wondered

. . . where salsa fits in the food groups? That depends on the ingredients. An all-vegetable salsa, perhaps made with beans, counts in the Vegetable Group. If the salsa has veggies, and perhaps mango or another fruit, your portion counts toward a little from both the Fruit and the Vegetable Groups.

. . . what cruciferous vegetables are? Members of the cabbage family, they get their name from their four-petaled flowers, which look like a crucifer, or cross. They include a diverse variety: arugula, bok choy, broccoli, Brussels sprouts, cabbage, cauliflower, collards, kale, kohlrabi, mustard greens, radishes, rutabaga, Swiss chard, turnip, turnip greens, and watercress. Cruciferous vegetables contain nutrients, as well as phytonutrients with unique health-promoting benefits. This vegetable family has something else in common: a strong cooking aroma. Proper food handling enhances their flavor without intensifying the aroma: (1) eat them soon after you buy them—raw or cooked, (2) cook them quickly, just until tender-crisp, and (3) eat leftovers within a day.

and pomegranates! *Check chapter 9, "Fresh Ideas: Uncommon Fruit," for starters.*

Any fruit or 100 percent fruit juice counts in the Fruit Group, whether it's fresh, canned, frozen, or dried. Fruit also may be whole, cut-up, or pureed. Make most of your fruit choices whole fruit, rather than juice. *Refer to page 165 in chapter 8 for more about juice.*

Why Eat Fruit?

Fit fruit in because it tastes good . . . and because fruit provides nutrients and phytonutrients for overall good health and disease prevention.

Key nutrients: Like vegetables, the nutrients in Fruit Group foods vary—the reason for varying your choices! Overall this food group supplies carotenoids, including those that form vitamin A, as well as vitamin C, folate, potassium, fiber, and many other phytonutrients. *To learn about the phytonutrients in fruit, refer to chapter 4, "Phytonutrients—A 'Crop' for Good*

DIFFERENT VEGETABLES AND FRUITS, DIFFERENT NUTRIENTS

Sources of vitamin A

● Bright orange vegetables like carrots, sweet potatoes, pumpkin

● Tomatoes and tomato products, and red sweet peppers

● Leafy greens such as spinach, collards, turnip greens, kale, beet and mustard greens, green leaf lettuce, romaine

● Orange fruits such as mangoes, cantaloupe, apricots, and red or pink grapefruit

Sources of vitamin C

● Citrus fruits and juices, kiwifruit, strawberries, guava, papaya, cantaloupe

● Broccoli, peppers, tomatoes, cabbage (especially Chinese cabbage), Brussels sprouts, potatoes

● Leafy greens, such as romaine, turnip greens, spinach

Sources of folate

● Cooked dry beans and peas

● Orange and orange juice

● Deep-green leaves such as spinach and mustard greens

Sources of potassium

● Baked white or sweet potatoes, cooked greens (such as spinach), winter (orange) squash

● Bananas, plantains, many dried fruits, oranges and orange juice, cantaloupe, and honeydew melons

● Cooked dry beans

● Soybeans (green and mature)

● Tomato products (sauce, pasta, puree)

● Beet greens

For a list of vegetables and fruits that are good to excellent sources of several key nutrients and dietary fiber, refer to "Produce 'Package'" in the Appendices.

help maintain quality. Most fruits are low in fat, sodium, and calories; all are cholesterol free. Often not thought of as fruits, avocados and olives contain monounsaturated fat. Avocados also supply beta carotene (forms vitamin A).

Important health benefits: As part of your overall healthy eating strategy, fitting in plenty of fruit delivers health benefits! Among the potential benefits: reduced risk for heart disease, type 2 diabetes, and some cancers. As a good potassium source, fruits may help maintain healthy blood pressure, and perhaps reduce the risk of developing kidney stones or possibly help reduce bone loss with age. Fruits' dietary fiber may help reduce heart disease risk, blood cholesterol levels, constipation, and diverticulosis in an overall healthful eating pattern.

Also on the plus side, fruits' vitamin C promotes growth and repair of all body tissues, helps heal cuts and wounds, and keeps teeth and gums healthy. Its fiber aids the digestive process. And its folate helps your body form red blood cells and, for many women, helps reduce the risk of birth defects.

Fruit is lower in calories per cup than many higher-calorie foods. For that reason, fruit may help lower calories in your meals and snacks. And fruit's fiber and water may help you feel full with fewer calories.

Fruit: How Much?

Sweeten your day with fruit! The specific amount depends on your age, gender, height and weight, and your level of physical activity. For 2,000 calories a day, you need about 2 cups of fruit a day. *Check "MyPyramid: Food Intake Patterns" in the Appendices for the amount that matches your calorie level.*

One Cup of Fruit Equals: As a rule of thumb, a cup

Health," and to "'Paint' Your Plate with Color" in chapter 13.

Citrus fruits, melons, and berries are excellent sources of vitamin C. Many deep-yellow fruits, such as cantaloupe, apricots, mangoes, and peaches, are rich in vitamin A. Fruits, especially edible peels on apples, pears, peaches, other fruits, and dry fruits provide fiber, too. Juices have little or no fiber. Many fruits also supply potassium and folate. Bananas, melons, and orange juice are among the better fruit sources of potassium.

Fruit's sweet flavor comes from its natural sugar called fructose. Sometimes sugars are added to canned and frozen fruits and fruit juice to enhance flavor or of fruit is 1 cup of fruit or 100 percent fruit juice, or ½ cup of dried fruit. Counting one cup with whole fruit takes more estimating:

- 1 cup cut-up fresh, frozen, or canned fruit, or applesauce
- 1 cup fruit juice
- 1 large (2¾-inch-diameter) peach
- 1 large (8- to 9-inch) banana
- 1 medium pear (2½ pears per pound)
- 3 medium or 2 large plums
- 1 medium (4-inch-diameter) grapefruit
- 32 seedless grapes
- 1 small (2½-inch-diameter) apple
- 1 small wedge (1-inch-thick) watermelon
- 8 large strawberries

MyPyramid Pointers

Versatile and "fast," whole fruits make great snacks, side dishes, or desserts. They may be sliced or pureed for salads; meat, poultry, or seafood dishes; desserts; toppings; or smoothies. Enjoy a variety of fruits and 100 percent fruit juices.

- Keep frozen and canned fruit on hand, especially when many fruits aren't in season.

- Go beyond basics: prickly pear, papaya, mango, star fruit, figs, kiwifruit, or guava. Try new-to-you varieties of apples, pears, plums, or melons.

- Keep dried fruits—apricots, apple slices, cranberries, raisins, and prunes (dried plums)—handy for healthful nibbling and pack-and-carry meals.

- Drink 100 percent fruit juice for snacks. Mix with sparkling water for a refreshing fizz.

- Enjoy a fruit smoothie from a smoothie bar, or make one at home. Whirl cut-up fruit (canned, fresh, or frozen), juice, and perhaps yogurt, frozen yogurt, or milk in your blender.

- Add fruits! Toss mandarin orange segments, grape halves, berries, and other fruit with garden salads. Add crushed pineapple, raisins, chopped apple, or pomegranate seeds to slaw.

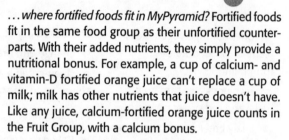

Have You Ever Wondered

. . . where fortified foods fit in MyPyramid? Fortified foods fit in the same food group as their unfortified counterparts. With their added nutrients, they simply provide a nutritional bonus. For example, a cup of calcium- and vitamin-D fortified orange juice can't replace a cup of milk; milk has other nutrients that juice doesn't have. Like any juice, calcium-fortified orange juice counts in the Fruit Group, with a calcium bonus.

. . . if fruit drinks (not 100 percent juice) count in the Fruit Group? No. Even if fruit juice is one ingredient, these drinks aren't nutritionally comparable to 100 percent juice. Many fruit-flavored drinks are actually water with fruit flavor and added sugars. Even a fortified drink made with a small percent of real juice usually won't supply all the nutrients, such as folate, that 100 percent juice contains.

. . . where supplements fit in? MyPyramid advice doesn't change if you take a multivitamin/mineral supplement. Supplements are merely what their name implies. They're intended to supplement nutrients from the foods you eat, not replace nutrient-rich foods. All healthy people need to follow MyPyramid guidelines first. Then a health professional may advise a supplement—generally not to exceed 100 percent of the Dietary Reference Intake for a nutrient.

- Sprinkle dried fruits on breakfast cereal, pudding, or frozen yogurt. Blend them with stuffing and rice dishes. Mix them in muffin batter and bread dough.

- Enjoy fruit as a sweet ending to your meals.

Milk Group: Get Your Calcium-Rich Foods!

Milk itself belongs in this food group—and so do the calcium-rich foods made from milk, such as yogurt and cheese. The most healthful choices—fat-free and low-fat dairy foods—are also the most nutrient-rich. If you choose dairy foods with more fat, those fat calories count as your "extra" discretionary calories. Added sugars in sweetened milk products, such as flavored milk, yogurt, drinkable yogurt, and desserts, also count as discretionary calories.

A few dairy foods—butter, cream, cream cheese, and sour cream—contribute fat, but few other nutrients. They're made from the cream that naturally separates from unhomogenized milk and don't count as Milk Group foods.

What about calcium-fortified foods and drinks, such as orange juice and soy beverages? While they may provide calcium and vitamin D, they may not provide other nutrients found in milk and milk products. These products supply calcium for those who don't consume milk and milk products and need other sources of calcium. *Refer to chapter 21 for handling lactose intolerance.*

Why Consume Milk and Other Calcium-Rich Dairy Foods?

For healthy bones, consume milk and milk products! Over a lifetime, an adequate amount from the Milk Group reduces the risk of low bone mass. However, any time is a good time to start consuming enough. Milk's other nutrients also keep your body in good working order.

Key nutrients: Milk Group foods are the body's best sources of calcium and riboflavin. Without dairy foods, getting enough calcium for bone health isn't as easy. Many dairy foods are also fortified with vitamins A and D, and they're good sources of protein, phosphorus, and potassium.

The fat and cholesterol content of dairy foods varies. Fat-free (skim) milk contains 0.5 percent fat or less. Low-fat or light (1 percent) milk has 50 percent less fat than whole milk. Reduced-fat (2 percent) milk has 25 percent less fat than whole milk. And whole milk contains 3.25 percent fat. These percentages refer to the amount of fat by weight, not calories. *For the calcium, fat, and cholesterol in various types of milk, refer to "Milk: A Great Calcium Source" on this page.*

Cheese varieties vary in their total fat, saturated fat, and cholesterol content. That said, fat-free and reduced-fat varieties with considerably less fat are sold. Dairy foods with less fat usually have less cholesterol, too. Regardless of their fat content, the amounts of other nutrients—calcium, protein, phosphorus, and vitamin D—remain about the same.

Dairy foods may contain two types of sugars: naturally occurring lactose and added sugars. Any added sugars in dairy foods come from flavorings added to ice cream, flavored yogurt, milk, and other dairy foods.

Important health benefits: The bone-healthy benefits—from childhood through adulthood—of milk and milk products are well known. Several nutrients in milk build and maintain bone mass and build healthy teeth, including calcium, phosphorus, and vitamin D. Consuming three cups or an equivalent from the Milk Group daily can improve or help retain bone mass.

Milk products, especially yogurt and milk, provide

MILK: A GREAT CALCIUM SOURCE*

MILK	CALORIES	CALCIUM (MG)	FAT (G)	SATURATED FAT (G)	CHOLESTEROL (MG)
8 ounces . . .					
buttermilk, low-fat	100	285	2	1.5	10
unflavored milk					
fat-free	85	300	<0.5	<0.5	5
1% low-fat	100	290	2	1.5	10
2% reduced fat	120	285	5	3	20
whole	150	275	8	4.5	25
chocolate milk					
1% low-fat	160	290	2	1.5	10
2% reduced fat	190	270	5	3	20
whole	210	280	8	5	30
4 ounces . . .					
eggnog	170	165	10	5.5	75
evaporated milk					
fat-free	100	370	<1	<0.5	5
whole	170	330	10	5.5	35
sweetened condensed milk	490	435	13	8.5	50

*Figures are rounded.

potassium, too, which helps maintain healthy blood pressure. These foods provide cell-building protein.

More health advice: most Milk Group choices should be fat-free or low-fat since they have little or no solid fat. To compare, cheese, whole milk, and products made from them are higher in saturated fats and cholesterol. High intake of saturated fats in particular raises LDL ("bad") cholesterol in blood, increasing heart disease risk. Using lower-fat dairy foods also helps you cut calories.

Milk: How Much?

How much from the Milk Group for you? And how do your choices stack up? The daily amount advised depends on your age. From age nine years on, the advice is 3 cups or its equivalent daily; for children ages two to eight years, the advice is 2 cups a day. Many people, teens and adult women especially, neglect the Milk Group.

One Cup of Milk or Its Equivalent Equals. Figure 1 cup of milk or yogurt, or 1½ ounces of natural cheese, or 2 ounces of process cheese as 1 cup from the Milk Group. To help keep your blood cholesterol levels healthy, make most of your choices fat-free or low-fat.

- 1 cup milk (flavored or unflavored) or buttermilk
- 1 cup (8 ounces) yogurt
- ½ cup evaporated milk
- 1½ ounces hard cheese (Cheddar, mozzarella, Swiss, parmesan)
- ½ cup shredded cheese
- 2 ounces process cheese (American)
- ½ cup ricotta cheese
- 2 cups cottage cheese
- 1 cup pudding made with milk
- 1 cup frozen yogurt
- 1½ cups ice cream

MyPyramid Pointers

Fit Milk Group foods in. Choose mostly fat-free or low-fat versions!

● Fit calcium-rich foods into everyday meals and snacks: milk on cereal, cheese on a sandwich, yogurt

dip with veggies, coffee "au lait" or "con leche" (with milk) or caffe latte, shredded cheese on soup or salad, or cottage cheese as a side dish. Try flavored milk (chocolate, strawberry, other flavors) if you prefer.

● Snack on calcium-rich dairy foods: perhaps yogurt, milk, or cheese cubes. For dessert try frozen yogurt or pudding. Or carry single portions of pudding in a packed lunch or snack.

● Use evaporated fat-free milk instead of cream in coffee, on cereals, whipped as a topping, and in recipes calling for cream. Although it's light yellow in color, evaporated fat-free milk has a creamy texture and less fat than cream.

● Use plain, low-fat, or fat-free yogurt or cottage cheese (pureed in a blender) as a sour cream substitute.

● Drink thick, creamy buttermilk, or use it in smoothies. Even with its "buttery" name, buttermilk is usually made from fat-free or low-fat milk.

● Start your day with dairy: yogurt or a yogurt-fruit smoothie with breakfast.

● Buy a milk jug or carton with deli or fast food.

● Make oatmeal, other instant cereal, and creamy soups with low-fat or fat-free milk, rather than water.

● If you're lactose intolerant, look for lactose-free and lower-lactose alternatives, such as hard cheese and yogurt, or take lactase enzyme capsules or tablets before eating milk products. Or add a few drops of it (available in stores) in liquid form.

● If you avoid dairy foods, choose calcium-fortified foods (soy beverages, juice, cereal, breads, and rice drinks); some are vitamin D-fortified, too. Choose other nondairy foods that contain more calcium: canned salmon or sardines with edible bones, some leafy greens (collard and turnip greens, kale, bok choy), some dried beans, and tempeh or soy yogurt.

Meat and Beans Group: Go Lean with Protein!

Even though we use its shortcut name, the Meat and Beans Group delivers much more than meat and beans! It's filled with many protein-rich foods: beef, veal, pork, chicken, turkey, finfish, shellfish, game, eggs, dry beans (legumes), lentils and peas, soybean products (tofu, tempeh, soyburgers, others), nuts, seeds, and nut butter. Beans actually lead a double life. They count toward the Meat and Beans Group or the Vegetable Group, but not both at the same time.

For good health, make most meat and poultry choices lean or low-fat. Nutrient-rich fish, nuts, and seeds contain healthy oils, making them a great meat alternate. Eggs are an economical protein source; just keep your day's cholesterol goal in mind. Enjoy meatless meals occasionally, too, with dry beans and peas as your "lean" protein.

Why Eat Meat, Beans, or Their Alternates?

Meat, poultry, fish, dry beans and peas, eggs, nuts, and seeds: they're all protein-rich. Important advice from the Meat and Beans Group—make your choices lean!

Key nutrients: Besides protein, foods in the Meat and Beans Group supply varying amounts of iron, zinc, magnesium, B vitamins (thiamin, niacin, vitamins B_6 and B_{12}), and vitamin E. Heme iron in meat, poultry, and fish is better absorbed than non-heme iron from eggs or plant sources of food.

The fat and cholesterol content of foods within this food group varies. *See page 61.* Lean meat and skinless (not fried) poultry are lower-fat choices, yet provide varying amounts of cholesterol. Many finfish have less fat, including less saturated fat, and cholesterol than meat and poultry do; shellfish tend to be low in saturated fat but higher in cholesterol than finfish. Fatty varieties of fish (such as salmon, mackerel, swordfish, and herring) have another benefit: more omega-3 fatty acids. *Refer to "Eat Your Omega-3s and 6s" in chapter 3.*

Soybeans contain high-quality proteins, with all essential amino acids. Other excellent protein sources—dry beans (legumes), lentils, nuts, and seeds—have nearly the high quality that meat, poultry, or fish have. Eating grain foods with these foods during the day completes the amino acid package. A great source of starches (complex carbohydrates), fiber, and other phytonutrients, legumes also are cholesterol free and virtually fat free! Nuts and nut butters are higher in fat (mostly healthy oils) and calories than legumes.

Important health benefits: Protein provided by this food group not only builds body cells, enzymes, and hormones; this nutrient also supplies food energy.

This food group has a vitamin and mineral package with more health benefits. For example, their B vitamins help with energy production, formation of blood cells and body tissues, and nervous system function. Their iron helps carry oxygen in your blood. Their magnesium aids in bone building and energy release in your muscles. Their zinc not only helps your immune system function, but it's part of other body processes, too.

Choose lean meat, skinless poultry, and fish since they have less saturated fat. A diet high in saturated fats raises LDL- ("bad") cholesterol levels in the blood, which increases the risk for heart disease. To help keep your blood cholesterol levels healthy, limit foods from this group with more saturated fat: fatty cuts of beef, pork, and lamb; regular (75 to 85 percent lean) ground beef; regular sausages, hot dogs, and bacon; some luncheon meats such as regular bologna and salami; and some poultry such as duck. Stearic acid, a saturated fat in meat, doesn't have the same cholesterol-raising effect.

Among other foods to limit: egg yolks (egg whites are cholesterol-free) and organ meats such as liver and giblets to help keep blood cholesterol levels healthy. Diets high in cholesterol can raise LDL- ("bad") cholesterol levels.

Fish, nuts, and seeds deliver other unique health benefits. Their fat is mostly heart-healthier mono- or polyunsaturated fats. *See "Oils: Go for Healthy Fats" later in this chapter.*

Even on a low-fat diet, nuts and seeds are generally okay. Although higher in fat than many other Meat and Beans Group foods, nuts and seeds contain mostly healthy oils. While high in calories, they're cholesterol-free and provide good sources of protein, phosphorus, zinc, magnesium, as well as vitamin E and selenium (two antioxidant nutrients). Their phytonutrients may have other health benefits. As long as portions are small, they're a healthful choice—especially for strict vegetarians. (Peanuts are actually a legume, not a tree nut; their phytonutrient benefits differ.)

Note: If you consume a high-fat diet overall, including foods from the Meat and Beans Group, it's hard to avoid consuming more calories than you need.

Meat and Beans: How Much?

How much do you need from the Meat and Beans Group? The equivalent of about 5 to 7 ounces a day may be enough for most people. This is often a surprise to people, who sometimes eat much more. That said, you may need to make leaner and more varied choices from this food group.

How much you need depends on your age, gender, height, and weight, and your level of physical activity. *Check "MyPyramid: Food Intake Patterns" in the Appendices for the amount that matches your calorie level.*

One Ounce of Meat and Beans Is: An ounce equivalent is generally 1 ounce of meat, poultry, or fish, or ¼ cup cooked dry beans, or 1 egg, or 1 tablespoon of peanut butter, or ½ ounce of nuts or seeds. For specifics:

- 1 ounce cooked lean beef, pork, or ham
- 1 ounce cooked chicken or turkey, without skin
- 1 sandwich slice (4½ x 2½ × ⅛ inches) turkey
- 1 ounce cooked fish or shellfish
- 1 egg
- ½ ounce nuts (12 almonds, 24 pistachios, 7 walnut halves)
- ½ ounce seeds
- 1 tablespoon peanut butter or almond butter
- ¼ cup cooked dry beans or peas
- ¼ cup baked beans or refried beans
- ¼ cup (about 2 ounces) tofu
- 1 ounce tempeh, cooked
- ¼ cup roasted soybeans
- 1 (4-ounce) falafel patty
- 2 tablespoons hummus

MyPyramid Pointers

Fit in a variety of foods from the Meat and Beans Group—not just lean meat and skinless poultry, but fish, legumes, eggs, nuts, and seeds, too.

● Prepare meat and poultry to keep it lean. Trim visible fat. Broil, grill, roast, or use other low-fat cooking methods.

● Enjoy fish at least two or three times a week. Include some fatty fish, such as salmon, herring, and trout. *Refer to chapter 12 for guidelines on eating fish during pregnancy and breast-feeding.*

● Be sensible with meat, poultry, and fish portions. As a rule of thumb, a portion that fills about one-quarter of your plate is enough. You probably need only about 5 to 7 ounces total from the Meat and Beans Group daily. Occasionally it's okay to eat larger portions, but a 12- to 16-ounce steak is more than enough at one sitting!

● Make dry beans, peas, lentils, tofu, or tempeh the "center of your plate" several times a week. Try vegetarian chili or lasagna, vegetable tofu stir-fry, or a bowl of bean soup. Or mix canned legumes with a vegetable salad. (Peanuts are legumes, not nuts.)

● Enjoy eggs as a meat alternate. To control cholesterol, eat egg yolks and whole eggs in moderation—up to one yolk a day *if* you keep your total cholesterol intake under 300 milligrams daily. That includes eggs used in prepared and baked foods. Since egg whites and egg substitutes have no cholesterol and little or no fat, use them freely. You can use egg substitutes or egg whites in recipes made with whole eggs.

● Eat nuts, seeds, and nut butters. A small handful adds flavor and nutrition. Vary your choices since their nutrients and phytonutrients differ: perhaps cashews in stir-fries; pecans, almonds, or sunflower seeds in salads, waffles, or sweet potatoes; pine nuts or pistachios in pasta sauces and casseroles; sesame seeds

Have You Ever Wondered

... if venison, rattlesnake, and buffalo are good choices from the Meat and Beans Group—or how about ostrich? Sure. Their nutrient content is similar to other meats. Their fat content varies. Many types of game—venison, bison, elk, moose, squirrel—are quite lean.

Ostrich tastes like red meat, even though it's poultry. From a nutritional standpoint, it's quite lean—fewer than 3 grams of fat in 3 ounces, which is less than beef round and chicken with skin. It's also a good source of protein and iron.

on green veggies, soups, and stews; walnuts and macadamia nuts in quick breads; or any nuts on cereal, lunchtime yogurt, or in trail mix.

● Try other alternatives: tofu, tempeh, veggie burgers, and other soy products.

Oils: Go for Healthful Fats

Like the vegetable oils you use in cooking, oils are simply fats that are liquid at room temperature. Oils mainly come from two sources: different plants, as well as fish. Among the plant sources, common oils include canola, corn, cottonseed, olive, safflower, soybean, and sunflower oils. Some other oils, such as walnut and sesame oils, make great flavorings. Several other foods are high in oils, too: avocados, nuts, olives, and fatty fish, such as salmon and tuna.

Mayonnaise, certain salad dressings, and soft (tub or squeeze) margarine are mainly oils with no *trans* fats. Use Nutrition Facts labels to find soft margarines with 0 grams of *trans* fat.

Caution: A few plant oils, including coconut oil and palm kernel oil, are high in saturated fats. For nutritional purposes, consider them as solid fats, instead of healthy oils. Other highly saturated solid fats that are solid at room temperature: butter, beef fat (tallow, suet), chicken fat, pork fat (lard), stick margarine, and shortening. These count toward discretionary calories, not as healthy oils!

Why Eat Healthy Oils?

Fat: it's an essential nutrient. For their health benefits, most should be monounsaturated and polyunsaturated, supplied mostly by foods' healthy oils.

Key nutrients: Not only high in heart-healthier monounsaturated or polyunsaturated fats, oils also are low in saturated fats. Coming from plant-based foods, including vegetable and nut oils, they're cholesterol-free. Fatty fish supply another type of polyunsaturated fat: omega-3s. Many oils also supply vitamin E.

Important health benefits: What makes monounsaturated or polyunsaturated fats healthful? They don't raise LDL- ("bad") cholesterol levels in blood as saturated fats do. Essential fatty acids (from some nuts

and seeds) are important for a healthy nervous system and skin, and for kids, they help keep skin healthy. Oils, your body's main source of vitamin E, are an important antioxidant. And the omega-3 fatty acids in fatty fish may help promote heart health.

Healthy Oils: How Much?

MyPyramid offers specific advice for oils—get enough to provide essential fatty acids for health. This advice differs from your discretionary calorie allowance.

The recommended amount depends on you: your age, gender, height and weight, and your level of physical activity. If you need 2,000 calories a day, the recommended daily amount is 6 teaspoons of healthy oils. *Check "MyPyramid: Food Intake Patterns" in the Appendices for the amount that matches your calorie level.* Most Americans consume enough oil from foods they eat normally.

Healthy oils: you need some for health. Yet, like solid fats, they still contain calories, about 40 calories a teaspoon, or about 120 calories per tablespoon. Limit the amount to balance your calorie (energy) intake with the calories your body uses.

One Teaspoon of Healthy Oils Equals: A teaspoon of vegetable oils (canola, corn, cottonseed, olive, peanut, safflower, soybean, and sunflower) is easy to measure. *See the chart "Sources of Healthy Oils" on page 230 for how other sources of healthy oils stack up.*

MyPyramid Pointers

Make the switch—to mostly oils, which have more unsaturated fats.

● Limit dressing on salads to 1 or 2 tablespoons of an oil-based dressing.

● Use mostly soft tub margarine and vegetable oils in place of solid fats in food prep and in spreads, e.g., herbed olive oil, pesto spread.

● Lighten up on shredded cheese on your pizza. Top with sliced olives or nuts.

● Go easy on fatty spreads, toppings, gravies, and sauces that add fat and calories to foods from all food groups. Count them as discretionary calories.

Sources of Healthy Oils

		IN ONE PORTION	
SOURCE	PORTION	AMOUNT OF OIL	CALORIES FROM OIL
Vegetable oil	1 tablespoon	3 teaspoons	120
Margarine, soft (*trans* fat free)	1 tablespoon	2½ teaspoons	100
Mayonnaise	1 tablespoon	2½ teaspoons	100
Mayonnaise-type salad dressing	1 tablespoon	1 teaspoon	45
Italian dressing	2 tablespoons	2 teaspoons	75
Thousand Island dressing	2 tablespoons	2½ teaspoons	100
Olives, ripe, canned	4 large	½ teaspoon	15
Avocado*	½ medium	3 teaspoons	130
Peanut butter*	2 tablespoons	4 teaspoons	140
Peanuts, dry roasted*	1 ounce	3 teaspoons	120
Mixed nuts, dry roasted*	1 ounce	3 teaspoons	130
Cashews, dry roasted*	1 ounce	3 teaspoons	115
Almonds, dry roasted*	1 ounce	3 teaspoons	130
Hazelnuts*	1 ounce	4 teaspoons	160
Sunflower seeds*	1 ounce	3 teaspoons	120

*Although they provide healthy oils, avocados fit in the Fruit Group, and nuts and seeds fit in the Meat and Beans Group.

Source: www.MyPyramid.gov.

● *Make MyPyramid yours.* Using your age, gender, and activity level, get an estimate of your daily calorie needs and how much food you need from each food group. *See "MyPyramid: Food Intake Patterns" in the Appendices.* The beauty of MyPyramid is its adaptability. As you get older or your activity level changes, simply adjust your plan to match your calorie target.

● *Stay within your day's calorie (food energy) budget.* Find your balance between the right amount of food and your physical activity to reach or maintain your healthy weight. Choose "extra" discretionary calories to keep within your calorie budget. Move more to "spend" more! And learn to fit foods you enjoy into your smart eating plan while sticking to your calorie budget.

● *Track your progress.* Go online, www.MyPyramid.gov, to use MyPyramid Tracker. Type in what you eat and drink and your physical activity level to see how your food choices and physical activity stack up against your goals.

● *Look inside MyPyramid.* Get familiar with foods in each food group, recommended amounts, and smart, easy ways to follow the advice.

● *Take it one step at a time.* Modify your food choices and physical activity gradually. That may be easier than overhauling your whole eating plan and lifestyle at one time. Perhaps start with a change in one meal or snack, just one food group, or one active living strategy today. Then move on gradually from there toward a healthier you.

Build MyPyramid Your Way!

Eating smart isn't just for today! To keep fit, you need to make wise food choices for a lifetime. A few thoughts before you start:

For some quick insights, give yourself a nutrition checkup with "Turning MyPyramid . . . Into Your Pyramid!" on page 232.

Pizza: What Food Group?

Pizza, fajitas, lasagna, and cioppino (fish stew) . . . many foods don't fit neatly into a single food group. Prepared with ingredients from several food groups, mixed foods can count toward your daily totals from two or more food groups. Use your best "guess-timate" to determine the amounts they represent. Be aware: some mixed dishes contain a lot of fat, oil, or sugar, which add calories.

The amounts of food group foods, fats and oils, and added sugars in any mixed dish depend on how it's prepared. Think about how you could change these dishes to add more vegetables, fruits, and whole grains, and perhaps lower the calories?

FOOD AND PORTION	GRAINS GROUP (OZ. EQUIVALENTS)	VEGETABLE GROUP (CUPS)	FRUIT GROUP (CUPS)	MILK GROUP (CUPS)	MEAT AND BEANS GROUP (OZ. EQUIVALENTS)	CALORIES
Cheese pizza-thin crust (1 slice from medium pizza)	1	1/8	0	1/2	0	215
Lasagna (1 piece 3½ inches by 4 inches)	2	1/2	0	1	1	445
Tuna noodle casserole (1 cup)	1½	0	0	1/2	2	260
Bean and cheese burrito (1)	2½	1/8	0	1	2	445
Beef stir-fry (1 cup)	0	1/2	0	0	1	190
Clam chowder—New England (1 cup)	1/2	1/8	0	1/2	2	165
Clam chowder—Manhattan (chunky—1 cup)	0	3/8	0	0	2	135

Source: www.MyPyramid.gov. You'll find more examples on this Web site.

Need more specific strategies for MyPyramid eating? Check here for "how-tos":

● Shop the food groups in the supermarket—chapter 11.

● Prepare food-group meals and snacks for the "health of it"—chapter 13.

● Offer healthful foods to kids—chapter 16.

● Adapt MyPyramid to vegetarian-style eating—chapter 21.

● See how ethnic foods (Chinese, Italian, Mexican) fit into MyPyramid—chapter 14.

Everyday Challenges: Smart Eating Strategies!

Do you prefer a hearty breakfast or a light morning bite? A big meal at lunchtime or at dinner? Snacks or no snacks? Three meals a day or several mini-meals? No approach is healthier than another if you follow your personal guidelines for smart eating and healthful living overall. That said, one meal,

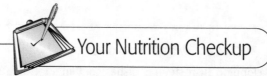

Your Nutrition Checkup

Turning MyPyramid . . . Into Your Pyramid!

MyPyramid.gov
STEPS TO A HEALTHIER YOU

Check how you did today. Set a goal to aim for tomorrow.

Food Group	Write in your goal. Check "MyPyramid: Food Intake Patterns" in the Appendices.	Jot down on paper: ● all the foods and beverages you consumed today ● the portion sizes.*	Estimate your total.
Grains	_____ ounce equivalents	_____	_____ ounce equivalents
Vegetables	_____ cups	_____	_____ cups
Fruits	_____ cups	_____	_____ cups
Milk	_____ cups	_____	_____ cups
Meat and Beans	_____ ounce equivalents	_____	_____ ounce equivalents
Physical Activity	_____ minutes	_____	_____ minutes

*Some foods don't fit into any group. These "extras" may be mainly solid fats or added sugars—limit your intake of these.

How do you think your food choices stacked up to your goals today?
☐ Great   ☐ So-so   ☐ Not so great

Think about some changes you could make. You can start small, perhaps just add a bigger spoonful of vegetables to your plate, or order a carton of milk to go with a fast-food lunch.

My food goal for tomorrow is: _____

My physical activity goal for tomorrow is: _____

For a detailed assessment of your food intake and physical activity level, click on www.MyPyramid.gov for MyPyramid Tracker.

Adapted from www.MyPyramid.gov.

one snack, or one day of less healthful food choices or high-calorie eating won't make or break your health. Your food choices on most days, over the long term, count!

Challenge One: Time-Pressed Lifestyles

Like most of today's consumers, you may spend 45 minutes or less preparing a family meal (compared with 2½ hours, 45 years ago). In fact, marketing research shows that 60 percent of American women want to spend less than 15 minutes preparing a meal! Like others, you may not decide on the menu until the end of the workday. Sound familiar? When time is short, don't give up on healthful eating. Just take short cuts to save time and energy!

● When you have time to cook, make a double or triple batch. For example, simmer enough pasta for two days. Serve it hot one night with meat sauce, then chilled in a salad with tuna, parsley, and low-fat salad dressing the next.

● Buy prepared foods for "speed-scratch" cooking: for example, grated cheese; precut stir-fry vegetables; shredded cabbage; skinless chicken strips; prewashed salad greens or spinach; and chopped onion. Even thin-sliced, lean deli meat is quick for stir-fried recipes.

Often more costly, prepared meals sold in many of today's supermarkets simply need to be cooked, heated, or assembled on your plate. Just make a simple side dish, perhaps a tossed salad—and you're ready to eat!

● Plan ahead: prepare ingredients ahead of time yourself. For example, wash and trim broccoli florets. Skewer kebobs with vegetable and meat pieces the night before. Cook lean ground meat ahead for soft tacos.

● Stock up with quick-to-fix foods: pasta, rice, frozen and canned vegetables, canned fruits, bread, lean deli meats, prewashed greens, presliced fruit or vegetables, salsa, canned beans, milk, yogurt, and cheese, among others.

● Cook on weekends; save food "prep" time on weekdays. Freeze leftovers in individual meal containers for quick thawing midweek.

● Use quick cooking methods. Stir-frying, broiling,

and microwaving are faster than baking or roasting. Slice meat and poultry thinly for faster cooking.

● Use cooking equipment to cut food preparation time. Rinse and dry vegetables in a salad spinner. Slice hard-cooked eggs and mash avocadoes with a pastry blender. Shred small amounts of cheese with a vegetable peeler. Thaw foods quickly in a microwave oven.

● Prepare meals that pack variety in just one dish. Try chicken fajitas in a soft taco. Stuff tuna, salmon, and vegetable salad into a pita pocket. Prepare a ham and spinach quiche. Make a chef's salad with no cooking at all. Or prepare risotto with seafood, Swiss chard, and shredded cheese, or stir-fry with noodles, tofu, and vegetables.

● Keep a variety of prepared foods on hand. Check the Nutrition Facts panel on the food label to choose those that match your family's nutrition needs. Prepare them with fresh foods: for example, prepared pasta sauce heated with cooked ground meat, then served over pasta or a microwave-baked potato. Or try a heat-and-eat pot roast sold in the meat case of the supermarket; just serve with a microwaved potato and green beans.

● Serve assemble-your-own menus: perhaps deli sandwiches, mini-pizzas on English muffins, or burgers with veggies and cheese toppings that your family can assemble to personal preference in your kitchen.

Challenge Two: Breakfast Dilemmas

"No time," "nothing to eat," "woke up too late," and "on a diet": people give many reasons for breakfast skipping or skimping. Despite its benefits, breakfast

WHAT'S ON THE DAY'S MENU FOR THE WHOLE FAMILY?

	ABOUT 1,600 CALORIES	ABOUT 2,000 CALORIES	ABOUT 2,400 CALORIES
Breakfast			
40% bran flakes topped with	1 cup	1 cup	1 cup
milk	½ cup, fat-free	½ cup, 1%	½ cup, 2%
banana	½ small	½ small	1 medium
whole-wheat toast with	1 regular slice	1 large slice	2 regular slices
soft margarine	1 teaspoon	1 teaspoon	2 teaspoons
orange juice	½ cup	¾ cup	1 cup
Lunch			
tuna fish sandwich with			
rye bread	2 regular slices	2 regular slices	2 regular slices
tuna, packed in water, drained	2 ounces	2½ ounces	3 ounces
celery, diced	2 teaspoons	1 tablespoon	1 tablespoon
romaine lettuce, shredded	¼ cup	¼ cup	¼ cup
tomato	2 medium slices	2 medium slices	2 medium slices
mayonnaise	1 teaspoon, low-calorie	2 teaspoons, regular	1 teaspoon, regular
pear	½ medium	1 medium	1 medium
milk	1 cup, fat-free	1 cup, 1%	1 cup, 2%
Snack			
dried apricots	¼ cup	¼ cup	¼ cup
fruit yogurt	½ cup, fat-free	¾ cup, low-fat	1 cup, low-fat
whole-wheat crackers	3	3	4
peanut butter	2 teaspoons	2 teaspoons	1 tablespoon
baby carrots	6	6	6
Dinner			
roasted chicken breast (skinless, boneless)	2½ ounces	2½ ounces	3 ounces
baked sweet potato	1 medium	1 large	1 large
peas and onions with	½ cup	¾ cup	¾ cup
soft margarine	1 teaspoon	1 teaspoon	1 teaspoon
leafy greens salad with	1 cup	1½ cups	1½ cups
sunflower oil and vinegar dressing	2 teaspoons	3 teaspoons	3 teaspoons
whole-wheat roll with	1 (2-inch)	1 (2-inch)	2 (2-inch)
soft margarine	1 teaspoon	1 teaspoon	1 teaspoon
milk	1 cup, fat-free	1 cup, 1%	1 cup, 2%

Calculated with www.MyPyramidtracker.gov.

Refer to chapter 16 for the benefits of family meals.

may the most neglected and skipped meal of the day. Some blame their body clock for not feeling hungry when they wake up. The excuse "not hungry" may instead be stress; stress hormones can affect hunger cues. With today's hectic lifestyles, others come up short on time and energy first thing in the morning. Some falsely believe that skipping breakfast is effective for weight control.

Yet breakfast is the healthful way to start the day. More than forty years of breakfast-related studies show that breakfast benefits children, teens, *and* adults.

Why Breakfast?

Breakfast is your body's early morning refueling stop. After 8 to 12 hours without a meal or snack, your body needs to replenish its glucose (blood sugar) with a new supply of food. The brain needs a fresh supply of glucose, its main energy source, because it has no stored reserves. Sustained mental work—in school or at work—requires a large turnover of glucose in the brain. Your muscles also need a replenished blood glucose supply for physical activity—even walking from your desk to the printer—throughout the day.

Actually, you may not feel hungry until midmorning if you skip breakfast. Conversely, you may feel hunger pangs even if you eat early in the day. Why? Your body reverts back to its normal metabolic response. Hunger pangs are a healthy signal. They mean your metabolism is working! Respond to, not deny, them. Denying often leads to bingeing later.

Are you a breakfast skipper, skimper, or eater? According to research, breakfast skippers often feel tired, irritable, or restless in the morning. On the flip side, breakfast eating has been associated with better attitudes toward work or school and higher productivity in the late morning, as well as better ability to handle tasks that require memory. Breakfast eaters tend to have more strength and endurance, and better concentration and problem-solving ability. What about breakfast skimpers? Eating even small food amounts helps restore glucose stores.

The Nutrient Connection. Often, meal skipping leads to missed nutrients. If you have to skip a meal, try to make up what you missed in other meals or with snacks.

Breakfast contributes to your food-group goals,

Kitchen Nutrition

"Jazz Up" Cooked Cereal

For a "great grain" breakfast, add flavor and nutrition to cooked cereals (instant or not), such as oatmeal, cream of wheat, grits, brown rice, or whole-grain couscous:

- Use fruit juice—apple, orange, or other 100 percent juice—or low-fat or fat-free milk as the cooking liquid.
- To cooked cereal, blend in grated cheese, chopped fruit (apple, peach, banana, kiwifruit), dried fruit (chopped apricots, papaya, dates, raisins), or nuts.
- Fortify cooked cereal with dry milk for more calcium.
- Liven it up with spices: cinnamon, nutmeg, allspice, or cloves.
- Top it with fresh fruit of any kind!

too. The good news: total nutrient intake for the day is usually higher for those who eat a morning meal, especially for children and women. A whole-grain cereal, milk, and citrus juice can provide 100 percent of the vitamin C, 33 percent of the calcium, thiamin, and riboflavin, and a good supply of fiber, iron, folate, and other nutrients for a day. Without a morning meal, breakfast skippers may not make up the missed nutrients.

Breakfast and Learning. Breakfast prepares children and teens to meet the challenges of learning. Those who regularly eat a morning meal tend to perform better in school, often scoring higher on tests. While adults may condition themselves to overcome symptoms caused by breakfast skipping, children cannot. They experience the very real effects of transient, or short-term, hunger.

Nutrition experts note that morning hunger significantly affects learning since it reduces concentration, problem-solving, and muscle coordination. That's especially hard on young children because basic skills—reading, writing, and arithmetic—are often taught first thing in the morning. Consider the long-term effect of transient hunger on learning. When children can't reach their learning potential day after day, they potentially can get further and further behind.

Kids who eat breakfast are more likely to be at school. Stomach aches or hunger pangs, caused by breakfast skipping or skimping, are the main reason for morning visits to the school nurse. And breakfast skippers tend to be tardy or absent from school more often. Breakfast eaters often behave better in school, too.

If your child doesn't eat breakfast at home, encourage school breakfast, if it's available to you. Many schools provide breakfast. *For more about school breakfast, see "For Kids Only—Today's School Meals" in chapter 16.*

Breakfast for Better Health. Among breakfast benefits: a jump start on fitting enough fruits, vegetables, and whole grains into your day. Orange juice for breakfast offers more than vitamin C; it's also a good source of potassium. Whole-grain and other fiber-rich cereals and breads can boost your fiber and folate intake.

Studies suggest two other reasons for eating breakfast: healthy weight and reduced risk for heart disease. Breakfast eaters are less likely to be overly hungry for mid-morning snacks or lunch; overall they tend to eat less fat during the day, too. Compared to breakfast eaters, studies show that those who skipped breakfast tend to have higher blood cholesterol levels, a risk factor for heart disease. Further research is needed to explore this link. For those who choose ready-to-eat breakfast cereals in the morning, their eating pattern typically has more vitamins and minerals, and less total fat, saturated fat, and cholesterol, and fewer calories.

An Energizing Start

Even if you've committed to eating breakfast, consider this: what you choose for breakfast can make a difference in your energy level for the morning. When a breakfast consists mostly of sugary foods, such as fruit, fruit juice, candy, or soda pop, a quick rise in your blood sugar occurs, causing a surge in energy. After about an hour, blood sugar and energy decline, bringing on symptoms of hunger.

With a varied breakfast of foods containing carbohydrates, proteins, and fats, a sustained release of energy occurs. This delays hunger symptoms for several hours and helps maintain blood sugar levels.

Have You Ever Wondered

... why protein foods seem to make meals more satisfying? For you, satisfaction may come in part from what you define as a meal, perhaps a protein food—such as meat, fish, poultry, eggs, or a soy burger—served with other foods (vegetables, fruit, whole-grain foods, and/or dairy foods). But the benefits of protein in meals extend beyond meal preferences.

Certainly your body needs enough of the high-quality protein that lean-protein foods can provide. In addition, recent research indicates that protein may be more satiating than fat or carbohydrate. So a lean-protein food may add satiety to a meal. By helping to stave off hunger longer, protein foods may aid weight management if your calorie intake remains within your energy budget and your overall approach to eating is healthful. In other research, eating enough protein, along with adequate physical activity, may also help people lose fat, not muscle, as they manage weight. Look for more emerging research in these areas.

The bottom line: include lean-protein foods in sensible amounts in your meals.

Beating Breakfast Barriers

For you or for children, every excuse or apparent breakfast barrier has a solution! If you have kids, you're their best role model. Children who see their parents eat breakfast more likely eat breakfast, too.

Not Hungry in the Early Morning? Start with a light bite, perhaps juice or whole-wheat toast. Later when you are hungry, eat a mid-morning food-group food: a hard-cooked egg, low-fat or fat-free milk or yogurt, cheese, or a whole-wheat bagel.

Short on Time? Keep quick-to-fix foods on hand: ready-to-eat breakfast cereal, instant breakfast mix, bagels, whole-grain toaster waffles, whole-grain bread for toast, yogurt, canned and fresh fruit, 100 percent juice, milk, cheese, and cottage cheese. Get breakfast foods ready the night before. Or plan on a breakfast that goes with you: a carton of yogurt; a bagel spread with peanut butter; or grapes, crackers, and cheese. If all else fails, set your alarm clock a few minutes earlier.

Think You'll Gain Weight? No evidence supports this belief. In fact, skipped meals often lead to overeating at snacktime or the next meal. A morning meal with lean protein and a whole-grain food may help with weight management. Choose mostly whole-grain breakfast foods, fruits, 100 percent juice, lean meat, and low-fat or fat-free dairy foods. Go easy on bacon, breakfast sausage, hash browns, and biscuits with gravy.

Don't Like Traditional Breakfast Foods? That's okay. Breakfast can be any food you like, even a slice of pizza, chicken or lean beef sandwich, or soup. Left-over macaroni and cheese, heated in the microwave

oven, makes a fine breakfast. Or make breakfast more interesting with a new yogurt flavor or an exotic fruit on cereal. *For more ideas, refer to "Easy Breakfasts for Kids to Make" in chapter 16.*

"Makes you feel more hungry." It may just take a few days for your body to adjust. In the long run, you'll likely eat fewer calories over the day because you'll be less likely to overeat at other meals.

For breakfast options away from home, refer to "Break-FAST" and "Breakfast on the Road" in chapter 14.

Challenge Three: That Snack Attack!

At the office, in the car, by the television set or computer, at a sports event, in the movie theater—snacking is part of American life. We often chide ourselves for between-meal nibbling, often with good reason. Too often, people snack mainly on energy-dense, low-nutrient foods, then skimp on nutrient-rich foods at meals—or perhaps overdo on calories.

Calcium is a case in point. Compared with moderate snackers, research suggests that people who frequently consume a lot of soft drinks and sugary snacks tend to take in less calcium. Likely, they're substituting these foods for calcium-rich Milk Group foods.

Carefully chosen, sensible snacks can be a key strategy for following food-group guidance from MyPyramid. They can supply nutrients that often come up short, including calcium, as well as fiber, phytonutrients, and other health-promoting food substances—without adding too many calories, added sugars, or solid fats. If you haven't eaten for three or more hours, a snack may even help bring up your blood sugar. For those higher-calorie snacks, choose them to fit as "extras," within your discretionary calorie allowance. *See "Extra Calories: Spend Wisely within Your Budget!" earlier in this chapter.*

For children and teens especially, snacks can supplement meals. Because their stomachs are smaller, children may need to eat more often than adults do, perhaps every three to four hours. Physically active, growing teens may need the added calories that snacks supply. *For more about snacking for kids and teens, refer to "Healthful, No-Cook Snacks for Kids" and "Great Snacking!" in chapter 16.* Adults may

"One-Minute" Breakfasts!

Each easy breakfast is packed with nutrients from three or more food groups.

- ready-to-eat cereal topped with sliced banana, sunflower seeds, *and* yogurt
- bran muffin *and* yogurt topped with berries
- peanut butter or hummus on whole-wheat toast or soft tortilla, *and* milk
- cheese or lean-meat pizza slice *and* orange juice
- instant oatmeal topped with dried cranberries *and* grated cheese
- breakfast smoothie (milk, fruit, and bran, whirled in a blender)
- toasted whole-wheat waffle topped with fruit, nuts, and ricotta cheese
- granola topped with canned peaches *and* yogurt
- whole-grain bagel topped with fruit chutney, baby carrots, *and* milk
- lean ham or deli meat on a toasted English muffin, vegetable juice
- low-fat yogurt with granola and cut-up fruit mixed in
- heated leftover rice mixed with beans, peppers and cilantro, *and* vegetable juice or milk
- heated leftover rice with chopped apples, nuts, and cinnamon, *and* fruit juice
- breakfast wrap with cut-up fresh or canned fruit and yogurt cheese (*see chapter 3*), rolled in a whole-wheat tortilla, *and* chocolate milk

enjoy a snack break to satisfy mid-day hunger. Older adults with small appetites or limited energy may find several small meals easier to handle. And many enjoy the social value of snacking with others.

Myths about Snacking

Snacking: a smart habit—or not? Actually, there's no need to feel guilty about snacking. In fact, here's the truth behind common snacking myths.

Myth: Snacking makes you fat!

Fact: There's no direct link per se between snacking and body weight. The issue is total calories in *and* out, not snacking itself, that determine whether you gain, lose, or maintain weight.

Snacking may have weight-control advantages. Eaten well before mealtime, snacks help take the edge off hunger, helping you avoid overeating at meals. For smart snacking choose foods carefully to fit with your day's calorie target. And be sensible with mega-size snacks and drinks.

Myth: Snacking causes cavities.

Fact: Frequent snacking can promote cavities. The longer teeth come in contact with food, particularly carbohydrate foods, the more time bacteria in plaque have to produce acids that damage tooth enamel.

To control a plaque attack, consume the whole snack at one time rather than constant nibbling. Brush and/or floss when you finish snacking to remove food that sticks to and between teeth—or rinse your mouth with water. *For more about oral health, refer to "Your Smile: Sugar and Oral Health" in chapter 5.*

Myth: Snacking gets in the way of good nutrition.

Fact: To the contrary, snacks can be *part* of good nutrition! Simply choose nutrient-rich snacks that fit within your healthful eating plan, perhaps to help fill in the food-group gaps in your day's meals. And choose snacks that help you stay within your discretionary calorie allowance.

Myth: Snacking isn't a good habit for kids to learn.

Fact: With their high-energy needs and small stomachs, most children need snacks. And so do teens. Three daily meals often aren't enough to provide all the nutrients and food energy they need. The advice for parents: help children learn good snacking habits. And keep nutrient-rich food-group snacks that kids enjoy on hand and encourage kids to snack to satisfy hunger, without overeating.

Myth: Snacks spoil your appetite.

Fact: Eaten two to three hours before meals, a small snack won't ruin your appetite. Snacks may quell hunger pangs so you are less likely to overeat at the next meal.

Myth: Healthful snacking means giving up some fun foods.

Fact: Any food can be eaten as a snack—even sensible amounts of chips, candy, and soft drinks. Again, use MyPyramid with its advice for your "extra" discretionary calories budget as your guide. And remember, the more physically active you are, the bigger your discretionary calorie budget!

Snacking Smart

Chosen wisely, snacks can work for you! As with other food and beverage choices, make between-meal eating a valuable part of your healthful eating style!

● Make snack calories count within your personal healthful eating plan—without overspending your day's calorie budget. Think of snacks as mini-meals that can contribute nutrient-rich food-group foods. *Refer to "A Food Group Plan—For You" and "Two Food-Group Snacks" in this chapter.* Go easy on

did you know

. . . munching on a handful of baby carrots can meet your day's vitamin A needs?

. . . preschoolers get nearly one-third of their energy from snacks?

. . . a planned snack can help prevent overeating?

. . . watching television tends to increase snacking— particularly high-calorie "goodies"?

. . . larger snack containers add up? People eat more when the package is bigger!

Source: American Dietetic Association.

energy-dense snacks (candy, juice drinks, soft drinks, others) with a lot of fat, especially saturated (solid) fat and/or added sugars; choose them appropriately so your day's food choices fit within your calorie budget. A little lean-protein food may add satiety.

● Snack only when you're hungry. Skip the urge to nibble when you're bored, frustrated, or stressed. "Feed" that urge to munch by walking the dog, checking your e-mail, or talking to your family instead.

● Snack on sensible portions. Choose a single-serve container; put a small helping in a bowl, rather than eating directly from the package; and skip "mega" or "super" size drinks and snacks.

● Use food labels to make snack decisions. Remember: If a snack package has two servings and you eat the whole amount, you double the calories, the saturated and *trans* fats, cholesterol, and sodium listed in one label serving, too! Check the ingredient list for added sugars. *For more on labeling reading, refer to "Today's Food Labels" in chapter 11.*

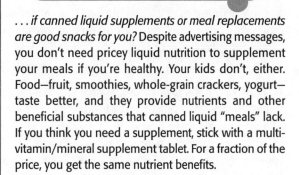

Have You Ever Wondered

. . . if canned liquid supplements or meal replacements are good snacks for you? Despite advertising messages, you don't need pricey liquid nutrition to supplement your meals if you're healthy. Your kids don't, either. Food—fruit, smoothies, whole-grain crackers, yogurt—taste better, and they provide nutrients and other beneficial substances that canned liquid "meals" lack. If you think you need a supplement, stick with a multivitamin/mineral supplement tablet. For a fraction of the price, you get the same nutrient benefits.

● Make snacking a conscious activity. Overeating is easy if you absentmindedly snack, perhaps while watching television or surfing the Internet.

● Plan your snacks. Keep a variety of tasty, nutritious, ready-to-eat snacks on hand at home, at work, or wherever you need a light bite to take the edge off hunger. That way, you won't be limited to snacks from vending machines, fast food restaurants, convenience stores, or your own randomly stocked kitchen.

● Eat small snacks well ahead of mealtime. A light bite, eaten two to three hours before meals, probably won't interfere with your appetite. Instead it may divert the temptation to overeat before dinner. To stave off hunger longer, pick snacks with protein and fat, such as peanut butter on celery, or cheese and crackers. Protein takes longer to digest; fat helps slow the release of food from your stomach to your intestines. Or pick carbohydrate-rich snacks, such as fruit, vegetables, and grain products, which digest quicker.

Check Your Snack Options . . . For Ease, Convenience, and Nutrition!

● Stock your fridge and freezer: fat-free or low-fat yogurt and milk, cottage cheese, cheese, lean deli meats, whole fruit, cut-up raw veggies, 100 percent fruit juice, frozen juice bars, frozen yogurt.

● Stash snacks at work—in case of late or busy workdays: instant vegetable or bean soup, pretzels, soy nuts, snack-size cereal boxes, mini-cans of water-packed

Two Food-Group Snacks

● whole-grain cereal and milk
● fruit smoothie (fruit or juice, with low-fat or fat-free milk or yogurt)
● yogurt and fresh fruit
● peanut butter on whole-wheat crackers
● pita bread and hummus (chickpea dip)
● apple or pear slices topped with cheese
● bagel chips (oven baked) and salsa
● dried cranberry and peanut mix
● whole-wheat pita stuffed with lettuce, tomato, cucumber, and low-fat dressing
● raw veggies with a cottage cheese or yogurt dip
● plain microwave popcorn and 100 percent fruit juice
● quesadilla (soft tortilla and cheese, folded and heated)
● flaked tuna or salmon and chopped celery, with low-fat mayonnaise
● microwave-baked potato topped with salsa and cheese shreds

tuna, boxes of raisins, instant oatmeal or couscous, dried fruit or single-serve fruit cups, whole-wheat crackers.

● Find vending machines with nutrient-rich food-group snacks: peanuts, raisins, trail mix, granola bars, whole fruit, 100 percent fruit juice, milk (flavored or unflavored).

● Stock up on microwaveable snacks: single-serving soups; whole-wheat pita bread or English muffins with tomato sauce, Italian herbs, and mozzarella cheese for instant pizza; bean dip or salsa, with tortillas; Cheddar cheese for a microwave-baked potato; plain sweet potato (great for microwaving).

● Pack a snack sack: canned or boxed juice, crackers and cheese, pretzels, soy nuts, air-popped popcorn, whole fruit, dried fruit, oatmeal-raisin cookies, fig bars, graham crackers, or raisin-nut mixes.

● Choose smart at convenience stores or malls: soft pretzels, bagel (go light with cream cheese), frozen yogurt, fruit smoothies (small size), fruit juice.

● Quench your thirst: water, low-fat or fat-free milk, 100 percent fruit juice or vegetable juice, juice spritzers (juice and mineral water), fruit smoothies (fruit or juice, blended with milk or yogurt), hot chocolate. (Fruit-flavored waters may be high in added sugars; check the label to be sure.)

Challenge Five: Grazing . . . A Healthful or Not?

Many Americans have moved away from "three square meals" a day. Instead, their series of mini-meals, called "grazing," matches their on-the-go lifestyle. That's okay—as long as they meet the nutrition goals for smart eating and active living. MyPyramid doesn't advocate a single meal and snack pattern. Instead, it's a guideline for what and how much to eat for the entire day or for several days. Eating five or six mini-meals can be as healthful as three meals a day.

Little meals—several small portions eaten throughout the day—are nothing new. Instead, they're part of the traditional eating style in many places outside the United States. A variety of small portions of traditional Spanish dishes are served as "tapas." In Greece,

Turkey, and Egypt they're called "mezze." A little meal, or "spuntino," in Italy might be a mini-pizza, grilled bread with tomatoes and cheese, or small skewers of meat and vegetables. And "dim sum," which means "to do (or touch) the heart" in Chinese, is a savory snack of spring rolls, pot stickers, and steamed dumplings, to name a few.

Eating several mini-meals may have several benefits. Like traditional eating styles, mini-meals can contribute nutrient-rich food-group foods. For some people, especially those with small appetites, little meals may match their personal needs and lifestyles. Eating fewer calories more frequently may burn a few extra calories; eating and digesting food has a thermogenic, or calorie-burning, effect for a short time. Some researchers also say that spreading the same number of calories over four to six meals throughout the day, rather than at three meals, may result in somewhat lower blood cholesterol levels, too. But these findings aren't conclusive.

For Healthful "Grazing" . . .

● Total it up. To avoid overeating, yet still satisfy your appetite, pay attention to your small helpings and to the overall amount you eat in *all* your mini-meals.

● Choose appetizer-size portions in restaurants and at home. That's about right for mini-meals.

● Use the power of MyPyramid to eat the right amount and food variety for you. Overgrazing can be your source of excess calories, added sugars, fats, especially saturated and *trans* fats, and sodium (or salt).

Challenge Six: Workplace Dilemmas, Eat Smart Solutions

Today's world of work demands increasing productivity. To reduce stress, yet increase your own productivity, eat for success!

● Start your workday with breakfast. You'll replenish your body's blood sugar stores, needed for sustained mental work and physical activity. You'll also stave off midmorning hunger that may reduce your concentration.

FUNCTIONAL FOODS: FAST, EASY, DELICIOUS!

Foods from every food group have functional health benefits that go beyond basic nutrition. Try these quick, easy, and convenient ways to fit functional foods in. *For more about functional foods (in italics below), refer to "Phytonutrients—A 'Crop' for Good Health" in chapter 4 and "Functional Foods: A New Wave" in chapter 9.*

BREAKFAST

- Top *oatmeal* with *blueberries*.
- Mix *yogurt* with *whole-grain dry cereal*.
- Spread *soy nut butter* on *whole-grain toast*.
- Drink sparkling *purple grape juice* with breakfast.
- Blend *soy beverage* with fresh *pineapple*.

HEALTHFUL MEAL IDEAS

- Mix *tuna* salad with grated *carrots, red peppers, onions*, and *garlic*.
- Serve *whole-grain pasta* with *tomato sauce* and fresh *herbs*.
- Cook *leeks* and *onions* with *tomatoes* as a side dish.
- Grill *salmon* and serve with fresh *greens* and *yogurt* salad dressing.
- Try low-fat cream of *carrot, spinach*, and *broccoli* soups.
- Enjoy *green tea* with a marinated *tofu* sandwich.
- Stir-fry fresh *vegetables* with extra *garlic*.

SNACK ON THE GO

- Grab a piece of fresh *fruit*.
- Mix *soy nuts* and *dried fruit* together and hit the trail.
- Grab a glass or box of *tomato, cranberry*, or *orange juice*.
- Try fresh *broccoli, cauliflower*, and *carrots* with *tofu dip*.
- Mix *bananas* with fresh *raspberries*.

Source: University of Illinois Functional Foods for Health Program.

● Take short stress breakers. Take a brisk, ten-minute walk. Stretch your muscles, and hold for 30 seconds. Relieve tension in your shoulders and neck by tilting your head from side to side, and front to back. Or switch tasks for a while. Avoid the urge to nibble for stress relief. Keep the snack bowl off of your desk— you'll be much less likely to overdo it!

● Take time for lunch—even when you're under pressure. Lunch may help you avoid a dip in your afternoon energy level, especially if the mix of foods has proteins, fats, and carbohydrates, including whole grains.

Feel sleepy in the afternoon anyway? Your overall sleep habits, age, and body cycle may cause drowsiness. New research also suggests that a midafternoon slump may be normal and induced by hormones. For some people, high-carbohydrate meals may increase serotonin, contributing to drowsiness. To stay alert all day, regularly rest well at night. If you feel sleepy, try a 10- to 20-minute nap (if your workplace allows).

● When you go out for lunch, sparkling water with a lemon twist makes a great "cocktail"—when you need to feel alert at work; alcoholic drinks can make you feel drowsy. Blood-alcohol levels from two drinks may stay with you the better part of the afternoon. When you handle potentially dangerous equipment or drive as part of your job, drinking and working is risky.

● Need a snack break? Stash nutritious foods in your desk drawer or in the workplace fridge. But control any urge for mindless nibbling at the computer.

● If you're caffeine-sensitive, limit coffee, tea, and soft drinks with caffeine. Enjoy a cup if that helps wake you up in the morning. But switch to "decaf," milk, water, or juice if caffeine bothers you.

● What about office celebrations? Enjoy just a small piece of cake. When it's your turn to bring doughnuts, bring bagels and fruit instead.

● Get your coworkers moving with you. Walk or take a fitness class over the lunch hour. Team up for an afterwork volleyball, baseball, or bowling league.

Healthy Eating from Your Home Office

Work from an office at home? Many do. If you're used to a company cafeteria or a nearby deli, you may need to redesign your eating approach. Start here:

● Keep routine in your life. Instead of rolling out of bed and into your home office at the computer, start with breakfast. And try to set a regular lunch time.

● Need a work break? Opt to walk outside, rather than check out the fridge.

● Make time to move. When you work at home, your chances for routine physical activity may go down. For example, there's no need to walk from the parking lot, bus, or train. Instead you take advantage of other ways to take an action break: for example, walk the dog, dig in the garden, swim in the neighborhood pool. Look for opportunities!

● Stock your kitchen for quick workday meals and snacks.

● Occasionally give yourself a treat. Make a workday lunch date with others who work at home, or with those who work in traditional settings. The social contact that goes with eating out is "good for your head."

● Take advantage of working at home for food prep. As a break, start afterwork meals. Perhaps simmer bean soup, or put a turkey breast or lean beef or pork roast in the oven.

VEGETABLE VARIETY: YOUR WEEKLY GOAL, TOO!

To get the nutrient variety that different vegetables provide, MyPyramid provides weekly advice from the vegetable subgroups.

GENDER AND AGE (YEARS)		DARK-GREEN VEGETABLES (CUPS)	ORANGE VEGETABLES (CUPS)	DRY BEANS AND PEAS (CUPS)	STARCHY VEGETABLES (CUPS)	OTHER VEGETABLES (CUPS)
Children	2 to 3	1	½	½	1½	4
	4 to 8	1½	1	1	2½	4½
Girls	9 to 13	2	1½	2½	2½	5½
	14 to 18	3	2	3	3	6½
Boys	9 to 13	3	2	3	3	6½
	14 to 18	3	2	3	6	7
Women	19 to 50	3	2	3	3	6½
	51+	2	1½	2½	2½	5½
Men	19 to 50	3	2	3	6	7
	51+	3	2	3	3	6½

Source: www.MyPyramid.gov.

CHAPTER 11

Savvy Shopping

With about fifty thousand items available in today's supermarkets, it's no wonder you have so many decisions to make! From food labels, to brochures and food TV, to "in-store" consumer affairs professionals, computer kiosks, and Web sites, you have more food facts at your fingertips than ever before. That's good for informed shoppers. With facts and plenty of choices available, you can shop for taste, nutrition, safety, price, and convenience, all at the same time. Food labels with Nutrition Facts appear on virtually all food products, and claims about nutrients and health, as well as food safety tips, appear on many.

Supermarkets comprise much of the retail food business, but that's not the only place where you can buy food to prepare and eat at home. Today, specialty stores, warehouse and bulk food stores, wholesale clubs, health food stores, restaurants, convenience stores, gas stations, department stores, drugstores, farm stands, farmers' markets, mail order, and even online shopping services sell food to eat at home.

No matter where you shop, look for qualities of excellence in a food store:

● The store should be clean—that means the display cases, the grocery shelves, and the floor. And it should have a pleasing smell.

● Produce, meat, poultry, fish, and dairy foods should show qualities of freshness. Read on for ways to spot the signs of freshness in a variety of foods.

● Refrigerated cases should be cold. Freezer compartments should keep food solidly frozen.

● Bulk bins, salad bars, and other self-serve areas should be clean and properly covered.

● Workers handling raw and unpackaged food should wear disposable gloves, and change them after handling nonfood items and again after handling raw food.

Beyond these minimum standards, today's supermarkets may offer other useful services: home delivery, electric carts, cooking classes, consumer newsletters, video rental, banking and postal facilities, pharmacies, photo finishing, florists, in-store restaurants, and recycling programs, to name just a few.

Today's Food Labels

At the store, food labels are your best sources of consumer information. Food labels tell the basics. They identify the food, the amount inside the package, an ingredient list, nutrition labeling, and the manufacturer.

If you need to eat fewer calories, less saturated or *trans* fat, more calcium, or more fiber, Nutrition Facts labels can help you. Nutrition information on labels helps you choose foods to meet recommendations of the Dietary Guidelines for Americans and MyPyramid. The ingredient list, safety guidelines, preparation tips, and freshness dating—food labels tell still more about food inside the package.

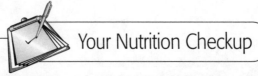

Your Nutrition Checkup

What's in Your Shopping Cart?

According to supermarket surveys done by the Food Marketing Institute, consumers rank taste, nutrition, safety, storability, and convenience as important reasons for making decisions in the store. If that's true for you, just how do your "supermarket smarts" stack up? Check here before you read this chapter.

Do You . . .	ALWAYS (3 PTS.)	USUALLY (2 PTS.)	SOMETIMES (1 PT.)	NEVER (0 PT.)
For nutrition . . .				
Read the Nutrition Facts on a food label?	_____	_____	_____	_____
Use nutrient content claims and health claims to quickly spot foods you want?	_____	_____	_____	_____
Check the % Daily Values to get specific information after you read a nutrient content claim?	_____	_____	_____	_____
Use food labels to compare the nutrients and ingredients in similar foods?	_____	_____	_____	_____
Look for nutrition information displayed near fresh foods: produce, meat, poultry, and fish?	_____	_____	_____	_____
Know how to use the "5–20 guide" to quickly check Nutrition Facts?	_____	_____	_____	_____
Use Nutrition Facts including serving sizes on food labels to plan healthful meals and snacks?	_____	_____	_____	_____
Subtotal for nutrition	_____	_____	_____	_____
For safety . . .				
Look for dates printed on packages to buy foods at their peak?	_____	_____	_____	_____
Check packaging and cans to be sure they're clean and not damaged?	_____	_____	_____	_____
Take perishable foods home within thirty minutes of shopping, and immediately refrigerate or freeze them?	_____	_____	_____	_____
Check to be sure that frozen foods are solid and that refrigerated foods are cold?	_____	_____	_____	_____
Know how to spot qualities of freshness in produce and raw meat, poultry, and fish?	_____	_____	_____	_____
Put fresh meat, poultry, and fish in separate bags when you can so they don't drip on other foods in your cart?	_____	_____	_____	_____
Put foods that need to be refrigerated in separate bags to help maintain a cooler temperature when they're bagged?	_____	_____	_____	_____
Subtotal for safety	_____	_____	_____	_____
For cost savings . . .				
Use unit price codes on shelves to compare the cost of similar products?	_____	_____	_____	_____
Take advantage of cents-off coupons and in-store specials?	_____	_____	_____	_____
Buy only the amount you'll use to avoid waste?	_____	_____	_____	_____
Shop for seasonal produce?	_____	_____	_____	_____
Pay attention to the price as the cashier scans each item?	_____	_____	_____	_____
Consider carefully before buying a new food after you sample it or see an attractive display?	_____	_____	_____	_____
Subtotal for cost savings	_____	_____	_____	_____
For convenience . . .				
Keep a shopping list to use as you shop?	_____	_____	_____	_____
Shop during off-hours to save time and avoid crowds?	_____	_____	_____	_____

Do You ...	ALWAYS (3 PTS.)	USUALLY (2 PTS.)	SOMETIMES (1 PT.)	NEVER (0 PT.)
Buy foods that are partly or fully prepared?	____	____	____	____
Buy single-portion or small-sized packages when you're feeding one or two?	____	____	____	____
Keep shopping trips to a minimum—no more than once or twice a week?	____	____	____	____
Subtotal for convenience	____	____	____	____

Count up your "supermarket smarts" category by category, then add up the total. *Total score* ____.

For nutrition and safety, a perfect score is 21 for each. For cost savings, it's 18; for convenience, 15. That adds up to 75 points.

If you come close to a perfect score in any category, count yourself as "supermarket smart" in that area. And make it your goal to be a well-rounded shopper—with top scores in every category! *Read on for more ways to shop smart and boost your score.*

What's on the Label?

Wrapped around almost every packaged food in the supermarket you'll find nutrition information. Today's food labels carry many types of nutrition and health information, to help you make choices and fit foods you like into your meals and snacks. Read on for more about ...

● A *nutrient content claim* such as "low-fat" or "high-fiber" helps you easily find foods that meet your specific nutrition goals. *See "Label Lingo" in this chapter for specific nutrient content claims.*

● The *Nutrition Facts* give specifics about the calories and nutrients, such as fat, saturated fat, *trans* fat, cholesterol, sodium, total carbohydrate, dietary fiber, sugars, and vitamins and minerals, in a single label serving of the food. This information must appear on virtually all food labels.

● The *ingredient list* on packaged food gives an overview of the "recipe," with the ingredients listed from most to least.

● A *health claim* describes the potential health benefits of a food, nutrient, or food substance, to reduce the risk of a chronic disease or condition.

● A *structure/function claim* describes the way a nutrient or a food substance maintains or supports a

normal body function, such as "helps maintain bone health" or "supports a healthy immune system."

Nutrition Facts and the ingredient list appear on almost every packaged food in the food market. Today many fresh fruits and vegetables, as well as meat, poultry, and seafood, may be labeled voluntarily with nutrition information, too, either on the package or on a poster or a pamphlet displayed nearby. If you don't find this information in your supermarket, ask the store manager to start providing it.

Food labels let you make nutrition-related decisions as you shop—and at home:

● Use labels to identify ingredients and compare calories and nutrients in similar foods.

● Use Nutrition Facts to pick nutrient-rich foods and make trade-offs to eat foods you enjoy.

● Use allergen labeling if food allergies are an issue.

The Language of Labels: Nutrient-Content Claims

Imagine rolling your shopping cart through the supermarket. Your eyes dart from one food product to another. Some canned peaches say "no added sugar." Certain breakfast cereals are "high in fiber"; others are "fortified." On packages of luncheon meat you see the term "lean." The words "high in calcium" on a milk carton catch your eye. You can choose "lite" salad dressing. And a box of cookies says "fewer calories." What does all this label language mean?

Known as nutrient content claims, these terms describe the amount of nutrients, cholesterol, fiber, or calories in food. But they don't give exact amounts. Usually they're on the front for quick comparisons.

For example, suppose you're comparing fat in salad dressing. Terms such as "reduced fat" and "fat-free" offer a general idea of the fat content. To find the exact amount in one label serving, check the Nutrition Facts.

Nutrient content claims mean the same thing for all foods, no matter what food or manufacturer. That's because they're defined strictly by regulation. Like Nutrition Facts, nutrient content claims are defined for

Label Lingo
What Nutrient Content Claims Mean

Label Term . . .	Means . . .
Free	It's an amount so small that it probably won't have an effect on your body—for example, "calorie-free," "fat-free," or "sodium-free." *Other terms:* "no," "zero," "without," "trivial source of," "negligible source of," "dietarily insignificant source of," "non" (nonfat only).
Low	It's an amount specifically defined for each term, such as "low-calorie," "low-fat," or "low-cholesterol." *Other terms:* "few," "contains a small amount of," "low source of," "low in," "little," "a little."
Reduced	It's an amount describing a food with at least 25 percent less calories, fat, saturated fat, cholesterol, sugars, or sodium than a regular food. Look for information about the food it's being compared to. *Other terms:* "reduced in," "___% reduced," "fewer," "lower," "lower in," "less."
High	It's an amount that's 20 percent or more of the Daily Value* for a nutrient—for example, "high in vitamin C" or "high-calcium." *Other terms:* "excellent source of," "rich in."
Good source	It's an amount that's 10 to 19 percent of the Daily Value* for a nutrient—for example, "good source of fiber." *Other terms:* "contains," "provides."
More	It's an amount that's 10 percent or more of the Daily Value*—for example, "more fiber" or "more iron." You won't find it on meat or poultry products. *Other terms:* "enriched," "fortified," "added," "extra," "plus."
Light	It's a food with a third fewer calories or 50 percent less fat than the traditional version. A "low-calorie" or "low-fat" food with 50 percent less sodium might also be called "light." *Other term:* "lite." When "light" describes a product characteristic, such as "light brown sugar," it isn't a nutrient content claim.
Healthy	It's a food that's low in fat and saturated fat, 60 milligrams or less cholesterol per serving, 480 milligrams or less sodium per serving, and at least 10 percent of the Daily Value per serving of vitamin A, vitamin C, calcium, iron, protein, or fiber. Fruits, vegetables and enriched cereal products can be labeled "healthy" without having 10 percent of the DV or more of these nutrients per serving. But they must meet low-fat, low-saturated fat, cholesterol, and sodium criteria. A meal or main dish product must have 600 milligrams of sodium or less.

On seafood, meat, or poultry, look for:

Lean	It's a food with less than 10 grams total fat, 4.5 grams or less saturated fat, and less than 95 milligrams cholesterol per 3-ounce (and per 100 grams) cooked serving.
Extra lean	It's a food with less than 5 grams total fat, less than 2 grams saturated fat, and less than 95 milligrams cholesterol per 3-ounce (and per 100 grams) cooked serving.

*When compared with a label serving size of the traditional food.
There are no FDA-defined nutrient content claims for *trans* fat.

a single serving. That's a standard label serving size set by the government—not necessarily what *you* may consider one helping.

Nutrient content claims are optional. Many foods that meet the criteria don't carry these terms on the label. If you see a product with a nutrient content claim, use the % Daily Value to compare it to a similar food that doesn't carry a claim. *For definitions of nutrient content claims, see "Label Lingo" on page 246. You'll find specific definitions in other chapters.*

Get All the Facts!

Let's get specific. Nutrition Facts differ from nutrient content claims. Nutrition Facts specifically state the amount of nutrients and calories in one label serving of a food, while terms such as "low in fat" or "more fiber" are quick-to-read descriptions.

Read the Nutrition Facts on food labels:

● To know the calorie and nutrient content of one label serving, and to compare similar foods.

● To keep these low: fat, saturated fat, *trans* fat, cholesterol, and sodium.

● To get enough of these: fiber, vitamins A and C, calcium, iron, and, if listed, potassium.

● To help you judge how your calorie and nutrient intakes change when you eat more or less than the label's serving size listed.

● To find foods that help you manage your weight; promote your health; reduce your risk for chronic diseases; or manage diabetes, cardiovascular disease, or hypertension.

● To help you make food trade-offs. (If you want one high-fat snack today, the label can help you trade off and find other foods with less fat.)

Nutrition Facts offer information in two parts: (1) specific information (standard serving size, calories, and nutrition content) for the food, and (2) general nutrition information in the footnote on the bottom.

Start with label servings. The label gives both the standard serving size and number of servings in the package. Given in both familiar kitchen measures (e.g., teaspoon, tablespoon, cup) and metric amounts, the serving size is a standardized amount for comparing similar foods. It's not necessarily the recommended amount for you or the portion you usually eat.

The Nutrition Facts apply to the amount in one label serving, not necessarily to all the food in the container. Some single-serving foods and drinks show the calories and nutrients in the whole package.

To know the calorie and nutrient amounts in your portion, compare your portion to a serving size on the label. If a label serving is one cup and you ate two cups, you consumed twice the amount of calories and other nutrients listed.

Check the calories. Calories are a measure of food energy. Look for the number of calories in a single label serving—and how many of those calories come from fat. *Tip:* Avoid confusing the number of "calories from fat" in one serving with the dietary advice "Eat 20 to 35 percent of total calories from fat." The dietary advice applies only to your overall food choices, not to a single food or meal. Percent of calories from fat does *not* appear on the food label.

Note the nutrients. Of all the nutrients in food, only a few are listed on the label—those that relate to important health issues. You'll find some you probably need to limit and others you may need in greater amounts.

Fats, saturated fats, *trans* fats, cholesterol, and sodium are nutrients people often consume in excess. The concern? Eating too much of them may increase your risks for some chronic diseases, including heart disease, some cancers, and high blood pressure.

Fiber, vitamins A and C, calcium, and iron are listed because they often come up short. So make food choices that help you eat enough of these nutrients. It's a way to help improve your health, stay healthy, and perhaps reduce your risk of some health problems such as osteoporosis or anemia.

Unless their amounts are insignificant, some nutrients must appear on the label: fat, saturated fat, *trans* fat, cholesterol, total carbohydrate, sugars, protein, vitamins A and C, calcium, and iron. Other nutrients may be listed voluntarily.

If you see a nutrient content claim, perhaps "fortified with vitamin D" or "high in folate," you'll find that nutrient on the Nutrition Facts panel. Nutrients added to a food such as fortified cereal must be listed.

Refer to the % Daily Values (DV). That's where you'll see if a single serving has a little or a lot of different nutrients. Percent DV isn't meant to calculate your individual nutrient needs. Instead, these percentages give you a general idea of how one label serving contributes nutritionally to a 2,000-calorie-a-day diet. Remember that % DV refers to a whole day, not to a single meal or a snack.

Depending on your age, gender, and activity level, you may need more or less than 2,000 calories a day, so for some nutrients, you may need more or less than 100% DV. *To estimate how much food energy, or calories, you need daily, see chapter 2.* Even if you don't know how many calories you need a day, the % DV offers a reference point. *For Daily Values used in food labeling, see the Appendices.* In your whole day's food choices, use the Nutrition Facts to help limit some nutrients and get enough of others:

● *For fat, saturated fat,* trans *fat, cholesterol, and sodium,* try to limit how much you consume. Total fat includes saturated fat and *trans* fat, as well as polyunsaturated and monounsaturated fats.

● *For fiber, vitamins A and C, calcium, and iron,* try to consume a variety of foods with more of these nutrients. Be aware that 100% DV may or may not be the optimal amount recommended for you. Daily Values are *not* based on the Dietary Reference Intakes (DRIs). For example, on food labels, the DV for calcium is 1,000 milligrams and the DRI for adults to

Use the "5–20 guide" as a quick guide to label reading. For any nutrient:

● *5% or less is low:* For nutrients you need to limit, eat plenty of foods with 5% or less Daily Value.

● *20% or more is high:* For nutrients you need more of, eat plenty of foods with 20% or more Daily Value.

age fifty is also 1,000 milligrams daily, teens through age eighteen are urged to consume 1,300 milligrams of calcium daily, and for adults over age fifty, the advice is 1,200 milligrams of calcium daily.

Choose foods with the lower combined saturated fat grams plus trans *fat grams.* Add up their amounts from the Nutrition Facts; for example, 1 cup of macaroni and cheese shown here has 6 grams of saturated and *trans* fats combined. *Note:* Similar foods may not be the same; Nutrition Facts may change if the ingredients (type of fats) change. For heart health, choose mostly foods with a lower combined saturated and *trans* fat and a lower amount of cholesterol.

Daily Values footnote. This reference chart shows some Daily Values. For two calorie levels (2,000 calories and 2,500 calories), it shows the maximum amounts recommended for total fat, saturated fat, cholesterol, and sodium—and the target amounts for total carbohydrate and fiber. Depending on your calorie needs, you may need less or more. This footnote is the same on every food label because it's general nutrition advice.

Calories-per-gram conversion. You may see the number of calories in 1 gram each of fat, carbohydrate, and protein. Notice that fat supplies more than twice the calories per gram (9 calories) than carbohydrate and protein (4 calories each).

How to Read a Food Label

Metric conversion key:

● 28 grams (g) = 1 ounce

● 1,000 milligrams (mg) =1 gram

A Word about Ingredients . . .

Imagine that you're reaching for a can of vegetable soup. The ingredient list, like a recipe, tells what's in the soup.

By regulation, any food made with more than one ingredient must carry an ingredient list on the label. Food manufacturers must list all ingredients in descending order by weight. Those in the largest amounts are first. For example, canned vegetable soup that lists tomatoes first contains more tomatoes by weight than anything else. Next time you reach for canned vegetable soup, check what ingredients are listed first, second, and third.

Have You Ever Wondered

. . . why you don't see % Daily Values for protein? Getting enough protein isn't a health concern for many people age four and over, so it usually isn't listed with a % DV. Adjustments for protein's digestibility makes calculating a % DV difficult. If the food is touted with a nutrient content claim—perhaps "high in protein"—then protein must be shown. Foods meant for infants and children under age four show % DV for protein on the Nutrition Facts.

. . . why a food with "no sugar added" shows grams of sugars on the Nutrition Facts? Fruits, vegetables, milk, grains, and legumes have naturally occurring sugars. "Sugars" in the Nutrition Facts include added and naturally occurring sugars. There's no DV for sugars because there's no daily recommendation. To find out about added sugars, check the ingredient list.

. . . if foods sold in health food stores or a supermarket's natural-food department are any more nutritious? The nutritional quality of foods sold as "health foods" isn't necessarily superior. In fact, the unregulated term "health food" is technically a misnomer. Check the Nutrition Facts and ingredient list to compare foods.

What's the difference? Perhaps price. Specialty stores or departments may charge more for similar foods. In most health food stores, the overall variety of foods is limited, too. But health food stores or natural-foods departments also may carry foods you may not easily find elsewhere: perhaps amaranth, quinoa, millet, or a wider variety of legumes.

The ingredient list is also useful for people with special food needs; for example:

● People with a food allergy, perhaps to peanuts or eggs, or a food intolerance, perhaps to lactose (milk sugar) or sulfites. If you're sensitive to artificial color, know that the colors are named individually, not just listed as "coloring." If the ingredient list isn't clear to you, write or call the food manufacturer. *See chapter 21, "Sensitive about Food," for more about food sensitivities, and page 251 on food allergen labeling.*

● People who avoid pork, shellfish, or other meat for religious or other reasons

● People who prefer vegetarian eating, including vegans who choose to avoid any food made with ingredients from animal sources

In some cases the ingredient list gives the source of the ingredients. For example, on the label for Mark's Cheese Pizza (*see below*), you'll see that "partially hydrogenated vegetable oil" is followed by "soybean and/or cottonseed oil" and that "tomato puree" is water and tomato paste. What is part-skim mozzarella cheese made from? The ingredient list says pasteurized milk, cheese cultures, salt, and enzymes.

See "Additives: Safe at the Plate" in chapter 9 and the list of additives and functions in the Appendices.

Nutrition Facts
Serving Size 1 pizza (184g)
Servings Per Container 1

Amount Per Serving

Calories 560 Calories from Fat 230

	% Daily Value*
Total Fat 25g	**38%**
Saturated Fat 13g	**65%**
Trans Fat 0g	
Cholesterol 45mg	**16%**
Sodium 1,090mg	**45%**
Total Carbohydrate 60g	**20%**
Dietary Fiber 4g	**16%**
Sugars 7g	
Protein 23g	
Vitamin A 45%	• Vitamin C 0%
Calcium 50%	• Iron 8%

* Percent Daily Values are based on a 2,000 calorie diet. Your daily values may be higher or lower depending on your calorie needs:

		Calories:	2,000	2,500
Total Fat	Less than		65 g	80g
Sat Fat	Less than		20g	25g
Cholesterol	Less than		300mg	300mg
Sodium	Less than		2,400mg	2,400mg
Total Carbohydrate			300g	375g
Dietary Fiber			25g	30g

Calories per gram:
Fat 9 • Carbohydrate 4 • Protein 4

MARK'S Cheese Pizza

MICROWAVE OVEN DIRECTIONS
1. Open pizza carton carefully. Remove frozen pizza and microwave disk; unwrap pizza. For best results, do not add additional toppings.
2. Reclose carton by inserting tab into slot. Place carton in center of microwave oven. Place disk silver side up on carton.
3. Center frozen pizza on top of disk. Microwave at HIGH 3 to 4½ minutes, or until most of cheese is melted, rotating carton ½ turn after 2 minutes.
4. Remove pizza from oven by holding sides of carton. Loosen pizza from disk with spatula.
CAUTION: Disk and pizza will be very hot.
NOTE: Microwave directions were developed using 600 to 700 watt ovens.

INGREDIENTS: CRUST: WHEAT FLOUR WITH MALTED BARLEY FLOUR, WATER, PARTIALLY HYDROGENATED VEGETABLE OIL (SOYBEAN AND/OR COTTONSEED OIL) WITH SOY LECITHIN, ARTIFICIAL FLAVOR AND ARTIFICIAL COLOR (BETA CAROTENE), SOYBEAN OIL, YEAST, HIGH FRUCTOSE CORN SYRUP, SALT, CALCIUM PROPIONATE ADDED TO RETARD SPOILAGE OF CRUST, L-CYSTEINE MONOHYDROCHLORIDE; **SAUCE:** TOMATO PUREE (WATER, TOMATO PASTE), WATER, GREEN PEPPERS, SALT, LACTOSE AND FLAVORING, SPICES, FOOD STARCH - MODIFIED, SUGAR, CORN OIL, XANTHAN GUM, GARLIC POWDER. **TOPPING:** LOW MOISTURE PART SKIM MOZZARELLA CHEESE (PASTEURIZED MILK, CHEESE CULTURES, SALT, ENZYMES.)

Manufactured by Mark's Pizza, Silver Spring, MD 20000

CONTAINS WHEAT, SOY, MILK.

Health Claims on the Label

Another bit of nutrition information might appear on food labels: a health claim. Health claims link food—or food components—in your overall eating plan with a lowered risk for some chronic diseases. Since this information is optional, many foods that meet the criteria don't carry any health claim on their label.

Strictly regulated by the U.S. Food and Drug Administration (FDA), health claims are supported by scientific evidence. So far these health claims have been approved on food, linking food, food substances, or nutrients to these health conditions:

● *Calcium* and osteoporosis

● *Sodium* and hypertension

● *Dietary fat* and cancer

● *Saturated fat and cholesterol* and the risk of coronary heart disease

● *Fiber-containing grain products, fruits, and vegetables* and cancer

● *Fruits, vegetables, and grain products that contain fiber, particularly soluble fiber,* and their risk of coronary heart disease

● *Fruits and vegetables* and cancer

● *Folate* and neural tube defects

● *Sugar alcohol or sucrolose* and dental caries (cavities)

● *Soluble fiber from certain foods* and the risk of coronary heart disease

● *Soy protein* and the risk of coronary heart disease

● *Plant sterol/stanol esters* and the risk of coronary heart disease

● *Whole-grain foods* and the risk of heart disease and certain cancers

● *Potassium* and the risk of high blood pressure and stroke

● *Moderate fat whole-grain foods* and the risk of coronary heart disease

(A few other health claims are approved for supplement labels; see chapter 23.) See the Appendices for specifics.

With so much emerging science on nutrition and health, some qualified health claims have been approved, too, showing the relationship between a food component and health or reduced disease risk. But a caveat, or qualifying language, must appear with it since scientific evidence isn't conclusive. *Check the Appendices for a Web site to find permitted qualified health claims.*

When you read health claims, remember: your food choices are just one factor that can reduce your risk for certain health problems. Heredity, physical activity, and smoking are among other factors that affect your health and risk for disease.

Structure/Function Claims on the Label

Structure/function claims such as "helps promote urinary tract health" describe how a nutrient or a food substance may affect your health; these claims *cannot* suggest any link to lowered risk for disease. Unlike health claims, structure/function claims don't need FDA approval or review, and they have no specific standards that regulate the wording. However, they still must be truthful and not misleading.

Dietary Guidance Statements

The FDA with the National Cancer Institute also may give dietary guidance. For example, "Diets rich in fruits and vegetables may reduce the risk of some types of cancer and other chronic diseases."

Food Labels: Food Safety and Handling Tips

For your good health, some food labels offer guidance on food safety and handling. To reduce the risk of foodborne illness, raw and partially cooked meat and poultry products must be labeled with guidelines for safe handling. *See the "Safe Handling Instructions" label.* Each of the simple graphics—a refrigerator, hand washing, fry pan, and meat thermometer—represents a safe handling tip.

Cartons of shell eggs also have safe-handling instructions to help control *Salmonella* contamination:

SAFE HANDLING INSTRUCTIONS: To prevent illness from bacteria: keep eggs refrigerated, cook eggs until yolks are firm, and cook foods containing eggs thoroughly.

Besides food safety, following these guidelines helps food retain its appealing flavor, texture, and appearance. *For in-depth information on food safety and handling, see chapter 12, "The Safe Kitchen."*

More Health-Focused Label "Info"

Food allergen labeling: As of 2006, the Food Allergen Labeling and Consumer Protection Act requires allergen labeling for foods containing a major food allergen or a protein from these allergens: milk, egg, fish, crustacean shellfish, tree nuts, wheat, peanuts, and soybeans. These allergens account for 90 percent of all food allergies. For example, it may say: "Contains milk, egg, peanuts."

Health warnings for more conditions: Warnings for people with special needs include:

● Foods and beverages made with aspartame (a non-nutritive sweetener) offer a warning for people with phenylketonuria (PKU). Aspartame contains the amino acid phenylalanine, which people with PKU can't metabolize.

● You'll find "Contains Sulfites" on beer and wine labels and on dried fruit and some salad seasonings, too, for those who are sulfite-sensitive.

● Alcohol-containing beverages also carry warnings for pregnant women.

Note: Any food with an allergen introduced through biotechnology must carry a statement of the food label.

See chapter 21 for more information on allergen labeling and on PKU and other food sensitivities.

Diet exchanges. Some foods provide diet exchanges for help in managing diabetes or weight. The label probably will say that these exchanges are calculated based on exchange lists from the American Diabetes Association and the American Dietetic Association.

More Reading on the Food Label

Taking a few more moments with food labels teaches even more about the food inside the package.

Type of food. The product name tells what's in the container. Besides naming the specific food, it tells the form, perhaps smooth or chunky, sliced or whole, or miniature—important to know when you're following a recipe.

Net contents. Food labels tell you the total amount in the container, either in volume, count, or net weight. Net weight refers to the amount of food inside the container, including any liquid.

For juice products, total percent juice content. This tells you how much juice and how much water the beverage contains. Keep reading for the Nutrition Facts. Compare nutrients, along with sugars and calories, before making your selection.

A "100 percent" juice may—or may not—supply 100 percent of the Daily Value for vitamin C. That said, juices offer more nutrients and phytonutrients than just vitamin C. Many juices are fortified with additional nutrients, too.

Juice "drinks," "beverages," or "cocktails" (with some juice, but not 100 percent juice) may be fortified to provide 100 percent of the Daily Value for some nutrients. Typically these beverages have added sugars, but probably not all the other nutrient and phytonutrient benefits of 100 percent juice. To the body, the sugar in fruit, called fructose, and added sugars in juice drinks can't be distinguished. They're used in the body in the same way. *For more on juice and juice drinks, see "Juicy Story: Fruit Juice, Juice Drink, Fruit Drink . . . or Just Plain Water?" in chapter 8.*

Safe Handling Instructions

This product was prepared from inspected and passed meat and/or poultry. Some food products may contain bacteria that could cause illness if the product is mishandled or cooked improperly. For your protection, follow these safe handling instructions.

Keep refrigerated or frozen.
Thaw in refrigerator or microwave.

Keep raw meat and poultry separate from other foods. Wash working surfaces (including cutting boards), utensils, and hands after touching raw meat or poultry.

Cook thoroughly.

Keep hot foods hot. Refrigerate leftovers immediately or discard.

Name and address of the manufacturer, packer, or distributor. With this information you can contact a food company with your consumer questions and concerns. Look for a consumer service phone number or Web site address, too. If the food is imported, the country of origin must be shown; this import regulation comes from the U.S. Department of the Treasury.

Food product dating. You can't see inside the package; how do you know if it's fresh? Many food packages, such as dairy products, have a date, often given as numbers, such as "12-15" or "1215" or as "Dec. 15" to mean December 15. Food manufacturers and retailers use three types of dates:

● *"Sell by" or pull date:* That's the last day a food should be sold to remain fresh for home storage.

● *Pack date:* That's when the food was manufactured, processed, or packaged.

● *"Best if used by" date:* For optimal quality, use food by this date; it's not a safety date. For example, the label may say, "Best if used by 12-31-07." Depending on the food and if it has been stored properly, it will likely be safe beyond this date.

Organic labeling. The Organic Foods Production Act and the National Organic Program ensure that the production, processing, and certification of organic foods are standardized. The term "organic" now has a legal label definition so you know what you're buying if you prefer organic foods. Foods may also bear the "USDA Organic" seal. Here's what the term "organic" means on food labels:

● *"100 percent organic":* The product must contain only organically produced ingredients (except for water and salt).

● *"organic":* The product must contain at least 95 percent organically produced ingredients (except for water and salt). The other 5 percent are ingredients that aren't available in organic form or that appear on an approved list.

● *"made with organic ingredients":* Processed foods may bear this label if they contain at least 70 percent organic ingredients—for example, "soup made with organic peas, potatoes, and carrots." The regula-

tion also identifies production methods that can't be used.

If it's labeled organic, you can find other label information. In the ingredient list look for the organically produced ingredient. The name and address of the certifying organization will appear, too.

Organic labeling regulations don't change food labeling regulations, administered by the U.S. FDA or the U.S.D.A.'s Food Safety and Inspection Service.

Organic foods aren't necessarily more healthful or more nutritious than other foods. Using them is really a consumer preference. *For more about organically grown foods, see chapter 9.*

Grading and inspection symbols on some products. These symbols indicate that foods have met certain standards set by the government:

● *Inspection stamps* on meat, poultry, and packaged meats mean the food is wholesome and was slaughtered, packed, or processed under sanitary conditions.

● *Food grades*—for example, on some types of meat, poultry, eggs, dairy foods, and produce—suggest standards of appearance, texture, uniformity, and perhaps taste. With the exception of marbling fat in meat, food grading does not suggest nutrient value. *Grading for meat, poultry, and eggs appears later in this chapter.*

Preparation instructions. Some products suggest oven or microwave times and temperatures, or perhaps other preparation or serving tips. Some offer recipes.

Kosher symbols. The term "kosher" means "proper" or "fit" in Hebrew. Kosher symbols indicate that the food has met the standards of a Jewish food inspector, done in addition to government safety inspection. The kosher code, which may appear on foods throughout the store, doesn't imply any nutritional qualities.

Often the word "Pareve" is written next to these symbols, meaning the food has neither meat nor dairy ingredients. During March and April a large "P" next to the symbols means it's kosher for Passover.

Star-K   **OU**   **OK**   **KOF-K**

Halal and Zabiah Halal symbols. Products prepared by federally inspected meat packing plants and handled according to Islamic dietary law and under Islamic authority may bear Halal and Zabiah Halal references.

Universal Product Code (UPC). These black bars, which identify the manufacturer and the food, are used by the food industry for inventory control and price scanning.

Country of origin. Fish and shellfish must be labeled with country of origin and how they are produced, for example, wild or farm-raised. This labeling is being considered for meat, peanuts, and other perishable commodities, too.

Labels—and You

What nutrition information do you use to make food selections—food labels or the MyPyramid? Use both!

● *MyPyramid* helps you choose from a variety of foods—and helps you know how much you need.

● *Nutrition Facts* on food labels offer nutrition information to help you choose foods wisely within each food group and the healthy oils.

Suppose you're shopping for dinner. You want a vitamin A-rich vegetable or fruit. Using food labels, you see that frozen broccoli fits the bill. But which

Label Lingo

Besides nutrition and health claims, some labels carry other label terms.

LABEL TERM ...	REFERS TO ...
Fresh	Food in its raw state. The term can't be used on food that has been frozen or heated, or on food that contains preservatives.
Fresh frozen	Food that is quickly frozen while very fresh shortly after harvest
Homogenized	Process of breaking up and separating milk fat. This makes the texture of milk smooth and uniform.
Natural	Product with no artificial ingredient or added color and that is minimally processed. The label must explain the use of the term "natural" (e.g., "no added colorings or artificial ingredients"; "minimally processed")
Pasteurized	Process of heating foods such as raw milk, raw eggs, and fresh juice to a temperature high enough to destroy bacteria and inactivate most enzymes that cause spoilage
Ultrapasteurized	Process of heating food such as cream to a temperature higher than pasteurization. This extends the time it can be stored in the refrigerator or on the shelf.
UHT (Ultra-High Temperature)	Process similar to ultra-pasteurization. With high heat and sterilized containers, food can be stored unopened without refrigeration for up to three months. Once opened, it needs refrigeration.

Have You Ever Wondered

... what the code on the lid or the bottom of canned foods means? A series of letters or numbers identifies the plant location, exact date, and perhaps work shift or time of processing. Codes differ from one processor to another. If you can't read the code but wish to, contact the food company, using the toll-free number, Web site address, or address on the label.

... what the term "wholesome" on food labels really means? Nothing legally. It may capture your attention, but it has no legal definition on a food package.

... if tattoos on eggshells and on produce peels are safe? Imprinted with a laser light beam, the tattoos provide codes for inventory, pricing, freshness, and tracking. They're safe and don't affect the quality of the food.

package of frozen broccoli? Read the label. Broccoli with sauce has more calories and fat than plain broccoli. Pick the one you prefer and that fits within your day's calorie (food energy) needs and fat budget.

Or suppose you're buying spaghetti sauce. Made with tomatoes, it counts toward the Vegetable Group. If you need to control your sodium intake, check the Nutrition Facts panel for the exact sodium content per label serving. The label also may offer other information, such as "reduced sodium" or "low sodium." And if you're curious, the ingredient list shows what ingredients contribute sodium.

Nutrition Facts help you make trade-offs. For example, a switch from regular to lean hot dogs likely saves both total fat and saturated fat grams and calories without giving up protein. The label tells how much. Feeling indulgent? "Spend" some of the savings on ice cream for dessert. *See "Quick, Easy Trade-offs" in chapter 10.*

Supermarket Psychology

Understanding food labels can help you shop for wellness and nutrition, but that's just part of your smart shopping strategy. Some practical tips can save you time, money, and hassle on grocery store trips.

Nutrition $ense

How can you get the most nutrition for those food dollars? Be an educated consumer and plan ahead. Know exactly what you need. And be aware of marketing ploys that may encourage you to buy beyond your shopping list.

● Keep a shopping list—and stick to it! A list jogs your memory and saves time as you walk the supermarket aisles. With a list, you're less likely to spend money on items you really don't need.

For time management, keep a running list in your kitchen of items you need to replace. Organize by category to match the store layout—for example, produce department, dairy case, meat counter, deli, bakery, frozen, and grocery shelves.

● Avoid extra shopping trips. If possible, shop just once or twice a week. You'll spend less on impulse items—and save time and gasoline expense, too.

● Check supermarket specials printed in newspaper inserts. Then plan menus around them. If the store runs out of an item on special, ask for a rain check. Be aware that "limit" signs ("limit three per customer") and messages such as "two for $5.00" (not "$2.50 each") are marketing ploys to get consumers to buy more. Research shows they work!

● Clip or download coupons for items you really need. Be aware that items with coupons aren't always the best buy. Another brand or a similar food might be cheaper, even without a coupon.

● Try not to shop when you're hungry. You'll less likely succumb to impulse items, including more expensive and less nutritious snack and dessert foods.

● Take advantage of seasonal produce. In season, the price for fresh fruit and vegetables may be lower, and the produce, more flavorful with more varietals. Depending on where you live, you might even go directly to the farm where they grow or to a local farmers' market.

● Use food labels to find foods that match your needs, provide Nutrition Facts for comparison shopping, and help you get the most nutrition for your food dollar.

● Decide what quality food you need. For example, if you're making a casserole, chunky tuna may be fine. But more expensive solid-pack tuna has more eye appeal in a tuna-vegetable salad.

● Buy the economy size or family packs only if you can use that much. There's no savings if food spoils and must be discarded. For foods that freeze, take time to repackage food into smaller amounts in freezer bags, then freeze for later use.

● Compare prices using unit pricing on supermarket shelves. To make comparisons easier, especially for similar foods in different-size containers, prices are given as cost per unit rather than price per package or container. The unit might be an ounce, a quart, or some other measurement. If the foods themselves and the units being compared are the same, the best value is the lowest price per unit.

● Compare the prices of national brands, store brands, and generic brands. Store brands and generic products may cost less than national brands since they

Unit Pricing

8 oz. Chunk Pineapple / Juice Pack

YOU PAY
83¢

UNIT PRICE
$1.66
PER POUND

don't have the same promotional costs. Convenient, innovative packaging such as squirt bottles and ready-to-serve pouches often add to the cost; decide if the benefits are worth any extra cost.

● If available, and if you qualify, take advantage of senior citizen discount days.

● Stock up on canned and other nonperishable foods when they're on sale. At home, rotate your food supply so that the "first in" is the "first out."

● Buy perishable foods in amounts that will be consumed during their peak quality. An extra bunch of broccoli that spoils in the refrigerator is no savings.

● Consider foods sold in bulk bins. Without the expense of packaging or branding, bulk foods often cost less, and they're usually the same foods you find on supermarket shelves. Perhaps the best advantage: you can buy just the amount you need. Foods such as dry fruits, rice, pasta, other grains, snack mixes, and spices are among those sold in bulk.

● Consider the cost for convenience. Prepared, pre-sliced, and precooked foods usually cost more. Depending on your schedule, labor-saving and step-saving ingredients may be worth the price.

● Remain flexible as you shop. If you see a better bargain or a new food (perhaps a vegetable or a fruit), adjust your menu.

● Shop during off-hours. If time is at a premium, shop when stores aren't crowded—often early in the morning, late in the evening, or midweek rather than on weekends. It may be a less stressful time to shop, too.

● Pay attention at checkout. See that prices ring up as advertised or as indicated on the shelf label, especially for sale items.

"Small-Scale" Shopping

How do small households maximize their food dollars? Besides general cost-saving tips, you might save in other ways if you're a household of one or two:

● Buy frozen vegetables and fruit in bags, not boxes. As long as they aren't thawed, you can pour out as much as you need, then reseal and return the package to the freezer.

● Look for foods sold in single servings: juice, yogurt, frozen meals, soup, and pudding, among others. In that way you can have a greater variety of food on hand. "Singles" may help with portion control, too. Because small households are a big consumer market segment, more and more products now are available in single-size servings.

● To save with economy-size packages, share your food purchases with a friend.

● Shop from bulk bins for small amounts.

● At home repackage meat, poultry, and fish into single portions in freezer wrap or plastic freezer bags. Freeze these portions to use later.

● Ask the butcher or the produce manager for a smaller amount of prepackaged fresh meat, poultry, or produce. Usually they can repackage food.

● Buy produce that keeps longer in the refrigerator: broccoli, Brussels sprouts, cabbage, carrots, parsnips, potatoes, sweet potatoes, apples, grapefruit, melons, oranges, pears, and tangerines.

● Shop for convenience. Often mixed salad greens (perhaps from the salad bar) or raw vegetables, already cut and mixed for stir-fry dishes or salads, cost less than individual foods in quantity.

● Buy small loaves of bread, or wrap and freeze what you won't use right away.

Your Shopping Guide

Filling your shopping cart? Choose plenty of nutrient-rich foods from the five food groups and then add a few extras with your discretion in mind. Overall, the foods you buy should allow you to make meals and snacks with variety, moderation, and balance.

Now let's tour the supermarket, department by department, focusing on shopping tips for high-

Shopping for Freshness!

For Fruit . . .

Apples: firm with smooth, clean skin and good color. Avoid fruit with bruises or decay spots.

Apricots: plump with as much golden-orange color as possible. Blemishes, unless they break the skin, will not affect flavor. Avoid fruit that is pale yellow, greenish-yellow, very firm, shriveled, or bruised.

Bananas: plump with uniform shape at desired ripeness level. Avoid produce with blemished or bruised skins.

Blueberries: plump, firm berries with a light-grayish bloom. The bloom is the thin coating on the surface.

Cantaloupes: slightly oval fruit, 5 inches or more in diameter, with yellow or golden (not green) background color. Signs of sweetness include pronounced netting on the rind and a few tiny cracks near the stem end. Smell the melon; it should be noticeably strong and sweet. At home, check for ripeness before you eat it; the stem area will be slightly soft when ripe.

Cherries: plump, bright-colored sweet or sour cherries. Sweet cherries with reddish-brown skin promise flavor. Avoid overly soft or shriveled cherries or those with dark stems.

Grapefruits: firm, thin-skinned fruit, full-colored, and heavy for their size. The best grapefruits are smooth, thin-skinned, and flat at both ends. Avoid fruit with a pointed end or thick, deeply pored skin.

Grapes: plump grapes firmly attached to pliable green stems. Color is the best indication of ripeness and flavor. Avoid soft or wrinkled fruits and those with bleached-looking areas at the stem end.

Honeydew melons: melons weighing at least 5 pounds, with waxy white rind barely tinged with green. Fully ripe fruit has a cream-colored rind; the blossom end should give to gentle pressure.

Kiwifruit: softness similar to a ripe peach. Choose evenly firm fruit.

Lemons: firm, heavy fruit. Generally, rough-textured lemons have thicker skins and less juice than fine-skinned varieties.

Mangoes: usually quite firm when sold and need to be ripened further at home before eating. Avoid those with shriveled or bruised skin. Once ripened, they will give to gentle pressure.

Nectarines: orange-yellow (not green) background color between areas of red. Ripe nectarines feel slightly soft with gentle handling, but not as soft as ripe peaches.

Oranges: thin-skinned, firm, bright-colored fruit. Avoid oranges with any hint of softness or whitish mold at the ends.

Papayas: fruit with the softness of peaches and more yellow than green in the skin. Most papayas need to be ripened further after purchase in a loosely closed paper bag at room temperature. Avoid bruised or shriveled fruit showing any signs of mold or deterioration.

Peaches: creamy or yellow background color. Ripe peaches feel slightly soft with gentle handling. Avoid green, extra-hard, or bruised fruit.

Pears: fruit with firm skin. Pears gradually ripen after picking.

Pineapples: large, plump, fresh-looking fruit with green leaves and a sweet smell. Avoid fruit with soft spots, areas of decay, or fermented odor.

Plums: fruit that is full-colored. Ripe plums are slightly soft at the tip end and feel somewhat soft when handled gently. Avoid fruit with broken or shriveled skin.

Raspberries or blackberries: firm, plump, well-shaped berries. If soft or discolored, they are overripe. Avoid baskets that look stained from overripe berries.

Strawberries: firm, plump berries that are full-colored.

Watermelons: fruit heavy for its size, well shaped, with rind and flesh colors characteristic of the variety. Ripe melons are fragrant and slightly soft at the blossom end. A melon that sloshes when shaken is probably overripe. The stem should be dry and brown, not green. When thumped, you should hear a low-pitched sound, indicating a full, juicy interior.

For Vegetables . . .

Artichokes: tight, compact heads that feel heavy for their size. Surface brown spots don't affect quality.

Asparagus: firm, brittle spears that are bright green almost their entire length, with tightly closed tips.

Beans (green or waxed): slender, crisp beans that are bright and blemish-free. Avoid mature beans with large seeds and swollen pods.

Beets: firm, smooth-skinned, small to medium beets. Leaves should be deep green and fresh-looking.

Bok choy: heads with bright white stalks and glossy

dark leaves. Avoid heads with slippery brown spots on the leaves.

Broccoli: compact clusters of tightly closed, dark green florets. Avoid heads with yellow florets or thick, woody stems.

Brussels sprouts: firm, compact, fresh-looking sprouts that are bright green. They should be heavy for their size.

Cabbage: firm heads that feel heavy for their size. Outer leaves should have good color and be free of blemishes.

Carrots: firm, clean, well-shaped carrots with bright, orange-gold color. Carrots with their tops still attached are likely to be freshest.

Cauliflower: firm, compact, creamy-white heads (without brown spots), with florets pressed tightly together. A yellow tinge and spreading florets indicate overmaturity. Leaves should be crisp and bright green.

Celery: crisp, rigid, green stalks with fresh-looking leaves. Avoid celery with limp stalks.

Corn: fresh-looking ears with green husks, moist stems, and silk ends free of decay or worm injury. When pierced with a thumbnail, kernels should give a squirt of juice. Tough skins indicate overmaturity.

Cucumbers: firm, dark green cucumbers that are slender but well shaped. Soft or yellow cukes are overmature.

Eggplants: firm, heavy for their size, with taut, glassy, deeply colored skin. Stems should be bright green.

Greens: fresh, tender leaves that are free of blemishes. Avoid bunches with thick, coarse-veined leaves.

Jicama: firm, well-formed tubers free of blemishes. Size does not affect flavor, but larger roots do tend to have a coarse texture.

Kohlrabi: young, tender bulbs with fresh green leaves. Avoid those with scars and blemishes. The smaller the bulb, the more delicate the flavor and texture.

Leeks: clean, white bottoms and crisp, fresh-looking green tops.

Mushrooms: blemish-free mushrooms without slimy spots or signs of decay.

Okra: small to medium pods that are deep green and free of blemishes. Pods should snap or puncture easily with slight pressure.

Onions: green onions with crisp, bright green tops and clean white bottoms. Choose firm, dry onions with brittle outer skin, avoiding those with sprouting green shoots or dark spots.

Parsnips: small to medium, smooth, firm, and well shaped. Avoid large roots because they may have a woody core.

Peas: small, plump, bright green pods that are firm, crisp, and well filled.

Peppers: bright, glossy, firm, and well shaped. Avoid those with soft spots or gashes.

Potatoes: firm, smooth, with no wrinkles, sprouts, cracks, bruises, decay, or bitter green areas (caused by exposure to light).

Rutabagas: small to medium, smooth, firm, and heavy for their size.

Salad greens: crisp, deeply colored leaves free of brown spots, yellowed leaves, and decay.

Sprouts: crisp buds still attached.

Summer squash: yellow squash and zucchini of medium size with firm, smooth, glossy, tender skin. Squash should be heavy for their size.

Sweet potatoes and yams: firm, well shaped, with bright, uniformly colored skin.

Tomatoes: smooth, well formed, firm, not hard.

Turnips: firm, smooth, small to medium size, that are heavy for their size.

Winter squash: hard, thick-shelled.

Source: Adapted from M. J. Smith, *The Miracle Foods Cookbook* (Minneapolis: Chronimed Publishing, 1995). This material is used by permission of John Wiley & Sons, Inc.

Produce Department

Today's supermarkets offer a great variety of fresh fruits and vegetables—about three hundred different types of produce in the average store. *See chapter 9 for new fruits and vegetables you might try.* Because fruit and vegetables are most nutritious and best-tasting at their peak quality, shop with savvy.

quality, nutritious, and safe foods—that match your needs.

● Check the produce department. Besides being clean, organized, and appealing, fresh fruits and vegetables should be held at a proper temperature. Most are chilled; a fine mist helps keep greens crisp; being soggy promotes growth of mold or rot.

● For fresh fruits, consider ripeness. Some fruits—for example, avocados, bananas, pears, peaches, pineapples—can ripen after picking. If you're buying fruits to eat today, buy ripe. If you don't plan to eat them until later in the week, buy fruits that aren't yet ripe. *Tip:* To hasten the ripening of some fruits such as pears and peaches, put them in a loosely closed paper bag at room temperature.

● Buy the amount you need. Even when properly stored, produce is perishable. Produce at peak quality contains the most nutrients.

● Look for nutrition information. If packaged, the label on produce may carry Nutrition Facts. If not, check for a poster or a pamphlet with this information nearby. Ask the store manager to provide this information if it's not available. *For fruits and vegetables that are good sources of beta carotene (which forms vitamin A), vitamin C, potassium, folate, and fiber, see "Produce 'Package'" in the Appendices.*

● Go for a colorful variety of fruits and vegetables. Rather than just the old standbys, add a new fruit or vegetable to your shopping cart each week or two; try some that are locally grown. The store may have preparation and handling tips for unfamiliar produce.

Explore different varieties of a familiar food. For example, try different apples: perhaps Cortland, Granny Smith, Newtown Pippin, and Rome Beauty. Or choose one of each variety of plums: perhaps Laroda, Queen Ann, Santa Rosa, and Wickson.

● Look for signs of quality. Bruised or wilted produce suggests that it hasn't been handled properly or that it's past its peak. Some nutrients may be lost as a result. *Refer to the chart "Shopping for Freshness!" earlier in this chapter for signs of quality in commonly eaten fruits and vegetables.*

● For flavor, buy small. Small fruit is often sweeter than larger pieces of the same fruit.

● Handle fresh fruits and vegetables gently. Damage and bruising hasten spoilage. Place produce in the shopping cart where it won't get bruised. At the checkout, make sure produce is packed on top or in separate bags.

● Pick up prewashed bags of salad greens, sliced stir-fry veggies, precut fruit, and packaged baby carrots and celery sticks for quick vegetables and fruit. Choose packaged fruit, such as melon and pineapple, without added sugars.

● Consider choosing your own produce rather than buying it prepackaged. In that way you can examine and pick out items at their peak of quality.

● Look for other items in the produce department, such as fresh herbs, herbs in jars, and sun-dried tomatoes. Fresh herbs are often prepackaged; choose those that look fresh, not wilted. Dried fruits are a non-perishable option, often sold in the produce department; they supply the same nutrients as fresh fruit. If you're sensitive to sulfites, check the label; sulfites prevent browning in many dried fruits.

Meat and Deli Case

Through advanced breeding and feeding practices, today's animals are leaner than ever. Leaner cuts are available also because of closer trimming of beef, veal, pork, and lamb cuts. The average thickness of fat around the edge of steaks and roasts has trimmed down from $\frac{1}{2}$ inch to $\frac{3}{4}$ inch twenty-five or more years ago to less than $\frac{1}{8}$ inch trim today. *See "Today's Meat" in chapter 9.* Choose mostly lean meat; higher-fat meats contribute more discretionary calories.

For the "lean advantage"—and the other nutrients that meat supplies (especially protein, B vitamins, iron, and zinc)—consider these shopping tips:

● *Shop for meat's lean cuts.* Certain cuts of meat are leaner than others. Use this rule of thumb in selecting lower-fat cuts of fresh meats: Look for the words "round" or "loin" in the name when shopping for beef, and the words "loin" or "leg" when buying pork or lamb. Here are some examples of lean cuts.

● *Beef:* eye of round, top round steak, top round roast, sirloin steak, top loin steak, tenderloin steak, flank steak, and chuck arm pot roast. *See page 320 for beef's lean cuts.*

● *Veal:* cutlet, blade or arm steak, rib roast, and rib or loin chop

● *Pork:* tenderloin, top loin roast, top loin chop, center loin chop, sirloin roast, loin rib chop, and shoulder blade steak

● *Lamb:* leg, loin chop, arm chop, and foreshanks

If you're not sure of the cut, check the meat label. It identifies the kind and cut, along with the net weight, unit price, and cost per package.

● Choose leaner grades of meat. "Select" grades of beef have the least marbled fat (or thin streaks of fat between the muscle) followed by "choice" cuts, then "prime" beef cuts. Veal and lamb use the same grading system; however, the term "good" is used instead of "select." Grading, which is determined by the U.S. Department of Agriculture, is based on fat content, appearance, texture, and the age of the animal. Pork is not graded.

The more costly "prime" grade of beef—more often on restaurant menus than sold in supermarkets—has more marbled fat, which helps make the meat juicy and flavorful. However, with proper methods of cooking and carving, the leaner "select" and "choice" meats can be tender, juicy, and flavorful, too.

Nutritionally speaking, nutrients in meat—protein, thiamin, niacin, iron, and zinc, among others—are the same, regardless of grade.

● Buy well-trimmed meat: ⅛-inch fat trim or less. "Trim" refers to the fat layer surrounding a steak or other cut of meat. *Note:* Marbled fat cannot be trimmed away. Only cooking methods can remove some, but not all, marbled fat.

● Check the "numbers" for ground meat—look for packages that have the greatest percent lean to percent fat ratio. Ground beef labeled as 95 percent lean also may include the nutrition description "Lean" because it meets the definition of a lean product. *Note:* "Percent lean" refers to the weight of the lean meat in relation to the weight of the fat.

● Buy enough meat without overdoing on portion size. For moderate-size portions (3 ounces cooked), figure 4 ounces of uncooked, boneless meat per person. *Refer to the chart "Meat Buying Guide" in this chapter to help you decide how much meat to buy.*

● Use nutrition labeling to find lean packaged meats. By regulation, packaged deli meats must carry nutrition labeling. That helps you find today's leaner hot dogs, luncheon meats, and sausage patties.

Also check out the lean options from the deli case. When buying ready-to-slice luncheon meats from a deli, ask for nutrition information if you're unsure of a product's leanness. Some lean products will be identified with a nutrient content claim such as "low-fat," "____% fat-free," or "lean."

● Look for nutrition information for fresh meat, poultry, and seafood. Single-ingredient raw meat, poultry, and seafood soon may be labeled voluntarily with nutrition information.

● When shopping for bacon, try Canadian bacon or turkey bacon. Canadian bacon is lean, much like ham. In contrast, traditional bacon is mainly fat, including saturated fat. Consider bacon, especially, among your discretionary calories. If you're watching your sodium intake, check the label.

● If you eat organ meats, also called variety meats, make them occasional choices. Brain, chitterlings (pig

Shopping at a Farmers' Market?

Make it a fun experience! With about 4,000 farmers' markets in operation in the United States and more every year, farmers' markets give you a chance to talk to growers and perhaps find local products you can't find elsewhere, local varietals of vegetables and fruits, artisan cheeses, fresh or potted herbs, cut flowers, homemade sauces, oven-fresh baked goods, organically certified foods, locally produced poultry, eggs, or meat, or fresh fish.

First, be aware that the produce sold may—or may not—be fresh from the field. Some markets feature only local growers. Others sell brokered products from the same commercial markets that supermarkets buy from. And some sell both. Ask the market manager or vendor.

For food safety and great shopping, bring a clean carry bag or two: separate ones for raw and cooked foods, or for meat, poultry, or fish. As you shop, pay attention to food safety practices of the vendor: cleanliness, gloves or clean utensils for food handling, covered garbage cans, clean bags. Go early for the best selection; check the market Web site ahead if there's one. Shop with flexibility; the market changes with the season and the local growers and vendors who come to market. Take time to talk to and learn from them. Pack your purchases so they don't crush; take perishables home right away.

intestines), heart, kidney, liver, sweetbreads (thymus gland), tongue, and tripe (stomach lining of cattle) are all organ meats. Organ meats are good sources of many nutrients; liver, in particular, is high in iron. However, most are higher in cholesterol than lean meat. And some, such as chitterlings, sweetbreads, and tongue, have more fat.

● For convenience, look for meat that's already seasoned, prepared, and ready to cook, such as meat and vegetable kebobs or marinated pork loin. You may also find precooked, packaged heat-and-eat meats in the refrigerated case. These meats may be higher in sodium.

● Recognize the qualities of fresh meat. The color of meat indicates its freshness. Beef is typically a bright red color. Both young veal and pork are grayish-pink. Older veal is a darker pink. And lamb can be light to darker pink, depending on how it was fed.

● Check food product dating on meat. Only buy fresh and processed meats that still will be fresh when you're ready to eat them. Or plan to freeze immediately for later use.

● Notice the safe food handling label. *A sample label is shown in this chapter. For more about the safe handling of meat, see chapter 12, "The Safe Kitchen."*

Meat Buying Guide

How much raw meat should you buy? If you figure about 3 ounces of cooked, lean meat per person, that's about 4 ounces of raw meat per person. For some meats you'll need to take the amount of bone and fat into account.

TYPE OF MEAT	SERVINGS PER POUND*
Boneless or ground meat	4
Meat with a minimum amount of bone (steaks, roasts, chops, etc.)	2 to 3
Meat with a large amount of bone (shoulder cuts, short ribs, neck, etc.)	1 to 2

*Three ounces of cooked trimmed meat equal one serving.

Source: Adapted from Nutrition, Health, and Food Management Division, American Association of Family and Consumer Sciences, *Food: A Handbook of Terminology, Purchasing, and Preparation* (Alexandria, Va.: American Association of Family and Consumer Sciences, 2001), pp. 139-143. Copyright 2001 by the American Association of Family and Consumer Sciences. Reprinted with permission.

Poultry Counter

Besides being economical, chicken and turkey offer high-quality protein, and they're usually very lean. As you choose poultry for your shopping cart:

● Choose mostly lean varieties of poultry—turkey and chicken. Domesticated duck and goose are higher in fat. A 3½-ounce cooked portion of roasted, skinless chicken (light and dark meat) has about 7 fat grams compared with 11 fat grams in the same portion of roasted, skinless duck. Pheasant and quail, especially without the skin, are lean, too.

● To trim fat, shop for skinless poultry—chicken and turkey. You'll cut the grams of total fat and saturated fat in half. Or buy poultry with the skin on if it costs less. Remove the skin before or after cooking it.

For less fat, choose light meat such as the turkey or chicken breast. Compare the difference: 3½ ounces of roasted, skinless, dark-meat chicken have about 10 fat grams and 3 grams of saturated fat; the same amount of roasted, skinless, light-meat chicken has about 3 fat grams and 1 gram of saturated fat. The cholesterol content is about the same.

Reading Meat Labels

1. The kind of meat—Listed on every label
2. The primal (wholesale) cut—Tells where the meat came from on the animal
3. The retail cut—Tells from what part of the primal cut the meat comes

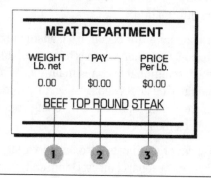

MEAT DEPARTMENT

WEIGHT Lb. net	PAY	PRICE Per Lb.
0.00	$0.00	$0.00

BEEF TOP ROUND STEAK

① ② ③

● When you buy whole turkey, know that self-basting varieties are higher in fat and sodium. Self-basting turkeys are moist because they're injected with fat—which may be high in saturated fatty acids. Instead, you can baste turkey regularly with broth, juice, or juices from the poultry. *Hint:* Roasting any whole bird with the breast side up makes it more moist.

● Is ground meat on your shopping list? Look for lean ground turkey breast, too. Ground turkey breast can be as lean as 99 percent fat-free. The fat content is higher if it's ground with dark meat and skin.

● Recognize the qualities of fresh poultry. Look for meaty birds with skin that's creamy-white to yellow and that are free of bruises, tiny feathers, and torn or dry skin. Check for product dating on food labels.

● Read the Nutrition Facts before you buy turkey dogs, turkey ham, or turkey bologna. They may—or may not—be low in fat. Compare the sodium content with that of traditional processed meats; processing typically adds sodium. For fresh cuts of poultry, look for Nutri-Facts, which may be posted in the retail case.

Poultry Buying Guide

How much poultry? Here's how many servings come from 1 pound of uncooked chicken, duck, goose, game hens, or turkey.

POULTRY	SERVINGS PER POUND*
Whole chicken (broiler-fryer or roaster)	2
Boneless chicken breast	4
Duck, whole	1
Goose, whole	1½ to 2
Rock Cornish game hen, whole	1
Whole turkey, bone in	2
Boneless turkey roast	3
Ground turkey	4

*Amounts are based on 3 ounces of cooked poultry without bone per serving.

Source: Adapted from Nutrition, Health, and Food Management Division, American Association of Family and Consumer Sciences, *Food: A Handbook of Terminology, Purchasing, and Preparation* (Alexandria, Va.: American Association of Family and Consumer Sciences, 2001), pp. 139-143. Copyright 2001 by the American Association of Family and Consumer Sciences. Reprinted with permission.

Have You Ever Wondered

. . . if free-range chickens have less fat? It's a common misperception that free-range chickens—those that "roam the barnyard and forage for food"—are always leaner than chickens raised in coops. Whether they're raised in a coop or a barnyard, their exercise level often is about the same. Genetic stock, age, and growth rate have greater influence on fat levels. Older, larger chickens and those that grow faster tend to have more fat. That's true of all chickens, no matter how they're raised.

According to the USDA's Food Safety and Inspection Service, which regulates poultry labeling, the terms "free-range" and "free-roaming" may be used on poultry labels if the producers can demonstrate that the poultry has been allowed access to the outside for a significant portion of their life. Some people are willing to spend more for free-range chickens because they perceive a taste difference; blind taste tests don't show differences in flavor perception.

. . . if the tiny red spots on finfish are safe to eat? These spots are bruise marks, not contamination. They occur when fish is not handled gently, either when it's caught or in the supermarket. It's safe to eat. But be aware that bruised areas often deteriorate faster.

. . . how the fat and cholesterol in surimi compare with crabmeat? Surimi is imitation crabmeat, made from pollock or another mild-flavored fish. The fish is processed by rolling "sheets" of fish and adding color so it looks like crab legs. The nutrient content reflects the fish it's made from. Surimi is comparable in fat content but lower in cholesterol than crabmeat.

● For cost savings, buy a whole bird. You'll usually save money if you carve a chicken yourself.

● Buy enough poultry for moderate portions. *The chart "Poultry Buying Guide" on this page shows how much to buy for 3-ounce cooked portions.*

● For safety, it's best not to buy fresh prestuffed poultry.

Fish Counter

There's increased attention to seafood these days, often for its nutritional benefits. Besides being a good protein source, most seafood is low in fat, especially saturated fat. Fatty fish offers potential health benefits from omega-3 fatty acids; that's partly why health experts recommend eating seafood several times a week. *See "Eat Your Omega-3s and -6s" in chapter 3.*

Fifty to 100 varieties of fish commonly on the market today can offer great taste and versatility in menu planning. Learn to shop for seafood confidently; choose high-quality, safe seafood that also matches your personal needs and preferences.

A few definitions before you start shopping: seafood includes both finfish and shellfish. Catfish, cod, flounder, haddock, mahimahi, salmon, snapper, tilapia, tuna, and trout are among the many types of finfish. Shellfish are both crustaceans (crab, crayfish, lobster, and shrimp) and mollusks (clam, mussel, oyster, scallop, octopus, squid, abalone, conch, and snail).

● Check the fish counter before you buy. Always buy fresh or frozen seafood from a reputable source. Fresh seafood should be displayed with food safety in mind: properly iced, well refrigerated, and in clean display cases. To reduce the chance of spoilage, fish should be displayed "belly down" to drain away melting ice. Be sure that the seafood is wrapped separately, in a leakproof package.

Check for general cleanliness and quality: clean look and smell; free of insects; employees wearing disposable gloves (changed after handling nonfood and again after handling raw fish); and knowledgeable workers who can answer your questions about the freshness of the seafood. Ask when and how often fresh and flash-frozen fish come in. Be flexible; buy the freshest fish if you don't need a specific type.

● Recognize the different fat contents of various fish. In general, most fish has less fat than many other protein-rich foods, including meat and poultry with skin. And most fat in seafood is polyunsaturated.

Fish that is firm and darker in color, such as king mackerel, salmon, and tuna, tends to have more fat and omega-3 fatty acids; omega-3s may offer heart-healthy benefits. Try to eat fatty fish twice a week.

● Choose fish that's best for the recipe. Lean fish is great for baking, microwaving, and poaching. Fish with more fat tends to be better for grilling and roasting because it doesn't dry out as quickly and because it holds its shape better. For example, salmon and tuna

are better for kebobs. Mild-flavored fish, such as cod, flounder, haddock, sole, snapper, and tilapia, tends to be the lowest in fat, while fish with more fat usually has a fuller flavor.

● Learn to recognize the qualities of fresh seafood.

● *Finfish.* At peak quality, whole finfish have a fresh ocean-breeze scent, not a fishy or ammonia-like smell. They're naturally firm to the touch, with stiff fins and scales that cling tightly to the skin. The skin is shiny and "metallic," not dull. The gills are pink or bright red and free from mucus or slime. If undamaged, their eyes are clear, bright, and protruding. Walleyes are among the few fish with naturally cloudy eyes. Fish fillets or steaks also have a mild scent, firm and moist flesh, a translucent appearance, and no browning around the edges. If wrapped, packaging should be tight and undamaged.

● *Shellfish.* Crustaceans and some mollusks are sold live. In fact, unless frozen, canned, or cooked,

Seafood Buying Guide

Type of Seafood	Approximate Amount of Raw Seafood Needed per Adult Serving*
Whole fish	¾ pound
Dressed or pan-dressed fish	½ pound
Fish fillets	¼ to ⅓ pound
Fish steaks with bone	½ pound
Fish steaks without bone	⅓ pound
Live clams and oysters	6 to 8
Shucked clams and oysters	⅓ to ½ pint
Live lobsters and crabs	1 to 1½ pounds
Cooked lobster or crabmeat	¼ to ⅓ pound
Scallops	¼ to ⅓ pound
Shrimp, headless and unpeeled	⅓ to ½ pound
Shrimp, peeled and deveined	¼ to ⅓ pound

*The smaller amounts in the ranges shown provide a cooked portion that is approximately 3 ounces when prepared by most common cooking methods.

Source: New York Seafood Council, 2004.

crabs, crayfish, and lobsters should be alive when sold. They'll move slightly if they're alive, and live lobsters curl their tails a bit when handled. For food safety, buy shellfish from a reputable source.

If their shells are still on, clams, mussels, and oysters must be sold alive, too, for food safety sake; shells shouldn't be damaged. When these mollusks are alive, their shells are slightly open, but they close tightly when tapped. As another test, hold the shell between your thumb and forefinger; press so that one part of the shell slides across the other. If the shells move, it isn't fresh.

Freshly shucked mollusks (shells removed) have a mild, fresh scent. A somewhat clear liquid, not too milky or cloudy, should cover shucked "meat."

Scallops are removed from their shells at sea. They vary in size and color, from creamy white to light orange, tan, or somewhat pinkish. When fresh, they're not dry or darkened around the edges.

Fresh, raw shrimp will have a mild odor. For all fish—finfish and shellfish—use your nose. A strong "fishy" odor is a sign that fish is no longer fresh. *Note:* "Previously frozen" (thawed for sale) fish—harvested and frozen in remote locations—may be superior in quality to fresh fish, transported for several days.

● Know the qualities of frozen fish. Frozen seafood should be solidly frozen, mild in odor, and free of ice crystals and freezer burn. Freezer burn is indicated by drying and discoloration. The package shouldn't be damaged or water-stained, and it should be stored below the frost line in the store's display freezer. These qualities apply to frozen fish and frozen prepared items such as crab cakes and breaded shrimp.

● Know what form you need: finfish—fillets, steaks, whole fish, or dressed (head, tail, and fins removed), or shellfish—whole live or just "meat."

● Check the food product dating on the label of frozen fish. Choose packaged seafood that doesn't show signs of thawing, then refreezing. Check the "sell by" date, if it has one. *Read about product dating earlier in this chapter.*

● Choose cooked shrimp, lobsters, crabs, and crayfish that are moist with a mild odor and a characteristic color. The shells of cooked shrimp should be pink

to reddish. For other crustaceans, the shells should be bright red. Some stores cook them for you

● For safety, don't buy cooked seafood that's displayed alongside raw seafood. Bacteria from raw fish can contaminate cooked fish, creating a potential for foodborne illness. *For more about cross-contamination, see "Checklist for a Clean Kitchen" in chapter 12.*

● Choose smoked fish, such as smoked salmon or smoked trout, that is bright, glossy, and free of mold. Since it may not be cooked before serving, smoked fish should be wrapped and kept away from raw fish to avoid cross-contamination.

● Substitute one fish for another. When the store doesn't have the seafood you want or if it costs more than you anticipate, make a switch. Sometimes lesser-known species cost less. For example, when a recipe calls for flounder, almost any mild finfish (perhaps haddock, halibut, or perch) can take its place.

Be aware of differences in nutritional content when you make substitutions. Squid, shrimp, and lobsters, for example, have more cholesterol than clams, crabs, mussels, and scallops do. Three ounces of boiled shrimp supply about 165 milligrams of cholesterol; the same amount of scallops has about 55 milligrams.

● Whether it's sold from the seafood counter or the freezer, go easy on breaded items such as shrimp and fish sticks, often containing more calories and fat.

● For nutrition information check the Nutrition Facts on packaged seafood products. For fresh seafood you'll find this information displayed nearby.

● Buy the amount of seafood you need. Because of waste, you need more when preparing whole or dressed fish. A dressed fish has the head, tail, and fins removed. Usually fish steaks, fillets, and shellfish, which have less waste, cost more per pound. Since you don't pay for waste, the price may equal out. *The chart "Seafood Buying Guide" on page 262 helps you estimate how much for a cooked 3-ounce portion.*

Refrigerated Case

Although you'll find tortillas, refrigerator rolls, and yeast among the many products in the refrigerated case, dairy foods and eggs are prominent. For both food categories, you have many choices.

Dairy Foods

Milk

● Choose milk that matches your needs. No matter what type, milk is an excellent source of calcium. Milk also provides protein, riboflavin, vitamins A and D, phosphorus, potassium, magnesium, and other vitamins and minerals. How do the various forms of milk differ? Fat content is the main difference. *"Milk: A Great Calcium Source" in chapter 10 makes nutrition comparisons. See "Which Milk for You?" in this chapter for types of milk.*

● If you're sensitive to lactose, or milk sugar, look for lactose-reduced or lactose-free milk. By adding the enzyme lactase, dairy foods have much less lactose. *See chapter 21 for more on lactose intolerance.*

Yogurt

Like milk, yogurt comes in whole, low-fat, and nonfat varieties. The calorie and fat content reflect the milk it's made from. Yogurt also may be flavored with fruit, fruit preserves, or extracts such as vanilla or coffee. If you're watching calories, reach for plain low-fat yogurt or yogurt flavored with a low-calorie sweetener, such as aspartame.

Yogurt is made with "friendly" bacteria, which give a distinctive taste and consistency. As an added benefit, active, live cultures may offer health benefits, perhaps in boosting immunity or in helping the body digest milk's sugar. However, the research on the health benefits of active, live cultures in yogurt isn't conclusive. *See chapter 4 for more on probiotics.*

Yogurt with labels that state "made with active cultures" may not contain live cultures if it's been heat-treated. Frozen yogurt may contain live active cultures; if they're present, freezing slows their action.

● If you want the potential benefit of active live cultures, look for the *"Live and Active Cultures"* seal, administered by the National Yogurt Association, on regular and frozen yogurt containers. The ingredient list shows the probiotic, or live, cultures; those most commonly used are *Lactobacillus acidophilus, L. casei, L. reuteri,* and *Bifidobacterium bifidum (Bifidus).*

● Look for different types of yogurt—fruit-flavored or plain, and whole, low-fat, or nonfat. Yogurt is another high-calcium, high-protein dairy food. In fact, 8 ounces of either yogurt or milk supply about 300 milligrams of calcium. If you don't drink much milk, you might buy more yogurt to get the calcium you need. Some yogurt is vitamin D fortified.

● Enjoy flavored yogurt-juice beverages or drinkable yogurt—another source of calcium. Or look for the yogurt drink called kefir. Ingesting thick and frothy kefir is somewhat like drinking yogurt. It's a cultured dairy beverage usually made from cow or goat milk and the active, "friendly" kefir bacteria.

Cheese

● Check out the wide variety of cheese sold today. Cheese is milk in concentrated form; about 10 pounds (5 quarts) of milk are used to make every pound of Cheddar cheese. That's why cheese is a great source of milk's nutrients: protein, calcium, phosphorus, zinc, vitamin A, riboflavin, and vitamin B_{12}.

● To moderate fat and perhaps calories, cut back on saturated fat, and still get plenty of nutrients, you might look for lower-fat cheeses such as low-fat ricotta, part-skim mozzarella, string cheese, or varieties of reduced-fat cheese. Many cheeses have considerably more fat per serving than a serving of milk does. As a rule of thumb, any cheese made with fat-free milk will likely have less fat and fewer calories.
  ● *Low-fat cheese* has 3 grams or less fat per serving; that's 1 ounce for most cheese and 4 ounces for cottage cheese.
  ● *Reduced-fat cheese* has 25 percent less fat than the same full-fat cheese.
  ● *Fat-free cheese* has less than 0.5 gram of fat per serving.
Cheese with less fat usually has less cholesterol, too, but check the label to be sure.

● Consider buying shredded cheese and sharp-flavored cheese. For cheese shreds you may pay a little more per ounce for the convenience of "pre-prep." When it's grated, you may use a little less cheese than if you had used sliced or chunk cheese. That's another way to savor the flavor yet control fat. *Tip:* Using stronger-flavored cheese such as Parmesan, feta, or sharp Cheddar delivers more flavor with less cheese.

● Look for reduced-sodium cheeses if you're watching your sodium intake. Traditional cheese has sodium because it's a key ingredient in cheesemaking.

● Look for cheese fortified with vitamin D, too!

Cream, Sour Cream, Spreads

● Buy them—go easy on how much you use. They're high in calories and fat and deliver little calcium.

● For less fat and fewer calories, try lower-fat and nonfat varieties. Try half-and-half rather than cream; another option is fat-free half-and-half (mostly made of fat-free milk). Choose sour half-and-half or fat-free sour cream. Read the labels; the fat content varies.

● Look for spreads—butter, margarine, and cream cheese—in the dairy case. From a fat and calorie standpoint, butter and margarine are the same, with about 35 calories and 4 grams of total fat per teaspoon. Both are primarily fat, but the source and type of fat differ. Butter contains more saturated fats than most margarines. Made from vegetable oil, margarine has no cholesterol, but may be high in *trans* fats.

● For a spread, buy soft tub margarine rather than stick margarine for less *trans* and saturated fats. Whipped versions of butter or margarine have less fat per tablespoon, too; air adds to the volume. However, they can't be substituted for regular butter or

Cream: How Much Fat? How Many Calories?

Cream	% Milk Fat Content	Total Fat Grams	Saturated Fat Grams	Calories
			Per Tablespoon	
Half-and-half	10.5 to 18	2	1	20
Light or coffee cream	18 to 29	3	2	30
Light whipping cream	30 to 36	5	3	44
Heavy cream	36 or more	6	3	52
Cream in aerosol cans		1	.5	8

Have You Ever Wondered?

. . . how cow milk and soy beverage compare? The nutrient content of soy beverage isn't the same as in cow milk. Unless fortified, soy beverage, made by pressing ground, cooked soybeans, is significantly lower in calcium. As a substitute for cow milk, choose soy beverage that's calcium-fortified. Soy drinks range from 80 to 500 milligrams of calcium per cup; read the Nutrition Facts.

The calcium absorbed from fortified foods varies. For example, the calcium from 1 cup of milk and 1 cup of soy beverage fortified with calcium carbonate is about the same. However, to get the same amount from soy beverage with tricalcium phosphate, you'd need to drink 1⅓ cups; this form of calcium isn't as bioavailable, or absorbed as well in the body.

Compared with cow milk, soy beverage is lower in protein and riboflavin, and has little vitamin A or D naturally; some soy beverage is fortified with vitamins A and D and riboflavin. As a phytonutrient, isoflavones in soy may offer unique benefits as phytoestrogens; *see "A Quick Look at Key Phytonutrients" in chapter 4.* Soy protein may have cardiovascular benefits. Soy beverage is cholesterol-free. The fat content of soy beverage is similar to 2 percent cow milk; also look for low-fat versions of soy beverage.

. . . why cottage cheese has less calcium than other cheese? During processing, the whey is drained away, along with 50 to 75 percent of the calcium. Check food labels for cottage cheese processed with extra calcium. Good news: it still provides plenty of protein and riboflavin, without much fat.

margarine in recipes that require baking or frying. Reduced-fat butter and margarine aren't suitable for some recipes because they have more moisture. Use them as spreads. Other less-saturated-fat options: squeezable, liquid margarine and spray margarine. Check labels for spreads with 0 grams *trans* fats.

● Enjoy small amounts of cream cheese, but don't confuse its nutrient content with other forms of cheese. Cream cheese is mainly milk fat, with very little milk solids. If you want the creamy texture with less fat, look for reduced-fat or fat-free cream cheese. Or buy regular cream cheese, then spread a little less

Which Milk for You?

From a nutritional standpoint, the differences among whole, 2 percent reduced-fat, 1 percent low-fat, and fat-free milk are the fat and the calorie contents. Because milk solids make up at least 8.25 percent of each of these types of milks, their nutrient content is about the same. (Milk solids are the part of milk that's neither milk fat nor water.) Keep in mind that the percentages of milk fat used to distinguish different types of milk refer to the percent milk fat by weight and not by calories. *See chapter 10 to compare the calorie, fat, and calcium differences.*

In the refrigerator case . . .

- *Whole milk* contains not less than 3.25 percent milk fat and may be fortified with vitamin D.

- *2 percent reduced-fat milk* has 2 percent milk fat. It's also fortified with vitamins A and perhaps D.

- *1 percent low-fat milk,* also called light milk, has just 1 percent milk fat. It must be fortified with vitamins A and D.

- *Fat-free, also referred to as nonfat or skim, milk,* has less than 0.5 percent milk fat. Like low-fat milk, fat-free milk must be fortified with vitamins A and D. Most labels now list fat-free or nonfat terms first and may or may not include the word "skim."

- *Chocolate milk* can be whole, 2 percent reduced-fat, 1 percent low-fat, or fat-free milk with added chocolate or cocoa, and sweetener. Fruit-flavored milk is available, too. Look for strawberry, orange, banana, and other flavors. These milks may not be vitamin D fortified.

- *Cultured buttermilk* is made by adding "friendly" bacteria cultures to milk, usually fat-free or low-fat milk. The bacteria cultures produce its unique flavor, aroma, acidity, and thick texture. Salt is often added for more flavor. Despite its name, butter isn't added.

- *Eggnog,* sold around certain holidays, is a blend of milk, pasteurized eggs, sugar, cream, and flavors. Because eggnog is higher in calories and fat, some people prefer eggnog-flavored milk, made with fat-free or 2 percent reduced-fat milk.

- *Acidophilus milk,* a fermented dairy food that's usually made from 1 percent low-fat or fat-free milk, is processed with "friendly" bacteria, which gives it a distinctive flavor. Although research isn't conclusive, "friendly" bacteria in fermented dairy foods may help improve lactose digestion and promote healthy bacteria in the gastrointestinal tract.

- *Lactose-free and lactose-reduced milks* (whole, 2 percent reduced-fat, 1 percent low-fat, and fat-free) are treated with the lactase enzyme. Because lactose, the sugar in milk, converts to glucose and galactose, people with lactose intolerance can drink it. To be considered "lactose-reduced," the lactose level must be reduced by 70 percent. Lactose-free milk is 100 percent lactose-reduced.

- *Protein-fortified milk* is milk that has nonfat milk solids added so the milk solids level reaches 10 percent. These solids are often added to fat-free or 1 percent low-fat milk for a fuller flavor and to improve the nutrient content. Often both protein and calcium are added.

- *Skim deluxe or skim supreme milk* is fat-free, but has the mouthfeel (from some added fiber) of 2 percent reduced-fat milk.

- *Organic milk* must comply with organic standards, *as explained earlier in this chapter and in chapter 9.*

On the grocery shelf . . .

- *Nonfat dry milk* is milk with the fat and the water removed. It has the same nutrients as fat-free milk.

- *Shelf-stable milk* has been processed quickly by very high heat to destroy bacteria. That allows it to be aseptically packaged and stored on a shelf until it's opened. Once opened, it needs refrigeration.

- *Sweetened condensed milk* is concentrated whole milk, with 8 percent or less milk fat, and added sweetener. You also can buy sweetened condensed fat-free milk.

- *Evaporated milk* has been concentrated with about 60 percent of the water removed. It's sold as both fat-free (skim) and whole evaporated milk and has no less than 20 percent milk solids. Evaporated milk is fortified with vitamins A and D. Once it's opened, it needs refrigeration.

Source: National Dairy Council.

on your morning bagel. Whipped cream cheese is often easier to spread, so you may be able to use less.

● As an alternative, look for cholesterol-lowering spreads with plant stanol and sterol esters. *See chapter 3.*

For fluid milk and other dairy foods, products that are properly refrigerated in the store won't spoil as quickly at home. Check the "sell by" date on the carton.

Eggs

For an economical, convenient, and easy-to-prepare source of high-quality protein, try eggs. A single egg supplies about 10 percent of the protein you need in a day, along with good amounts of vitamins A, D, and B_{12} choline, as well as phytonutrients (lutein and xeaxanthin). Although eggs are high in cholesterol, 213 milligrams per large egg, they have 5 grams of fat—no more than an ounce of cheese. Shell color—brown or white—doesn't affect the nutritional quality of eggs; the color varies with the breed of hen. The color of the yolk depends on the feed and doesn't affect the quality, flavor, nutritive value, or cooking characteristics.

From jumbo to small eggs: What size to buy? The bigger the egg, the more it has of everything: nutrients, cholesterol, and calories. *As a shopping and food preparation tip:* Four jumbo eggs equal five large eggs or six small eggs. Most recipes are written for large eggs.

The size is different from the grade printed on the label. Eggs are graded AA, A, and B. Grading refers to the interior and exterior quality of eggs when they're packed. Most eggs sold in supermarkets are Grade A; they're almost the same as Grade AA eggs, which are considered slightly higher in quality.

● To check the freshness of shell eggs, look for the date on the carton. If the egg carton comes from a USDA-inspected plant, it displays a number (called a Julian date) for the packing date. A Julian date will be between 1 (January 1) and 365 (December 31). You can refrigerate fresh shell eggs for four to five weeks beyond the Julian date, in their carton, without losing quality. The carton also may carry an expiration date; after that it can't be sold. When you use eggs, the yolks of fresher eggs hold their shape when they're cracked open. As eggs age, the white thins and the yolk flattens. However, the nutrition and functional qualities of eggs don't change.

● Open egg cartons before you buy. Are the eggs clean and whole? Avoid cartons with cracked eggs. They may be contaminated with *Salmonella*.

● Buy eggs that are refrigerated, not kept at room temperature in the aisle. Even though eggs are stored in their own natural package, they spoil quickly when they're not refrigerated.

● Need to limit yolks to cut cholesterol? Try cholesterol-free or reduced-cholesterol egg substitutes. The yolk, which contains the cholesterol, is left out. Other ingredients, such as nonfat milk, tofu, and vegetable oils, take its place; for coloring, it may contain beta carotene. Find egg substitutes in the store's freezer or the refrigerated section.

Since cholesterol is in the yolk and not the white, you also can buy eggs and use just the whites to replace some or all of the whole eggs. *For more on cutting cholesterol in egg cookery, refer to chapter 13.*

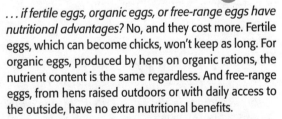

Have You Ever Wondered

. . . if fertile eggs, organic eggs, or free-range eggs have nutritional advantages? No, and they cost more. Fertile eggs, which can become chicks, won't keep as long. For organic eggs, produced by hens on organic rations, the nutrient content is the same regardless. And free-range eggs, from hens raised outdoors or with daily access to the outside, have no extra nutritional benefits.

. . . if modified-fat eggs or lower-cholesterol eggs are worth the extra cost? That depends on your overall food choices. Hens on feed that's high in flaxseed can produce eggs with more omega-3 fatty acids; flaxseed is a great source of omega-3 fatty acids, which may offer health benefits. *See "Eat Your Omega-3s and -6s" in chapter 3 for more about omega-3 fatty acids.* Shell eggs produced with less cholesterol are available as well; however, you may save money by buying whole eggs and tossing out some yolk. Look for other specialty eggs, including lutein-enriched eggs and high-vitamin E eggs.

● Want convenience? Consider frozen and refrigerated whole egg products. They're pasteurized; use them immediately after you open the container.

Freezer Case

Bagels and bread dough, waffles and cookies, fruit and fruit juice, pizza and burritos, vegetables and full dinners, fish and poultry, ice cream and frozen yogurt—the freezer case is stocked with every kind of convenience food. Many of these foods are preportioned, or partly or fully cooked, so you can serve these foods with little or time or effort.

Frozen Vegetables and Fruits

Stock up for quick, easy microwave cooking!

● To control fat and perhaps calories, choose frozen plain vegetables or those made with low-fat sauces. Some sauces mixed with frozen vegetables add fat, saturated fat, and calories; check the Nutrition Facts on the label.

● Look for frozen fruits as an option when fresh berries and other fruits are out of season; they're sold in both sweetened and unsweetened varieties. To help frozen fruit keep its shape, serve while it's somewhat frozen. Frozen fruit bars make a nutritious snack, too; read the label to know if they're made with juice or just flavored water with sweeteners.

● Buy fruit and vegetables in loose-pack plastic bags. You'll only need to pour out what you need; then immediately return what you don't use to the freezer.

● Choosing frozen juice concentrate? *The tips in "More Reading on the Food Label" in this chapter apply.* Read the label to compare products. Juice concentrates often cost a bit less than juice sold in cartons—and you can store them longer.

Frozen Meals and Entrées

● Use nutrition labeling to compare frozen prepared meals, bowl meals, and entrées. Along with traditional foods, you'll find many products with fewer calories and with less fat, including saturated fat and *trans* fat, cholesterol, and sodium—even pizza, lasagna, enchiladas, and burritos! When you're comparing the nutrients in one frozen dinner with another, check the label

serving size. For example, some may be 7-ounce dinners; others, 11 ounces.

● Whether vegetables, fish, or poultry, go easy on breaded and fried frozen foods. They supply more calories and fat. When you buy them, check the package directions for oven heating rather than deep-fat frying, to control calories and fat.

Frozen Desserts

● For frozen desserts, compare frozen yogurt, various ice creams, sherbet, and sorbet. The calories and fat in frozen yogurt (hard-frozen or soft) depend on its main ingredient: whole, 1 percent low-fat, or fat-free milk. Although frozen yogurt is made with lactic acid cultures, it may or may not have active, live cultures; to find out, look for the seal administered by the National Yogurt Association indicating active, live cultures.

Most frozen yogurt has less fat than ice cream—although you'll also find lower-fat brands of ice cream in today's freezer section, too. In a half-cup serving:

● *Reduced-fat (2 percent) ice cream* has at least 25 percent less fat than regular ice cream.

● *Low-fat (1 percent) ice cream* has 3 grams or less of fat.

● *Light ice cream* has at least 50 percent less fat.

● *Fat-free ice cream* has less than 0.5 fat grams per serving.

To get the whole story, check the Nutrition Facts for the calories and fat grams in one serving.

You may prefer the creamy texture and rich flavor of premium ice cream, which contains more fat and thus more calories. If so, cut back on calories and fat elsewhere so you can enjoy premium ice cream, or eat a smaller helping.

Sold alongside ice cream and frozen yogurt, sherbet is sweetened fruit juice and water, 1 to 2 percent milk fat, and 2 to 5 percent milk solids, and stabilizers such as egg white and gelatin. While it has less fat, it contains more sugar than ice cream. Fruit sorbet—whipped and frozen fruit juice—is sold commercially. It may be counted in the Fruit Group.

● Buying a whipped topping? Frozen whipped toppings are convenient to keep in the freezer. Many have the same calories and contents as real whipped cream. If they're made with palm and coconut oils, frozen whipped toppings are high in saturated fat. If you enjoy the taste of whipped cream, buy it—then use just a dollop, not a heaping spoonful. Or look for light or low-calorie versions of frozen whipped toppings.

Grocery Aisles

Up and down the inside aisles of the supermarket, you'll find convenience foods, ethnic foods, baking ingredients, snack foods, seasonings, and beverages.

Canned Fruits and Vegetables

● For a nonperishable supply of fruit and vegetables, buy canned and jarred varieties. They're great to have on hand for boosting vegetables and fruits in mixed dishes and for convenience—especially when their fresh counterparts aren't in season. Besides common items, you'll find beets, collards, hominy, zucchini, blueberries, mangoes, and papaya, among others. (*Tip:* In many mixed dishes such as in soups, stews, other cooked dishes, and smoothies, the flavor and appeal from canned and fresh ingredients are comparable, according to consumer research.) Canned beans are faster to prepare than soaking dry beans overnight. Look for flavorful, newer products, too, such as raspberry-flavored peaches, cinnamon-flavored pears, tomatoes with cilantro, and corn with chopped peppers. Stock up on some "gourmet" items—perhaps canned or jarred artichokes, olives, and roasted peppers.

● For canned fruit, examine the label. You'll find descriptions such as "packed in its own juices," "packed in fruit juice," "unsweetened," "in light syrup," or "in heavy syrup." Fruits packed in juices have less added sugar and so fewer calories than fruits packed in syrup. If you prefer the flavor of fruit packed in syrup, just be sure the extra calories fit within your own calorie target.

● Juice, juice cocktail, or juice drinks—which should you buy? *See "More Reading on the Food Label" in this chapter. Tip:* Juices may cost less per serving than soft drinks—and juice is more nutritious.

● Canned vegetables: if you're cutting back on sodium, which should you buy? Read the Nutrition Facts for sodium content, or look for descriptions such as "no salt added" and "reduced sodium."

● For less fat, buy vegetarian or fat-free baked beans

Have You Ever Wondered

... how frozen custard differs from ice cream? It's about the same. The only difference is that more egg yolks are used in custard.

and refried beans. Compared with traditional products, you may cut the fat by 50 percent or more. Some are sodium reduced, too. Refried beans may be made with lard, which contains saturated fat and cholesterol.

Canned Fish

● Be aware that tuna, salmon, sardines, crabs, clams, mackerel, and other fish are canned in water or oil (typically vegetable or olive oil). Even when the oil is drained, fish in oil have significantly more (mostly unsaturated) fat than water-packed varieties. With oil-packed canned fish, some omega-3 fatty acids transfer to the oil, which may be discarded. *For more about omega-3 fatty acids, see "Eat your Omega-3s and -6s" in chapter 3.* Besides the fat and calorie difference, fish packed in spring water have a milder flavor, but a drier texture. Also look for fish in shelf-stable pouches.

Compare the calories and fat in 3 ounces of water-packed and oil-packed tuna.

3-OUNCE SERVING	CALORIES	FAT GRAMS
Water-packed tuna, drained	100	1
Oil-packed tuna, drained	165	7

● For calcium, buy canned fish (salmon and sardines) with edible bones. Three ounces of salmon eaten with the bones have about 200 milligrams of calcium, almost as much as 6 ounces of milk. (Not all canned salmon has edible bones—check the ingredient list.) Canning softens bones, making them edible. Canned tuna and crabmeat don't have edible bones.

● Although tuna outsells other canned fish, give yourself a change in flavor with canned salmon or sardines. Besides adding variety to your eating pattern, salmon is higher in omega-3 fatty acids. Use it in salads, stir-fries, soups, and pizza toppings.

Soups, Stews, and Convenience Foods

● As a main dish, choose stews and hearty soups; because they're made with nutrient-rich foods, they usually provide plenty of nutrients. Use the Nutrition Facts and the ingredient list to find out. Clear soups and stews are usually lower in calories and fat than creamy varieties or stew with gravy. For creamy soups: low-fat and fat-free versions of cream of celery soup and cream of mushroom soup, among others.

● If you're heating a quick meal at the office, look for ready-to-eat soup or dehydrated soup. Unlike condensed soup, ready-to-eat soup doesn't need added liquid—open the can, heat, then serve. For dehydrated soup, just add hot water.

● For quick meals, buy canned and shelf-stable microwaveable entrées: perhaps pasta with meat or cheese, or chili con carne. If you eat them regularly, look for varieties with less fat and, depending on your needs, less sodium.

● If you're watching how much sodium you eat, read the Nutrition Facts for sodium content. Many canned and instant soups, as well as canned stews, are high in sodium. Check grocery shelves, though; you'll see many prepared with less sodium or no salt added.

For instant noodles (Oriental noodles) and entrée mixes (macaroni and cheese), use half of the seasoning packet to cut back on sodium. Depending on your overall food choices, you might toss in some chopped vegetables for more vitamins and fiber, too. To reduce fat, use less butter or margarine than the directions call for.

● To cut back on fat, look for defatted broth. Or put a canned soup or stew in the refrigerator prior to use. The fat will congeal so you can skim it off.

Pasta, Rice, and Other Grains

● For meal appeal, buy a variety of pasta shapes. For thick sauces, use thicker pastas: fettuccine, lasagna, and tagliatelle. Chunky sauces are best with sturdy pasta shapes: fusilli (twists), farfalle (bow ties), macaroni, rigatoni, and ziti. With smooth, thin sauces, use thinner strands of pasta: cappellini (angel hair), vermicelli, and spaghetti. The refrigerated section of the store also sells fresh pasta; use it right away or freeze it.

● Look for whole-grain pasta: spaghetti, lasagna,

How Much Pasta? How Much Rice?

Because dry pasta and rice cook to a larger volume, use these guidelines when deciding how much to buy.

Pasta or Rice	Uncooked	Equal Cooked
Egg noodles	8 oz. (2 cups)	4 cups
Spaghetti, fettuccine, other long shapes	8 oz. (1½-in. diameter bunch)	4 cups
Macaroni, shells, bow ties, penne, other small to medium shapes	8 oz. (2 cups)	4 cups
Brown rice	½ lb. (1¼ cups)	4⅓ cups
Polished, long-grain white rice	½ lb. (1¼ cups)	3¾ cups
Converted white rice	7 oz. (1 cup)	3½ cups
Instant white rice	8 oz. (2 cups)	4 cups

macaroni, and fettuccine. Like traditional pasta, whole-wheat pasta is high in starches (complex carbohydrates). The fiber content is almost three times higher; half a cup of whole-wheat pasta has about 3 grams of fiber, compared with about 1 gram of fiber in traditional pasta. *See page 277 for more about whole grains.* Other options: soy pasta for soy protein benefits and pasta made with other grains and with legumes.

For more variety, savor the appeal of vegetable and herbed pasta. The addition of tomatoes, beets, carrots, spinach, and other vegetables adds a variety of colors and flavors to pasta. And herbs add a delicate flavor. What about the nutrients? Tomato pasta and spinach pasta don't count toward your goal for the Vegetable Group. The nutritional contribution of vegetable purees used to make commercially flavored pasta is quite small. It's the vegetables or tomato sauce tossed with pasta that carry extra nutrients.

● Experiment with Asian-style noodles. They're made with many ingredients besides wheat flour, including potato flour, soybean starch, rice flour, and buckwheat flour. Japanese soba noodles are made with buckwheat and wheat flour; Japanese wheat noodles are udon (thick noodles) and somen (thin noodles). Look for rice noodles, mung bean noodles, wonton wrappers (sheets of wheat dough), and rice paper (a thin dough used somewhat like a tortilla). Ramen noodles, which are Japanese instant-style deep-fried noodles, are often packaged with dehydrated vegetables and broth mix; the mix is typically high in sodium.

● Wonder about the fat in egg noodles? While pasta is made from flour and water, noodles also contain eggs, egg yolks, or egg whites. Nonegg pasta contains no cholesterol and very little fat. Egg noodles may have small amounts of cholesterol and a little more fat but still are low in fat and cholesterol.

● Try different forms of rice. Use the label to compare their nutrients. Brown rice contains slightly more nutrients, followed by polished white rice, then instant white rice. Because it's a whole grain, brown rice—with 1.5 grams of fiber per half cup—has about three times the fiber of white rice. When you read the label, check for uncooked and cooked rice; it may give the nutritional content for prepared rice with added butter or salt.

Change the flavor and the texture with specialty rices. Jasmine and basmati rice have a fragrant flavor and aroma, especially nice with Thai and Indian food. Arborio rice, a short-grain rice, gives Italian risotto its creamy texture.

Despite its name, wild rice is actually a long-grain marsh grass. From a nutritional standpoint, wild rice has a little more protein, riboflavin, and zinc, and a little less carbohydrate than brown rice. The fiber content is about 0.5 gram per half cup. For its nutty flavor, serve wild rice in salads, stir-fries, soups, stuffing, and side dishes. Or mix it 50–50 with regular or brown rice.

What about rice mixes? If you need to watch sodium, consider using just half the dry seasoning mix.

● Browse the grocery shelves for other grain products: barley, bulgur, couscous, kasha, and quinoa, to name a few. *See "Today's Grains" in chapter 9. In "Cooking Grain by Grain" in chapter 13 you'll find guidelines for cooking with other grains.*

● How much should you buy? Base the amount of dry pasta and rice on their cooked volume. And remember, you may eat more than one serving, so figure the nutritional contribution based on the amount you really eat.

Breakfast Cereals

● Stocking up for quick breakfasts? Choose from the huge variety of ready-to-eat breakfast cereals. Besides being fortified with vitamins and minerals, you'll also find many high-fiber cereals. Because cereals use different parts of the grain—bran, germ, and endosperm—in differing amounts, their nutritional content varies. Use the Nutrition Facts to compare.

Adding milk or yogurt makes cereal a great vehicle for delivering calcium and other nutrients in milk. For this reason, cereal labels often give the Nutrition Facts for cereal only and for cereal with added milk.

When buying sweetened cereals, use the same criteria for choosing any cereal—sweetened or unsweetened. Read the Nutrition Facts for the nutrient and fiber content in one serving, then make your choice. Sweetened cereals are no more cavity-promoting than unsweetened cereals; both starches in all kinds of cereal and sugars can linger on tooth surfaces and promote cavities. Choose the cereal that matches your family's preferences and needs, and encourage good oral hygiene.

● Look for clues to breakfast cereals with more fiber. They may carry label terms such as "high fiber," "whole grain," or "bran." If the label gives a nutrient content claim, check the Nutrition Facts for specific nutrient information. Cereals that are good fiber sources supply at least 2.5 grams of fiber per serving; whole-grain cereals typically have more. The ingredient list reveals the whole grains and bran in the cereal's "recipe."

● Check the nutrients in fortified cereals. Most supply about 25 percent of the Daily Value for vitamins and minerals. And some have much more—100 percent—making these cereals comparable to a nutrient supplement. Remember, a variety of other foods supply these nutrients, too. Like any food, consider fortified cereal as part of your whole day's eating plan.

Like many other breakfast cereals, bran cereals usually are fortified. Although high in fiber, bran lacks the vitamins and minerals supplied by the germ portion of grain.

Tip: Because many vitamins and minerals may be sprayed onto cereals, they can be lost if all the milk in the bottom of a cereal bowl isn't eaten along with the cereal. Drink your "cereal milk"!

● Check the variety of cooked cereals, too: Cream of Rice, grits, rolled oats, and toasted wheat. Many are whole grain.

Think cooked cereals take too long to prepare? With today's packaging, you'll find microwave instructions for quick prep. Many to-be-cooked cereals—oatmeal, grits, Cream of Wheat—are "instant" varieties. The nutritional content is comparable to their traditional counterpart, although sodium may be higher in instant cereals. Read the label to compare.

● Check the Nutrition Facts on cereal labels. The nutritional content varies from product to product, brand to brand. "Natural" cereals or granola may have more fat, sugars, or sodium than you'd think; many contain more saturated fats from palm and coconut oils. For something different, try muesli, made with grains, nuts, and dried fruit.

Beans, Nuts, and Peanut Butter

● Add a variety of legumes (beans and lentils) to your shopping list: adzuki, cannellini, garbanzos, navy beans, soybeans, and pinto beans, to name a few. With the demand for nutrient-rich, high-fiber recipes and the interest in ethnic cooking, today's stores stock a greater variety of beans and lentils—dry, canned, and frozen. You may find fresh legumes in the produce department and frozen beans in the freezer case.

If the store doesn't carry the type you're looking for, you usually can substitute another. For example, pinto, adzuki, and black beans can substitute for kidney beans, giving a dish a slightly different look. Cannellini, lima beans, and navy beans are the same color, just a different size. Nutritionally, most legumes are about the same, even though their appearance, texture, and flavor may differ somewhat. *To explore the varieties of legumes, see "Bean Bag" in chapter 6.*

● For freshness, look for these qualities in dry beans:

no pinhole marks or discoloration, beans with a bright color, and bags that aren't torn.

● When food preparation time is short, opt for canned, rather than dry, beans. Unlike canned varieties, dry beans require cooking and perhaps soaking time. If your blood pressure is sodium-sensitive, be aware that salt is added to canned beans; check the Nutrition Facts and the ingredient list to compare similar products. *Tip:* Rinse canned beans under cold running water to reduce sodium.

● Read labels on peanut butter. Peanut butter is simply roasted peanuts ground into a paste. The style—smooth, chunky, or crunchy—doesn't affect the nutritional content. All are good sources of protein, but the added ingredients may make a difference. To the ground peanuts, salt or small amounts of sugar may be added for flavor; unsalted and sugar-free varieties also are sold. You'll also see reduced-fat varieties, which may not be lower in calories; sugar and other ingredients may be added to enhance flavor and texture. The small amount of naturally occurring oils in peanut butter may be hydrogenated for spreadability, adding *trans* fats. *For more about partially hydrogenated (*trans*) fats, see "About* Trans *Fats" in chapter 3.*

To keep oil and solids from separating, stabilizers usually are added to peanut butter. However, in "natural" peanut butter, the oil separates out. At home, avoid the urge to make peanut butter lower in fat by pouring that fat away. Your peanut butter will become too stiff to spread. Instead mix it well, or turn the jar upside down to let the oil run through.

● Buy a variety of tree nuts—almonds, cashews, hazlenuts, pecans, pine nuts, pistachios, walnuts, among others. Their nutrient and phytonutrient benefits differ, and their fats are mostly polyunsaturated. Be aware that nuts often are sold in salted and unsalted varieties. Unsalted nuts typically are found in the baking aisle; salted nuts, with snack foods.

Beverages

● Enjoy flavored waters. Peach, lemon, mango, and other fruit-flavored waters are refreshing. For the "fizz," some are made of sparkling water and juice. Others are flavored with sweeteners but contain little juice. Unlike plain water, they may not be calorie-free. *See "What about Bottled Water?" in chapter 8.*

● For a no-calorie beverage, look for club soda, mineral water, and plain seltzer. Don't confuse these beverages with tonic or quinine water, which has 125 calories per 12 ounces.

● For carried meals, camping, and emergencies, stock up on boxed, or UHT, milk. Because boxed milk is ultrapasteurized, or heated to an ultrahigh temperature (UHT), then sealed in a sterile container, it can be stored unopened at room temperature for about three months without spoiling or nutrient loss. For added appeal, simply chill it before drinking. Once opened, UHT milk is as perishable as milk sold in the refrigerated dairy case.

● For more convenience, try nonfat dry milk or evaporated, canned milk. They're both shelf-stable. When reconstituted, nonfat dry milk powder has the same amount of nutrients as fat-free fluid milk. *Tip:* For 1 cup of fluid milk, combine ¾ cup of water with ⅓ cup of dry milk powder. Use dry milk powder also to fortify casseroles and other mixed dishes with calcium and other nutrients from milk. It costs less than fat-free fluid milk, too.

Evaporated milk has about 60 percent of the water removed, so its nutrients are more concentrated than regular fluid milk. If reconstituted, the nutrients are equivalent to the same-size serving. Evaporated milk may be whole or fat-free (skim). Sweetened condensed milk—whole or fat-free—is concentrated, too, but because sugars are added, it's higher in calories. *See the chart "Milk: A Great Calcium Source" in chapter 10 to compare the calories, fat, cholesterol, and calcium in evaporated milks.*

Tip: Once evaporated milk is opened and dry milk is reconstituted, both should be refrigerated.

● *Be aware:* Nondairy creamers, either dry or liquid, may be high in saturated fat or *trans* fat. Although nondairy creamers are made with vegetable oil, the fats—often coconut or palm oil—are highly saturated. To lighten your coffee or tea, nonfat dry milk or evaporated fat-free (skim) milk are both good substitutes from the grocery aisle—or use fluid milk or fat-free half-and-half instead.

● Sensitive to caffeine? Then look for decaffeinated

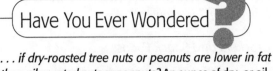

. . . if dry-roasted tree nuts or peanuts are lower in fat than oil-roasted nuts or peanuts? An ounce of dry- or oil-roasted tree nuts has about the same amount of fat and calories—almost 14 fat grams per ounce. Nuts and peanuts don't absorb much oil when they're roasted. The fat comes from the nuts and peanuts themselves. They also are a good protein source and provide fiber and varying amounts of different phytonutrients.

coffee and tea, and caffeine-free soft drinks. Also, seltzer, sparkling water, and most fruit-flavored soft drinks have no caffeine. *See "Drinks: With or Without Caffeine?" in chapter 8.*

● *Note:* Flavored coffee mixes may contain sugars and coconut oil, which are high in saturated fatty acids.

● For soft drinks, know the calorie differences as you shop. A regular soda has 150 to 200 calories per 12-ounce can—with carbohydrates and water as the only significant nutrients. Buy sensibly sized cans or bottles, perhaps 8-ounce cans to control your portions. Diet sodas may quench thirst, too, and they're essentially calorie-free. *For more about including soft drinks in your overall eating plan, see "Soft Drinks: Okay?" in chapter 8.*

Soft drinks and other beverages with non-nutritive, or intense, sweeteners, carry nutrition labeling. If you're sensitive to their non-nutritive sweetener, avoid these products. In moderation, non-nutritive sweeteners are fine. *See "Aspartame" in chapter 5.*

● Buy single-serving containers of juice and boxed milk. They're handy for packing along to lunch, meetings, or a spectator sport, rather than rely on a vending machine. Be aware that single soft drinks have gotten bigger; 20-ounce plastic bottles are as common in vending machines as 12-ounce cans. Ask yourself if you need that much.

● If you enjoy the taste of alcohol-containing drinks but choose to cut back, look for low-alcohol versions of beer and wine. The taste compares favorably. For single serve, buy 12-ounce cans or small bottles of beer instead of a bigger size. Regarding calories, you'll need to check the label. *For more about alcoholic beverages, see "Alcoholic Beverages: In Moderation" in chapter 8.*

Crackers and Snack Foods

● For meals or snacks, consider the growing array of crackers, including those with "less fat," "0 grams *trans* fat," or "less sodium." Typically low in fat, or even fat-free: packaged bread sticks, graham crackers, melba toast, rice crackers, matzos, rusk, saltines, and zwieback. For more fiber, look for whole-wheat crackers, too!

● Many snack foods are made with oil—but what kind of oil? Check the ingredient list and the Nutrition Facts. Those made with partially hydrogenated vegetable oils have more *trans* fats.

● For a low-fat, crunchy snack food, buy pretzels or plain popcorn. They have less fat than potato chips, corn chips, bagel chips, or buttered popcorn. To eat less salt, look for unsalted snack foods such as unsalted pretzels. For a lower-fat option, look for oven-baked tortilla and potato chips; 1 ounce of baked tortilla chips has about 1 fat gram compared with about 7 fat grams in the same amount of regular tortilla chips. And check the label on microwave popcorn. Some contain high-fat flavorings.

● When it comes to cookies, explore the growing variety of reduced-fat, fat-free, and "0 grams *trans* fat" varieties. If calories are your challenge, read the label for calorie content, too, to see if the calories really are less. Even fairly small calorie and fat savings can be significant if you eat these cookies frequently. On the other hand, bigger helpings may "spend" any calorie or fat savings! Some types of commercial cookies are typically lower in fat: animal crackers, fig bars, gingersnaps, and vanilla wafers.

● If you buy candy and other snacks, look for small, portion-controlled packages (perhaps 100-calorie packs). In that way, it's not as easy to overindulge. To check the calories, read the Nutrition Facts. Some sugar-free candies have calories. And remember, candy bars may have fat, too.

Dressings, Sauces, Oils, and Condiments

● Mayonnaise or salad dressing? For less fat, choose "light," "reduced-fat," "low-calorie," or "fat-free"

varieties. Fat-free dressings typically have 5 to 20 calories per tablespoon, compared with 75 calories and 6 to 8 fat grams in 1 tablespoon of regular salad dressing. Vinegar and water usually are the first two ingredients in fat-free dressing.

● Buy dry blends for mixing your own salad dressing. Then you can control the amount and type of oil and vinegar you add. Often you can use less oil and more vinegar, water, or other flavorful liquid than the package directions call for.

● Shopping for prepared pasta sauce? Alfredo, clam, meat, marinara, and primavera: the type of sauce doesn't indicate nutrient content (although creamy sauces such as alfredo and clam usually have more fat). Read the Nutrition Facts. *See "Gourmet's Guide to Sauces" in chapter 14.*

● If you're trying to cut back on sodium, look for soy sauce, teriyaki sauce, chile sauce, and marinades that are "reduced-sodium." Their traditional counterparts may be quite high in sodium.

● Look for oil (canola, olive, vegetable) sprays. With these sprays you can use less oil in a fry pan or casserole dish, or on a baking pan.

● Remember that all vegetable oils contain the same amount of calories: about 120 calories per tablespoon. And while the amounts of saturated, monounsaturated, and polyunsaturated fatty acids differ, all vegetable oils are cholesterol-free. "Light" oil refers to the color or mild flavor, not the fat content.

● Make healthy oils a main source of your discretionary fat calories. Oils high in polyunsaturated fatty acids include corn, safflower, and sunflower oils. And those high in monounsaturates include olive, flaxseed, and canola oils. *See "Fats and Oils: How Do They Compare?" in chapter 3.*

● Experiment with stronger-flavored oils: for example, sesame, walnut, herb-infused, or chile-flavored oils. These are finishing oils, not cooking oils. Just a splash adds a distinct flavor to salads, stir-fries, pasta, rice, and other dishes.

● Stock your kitchen with a variety of vinegars to pair with oils in saladmaking: red wine vinegar, herb vinegars, apple cider vinegar, and fruit-flavored vinegars. The strong flavor of sweet balsamic vinegar complements salad greens. Vinegars are fat-free.

● Buy ketchup, mustard, and pickle relish as tasty spreads, with just 2 fat grams or less per tablespoon. Check the label for sodium content to watch your sodium intake. Unless prepared with less salt or sodium, most of these condiments provide 150 to 200 milligrams of sodium per tablespoon. For more flavor with fewer calories, buy prepared horseradish. And look for chutney—a condiment made with fruit or vegetables, vinegar, spices, and sugar—that's low in sodium and fat.

● Remember salsas. They're low in calories and bursting with flavor. Experiment with the different levels of spiciness—usually labeled as mild, medium, or hot—to see which you like best.

● Fruit jams and jellies—nutritionally they're much the same. Check the label. Both have relatively small amounts of nutrients. *Hint:* Fruit jams and jellies supply extra calories from added sugars. Fruit spreads— sweetened with juice—can have the same number of

calories as jam or jelly, or they may have less sugar. And they provide some nutrients. Check the label's Nutrition Facts.

Baking Aisle

Flour

● Recognize different types and qualities of wheat flour before you buy. Whole-grain flour contains more fiber than refined wheat flour because the bran layer of the grain is still intact; that's where most of the fiber comes from. Whole-grain flour also contains the germ layer, which provides many vitamins and minerals. *See "What Is a Whole Grain?" in chapter 6.*

Refined flour, used in about 80 percent of baked goods, including most white bread, is made only from the endosperm of the grain. While the flour has a snowy-white appearance, almost all of the fiber and many of the vitamins and minerals are lost. Refined flour may be bleached or unbleached. Bleaching simply whitens the somewhat yellowish unbleached flour. From a nutritional standpoint, bleached and unbleached flours are almost the same.

When flour is enriched, four nutrients that were lost in processing—thiamin, riboflavin, niacin, and iron— are added back. The amounts of these nutrients compare to those of whole-grain flour. Enriched flour also is fortified with folic acid; whole-wheat flour may or may not be folic acid fortified.

The label also may describe the flour as "all-purpose," "bread," "cake," or "self-rising."

● *All-purpose flour* is a mixture of high-gluten hard wheat and low-gluten soft wheat.

● *Bread flour* is mainly high-gluten hard wheat, suitable for yeast bread.

● *Cake, or pastry, flour* made from low-gluten soft wheat has a finer texture that makes pastry and cakes more tender.

● *Self-rising flour* is all-purpose flour with baking powder and salt added for making quick breads.

Although bread can be made with only 100 percent whole-wheat flour, the result will be a dense, heavy loaf. For a lighter texture, use a combination of whole wheat and refined white flour.

● Look for other types of whole-grain flour in the supermarket and specialty stores: barley, buckwheat,

Have You Ever Wondered ？

... if virgin olive oil has fewer calories than pure olive oil? No matter what the type, olive oil is high in monounsaturated fatty acids, and the calories are the same. Terms that may confuse consumers, such as "virgin" and "extra virgin" olive oil, refer to the acid content—not the nutrient content. Extra virgin olive oil has less acid and a fruitier flavor than "pure" or "virgin" olive oil. Because it has more aroma and flavor, you can use less.

What about light olive oil? The term "light" refers to the color and fragrance, not to the calories, fat content, or if it has an olive-oil flavor.

corn, oats, brown rice, rye, and triticale. Triticale flour, with less gluten than all-purpose flour, makes a denser bread; triticale is a blend of wheat and rye flour. To lighten the texture of baked goods, go "50–50" with triticale and bread flour. Corn flour, made from the whole kernel, is finely ground cornmeal; masa harina is a specialty corn flour used to make tortillas. Yellow corn flour—and other yellow cornmeal—have more vitamin A than white corn flour.

● Try other types of flour, such as corn and rice flours, especially useful for people who have a wheat allergy or are sensitive to gluten. *See "Gluten Intolerance: Often a Lifelong Condition" in chapter 21.*

Sugar

● Know the difference in various types of sugar. Most cooking and baking are done with granulated, refined sugar. Superfine sugars, more finely granulated, may be used in meringues or in recipes that call for granulated sugar. Powdered or confectioners' sugar is granulated sugar that's been crushed into a fine powder. *See chapter 5 for information on honey, brown sugar, and raw sugar as well as sugar replacers.*

Baking Mixes

● Choose baking mixes—cakes, breads, waffles, muffins, etc.—that allow you to add ingredients. When you add the fat, eggs, and liquid, you can control the type you use. If you need to watch cholesterol carefully, you might add an egg substitute rather than an egg. Or to cut back on saturated fats, you could use soft margarine rather than butter. Check the label; some manufacturers provide tips for preparing mixes with less fat and less cholesterol. Look for whole-grain mixes for more fiber.

Breads and Bakery Items

● Make an effort to buy more "whole grain" and "whole wheat" bakery products. Other label terms may suggest whole grain—for example, oatmeal and multigrain—but check the label to be sure.

Just because it's called "wheat bread" doesn't mean it's whole grain. Instead it may be made mostly from refined wheat flour. Terms such as "stone ground," "multigrain," "cracked wheat," or "100 percent wheat" don't mean whole wheat. And most store-bought rye and pumpernickel breads are made mostly from refined white flour. For more fiber, check the Nutrition Facts and the ingredient list for those made with mainly whole-wheat flour.

On the Nutrition Facts you'll see that a 1-ounce slice of whole-wheat bread has about 1.6 fiber grams compared to 0.5 to 1 gram of fiber in the same-size slice of enriched white bread. Bakery products that supply 2.5 or more grams of fiber per serving are a good fiber source. *Refer to page 142 in chapter 6.*

● For white bread and rolls, look for "enriched" products. Bread made from enriched flour is a good source of starches (complex carbohydrates), B vitamins (including folic acid), and iron. When flour is enriched, B vitamins and iron are added back—but not fiber or other vitamins and minerals. Most other products made with refined grains also are fortified with folic acid.

● Choose mostly bread and other bakery products with less fat. Most Italian bread, French bread, bagels, pita bread, kaiser rolls, English muffins, rye bread, corn tortillas, and pumpernickel bread have 2 grams of fat or less per serving. Check the Nutrition Facts for serving size and nutrient content.

● Go easy on bakery products with more fat: croissants, many muffins, doughnuts, sweet rolls, and many cookies and cakes. Although croissants make a tasty sandwich bread, half of a croissant has about 5 fat grams compared with 1 fat gram in half of an Italian roll. And a doughnut has about 10 fat grams. Be portion savvy; just the amount you need!

● Use food labels—the ingredient list and the Nutrition Facts–to find bakery products with fewer calories and added sugars and less salt, too.

● Check the product date on the label for freshness. Packaged bakery products, with preservatives added, may have a longer shelf life than from the in-store bakery. *See "Additives: Safe at the Plate" in chapter 9.*

Seasonings: Dry or Fresh

Herbs and spices enhance the flavor of food without adding sodium. Dry or fresh, add them to your list.

Is It Really Whole Grain? Check the Label!

- Does the package claim link whole grains to a reduced risk for heart disease or some cancers? If so, the food must contain at least 51 percent whole grain by weight and meet specific levels for fat, cholesterol, and sodium. A new FDA labeling guideline: a "whole-grain food" must contain the bran, endosperm, and germ in natural proportions.

- Is the first ingredient on the ingredient list whole grain? That's the ingredient in the greatest amount. That said, even if a refined grain is listed first, the sum of several whole grains listed next add up. To address this issue, the package may have a voluntary Whole Grain Stamp sponsored by the Whole Grain Council, indicating whether one label serving of the food contains at least 8 grams of whole grain. To meet MyPyramid advice, you'd need to eat at least 48 grams of whole grain daily. Some food companies have their own whole-grain symbol, too.

- Buy herbs and spices in the amounts you need. Fresh herbs last in the refrigerator for only a short time. Dry herbs can be stored for up to a year to retain their peak flavors. *Tip:* Ethnic food stores often sell herbs and spices in bulk at lower prices.

- Know that seasoned salts are high in sodium. This includes garlic salt and onion salt. As an alternate, look for garlic powder and onion powder. To check the sodium content, read the Nutrition Facts.

- Look for salt-free herb blends. Italian herb blend or herbs de Provence (typical in French cooking) take the guessing out of seasoning.

- Be adventuresome—buy seasonings that may be new to you: perhaps sage for chicken soup, tarragon with peas, fresh ginger for sweet potatoes, or cumin in chili.

- Try liquid smoke. It adds the smoky flavor of cured meat without the salt that's added during curing.

See "A Pinch of Flavor: How to Cook with Herbs and Spices" in chapter 13; check "Salty Terms" in chapter 7 for more about types of salt.

Take-out Foods

Consumers increasingly shop at supermarkets for the most convenient home-served meals of all, foods that are ready to eat: salad bars, rotisserie chicken, steamed shrimp, sushi bar, and deli sandwiches, as well as a variety of heat-only main dishes, appetizers, and side dishes. The food industry puts these foods in a broad category of "meal solutions."

If you're time-pressed, buy your main dish—or a whole meal—already prepared. Then just heat and serve as your own healthful eating solution on a hectic day! For food safety, eat them the same day you buy them. Guidelines for supermarket take-out foods are similar to buying and handling foods from a carry-out restaurant. *See "Safe Take-out" in chapter 14.*

Food Safety: Start at the Store

While the safety of the food supply has been monitored and regulated all along the food chain, it's your responsibility to select foods carefully at the store, then keep them safe until they're eaten.

- Only buy food from reputable food businesses that follow government regulations for food safety.

- Check the package. It shouldn't have holes, tears, or open corners. Frozen foods should be solid, and refrigerated foods should feel cold. Frozen foods shouldn't show signs of thawing.

- Check safety seals and buttons. Safety seals often appear on milk, yogurt, and cottage cheese. Jars of foods often are vacuum-sealed for safety. Check their safety buttons or seals with your finger. If the indented safety button on the cap pulls down, it's still in place; if it's up, don't buy or use the food. Report the incident to the store manager.

- Reject cans that are swollen, damaged, rusted, or dented. These are warning signs for bacteria that cause botulism. *See "Bacteria: Hard Hitters" in chapter 12.*

- If you suspect food tampering, report it to the store manager. Once you're home, contact a public health authority, the local police, or, for meat and poultry, the USDA's Meat and Poultry Hotline (800-535-4555) or for other foods, the U.S. Food and Drug Administration (888-SAFEFOOD).

What's "Soy" Good?

Soybeans! Made into many food products, they're very versatile and nutritious. Compared with many other legumes, soybeans are a rich, unique source of high-quality, plant-based protein—unique because soybeans contain complete protein as does meat, with all nine essential amino acids needed to build and repair body cells. That's why many soy products make good protein alternatives in meatless meals!

Beyond that, soybeans are a good source of B vitamins. A source of essential fatty acids (including some omega-3s), soybeans' fat is mostly poly- and monounsaturated. Tofu made with calcium sulfate, and calcium-fortified soy beverage and soy yogurt, deliver calcium.

Health benefits of soy may go beyond nutrients. Many soy foods contain isoflavones that may help lower risks for some diseases. Their two main isoflavones—genistein and daidzein—have weak estrogenlike effects. Current soy research is looking at potential benefits to heart health, blood pressure, and cancer protection, among others.

Fresh, canned, dried, or frozen . . . soybeans fit in soups, stews, casseroles, salads, pasta sauces, and Mexican dishes. And look for these soy foods next time you shop:

- *Produce Department:* tofu, tempeh, edamame (ed-ah-MAH-may) (in the pod or shelled), soy sprouts
- *Grocery Aisle:* canned black and yellow soybeans, dried soybeans, soy pasta (sold in many shapes), soy pudding, soy jerky, soy-nut butter (like peanut butter), soy cereal (soy flakes, granola, soy mixed with other cereals, soy grits), soy flour, soy baking mixes (for pancakes, muffins, brownies), soy protein and soy beverage powders (to add to drinks and other foods), seasoning mixes for burgers, chili and tacos with soy
- *Dairy Case:* soy beverage, soy cheese, soy eggnog, soy yogurt, soy smoothies, dairy milk and dairy yogurt with soy protein, soy beverage–juice blends, soy sour cream. Although cholesterol free, these soy foods don't have the same characteristics as milk products.
- *Frozen Foods:* edamame, soy entrées, soy sausage and patties, soy bacon, soy-based burgers, soy crumbles, soy ice cream
- *Snack Aisle:* soy nuts, soy-nut trail mix, soy protein bars

Some notes about a few soy foods:

- *egg replacers:* made from potato starch and lecithin, a soy-based product
- *miso (MEE soh):* fermented soybean paste, most commonly used as a flavoring in Japanese cooking. With a consistency like peanut butter, miso can be used as a condiment. But it's also prepared in dips, marinades, sauces, and soups. Depending on the amount used, miso adds protein, calcium, and some B vitamins to dishes. Unless it's a low-salt variety, miso tends to be high in sodium.
- *soy flour:* flour that's much higher in protein but lower in carbohydrate than wheat flour. In baking, it's usually mixed with other types of flour.
- *soy mayonnaise:* typically made with tofu. Read the ingredient list to find out if it's made with eggs.
- *soy oil and margarine:* unsaturated fat extracted from whole soybeans. The most commonly available vegetable oil is made from soy. (Partially hydrogenated soy oil has more *trans* fat.)
- *soybeans (in the pod):* picked immature and sold frozen or fresh. Edamame (ed-ah-MAH-may) are soybeans cooked in the pod and eaten as a snack.
- *soy sauce:* a condiment in many Asian dishes, it comes from fermented soybeans. Although it adds flavor, it's not a significant protein source. Tamari is a wheat-free variety; shoyu is not.
- *tempeh (TEHM-peh):* soybeans, mixed with rice, millet, or other grain, then fermented into a rich soybean cake. Tempeh has a smoky or nutty taste that adds flavor to soups, casseroles, chili, or spaghetti. It can be grilled or marinated. Like tofu, tempeh is a good protein source, but it has somewhat less calcium.
- *textured soy protein, or TSP:* soy flour that's high in protein and often sold as granules, flakes, or chunks. You can use TSP to replace or extend meat or poultry. Vegetable burgers and sausages often are made with TSP, too.
- *tofu (TOH-foo), or soybean curd:* a cheeselike curd, made from curdled soybean milk and pressed into

soft cakes. Tofu easily takes up the flavor of other ingredients in a dish, including stir-fries, chili, tacos, salads, noodle dishes, and pizza. You can also buy flavored tofu, such as smoked, teriyaki, Mexican, and Italian tofu.

Tofu is sold in several forms: soft or silken for dressings, smoothies, soups, dips, shakes, and sauces; medium-soft for puddings, cheesecakes, pie fillings, and salads; and firm or extra firm for grilling, marinating, slicing, and stir-frying and in casseroles, soups, and sandwiches; baked for stir-frying and grilling. Tofu sold in bulk (not packaged) or in water needs to be refrigerated and used within a week because it's very perishable. It should be kept in water that's changed daily. Bought in an aseptic package, tofu doesn't need refrigeration until opened. You can freeze tofu for up to three months for a chewier texture.

Tofu is a good source of protein. Its calcium content is highest when it's calcium fortified. Look for calcium sulfate on the ingredient list and on the label.

● When possible, put raw poultry, meat, and fish in separate plastic bags before placing them in your cart. Occasionally their packaging may leak and drip onto unprotected foods.

● Pay attention to "sell by" and "use by" dates on perishable foods. If the "sell by" date has passed, don't buy the product. The "use by" date applies to its use at home. Purchase only those that will be fresh when you're ready to eat them. *See "More Reading on the Food Label" earlier in this chapter for more about food product dating.*

● Select perishable foods such as meat, poultry, and seafood last before checkout, if possible.

● In the checkout line, pack cold foods together, preferably in paper bags, which keep foods cold longer than plastic bags do. They'll stay chilled longer for the trip home.

● Take groceries home immediately, and store them right away. If you must run a few quick errands, bring a cooler with chill packs for perishable foods if you'll be longer than thirty minutes. That's especially important in warm weather. The temperature of refrigerated food can go up 8 to 10 degrees Fahrenheit on a typical trip home from the store. That goes higher as the time gets longer. *For guidelines on keeping food safe at home, see chapter 12, "The Safe Kitchen."*

Have You Ever Wondered

. . . how safe are the refrigerated juices purchased from the store? Most packaged juices and juice drinks—refrigerated, frozen, and shelf-stable—have been heat-treated (pasteurized) or processed in other ways to destroy harmful bacteria and naturally occurring enzymes that hasten spoilage.

If sold in interstate commerce, fresh juice and juice products that have *not been pasteurized* or appropriately treated must show this warning on the package label.

> WARNING: this product has not been pasteurized and, therefore, may contain harmful bacteria that can cause serious illness in children, the elderly, and persons with weakened immune systems.

Juices made locally, such as apple cider from a nearby orchard, aren't required to provide this warning unless there is a state ruling. Juice bars and restaurants that sell freshly squeezed juice in glasses to drink right away don't need to provide this warning, either.

CHAPTER 12

The Safe Kitchen

America's food supply is one of the safest in the world. All those along the food chain—farmers, food manufacturers, supermarkets, and restaurants—are required by law to follow strict food safety regulations, which are carefully monitored. Once food leaves the grocery store, the responsibility for food safety is up to you. Because of the risks posed by foodborne illness, the Dietary Guidelines for Americans provide advice for keeping food safe to eat. Read on!

We've all heard the most important rules for handling food safely: Keep all food clean, keep hot foods hot, and keep cold foods cold. But just what is the temperature connection? How can you keep foods clean and safe . . . for "goodness sake," wherever you eat: home, work, picnic, on the road? And most important, how does food safety affect your health?

Foodborne Illness: More Common than You Think!

Imagine . . . an upset stomach, diarrhea, and fever. Do you have the flu? Your illness actually may be foodborne illness, not flu (a respiratory viral infection).

Foodborne illness, sometimes called food poisoning, comes from eating contaminated food. But the symptoms can easily be mistaken for other health problems. In fact, symptoms vary from fatigue, chills, a mild fever, dizziness, headaches, an upset stomach, and diarrhea, to dehydration, severe cramps, vision problems, and even death. Although actual incidence is unknown, foodborne illness may lead to a small percentage of some long-term health problems, too, including arthritis and Guillain-Barré syndrome.

Food safety and health experts at the Centers for Disease Control and Prevention (CDC) have estimated that seventy-six million people get sick, more than three hundred twenty-five thousand are hospitalized, and five thousand Americans die each year as a result of foodborne illness. Foodborne illnesses that result in more severe symptoms and death usually are diagnosed. However, the less severe "nuisance" symptoms more likely go unreported. While many reported cases are caused by food prepared outside the home, small outbreaks in home settings are considered to be far more common.

The ways people react to foodborne bacteria and contaminated food differ. One person may show no symptoms; another may get very ill. The reaction depends on the type of bacteria or toxin, how extensively the food was contaminated, how much food was eaten, and the person's susceptibility to the bacteria.

Anyone can be a victim of foodborne illness, but some people are at increased risk. They may include friends and families you entertain, perhaps at holiday parties or casual gatherings. You may not be aware that someone you offer food to is at high risk; always make food safety a high priority! *See "Who Is at High Risk for Foodborne Illness?" in this chapter.*

Bacteria cause most cases of foodborne illnesses, usually due to improper food handling. But foods also can be contaminated by viruses, parasites, and toxic chemicals such as cleaning supplies stored near food. With proper hand washing when preparing and handling food, nearly half of all cases of foodborne illness can be prevented. (With government, industry, and consumer food safety efforts, CDC reported that the incidences of foodborne illness may be declining. But there are ups and downs.)

Bacteria Basics

Life begins at 40! Between 40° F and 140° F, a single bacterium can multiply to become trillions in just

Have You Ever Wondered

. . . how much you need to worry about mayonnaise in picnic foods and brown-bag lunches? Mayonnaise is a perishable spread, so it must stay chilled. Homemade mayonnaise, made with uncooked eggs, is potentially more hazardous than its commercial counterpart and isn't considered appropriate for people at high risk. Commercial mayonnaise and salad dressings, made with pasteurized ingredients, also contain salt and more acid, which slow bacteria growth. In unrefrigerated mayonnaise-based salads such as chicken, tuna, or egg salad, it's usually not the mayonnaise that poses the risk but the chicken, tuna, or eggs.

. . . if fish you catch are safe to eat? About 20 percent of fish eaten in the United States are caught for personal use. They're okay if caught in safe waters. However, seafood toxins, which occur naturally in some waters, and fish contaminated by chemicals in the water pose health risks. Check with authorities from your local and state health department, state fishery agency, or Sea Grant office for a current safety status. Follow advisories.

. . . how food irradiation affects food safety? Food irradiation breaks down the DNA molecules in harmful organisms such as *Salmonella, E. coli,* and other foodborne bacteria. In that way it can dramatically reduce or eliminate disease-causing bacteria and other harmful bacteria, and so reduce or prevent outbreaks of foodborne illness. With that in mind, you still need to handle food properly to keep it safe to eat. *See "Irradiated Foods: Safe to Eat? in chapter 9.*

twenty-four hours! Why the exponential leap? Under the right conditions, bacteria double in number every twenty to thirty minutes.

Even with so many, you can't see bacteria without a microscope. Unlike microorganisms that cause food to spoil, you can't taste or smell most bacteria. Yet they live everywhere—in many foods, on your skin, under your fingernails, on other surfaces, and on pets and other live animals. Foods of animal origin—raw meat, poultry, fish, eggs, raw (unpasteurized) milk—are the most common food sources of bacteria. Although less common, harmful bacteria also can be transferred to fresh produce, perhaps through contaminated water or soil residue.

Because they're everywhere, you can't avoid harmful bacteria completely. Fortunately, from a food safety standpoint, most adults don't need to worry about harmful bacteria—at least not in small numbers. Your body can handle small amounts with no threat to your health. However, you are at risk for foodborne illness when bacteria multiply to very large numbers—which can happen when you mishandle food. **Caution:** Young children, pregnant women, older adults, and people whose immune systems don't function normally are at greater risk, even for small amounts of harmful bacteria.

To survive and multiply, bacteria need time and the right conditions: food, moisture, and warm temperature. Many need oxygen, too. Bacteria thrive on protein. Foods with protein—meat, poultry, fish, eggs, milk—offer the medium for bacteria to grow. The ideal temperatures for bacterial growth are between 40° F and 140° F. Above 160° F, heat destroys bacteria. Refrigerating foods below 40° F slows their growth. Freezing stops but doesn't kill bacteria. *Check "The Danger Zone" on page 282.*

Mishandling food—improper preparation, cooking, or storage—is the culprit action that allows bacteria to grow and multiply in your kitchen. With its rich supply of nutrients and often moist quality, food offers the perfect medium for bacteria to grow in.

Most bacteria won't harm you. Some, such as those used to make yogurt, some cheeses, and vinegar, are helpful. Yet harmful bacteria are the main sources of foodborne illness in the United States. That's why keeping bacteria under control is so vital to your health.

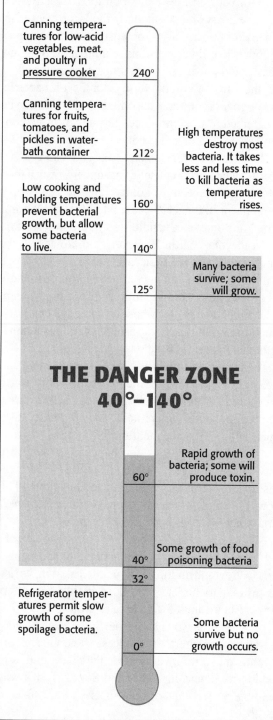

The Danger Zone

Effects of temperature (°F) on growth of bacteria in food. The most dangerous zone of temperature is between 40° and 140° F.

Canning temperatures for low-acid vegetables, meat, and poultry in pressure cooker — 240°

Canning temperatures for fruits, tomatoes, and pickles in water-bath container — 212°

High temperatures destroy most bacteria. It takes less and less time to kill bacteria as temperature rises.

Low cooking and holding temperatures prevent bacterial growth, but allow some bacteria to live. — 160° / 140°

125° — Many bacteria survive; some will grow.

THE DANGER ZONE 40°–140°

60° — Rapid growth of bacteria; some will produce toxin.

40° — Some growth of food poisoning bacteria

32°

Refrigerator temperatures permit slow growth of some spoilage bacteria.

0° — Some bacteria survive but no growth occurs.

If you suspect that food is contaminated, don't even taste it! You can't see, smell, or taste bacteria that cause foodborne illness. Securely wrap the suspected food, and discard it where neither humans nor animals can get at it.

Bacteria: Hard Hitters

Although as many as a hundred bacteria cause foodborne illness, these are among the worst troublemakers: *Salmonella, Staphylococcus aureus, Campylobacter jejuni, Clostridium perfringens, Clostridium botulinum, Escherichia coli O157:H7,* and *Listeria monocytogenes.* You also may hear about *Shigella, Vibrio vulnificus,* and *Yersinia enterocolitica,* three other bacteria that cause foodborne illness.

Salmonella, the second most common cause of foodborne illness, is found mostly in raw or undercooked poultry, meat, eggs, fish, and unpasteurized milk. Control is simple enough—proper cooking kills *Salmonella.* Combat this bacterium by cooking foods thoroughly, especially eggs, poultry, and meat; by keeping foods clean; and by consuming only pasteurized milk.

Raw milk, even if it's certified, may not be a wise choice because it isn't pasteurized. Pasteurized milk is quickly heated to a temperature high enough to kill harmful bacteria such as *Salmonella.* Raw milk and unpasteurized cheese are sold in gourmet and specialty stores.

Staphylococcus aureus (staph) spreads from someone handling food. It's carried on the skin, nose, and throat and in skin infections; then it spreads to food. Toxins, or poisons, produced by staph aren't killed by ordinary cooking. That's why personal hygiene and cleanliness in the kitchen are so important!

Campylobacter jejuni is estimated to be the major bacterial cause of diarrhea in the United States. Like *Salmonella, Campylobacter jejuni* can be transferred to raw and undercooked poultry and meat, unpasteurized milk, and untreated water.

The good news is that *Campylobacter jejuni* can be destroyed easily through safe food handling and water treatment systems. To protect yourself, always cook food thoroughly and avoid cross-contamination by washing utensils, cutting boards, and hands after handling raw poultry or meat. Avoid raw, unpasteurized milk. And if you're camping, always treat water from streams or lakes.

Clostridium perfringens is present everywhere, growing where there's little or no oxygen. Sometimes called the "buffet germ," it grows fastest in large portions—such as casseroles, stews, and gravies—held at low or room temperatures in "the danger zone." Chafing dishes that aren't hot enough and large portions that don't cool quickly in the refrigerator are breeding grounds. To slow bacterial growth, replace buffet food often, rather than put out large portions for an extended time. Refrigerate leftovers quickly.

Clostridium botulinum is rare. Yet, left untreated, botulism is often fatal! It requires immediate medical attention. Botulism-causing bacteria can come from home-canned or commercially canned foods. Usually these are low-acid canned foods such as meats and vegetables that haven't been processed or stored properly. Foods improperly canned at home, as well as improperly handled home-prepared herbal oils, pose a higher risk.

Look for warning signs: swollen or leaking cans or lids, cracked jars, loose lids, and clear liquids turned milky. Beware of cans or jars that spurt when they're opened. Never eat—or even taste—these foods. For home canning, always use approved methods. Heat home-canned meats and vegetables thoroughly, about fifteen to twenty minutes, before serving. And serve or refrigerate baked potatoes and grilled vegetables right away. Cooked root vegetables held at room, instead of refrigerated, temperature can be a problem. That's especially true when they're wrapped in foil; botulinum spores thrive without the air!

Escherichia coli (E. coli), a common bacterium, exists in your intestinal tract. For the most part, it's harmless. However, some strains are associated with travelers' diarrhea caused by contaminated drinking water, as well as with diarrhea among infants.

One strain—*E. coli O157:H7*—has received attention because its effects can be so severe. This strain, associated with eating raw or undercooked ground beef, or drinking unpasteurized milk or unpasteurized cider, can cause life-threatening health problems: hemorrhagic colitis with severe abdominal cramps, bloody diarrhea, nausea, and vomiting and perhaps hemolytic uremic syndrome (HUS), which may cause kidney failure, brain damage, strokes, seizures, and

Who Is at High Risk for Foodborne Illness?

- Pregnant women
- Young children
- Older adults
- People with weakened immune systems or certain chronic illnesses

If you're at high risk, follow general advice for food safety and take *extra* precautions:

- Do not eat or drink unpasteurized juice, raw sprouts, raw (unpasteurized) milk, and products made with unpasteurized milk.
- Do not eat raw or undercooked meat, poultry, eggs (or foods made with them), fish, and shellfish (clams, oysters, scallops, and mussels).
- Avoid soft cheeses such as feta, Brie, Camembert, blue-veined, and Mexican-style cheeses.
- Eat only certain deli meats and frankfurters, reheated to steaming hot.

New information on food safety is constantly emerging. Recommendations and precautions for people at high risk are updated as scientists learn more about preventing foodborne illness. *If you are among those at high risk,* be aware of and follow the most current information on food safety. For the latest information and precautions, talk to your healthcare provider, check the government's food safety Web site *(http://www.foodsafety.gov),* or *call the government information numbers listed in the Appendices.*

Source: Dietary Guidelines for Americans (2005).

If you or someone you know is at high risk and needs help with meals, find out about services such as home-delivered meals in your community. Check to be sure that the service follows food safety regulations. *To find services in your community, see "To Find Food and Nutrition Services" in chapter 24.*

death, especially in young children and the elderly.

To combat all strains of *E. coli,* cook and reheat meat thoroughly. Be especially careful of ground meat—for example, hamburgers—because bacteria on the surface of the meat get mixed into the center of the meat, which takes longer to cook. Keep cutting surfaces clean. Avoid cross-contamination of raw food, or transferring bacteria from one food to another with dirty utensils, cutting boards, plates, and hands. Raw milk and produce also may be sources.

Listeria monocytogenes can cause a less common but potentially fatal foodborne illness called listeriosis. Pregnant women, infants, older adults, and those with weakened immune systems are more susceptible. *Listeria* are part of your everyday surroundings, including places where food is processed. It can grow even under proper refrigeration.

Because *Listeria* is common in unpasteurized milk and in cheese made from unpasteurized milk, avoid unpasteurized milk products. *Listeria* also can be found in raw and undercooked meat, poultry, seafood, and eggs, and in produce. As with any packaged food product, follow the "keep refrigerated" advice on the label, the "use by" date on the package, and the reheating instructions.

To avoid *Listeria*, high-risk individuals are advised by the U.S. Food and Drug Administration to avoid soft cheeses (such as Brie, Camembert, feta, and Mexican-style cheeses); refrigerated pâtés and meat spreads; and smoked seafood (such as lox, jerky, or nova-style) that require refrigeration. When they haven't been reheated to a safe internal temperature, frankfurters and deli meat (except for very salty ham or hard salami) are considered very high risk for listeriosis.

Shigella, one source of bacterial diarrhea, is transmitted from improper handling of either food or water. It originates in the feces of infected humans and easily passes from one person to another through improper hand washing. Proper cooking eliminates it; uncooked food such as potato, tuna, or chicken salad is more likely the source.

Vibrio vulnificus, a bacterium in shellfish, especially in mollusks, can be fatal within two days of developing the condition. Symptoms include sudden chills, fever, nausea, vomiting, and stomach pain. Although this bacterium is destroyed in the intestinal tract or in the immune system of most healthy people, this form of foodborne illness can be very serious, even fatal for high-risk individuals. These bacteria multiply even during refrigeration. Thoroughly cooking shellfish destroys them.

Yersinia enterocolitica is most often found in contaminated raw or undercooked pork products (including chitterlings, or pork intestines). The most common

symptoms: for young children, fever, abdominal pain, and diarrhea, often bloody, and for older children and adults, fever and abdominal pain that feels like appendicitis. Unpasteurized milk or untreated water also may transmit this bacterium. In most cases the body can handle a yersiniosis infection without antibiotics. As prevention, avoid eating raw or undercooked pork and unpasteurized dairy foods, wash hands well, avoid cross-contamination, and dispose of animal feces in a sanitary way. If you're making chitterlings, have someone else care for your children. *For cooking pork, see "Safe Internal Temperatures" in this chapter.*

Parasites and Viruses, Too

Bacteria cause most foodborne illness. However, parasites and viruses—other tiny organisms that contaminate food—are culprits, too. Parasites such as *Trichinella spiralis, Toxoplasma gondii, Cryptosporidium parvum, Entamoeba histolytica,* and *Giardia lamblia* survive by drawing on the nutrients of a living host. Viruses such as hepatitis A and *Calcivirus,* or Norwalk-like virus, act like parasites. Through the food chain, parasites and viruses can infect humans.

Trichinosis is contracted by consuming undercooked pork or game that has been infested with trichina larvae. With careful controls in the food industry, trichinosis is much less common today. However, still cook pork, game, and other meat to the recommended internal temperature to destroy any live trichina larvae. *See "Safe Internal Temperatures."*

Toxoplasmosis is caused by a parasite indirectly linked to raw and undercooked meat or poultry, unwashed fruits and vegetables, and contaminated water. It's also directly transferred to humans from cat feces. Pregnant women are at special risk because they can pass the parasite to their unborn baby. The disease can severely affect the central nervous system, causing mental impairment and visual disorders. To combat this parasite, cook meat, especially pork, lamb, and poultry, thoroughly. For pregnant women, avoid handling a cat's litter box; have it cleaned daily. Keep your cat indoors. If you do handle cats, wash your hands well with soap and water.

Cryptosporidium, traditionally linked to travelers' diarrhea in developing nations, has become a more common parasitic illness in the United States. It enters

Have You Ever Wondered

. . . if you need to be concerned about "red tide"? No, unless you harvest your own shellfish. "Red tide" happens when marine algae are in a time of excessive growth. That's when they produce shellfish toxins that may cause illness. These areas are carefully monitored to protect the shellfish supply. Heed "red tide" warnings issued by local authorities if you harvest your own shellfish.

. . . if mercury in seafood is risky? Mercury is naturally present in all living things as well as in soil, air, and water. Pollution also releases into the air mercury that falls into water or on land, then washes into lakes, rivers, and oceans. Bacteria in water change mercury to methyl mercury, which is toxic. Over time methyl mercury can build up in long-lived larger fish.

Because methyl mercury is a potential risk to the developing nervous system of the fetus or the child, the U.S. Food and Drug Administration (FDA) and the Environmental Protection Agency advise: Women who are pregnant or who might become pregnant and nursing mothers should avoid eating shark, swordfish, king mackerel, and tilefish. Eat up to 12 ounces (2 average meals) a week of a variety of fish, lower in mercury (for example, shrimp, canned light tuna, salmon, pollock, and catfish), that can include up to 6 ounces of albacore ("white") tuna. Check local fishing advisories about fish you catch. No advice? You can eat up to 6 ounces of locally caught fish, if that's all the fish you eat that week. This advice also applies to young children, but serve smaller portions. *Note:* Fish in fish sticks and "fast-food" sandwiches are usually made with fish that is low in mercury.

. . . if your food is safe from "mad cow disease" and "foot-and-mouth" disease? These are different diseases. Although foot-and-mouth disease (FMD) is highly contagious among livestock and is economically disastrous, it poses no human risk, and FMD hasn't been found in U.S. livestock for about 75 years. Because travelers who visit agricultural areas can bring it back, the government prohibits import of agricultural products by people entering the United States who've been on a farm abroad or in contact with livestock abroad, and inspects their baggage. Before returning to the United States from FMD-infected areas, the U.S. Department of Agriculture (USDA) advises: Avoid agricultural areas five days before returning to the United States; clean and disinfect footwear with detergent and bleach; wash or dry-clean clothing; and avoid contact with livestock or wildlife for five days after returning to the United States. As other safety measures, the USDA regularly monitors U.S. cattle herds and has banned animals and animal products from infected areas. *Note:* FMD is different from hand, foot, and mouth disease (HFMD), common among infants and children.

"Mad cow disease," or bovine spongiform encephalopathy (BSE), affects the nervous system in cattle; it may be linked to a brain-wasting illness in humans known as Creutzfeldt-Jakob disease. To protect the U.S. food supply, government regulations have imposed import bans to make sure no live cattle or products from these animals are imported from areas where BSE is known to exist or is at risk, a ban on most mammalian protein in cattle feed, and a USDA surveillance program. Since 2004, FDA and, similarly, USDA regulations exclude potentially risky cattle products from human food, dietary supplements, and cosmetics. No research indicates that BSE is transmitted to cow milk. If you travel to Europe, where BSE is known to exist, your risk for getting this disease is very small, according to the National Institutes of Health. If you're concerned, however, avoid beef or beef products, or eat only solid pieces of meat rather than ground-beef products such as burgers or sausage when you travel there.

---

the environment through the feces of warm-blooded animals, including humans. Contaminated water or ice usually is the source. Municipal water filtration controls this parasite; chlorine doesn't destroy it. Proper hand washing and food handling are extra controls you can take at home. People with compromised immune systems and children are among those at higher risk. *See "Drinking Water: For Special Health Needs" in chapter 8.*

Giardiasis, most often caused by drinking untreated water, also may be transmitted by uncooked food contaminated with *Giardia* or by passing the parasite from hand to hand on surfaces. In recent years, giardiasis has become one of the most common causes

Need more strategies for food safety? Check here for "how-tos":

- Purify unsafe water—see chapter 8.
- Buy pasteurized juice—see chapter 11.
- Learn to eat out safely—see chapter 14.
- Take food safety precautions when you travel—see chapter 14.

of waterborne disease among humans in the United States. Another source of gastrointestinal symptoms, it more likely strikes campers and hikers, travelers, diaper-age children who go to day-care centers, and others who drink untreated water from contaminated sources. Symptoms typically appear one to two weeks after infection and may last several weeks. Boiling

Should You Call Your Doctor?

Suppose you suspect foodborne illness. You or a family member has an upset stomach, diarrhea, vomiting, fatigue, abdominal discomfort, or a fever. Symptoms of foodborne illness can appear from thirty minutes to three weeks after eating contaminated food. Most often, though, symptoms appear within four to forty-eight hours after eating. Symptoms usually pass within twenty-four to forty-eight hours; rest and plenty of fluids are the best ways to treat most cases. Some foodborne illnesses can affect your health for weeks, months, even years. Talk to your healthcare provider if you think that food has made you sick. In some circumstances it's very important that you receive care from a doctor:

- When diarrhea is bloody. This may be a symptom of *E. coli O157:H7.*
- When diarrhea or vomiting is excessive. This may lead to dehydration if fluids aren't replaced.
- When these three symptoms all appear: stiff neck, severe headache, and fever. The victim may have *Listeria,* which can be life-threatening.
- When you suspect illness from *Clostridium botulinum* or *Vibrio vulnificus,* which can be fatal.
- When the victim is at high risk—perhaps a young child, an elderly person, or someone whose immune system is compromised due to illness.
- When symptoms persist longer than three days.

What Do You Do if You Suspect Foodborne Illness?

- Call or see a medical professional. Physicians and laboratories are responsible for contacting the appropriate health department to report diagnosis of foodborne illness. However, most cases of foodborne illness aren't diagnosed; the symptoms simply are treated to relieve discomfort.
- Report the incident to your local health department as soon as possible if the suspected food came from a public place or large gathering—a restaurant, sidewalk vendor, employee cafeteria, company picnic, or grocery store, among others.
- If you are reporting the incident, try to preserve the suspected food. Ask authorities for instructions for packaging and storing the food until it can be collected by them. If you can, keep the packaging; it identifies where the product was produced. Mark it with a warning label so no one consumes it.

If you suspect that a food has been contaminated by a household chemical:

- Check the label for an antidote or a remedy. Likely you'll find an "800 or other toll-free" number for first-aid advice, too. Follow the advice.
- Call the national hotline to reach a poison control center: 1-800-222-1222. This number will automatically link you to the closest poison control center. Another option: Contact your local health department or use a local poison control center number. As a precaution, post their phone numbers by your telephone. You'll have them handy if needed.

destroys *Giardia* in water; chlorine may not if the chlorine concentration isn't high enough. Good hand-washing habits are essential to its control. If you travel or camp, only drink from a safe water supply, and wash and peel produce before eating it.

What if there's a giardiasis outbreak in your child's day-care center? If it continues despite control efforts, children with or without symptoms might be screened and perhaps treated. If your child has symptoms (diarrhea, abdominal cramps, nausea), contact your healthcare provider. The American Academy of Pediatrics doesn't advise treatment for children diagnosed with giardiasis who don't have diarrhea—unless poor appetite, weight loss, or fatigue are observed.

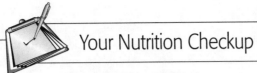

Your Nutrition Checkup

Kitchen Safety

How's your food safety savvy? Are you clean and careful enough to keep foodborne illness out of your kitchen? Take this kitchen safety checkup to find out.

Do You . . .	ALWAYS	USUALLY	SOMETIMES	NEVER
Wash your hands with warm, soapy water before and after handling food? Dry them with a clean cloth?	_____	_____	_____	_____
Change your dishtowels and dishcloths every few days?	_____	_____	_____	_____
Clean up splatters in your microwave oven immediately with hot, soapy water?	_____	_____	_____	_____
Sanitize cutting boards after each use with a chlorine bleach-water solution?	_____	_____	_____	_____
Clean your refrigerator each week, discarding foods that are too old?	_____	_____	_____	_____
Wash fresh vegetables and fruit?	_____	_____	_____	_____
Thaw foods in the refrigerator, not on the counter?	_____	_____	_____	_____
Rotate foods in your freezer and cupboards, with the oldest foods in front?	_____	_____	_____	_____
Check foods in cans and jars for bulging or leaking before opening?	_____	_____	_____	_____
Marinate meat, poultry, and seafood in the refrigerator?	_____	_____	_____	_____
Grill food so it cooks evenly inside and outside?	_____	_____	_____	_____
Use a clean plate and fork to take cooked food from the grill to the table?	_____	_____	_____	_____
Clean your picnic cooler with hot, soapy water before you use it?	_____	_____	_____	_____
Use leftovers within three or four days?	_____	_____	_____	_____
Remove stuffing from chicken and turkey before refrigerating leftovers?	_____	_____	_____	_____
Avoid the urge to use the stirring spoon for a quick taste?	_____	_____	_____	_____
Use a clean knife and cutting board for vegetables after cutting meat, poultry, or seafood?	_____	_____	_____	_____
Use a meat thermometer to cook meat and poultry to a safe internal temperature? Cook eggs thoroughly?	_____	_____	_____	_____
Use pasteurized eggs in recipes calling for eggs that won't be cooked?	_____	_____	_____	_____
Put leftovers in the refrigerator within two hours of cooking?	_____	_____	_____	_____
Cook hamburger patties until they're 160° F and no longer pink inside?	_____	_____	_____	_____
Heat leftovers until they're steaming hot?	_____	_____	_____	_____
Clean the outdoor grill after every use?	_____	_____	_____	_____
Remove perishable foods from a buffet after two hours?	_____	_____	_____	_____
Store poultry, meat, and fish on the bottom of your refrigerator in containers that won't leak?	_____	_____	_____	_____
Subtotal	_____	_____	_____	_____

Now score yourself:

"Always": 4 points

"Usually": 3 points

"Sometimes": 2 points

"Never": 1 point

Your total score _____

When it comes to food safety, you need a perfect score—100 points! Anything less and you're putting yourself—and anyone who eats with you—at risk for foodborne illness. It's safe to assume that the higher your score, the lower the risk.

For any item on which you scored "3" or less, exert a conscious effort to make a change to "always." Keep reading—for more advice on food safety!

Take Control of Home Food Safety

1. Wash hands often.
2. Keep raw meats and ready-to-eat foods separate.
3. Cook to proper temperatures.
4. Refrigerate promptly below 40° F.

Source: Home Food Safety . . . It's in Your Hands (American Dietetic Association and ConAgra, Inc.

Amebiasis (*Entamoeba histolytica*) also comes from polluted water and vegetables grown in soil polluted with human feces. It's a problem mostly for travelers in less-developed areas. Symptoms include intestinal cramps and diarrhea.

Calicivirus, or Norwalk-like virus, is very common, but rarely diagnosed. It causes acute gastrointestinal illness, usually lasting two days. This virus is passed primarily from one infected person to another, often on the hands of kitchen workers who handle salads and sandwiches.

Hepatitis A virus comes from food contaminated by feces. The conditions caused by hepatitis, such as jaundice and liver problems, can be severe. Sometimes hepatitis A comes through the food chain from shellfish harvested from contaminated waters—perhaps where raw sewage is dumped. More commonly, an infected person who handles food without properly washing his or her hands can transmit the disease—often from a food-service operation. Cooking may not kill the virus. As a precaution, always choose a restaurant that looks clean. Eat only well-cooked seafood.

Checklist for a Clean Kitchen

From top to bottom, a clean kitchen offers a main line of defense against the spread of colds, flu, and foodborne illness. Before you work with food, eliminate the breeding grounds for harmful bacteria:

Hands. Wash your hands—front and back, between your fingers, under your fingernails—in warm, soapy water for at least twenty seconds before and after every step in preparing foods. That includes your kitchen helpers, including children. Teach kids to sing "The Alphabet Song" while they wash their hands; that

takes about twenty seconds. Use disposable paper towels or a clean cloth to dry your hands completely.

Why is hand washing so important? Bacteria live and multiply on warm, moist hands. Hands pick up germs, spreading them from surface to surface, food to food, and person to person. One of the best ways to control the spread of illness is thorough proper hand washing—even while you're multitasking! That includes desktop and drive-time dining.

Work surfaces. Clean them often to remove food particles and spills. Use hot, soapy water. Keep nonfood items—mail, newspapers, purses—off the counters and away from food and utensils. Wash the counter carefully before food preparation.

Utensils. Wash dishes and cookware carefully in the dishwasher or in hot (at least 140° F), soapy water. Rinse well. Chipped dishes can collect bacteria.

Towels and dishcloths. Change them often. Wash them in the hot cycle of your washing machine. Dry them between each use. Being damp, they're the perfect

Wash Your Hands More Often

Before you:
- Handle or prepare food
- Eat meals
- Feed children

After you:
- Prepare food
- Touch raw food, especially meats and poultry
- Switch food preparation tasks
- Touch eggs and egg-rich foods
- Use the rest room
- Change a diaper
- Clean an appliance
- Handle garbage or dirty dishes
- Smoke a cigarette
- Pet animals and scoop animal feces
- Use the phone or computer
- Touch face, hair, body, other people
- Touch a cut or a sore, cough, or sneeze
- Clean or touch dirty laundry

Adapted from: Home Food Safety . . . It's in Your Hands (American Dietetic Association and ConAgra, Inc.).

breeding ground for bacteria. Throw out dirty sponges, or wash them in a bleach-water solution.

Appliances. On any appliance, clean spills right away including liquids from opened packages of hot dogs and deli meat. Wash appliance surfaces with hot, soapy water. Pay attention to the refrigerator and the freezer—shelves, sides, and door—where foods are stored. (Pack perishables in coolers while you clean or defrost your refrigerator and freezer.) Splatters inside your microwave oven harbor bacteria. Keep it clean!

Safe from Cross-Contamination

Cross-contamination happens when bacteria in one food spread to another, often from a cutting board, knife, plate, spoon, or your hands. For example, drippings from raw meat, poultry, and seafood left on a cutting board can transfer bacteria to vegetables, which are being sliced next.

Cutting boards. Use cutting boards that clean easily: smooth hard maple, acrylic, plastic, marble, or glass, free of cracks and crevices. Avoid boards made of soft, porous materials. After each use, wash them in hot,

soapy water, rinse, and dry well, perhaps in the dishwasher. Rinsing or wiping isn't enough!

Clean a cutting board after using it to cut raw meat, poultry, or seafood. If you prefer wooden cutting boards, keep one just for raw meat, poultry, and seafood. Mark it to avoid confusion. Discard wooden boards with deep grooves and knife scars that can't be cleaned easily.

Sanitize cutting boards with a chlorine bleach-water solution after each use: mix 2 teaspoons of bleach in a quart of water. Let the boards air-dry. Brush to reach grooves and other hard-to-reach places.

Utensils. Unless it's cleaned well in between, avoid using the same knife to slice meat and chop vegetables.

Although hard to resist, remind everyone who ventures in the kitchen—never taste with the stirring spoon! If children reach for a finger-licking taste, be sure they wash their hands before continuing to help in the kitchen. There's another reason to resist tasting: if food (perhaps meat sauce) isn't cooked through yet, it may still harbor harmful bacteria!

Other reminders. Store produce in clean bags or containers after you wash it, not in the store bag. If you

Have You Ever Wondered

. . . if you make any common food mistakes? Here they are: countertop thawing, leftovers left out of the fridge, unclean cutting board, store-to-refrigerator lag time, room-temperature marinating, grilling blunder (same platter for raw and grilled meats), "doggie bag" delay, stirring-and-tasting spoons, shared knife for trimming raw meat and chopping vegetables, undercooked high-risk foods such as eggs, meat, poultry, and fish, hide-and-eat Easter eggs.

. . . if acrylamide is a health risk? In your own kitchen and in food processing, acrylamide forms naturally in foods such as fries, browned breads, and toasted cereals. That happens as sugars react with certain amino acids as some foods are cooked at high temperatures: perhaps fried, baked, or toasted. Likely around since cooking began, acrylamide has been detected only recently at very low levels in food. There's not enough research to conclude that acrylamide, a potential carcinogen, is a human health risk. Yet FDA is one of many

institutions involved in long-term research. The best advice based on what's known now: there's no reason to change your food or cooking habits. Eat a variety of healthful foods, plenty of fruits and vegetables, and go easy on fatty and fried foods.

. . . if you can catch bird flu from eating chicken? The U.S. Department of Agriculture (USDA) advises: proper food handling and cooking (*described in this chapter*) protect against avian influenza and other viruses and bacteria such as Salmonella. Cooking eggs properly and cooking poultry to safe internal temperatures (*see page 298*) should destroy any possible foodborne virus. The chance of catching avian influenza from cooked poultry and eggs is extremely low. The USDA and other government agencies are working to protect poultry and eggs and prevent infected poultry and eggs from reaching consumers. If you travel to places affected by bird flu (avian influenza), check with the Centers for Disease Control for current traveler's advice.

have an open cut or sore, wear latex gloves to handle food. Open food bags with a clean knife or scissors.

Safekeeping

Store food in the right container, in the right place, at the right temperature, for the right length of time. Foods maintain their quality, safety, and nutrients when they're stored properly and used within a certain time. Besides, you stretch your food dollar when you don't need to discard spoiled food. *To determine the freshness of a packaged food, see chapter 11.*

In the Cupboard

How long do nonrefrigerated foods keep their quality? That depends on how carefully you store them. For safe, dry storage, store food for keeps!

● Keep your cupboards and pantries clean, dry, dark, and cool—preferably away from heat-producing appliances. Ideally 50° F to 70° F is the best storage temperature range. High temperatures (over 100° F) lower the quality of canned foods.

● Organize your cupboards with older cans up front for first use. The good news is: canned foods do have a long shelf life. Stored properly, most unopened canned foods stay edible and keep their nutritional quality well beyond two years. Although the food is still safe to eat for a long time, the color and texture of the food may change after a while.

● Be alert for food spoilage. Never use food from cans that are cracked, bulging, or leaking or that spurt liquid when opened. Food may be contaminated with deadly botulism organism. Toss—don't taste!

● Store opened packages of food in dry, airtight containers. That keeps out insects and rodents and keeps food from absorbing odors.

● Store foods away from kitchen chemicals and refuse. As important, keep chemicals and refuse away from places where food is prepared and eaten.

In the Fridge

Do "science experiments" ever grow in your refrigerator? Is yesterday's meat loaf hiding behind tomorrow's juice carton? Has that special cheese become as

Have You Ever Wondered

... if molds on cheese are dangerous? Not usually. Few molds on cheese produce toxins, or poisons. But just to be on the safe side, discard one inch of the cheese on all sides where mold is visible. Re-cover the food with fresh, clean wrap. Soft cheeses such as cream cheese, Brie, and cottage cheese, and other foods with mold on them, should be discarded. The exceptions are mold-ripened cheeses such as blue, Gorgonzola, Roquefort, and Stilton. Check the color and the pattern of the mold. If it's different from the usual blue or green veins and you see furry spots or white, pink, blue, green, gray, or black flecks, discard the cheese. Mold spores may have spread throughout the cheese.

dry as old leather? With the hustle and bustle of today's living, these things happen, even in the best kitchens. To keep perishable food safe and out of the "danger zone," wrap it and store it right. Follow safe handling instructions on food packages and labels. *For a safe food handling label found on fresh meat and poultry, see "Safe Handling Instructions" on page 250.*

● Keep your refrigerator cold—between 34° F and 40° F. In this range, bacteria that spoil food grow slowly. Below 32° F, which is freezing, bacteria survive but won't grow. Keep a refrigerator thermometer inside on the middle shelf; buy one at the supermarket. Remind your family to make their refrigerator raids quick so the door doesn't stay open too long.

● Store all foods wrapped or in covered containers. Seal storage containers well to prevent moisture loss and absorption of off-odors. Unless the package is torn, leave food in its store wrapping. The less you handle food, the better. Store washed produce in a clean container, not the store bag.

● Transfer opened canned food to a clean container. It's safe to refrigerate food in covered cans after opening, but off-flavors may develop.

● Keep packages of raw meat, poultry, and fish in separate plastic bags, in a bowl or a pan, on the lowest refrigerator shelf so juices won't drip onto other foods. The lowest shelf usually is the coldest.

● Store food quickly. Avoid keeping perishable foods at room temperature for long. Cool leftovers and food cooked for later use in the refrigerator or freezer, not on the counter. Leftovers shouldn't be left at room temperature for longer than two hours.

● For faster cooling, store cooked food in small portions and in shallow containers. Large portions can take a long time to drop below 40° F.

● Keep leftovers where you'll see them. Then use them up within three or four days at the most. Toss them out if you can't remember when you stored them.

● Avoid overloading your refrigerator. Cold air needs room to circulate.

● Use refrigerator compartments. The meat keeper keeps meat extra cold so it stays fresher longer. Crisper bins help produce retain its moisture. Keep eggs, however, in their carton, not in the egg tray or door shelf, to keep them fresher longer. Use them within four to five weeks of the Julian date on the carton. *See "Eggs" in chapter 11 to read the date on an egg carton.*

● Eat perishable foods while they remain at peak quality. Discard foods, rather than risk foodborne illness, after they've passed their prime. Use fresh (unfrozen) beefsteaks, roasts, deli meats, and poultry within three to four days. Use ground meat, ground poultry, and fish within one to two days. You may notice that the interior of ground beef often is purplish-red in color. The color doesn't mean the meat is spoiled. Instead, it has not been in direct contact with oxygen. As it's exposed to air, meat will turn the familiar bright red. Toss meat and poultry with an off odor, a sticky or slimy surface, and perhaps a color change. *Check the chart "The Cold Truth: How Cold, How Long?" in this chapter.*

● Refrigerate cut, peeled, or cooked fresh fruits and vegetables within two hours.

● If you're not sure about a food's safety, toss it out! Never trust the odor or the appearance. Food may look, taste, and smell okay—even when it's no longer safe to eat. When in doubt, throw it out!

● Discard moldy food "under wraps." Put food in a bag or a wrapper so mold spores don't spread. Then clean the container and the refrigerator well.

Caution—Decorative Dishes

For years lead has been an ingredient in the glaze, or coating, on ceramic bowls, dishes, and pitchers. With proper firing, or heating in a kiln, glazes with lead are safe. However, when dishes are fired incorrectly or when copper is added to the glaze, hazardous amounts of lead can leach from dishes into food. Lead is harmful to health, collecting in bones and some soft tissues. Among other problems, lead poisoning can cause learning disabilities, organ damage, and even death. Children and pregnant women are particularly sensitive to the toxic effects of lead. *Check chapter 16.*

To be sure your dishes are safe enough for food, follow these guidelines:

● Inspect the surface of ceramic dishes. The surface that contacts food should be smooth and shiny, not rough or painted on top of the glaze.

● Check both sides of dishes, bowls, and pitchers. If it says "Not for Food Use" or "For Decorative Purposes Only," don't use it for food!

● Don't store food in ceramic dishes or leaded crystal. Lead can leach out when acidic foods and beverages such as coffee, juice, fruit, or wine come in contact with glaze or leaded crystal over time.

● Beware of ceramicware made by untrained potters. For the most part, today's hobbyists are well aware of the problems of lead glazes.

● Beware of ceramicware brought back from foreign travel and of older dishes, imported before government monitoring.

● To check your own dishes, purchase a lead-test kit. Find one at hardware or hobby stores.

● Refrigerate or freeze whole-grain foods since they tend to get rancid faster than refined grains.

In the Freezer

In freezer storage, the colder, the better. Freezing extends the shelf life of all kinds of foods.

● Keep your freezer "iceberg" cold! For long-term storage, maintain a freezer temperature of 0° F or less. A freestanding freezer can stay that cold. However, the freezer compartment of most refrigerators usually won't; plan to use foods stored there more quickly. To check the temperature, install a freezer thermometer, available at many kitchen stores or supermarkets.

● Store foods purchased frozen in their original packaging. Commercial packaging usually is airtight.

● Freezing home-prepared foods? Properly package them. Use freezer containers, foils, and moistureproof paper, plastic bags, or other wraps. Traditional plastic wraps aren't suitable. Use freezer tape to help keep the package airtight and free of freezer burn. For storage that's longer than a few days, fresh meat retains its quality best when it's rewrapped or overwrapped.

● Before freezing, label each package with the food, date, and the amount.

● Organize your freezer. Rotate foods, keeping the oldest foods in front so they're used first. Stack similar foods together—they'll be easier to find.

● Remember that some foods don't freeze well: bananas, fresh tomatoes, lettuce, celery, gelatin salads, custard, mayonnaise, hard-cooked eggs, sour cream, cream (unless it's whipped), raw potatoes, unblanched vegetables, and foods made with these ingredients. Freezing affects their quality, not the safety.

● Blanch vegetables to lengthen their freezer life: immerse foods in boiling water for one to three minutes, then plunge them in cold water to stop the cooking. Freeze in airtight plastic bags after draining well.

To Thaw Safely

● Thaw foods in the refrigerator, not on the counter. Bacteria thrive at room temperature. Put thawing food in a plastic bag or on a plate to collect any juices. If you need a fast thaw, remove the store wrap first; put meat, poultry, or fish in a microwave-safe container; and defrost on "low" or "defrost" settings in your microwave oven. Or thaw frozen meat, poultry, or fish in cold water that's changed every thirty minutes. Cold water chills the surface. Then cook the food right away!

● Plan ahead to defrost frozen meat in the refrigerator. Here's how long it takes:
- ● Large roast—four to seven hours per pound
- ● Small roast—three to five hours per pound
- ● 1-inch-thick package of ground beef—twenty-four hours
- ● 1-inch-thick steak—twelve to fourteen hours

● To thaw, especially small amounts, in a microwave oven, use the "defrost" setting. Once thawed, cook food right away. The time for microwave thawing depends on the amount of food you need to thaw.

When Your Power Goes Out

Suppose a storm, an accident, or another event shuts off power to your home—along with your refrigerator and freezer. You may not need to toss out food if you take a few precautions.

Keep the refrigerator and freezer doors closed so heat stays out and cold stays in. Unopened, most refrigerators stay chilled for about four hours, depending on the warmth of your kitchen. If the power is out longer, you might get dry or block ice to keep the refrigerator and freezer as cold as possible.

Frozen foods can hold for about two days in a full, freestanding freezer if it stays closed. Half full, a freezer remains cold for about one day. Freezers are well insulated; each frozen food package is an ice block, protecting foods around it.

Once the Power's Back On

Avoid using appearance or odor as your guide to food safety. Instead, follow these guidelines:

● If foods in the freezer still have ice crystals, or are at 40° F or less, refreeze them right away. Then use them as soon as you can.

THE COLD TRUTH: HOW COLD, HOW LONG?

How long can refrigerated and frozen food keep safely and remain at top quality? Freezer and refrigerator times vary. As long as the food is properly packaged, these are basic guidelines:

FOOD	REFRIGERATOR (40° F)	FREEZER (0° F)
Eggs		
Fresh eggs, in shell	4 to 5 weeks	Don't freeze
Hard-cooked eggs	1 week	Doesn't freeze well
Liquid pasteurized eggs or egg substitutes,		
Opened	3 days	Don't freeze
Unopened	10 days	1 year
Dairy products		
Milk	1 week	3 months
Cottage cheese	1 week	Doesn't freeze well
Yogurt	1 to 2 weeks	1 to 2 months
Commercial mayonnaise		
(refrigerate after opening)	2 months	Don't freeze
Vegetables	*Raw*	*Blanched/cooked*
Beans, green or waxed	3 to 4 days	8 months
Carrots	2 weeks	10 to 12 months
Celery	1 to 2 weeks	10 to 12 months
Lettuce, iceberg	1 to 2 weeks	Don't freeze
Lettuce, leaf	3 to 7 days	Don't freeze
Spinach	1 to 2 days	10 to 12 months
Squash, summer	4 to 5 days	10 to 12 months
Squash, winter	2 weeks	10 to 12 months
Tomatoes	2 to 3 days	2 months
Deli and Self-Serve Foods		
Store-prepared or homemade salads: egg,		
ham, chicken, tuna, macaroni salads	3 to 5 days	Don't freeze
Entrées, cold or hot	3 to 4 days	2 to 3 months
Frozen Dinners and Casseroles		
Keep frozen until ready to serve		3 to 4 months
*Hot Dogs**		
Opened package	1 week	Don't freeze
Unopened package	2 weeks	In freezer wrap, 1 to 2 months
Lunch Meats		
Opened	3 to 5 days	1 to 2 months
Unopened	2 weeks	1 to 2 months
Fresh Meat		
Beef—steaks, roasts	3 to 5 days	6 to 12 months
Pork—chops, roasts	3 to 5 days	4 to 6 months
Lamb—chops, roasts	3 to 5 days	6 to 9 months
Veal—roast	3 to 5 days	4 to 6 months

THE COLD TRUTH: HOW COLD, HOW LONG? *(continued)*

FOOD	REFRIGERATOR (40° F)	FREEZER (0° F)
Fresh Poultry		
Chicken or turkey, whole	1 to 2 days	1 year
Pieces	1 to 2 days	9 months
Giblets	1 to 2 days	3 to 4 months
Fresh Fish		
Lean fish (cod, flounder, etc.)	1 to 2 days	6 months
Fatty fish (salmon, etc.)	1 to 2 days	2 to 3 months
Ham and Corned Beef		
Canned ham (label says keep refrigerated)	6 to 9 months	Don't freeze
Ham, fully cooked, and corned beef (half and slices)	3 to 5 days	1 to 2 months
Corned beef, in pouch with pickling juices	5 to 7 days	Drained, wrapped, 1 month
Hamburger, Ground and Stew Meats		
Hamburger and stew meats	1 to 2 days	3 to 4 months
Ground turkey, veal, pork, lamb, and mixtures	1 to 2 days	3 to 4 months
Bacon and Sausage		
Bacon	1 week	1 month
Sausage, raw (pork, beef, turkey)	1 to 2 days	1 to 2 months
Precooked, smoked breakfast links, patties	1 weeks	1 to 2 months
Hard sausage (pepperoni, jerky sticks)	2 to 3 weeks	1 to 2 months
Leftovers		
Cooked meat, meat dishes, egg dishes, soups, stew, vegetables	3 to 4 days	2 to 3 months
Gravy and meat broth	1 to 2 days	2 to 3 months
Cooked poultry and fish	3 to 4 days	4 to 6 months

Fresh Produce

● The quality of certain perishable fresh fruits and vegetables (such as strawberries, lettuce, herbs, and mushrooms) can be maintained best by storing in the refrigerator. If you are uncertain whether an item should be refrigerated to maintain quality, ask your grocer.

● All produce purchased precut or peeled should be refrigerated for safety as well as quality.

● Produce cut or peeled at home should be refrigerated within two hours.

● Any cut or peeled produce that is left at room temperature for more than two hours should be discarded.

*Some may have package dates that may not be consistent with these guidelines.

Adapted from: To Your Health: Food Safety for Seniors (Washington, D.C.: U.S. Food and Drug Administration and U.S. Department of Agriculture, 2004).

● Discard perishable foods if the power has been out for more than four hours: meat, poultry, fish, milk, soft cheese, eggs, leftovers, and deli items. In that time, bacteria can multiply enough to cause illness. Dispose of them safely—where animals can't eat them. For more about what foods to keep and discard after an emergency, check USDA's: www.fsis.usda.gov.

● If the power's been out for only a few hours, keep less perishable foods. Fresh whole fruits and vegetables, hard and process cheeses, condiments, butter, and margarine often keep for several days at room temperature. Toss food out, however, if it turns moldy or smells bad.

Plan for Unexpected Emergencies

Wherever you live, keep a three-day supply of food and water for you, your family—and your pets.

● Stock up on nonperishable foods: ready-to-eat canned meat, fruits, juices, milk, soups, and vegetables. Canned foods are better than foods in glass bottles or jars because they won't break in a disaster. Choose single-serving portions, too; you may have no way to keep leftovers cold. Keep high-energy foods on hand, such as peanut butter, nuts, and trail mix.

● Rotate your emergency food and water supply every year or so. In that way it's fresh when you need it.

● Buy commercially bottled, well-sealed water, or store your own water in sanitized, food-grade containers (not milk cartons or jugs). Plan for 1 gallon of water per person per day. *See "Safe Enough to Drink" in chapter 8 for making contaminated water safe to drink.*

● Keep manual can openers on your emergency shelf. A well-stocked emergency shelf with no way to open food cans doubles any disaster!

For more advice about handling and perhaps discarding food and kitchen equipment after disasters (fires, floods, hurricanes) and power outages, contact experts: the U.S. Food and Drug Administration (FDA) Food Safety Hotline (1-888-SAFE-FOOD), the U.S. Department of Agriculture's Meat and Poultry Hotline (1-800-535-4555), your local American Red Cross, Cooperative Extension Service, Civil Defense, or emergency management office.

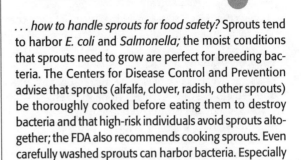

Have You Ever Wondered

. . . how to handle sprouts for food safety? Sprouts tend to harbor *E. coli* and *Salmonella;* the moist conditions that sprouts need to grow are perfect for breeding bacteria. The Centers for Disease Control and Prevention advise that sprouts (alfalfa, clover, radish, other sprouts) be thoroughly cooked before eating them to destroy bacteria and that high-risk individuals avoid sprouts altogether; the FDA also recommends cooking sprouts. Even carefully washed sprouts can harbor bacteria. Especially if you're at high risk, be aware that sandwiches and salads in restaurants may be made with raw sprouts.

To reduce your risk for foodborne illness if you choose to eat them raw, handle sprouts with care: refrigerate to slow bacterial growth; wash under cold, running water; and buy them fresh, with the buds on.

. . . about the safety of wild mushrooms? Stick with exotic mushrooms from the store if you're a mushroom-lover. Telling the difference between edible and poisonous (some deadly) mushrooms takes a lot of expertise. Unless they're gathered by a trusted mushroom expert, the best advice is to avoid them.

. . . if blood spots on eggs are okay? Yes, they happen naturally while the egg is forming, sometimes when a blood vessel on the yolk ruptures. You can remove them.

. . . if you need to wash bagged produce that's labeled "ready-to-eat, prewashed"? It's okay without further washing if kept refrigerated and used by the "use by" date.

Safe Preparation and Service

Preparing, cooking, and serving can't make your food safe—if it hasn't been handled properly from the very start. But, cared for safely all along, you can ensure its quality as you prepare and serve it.

"Prep" It Safe

● Wash fresh fruits and vegetables to remove any pathogens from dirt or handling—even if you discard rinds or peels—just before cooking or eating. Remove any outer leaves. Wash with clean, running water, but not soap. Porous surfaces of produce can absorb ingredients in soap products. If appropriate, use a brush. Dry produce with a clean towel; moisture left on pro-

duce may attract bacteria and promotes its growth if produce isn't eaten right away.

Cutting through unwashed produce can carry bacteria from its surface into the inside flesh. Remove bruised or damaged spots because they may harbor bacteria or mold. "Rust" spots on lettuce aren't harmful; they occur as cells in the leaf break down naturally after harvest.

● Check canned and jar foods before opening them. Make sure that safety buttons on jar lids are depressed and that canned goods are still safe, not bulging or leaking. Wash the tops of canned goods before opening them so particles don't fall into food. Vacuum-packed canned foods may hiss softly when they're opened. That's probably the normal release of air

Disaster Planning: Emergency Supply Checklist

Stocking up now on emergency supplies—and rotating them regularly—can add to your safety and comfort during and after a disaster. Store enough supplies for at least seventy-two hours. If you're in a flood area, store foods and eating utensils where they'd likely be away from contaminated water

FOOD AND WATER*

- Water: 1 gallon per person per day (for pets, too)
- Ready-to-eat canned meats (tuna, chicken, beef, chili), beans, soups, spaghetti
- Canned fruits, vegetables, juice; dried fruit, raisins; other dry foods
- Evaporated, powdered or ultrapasteurized milk
- Boxed soy beverage
- Crackers, ready-to-cereals, pretzels, instant oatmeal, pasta, rice
- Peanut butter, jelly, granola bars, trail mix, nuts
- Instant coffee, teabags, hot chocolate, meals, pudding, cookies, candy
- Staples: sugar, salt, pepper, mustard, catsup, mayonnaise, creamer
- Ready-to-eat infant formula, infant foods, food for elderly people and those with special needs, if appropriate
- Pet food, if appropriate

Avoid salty foods since they'll make you thirsty, a problem when water is in short supply.

COOKING

- Barbecue grill, camp stove, pots/pans
- Fuel for cooking (charcoal, propane, etc.)
- Plastic knives, forks, spoons
- Paper plates and cups
- Paper towels
- Heavy-duty aluminum foil
- Matches in a waterproof container
- Can opener (manual)
- Appliance (refrigerator) thermometer

The National Disaster Education Coalition provides more food and water related advice: www.disastereducation.org

SANITATION SUPPLIES

- Large plastic trash bags for trash, waste, water protection
- Large trash cans
- Bar soap and liquid detergent
- Hand sanitizer, wet wipes
- Shampoo
- Toothpaste and toothbrushes
- Feminine and infant supplies
- Toilet paper
- Household bleach
- Newspaper (to wrap garbage and waste)

SAFETY AND COMFORT

- Sturdy shoes, socks
- Heavy gloves for clearing debris
- Candles and matches in a waterproof container
- Change of clothing, sweatshirts
- Knife or razor blades
- Garden hose for siphoning and firefighting

OTHER SUPPLIES

- Copies of personal identification, medication prescriptions, and credit cards
- Medication that doesn't need refrigeration
- Extra keys for car and house
- Map with places you could go and phone numbers
- First-aid kit—freshly stocked
- First-aid book
- Suntan lotion, hats
- Blankets or sleeping bags
- Portable battery-powered radio or television, flashlight, and spare fresh batteries
- Essential medication and spare glasses
- Fire extinguisher: A-B-C type
- Ax, shovel, broom
- Crescent wrench for turning off gas
- Screwdriver, pliers, hammer
- Coil of 1/2-inch rope
- Plastic tape
- Tent
- Money
- Essential medication for pets
- Toys for children

*In case distribution is disrupted after an emergency, store a two-week supply if you have special food or medical needs.

Source: Adapted from American Red Cross WIC Program, San Diego, CA. "Emergency Supply Checklist." Governor's Office on Emergency Services, Sacramento CA, and the National Disaster Education Coalition.

pressure. A loud hiss or spurting may indicate food spoilage. Wash can openers after each use.

● Avoid washing raw meat and poultry. Besides being unnecessary, it increases the chance of cross-contamination.

● Devein shrimp if you want to. Cooking destroys any bacteria in shrimp, including in the intestinal vein. For cosmetic purposes you may want to remove it. In large shrimp the vein may contain a lot of grit.

● Keep juices from raw meat, poultry, or fish from coming in contact with other foods—cooked or raw. Use separate cutting boards, plates, trays, and utensils for cooked and uncooked meat, poultry, and fish.

● Marinate meat, poultry, and seafood in covered, nonmetallic containers—in the refrigerator! Many marinades have acid-containing ingredients—wine, vinegar, and citrus juice—that react with metals. These metals can leach into food.

● If you want to use marinade as a dip or sauce, make a double batch. Use half to marinate, then discard it after marinating. Use the rest for a sauce at serving time.

● Avoid mixing dark-colored sauces into ground meat or poultry. Dark-colored sauces such as teriyaki sauce, soy sauce, barbecue sauce, and Worcestershire sauce make it hard to judge the doneness of ground meat. Instead, brush sauces on cooked patties when they're almost cooked. When ground beef is cooked to the proper and safe inside temperature, the juices run clear; use a meat thermometer to check.

● Avoid eating raw seafood, meat, poultry, and eggs, or foods containing these foods. Foods with raw eggs include some recipes for homemade mayonnaise, homemade eggnog, homemade ice cream, Hollandaise sauce, and Caesar salad dressing. For people with a compromised immune system, even lightly cooked egg dishes such as soft custards and French toast can be risky. *See "Is Raw Seafood Safe to Eat?" if you choose to enjoy raw seafood occasionally.*

● If you stuff poultry, do so just before roasting, and stuff loosely. Be sure that the internal temperature of the meat reaches 180° F and the center of the stuffing reaches 165° F before removing from the oven. As an option, cook stuffing separately from chicken or

turkey, especially if you don't have a meat thermometer. Never cook stuffed poultry in a microwave oven. Refrigerate leftover poultry and stuffing separately.

● If you infuse oil with herbs or garlic, use it right away rather than store it. Botulism has been linked to consuming some home-prepared herb and garlic oils. Commercially prepared herb and garlic oils are required to contain protective additives to prevent possible foodborne illness. As an added precaution,

Is Raw Seafood Safe to Eat?

With sushi bars and with seviche (a popular Mexican and Caribbean appetizer), many people have come to enjoy raw and uncooked marinated seafood. With careful control, they can be safe; read on to learn how.

Shellfish, especially mollusks (oysters, clams, mussels, and scallops), may carry the bacterium *Vibrio vulnificus,* which multiplies even during refrigeration. Other viruses in uncooked or partly cooked mollusks also can cause severe diarrhea. *See the early part of this chapter for more about the risks related to* Vibrio vulnificus. Precautions reduce the risks:

● High-risk individuals—those with HIV, impaired immune systems, liver and gastrointestinal disorders, kidney disease, inflammatory bowel disease, cancer, diabetes, hemochromatosis, stomach problems, or steroid dependency—should avoid eating any raw or partly cooked fish. Pregnant women, infants, young children, older adults, and those with alcohol problems also are considered at high risk.

● If you prepare raw fish at home, start with high-quality seafood—very, very fresh, and use it within two days. Buy from a licensed, reputable dealer. For mollusks (clams, mussels, oysters), you can ask to see the certified shipper's tag. If you harvest your own, make sure the waters of origin are certified for safety. Follow the rules for safe food handling in this chapter. Even at that, eating raw fish at home isn't advised. You're wiser to cook fish to an internal temperature of 145° F to destroy parasites.

● If fish is sushi-grade or high-quality, sushi, sashimi, seviche, and oyster bars are generally safe. Reputable restaurants have highly trained chefs who not only know how to buy fish for safety and sanitation standards but also know how to handle fish safely.

See chapter 11 about buying fresh seafood.

always store commercial herb and garlic oil products in the refrigerator.

● Direct your coughs and sneezes away from food. Coughs and sneezes spread germs. Cover your mouth and nose with a tissue when you sneeze or cough. Then wash your hands with warm, soapy water.

Cook It Safe

● Keep hot food hot. Cook and hold cooked foods at temperatures higher than 140° F. High temperatures (160° F to 212° F) kill most bacteria. Temperatures between 140° F and 159° F prevent their growth but may let bacteria survive.

● Get the right tools for the job: a meat or "instant-read" thermometer to see when foods are thoroughly cooked; an oven thermometer to check your oven heat; and a timer to time the cooking accurately. Regularly check nondigital food thermometers; calibrate according to the manufacturer's directions.

● Check the internal temperature of food, especially roasts, thick steaks (more than 2 inches thick), large cuts of meat, whole chickens or turkeys, and large casseroles. Put the thermometer or oven temperature probe into the center of the thickest part of the food, but not near the bone or fat. After each use, wash the thermometer stem well in hot, soapy water. *See "Safe Internal Temperatures" and "Using a Meat Thermometer" in this chapter.*

● Cook ground meat and poultry thoroughly—until no longer pink inside, juices run clear, and the internal temperature reaches 160° F. Thorough cooking is especially important with ground meat; bacteria on the

Have You Ever Wondered

. . . how you store live mollusks? For the very short time you may keep them (within two days), refrigerate them in a container with a damp cloth over the top. Be sure other foods don't drip on them. Do not store them in an airtight container or in water. They're salt-water fish that need air to stay alive. Scrub them with a stiff brush just prior to shucking or cooking them.

Safe Internal Temperatures

For food safety—and the best flavor—cook meat and poultry to the right internal temperature. To check, use a meat or "instant-read" thermometer.

FOOD ITEM	INTERNAL, COOKED TEMPERATURE (° F)
Beef, Veal, and Lamb	
Ground products such as hamburger (as patties, meat loaf, meatballs, etc.)	160
Nonground products such as roasts and steaks	
Medium rare	145
Medium	160
Well done	170
Fresh Pork	
All cuts, including ground products	
Medium	160
Well done	170
Ham	
Fresh, raw ham	160
Fully cooked ham, to reheat	140
Fish	145
Poultry	
Ground chicken, turkey	165
Whole chicken, turkey	180
Boneless turkey roasts	170
Poultry breasts and roasts (white meat)	170
Poultry thighs, wings and drumsticks (dark meat)	180
Duck, goose	180
Stuffing (cooked alone or in bird)	165
Eggs	Yolks and whites are firm.
Egg dishes, casseroles, and cheesecakes	160
Leftovers, reheated	165
Sauces, soups, gravy	160

Source: Adapted from and consistent with guidelines from the U.S. Department of Agriculture, the U.S. Food and Drug Administration, and the 2005 Dietary Guidelines for Americans.

outside get mixed inside as meat and poultry are ground and mixed.

● Instead of "rare," cook beef until "medium rare" (to an internal temperature of 145° F) for safety.

● When in doubt, cook ham. If the label says "cooked ham," it's okay to eat without cooking or heating. If not, don't take chances; cook it before eating it. Words such as "smoked," "aged," or "dried" are no guarantee of safety without cooking. The smoked flavor may come from added flavoring, not curing.

● Follow the "ten-minute" rule for cooking finfish—whole fish, steaks, and fillets. For every inch of thickness, cook fish for ten minutes at 425° F to 450° F. If the fish is cooking in a sauce or foil wrap, cook for five minutes longer. The internal temperature should reach 145° F. If one end is thinner than another, fold it underneath so the thickness is uniform. This rule applies to broiling, grilling, steaming, baking, and poaching. Cooking times for frying and microwaving are generally faster ways to cook. If fish is cooked from a frozen state, double the cooking time. Cooked fish is opaque and flakes easily with a fork.

● Cook shellfish properly. Scallops and shrimp take three to five minutes, depending on size. Scallops turn white and firm; shrimp turn pink. Boiling lobsters takes five to six minutes per pound after the water comes back to a boil; when fully cooked, they turn bright red.

● Be sure that mollusks are still alive before you cook them. If the shells don't close tightly when you tap them, toss them! Cook them in a pot that's big enough to cook all the shellfish thoroughly—even the shells in the middle. Discard any that don't open during cooking. For live clams, mussels, and oysters: boil water for three to five minutes after the shells open, or steam them for four to nine minutes. *If they're shucked:*

   ● Bake them for about ten minutes at 450° F.
   ● Boil for at least three minutes or until the edges curl.
   ● Fry for at least ten minutes at 375° F.
   ● Broil them for at least three minutes.

● Know the visual signs of doneness: egg yolks and whites that are firm; fish that is opaque and flakes easily; juices from meat and poultry that aren't pink; and poultry joints that move easily.

● If you've been basting or brushing sauces on food as you cook, switch to a clean brush and fresh sauce for cooked foods. In that way you won't transfer bacteria from raw to cooked foods. Discard the marinade used for raw meat, poultry, or fish, or boil it for at least one minute before using on cooked food.

● Avoid very low oven temperatures (below 325° F) for roasting meat, or long or overnight cooking for meat. With oven cooking, these low temperatures encourage bacterial growth before the meat is cooked.

● Know how to use a slow cooker safely. Even though the food is cooked at a lower temperature, food prepared in a slow cooker is safe because the moist heat used to cook foods in this way is more lethal to bacteria than dry heat, such as oven cooking. Set the cooker on high until the food begins to bubble, then turn to a simmer or "low" setting to continue cooking. Cover and check the internal temperature, which should be at least 160° F. Always choose a recipe that contains a liquid. When adding meat, use small pieces of thawed meat. Avoid filling the cooker to more than two-thirds of its capacity. A slow cooker is not for reheating.

● Cook food through at one time. Don't cook it partially, then finish later. Partially cooked food may not get hot enough inside to destroy bacteria; these conditions may encourage bacteria to grow.

● Heat leftovers to 165° F or until steaming hot. That includes precooked foods such as stuffed chicken breasts and preroasted chickens from takeout; eat them the same day you purchase them. Reheat sauces and gravies to a rolling boil for at least one minute.

Play It Microwave-Safe

Today, a microwave oven is as common as a television set in our homes, workplaces, schools, and even recreational vehicles! For most people, the main reason is

For the Mile-High Cook

If you live at an altitude of 1,000 feet or more, you may need to cook food longer to kill bacteria. At higher altitudes, water boils at a lower temperature, which makes it less effective for killing bacteria. Most cooking and canning temperatures are based on food preparation at sea level.

cooking speed. However, microwaving also has nutrition benefits. Faster cooking helps retain nutrients and allows food to be cooked without added fat.

General cooking guidelines apply to microwave cooking. Since foods cook differently in a microwave oven, follow these special precautions:

● Use only microwave-safe containers. To see if your glass bowls, dishes, or cups are safe, place each one empty in the microwave oven with a separate cup of tap water. Microwave it on high for one minute. If the empty container stays cool, it's microwave-safe; slightly warm, use it for reheating only. Any bowls, dishes, or cups that get hot shouldn't be used in a microwave oven. Unless it says "microwave safe," avoid microwaving food in the container it came in. That includes margarine or butter tubs, other plastic tubs, polystyrene boxes or trays, plastic bags, brown paper bags, paper towels, paper plates, and paper napkins. Chemicals from these products may transfer to food. Containers from store-bought microwave meals are meant for one-time use; toss them.

● Cut food so the pieces are the same size. This helps ensure even cooking.

● Keep food well covered while cooking. Use waxed paper, microwave-safe plastic wrap, or a lid that fits. This keeps food from drying out and helps ensure even cooking. For safety, allow a little space for some steam to escape.

● Rotate food for even cooking. Halfway through cooking, do one of the following: turn the dish; stir or reposition the food on the plate or bowl; turn large foods over; or reposition the dish on the turntable. Check for cold spots.

● Allow for standing time. Food keeps cooking after the microwave oven turns off, spreading the heat more evenly. In fact, the internal temperature can go up several degrees as food stands.

● Check for doneness—after the standing time. Then, as with food cooked in the oven, check the internal temperature and the visual signs of doneness. Check in several places, but not near the bone.

● Be aware of differences in the power, or wattage, of microwave ovens. Cooking times may differ. Use a thermometer to check for doneness.

● Follow microwave instructions on food packaging. By law, package directions are approved by the U.S. Food and Drug Administration; however, recipes on packages may not be approved.

● Avoid using your microwave oven for canning. The pressure that builds up inside the jar may cause it to explode.

For more on microwave oven safety, see "Play It Safe: Warming Baby's Bottle and Food" in chapter 15 and "Microwave Oven Safety for Kids" in chapter 16.

Grill It Safe

Before you put a burger on the grill, take precautions:

● Adjust the grill so the food cooks evenly—inside and outside. When meat or poultry are too close to the heat, the outside surfaces cook quickly and may appear to be done, but the inside may not be cooked well enough to destroy bacteria.

● Transfer food to a clean plate once it's cooked—with a clean utensil! Don't use your fingers. To avoid cross-contamination, carry cooked meat to the table on a clean dish—not the unwashed dish you used to bring raw meat to the grill.

● Clean the grill between each use. Removing charred food debris from the grill reduces exposure to bacteria and possible cancer-causing substances.

● If you're grilling at a picnic site, do all the cooking there—from start to finish. Partially cooked meats transported there may contain bacteria.

● Grill on both sides. Turn meat, poultry, and fish over at least once for even cooking. If fish is less than ½ inch thick, you don't need to turn it.

Have You Ever Wondered

. . . if liquid smoke is safe to eat? Bottled liquid smoke is sold alongside herbs and sauces in many supermarkets. It gives a smoky flavor without grilling. The flavoring is created by burning wood, then trapping the smoke; most potential carcinogens are removed. About 60 percent of processed meats sold in supermarkets are "smoked" with liquid smoke.

• Grill meat, poultry, and fish until they're cooked through but not charred. The charring—for example, on a well-done steak—is a possible cancer-causing compound called heterocyclic amines, or HCAs. While the research on health effects is inconclusive, you're smart to avoid the "black stuff." Instead, cook meat to medium, rather than well done. Marinating meat first may help reduce HCAs; precooking meat, then quickly grilling for flavor, may, too. Grill poultry and fish until the internal temperature reaches its target but the surface isn't blackened. Scrape off charred areas before you eat.

• Control hot coals to avoid flame flare-ups. The smoke caused by fat dripping on hot coals contains another possible cancer-causing compound, called polycyclic aromatic hydrocarbons. The research as a health risk isn't conclusive. These compounds may not pose a cancer risk, but you're wise to trim visible fat from meat before cooking, drain any high-fat marinades, and have a spray bottle with water for flare-ups. Never use water to control flames on a gas grill!

Where to Place the Meat Thermometer?

Poultry (Whole Bird)

Insert the meat thermometer into the inner thigh area of the breast but not touching bone.

If stuffed, stuffing temperature must reach 165° F. Do this near and at the end of the stand time.

Ground Meat and Poultry

The thermometer should also be placed in the thickest area of ground meat or poultry dishes such as meat loaf. The thermometer may be inserted sideways in thin items such as patties, reaching the very center with the stem.

Beef, Pork, Lamb, Veal, Ham (Roasts, Steaks, or Chops), and Poultry Pieces

The thermometer should be inserted into the center of the thickest part, away from bone, fat, and gristle.

Casseroles and Egg Dishes

The thermometer should be inserted into the center or thickest part.

Using a Meat Thermometer

Using a meat thermometer takes the guesswork out of cooking. Besides helping to prevent foodborne illness, a meat thermometer helps to prevent overcooking and can help to hold foods at a safe temperature. Use a meat thermometer every time you prepare poultry, roasts, ham, casseroles, meat loaves, and egg dishes.

Types of Meat Thermometers

- *Regular, ovenproof:* Inserted into food at the beginning of cooking and remains there throughout cooking. Easy to read; placement is important.
- *Instant-read and digital:* Not intended to stay in food while cooking; gives a quick reading when the stem is inserted into food about 2 inches. For very thick foods, these thermometers cannot measure temperature accurately because they cannot reach the cold center.
- *Pop-up:* Often found already inserted into poultry; also may be purchased for other types of meat. Verify that meat is done by checking the temperature with a conventional thermometer as well.
- *Microwave-safe:* Designed for use in microwave ovens only.
- *Disposable thermometer:* Use once and toss. Meant for grilling at picnics and tailgate parties, they're inexpensive. Find these thermometers for burgers or chicken in the meat case of your supermarket.

Note: When buying a meat thermometer, read the package label carefully to be sure you buy the type designed for use with meat, not other food items such as candy. Look for a thermometer made of stainless steel, with an easy-to-read dial and a shatterproof clear lens.

"Egg-Stra" Cooking Tips for Food Safety

If handled improperly, eggs and egg-rich foods are a perfect medium for *Salmonella* to grow.

- Avoid washing eggs. You'll remove the edible coating that protects eggs from bacteria after they're routinely washed during processing.
- Toss any cracked or dirty eggs.
- Cook eggs until they're done—slowly over gentle heat. *See "How Do You Know When Cooked Eggs Are Done?" on this page.*
- Prepare soft meringues and mousse made with slightly cooked eggs to destroy any *Salmonella*. To

prepare, put the egg whites in a double boiler or a heavy pan. Add 2 tablespoons of sugar for each egg white. Cook over low heat, beating on low speed as you cook until the whites reach 160° F, then turn the speed to high and beat until soft peaks appear. Then proceed with the recipe as directed.

- Avoid foods with raw eggs, such as Caesar salad or homemade ice cream, mayonnaise, or eggnog—unless they're made with an unopened carton of pasteurized eggs. However, once pasteurized eggs are open, they must be treated like any other eggs because they can be contaminated by bacteria. How about homemade

How Do You Know When Cooked Eggs Are Done?

Cooking eggs? Look for these signs of doneness to ensure that *Salmonella* are destroyed.

COOKING METHOD	SIGNS OF DONENESS
Scrambled, omelettes, frittata	No visible liquid egg remains
Poached, fried over easy, sunny side up	White completely set; yolk starting to thicken but not hard (*Hint:* For sunny-side-up eggs, cover with lid to ensure adequate cooking.)
Soft-cooked	White completely set; yolk starting to thicken but not hard (Bring to a boil; turn off heat. Let eggs stand in water for four to five minutes.)
Hard-cooked	White and yolk completely set (Bring to a boil; turn off heat. Let eggs stand in water for fifteen minutes.)
Stirred custard, including ice cream and eggnog	Mixture coats the spoon; temperature reaches 160° F
Baked custard, including quiche	Knife placed off-center comes out clean (*Note:* Cheese in a properly cooked quiche will leave particles on the knife, too.)

FOR SAFETY'S SAKE: HOW LONG CAN YOU REFRIGERATE LEFTOVERS?

PERISHABLE FOOD	KEEPS REFRIGERATED UP TO
Cooked fresh vegetables	3 to 4 days
Cooked pasta	3 to 5 days
Cooked rice	1 week
Deli counter meats	5 days
Greens	1 to 2 days
Meat	
● Ham, cooked and sliced	3 to 4 days
● Hot dogs, opened	1 week
● Lunch meats, prepackaged, opened	3 to 5 days
● Cooked beef, pork, poultry, fish and meat casseroles	3 to 4 days
● Cooked patties and nuggets, gravy, and broth	1 to 2 days
Seafood, cooked	2 days
Soups and stews	3 to 4 days
Stuffing	1 to 2 days

When in doubt, throw it out!

Source: Home Food Safety ... It's in Your Hands (American Dietetic Association and ConAgra, Inc., 2000).

---

other sources of bacteria. Toss any that get cracked or dirty or go unfound (unrefrigerated) for more than two hours. Hard-cooked eggs don't keep as well as raw shell eggs; use hard-cooked eggs within a week. Like other high-protein foods, hard-cooked eggs shouldn't sit out at temperatures of 40° F or higher for longer than two hours. If they do, toss!

Plate It Safe

● Use clean dishes and utensils for serving—use nothing that touched raw meat, fish, or poultry unless it was cleaned in hot, soapy water first.

● Avoid keeping perishable foods on a serving table or at room temperature for longer than two hours (one hour in hot weather 90° F or above). That includes cooked meat, poultry, fish, eggs, and dishes made with these ingredients.

● For buffet-type service keep cold foods cold and hot foods hot. Serve cold foods on ice, at a temperature of 40° F or below. Use heated servers such as a chafing dish to keep hot foods hot. After two hours discard even these foods.

● When replenishing serving dishes, don't mix fresh food with food that's been sitting out. *For more about Clostridium perfringens contamination on buffets, see "Bacteria: Hard Hitters" earlier in this chapter.*

● Refrigerate leftovers as soon as you're done eating. That includes leftover pizza!

Carry It Safe

Picnic Foods

It's summertime. The season's "ripe" for picnics—and foodborne illness. Keep food fit to eat in your fresh-air kitchen. Keep food clean, keep hot food hot, and keep cold food cold.

● For perishables, use clean, insulated coolers chilled with ice or chemical cold packs. As a rule of thumb, pack your cooler with 75 percent food and 25 percent ice or frozen cold packs. Freeze cold packs at least twenty-four hours ahead so they stay cold as long as possible. Chill the cooler ahead, too. Secure the lid. Then keep the cooler closed—no peeking!

● Store nonperishable foods in a clean picnic or laundry basket—with the heaviest foods on the bottom.

cookie dough? If it contains raw eggs, there can be risk. Commercially prepared dressing, mayonnaise, cookie dough, and cookie dough ice cream all use pasteurized eggs.

● As another option, use cooked yolks in recipes that call for raw eggs. Cook the yolks in a double boiler or a heavy skillet with liquid from the recipe: 2 tablespoons of liquid for each yolk. Beat it while it cooks until the yolk coats a spoon, or bubbles form around the edges, or the temperature reaches 160° F.

● Keep eggs and egg-rich foods, including pumpkin and custard pies, at 40° F to 140° F for no longer than two hours, including serving time. Otherwise, keep them refrigerated. Use leftovers made with eggs within two or three days.

● Store Easter eggs in the refrigerator. Handle eggs carefully while decorating; cracked eggs invite bacteria. Hide them so they stay clean from pets, dirt, and

If You or Someone Else Is Choking

Perform the Heimlich Maneuver. If a victim can't talk, can't breathe, is turning blue in the face, or is clutching at his or her throat, get behind the person and wrap your arms around his or her waist. Making a fist, put the thumb side of the fist against the victim's upper abdomen, below the ribs and above the navel. Grasp your fist with your other hand and press into the victim's upper abdomen with a quick upward thrust. Repeat until the object is expelled. (Don't slap the victim's back. This can make matters worse.)

When you choke and no one is there to help, use the same technique as described above. You can also lean over a fixed horizontal object (a chair, a table edge, a railing), pressing your upper abdomen against the edge until the object is expelled.

Source: Courtesy of The Heimlich Institute, Cincinnati, Ohio.

Refer to chapter 15 for choking prevention for young children.

● Seal all foods tightly in bags, jars, or plastic containers. That keeps out moisture and bugs.

● Pack foods already cold or frozen. Don't assume your cooler can cool foods adequately if they're packed at room temperature. Pack perishables between ice or cold packs; they'll stay cold longer.

● Pack uncooked meat, poultry, or fish carefully— in well-sealed containers—for grilling at the picnic spot. Put them in the bottom of the cooler so any juices won't leak onto other foods. Bring a meat thermometer in your picnic basket.

● Keep your cooler in a cool place (under a tree or a picnic table)—not in the hot trunk or in the sun.

● Keep ice for drinks in a sealed bag. Loose ice used to chill foods and drinks isn't safe in drinks.

● Return perishable foods to the cooler immediately after serving, and serve only the amount of food you'll eat right away. Keep the rest in the cooler.

● For picnics nearby that will be eaten right away, consider a hot dish—covered and wrapped well. Wrap the dish in several layers of newspaper, then in an insulated container. Baked beans are a popular choice.

● Bring premoistened towelettes to wash up after handling meat, poultry, or chicken—or any food, for that matter. Or bring soap and a bottle filled with clean water to wash your hands and cooking surfaces. *Another option:* a hand sanitizer, usually formulated with alcohol, which kills bacteria on your hands.

● Be prepared to clean the grill at the picnic site— unless you bring your own clean grill. Pack a brush, soap, and perhaps water.

● After the picnic, toss perishable leftovers. Or repack them in a cold cooler if they have been out for less than two hours (one hour at 90° F or warmer) and are clean (no flies, dirt, or improper handling).

Carried Meals and Snacks

Whether you pack it at home or buy ready-to-eat take-out foods, any time perishable foods are left at room temperature for two hours or more, there's risk for foodborne illness. That's especially true when it's stuffed in a school locker with a dirty gym bag or left on a warm windowsill at the office!

● Order take-out food just before lunch or dinner, then eat it right away. Or keep it in the refrigerator.

● Use a clean insulated bag or a lunch box. Tuck in a small refreezable ice pack to keep food cold. Or freeze a juice box or small plastic container of water to keep the lunch box and the food cold. Pack a hand sanitizer, too, if there's no chance for hand washing.

● For cold beverages, refrigerate an insulated vacuum bottle ahead. Then fill it with milk or juice to carry with you. Keep juice or milk in the fridge at work.

● For hot soups, stews, and chilis, heat an insulated container ahead. Fill it with boiling water, then let it sit for several minutes before pouring it out. Be sure the food is very hot when it's put into the container. Then keep the container closed until you eat the food.

● Assemble your meal the night before; chill well.

● Keep carried, perishable food in a clean, cool place—away from sunlit windowsills, radiators, or warm vehicles. If a refrigerator is available, use it.

● Pack nonperishable foods: unopened canned soup or stew to heat up in the microwave oven at work, dried raisins or apple slices, crackers and peanut butter, boxed juice or milk, beef jerky, to name a few. For canned foods with no pop top, tuck in a can opener!

● Discard any perishable, carried food that isn't eaten.

● Launder your lunch bag or wash your lunch box with soapy water after every use.

Ship It Safe

Food safety is an issue if you buy food online or mail order, call for home-delivered groceries, or ship perishable food as a gift.

● *To place an order,* ask how and when perishable foods will be sent. Ask that the food be packed with dry ice or cold packs, and order for overnight delivery. Record the order number for tracking—just in case!

● *If you're packing a perishable food gift,* freeze it solid or refrigerate until cold before packing it. Pack food in an insulated cooler or a heavy corrugated box with cold packs or dry ice. (Check the phone book for a place to buy dry ice; talk to your shipper or the post office about proper forms and warning labels for shipping packages with dry ice.) Mark the properly addressed package as "Perishable—Keep Refrigerated." Use overnight delivery. And let the recipient know it's coming so it won't sit on the doorstep.

● *If you receive a food gift,* open it right away. Some mail-order foods, such as dry-cured ham and hard salami, don't require refrigeration. Other meats (including most hams), poultry, fish, and other perishable foods should arrive just as cold as they would be in your refrigerator. If it's cold enough, put the food in the freezer or the refrigerator. If it's not, toss it out, and contact the mail-order company for a replacement or a refund.

Quick Tips for Injury Prevention

Kitchen safety is more than preventing foodborne illness. Keep your kitchen safe from injury:

● Wipe up spills immediately. Someone who enters the kitchen may not notice water or grease on the floor before he or she slips.

● Avoid teetering on a chair or a bar stool to reach a high cabinet. Invest in a stable stool.

● Keep cabinets, drawers, and doors closed so you don't bump into them. Put safety catches on drawers so they won't fall out when they're opened too far.

● Keep pot holders handy—and use them. Be careful if they get wet; water conducts heat.

● Turn the handles on pots and pans inward and away from the edge of the stove where they may be knocked . . . or where children can grab them.

● Avoid overfilling pots and pans. Too much hot soup, stew, or pasta can quickly burn if it spills on you.

● Be careful with the hot-water tap, especially if you have small children.

● Allow enough time for the pressure to release if you use a pressure cooker.

● Avoid dropping water into hot oil. The splatters may burn you. Remember: Water and oil don't mix!

● Douse grease fires with baking soda—not water! Or "put a lid on it" to control the flame.

● Keep electrical cords away from stove burners.

● Use a safety latch on cabinets with household chemicals, alcoholic beverages, matches, plastic bags, and sharp utensils (knives, toothpicks) so they're out of reach of children.

● Handle knives for safety. Store them carefully, perhaps in a knife holder. Avoid leaving them in the dishpan where you can't see them. Use sharp knives; dull knives are harder to use and promote injury. Always cut away from you, using a cutting board.

● Watch out for broken glass. Remove it immediately. If glass breaks in the sink, empty the water so you find all the pieces before you cut yourself.

● Watch your fingers near your garbage disposal! Teach children to use it safely.

The "Eco Kitchen"

Along with food safety, go "green" with kitchen ecology—conserving fuel, energy, and water and minimizing waste.

Water in the "Eco Kitchen"

● Choose the proper size pots and pans for cooking. Utensils that are too big use more cooking water.

● Cook in a microwave oven or a pressure cooker to conserve water—and time.

● Time foods that need to boil or simmer so you don't lose too much water through evaporation.

● Washing dishes? Turn the faucet on and off as you rinse, rather than allowing the water to run continually.

● Run your dishwasher only when full.

● Repair your faucet if it leaks.

Energy Savers

● Preheat your oven right before you use it.

● For energy-efficiency, defrost your freezer regularly.

● Turn off lights when you leave the kitchen.

● Avoid the habit of leaving the heat under the coffeepot all day. Turn it off when it's no longer needed.

● Buy energy-efficient appliances. Dishwashers that use less hot water save energy, too.

● Keep the oven and the refrigerator doors shut. Each time you peek inside, your appliance needs to use power to regain its set temperature. For the refrigerator, decide what you want before you open the door. When using the oven, use a timer. *Tip:* An open oven isn't efficient or safe for heating your kitchen!

● Keep appliances in good condition: tight gaskets around the oven and refrigerator doors. For efficiency, a gas stove should burn with a blue, not a yellowish, flame in the pilot light.

● Use equipment to cook faster, such as a microwave or convection oven, a pressure cooker, or ovens that also use radiant or halogen heat.

● Trim the flame. Use a burner that matches the cooking pot.

● Arrange baking pans in the oven so air circulates. You'll get more even baking, and your food will cook faster and more efficiently.

● Use the self-cleaning feature on your oven judiciously—when it really needs cleaning. For a head start, start it while the oven is still hot from baking.

Resource Conservation

● Resist the urge to buy food you don't need. Buy only the amount your family will eat.

● Look for products in packaging that can be recycled, such as aluminum cans, steel cans, glass containers, recycled plastic, and paperboard cartons that are gray on the inside. On plastic containers, look for the recycling symbol with a number in the center. Lower numbers are recycled more easily.

● Recycle. Keep a recycling bin. Dispose of recyclables according to municipal regulations and services.

● Reuse glass or plastic food packages. Clean them well with hot, soapy water if used for food storage.

● If you grow your own vegetables, make a compost heap. Add kitchen waste—for example, corn husks and melon rinds—to your compost heap.

● Keep your refrigerator in check. Use perishable foods before they spoil and need to be discarded.

CHAPTER 13

Kitchen Nutrition
Delicious Decisions

Kitchen nutrition—cooking for health—isn't new. About 150 years ago, *The Book of Household Management* described the kitchen as "the great laboratory of the household . . . much of the 'weal and woe' as far as regards bodily health, depends on the nature of the preparations concocted within its walls."

Now, in this new century, the kitchen is still where foods are transformed into nourishment. Yet foods, food preparation methods, and recipes have changed dramatically, as have lifestyles.

"Resetting" Your Table . . . for Flavor and Health

Flavor is a bigger nutrition issue than many realize. According to consumer research, taste tops nutrition as the main reason why consumers buy one food over another. There's a lot wrapped up in why you prefer certain foods, including many social, psychological (emotional), and health reasons. In any case, the foods you enjoy are likely the ones you eat most. The more often you eat them, the more important their nutritional impact on your overall health.

For most Americans, enjoyment is an important reason for eating; it may even be *the* reason. If you're nutrition-savvy, it's great to make food appeal a major kitchen priority. When it comes to nutrition, think flavor . . . and when it comes to flavor, think nutrition!

"Flavor" the Difference

Imagine . . . the aroma of homemade, whole-wheat bread baking in your oven . . . the sweet, juicy taste of a ripe peach—just picked . . . the cool sensation of ice-cold milk . . . the crispy crunch of a raw carrot; the smooth, creamy texture of chocolate ice cream; or the fiery feeling of a hot chile pepper!

There's no question: foods that appeal to your senses are probably those you enjoy most! Sensory stimulation evokes food memories. The more senses a food or meal affects, the more vivid the flavor memory, positive or not. What is flavor? And how does it contribute to nutrition?

Flavor is actually several sensations closely linked together: taste plus smell, as well as touch (temperature and mouth feel). Sound, perhaps the crunch of an apple, and sight may contribute to flavor, too. With one sensation diminished, your flavor experience is entirely different. As an experiment, hold your nose so you can't smell, then bite an onion. It may taste somewhat sweet, more like an apple. Or think about food's taste when your nose is stuffed up—not much flavor, not much pleasure either. About eighty percent of food's flavor is aroma.

As an average adult, you have about ten thousand taste buds, which respond to different tastes: sweet, sour, salty, bitter, and also umami (the brothy, meaty, and savory flavor of glutamate). You can sense *all* these tastes on *every* part of your tongue. Some parts of the tongue may be especially sensitive to certain tastes—

for example, bitter will taste stronger at the back of the tongue. Even the lining of your mouth, the back of your throat, your tonsils (if you still have them), and your epiglottis (a flap of tissue that covers your larynx, preventing food and liquids from entering the airway) have some taste buds, especially in childhood.

Aromas that waft through the room get picked up by smell receptors high up in your nasal passages. Temperature, mouth feel, even the "irritation" from a jalapeño pepper or the "numbing" effect from a persimmon also affect your perceptions of food and its flavor—and what you may describe as its "taste."

Not surprisingly, we're born with an ability to perceive, and a preference for, sweet tastes. To some degree, we can perceive all tastes at birth—sweet, sour, bitter, salty, and umami. Flavor preferences are learned—starting from the early years.

Why does the same food taste too spicy for some

Are You a Supertaster?

Why do you like the foods you like? The reasons are partly genes and age. Even in the same family, people experience tastes differently. The intensity of taste depends partly on how many fungiform papillae (tiny, smooth red bumps with clusters of taste receptor cells, or tastebuds) a person has on his or her tongue.

Supertasters have a lot of papillae, and tend to strongly like or dislike certain foods. They pick up bitter flavors, perhaps in pungent vegetables, tea, coffee, and grapefruit juice, and sweet flavors more intensely, too. Those with few papillae tend to be indifferent to one flavor over another, and those in the middle are likely to enjoy all kinds of food if prepared well.

Children have more papillae than adults, perhaps one of many reasons why a child may be a picky eater. Taste sensitivity seems to decline with age, which is explained by the decrease in the number of papillae.

Have you ever burned your tongue on steamy hot soup, or the roof of your mouth on cheese topping a hot pizza? Hot foods may damage papillae. Fortunately, your body repairs its papillae fairly quickly.

Are you a supertaster? Find out. First punch a hole (with a hole punch) in a small piece of wax paper. Put the hole on the tip of your tongue; wipe it with blue food coloring. With a mirror, magnifying glass, and flashlight, count the papillae. Nontasters only have five or six, but supertasters have dozens of them! (More women are supertasters than men are.)

Have You Ever Wondered

. . . what makes chile peppers taste "hot"? Capsaicin in chile peppers stimulates pain receptors in your mouth. The irritation, or "heating" effect, depends on the amount of capsaicin, measured in Scoville heat units (SHU)—anywhere from 1 to 300,000 SHU (mild to very hot). A sweet bell (pimento) pepper is rated at 0 to 5; an anaheim pepper at 500 to 1,000; ancho or poblano pepper at 1,000 to 1,500; jalapeño or chipotle pepper at 2,500 to 5,000; a Serrano pepper at 5,000 to 15,000; and a habañero (Scotch bonnet) pepper from 80,000 to 300,000!

. . . how to reduce the "fire" caused by eating hot chile peppers? Try dairy foods! Caesin, the main protein in milk, washes away capsaicin that makes your mouth and throat "burn." Hot chile peppers do "fire up" the flavors of Thai dishes, Mexican salsas, and Cajun foods, among others. To tone down the heat, remove the seeds and inner membranes of hot chiles. To avoid a burning sensation on sensitive skin as you handle hot chiles, use rubber gloves. Never touch or rub your eyes—or any other sensitive areas—when you're handling them.

but not for others? People sense the same foods differently. Among the factors that make a difference: saliva (affected by diet, heredity, and other factors), the number of taste buds, medications, some illnesses, and smoking. The senses of taste and smell diminish with age. That's partly why older people may say: foods just don't taste the way they remember. *For more about flavor and older adults, see chapter 18.*

Today, taste and smell are getting more attention in the scientific world—in part because flavor is a priority for food choices. Since people eat for flavor, there's good reason to think of nutrition and taste together. That's why research is being done—for example, to make food more flavorful for older adults; to find ways to magnify salty perception while lowering levels of sodium in food; and to use biotechnology to develop more flavorful fruits and vegetables.

To get the most flavor from foods and stimulate the senses:

● Enjoy ingredients at their peak of quality.

● Take time to chew! Chewing stimulates saliva flow, enhancing flavor as food's components

Paint Your Plate with Color!

Toss blueberries in your yogurt. Garnish your salad with sliced beets. Tuck spinach leaves in your sandwich. Color offers much more than eye appeal to a wonderful meal! A rainbow of fruits and vegetables creates a palette of nutrients and phytonutrients on your plate, each with a different bundle of potential benefits in a healthful diet: from oxidizing free radicals that may damage healthy cells, to having anti-inflammatory qualities, to lowering LDL cholesterol. *See "Phytonutrients—a 'Crop' for Good Health" in chapter 4.*

Research is uncovering the benefits of the pigment-related phytonutrients—and the colorful fruits and vegetables that supply them.

- *Green: fruit*—avocado, green apples, green grapes, honeydew, kiwifruit, lime, green pears; *vegetables*—artichokes, asparagus, broccoli, Brussels sprouts, green beans, green cabbage, leafy greens, okra, green pepper, snow peas, zucchini. Their lutein and indoles have antioxidant potential and may help promote healthy vision and reduce cancer risks.

- *Orange and deep yellow: fruit*—apricot, cantaloupe, grapefruit, mango, papaya, peach, pineapple, yellow apple, yellow fig; *veggies*—carrot, yellow beets, yellow pepper, sweet corn, sweet potato, winter squash. Carotenoids, bioflavonoids, and the antioxidant vitamin C may promote a healthy heart, vision, immunity, and reduced risk for some cancers. The deeper the yellow/orange color, the more carotenoids these foods have!

- *Purple and blue: fruit*—blackberries, blueberries, plums, purple figs, raisins; *veggies*—eggplant, purple cabbage, purple-fleshed potato. Anthocyanins, which give a blue-purple color, and phenolics, may have antioxidant and anti-aging benefits, and may help with memory, urinary tract health, and reduced cancer risks.

- *Red: fruit*—cherries, cranberries, pomegranate, red/pink grapefruit; red grapes, strawberries, watermelon; *veggies*—beets, red onions, red peppers, red potatoes, rhubarb, tomatoes. This color group delivers lycopene, a powerful carotenoid, as well as anthocyanins. They may help maintain a healthy heart, vision, immunity, and may reduce cancer risks. When cooked or canned, lycopene is more available to your body.

- *White, tan, brown: fruit*—banana, brown pear, dates, white peaches; *veggies*—cauliflower, jicama, kohlrabi, mushrooms, onions, parsnips, turnip, white-fleshed potato, white corn. Of particular interest: allicin in garlic and onion, and selenium in mushrooms may promote heart health and reduce cancer risks.

For more about colorful vegetables and fruits, see chapter 10.

---

dissolve. Aromas and tastes need time to blend. Textures change as you chew, too!

- Handle and cook foods with care. Overcooking and poor storage destroy flavor.

- Serve food hot—or cold. Enticing flavors come partly from aromas released with heat. Coldness can give a refreshing mouthfeel.

See "Flavor on the Menu" in chapter 14.

Variety: A Meal with Appeal

Like a well-decorated room or a beautifully landscaped garden, an appealing meal follows basic principles of design. Different foods add a variety of color, flavor, texture, shape, and temperature to meals or snacks. At the same time, food variety supplies different nutrients and phytonutrients.

Vary the color. Contrast the visual differences: meat loaf, mashed potatoes with gravy, corn, and applesauce . . . compared with meat loaf, baked sweet potato with chopped chives, asparagus, and spinach salad with orange slices. Which one has more interest? The meal with an artist's palette of color! Phytonutrients that give fruits and vegetables their colorful appeal and health benefits also deliver flavor appeal. Your eyes tell your brain that great-tasting food is on its way.

Vary the flavors. Different ingredients and seasonings in a dish or meal add layers of flavor. Instead of orange-glazed chicken, candied sweet potatoes, and fruit compote, complement the chicken with wild rice pilaf and a crisp spinach salad with herbed balsamic dressing.

Vary the texture. Crunchy foods contrast soft foods— for example, chopped nuts in brown rice, or raw veggies with herbed cottage cheese dip. Variety of texture adds appeal as much as variety of color!

Vary the shape. Round meatballs, round peas, round new potatoes, and round grapes may look somewhat boring if plated together. Add variety to the plate with baby carrots or pea pods instead of peas, pasta spirals instead of potatoes, or sliced peaches instead of grapes.

Vary the temperature. Hot and cool in the same meal maximizes the flavor perception of a meal. For example, a cold summer supper or a picnic from the cooler can be refreshing. However, a warm whole-wheat roll offers a nice contrast to a cool chef's salad. And frozen yogurt makes a nice ending to a hot dinner.

For a Taste Lift

- Grill or roast your veggies in a very hot oven or grill for a sweet, smoky flavor. Brush or spray them lightly with oil so they don't dry out. Sprinkle with herbs.

- Caramelize sliced onions to bring out their natural sugar flavor. Just cook them slowly over low heat in a small amount of oil. Use them to make a rich, dark sauce for meat or poultry.

- Spark up sauces, soups, and salads with a splash of flavored, balsamic, or rice vinegar. *See "Herbed Vinegars" in this chapter for ways to make your own herb and fruit vinegars.*

- Add a tangy taste with citrus juice or grated citrus peel: lemon, lime, or orange. Acidic ingredients help lift and balance flavor.

- Pep it up with peppers! Use red, green, and yellow peppers of all varieties—sweet, hot, and dried. Or add a dash of hot pepper sauce.

- Give a flavor burst with good-quality condiments such as horseradish, flavored mustard, chutney, wasabi, and salsas of all kinds!

- Simmer to make reduction sauces. Concentrate the flavors of meat, poultry, and fish stocks. Reduce the juices by heating them—don't boil! Then use them as a flavorful glaze or gravy.

More Taste Lifters

- For grains that absorb fluid (rice, buckwheat, and barley), cook them in defatted, perhaps reduced-sodium, chicken or beef broth. Risotto, an Italian rice specialty, typically is prepared by cooking arborio or white short-grain rice in broth, along with herbs and other ingredients.

- Blend herbs, spices, sun-dried tomatoes, and shredded cheese into bread dough before baking it.

- Experiment with herbs and spices: basil, chives, cilantro, rosemary, garlic, ginger, caraway, cumin.

- Sharpen up the flavor with cheese. Add a little Parmesan, sharp Cheddar, Romano, feta, Asiago, or blue cheese—on vegetables, rice, or pasta.

- Intensify flavor with dried ingredients: sun-dried tomatoes, dried mushrooms, dried cranberries, dried apricots, dried plums (prunes), dried figs, and red pepper flakes. Plump sun-dried tomatoes and dried mushrooms in broth or cooking wine, and dried cranberries or dried plums in apple juice.

- Marinate with tangy, sweet, or savory sauces to infuse flavor from the outside in.

- Use a little nut oil: hazelnut, almond, or walnut oil. A little drizzle will do!

Food "Prep": The Nutrition-Flavor Connection

Nutrition and flavor go hand in hand. You don't need to sacrifice one for the other. Proper food storage and handling enhance the natural flavors of food and keep nutrient loss to a minimum.

- Start with high-quality ingredients. These don't need to be the most expensive foods in the store. But they do need to be handled properly all along the food chain—right to your kitchen. *Refer to "Shopping for Freshness" in chapter 11.*

- Store foods properly until they're prepared. Cooking can't improve poor-quality food, but it can enhance the flavors of already high-quality foods. *Chapter 12, "The Safe Kitchen," offers many culinary tips for freshness.*

- Cook to retain nutrients, flavor, color, texture, and overall taste appeal. *For quick flavor enhancers, see "For a Taste Lift" and "More Taste Lifters."*

High temperatures and long cooking times can destroy heat-sensitive nutrients such as B vitamins, vitamin C, and folate. Some minerals and water-soluble vitamins dissolve in cooking water; they're lost when cooking water is discarded. And light destroys riboflavin (vitamin B_2) and vitamin A. Proper cooking techniques keep nutrient loss to a minimum and food quality at its peak. *See "Simple Ways to Keep Vitamins in Food" later in this chapter.*

Beyond Parsley . . . Quick, Easy Garnishes

Garnishes do more than add eye appeal to food; they also offer flavor, color, and texture contrasts and, if eaten, some nutritional value. Garnish food with edibles that complement the ingredients in the food. For example, a sprig of basil goes with many Italian dishes; a slice of lemon or lime complements many seafood dishes; and a sliced vegetable garnish adds more veggies to a meal! Arrange the garnish artistically around, under, or on top of the food.

Parsley, which may be the most common garnish, dresses up a plate and serves as a natural breath freshener. While having less flavor than flat-leafed varieties, curly parsley adds texture to the plate, too, and both varieties have some beta carotene (which forms vitamin A) and vitamin C! To garnish, go beyond parsley and "paint your plate" with other foods, too:

Give It a Little Salsa

Salsa is the Spanish word for "sauce." With today's cuisine, salsa has become a lot more sexy! By combining a variety of chopped vegetables, fruits, herbs, and even hot sauce, there's a salsa for every flavor mood.

Tomato salsa: Combine chopped plum tomatoes, onions, canned green chiles, cilantro, and lime juice. Add red pepper flakes or hot sauce for more zip. Chill. *Tip:* Plum tomatoes, especially when they're in season, often have more flavor than salad tomatoes.

Pineapple salsa: Combine chopped, fresh, or canned pineapple with chopped cilantro, fresh lime juice, and a touch of sugar and minced garlic. Chill.

Black bean salsa: Combine canned, drained black beans with chopped tomato, chopped onion, chopped cilantro, and a little jalapeño and red wine vinegar. Chill.

On salads . . . capers; fennel slices; pomegranate seeds; red onion slices; red, green, and yellow pepper strips; toasted, chopped walnuts or pecans; chopped apple (tossed with lemon juice to prevent browning); watercress; orange sections; blueberries or raspberries; grated cheese; snow peas; shredded jicama; or marigold petals. *For edible flowers as garnishes, see "Please Don't Eat the Daffodils" in this chapter.*

On soups . . . an avocado slice dipped in lemon; shredded carrot; minced chives; sprigs of herbs; minced fresh herbs; snow peas; a dollop of plain yogurt; orange peel strips; a lemon slice; croutons; pesto sauce; edible flowers; shredded green, yellow, and red peppers; grated cheese; or plain, air-popped popcorn.

On cooked vegetables . . . toasted, sliced almonds; toasted pine nuts; grated Parmesan cheese; stir-fried onion slices; stir-fried mushroom slices; chopped lean ham; chopped olives or pimiento; or fresh herbs.

In beverages . . . a mint sprig; scented geranium leaves; orange, lime, or lemon slices; fresh, whole berries; sliced starfruit (carambola), apple, or kiwifruit; or a cinnamon stick.

With meat, poultry, or fish . . . tomato slices; a small bunch of grapes; lemon and lime wedges; crab apple slices; a grilled peach or pear half; baby corn; baby beets, squash, and carrots; or chutney or salsa in endive, a lettuce cup, or a lemon slice.

Recipes: Judge for Yourself!

Each year, hundreds of new cookbooks appear on bookstore shelves. Many focus on healthful eating. Besides cookbooks, you find recipes in magazines and newspapers; on supermarket racks, package labels, and computer software; and on Web sites. To find a cookbook or a food magazine that matches your needs, read its introduction. How can you sort through their recipes and endless combinations of ingredients?

Look at the main ingredients and the portions. You'll get an idea of how just one recipe portion fits within your day's eating plan and whether it's high or low in fat, sugar, or salt. *Use MyPyramid, described in chapter 10, for your healthy eating plan.*

Check the nutrient analysis of the recipe—if it's provided. Unlike food labels, nutrition information and serving sizes for recipes aren't standardized.

Please Don't Eat the Daffodils

Edible flowers add a distinctive flavor (*sweet* lilac, *spicy* nasturtium, *minty* bee balm) and a unique splash of color to foods. But you can't eat just any flower!

Some are poisonous; even edible flowers may be contaminated by chemicals if they weren't grown for eating. Don't eat flowers you buy from a florist or a greenhouse—or that you pick along the road. Don't use them as a garnish, either. There's a long list of flowers that aren't edible: buttercup, delphinium, lily of the valley, foxglove, goldenseal, periwinkle, oleander, sweet pea—and daffodils, to name just a few!

For edible flowers, grow your own or buy them in the produce section of your store. They should be labeled as "edible flowers." Only eat flowers if you're *absolutely* sure of their safety! *Tip:* If you have hay fever, allergies, or asthma, be cautious about eating flowers.

Try growing these edible flowers in the kitchen garden outside your back door: bee balm, calendula (pot marigold), borage, chrysanthemum, day lilies, dianthus, marigolds, nasturtiums (enjoy leaves and blossoms), pansies, roses, scented geraniums, squash blossoms, sunflowers, tulips, and violets. Enjoy the blossoms from any herb plant, too; try basil, chive, lavender, oregano, sage, savory, and thyme blossoms.

Fertilize your flowers as you would a vegetable garden. Then, when harvesting, wash them well, and gently pat them dry.

To keep edible flowers for a few days, refrigerate them. Just keep the stems in water, or put short-stemmed blossoms in a plastic bag or between damp paper towels. For most flowers, enjoy the petals.

Recipes may list some, but not all, the nutrients you find on a label. Sometimes the nutrient analysis in a recipe is provided for a single portion, but not always. A portion, perhaps of lasagna, in one recipe might be bigger or smaller than a portion of the same food in another recipe. And neither one might equal one label-size serving of a frozen version. Computerized cookbooks offer the advantage of technology. With some, you can plan meals for the day—with recipes from the cookbook—then total the calories and nutrients. Changing the menu for your nutrient and calorie needs takes just a few computer keystrokes!

Choose recipes to complement the whole meal—in fact, meals and snacks for the whole day! Consider variety of color, flavor, texture, taste—and nutrition. Nutrients and calories in any one recipe aren't the whole picture. If the recipe you choose has more fat or sodium, plan your menu with other foods with less.

Most important, choose recipes that appeal to you. No matter how nutritious a recipe sounds, the end result should be something you enjoy—or a food you're willing to experience, perhaps for the first time.

Recipe Makeovers

Ready to decrease calories, fat, especially saturated fat, *trans* fat, or sodium . . . or boost calcium, fiber, or other nutrients? You can transform almost any recipe, even Mom's specialties. A few subtle modifications may improve their nutrition content without much flavor change. Experiment more dramatically by adding more fruits, vegetables, or whole grains to recipes!

Chefs and test-kitchen experts change recipes all the time. There's nothing sacred about most recipes (except perhaps Mom's). Recipes get altered when new ingredients come on the market, when cooking equipment changes, when consumers want recipe shortcuts, when ingredients are in or out of season or become more or less costly, when consumers shift food preferences, and when nutrition and health issues arise.

In your own "test kitchen," you can modify recipes in several ways: change the ingredients, modify the way the recipes are prepared, cut portion sizes, or do all three. Even one or two small recipe changes can net a significant difference in the nutrition content. This chapter has plenty of ideas to get you started!

Whatever your approach to recipe makeovers, keep flavor, texture, and appeal as priorities. Remember that moderation in your overall food choices counts, not what's in one dish. A single dish that's high in fat, sugar, or salt may not need a makeover—*if* you don't eat it often; *if* the rest of your day's choices have less fat, sugar, or salt; or *if* you eat just a small amount.

1. *Change the ingredients or switch proportions.* You might use less of one or more ingredients . . . or substitute one ingredient for another . . . or take an ingredient out entirely . . . or add something new.

● *Start by reviewing the recipe and the ingredient list.* Does it need to be adjusted? Decide what ingredients might be changed to achieve your goals, perhaps to switch the type of fat, boost calcium,

An Easy Makeover: Tuna-Noodle Bake

Compare these two recipes for Tuna-Noodle Bake. How has the traditional recipe been changed to make it lower in fat, cholesterol, and sodium, yet higher in vitamins A and C and fiber?

ORIGINAL RECIPE

8 oz. egg noodles
2 tbsp. butter
2 cans (7 oz. each) tuna, packed in oil, drained

1 cup sour cream

¾ cup whole milk
1 can (3 oz.) sliced mushrooms

1 tsp. onion salt
½ tsp. salt
¼ tsp. pepper
¼ cup plain, unseasoned bread crumbs
⅓ cup grated Parmesan cheese
2 tbsp. butter, melted

Preheat oven to 350° F. Cook noodles in salted water as directed on package. When cooked, drain and rinse. Return noodles to pot; add butter or margarine. Stir in tuna, sour cream, milk, mushrooms, onion salt, salt, and pepper. Pour into a greased 2-quart casserole. Combine bread crumbs, Parmesan cheese, and melted butter. Sprinkle over casserole. Bake uncovered for thirty-five minutes. Makes six servings.

Nutrition information per serving:
480 Calories (235 Calories from Fat)

	% Daily Value
Total fat: 26 g	39%
Saturated fat: 13 g	64%
Cholesterol: 102 mg	34%
Sodium: 1,100 mg	46%
Total carbohydrate: 34 g	11%
Dietary fiber: 0 g	1%
Sugars: 3 g	
Protein: 28 g	
Vitamin A	21%
Vitamin C	1%
Calcium	19%
Iron	15%

MAKEOVER RECIPE

8 oz. whole-wheat noodles

2 cans (7 oz. each) tuna,* packed in spring water, drained
½ can (10½- oz.) cream of mushroom soup
½ cup pureed low-fat (1%) cottage cheese
¾ cup fat-free milk
½ cup chopped celery
½ cup shredded carrot
¼ cup chopped green pepper
1 tsp. onion flakes
¼ tsp. each paprika and tarragon
¼ tsp. pepper

⅓ cup grated Parmesan cheese

Preheat oven to 350° F. Cook noodles in unsalted water as directed on package. When cooked, drain. Return noodles to pot; add tuna, soup, cottage cheese, milk, celery, carrot, green pepper, onion flakes, paprika, tarragon, and pepper. Pour into a nonstick 2-quart casserole. Sprinkle with Parmesan cheese. Bake uncovered for thirty-five minutes. Makes six servings.

Nutrition information per serving:
295 Calories (45 Calories from Fat)

	% Daily Value
Total fat: 5 g	8%
Saturated fat: 2 g	10%
Cholesterol: 25 mg	8%
Sodium: 640 mg	27%
Total carbohydrate: 35 g	12%
Dietary fiber: 2 g	8%
Sugars: 3 g	
Protein: 29 g	
Vitamin A	32%
Vitamin C	19%
Calcium*	17%
Iron	16%

*Use canned salmon in place of canned tuna to increase calcium to 32% Daily Value.

Daily Values are used with food labeling. To help you compare these two recipes, Daily Values are used with this nutritional analysis. *To learn about Daily Values on the Nutrition Facts of food labels, see chapter 11.*

use leftovers, add flavor, take advantage of a super-market sale, or match a family preference.

● *Consider the ingredients' functions before you switch.* To get an appealing result, make suitable substitutions. For example, in meat, poultry, fish, and vegetable dishes, salt enhances taste; herbs make flavorful substitutes. Regular ground beef is a key ingredient in hot chili, but lean ground turkey works just as well. Low-fat yogurt can replace sour cream in dips, potato toppers, and some creamy sauce.

You can learn more about the functions of:

1. *Fat: "Why Foods Contain Fat," in chapter 3*
2. *"Sugars: Their Roles in Foods," in chapter 5*
3. *Salt: "Salt and Sodium: More than Flavor," in chapter 7*

● *Reduce or eliminate some ingredients.* In many baked foods, you may cut back on sugar by a third and still enjoy good results. With sautéed foods or with foods cooked in a small amount of oil, try using less cooking oil. Optional ingredients are easy to take out; removing others may alter the appearance or the flavor. Season with extra herbs or spices if you cut back on salt.

● *To boost nutrients, decide what ingredients to add.* Fortifying casseroles with wheat bran or dry milk powder may go unnoticed. Adding shredded carrots to mashed potatoes, legumes to salads, or dried cranberries to muesli, gives extra flavor and color, along with more nutrients and phytonutrients.

● *As easy substitutions, try modified ingredients.* For example, use cholesterol-free egg products, reduced-fat cheese, or sodium-reduced chicken broth in some recipes. Follow package directions if the product needs to be prepared differently.

● *Experiment a little at a time, perhaps with just one ingredient.* That's especially important when the ingredient has functional purposes, such as eggs or sugar in baked foods. When the recipe makeover works, jot it down—in your cookbook or your file.

● *Make an ingredient switch:* perhaps to a healthy oil (perhaps canola or olive oil) for less saturated fat.

2. *Modify food prep.* Simple changes in cooking tech-niques may require little or no extra time investment—

Culinary Lingo

Braise: to simmer over low heat in liquid—water, broth, or even fruit juice—in a covered pot for a lengthy time

Broil: to cook with direct heat, usually under a heating element in the oven

Grill: to cook with direct heat directly over hot coals or another heat source

Panbroil: to cook uncovered in a preheated, nonstick skillet without added fat or water

Poach: to cook gently in liquid, just below boiling

Roast: to cook uncovered with dry heat in the oven

Sauté: to cook quickly in a small amount of fat, stirring so the food browns evenly

Simmer: to cook slowly in liquid, just below boiling

Steam: to cook with steam heat over (not in) boiling water, or wrapped in foil or leaves (such as lettuce or banana leaves) packets, over boiling water or on a grill

Stew: to cook in liquid, such as water, juice, wine, broth, or stock, in a tightly covered pot over low heat

Stir-fry: to cook small pieces of meat, poultry, fish, seafood, and/or vegetables in a very small amount of oil, perhaps with added broth, over very high heat, stirring as you cook

just know-how. For example, skim fat that collects on stews, scrub rather than peel fiber-rich potato skins, skip salt in cooking water, or oven-bake frozen French fries rather than fry them.

3. *Reduce portion sizes.* If a recipe is high in calories, fats, or sugars, try serving less. For example, instead of ¼ cup of cheese sauce on a baked potato, use just two tablespoons—and add some steamed, chopped vegetables and/or herbs for flavor. Trick the eye so less looks like more. Serve smaller portions on smaller plates. That's a calorie trimmer!

Simply Nutritious, Simply Delicious

Modifying recipes without compromising taste doesn't require extra time—just quick, easy kitchen know-how. Tips here offer many ways to prepare foods with less fat (including saturated and *trans* fats), cholesterol, added sugars, and sodium. You'll also find ways to add fruits, vegetables, whole grains, fiber, and calcium to your food preparation—and keep vitamins in. Trimming fat and added sugars can cut calories, too! Now cook for the health (and flavor) of it!

Fruits and Vegetables: Fitting More In!

As a child, you probably enjoyed fruits and vegetables for their vibrant colors, crunch, and wonderful flavors. You probably also learned that fruits and

Stocking the Kitchen . . . with Easy Nutrition

Keep a variety of foods on hand—and make nutritious meals and snacks quick and easy to prepare. Buy fresh ingredients as you need them! Many of these foods are sold with reduced amounts of fat or sodium—or they're fat- or sodium-free. Decide which form to buy to fit your overall goals for your meal and snack choices.

To Store in Your Kitchen Cabinet . . .
Whole-grain breakfast cereal
Rice (brown and white)
Brown and wild rice pilaf mix
Pasta (spaghetti, macaroni, others)
Couscous (perhaps whole-wheat couscous)
Bulgur or whole barley
Gingersnaps or vanilla wafers
Whole-wheat or mixed grain bread and rolls
Beans (dry and canned)
Peanut butter
Tuna or salmon (canned, packed in spring water)
Refried beans (canned, fat-free, reduced-fat, vegetarian)
Fruit (canned in own juice or light syrup)
Vegetables (canned, perhaps sodium reduced)
Fruit (dried)
Vegetable soup (canned and dry mix)
Nonfat dry milk powder
Evaporated fat-free (skim) milk
Salsa or picante sauce
Pasta sauce
Chicken or beef broth (canned, reduced sodium and fat)
Fruit spread
Mustard
Ketchup
Vinegar
Vegetable or olive oil (peanut, canola, soybean, others)
Salad dressing (perhaps reduced fat)
Vegetable oil cooking spray
Herbs and spices
Flour (whole-wheat, bleached white)
Sugar (granulated, powder)

Brown sugar
Cornstarch
Baking powder
Baking soda

To Keep in a Cool, Dry Place . . .
Potatoes
Onions

To Store in Your Refrigerator . . .
Apples
Oranges
Tortillas
Milk (fat-free, low-fat, perhaps whole milk)
Yogurt
Parmesan cheese
Cheese (regular, reduced-fat)
Sliced smoked turkey breast or chicken, deli meat
Eggs (egg substitute in your freezer)
Bottled lemon juice
Bottled garlic (minced)

To Keep in Your Freezer . . .
Fruit juice concentrate (or fresh juice in your refrigerator, or juice boxes on the shelf)
Frozen vegetables
Frozen green pepper (chopped)
Frozen onion (chopped)
Frozen waffles or whole-wheat bagels
Frozen fish fillets
Lean ground beef
Pork loin chops
Chicken breast (perhaps skinless)
Frozen yogurt or fruit sorbet

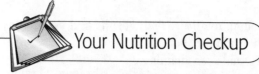

Your Nutrition Checkup

Kitchen Nutrition IQ

Do you cook with nutrition, as well as flavor, in mind? Test your kitchen nutrition IQ to see if what you know shows up in how you cook!

Do You . . .	ALWAYS	USUALLY	SOMETIMES	NEVER
Trim visible fat from meat and poultry?	___	___	___	___
Keep edible peels on fruits and vegetables—just wash, not peel them?	___	___	___	___
Remove the skin from poultry before eating it?	___	___	___	___
Use garnishes to make food look more appealing?	___	___	___	___
Cook vegetables until they're just tender-crisp?	___	___	___	___
Plan meals with many different fruits and vegetables?	___	___	___	___
Cook mostly with healthy oils?	___	___	___	___
Cook with whole grains such as brown rice or whole-wheat pasta?	___	___	___	___
Try to include foods with different colors and tastes in a meal?	___	___	___	___
Add canned or cooked legumes to salads, soups, or other foods?	___	___	___	___
Sprinkle cheese on salads, soups, and vegetables for more calcium?	___	___	___	___
Cook vegetables with the lid on the pot—in just a small amount of liquid, or steam or microwave them?	___	___	___	___
Sweeten foods with fruit, fruit juice, or fruit purees?	___	___	___	___
Use ingredients with less fat, such as low-fat yogurt, lean ground meat, and defatted broth?	___	___	___	___
Boost calcium in soups, cooked cereals, and casseroles with dry milk powder?	___	___	___	___
Drain fat off meat after it's cooked?	___	___	___	___
Use herbs, spices, or lemon juice and ease up on salt to flavor food?	___	___	___	___
Use lower-fat cooking methods: broil, grill, roast, stir-fry, steam, microwave, or braise?	___	___	___	___
Taste before deciding to add salt to foods?	___	___	___	___
Use cooking water from vegetables for soups, stews, or sauces?	___	___	___	___
Subtotal	___	___	___	___

Now score yourself:

"Always":   3 points

"Usually":   2 points

"Sometimes": 1 points

"Never":   0 point

Your total score _____

With 50 to 60 points, you're "kitchen nutrition-savvy."

With 40 to 49 points, improving your food preparation skills would make a nutrition difference! Read on.

With 21 to 39 points, you're starting to get the hang of it. Now turn those "sometimes" answers to "usually" and "always." Read the rest of the chapter for "food prep" tips.

With 20 points or less, read the chapter. There's lots to learn!

vegetables were good for you. Today, science better understands why they should be part of a personal eating plan with variety, balance, and moderation built in. Although their nutrient content varies, fruits and vegetables:

● Supply many essential nutrients: beta carotene (which becomes vitamin A), vitamin C, folate, vitamin B_6, potassium, calcium, magnesium, and selenium, as well as naturally occurring sugars, starches, and fiber.

● Are naturally low in total fat, saturated fat, *trans* fat, and sodium. They're also cholesterol-free.

● Provide an array of health-promoting phytonutrients, or plant chemicals.

● Get bulk from water, which is calorie-free!

Follow advice from MyPyramid on amounts: 2½ cups of vegetables and 2 cups of fruits daily if you eat 2,000 calories day—and make them colorful! If your calorie level is different, *check the Appendices for amounts*. Here's how you might fit a rainbow of fruits and vegetables in your food prep:

● *Try "grate" ways.* Add grated, shredded, or chopped vegetables such as zucchini, spinach, and carrots to lasagna, meat loaf, mashed potatoes, and meat, poultry, pasta, rice, and other grain dishes. Try shredded carrot or zucchini in muffins and other quick breads.

● *Be saucy with fruit.* Puree berries, apples, peaches, or pears for a thick, sweet sauce on grilled or broiled seafood or poultry, pancakes, French toast, or waffles.

Have You Ever Wondered ?

. . . if cooking ever makes vegetables or fruits more nutritious? Cooking won't add nutrients (unless ingredients are added) to a food, but can make food safer and perhaps more edible and appealing. For example, you probably prefer eating a potato that's cooked, not raw.

Sometimes cooking enhances nourishment. For example, lycopene, a phytonutrient in tomatoes, is absorbed in the body better from cooked or processed tomatoes; lycopene may offer protection from some cancers. Carotenoids (form vitamin A) are more available for absorption when cooked, as is lutein, a phytonutrient in corn.

● *Get creative with pizza.* Order or make it "deluxe" with vegetable toppings: asparagus, broccoli florets, carrot shreds, thinly sliced zucchini, chopped spinach, red and green bell pepper strips, chopped tomatoes, roasted peppers, or other firm veggies!

● *Bake with fruits and vegetables.* Use pureed fruit such as applesauce, dried plums (prunes), bananas, or peaches in place of about half the fat in recipes for homemade breads, muffins, pancakes, and other baked goods. For flavor, texture, and nutrients, blend in shredded zucchini, carrots, or dried fruits.

● *"Sandwich" in fruit and vegetables.* Add pizzazz to sandwiches by layering on sliced pineapple, apple, raisins, peppers, cucumbers, sprouts, or tomatoes.

● *Combine with veggies or fruit.* Make a quick stir-fry or combine pasta or rice with just about any vegetables, or add them to soup—great ways to use fresh vegetables before they spoil. Add apricots, pineapple, other fruit, or fruit chutney to meat or poultry dishes. *Hint:* Add canned, frozen, or cooked legumes.

● *Experiment.* Substitute a new-to-you fruit or vegetable in a favorite recipe. Try broccoli rabe (broccoli variety with smaller heads, also called rapini) in stir-fries, fennel in salad, or yautia (a starchy vegetable) in stew. Or try a new fruit or vegetable recipe.

● *Take a fruit to lunch!* Make a habit of tucking an apple, a tangerine, two plums or kiwifruit, grapes, cherries, dried fruits, or other fruit into your briefcase, tote, or lunch bag. Fruit is a great traveling snack.

● *Stuff an omelette with veggies.* For a hearty meal, fill it with crisp, tasty vegetables like broccoli, squash, carrots, peppers, tomatoes, spinach, or onions.

● *Toss up a vegetable salad.* Add colorful vegetables, legumes, and fruits (such as berries, kiwifruit, or mandarin oranges). Even if you prefer iceberg lettuce, which delivers less nutrients than other greens, pair it with other veggies—sliced beets, shredded red cabbage, spinach leaves, baby carrots.

● *Count your beans.* If you consume enough protein-rich foods from the Meat and Beans Group, legumes can count in the Vegetable Group. Add cooked, canned, or frozen beans, peas, or lentils to salads, casseroles, and pasta dishes. Puree cooked beans as a low-fat base for spreads, sauces, and soups.

Simple Ways to Keep Vitamins in Food

- Clean thick-skinned vegetables and fruits well with a soft brush and water. Avoid soaking them as you wash. Some vitamins dissolve in water.

- Leave edible skins on vegetables and fruits—for example, on carrots, potatoes, or pears. And trim away as little as possible. Most vitamins and minerals are found in the outer leaves, skin, and area just below the skin—not in the center. Peels also are natural barriers that help protect nutrient loss.

- Cook vegetables or fruits in a small amount of water—or better yet, steam them in a vegetable steamer or a microwave oven. Steaming retains most of the nutrients because vegetables usually don't come in contact with cooking liquids.

- Cut vegetables that need to be cooked longer into larger pieces. With fewer surfaces exposed, less vitamins are lost.

- Eat vegetables and fruits raw. Or cook many vegetables, such as asparagus, green beans, broccoli, and snow peas, quickly—just until tender-crisp. Some nutrients, such as B vitamins and vitamin C, are destroyed easily by heat. The shorter the cooking time, the more nutrients are retained.

   Short cooking times help vegetables keep their bright color and flavor, too. The flavors of strong-flavored vegetables, such as Brussels sprouts and turnips, can get even stronger when overcooked.

- Cook vegetables and fruits in a covered pot. Steam doesn't escape, and cooking time is faster.

- Just reheat canned vegetables on the stovetop or in the microwave oven. Canning is cooking, so canned vegetables don't need to be cooked again. They would lose flavor and nutrients!

- Save liquid from cooking vegetables for soups, stews, and sauces; perhaps freeze it for later use. That's one way to "recycle" water-soluble vitamins and minerals that otherwise would be tossed with the cooking water.

- For beets and red cabbage, add a little lemon juice or vinegar to the cooking water. This helps retain their bright-red color. Don't add baking soda! Although the alkali in baking soda keeps vegetables looking greener, it also destroys some vitamins.

- Microwave! Why? First, because microwaving is so fast, heat-sensitive nutrients aren't subjected to heat for long. Second, microwaving doesn't require added fat. There's a flavor advantage, too: unless overcooked, vegetables retain the color and tender-crisp qualities that make them appealing.

- Keep milk in opaque containers in the fridge. Leaving it in a clear, glass pitcher on the table allows some riboflavin to be destroyed by sunlight.

- Skip the urge to rinse grains, such as rice, before cooking. That may wash nutrients down the drain.

- *Make dips and spreads with vegetables and fruit.* Spicy salsas can be made with tomato, bell peppers, onions, and cilantro. For a tangy twist, also look for salsas with pineapples, mangoes, papayas, or peaches. Try hummus, made with mashed chickpeas; or caponata, made with eggplant and tomato; or baba ghanouj, made with eggplant.

- *Toss in dried fruits:* dried cranberries, apples, dried plums (prunes), bananas, papayas, mangoes, apricots, pears, pineapples, or raisins. They're great in stuffing, rice dishes, tossed salads, main dish salads, homemade breads, and casseroles; even desserts!

- *Focus on veggies.* Enjoy 3-ounce cooked portions of meat, poultry, and fish; fill the rest of the plate with vegetables, fruits, and grain products. A vegetable-meat kebob is one way to do it. It's great for grilling!

- *Feature veggies with grains in casseroles.* Let meat, poultry, or fish add flavor but not take center stage.

- *Stock up.* Fill your fridge with raw vegetables and fruits—"nature's fast food"—cleaned, cut up, and ready to eat in a see-through container. Try baby carrots! Keep canned and frozen vegetables and fruit on hand for convenience.

For more ideas, see "Garden of Eatin': Uncommon Vegetables" and "Fresh Ideas: Less Common Fruit" in chapter 9, and "MyPyramid Pointers" in chapter 10.

Fat (and Cholesterol): Trim or Switch

Hardly a day goes by without a new magazine or newspaper article giving tips for trimming total fat, saturated fat, *trans* fat, and cholesterol in foods prepared at home. And with good reason—many people consume more fat, especially saturated fat, than their bodies need for health. And there's no known need for *trans* fats.

Many health conditions can be linked to high-fat diets, especially those high in saturated fat. Instead learn to prepare foods with healthy oils (such as canola, olive, and sunflower oils), which contain less saturated fat and *trans* fats. Cook so your overall food choices provide 20 to 35 percent of your total calories. *Refer to chapter 3 with more ways to moderate fat.*

Fats have many roles in recipes. For one, they carry, blend, and stabilize flavor. With less fat, flavors may be more volatile, and not hold up as long as you might like. In baked foods, fat tenderizes, adds moisture, holds air in so they're light, and affects the shape—

Meat, Poultry, and Fish: Lean Cuts and Low-Fat Cooking Methods

	Dry Heat					Moist Heat			
	Roast	Broil	Grill	Panbroil	Stir-fry	Braise	Stew	Steam	Poach
Beef									
Eye round*		X				X	X		
Top round*	X	X	X	X	X				
Round tip*	X	X	X	X	X	X	X		
Bottom round*	X					X	X		
Sirloin	X	X	X	X	X				
Top loin	X	X	X	X	X				
Tenderloin	X	X	X	X	X				
Flank*		X	X		X				
95% lean ground beef	X	X	X	X	X				
Pork									
Tenderloin	X	X	X	X	X				
Boneless top loin roast	X	X	X						
Loin chop		X	X	X					
Loin strips					X				
Boneless sirloin chop		X	X	X					
Boneless rib roast	X		X			X	X		
Rib chop		X	X	X					
Boneless ham	X	X	X	X	X				
Poultry†									
Whole chicken	X		X			X	X		
Whole turkey	X		X			X			
Cornish game hen	X		X			X	X		
Breast	X	X	X	X	X				X
Drumstick	X	X	X						
Fish									
Cod	X	X	X	X	X		X	X	X
Flounder	X	X	X	X				X	X
Halibut	X	X	X	X	X		X	X	X
Orange roughy		X	X	X	X			X	X
Shrimp		X	X	X	X		X	X	X

*May be cooked by dry heat methods if they are tenderized first by marinating or pounding.
†White meat has less fat than dark meat. Skin should be removed before eating.
Source: ©Cattlemen's Beef Board and National Cattlemen's Beef Association Culinary Center.

for example, in cookies. In sauces, fats keep foods from curdling and form part of an emulsion, so water and fats combine smoothly. Fat in recipes conducts heat—for example, when sautéeing and stir-frying. Fat lubricates so food doesn't stick to the pan and seals in moisture when foods are basted. Fat also carries some nutrients from food into your body.

Good cooking and good health rely on moderate amounts of total fat. To trim saturated and *trans* fats and calories, too, use more oils and fewer solid fats, and more lean meats and low-fat or fat-free dairy foods. And trim fat in food prep. With these changes, you can serve great-tasting food!

Lean Tips . . . for a Variety of Foods

● Use cooking methods that require little or no added fat; try to boil, broil, grill, roast, braise, stew, steam, poach, stir-fry, or microwave foods, rather than fry them, most of the time. *For more about these cooking techniques, see "Culinary Lingo," "Meat Cookery: Moist-Heat Methods," and "Meat Cookery: Dry-Heat Methods" in this chapter.*

● Stretch higher-fat ingredients. For example, grate cheese so less looks like more. Spread 1 tablespoon of peanut butter on toast rather than 2 tablespoons.

● Use tempeh, tofu, or legumes as a low-fat but high-protein ingredient in stews, soups, pasta dishes, and other mixed foods. *For more about tempeh and tofu, see "What's 'Soy' Good?" in chapter 10.*

● Substitute reduced-fat and fat-free products in many recipes. *See chapter 11, "Shopping Savvy," for suggestions throughout the supermarket.*

How Much Fat and "Sat-Fat" in the 29 Lean** Beef Cuts?

BEEF CUT	CALORIES	SATURATED FAT (GRAMS)	TOTAL FAT (GRAMS)
Eye Round Roast and Steak*	144	1.4	4.0
Sirloin Tip Side Steak	143	1.6	4.1
Top Round Roast and Steak*	157	1.6	4.6
Bottom Round Roast and Steak*	139	1.7	4.9
Top Sirloin Steak	156	1.9	4.9
Brisket, Flat Half	167	1.9	5.1
95% Lean Ground Beef	139	2.4	5.1
Round Tip Roast and Steak*	148	1.9	5.3
Round Steak	154	1.9	5.3
Shank Cross Cuts	171	1.9	5.4
Chuck Shoulder Pot Roast	147	1.8	5.7
Sirloin Tip Center Roast and Steak*	150	2.1	5.8
Chuck Shoulder Steak	161	1.9	6.0
Bottom Round (Western Griller) Steak	155	2.2	6.0
Top Loin (Strip) Steak	161	2.3	6.0
Shoulder Petite Tender and Medallions*	150	2.4	6.1
Flank Steak	158	2.6	6.3
Shoulder Center (Ranch) Steak	155	2.4	6.5
Tri-Tip Roast and Steak	158	2.6	7.1
Tenderloin Roast and Steak*	170	2.7	7.1
T-Bone Steak	172	3.0	8.2

*Cuts combined for illustration purposes.

**Less than 10 grams of total fat, 4.5 grams or less of saturated fat, and less than 95 milligrams of cholesterol per 3-ounce cooked serving (per 100 grams)

Calories and fat are based on 3-ounce cooked servings, visible fat removed.

Source: ©Cattlemen's Beef Board and National Cattlemen's Beef Association Culinary Center.

● Coat pans with a thin layer of oil, then wipe with a paper towel. Two tablespoons of oil add 240 calories and 28 fat grams; a thin coating of vegetable oil spray has just 10 calories and 1 fat gram. Using nonstick pans makes it easier to use less fat.

● Substitute yogurt cheese for higher-calorie, higher-fat spreads. *To learn to make it, see chapter 3.*

● Skip or limit breading, which adds fat and calories. It makes food soak up more fat during frying.

● Drain pan-fried foods on a paper towel to absorb extra grease. Go easy on the oil.

● When adding ingredients to packaged mixes (such as macaroni and cheese, scalloped potatoes, or brownies), try soft margarine or oil instead of stick

---

Meat Cookery: Dry Heat Methods in Three Easy Steps

Roasting

1. Heat oven to recommended temperature (varies based on cut of meat).

2. Place roast (straight from refrigerator) fat side up, on rack in shallow roasting pan. Season before cooking as desired. Insert an ovenproof meat thermometer so tip is centered in thickest part of roast, not resting in fat or touching bone. Do not add water; do not cover.

3. For beef, pork, veal, and lamb, roast to 5 to 10° F below desired doneness.* Transfer to carving board; tent loosely with aluminum foil. Let stand fifteen to twenty minutes. (Temperature will continue to rise 5 to 10° F to reach desired doneness.) For whole poultry, cook until desired temperature is reached.*

Broiling

1. Preheat broiler for ten minutes.

2. Place meat, poultry, or fish on rack in broiler pan. Season with herbs or spices as desired. Position thinner pieces (¾ to 1 inch) so that surface of meat is 2 to 3 inches from the heat; thicker pieces, 3 to 6 inches from the heat.

3. Broil to desired doneness, turning once.* After cooking, season with salt if desired.

Grilling

1. For gas grilling, set heat to medium. For charcoal grilling, coals should be ash-covered and medium temperature; allow about thirty minutes. (To test cooking temperature for charcoal grill: spread coals out in single layer. Carefully hold palm of hand above the coals at cooking height. Count the number of seconds you can hold your hand in that position before the heat forces you to pull it away—approximately four seconds for medium heat.)

2. Season meat, poultry, or fish with herbs or spices as desired. For smaller pieces of meat, poultry, or fish (chops, steaks, burgers, breasts, fillets, or kebobs), place on cooking grid directly over coals. For roasts, thick steaks, or chops, whole chicken or turkey, the meat is placed on the grid, with coals or heat source on each side.

3. Grill to desired doneness, turning occasionally.* After cooking, season with salt if desired.

Panbroiling

1. Heat heavy nonstick skillet over medium heat (meats ¾ inch or thicker) or medium high heat (meats ½ inch or thinner) until hot, about five minutes.

2. Season meat, poultry, or fish with herbs or spices as desired. Place in preheated skillet. Do not crowd. Do not add oil or water. Do not cover.

3. Cook to desired doneness, turning once.* For thicker pieces, turn occasionally. Remove excess drippings as they accumulate. After cooking, season with salt if desired.

Stir-Frying

1. Partially freeze meat, poultry, or fish (about 30 minutes) for easier slicing. Cut into thin, uniform strips or pieces. Marinate to add flavor or tenderize while preparing other ingredients if desired.

2. Heat small amount of oil in wok or large heavy nonstick skillet over medium high heat until hot.

3. Stir-fry in ½-pound batches (do not overcrowd), continuously turning with a scooping motion, until cooked to desired doneness. Add additional oil for each batch if necessary. (Cook meat and vegetables separately, then combine and heat through.)

*See "Safe Internal Temperatures" in chapter 12.

Source: ©Cattlemen's Beef Board and National Cattlemen's Beef Association Culinary Center.

margarine or butter. Or use half the fat, 95% lean ground beef in casserole mixes, or fat-free milk in brownies or instant pudding.

● In place of butter only, use half butter and half oil for less saturated fat.

Lean Tips . . . for Meat, Poultry, and Fish

● Cook with lean meats (*see page 319*), skinless poultry, and fish. *See chapter 11 for buying tips. To decide how to cook them, see "Meat, Poultry, and Fish: Lean Cuts and Low-Fat Cooking Methods" in this chapter.*

Have You Ever Wondered?

. . . how the fat content of deep-fried turkey compares to roasted turkey? If the cooking oil stays high enough— 350°F for the entire frying process—it makes little difference. A 3½-ounce portion of deep-fried turkey with the skin on has about 12 grams of fat, compared with 10 grams in a 3½-ounce portion of roasted turkey (white and dark meat) with the skin on. However, if the cooking oil remains at 340°F or less, more oil seeps into the turkey meat, adding to the fat content. For the record, without the skin, the same amount of roasted turkey (white and dark meat) has 5 fat grams.

Meat Cookery: Moist-Heat Methods in Three Easy Steps

Braising

1. Slowly brown meat or poultry on all sides in small amount of oil in heavy pan. Pour off drippings. Season as desired.
2. Add small amount (½ cup to 2 cups) of liquid such as broth, water, juice, beer, or wine.
3. Cover tightly and simmer gently over low heat on top of the range or in a preheated 325° F oven until meat or poultry is fork-tender. (The cooking liquid may be reduced or thickened for a sauce after removing fat as desired.)

Stewing

1. Lightly coat meat, poultry, or fish with seasoned flour if desired. Slowly brown on all sides, in small amount of oil, if necessary, in heavy pan. Pour off drippings. Season as desired.
2. Add liquid such as defatted broth, water, juice, beer, and/or wine to pan. (Use ½ cup to 2 cups liquid for chili type/shredded beef dishes; enough liquid to cover for stews and soups.) Bring to a boil; reduce heat.
3. Cover tightly and simmer gently over low heat on top of the range, or in a preheated 325° F oven until meat, poultry, or fish is fork-tender. (Cooking soups in the oven is not practical.) Thicken or reduce defatted liquid as desired.

Poaching

1. Season meat, poultry, or fish as desired. For roasts, tie with heavy string at 2-inch intervals if needed. Brown on all sides in nonstick pan. Pour off excess drippings.
2. Cover meat, poultry, or fish with liquid such as defatted broth, juice, water, beer, or wine. Season with additional ingredients if desired.
3. Bring to a boil. Reduce heat, cover, and simmer until fork-tender.

Steaming

1. Place fish on a steamer pan or a perforated tray. Vegetables, such as onions, leeks, celery, and bok choy, can be added.
2. Set steamer into pan above simmering liquid.
3. Cover pan and continue simmering over low heat until fish flakes.

Microwave

1. Place fish in a microwave-safe dish in spoke fashion for even cooking.
2. Add a small amount of liquid or seasoned vegetables if desired. (Some vegetables may take longer to cook; choose vegetables with similar cooking times, or cook vegetables separately.)
3. Cover with microwave-safe plastic wrap, venting or lifting one corner.
4. Following manufacturer's directions, microwave on high until fish flakes and any added vegetables are tender.

Source: ©Cattlemen's Beef Board and National Cattlemen's Beef Association Culinary Center.

Degreasing Pan Juices, Soups, and Gravies

Remember your science lessons? Fat rises to the top because it's lighter than water. The same thing happens in cooking. Fat in pan juices, soups, gravies, and canned broth collects on top, making it easy to skim off. Every tablespoon of fat you discard removes about 120 calories and 13 fat grams from the dish you're preparing.

- Remove fat from meat and poultry juices with a wide-mouthed spoon or a fat-separating pitcher.

- Refrigerate soups and stews before they're served. Do the same with homemade and canned broth, soups, and chili. Fat, which hardens when chilled, is easy to remove with a spoon.

- When time is short, add a few ice cubes to the broth. Fat will rise and congeal around the ice, but the ice may dilute the broth slightly.

- Use smaller amounts of processed meats that tend to have more fat: bacon, hot dogs, and luncheon meats. Or use leaner versions, at least "90 percent lean."

- When recipes call for bacon, use lean ham, Canadian bacon, or smoked turkey for the smoky flavor.

- Trim off visible, solid fat on meat and poultry before cooking. Even on lean meat, you'll find some fat. Trimming fat from the edges removes some, but not all the cholesterol; cholesterol is in both the lean tissue and the fat in meat, poultry, and fish. On whole birds most fat appears near the cavity opening.

- Go "skinless" on poultry. Under the skin there's a layer of fat. Remove the skin before or after cooking it to cut the fat content about in half; there's not much difference, as long as you remove the skin before you eat it! *Tip:* Cooking poultry with the skin on helps keep it tender and moist. The same is true for beef and pork; trim remaining fat after cooking.

- Drain off fat from ground-meat crumbles as they're cooked. To reduce fat further, transfer cooked ground-meat crumbles to a large plate lined with 3 layers of white, recycled paper towels. Blot top of meat and let sit one minute. Place meat in a strainer or a colander. Pour about 1 quart of hot tap water over the meat. Drain five minutes. You can rinse away 2 to 5 grams of fat per 3-ounce cooked serving.

- Blot cooked ground-meat burgers, meatballs, and meat loaf with several layers of clean paper towels.

- Brown meat, poultry, and seafood in a nonstick skillet with little or no added fat, except for vegetable oil spray, or use a little oil. Compare: 2 tablespoons of oil to brown meat carry an extra 240 calories from 28 fat grams, compared with less than 10 calories (1 fat gram) from oil spray. Browning adds flavor.

- Grill, broil, or roast meat and poultry on a rack so fat drips through and drippings aren't reabsorbed. Drain away any fat that appears during cooking.

- Marinate meat, poultry, and fish in marinades with little or no fat: orange, lime, or lemon juice; defatted broth; wine; tomato juice; salsas; fat-free or reduced-fat salad dressings; plain, low-fat yogurt; or buttermilk. Add fresh herbs to the marinade.

- To keep fish or chicken moist, steam fillets in heavy aluminum foil with fruit, herbs, onions, vegetables, and other flavorings. Secure the "package" and then bake it in the oven or on the grill. For the oven, you can also wrap and cook meat, fish, or poultry in parchment paper (chefs call this *en papillote,* or paper package) or leaf packets (such as banana leaves).

- Oven-fry fish or chicken. Dip it first in egg whites, then coat with seasoned bread crumbs. Bake on a nonstick baking pan coated with vegetable oil spray.

- As a quick, low-fat dish, bake fish with a splash of white wine, tomatoes, and fresh herbs.

Lean Tips . . . for Egg Dishes

A great meat alternative, eggs supply protein, iron, and lutein to the diet. While nutritious, health experts advise healthy Americans to eat whole eggs and yolks in moderation to control dietary cholesterol (to keep cholesterol intake less than 300 milligrams daily).

Egg yolks, not whites, contain fat and cholesterol. (A yolk from one large egg has about 215 milligrams of cholesterol.) That's why you can use egg whites liberally in place of egg yolks in many foods. Here's how to enjoy eggs in moderation:

- Use two egg whites in place of one whole egg in breads, pancakes, casseroles, French toast, cookies, cheesecake, pudding, and other recipes that call for whole eggs. Although one egg white can substitute for one yolk, recipes that require egg yolks, such as puff pastry, are best made with whole eggs.

● Use a cholesterol-free liquid egg product in place of whole eggs. Usually ¼ cup egg product equals one whole egg; check the package label.

● In recipes that call for two or more eggs, substitute just some of the whole eggs with egg whites. For example, for two whole eggs, instead use two egg whites and one whole egg. That way you'll get the color and the flavor of the yolk, but less cholesterol and less fat. This idea works well for scrambled eggs, quiche, and omelettes.

Lean Tips . . . for Vegetables

● For vegetables, "sauté" with just a little oil. Or cook them in a little defatted broth, juice, wine, or water in a covered, nonstick pan. It's great for onions and mushrooms, which are sautéed for many recipes!

● Cook vegetables by steaming, stir-frying (in a nonstick wok or skillet), simmering, or microwaving. If you really enjoy the crispiness of French fries and fried onion rings, oven-bake them instead of frying them. Skip added fat, such as bacon, on legumes (dry beans) and other vegetables.

EASY SUBSTITUTIONS TO CUT FAT, SATURATED FAT, *TRANS* FAT, AND/OR CHOLESTEROL

WHEN COOKING CALLS FOR . . .	USE . . .
Sour cream	Plain low-fat yogurt, or ½ cup cottage cheese blended with 1 ½ tsp. lemon juice, or light or fat-free sour cream
Whipped cream	Chilled, whipped evaporated fat-free (skim) milk, or nondairy whipped topping
Cream	Evaporated fat-free (skim) milk, fat-free half-and-half
Whole milk	Fat-free (skim), 1 percent, or 2 percent milk as a beverage or in recipes
Full-fat cheese	Low-fat, part skim-milk cheese, cheese with less than 5 grams of fat per ounce, or fat-free cheese (be aware that cooking qualities differ)
Ricotta cheese	Low-fat or fat-free cottage cheese or nonfat or low-fat ricotta cheese
Ice cream	Low-fat or fat-free ice cream, or frozen low-fat or fat-free yogurt, frozen fruit juice products such as sorbet
Ground beef	95% lean ground beef, or lean ground turkey or chicken
Bacon	Canadian bacon, lean ham, or smoked deli turkey
Sausage	Lean ground turkey, or 95% fat-free sausage
Whole egg	Two egg whites, or ¼ cup cholesterol-free liquid egg product, or 1 egg white plus 2 tsp. oil
One egg yolk	One egg white
One egg (as thickener)	1 tbsp. flour
Mayonnaise	Low-fat, reduced-fat, or fat-free mayonnaise or whipped salad dressing, or plain low-fat yogurt combined with pureed low-fat cottage cheese
Salad dressings	Low-fat or fat-free dressings, or homemade dressing made with less saturated oil (peanut, soy, olive, canola, others), water, and vinegar or lemon juice
Cream soups	Defatted broths, or broth-based or fat-free milk-based soups
Nuts	Dried fruit such as raisins, chopped dried apricots, or dried cranberries
1 ounce unsweetened baking chocolate	3 tbsp. cocoa powder and 1 tbsp. oil
Butter, lard, stick margarine	Soft, tub margarine, squeeze margarine

KITCHEN NUTRITION: DELICIOUS DECISIONS

● Puree or mash potatoes, sweet potatoes, and other vegetables with milk, reduced-sodium broth, or liquid from cooking potatoes. Go easy on butter or margarine. Boost the flavor and the nutrients by blending in shredded carrots or zucchini or a little olive oil!

● For the flavor of butter on vegetables, add a small amount of butter—but just before serving. (Add herbs and garlic, too.) Cooking dilutes the flavor. You need less if you add it last. Or try a butter-flavored spray or powder.

● Sprinkle some Parmesan or Romano cheese on vegetables for flavor but not much fat or calories.

● Roast or grill vegetables and fruit (sliced eggplant, pineapple slices, bell pepper chunks, sliced zucchini) as a low-fat way to bring out the flavor. They're great as kebobs! Coat them lightly with vegetable oil spray or olive oil. Then roast in the oven at 400° F or grill for about 15 minutes until tender-crisp.

Lean Tips . . . for Salads

● Flavor salads with lower-fat commercial dressings, or make your own with less oil and more vinegar. Use healthy oils! *See Chapter 10.*

● On taco salads, use lots of salsa with tomatoes, chiles, onions, herbs, and lime juice. Use a lighter touch with sour cream by going "50–50": 50 percent sour cream, 50 percent plain, low-fat yogurt. Or use reduced-fat or fat-free sour cream.

● Instead of creamy coleslaw made with regular mayonnaise, moisten cabbage and other shredded vegetables with low-fat or fat-free yogurt or mayonnaise with seasonings. Or use vinaigrette dressing.

● Adjust the proportions in homemade vinaigrette. Make it with three parts vinegar to one part oil (e.g., ¾ cup vinegar to ¼ cup oil) instead of the other way around. Experiment with different types of flavored oils and vinegars or make your own herbed vinegars. *See "Herbed Vinegars" later in this chapter.*

Lean Tips . . . for Grain Dishes and Breads

● Skip the oil or use just a little when cooking pasta, but use plenty of water. Don't rinse, just drain cooked pasta; toss with sauce immediately so pasta won't stick together; use a lower-fat sauce such as tomato-based or other vegetable sauces. For more flavor, add herbs or flavored pastas, such as basil or garlic.

● Cook couscous, rice, and other grains with herbs, defatted broth, or juice instead of fat. Don't rinse rice; you'll wash away some vitamins, especially B vitamins, added to enriched and fortified grain products.

● Serve breads, rolls, muffins, bagels, and biscuits with low-fat spreads—fruit butter, chutney, jam, mustard, reduced-fat margarine spread, nonfat mayonnaise, reduced-fat or nonfat cream cheese, or pureed beans such as hummus. *For condiments with less fat, see "Lighter Condiments" in this chapter.*

Lean Tips . . . for Soups, Stews, and Sauces

● Skip gravy and rich sauces; enhance the flavors with fat-free ingredients: garlic, ginger, lemon juice, onions, tomatoes, herbs, and spices, among others. Before cooking, use a herb rub on meat, poultry, or fish; for a spicy taste, rub a mixture of cumin, chile powder, coriander, red and black peppers, and cinnamon on a pork roast. Or coat meat, poultry, or fish with salsas or chutneys. *See "Rub Combos" in this chapter for herb rubs and salsa ideas.*

● Cut back on oil in homemade marinades. Or marinate with reduced-fat or fat-free salad dressing.

● "Sauce" up the flavor of vegetables, poultry, fish, and pasta with pureed vegetables or reduction sauces rather than cream-based sauces. For a creamy texture, add milk, yogurt, or low-fat cottage cheese to vegetables as you process them in the blender or food processor. To warm, reheat gently.

● Try these "creamy" sauces. Blend fresh dill or other herbs into fat-free, plain yogurt as a sauce for seafood or chicken. Blend horseradish with plain yogurt to serve with lean beef. For an easy sauce, braise poultry, fish, and meat in low-fat canned soups. Then heat to reduce the liquid to sauce consistency.

● Skim fat from pan juices, soups, and stews. *For quick techniques, see "Degreasing Pan Juices, Soups, and Gravies" in this chapter.*

● Thicken soups and stews with pureed beans, potatoes, or other vegetables and nonfat dry milk. Or puree part of the soup and add it back as a thickener. Added vegetables can boost the vitamin and phytonutrient content; adding dry milk powder "ups" the calcium. Neither adds fat. For another "creamy" ingredient, try buttermilk or evaporated fat-free (skim) milk.

● If the recipe calls for a rich sauce, go easy. You want to add flavor, not overwhelm the food, with sauce.

Lean Tips . . . for Baked Goods

● Experiment a little. Take out some fat—but not all. In baked breads, cakes, muffins, and brownies, try substituting an equal amount of applesauce, mashed bananas or dried plums (prunes), other pureed fruit, mashed garbanzos, or cottage cheese for at least half the oil, margarine, or butter in recipes. For bar and drop cookies, this substitution often works well.

Try buttermilk or nonfat or low-fat yogurt in place of sour cream, butter, and margarine in biscuits, muffins, and other breads. Some recipes work well with less fat; others don't. For example, with less fat, baked goods may not brown as well. Shortbread, butter cakes, butter cookies, and many pound cakes need fat for the flavor and texture you expect.

● Enjoy a nutty flavor? So less nuts taste like more, toast or chop them for the most flavor. For even more flavor (or to extend it), yet no more fat, mix in chopped dried fruits, too: dried apricots, dried apples, raisins, dried cranberries, or dried plums (prunes).

● Coat baking pans very lightly with nonstick vegetable oil spray rather than margarine, butter, or oil.

● Instead of whipped cream toppings, whip chilled evaporated fat-free milk—with a touch of sugar—for a creamy topping. Serve it right away since it's less stable and may get runny! Evaporated fat-free milk can be substituted for heavy cream in many recipes.

● Skip the frosting on a cake, or frost it lightly. Why not dust it with powdered sugar, or top with fresh fruit or fruit puree?

● Instead of flaky pastry shells with their high-fat content, make desserts with graham cracker crumb crusts. Prepare crumb crusts with half the margarine or butter called for in the recipe. If the crumbs seem dry, add just a little liquid to moisten.

● Prepare single-crust pies. Either make an open-face pie, or arrange the fruit in the pie pan first, then put the crust on top. *Another tip:* Top with uncooked oatmeal mixed with a few finely chopped nuts.

Try This: Give It a Shake!

How much salt do you typically add to food? Take the "shaker test" to find out. Cover a plate or a bowl with foil or plastic wrap. Now pretend your dinner is on the plate—or that the bowl is filled with popcorn. Salt your "food" just as you would if the bowl or plate was full of food. Now measure how much salt you added. If you shook as much as ¼ teaspoon of salt, you added almost 600 milligrams of sodium to your meal or popcorn.

● As easy substitutions, use low-fat and fat-free dairy products to trim calories, too.

● To cut down on saturated fat and *trans* fat, experiment with cooking oil instead of margarine, butter, or lard. However, the texture of baked goods will differ, being coarser, mealier, and perhaps more oily. This substitution isn't suggested for quick breads, pastry, or sweet baked goods that are higher in fat to start.

Oil has more shortening power than solid fat, without the small amount of water that most solid fats contain. The recipe probably needs less oil than the amount of solid fat called for. Use this substitution:

FOR SOLID FAT . . .	TRY LIQUID OIL . . .
1 tbsp.	¾ tbsp.
⅓ cup	4 tbsp. (¼ cup)
½ cup	6 tbsp.
¾ cup	9 tbsp.
1 cup	12 tbsp. (¾ cup)

● Replace some (not all) whole eggs with whites. Baked goods can be rubbery with only whites.

Salt "Shakers"

Cooking with salt may seem so natural that it goes unnoticed. As an average American, about 11 percent of your sodium comes from food prep or salt you add at the table. A salt preference and the habit of cooking with salt are learned. You can unlearn them, too.

You don't need to eliminate sodium from your cooking. In fact, you probably can't—and you shouldn't! Sodium occurs naturally in many foods, and it's a nutrient your body needs in limited amounts. *See chapter 7, "Sodium and Potassium: A Salty Subject."*

Learn to choose and prepare food with little salt. Do

so gradually . . . especially if you're a salt lover. After a while, your taste for salt probably will change. You might be surprised when some foods seem too salty! Except for recipes with yeast, you can cut back on salt, in most traditional recipes, perhaps by 50 percent—or even eliminate it. Baked goods made with yeast need salt to control the rising of the dough.

● Taste before you reach for the salt shaker. Food may taste great just as it is!

● Shake the habit! Remove the salt shaker from the kitchen counter and the table. A ⅛-teaspoon "salt shake" adds about 300 milligrams of sodium to your dish. Many health experts advise a limit on sodium intake for the general population: less than 2,300 milligrams a day.

● Instead of added salt, spark up the flavor with herbs and spices, garlic, onions, balsamic vinegar, and citrus juice. *See "A Pinch of Flavor: How to Cook with Herbs and Spices" in this chapter.*

● Make a little salt go further. Salt your food lightly just before serving. When it's on the surface of food, the salty taste seems more intense. Get a bigger flavor burst (and use *less* salt) with a large-granule, coarse salt, such as kosher or sea salt. Instead of salt, add a touch of flavor with foods that contain some salt and a little fat, such as olives, Parmesan or Romano cheese, and salted nuts. The fat helps keep the salty taste in your mouth longer.

● Drain liquid and rinse some canned vegetables such as canned beans to reduce salt. Cook in tap water or defatted sodium-free broth.

● Reduce or skip salt in cooking water . . . even if a package label says to add it. Salt won't make water boil any faster. Instead, season pasta, rice, vegetables, and cereals with spices or herbs *after* they're cooked.

● Use prepared ingredients with less sodium—perhaps low-sodium broth, no-salt-added canned vegetables, light soy sauce, and salt-free seasoning mixes. Read the label. If foods have ingredients with salt or sodium already, you likely don't need more in a recipe.

Fiber Boosters

Does your plate lack much fiber? You're not alone. With so many refined ingredients in breads, pasta, and

other grain products and too few fruits and vegetables, many people come up short. Yet a few easy changes—more vegetables, fruits, and whole grains—in your cooking style can boost your fiber factor—and add interest and flavor, too!

Why boost fiber? Besides fiber's many health benefits, it's often bundled with other important nutrients and phytonutrients. And many fiber-rich foods have fewer calories and less fat. *To learn more, see chapter 6, "Fiber: Your Body's Broom."*

More Fiber with Grains . . . Especially Whole Grains

MyPyramid advice: make at least half your grains whole! Although fiber content varies, many whole grains are great sources of fiber (and they deliver many more nutrient and phytonutrient benefits, too). *See chapter 5, "Carbs: Simply Complex."*

● Substitute whole-grain pasta—lasagna noodles, macaroni, spaghetti, and other whole-grain pastas—in all kinds of dishes. Use brown or wild rice (2 grams and 1.5 grams of fiber, respectively, per ½ cup cooked) in place of white rice (<0.5 fiber grams per ½ cup cooked), too—or use a combination.

● Experiment with unfamiliar whole grains: perhaps whole barley, buckwheat, bulgur, millet, quinoa, rye berries, and wheat berries. *Refer to "Today's Grains" in chapter 9. The chart "Cooking Grain by Grain" in this chapter shows how to prepare them.*

● In dough and batter, substitute whole-wheat flour for half of the refined white flour. Don't go 100

Have You Ever Wondered

. . . how to cook with flaxseed? To get the benefit of flaxseed, you need to grind it in a blender, food processor, or coffee grinder. Then add it to dough and batter, or use it as a topping on puddings, cereal, and other food. Flaxseed is high in fiber and supplies omega-3 fatty acids, yet has little saturated fat.

. . . if you should soak ham, bacon, or salt pork to get rid of some salt? No. Very little salt is removed. More important, for food safety, washing meat is not advised.

Cooking Grain by Grain

Wonder how to cook whole grains? You can use the same simple steps for all these whole grains. Bring the cooking water to a boil; stir in the grain. Cover, reduce heat, and simmer. Let stand, covered, if indicated below. Then use these wonderful cooked grains in salads; as side dishes flavored with sauces or seasonings; or in soups.

1 Cup Uncooked Grain	Cooking Water (Cups)	Cooking Time (Minutes)	Standing Time (Minutes)	Yield (Cups)	Common Uses
Amaranth	3	25	—	3½	Cereal, side dish
Buckwheat (kasha)	2	20	10	3	Side dish (buckwheat groats flour also used in baked foods)
Bulgur	1½	*	30	2½	Side dish, stew, salad (tabbouleh)
Hominy (corn) (soak 8 hours)	4	30	5	3½	Side dish, stew, soup, cereal
Millet	2¾	30	15	3	Side dish, bread
Pearl barley	3	40	5	3½	Side dish, cereal, soup
Quinoa (rinsed)	2	15	—	3	Side dish, stuffing, soup, salad, stew
Rice, brown	2½	45	5	3	Wherever rice is used
Rice, wild[†]	3	55	—	3½	Side dish, stuffing, soup, salad
Rye berries	2	60	—	2¾	Side dish, bread
Triticale (wheat and rye) (soak overnight)	2½	40	—	4	Side dish, soup, cereal, bread
Wheat berries (soak overnight)	2	45	—	2½	Side dish, bread

*Bulgur isn't cooked. Put bulgur in a bowl, pour boiling water over it, and let it stand until the water is absorbed.
[†]Wild rice is actually a seed, not rice.

Sources: Compiled from L. C. Peterson, "The ABC's of Whole Grains," *Food Management* (March 1993):108; J. E. Brody, *Jane Brody's Good Food Book* (New York: Bantam Books, 1987).

percent, though; the texture will be too dense. Try the new whole-grain white flour.

● Try oat flour in baking, too. Whirl dry oatmeal in a blender to make oat flour. Use it to replace up to ⅓ of white flour in a recipe.

● Stack your sandwiches with whole-grain goodness. Use whole-grain breads, whole-grain English muffins, and whole-grain pita pockets.

● Add wheat or oat bran to casseroles, meat loaf, and dry or cooked cereal. Or blend some with yogurt for a little crunch. Each tablespoon of bran adds a little more than 1 gram of fiber.

● Use whole-grain breakfast cereals. Look for the words "whole-grain" on the package. Other label clues are a "good source of fiber" or "rich in fiber." Oats in cereal are whole grain, too. *Note:* Bran cereals are high in fiber, but they aren't whole grain. *Refer to chapter 11 for more on label reading.*

● Add oatmeal, nuts, and seeds (sesame seed, poppy seed) to mixed dishes: pudding and fruit toppings, meat loaf, stuffing, salmon patties, crab cakes, burgers.

More Fiber with Fruits and Veggies

● Keep peels on fruits and vegetables. A medium baked potato with the skin on has about twice the fiber of a "naked" potato: 5 fiber grams compared to 2.5 fiber grams!

● Add legumes and lentils to all kinds of dishes. For

convenience, use canned or frozen. *Check "A Word about Legumes . . ." in this chapter for ideas!*

● Add extra vegetables to casseroles, soups, salads, pizza, sandwiches, and pasta and rice dishes. For example, adding ½ cup of broccoli to a pasta dish adds 2 grams of fiber. A quarter cup of cooked spinach, mixed in soup or risotto, adds 2 grams of fiber. And half a medium-size carrot, shredded as a salad topper, adds 1 gram of fiber.

● Enjoy the fiber factor of fruits. Use all kinds of fruit in salads, cooked cereals, and as toppers on frozen desserts and angel food cake. For example, try sliced berries, pears, or peaches. A half cup of strawberries and a half of a pear (skin on) each add 2 grams of fiber!

● Mix dry fruit—raisins, dried cranberries, apricots, figs, and plums (prunes)—into breads, cookie dough, salads, and other dishes. One-quarter cup of raisins adds 2 grams of fiber; three dried plums (prunes) have almost as much!

A Word about Legumes . . .

Legumes—dried beans, peas, and lentils—are packed with fiber! A half-cup serving of cooked legumes supplies 4 to 10 grams of fiber. (As a healthy adult, you need 21 to 38 grams of total fiber a day, depending on your age and gender.) Legumes also are packed with protein, other nutrients, and phytonutrients, yet little fat and no cholesterol. So adding them to meals and snacks several times each week is well worth it. Canned beans take little effort.

When boiled and served plain, beans don't have much flavor. But when combined with other foods, they're versatile, taking on many flavor dimensions.

● Make minestrone soup with drained, canned kidney or garbanzo beans and vegetables. Add beef or chicken broth or canned tomatoes for flavor.

● Fill tacos or burritos with drained, cooked or canned pinto beans. Accent the flavor with a little grated cheese and lots of salsa, tomatoes, onions, and/or chopped lettuce or cabbage.

● Top green salads with drained, canned or cooked beans. Or mix up a three-, four-, or five-bean salad!

● For an easy lunch, serve split pea, navy bean, or lentil soup. Top with shredded carrot or apple!

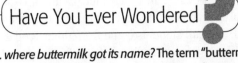

Have You Ever Wondered

. . . where buttermilk got its name? The term "buttermilk" sounds like a misnomer. Its name refers to the way buttermilk was first made—from the whey, or liquid, left after butter was churned from cream. Today most buttermilk is made from fat-free or low-fat milk.

● As an easy side dish, baked potato topping, or pasta sauce, simply heat frozen or canned beans with a tasty sauce of tomatoes, molasses, or jalapeño peppers.

● Use legumes as a meat substitute in many mixed dishes: kidney beans in chili, lentils in meat loaf, pinto beans in enchiladas, black beans in chunky soups, mashed kidney or pinto beans in meatballs, soybeans in casseroles, and white beans in stews.

● Create a high-fiber pasta sauce that's low in fat, too! In a blender or a food processor, puree cooked or drained, canned beans with beef or chicken stock. White cannellini beans make a creamy white sauce, but any variety of beans will do. Add fresh herbs: basil, chives, garlic, marjoram, and oregano, among others. Fresh tomatoes or tomato sauce add a nice flavor and color.

See "Kitchen Nutrition: Cooking a Pot o'Beans" in chapter 6 and "Vegetarian Way: Legumes and Other Meat Alternates" in chapter 20 for more tips.

Calcium Boosters

If you're like many Americans, the calcium in your diet needs a boost! People of all ages need calcium for healthy bones and teeth, and for other body functions. Yet too many of us just don't consume enough calcium-rich foods, especially milk and other dairy foods. *See chapter 4 for daily recommendations for calcium.*

How Much Cheese?

1 cup shredded cheese = 4 ounces*
1 cup grated cheese (Parmesan, Romano) = 3 ounces

*Eight ounces of milk is equivalent to ½ cup (2 ounces) of shredded processed cheese, or about ⅓ cup (1½ ounces) of natural cheese such as Cheddar or mozzarella.

Dairy foods are the best source of calcium—in fact, about 72 percent of the calcium in the U.S. food supply. But small amounts come from other food groups too. *See "Calcium: A Closer Look" in chapter 4.*

Calcium . . . From Dairy Foods

To boost the calcium, consume three cups or the equivalent from the Milk Group daily. Fat-free and lower-fat products are good choices. Use these food preparation tips to add a little more calcium here and there.

● Fortify mashed potatoes, casseroles, vegetable purees, and thick soups with nonfat dry milk, evaporated fat-free milk, or plain yogurt. Dry milk in meat loaf won't be noticed! One-quarter cup of dry milk powder adds 375 milligrams of calcium to a recipe.

● Sprinkle shredded cheese on salads, soups, stews, baked potatoes, and vegetables. One ounce of Cheddar cheese (¼ cup) has 200 milligrams of calcium.

● Make oatmeal, hot cereal, and hot cocoa with milk instead of water. One-half cup of milk adds 150 milligrams of calcium to your meal. You might fortify them with extra nonfat dry milk powder, too. Calcium-fortified soy beverage also adds calcium.

● Puree cottage cheese in a food processor or a blender. Add herbs; use it as a dip or a spread.

● Instead of black coffee (regular or decaffeinated) in the morning, try caffe latte (made with milk, perhaps fat-free). It's made with steamed milk. One-half cup (4 ounces) of milk added to coffee adds 150 milligrams of calcium.

● Use plain yogurt for some or all of the mayonnaise in salad dressings, sandwich spreads, and dips.

● If you boost calcium with reduced-fat or fat-free cheese, recognize that it doesn't blend or melt as well as whole-milk cheese. For best results shred lower-fat cheeses finely or use them in a mixture with whole-milk cheese. Blend them with other ingredients rather than just sprinkling them on top.

● Boost calcium, not fat, with yogurt cheese. Made by draining the whey from the solids in yogurt, it may substitute for cream cheese or sour cream. *See "Kitchen Nutrition: Yogurt Cheese" in chapter 3.*

If you're lactose intolerant, refer to "Lactose: Tips for Tolerance" in chapter 21.

● For something different, try goat cheese. It has a strong and unique flavor. A half-ounce portion of semisoft goat cheese has about 42 milligrams of calcium. Serve it on crackers, on salads, or as a vegetable garnish. A half ounce of hard goat cheese has 127 milligrams of calcium. *Hint:* You might find herb-flavored goat cheese in your supermarket.

Calcium . . . From Other Foods

● Add vegetables that have more calcium to many dishes: soups, salads, and stews, for example. One serving of broccoli, collard greens, kale, mustard greens, okra, and turnip greens all provide calcium, although not as much as milk.

● For main dish salads and sandwich spreads use salmon with bones as an occasional change from tuna. Fish with edible bones—salmon, sardines, perch—all supply calcium to the diet.

● Make stir-fried dishes with tofu (soybean curd), preferably made with calcium sulfate. One-quarter cup of tofu with calcium sulfate has about 130 milligrams of calcium. The same amount of tofu without calcium sulfate has 65 milligrams of calcium.

● Blend a delicious fruit smoothie with calcium-fortified beverages: soy beverage and/or orange juice.

Sugar Savers

"Just a spoonful of sugar," as Mary Poppins knew, adds flavor! Besides the taste, sugar adds aroma, texture, color, and body to a variety of foods. Sugar is

---

BAKING WITH SUGAR

To ensure good results when reducing sugar in baked foods, use this guideline.

BAKED FOODS	FOR EACH CUP OF FLOUR USE
Cakes and cakelike cookies (cookies made with juice, milk, water)	½ cup sugar
Muffins and quick breads	1 tbsp. sugar
Yeast breads	1 tsp. sugar

the "food" for yeast that helps bread rise. In baked foods it contributes to the light brown color and crisp texture. In canned jams and jellies, sugar helps inhibit the growth of molds and yeasts. In many foods sugar contributes to a food's bulk and texture.

Choosing and preparing food with little added sugars is part of a healthful eating plan. Sugars are one source of food energy. For some people, moderation means controlling sugar they add to foods, perhaps to cut back on calories. *For a quick review of sugars, see Chapter 5, "Carbs: Simply Complex."*

Before you change the sugar in a food you're preparing, think about its function and whether reducing or eliminating sugars will give the baking or cooking result you want. Then if you need to cut calories, use sugars in moderation in your cooking:

● In cakes, cookies, breads, and other baked goods, try using less sugar. Often you can reduce sugar by a fourth to a third, yet hardly notice the difference. *Be aware: many recipes already have done this. Check "Baking with Sugar" on page 330 as your guide.*

● "Sweeten" recipes with extracts such as vanilla or peppermint, or so-called sweet spices such as cinnamon or allspice. This enhances the sweetness of food. Warm spicy foods; they'll taste sweeter! Other spices that give the sweet perception include cardamom, coriander, ginger, mace, and nutmeg. *For more tips, see "Kitchen Nutrition: Sweet Seasons" in chapter 5.*

● Briefly broil or microwave peach, pear, or grapefruit halves. Sprinkle with a small amount of sweetener or sweet spice . . . or just enjoy the natural flavor. The warm temperature enhances their sweet flavors!

● Sweeten with fruit pureed in a blender or a food processor. Too thick? Add a little fruit juice. Fruit purees are great on pancakes, waffles, French toast, fruit salads, angel food cake, and frozen desserts. They're also a tasty glaze for meat, fish, and poultry! Use applesauce or pureed baby-food fruits, too.

● Instead of fruit-flavored yogurt, add your own fruit flavoring to plain yogurt with fresh, canned, or frozen fruit. Blend in chopped fruit, berries, or fruit puree.

● To fit more fruit in, enjoy a baked apple or a pear for dessert, poached in fruit juice and any "sweet" spice.

● Buy processed foods with less added sugars— frozen fruit without added sugar, canned fruits in natural juices, and unsweetened cereals. Skip sugar from your sugar bowl.

● In some foods you can use intense sweeteners such as aspartame or saccharin. They're almost calorie-free! However, because they don't function in food like sugars do, their use is limited. *See "Cooking with Intense Sweeteners" in chapter 5 for more about cooking with these sweeteners.*

● Making a gelatin salad or a dessert? Rather than using flavored gelatin, dissolve unflavored gelatin in fruit juice. Then sweeten with an intense sweetener.

Well Equipped—for Healthful Cooking!

To cook the healthful way, equip your kitchen.

Cheese grater. With a grater, a little cheese goes a longer way. When cheese is grated, a smaller portion still adds plenty of flavor. It's also a "grate" idea for shredding vegetables such as carrots and summer squash, or for grating citrus rinds for flavor.

Coffee grinder. It's great for grinding small amounts of nuts, seeds, and grains as well as dry herbs and spices.

Egg separator. An egg separator helps you easily separate the yolks from the whites. That's important when you're cutting back on dietary cholesterol. Using an egg separator has a food safety benefit, too. Compared to the technique of transferring the yolk back and forth between the two shell halves, using an egg separator reduces the chance of transferring bacteria from the outside of the shell to the uncooked egg.

Fat-separating pitcher. With the position of the spout, a fat-separating pitcher lets you pour out the liquid from the bottom, leaving the fat behind.

Food processor or blender. You can puree low-fat cottage cheese to the consistency of thick cream; chop, grate, or puree vegetables for use in soups, sauces, salads, and side dishes; or puree fruit, yogurt, and milk for a thick yet lower-calorie milk shake.

Hot-air popcorn popper. This popper requires no oil, so popcorn can be a quick, low-fat, low-calorie snack.

Indoor grill. Indoor grills either fit over the burners on your stove, or they may be freestanding appliances. Either way, you can easily discard the excess fat, which drips through the grates into a drip pan.

Instant-read thermometer. An instant-read thermometer helps you cook food to a safe internal temperature. *See chapter 12 for tips on using a meat thermometer.*

Kitchen scale. A scale that measures in ounces helps you figure portion sizes. If you have a hard time determining the size of your meat, poultry, fish, or cheese servings, a kitchen scale is helpful.

Kitchen scissors. Along with knives, kitchen scissors can trim visible fat from meat and poultry.

Microwave oven. A microwave oven cooks food fast, without the need for added fat. The fast cooking time also helps food retain vitamins and minerals. Why so speedy? Microwaves, which cause food molecules to vibrate and create friction, travel fast; the friction heats and cooks food.

Nonstick pots and pans. Some cookware is specially coated, allowing you to cook with little or no added fat. Although today's nonstick finishes last a long time, care for them properly. Use nonmetal utensils to prevent scratching; avoid abrasive cleaners that strip away coatings. Many are dishwasher-safe.

Pastry brush. A small pastry brush lets you just lightly coat meat, poultry, fish, and baked goods with oils.

Pressure cooker. To save time, you can cook dry beans in it quickly. (Cooked dry beans have less salt than canned beans.) It cooks food quickly without much water, helping with vitamin retention.

Pump spray bottle. A refillable oil pump can be filled with the type of oil you like, for use as a vegetable oil spray. By spraying olive oil on bread you may use less.

Ribbed frypan. The ribs on the bottom surface let meat or poultry cook above the fat drippings so less fat gets absorbed.

Rice cooker. With this countertop appliance, rice cooking is easy! Just add rice, the liquid of your choice (perhaps juice or broth), and herbs, and flip a switch. It turns off automatically when the rice is cooked.

Roasting pan with a grate. With a grate, roasted and broiled meat or poultry can't absorb fat drippings. They collect in the pan below.

Slotted spoon. A slotted spoon allows you to lift food out of the pan, leaving any fat drippings behind.

Slow cooker. This countertop appliance cooks food with low, steady, moist heat. It can be used to make tougher cuts of meat more tender. Casserole-type dishes and soups work well in a slow cooker.

Steamer. Rather than fry foods, steam them. There are several kinds of steamers: an electric steamer for vegetables, rice, fish, or chicken; a stackable bamboo steamer set that fits in a wok or a stockpot; or a small aluminum vegetable steamer that fits in a saucepan.

Strainer. With a microwave-safe plastic strainer you can cook ground meat in a microwave oven, collecting fat drippings in a container underneath.

Wok. A wok's sloped sides allow food to cook fast without much oil. Unless it has a nonstick surface, "season" a new stainless-steel wok to keep food from sticking. Here's how: first coat the cooking surface with vegetable oil, then heat in a 350° F oven for about an hour. Oil will work its way into the porous surface.

Yogurt cheese strainer. A fine mesh strainer allows you to drain away the liquid in yogurt and use the thickened yogurt as a substitute for sour cream. *See chapter 3 for tips on making yogurt cheese.*

Add Life to Your Spices— and Herbs, Too!

With today's cuisine, we've discovered a new world of taste. Innovative uses of herbs and spices offer a flavor advantage as we trim fat and sodium from cooking. And the result is a new fusion of flavors!

Have You Ever Wondered

. . . what a flavor extract really is? Extracts are concentrated flavorings from foods and plants. Some are made by distilling fruits, seeds, or leaves; anise, vanilla, peppermint, and almond extracts are made this way. Because they are so concentrated, use just a few drops. Meat, poultry, and vegetable extracts (such as Kitchen Bouquet) are made by concentrating the stock, or cooking juices; use them in marinades and sauces.

Herbs and spices have a long culinary tradition. If you're a history buff, you know that spices have been traded throughout the Mediterranean and the Middle East for more than two thousand years. In the first century, Apicus, who was a Roman epicure, described herb combinations to enhance flavor. Spices were the motive for Christopher Columbus's forays across the ocean. Now, with our nutrition interest and a flavor world that's smaller than ever, we use more herbs and spices—in new combinations—than ever before.

Many people confuse the terms "spice" and "herb." Spices, which grow in tropical areas, come from the bark, buds, fruit, roots, seeds, or stems of plants and trees. Usually they're dried; garlic and gingerroot are two common exceptions. Herbs, which grow in temperate climates, are the fragrant leaves of plants. The same plant may supply both. For example, the seeds of coriander are used in curry powder, while the leaves of the same plant are called cilantro, a favorite seasoning in Mexican dishes.

Locking in Flavor: Storing Herbs and Spices

Your herbs and spices won't keep indefinitely—even dried! To lock in the aromatic flavors, store carefully.

● Store dry herbs and spices in tightly covered containers—in a cool, dry, dark place (not the refrigerator). Avoid placing your spice rack near a window or above the stove. Heat, bright light, and air destroy flavor. Moisture can promote mold.

● Date dry herbs and spices when you buy them. Then use them preferably within a year. After a while, even properly stored seasonings lose their full "bouquet."

● To check the freshness, rub seasonings between your fingers, and smell the aroma. If there's not much, get a new supply. Buy just enough dry herbs for a few months for the most freshness.

● To keep fresh herbs longer, treat them like a bouquet of flowers! Snip the stem ends, then stand them in water. Cover them with a plastic bag, and store in the fridge. Change the water every couple of days.

● Growing your own herbs? Preserve them for those long, cold weather months. Either freeze, dry, or add fresh herbs to oils and vinegars. Be aware that some herbs are better dried—for example, bay leaves, marjoram, oregano, and summer savory.

● *To freeze herbs* . . . Wash and dry them well; then seal them in plastic freezer bags. Or snip herbs, then freeze them with water in ice cube trays. Adding a "herb ice cube" to soups and stews is easy! Basil, chives, dill, fennel, parsley, rosemary, and tarragon are among the herbs that freeze well.

● *To dry herbs in the oven* . . . Wash the herbs first, blot them dry, and remove the leaves from the stems. Place the herbs on baking trays in a single layer. Heat them in the oven at 100° F for several hours with the door slightly open. Remove the leaves before they get browned. Cool, then store in tightly covered containers.

● *To dry herbs in the microwave oven* . . . Wash the leaves first, then place them between paper towels. Then dry the herbs on the lowest setting for two or three minutes.

A Pinch of Flavor: How to Cook with Herbs and Spices

Add a pinch of this and a pinch of that. Used carefully, herbs and spices make many foods distinctive and "simply flavorful"!

Dry or fresh—which herbs should you use? Nothing beats the delicate flavor of fresh herbs. But they're not always available. And unless you have your own herb garden, fresh herbs can be expensive. Whether you use fresh or dry seasonings, use them carefully for their best flavor advantage:

● Before using fresh herbs, wash them! Then pat them dry with paper towels.

● If fresh herbs have woody stems, strip off the leaves before using them. Discard damaged leaves. If the stems are soft and pliable, use them, too. Stems often carry a lot of flavor and aroma.

● To harvest herbs, pick them at their peak of flavor. That's just before they bloom. Remember: The flowers on many herb plants are very flavorful, too.

● To release more flavor and aroma, crumble dry, leaf herbs—basil, oregano, savory, and tarragon, among others—between your fingers. Or use a mortar and pestle or coffee grinder. Finely chop fresh herbs.

Flavor Profile!

Would you combine tomato with basil, or with cinnamon, or with chile powder? The subtle blend of the two ingredients often defines the distinctive flavor of an ethnic cuisine . . . in this case, Italian, or Middle Eastern, or Mexican.

Many ethnic cuisines are defined partly by their mix of seasonings.

Italy	Tomato, olive oil, garlic, and basil
Mexico	Tomato and chile
West Africa	Tomato, peanut, and chile
Middle East	Lemon and parsley
Greece	Olive oil, lemon, and oregano
India	Curry, cumin, ginger, and garlic
Hungary	Onion and paprika
China	Soy sauce, rice wine, and ginger
Morocco	Cinnamon, cumin, coriander, ginger, and fruit
France	Thyme, rosemary, sage, marjoram, and tomato

● In dishes that require a long cooking time, such as soups, stews, and braised dishes, add herbs toward the end of cooking. In that way their flavor won't cook out.

● For chilled foods such as salads and dips, add seasonings several hours ahead so flavors blend.

● When substituting fresh for dry herbs, figure: 1 tablespoon of fresh herb equals 1 teaspoon of dried herb. Dry herbs are stronger than fresh; powdered herbs are stronger than crumbled herbs.

● Add dry herbs and spices to liquid ingredients. They need moisture to bring out their flavors.

● Chop fresh herbs very fine. Kitchen shears are great for mincing and snipping. With more cut surfaces, more flavor and aroma are released.

● Use seasonings with care—especially if you're not familiar with their flavor. They should enhance, not disguise, the aroma and taste of food. Start with ¼ teaspoon of dry herbs for 1 pound of meat or 1 pint of sauce. You can always add more herbs and spices, but you can't take them away!

● Avoid overwhelming a dish with seasonings. A few simple herbs and spices bring out the flavor of food without confusing your taste buds.

● If you're doubling a recipe, you may not need to double the herbs. Use just 50 percent more. If you triple the recipe, start by doubling the seasonings.

● Toast dry spices in a dry nonstick skillet to enhance their flavor.

● Use seasoning blends, including curry, fine herbes, and bouquet garni. Each one is really a blend of herbs—and maybe spices, too. *Curry powder* is a pulverized mixture of as many as twenty different spices, herbs, and seeds. The spice turmeric is the ingredient that makes curried dishes yellow. *For a recipe to make your own curry, see "Kitchen Nutrition: Salt-Free*

Herbed Vinegars

Although today's supermarket shelves are stocked with herbed vinegars, why not make your own? They're less costly—and very satisfying to make. They also make great gifts from your kitchen!

● To sterilize, simmer the bottle for ten minutes, and let it cool. Wash the cap or obtain a clean cork.

● Insert a combination of fresh herbs (stems and leaves) and spices into the bottle. Three or four herb sprigs per pint are usually enough.

● Fill the bottle with vinegar. You can use any vinegar as a base: white, red wine, or cider vinegar. Herbs and spices may go better with some vinegars than others. For example, try tarragon and garlic cloves in red or white wine vinegar, and delicate herbs in distilled white vinegar.

Is wine or rice wine vinegar okay to use? Be aware that a protein they contain may promote bacteria growth if the herbed vinegar isn't stored properly.

● Put on the cap, or insert the cork. Store the bottle in a cool, dark place. Allow the flavor to develop for two to three weeks.

● Try these flavorful combinations: fresh tarragon in cider vinegar; garlic cloves, fresh rosemary or sage, and lemon peel in white wine vinegar; and fresh mint and orange peel in cider vinegar. For fun, make herbed vinegar with edible flowers—for example, nasturtiums with peppercorns, garlic cloves, whole cloves, and cider vinegar.

See "Flavor Profile!" on page 334 for seasonings that define various ethnic cuisines. Also see "Kitchen Nutrition: Salt-Free Herb Blends" in chapter 7.

Have You Ever Wondered

. . . if homemade herbed oils and garlic oils can pose a food safety risk? Yes, for *Clostridium botulinum* bacteria! *(See chapter 12.)* If you make them at home, use immediately! The U.S. Food and Drug Administration advises that home-prepared mixtures of garlic in oil be made fresh for any meal or snack and not be left at room temperatures. Refrigerate and use leftovers within ten days; after that, discard.

Herb Blends" in chapter 7. *Fine herbes* usually refers to a mixture of chopped herbs, such as chervil, chives, parsley, and tarragon. *Bouquet garni* is a bundle of fresh and/or dried herbs, often parsley, bay leaf, and thyme, that's added to soups, stews, and braised meat or poultry. Usually they're tied up in cheesecloth or placed in a metal teaball to easily remove later.

● If you grow herbs, experiment with less common varieties: pineapple sage, orange mint, burnet, lemon basil, culinary lavender, and coriander, among others.

● Grow scented geraniums: apple-, lemon-, peppermint-, and rose-scented geraniums, to name a few. Their aromatic leaves and flowers offer a nice garnish and flavor to sauces, salads, vinegars, and baked foods.

Rub Combos

Experiment with your own favorite blend of herbs and spices for all sorts of great rubs. You don't need a recipe; just combine flavors that taste good together. Use rubs on tender cuts of meat, poultry, and fish. To apply the rub, gently press the mixture onto the surface of the meat prior to cooking. Flavors usually become more pronounced the longer the seasoning is on the meat.

Citrus rub. Combine grated lemon, orange, and/or lime peel with minced garlic and cracked pepper.

Pepper-garlic rub. Combine garlic powder, cracked black pepper, and cayenne pepper.

Italian rub. Combine fresh or dried oregano, basil, and rosemary with minced Italian parsley and garlic.

Herb rub. Combine fresh or dried marjoram, thyme, and basil.

Foods for All "Seasons"!

Use herbs and spices in food preparation.

● For baked chicken, fill the cavity with herbs and citrus peel—perhaps rosemary and sliced lemon—then roast it in the oven. Lemongrass or lemon-scented geranium leaves are nice, too.

● Cook strong-flavored vegetables, such as cabbage, with savory to cut down on the strong aroma yet enhance the flavor.

● Add flavor with herb and spice rubs. *See "Rub Combos" on this page.* For a simple rub, just combine garlic and lemon pepper. Use herbed yogurt as a flavorful dip or vegetable topping. To get started, blend dill, parsley, chives, and garlic into low-fat yogurt.

● Make no-fat marinades with an acid ingredient—vinegar or fruit juice—and herbs or spices. For example, combine orange juice and nutmeg. Splash herbed vinegar on salads and soups.

● Flavor mineral water, iced tea, lemonade, and spritzers with the leaves of scented geraniums, sprigs of fresh herbs, or edible flowers. Allow enough time for the flavor infusion. *For more about edible flowers, see "Please Don't Eat the Daffodils" in this chapter.*

● Experiment with "reverse" flavors. Use a "sweet spice" with meat or poultry, and a savory herb in dessert. Try cinnamon in tomato sauce and rosemary in pound cake.

Looking for more food preparation tips for healthy eating? Check here for "how-tos:"

● Find more creative food "prep" ideas—see "Kitchen Nutrition" in many chapters.

● Add nutrition to speed scratch meals—see chapter 10.

● Cook healthy and "small" for one or two—see chapter 18.

● Cook with kids—see chapter 16.

Quick Reference: Herbs and Spices

Not sure what herbs and spices to use? Use this quick reference to enhance the flavor of foods in every part of your meal. This is just a partial list—add your flavor creativity to this list, too.

IN THESE FOODS . . .	TRY THESE HERBS AND SPICES!
Bread	
Sweet breads, rolls	Allspice, cinnamon, cloves, ginger, lavender, nutmeg
Other breads, rolls	Any herb, spice, or seed
Eggs	Basil, black pepper, chervil, chives, cilantro, garlic marjoram, oregano, tarragon, thyme
Fish and Seafood	
Finfish	Basil, bay leaf, chile powder, dill, fennel, ginger, oregano, paprika, sage, tarragon, thyme
Shellfish	Basil, black pepper, curry powder, dill, garlic, ginger, tarragon
Fruit	Cinnamon, cloves, ginger, lavender, mint, nutmeg, rosemary
Meat	
Beef	Bay leaf, basil, black pepper, celery seeds, curry powder, fennel (in sausage dishes), marjoram, oregano, onion, savory, thyme
Ham	Cloves, ginger, mustard seeds, tarragon
Lamb	Garlic, marjoram, mint, oregano, rosemary
Liver	Basil, onion
Pork	Cayenne pepper, chile powder, cinnamon, cloves, fennel (in sausage dishes), sage, thyme
Veal	Basil, curry powder, lemongrass, oregano, rosemary, sage, thyme
Poultry	
Chicken, turkey	Curry powder, ginger, marjoram, sage, tarragon
Stuffing	Basil, marjoram, onion, parsley, sage, savory
Pasta, Rice	
Pasta (including couscous)	Basil, chives, marjoram, oregano, saffron
Rice (white)	Cumin, fennel, onion, parsley, saffron, turmeric
Rice (brown and wild)	Ginger, onion, parsley
Salads	
Chicken or turkey	Chives, celery seeds, oregano, tarragon
Egg	Marjoram, onion, parsley, tarragon
Fish or seafood	Chives, curry, powder, ginger, marjoram, oregano, tarragon
Fruit	Cinnamon, ginger, lavender, mint
Greens	Basil, black pepper, chervil, chives, cilantro, garlic, marjoram, mint, onion, parsley, tarragon, thyme
Vegetables or legumes	Basil, oregano, onion, parsley, tarragon

IN THESE FOODS . . .	TRY THESE HERBS AND SPICES!
Sauces	
Cheese	Chervil, chile powder, chives, paprika, parsley
Cream (milk-based)	Basil, curry powder, marjoram, tarragon, thyme
Tomato	Basil, bay leaf, cayenne pepper, cilantro, fennel seed, oregano, paprika, parsley, sage, thyme
Soups	
Chicken or poultry	Bay leaf, lemongrass, mace, marjoram, paprika, parsley, sage, savory, thyme
Clear broth	Basil, lemongrass, paprika, parsley
Cream (or milk based)	Chervil, chives, rosemary, sage, tarragon, white pepper
Fish or seafood	Bay leaf, celery seeds, chives, curry powder, ginger, saffron, tarragon, thyme
Legume	Bay leaf, celery seeds, saffron, tarragon, thyme
Meat	Basil, clove, coriander (cilantro), oregano, rosemary, savory, thyme
Mushroom	Basil, bay leaf, garlic, marjoram, onion, oregano, parsley, tarragon, thyme
Potato	Chives, curry powder, dill
Vegetable	Allspice, basil, bay leaf, black pepper, cloves, garlic, marjoram, sage
Vegetables	
Asparagus	Chervil, savory
Baked beans	Allspice, chile powder, cinnamon, cloves, mace, parsley, red pepper
Broccoli	Oregano
Brussels sprouts and cabbage	Caraway, celery seeds, dill, marjoram, mint, sage, savory, tarragon
Carrots	Basil, bay leaf, ginger, marjoram, mint, oregano, parsley, thyme
Cauliflower	Marjoram, nutmeg, parsley
Corn	Chile powder, chives
Green beans	Basil, cloves, marjoram, parsley, sage, savory
Lima beans	Marjoram, sage, savory
Mushrooms	Marjoram, oregano, parsley, tarragon, thyme
Onions	Basil, oregano, sage, thyme
Peas	Basil, chervil, marjoram, mint, oregano, parsley, sage, tarragon, thyme
Potatoes	Basil, caraway, chives, dill, garlic, parsley
Spinach	Marjoram, ginger, nutmeg, parsley, savory
Tomatoes	Basil, bay leaf, cilantro, cloves, marjoram, nutmeg, oregano, sage
Winter squash and sweet potatoes	Allspice, cinnamon, cloves, ginger, nutmeg, savory, thyme
Sweet desserts	Allspice, cinnamon, cloves, ginger, lavender, mace, mint, nutmeg

Lighter Condiments

Add chutneys and sauces, made with little or no fat, to your cupboard to spice up light menus. Some are high in sodium.

Barbeque sauce	Pickle relish	Chili sauce	Seafood cocktail sauce
Cranberry-orange chutney	Soy sauce	Horseradish	Teriyaki sauce
Ketchup	Worcestershire sauce	Dijon mustard	

CHAPTER 14

Your Food Away from Home

Whether it's a rushed, fast-food meal, lunch in the company cafeteria, an order of pizza, a casual dinner at a family restaurant, or an elegant evening of fine dining in a relaxing atmosphere, eating out is no longer just for special occasions. It's become part of our everyday lifestyle!

According to the National Restaurant Association, Americans eat about 76 percent of meals at home. Looked at another way, Americans dine out for about 24 percent of their meals, or more than four meals each week. Overall, food service currently gets about 47 percent of every dollar that U.S. consumers spend on food, with projections expected at 53 percent by 2010. In fact, in 2006, about $511 billion are expected in restaurant industry sales. *The data are clear: there's good reason to give eating out your careful attention!*

Food service includes any food that's not prepared in the home kitchen. So who's cooking for us?

In growing numbers, consumers want fast, easy, and flavorful food to fit their busy lifestyles. Take-out, delivered food, and fast-food restaurants do the job so you have time for other things. In the late 1970s, fast-food sales amounted to about $9 billion annually in the United States. In 2006 that figure was projected at over $142 billion.

Despite our reliance on quick food, consumers also flock to full-service restaurants, which are projected to take in over $173 billion in 2006. Why? Chances to socialize with family, friends, and coworkers; to enjoy their leisure time; and to experience flavors that aren't prepared at home.

Hungry or not, food bombards our senses almost everywhere we go today. The broad array of restaurants offers an explosion of dining-out options to choose from: traditional family cuisine; regional, ethnic, and fusion cuisine; vegetarian cuisine; coffee and tea cafés; bagel and doughnut shops; and sushi and tapas bars, to name a few.

Supermarkets cook, letting us "take out" to "eat in." We also eat from convenience stores, bookstores, drugstores, recreational centers, institutions (schools, hospitals, businesses, and others), sports and cultural events, hotels and cruise ships, airlines, and vending machines, among others.

Where do you typically eat out—how often and what do you order? Whatever your answers, the more you eat away from home, the greater the impact food-service meals and snacks make on your overall food choices, health, perhaps your weight, and well-being.

Dining Out for Health and Pleasure

Eating out? You've got choices—plenty of them! It's up to you decide what foods to enjoy, where, and how much. With a little forethought and menu savvy, the meals and the snacks you eat away from home can be great-tasting, enjoyable, even adventuresome—and healthful, too.

What are your eating-out challenges: "too big" portions, the urge to splurge, no time to eat smart away from home?

What are your eating-out pleasures? Dining out offers easy access to unique, delicious flavors. *See "Flavor on the Menu," page 369.* Flavor sells, flavor entices!

Restaurant Eater's Tip List

No matter where you choose to eat, the same smart-eating strategies can guide you: plan ahead, consider the menu, and choose foods carefully. An occasional meal with elegant, creamy sauces or a rich dessert pastry needn't upset your overall plans for healthful eating. What and how you eat over time is what counts.

Plan Ahead

How can your restaurant choices fit into your whole day's eating plan—without overdoing on calories or "underdoing" on vegetables, fruit, whole grains, or milk? How can you enjoy the variety of food available in today's restaurant scene?

● Map out your restaurant plan of action. Perhaps plan for a light dinner out if you just ate a big lunch, or decide ahead to split a dessert, even before you see the menu. If you know ahead that your restaurant meal will have more calories or fat, just trade off: cut back during other meals that day or the next.

● Eat small meals earlier, rather than skip breakfast or lunch to "save up" for a fancy restaurant dinner. This meal-skipping strategy often backfires. It's easy to overindulge at a restaurant when you're over-hungry.

● Looking for convenience, saving time, a flavor adventure, or a lower-calorie meal? Some restaurants offer more food variety, ethnic cuisine, unique dishes, smaller portions, and lighter cuisine than others. A restaurant that prepares food to order allows more control for any special requests; call ahead to find out. A handful of today's restaurants let you call or fax your order ahead so the kitchen is ready for you.

● Go with a "smart eating" mind-set, which may help you sort through the menu faster and avoid straying from your goals. Use the menu on the restaurant's Web site to plan your order ahead.

Did You Know

... dietitians with chef training have entered the restaurant scene, blending flavor and healthful eating into their menus?

... many adult restaurantgoers like display cooking, where they can see their food prepared?

... personal chefs are a growing trend for busy professional families; it's one way to match food preferences and plan for healthful eating, while offering a convenient and time-saving alternative to eating out?

... the restaurant trend toward simple foods and flavors is putting basic, "comfort" foods back on the table—more stews, mashed potatoes, steamed or grilled vegetables, macaroni and cheese, and meat loaf?

... chefs and farmers are collaborating to put more local and regional foods on many restaurant menus?

... a cooking class can be a great way to dine out, sharpen your culinary skills—and help you learn more ways to prepare the flavors of good health?

... kitchen "workshops" with personal chefs help customers assemble meals to freeze at home and eat later at the family table? Worth the time and money? That depends on you.

Learn Menu Language

Primavera, béarnaise, al dente. What do all these menu terms mean? Knowing menu terms and cooking basics makes ordering easier, especially if you need to control calories, fat, and other nutrients, or handle any food sensitivity such as a food allergy. And menu literacy also makes eating out more fun! *For terms, check "Menu Language" in this chapter.*

● Generally, look for foods with simple preparation, such as steamed vegetables or broiled chicken, if you need to lower calories and fat. For instance, the term "al dente" describes how pasta and vegetables are cooked—only until firm when bitten, not soft or overdone. Literally translated, it means "to the tooth." Vegetables cooked "al dente" retain more nutrients.

● Check menus for voluntary nutrient content claims. With government regulations, terms such as "lean," "low-fat," and "light" are defined consistently. Used on menus, these terms have roughly the same meaning as the same terms on food labels. *For more on label terms, see "Label Lingo" in chapter 11.*

Have It Your Way!

Do you have unique food and nutrition needs or preferences? Customize your order. You have the right to substitute. It's up to you to be assertive, ask menu questions, make special requests—and be realistic. Service-oriented restaurants are eager to please. They want you back!

Ask how the food is prepared or served, especially if the description isn't clear or the food is unfamiliar. Today's servers expect questions from more sophisticated diners. Find out about ingredients and any substitutions. You might ask:

● How are the vegetables seasoned? Are they salted? Is butter or margarine added?

● Is the fish grilled, broiled, breaded, or fried? Is it cooked with butter, margarine, or some other fat?

● How is the sauce prepared?

● Can I have the sauce (or salad dressing or whipped topping) on the side?

● Is the soup clear (broth) or cream-based?

● Can I substitute a baked potato, rice, vegetables, or a salad for the fries?

● What is mole (in a Mexican dish)? Galangal (in a Thai dish)? Cassava (in a Caribbean dish)?

● Does the dessert have nuts (if you're allergic to them)?

Have You Ever Wondered

... what's "slow food"? It's the idea of enjoying food traditions and high-quality food, and taking time in your busy life to enjoy it. Consider how time at the table may add pleasure, great flavors, and social time to your lifestyle! Eating slower may also help you eat less as you pay attention to satiety cues.

... if Caesar salad on the menu is safe to eat? Probably so, but ask how it's prepared. In the past, a Caesar salad, made with a raw egg, was often prepared right at your table. Today most Caesar salads are made in the kitchen with a pasteurized egg product or cooked salad dressing, following safe food-handling techniques. Some Caesar salads are eggless.

On the "Leaner" Side

Not sure what to order? For lower-calorie, perhaps lower-fat cuisine, try this:

Appetizers	Fresh fruit cup, broth, bouillon, or consommé, fruit or vegetable juice, marinated vegetables, crudités, or raw vegetables, with a yogurt or salsa dip, seafood cocktail
Breads	Hard rolls or whole-wheat buns, French or Italian bread, bread sticks, melba toast, or saltine crackers
Salads	Salads with dressing on the side
Vegetables	Steamed vegetables, plain or with a lemon wedge, grilled or roasted vegetables
Entrées	Lean meat, fish, and poultry that are broiled, grilled, or roasted, with any sauces served on the side (remove visible fat and poultry skin); vegetarian dishes that go easy on cheese or cheese sauces
Desserts	Fruit ice or sorbet, fresh fruit, angel food cake with fruit, low-fat frozen yogurt, cappuccino

Ingredients in sauces confuse many restaurant-goers. What, for example, is the difference between béarnaise and bolognese sauce? Which is apt to be lower in fat? What's a reduction sauce? *For a quick description, see "Gourmet's Guide to Sauces" on page 343.*

● Find out about portion sizes. Big portions do not mean restaurant quality. For example, a 5- to 6-ounce portion of meat, poultry, or fish probably is enough for the whole day, especially if you eat other Meat and Beans Group foods during the day. A 12-ounce steak or a 6-ounce filet mignon? Go for the smaller portion. You'll save on calories, fat, and perhaps money. *See "Restaurant Portions: You're in Control" in this chapter.*

● Don't see anything that's right for you? Ask to order "off the menu." For less fat and calories, you might request broiled fish or chicken breast seasoned with herbs and lemon juice, or fresh fruit for dessert, or low-fat milk. *See "On the 'Leaner' Side" above for common menu items with less fat.*

● Choose a meal with food variety when you eat out: more variety often means more flavor! That's easy to do with an à la carte menu. À la carte means that each item is separately ordered and priced. Be specific about a special menu request—for example, rather than ask for a "low-fat plate," ask if the chef can "broil fish without butter," "bring dry toast," or "serve dressing on the side."

● If you don't plan to eat a side dish or sauce, ask to have it left off your plate—perhaps skip tartar sauce served with fish, or chips served with a sandwich.

● If you choose a higher-calorie entrée, balance it with a lower-calorie side dish and dessert. Perhaps balance fettuccine alfredo, which is high in calories and fat, with fresh fruit to end the meal. Just make trade-offs: if you eat foods with more calories, fat, or sodium when you dine out, cut back at home.

● If the food isn't prepared as you ordered, send it back. Ask for something else if necessary.

Help Yourself

Practice the art of enjoying food variety, balance, and moderation when you eat out.

● Can't resist the urge to overindulge on tortilla chips or bread served when you're seated? Do you nibble mindlessly on pretzels and chips, brought with a beverage order? Take a few on a plate or napkin, and then move them, or ask to have them removed from the table.

● Go easy on dipping oils—even though they're usually olive oils (healthy oils). A slice of bread may soak up 3 or 4 teaspoons of oil, or 14 to 19 fat grams, compared 4 to 8 fat grams in 1 to 2 teaspoons of butter or margarine spread on a bread slice.

● If you need help in curbing a big appetite, order a salad or broth-based soup, or appetizer crudités (raw vegetables) right away. Go easy on dressings and dips.

● Eat slowly, and stop eating before you feel too full.

MAY I TAKE YOUR ORDER?

Variety on the menu? The choices on the left have fewer calories and fat than their counterparts on the right.

ENJOY MORE OFTEN	ENJOY SOMETIMES
Consommé, gazpacho, clear soups	Cream soups, soups topped with cheese, bisques
Vegetable plate with salsa, steamed vegetables	Pâté, quiche lorraine, stuffed appetizers
Garden, tossed, or spinach salad with dressing on the side, crisp and crunchy vegetables	Salads with large amounts of dressing, bacon, cheese, croutons, and mayonnaise-laden salads such as potato, macaroni, and tuna
Grilled meats, broiled or flame-cooked	Breaded or batter-dipped meat or extra gravy
Broiled, steamed, poached, roasted, baked, Cajun, or blackened	Breaded, fried, sautéed, au gratin, escalloped, en croûte, creamed, en casserole, or Kiev entrées
4- to 6-oz. steak	More than 8-oz. steak
Au jus, Provençal or fruit sauces	Gravy, alfredo, béarnaise, béchamel, beurre blanc, carbonara, hollandaise, pesto, and velouté sauces
Baked potatoes (plain or with a small amount of margarine or sour cream), red skin potatoes	Home-fried and deep-fried potatoes, twice-baked potatoes, croquettes, buttered noodles
Sandwiches on whole-wheat, pita, or rye with mustard or low-fat mayonnaise	Sandwiches on croissants or biscuits
Plain whole-wheat or multigrain rolls or bread sticks	Garlic bread, cheese spreads, flavored butters
Fruit, fruit sorbet	Cheesecake, French pastries, pie, ice cream
Colorful vegetable side dishes	Mashed potatoes with gravy, fries

That gives you time to get in touch with your satiety cues. Ask the server to remove your plate when you're done, even if a little food is left.

● If you drink, enjoy alcoholic beverages, including wine and beer, in moderation. Healthful eating guidelines advise no more than one (if you're a woman) or two (if you're a man) alcoholic drinks per day. Besides their calories, a drink or two may increase your

---

MENU LANGUAGE

Looking for foods with less calories, fat, or sodium? Check the menu. Although they offer no guarantee, descriptive terms often give clues to more or less fat, perhaps calories, or more sodium. *See "Eating Out" in chapter 7.*

Menu Clues: Less Calories and Fat

Baked	Grilled
Braised	Lightly sautéed
Broiled	Poached
Cooked in its own juices	Roasted
Dry broiled (in wine or lemon juice)	Steamed
	Stir-fried

Menu Clues: More Calories and Fat

Au gratin or in cheese sauce	French-fried
Batter-fried	Hollandaise
Béarnaise	Marinated (in oil)
Breaded	Pan fried
Beurre blanc	Pastry
Buttered	Prime
Creamed	Rich
Crispy	Sautéed
Deep-fried	Scalloped (escalloped)
Double crust	With gravy
En croûte	With mayonnaise
Escalloped	With cream sauce

Menu Clues: More Sodium

Barbecued	Smoked
Cured	Teriyaki
In broth	With cocktail sauce
Marinated	With creole sauce
Pickled	With soy sauce

Restaurant Portions: You're in Control!

If restaurant portions seem too big for you, remember this: you have choices. You control portions by what you order and how you handle what comes on your plate.

● First think, just how hungry are you?

● Order first, before your meal companions do, if possible. Then you won't be influenced by their order.

● Choose the portion size you want. Many restaurants offer appetizer portions, half portions, and full portions. Or try tapas, "little plates," or dim sum, and just order one or two dishes to share at a time.

● Split a dish with someone. Ask for two plates.

● Order two appetizers, or an appetizer and a salad, instead of the full entrée and other courses.

● Order à la carte. You won't be tempted by more food than you need.

● Turn today's dinner into tomorrow's lunch. Most restaurants have take-away containers—a time-saving strategy for your next meal. *Tip:* Store perishable foods in the refrigerator within two hours, or within one hour if the temperature is over 90° F.

● For double benefits, look for "early bird" specials. They may offer smaller portions for a lower price. Or eat out midday for a lunch-size portion.

● Leave some food on the plate; it's okay to do this. Why pay twice: your pocketbook *and* your waistline?

● Plan ahead for a trendy, multicourse tasting menu. Enjoying many small portions can add up to a lot of food!

● Pass on all-you-can-eat specials, buffets, and unlimited salad bars if you tend to eat too much. Food bars can easily add up to too many calories.

● If buffet-style eating is your choice, fill up on salad (easy on dressing) and vegetables first to appease your appetite. Take only two trips to the buffet: one for veggies, fruit, and salads, one for anything else. Use the small plate, which holds less.

● Before it's served, ask your server to put half in a take-away container.

---

appetite and lessen your personal discipline at the table. As an option, try mineral water or club soda with a twist of lemon or lime.

● What about menus featuring several wine or beer pairings in a meal, or flights (several smaller portions

Gourmet's Guide to Sauces

What's in the sauce? Use this list as a quick reference to make you a savvy restaurant patron.

Alfredo. Creamy Italian sauce, typically prepared with butter, heavy cream, and Parmesan cheese.

Béarnaise. Thick French sauce made with white wine, tarragon, vinegar, shallots, egg yolks, and butter.

Béchamel. Basic white sauce made with flour, milk, and butter, and flavored with onion.

Bolognese. Italian meat sauce made with ground beef and sometimes pork and ham and sautéed in a small amount of butter and/or olive oil with tomatoes, other vegetables, herbs, and sometimes wine. Also referred to as a ragú bolognese sauce.

*Bourguignonne.** French sauce made with red wine, carrots, onions, flour, and a little bacon.

Buerre blanc. Thick, smooth sauce whisked with wine, vinegar, shallot reduction, and cold butter.

Carbonara. Italian sauce made of cream, eggs, Parmesan cheese, and bits of bacon.

*Coulis.** Thick puree or sauce, such as tomato or squash coulis.

*Demi-glace.** Reduction sauce that gets its intense flavor by slowly cooking beef stock and Madeira or sherry to a thick glaze.

Hollandaise. Thick sauce with white wine, vinegar, or water, egg yolks, melted butter, and lemon juice.

*Marinara.** Italian tomato sauce made with tomato and basil and perhaps other seasonings such as onions, garlic, and oregano.

Pesto. Uncooked sauce made of fresh basil, garlic, pine nuts, Parmesan or Pecorino cheese, and olive oil. It's a favorite with Italian pasta.

*Reduction sauce.** Sauce of usually broth or pan juices boiled down to concentrate the flavor and thicken the consistency. Unlike in many other sauces, flour or other starches aren't used as thickeners.

*Sweet-and-sour.** Sugar and vinegar added to a variety of sauces; typically added to Chinese and German dishes.

Velouté. Light, stock-based white sauce. Stock is the broth left from cooking meat, poultry, fish, or vegetables. It's thickened with flour and butter; sometimes egg yolks and cream are added.

*Vinaigrette.** Oil-and-vinegar combination.

*These sauces tend to be lower in fat. But the ingredients vary, and so does the fat content.

---

of beer, sake, or other distilled spirits)? Go easy on drinks. Enjoy them with your meal—slowly; share if you can. Have a designated driver.

● Trying to control calories? If you choose to resist rich desserts, don't even peek at the dessert tray. If you're tempted, share it with someone else. Order seasonal fruit, cappuccino, or sorbet instead.

Enjoy, Enjoy, Enjoy!

Eating can "nourish" the soul as well as the body. In fact, eating out can be one of life's pleasures.

● Take your palate on a taste adventure. Order something you've never tried before—or that you usually don't eat at home. Feeling cautious about something new? Try an appetizer portion.

● Savor each bite and enjoy food—and the layers of flavor—at a leisurely pace.

● If you eat with others, enjoy the social time. Make

it a relaxing chance to be with your family and friends. *Check "Eating Out with Kids" in chapter 16.*

● Seize the chance for culinary insights. Ask about the ingredients, flavors, and preparation of dishes on the menu.

Sizing Up Salad Bars

A salad bar can serve up a healthful meal all by itself—or as a great side dish. The rainbow of vegetables and fruits often is loaded with vitamins A and C, folate, fiber, and an array of phytonutrients.

Did you know: A do-it-yourself salad, chosen from the salad bar, often has more calories than a deluxe burger, fries, and a shake, or a steak-and-potato dinner? An average salad bar plate can top out at more than 1,000 calories, depending on your choices and portions. Not so surprisingly, then, salads have been reported to be a main source of dietary fat for many women.

BUILD A HEALTHFUL SALAD

Imagine a salad bar with bowls and bowls of ingredients. Your plate is empty. How would you build your salad? Choose the ingredients from the list below—and decide how much you'd take of each one. When your salad plate is full, add up the calories and the fat. You may be surprised.

Food	Amount	Calories*	Fat (g)
Greens			
Bean sprouts	¼ cup	8	trace†
Lettuce	1 cup	8	trace
Spinach	1 cup	7	trace
Other Veggies			
Artichoke hearts	¼ cup	20	trace
Beets	¼ cup	20	0
Bell peppers	2 tbsp.	5	trace
Broccoli	¼ cup	8	trace
Carrots, shredded	¼ cup	10	trace
Cauliflowers	¼ cup	6	trace
Cucumbers	¼ cup	4	trace
Green peas	2 tbsp.	15	trace
Mushrooms	¼ cup	4	trace
Onions	1 tbsp.	4	0
Radishes	2 tbsp.	2	trace
Tomatoes	¼ cup	8	trace
Fruits			
Avocados	¼ cup	60	6
Canned peaches, in juices	¼ cup	25	trace
Fresh melons	¼ cup	15	trace
Fresh strawberries	¼ cup	10	trace
Mandarin oranges, segments in juice	¼ cup	20	trace
Olives, ripe	2 tbsp.	20	2
Raisins	2 tbsp.	60	trace
Beans, Nuts, and Seeds			
Almonds, sliced	1 tbsp.	55	5
Chickpeas	¼ cup	65	1
Kidney beans	¼ cup	55	trace
Sunflower seeds	1 tbsp.	45	4
Tofu (raw, firm)	¼ cup (about. 3 oz.)	90	6

Food	Amount	Calories*	Fat (g)
Meat, Poultry, Fish, and Eggs			
Eggs, chopped	2 tbsp.	25	2
Lean ham, chopped	1 oz.	40	2
Popcorn shrimp	1 oz.	30	<1
Surimi	1 oz.	30	<1
Tuna in spring water	1 oz.	35	<1
Turkey in strips	1 oz.	40	<1
Cheese			
Cheddar cheese, grated	2 tbsp.	55	5
Cottage cheese, creamed	¼ cup	60	2
Cottage cheese, 1% low-fat	¼ cup	40	<1
Feta cheese	2 tbsp.	50	4
Mozzarella cheese, grated (part skim)	2 tbsp.	45	3
Parmesan cheese	2 tbsp.	45	3
Others			
Bacon bits	1 tbsp.	25	2
Chow mein noodles	1 tbsp.	15	<1
Croutons, seasoned	2 tbsp.	25	1
Mixed Salads			
Potato (with mayonnaise)	¼ cup	90	5
Three-bean (in vinaigrette)	¼ cup	60	0
Tuna salad (with mayonnaise)	¼ cup	95	5
Dressings			
Blue cheese, regular	2 tbsp.	150	16
French, regular	2 tbsp.	145	14
Italian, fat-free	2 tbsp.	15	<1
Italian, regular	2 tbsp.	85	8
Lemon juice	2 tbsp.	6	0
Oil and vinegar	2 tbsp.	145	16
Thousand Island, regular	2 tbsp.	120	11
Vinegar	2 tbsp.	6	0

*Nutrient values have been rounded.

†"Trace" on all the vegetables and fruits is about .05 to 0.2 gram of fat.

Source: U.S. Department of Agriculture, Agricultural Research Service, 2005. *USDA National Nutrient Database for Standard Reference,* Release 18.

Where do excessive calories, fat, even sodium come from? Not from the lettuce, tomatoes, cucumbers, and other fresh vegetables. Depending on the amount, regular salad dressings, along with many higher-fat toppings such as cheese, croutons, bacon bits, nuts, chow mein noodles, and olives, can heap calories on a bed of raw vegetables. "Dressed" side dishes (potato salad, pasta salad, ambrosia, and macaroni salad), creamy soups, cheese and crackers, even desserts—all with more calories—line up on the salad bar, too.

To control calories and fat in your salad concoctions and to fill your plate with nourishment:

● Pace yourself. Check out the salad bar from end to end before you even begin filling your plate.

● Use a small salad plate, not a dinner plate, if you're tempted to overdo.

● Start with greens. Dark-green leafy vegetables such as spinach and romaine supply more nutrients and phytonutrients than iceberg lettuce does.

● Spoon on plenty of brightly colored vegetables (broccoli, peppers, beets, carrots, to name a few), legumes (such as kidney and garbanzo beans), and fruits for their nutrient, fiber, and phytonutrient benefits. They're low in fat, too.

● Make it a hearty salad with protein-rich ingredients: legumes, lean meat, turkey, crabmeat or surimi, tuna, eggs, and cheese. Cottage cheese, other cheese, and yogurt on the salad bar also add calcium.

● Lighten up on higher-fat toppings and mayonnaise-based side salads.

● Dress your salad for success! A 2-tablespoon ladle of French, Italian, blue cheese, or Thousand Island dressing adds about 150 calories to an otherwise low-calorie salad. Too often, people spoon on double or triple that amount and overpower the delicate flavor of the salad ingredients. Go easy, try a low-fat or fat-free dressing—or sprinkle on just a splash of flavored vinegar or lemon juice.

Eating Out Safely!

Almost nothing can ruin a trip or a pleasant meal out more than foodborne illness. Although restaurants in the United States, Canada, and many other developed nations must pass strict public health regulations,

you're still wise to double-check for cleanliness. Any restaurant can have an occasional lapse in sanitation procedure, and in some parts of the world, these regulations may not exist. Hotel staff often can recommend restaurants with high standards.

These tips can help ensure that the meal you eat away from home won't come back to "bite you":

● Check for cleanliness. Although you probably can't see into the kitchen, you can learn a lot about a restaurant by looking at the public areas. Look for:
  ● Tables that are wiped clean—using clean cloths
  ● Well-groomed servers
  ● Clean silverware, tablecloths, glasses, and dishes
  ● Adequate screening over windows and doors to keep out insects
  ● No flies or roaches, which can spread disease
  ● Clean rest rooms with soap, hot water, and towels or air dryers
  ● A clean exterior with no uncovered garbage

● Before you eat from a food bar, check the temperature. A hot buffet should be piping hot. And a cold salad bar should be well chilled or placed on ice.

● Order food from food bars and displays only if the food is properly covered with a sneeze guard or a hood. This includes desserts and appetizers.

● Be cautious about raw meat and fish; they may carry bacteria and parasites. These menu items are served raw: steak tartare (raw ground beef and raw eggs), carpaccio (thin-sliced raw beef), and sashimi (raw fish). Sushi, often made with raw fish, is popular among many restaurantgoers. *See "Is Raw Seafood Safe to Eat?" in chapter 12 for guidance on sashimi.*

● Check your burger. It should be cooked until the center is no longer pink and the juices run clear, usually "medium" or "medium-well." If it's not cooked thoroughly, send it back!

Safe Take-out

From restaurants, delis, and supermarkets, take-out foods are becoming essential to today's busy lifestyles. Because many buy-and-go foods are perishable, you need to handle them with care to avoid foodborne illness. Keep hot foods above 140° F and cold foods at 40° F or below. Discard perishable foods kept at room temperature for more than two hours. If the temperature inside or outdoors tops 90° F, toss after one hour.

For hot foods . . .

● Make sure the food is hot when you get it. Then eat it within two hours, or one hour if the temperature is 90°F or more.

● If the food won't be eaten for more than two hours, refrigerate it in shallow, covered containers. Then reheat it to a temperature of 165° F, or until it's hot and steaming. Check the temperature with a meat thermometer. *See "Using a Meat Thermometer" in chapter 12.* Or reheat it, covered and rotated for even heating, in a microwave oven. Then let the food stand for two minutes for more thorough heating.

● Keep hot take-out food in the oven or in a slow cooker at 140° F or above—but not if you'll hold it much longer than two hours. Food loses its appeal if it's held longer. Cover it with foil to keep it moist. And check the temperature with a meat thermometer.

For cold foods . . .

● If you don't eat cold take-out foods right away, refrigerate them, or store them in chilled, insulated coolers.

● For deli platters that stay on the buffet, keep the platters on bowls of ice.

For more information on foodborne illness—and how to prevent it—see chapter 12, "The Safe Kitchen."

Fast Food, Healthful Food

Dependence on fast foods goes back thousands of years. In the Roman Forum more than two thousand years ago, urban consumers ate sausages and honey cakes. The Chinese ate stuffed buns in the twelfth century. Five hundred years ago, Spaniards encountered tacos in the markets of today's Mexico.

Fast food has been part of American food culture for many more years than most people realize. If your great-grandparents traveled by train in the early 1900s, they likely devoured "fast food," or quick meals, from the dining car. When the automobile took over, the dining-car concept was reinvented as fast-food restaurants, dotting the roadside. Eating in the car isn't new; the popular "drive-in" restaurant of

the 1950s evolved into the "drive-through" window.

As we know it today, the so-called fast-food chain, or quick-service restaurant, is a phenomenon that's only about fifty-five years old, launched for a post–World War II, fast-oriented, mobile society. At that same time, eating out became more than an occasional treat. At the start, fast food was limited to mainly fried chicken, hamburgers, French fries, ice cream, shakes, and soft drinks.

Today's fast-food menus offer far more options than traditional fare. From grilled chicken sandwiches, wraps, and broiled fish, to salads, to low-fat milk and fruit smoothies, you have plenty to choose from, including lower-calorie, lower-fat, and fresh menu items. You might even find pizza, seafood, pasta, Tex-Mex food, stuffed baked potatoes, noodles, and deli items along with quick ethnic cuisine. Breakfast also has become a big fast-food business. Even convenience stores where you gas up your car sell fast food—truly the "dining car" of the highway!

Are fast-food meals healthful? Overall, yes—if you choose wisely. Because menus are so varied, no overall comment can describe their nutritional value. Traditional meals—a burger, fries, a fried fruit turnover, and a soft drink, or fried chicken, biscuit, creamy slaw, and mashed potatoes with gravy—remain *high* in calories and fat, including saturated fat, and sodium, but *low* in vitamins A and C, calcium, and fiber, and *short* on fruits and vegetables. In response to consumer demand, many of today's fast-food restaurants offer more varied menus with more vegetables and fruits; lower-calorie, lower-fat options; and smaller portions.

Fast-Food Pointers

If you're a fast-food regular, keep these pointers in mind. As general advice for healthful eating, order more fruits and vegetables, more foods with bone-building calcium, less foods with fat, saturated fat, and added sugars, and reasonably sized portions.

To watch your portions . . .

● Be aware of portions that may be larger than you need: "deluxe," "super," and "mega" may be different sizes of "big." Whether it's a sandwich, fries, a shake, or another menu option, bigger portions mean more calories and likely more fat, cholesterol, and sodium. For most people, the small or regular size is enough.

● Think before you buy. Order takers often promote with marketing questions—for example, "Would you

Your Nutrition Checkup

How Do Your Fast-Food Meals Measure Up?

Reflect back on your last fast-food meal or snack. What did you order? Did you consider how your menu choices fit within your overall diet? Take a moment to rate your food choices.

● On the following chart, write in the last fast-food meal or snack you ordered and the portion size for each menu item.

● *Using the chart "FFF—Fast Food Facts" in this chapter,* find out how your food choices measured up. Write in the amount of calories, fat, saturated fat, cholesterol, and sodium for each menu item you ordered. Then total the amounts at the bottom of

the chart. Check the restaurant's Web site for the nutritional breakdown of their current menu.

● Go a little farther. *Using information from MyPyramid in chapter 10,* write the food group and the amounts from each menu item.

● Surprised by the results? What did you learn about your fast-food choices? What might you change if you order this meal or snack again?

There's no right or wrong answer to fast-food eating. The best meal or snack for you depends on you—your needs, your health, and the overall food choices you make every day!

WRITE IT DOWN

MENU ITEM	YOUR PORTION SIZE	CALORIES	FAT (G)	SATURATED FAT (G)	CHOLESTEROL (MG)	SODIUM (MG)	FOOD GROUP/AMOUNT
TOTALS:							

Fast Food: Beyond Burgers

If you're in a fast-food rut, look around for some quick and different approaches to fast-food eating:

- Sushi bar
- Submarine sandwich spot
- Wrap restaurant
- Bakery-shop deli
- Noodle shop

like fries with that?" or "Do you want the value size?" It's okay to say "no."

- Go easy on snacks. A large order of fries and a large soft drink can add up to a hefty 650 or more calories!

- Split your order. Halve the calories and double the pleasure—share your fries or sandwich with a friend!

- Decide *before* you order whether the "value meal" is a good deal. If you don't need the extra food, there's really no extra value; smaller may cost less. Sharing may be a good deal.

For more food variety . . .

- For flavor and nutrition, consider the other foods you have eaten—or will eat—during the day. Order fruits, vegetables, calcium-rich foods, and even whole grains if you can.

- Select a side of salad, raw vegetables, or coleslaw for added vitamins A and C, and fiber. Boost your calcium intake with reduced-fat, low-fat, or fat-free milk.

- Try different types of fast foods, not the same foods every day.

- Enjoy fast-food outlets that serve ethnic foods: perhaps Chinese stir-fry dishes, a Mexican burrito, Japanese domburi, or a vegetable-stuffed pita with cucumber-yogurt dressing. Often food courts in shopping malls allow you to travel the world of flavor without leaving home.

Trim the calories and fat . . .

- Learn to spot high-fat foods—then go easy.

- On sandwiches and salads, go easy on condiments, special sauces, and dressings. Just one packet of mayonnaise (about 1 tablespoon) adds about 60 calories and 5 fat grams. The same size packet of tartar sauce has about 70 calories and 8 fat grams. And a 1½-ounce packet of French dressing contains about 185 calories

and 17 fat grams. Ask for mustard, catsup, salsa, or low-fat or fat-free condiments, spreads, and dressings (mayonnaise, sour cream, or cream cheese).

- For fried foods, pay attention to the oil used for frying. Most fast-food chains use 100 percent vegetable oil, which may be identified on the menu. Vegetable oil is cholesterol-free and high in polyunsaturated fatty acids; the oil used for frying in the fast-food industry is often high in *trans* fatty acids. *See "About* Trans *Fats" in chapter 3.* And when French fries and other foods are fried in fat that's partly beef tallow, these foods contain more cholesterol and saturated fats.

- Better yet, choose fried foods only as "sometimes" foods. Rely mostly on grilled, broiled, steamed, or microwaved fast foods instead.

- Read on for more fast-food tips. *Check "FFF— Fast Food Facts" in this chapter,* or look for nutrition information on posters, in brochures, or online.

Lighten up on salt . . .

Many fast foods are high in sodium—a challenge if you're sodium-sensitive. For less salt and sodium, ask for unsalted fries. Skip special sauces, pickles, olives, relish bacon, sausage, ham, and deli meat.

Eating and Driving: A Safety Issue?

With Americans' hectic lifestyles, more people eat in the car—and more than 70 percent use the drive-through window, according to the National Restaurant Association. And cars and fast-food packaging are being designed to do that.

When time is short, many people assume that the fastest food comes from the drive-up window. Not so. Many times the drive-through line is longer than that for counter service. Beyond that, eating or drinking while driving not only can be messy, it's also dangerous when one hand is on the wheel and the other hand is holding a burger or a steaming hot beverage. If the cell phone rings at the same time, you may really be in trouble!

If you do eat in the car, pull over in a parking lot, city park, or by the curb. Then enjoy those few minutes of eating without thinking about driving, too. Better yet, relax with your food in a mall or on a park bench. Then take a brisk walk.

Break-FAST

With the more hectic pace today, more and more consumers, particularly those heading to work, buy breakfast on the run: a quick breakfast sandwich from the drive-up window; a sit-down meal of eggs and hash browns, or pancakes from the fast-food counter; or coffee and a deli muffin or a bagel to eat at the desk. When these quick breakfasts become a regular eating pattern, it's time to take stock of their nutritional impact!

Fast-food menus usually offer fewer options for breakfast than for lunch and dinner. Many of the choices are high in calories, fat, saturated fat, cholesterol, and sodium. Here's some breakfast menu savvy:

● Order the fastest breakfast of all: dry cereal and milk. Cereal offers a serving from the Grains Group, along with starches (complex carbohydrates) and B vitamins and almost no fat. If you choose a whole-grain or bran cereal, you get more fiber, too. An 8-ounce carton of milk supplies about 300 milligrams of calcium; that's about 25 percent of the calcium you need daily. Pour some on your cereal, perhaps some in your coffee—and drink the rest!

● Order a stack of pancakes. For less fat, use syrup and skip the margarine or the butter. Enjoy half the bacon, or ask for Canadian bacon, which is leaner.

● Look for other options: egg-white omelets, fruit plates, and fruit and yogurt.

Breakfast: Cut Down on Fat and Sodium

● Go easy on breakfast sandwiches. A typical bacon, egg, and cheese biscuit sandwich has about 440 calories, 24 fat grams, and 1,250 milligrams of sodium. Go for a breakfast (bean and cheese) burrito with 375 calories, 12 fat grams, yet 1,170 milligrams of sodium.

● Skip bacon or sausage on your breakfast sandwich. Or substitute ham or Canadian bacon for less fat.

● Order your sandwich on an English muffin, bagel, or even a hamburger bun. To compare, a typical fast-food breakfast biscuit can have about 18 fat grams, and a croissant, about 10 fat grams, compared to 1 fat gram in an English muffin.

● Instead of a doughnut, order an English muffin, bagel, toast, or a plain soft baked pretzel. To save on fat grams, order cream cheese, margarine, or butter on the side, and spread it on lightly. Or use jam or jelly.

● Be sizewise about muffins and bagels, as well as croissants and biscuits. Muffins can be higher in fat than you'd think when they are big. A typical 2-ounce muffin has about 5 fat grams—10 to 15 fat grams or more if it's jumbo-size! A large bakery bagel can count toward as many as 6 ounces from the Grains Group.

● If you're a fast-food regular, go easy on egg entrées. The reason? A large egg has 213 milligrams of dietary cholesterol. Health experts advise that healthy people consume 300 milligrams of cholesterol or less per day, and eat yolks and whole eggs in moderation. A two-egg breakfast has at least 425 milligrams of cholesterol!

● Order juice as your breakfast beverage. With an 8-ounce carton of orange juice, you'll get more than 100 percent of the vitamin C you need in a day.

● At a deli? Ask for yogurt to go with your bagel and juice. An 8-ounce carton of low-fat fruit yogurt supplies about 315 milligrams of calcium, 225 calories, and just 2 to 3 fat grams. Or order a fruit cup!

Burgers, Chicken, or Fish?

Hamburgers may be America's all-time favorite fast food. But chicken and fish have gained a significant market share, in part because consumers perceive them as lower in calories and fat. Chicken and fish sometimes have a lean advantage. However, fast-food preparation—breading, battering, and frying—bump up the calorie and fat content significantly. A fried fish or fried chicken sandwich may supply more calories and fat than a burger!

To keep the lean advantage of hot sandwiches and to boost other nutrients, consider this advice:

● Boost the nutrients in all kinds of hot sandwiches—burgers, chicken, or fish—by adding tomato slices and other vegetables. If you're short on calcium, add cheese. For a fiber boost, ask for a whole-wheat bun.

● Cut calories by ordering sandwiches without higher-fat condiments and special sauces, such as mayonnaise-based spreads and tartar sauce. Instead use mustard, relish, or ketchup. As a rule of thumb: calories go up with the number of "extras."

● Skip the super-size sandwich; go for the regular, junior, or single size instead. The bigger size can about double everything, including the calorie, fat, and sodium content. A large hamburger, for example, supplies about 510 calories and 28 fat grams compared with 275 calories and 12 fat grams in a regular hamburger. A regular burger has about 2 ounces of cooked meat, compared with 3 to 4 ounces in a larger sandwich. Double patties are bigger still.

● To lower the calories and the fat, remove the crispy crust from fried chicken and the skin from rotisserie chicken. Get grilled, skinless chicken. If you prefer fried chicken, order the regular variety rather than "extra-crispy," which soaks up more oil when cooked. The batter or the breading may have a high-sodium seasoning, too, so you can lower the sodium by removing the crust. And eat just one piece, rather than a two- or three-piece order. Chicken nuggets are usually fried and may contain skin and meat (white and dark). Poultry skin is high in fat.

● Choose broiled or baked fish if you have a choice. But be aware that the fillets on most fish sandwiches are battered and fried. Go easy on tartar sauce; ask for tomato-based cocktail sauce instead.

On the Side

Food variety adds nutrients, so round out your fast-food meal with veggies, fruit, and calcium-rich foods —perhaps a salad, baked potato, carrot sticks, fruit, juice, milk, or frozen yogurt. In most fast-food restaurants your options are limited. Get the most nutrition mileage from the choices you have.

Spuds

● Order a baked potato as a side dish or an entrée. Served plain, a baked potato is fat-free and cholesterol-free, with almost no sodium. It also supplies starches (complex carbohydrates), fiber, vitamin C, and other vitamins and minerals.

● Go easy on higher-fat toppings: bacon, sour cream, and butter. For more nutrients and usually less calories and fat, top with broccoli, salsa, chili, or cottage cheese. Along with a salad and milk, a broccoli-cheese spud or a chili spud make a nutritious meal!

● Go easy on fries to limit calories and fat in an already higher-fat meal. Or ask for the small order, then share. French fries offer some vitamin C.

● If you have the option, ask for a plain baked potato or mashed potatoes to control calories and fat. Ask for gravy on the side to control how much you add. Find out how mashed potatoes with gravy are prepared; check the nutrition information if it's posted.

● As alternative to fries, fried onion rings, fried okra, and hush puppies, order corn on the cob, green beans, or baked beans. For corn, ease up on butter and salt.

Salads

● Order a garden salad with dressing on the side. Use a reduced-fat or fat-free dressing. *For salad bar tips, see "Sizing Up Salad Bars" earlier in this chapter.*

● Go easy on prepared salads with a lot of mayonnaise or salad dressing, such as creamy coleslaw, potato salad, or macaroni salad. They have more fat than salads with a vinaigrette dressing, such as coleslaw or three-bean salad.

● Order a container of raw veggies or fruit chunks, or whole fruit if you can.

● Enjoy flavorful entrée salads (easy on the dressing) from most fast-food chains.

Beverages

● Make beverages count! For flavor and nutrients, round out your meal with milk or juice. Many fast-food chains offer reduced-fat and fat-free milk. For a flavor switch, try chocolate or other flavored milk.

　● An 8-ounce carton of milk supplies about 300 milligrams of calcium as well as protein, riboflavin, vitamin D, and other nutrients.

　● An 8-ounce carton of orange juice supplies 75 milligrams of vitamin C, which more than meets your daily need.

● Go easy on soft drinks. Reasonable amounts are okay sometimes for their fluids, food energy, and enjoyment. They don't, however, contribute other nutrients supplied by milk, or fruit or vegetable juice. Large-size drinks can add up to a lot of calories: 150 for every 12 ounces of regular soft drinks, or 800 calories for a 64-ounce cup! Diet drinks supply essentially no calories—and no nutrients (except water).

● If the added calories match your eating plan, enjoy a milk shake as part of your fast-food meal or snack. A shake of any flavor is a good calcium source—if it's made from milk. A 10-ounce strawberry shake contains about 320 calories. It can serve double duty—as both your beverage and dessert. Super-size shakes, with their 18 ounces, may supply a hefty 575 calories.

● Try a smoothie bar for a thick blend of juice, fruit, and perhaps yogurt. Consider size. A smoothie that's 20 ounces or more may supply more than you need—including calories. Beware that some smoothies are made with fruit syrup that adds sugar, but not all the nutrients that fruit contains; ask about the ingredients before you order.

● Order a latte, cappuccino, or coffee or hot tea (chai) with low-fat or fat-free milk. Milk, rather than cream, is the calcium booster. Creamers are typically high in saturated fats, too. Remember: Sweetened ice tea and many flavored coffee drinks have added sugars, too.

● For an ideal thirst quencher, choose water. For added flavor, add a lemon wedge. Unless bottled, it's usually offered free as a customer service—ask!

Desserts

● Go easy on fried fruit fritters or turnovers—eat them only if they fit within your daily calorie and fat budget. They're usually more sugar and fat than fruit.

● Check to see if fresh whole or cut-up fruit is available. As another option, bring fresh fruit from home, perhaps an apple, banana, pear, or grapes.

● For a refreshing dessert, enjoy frozen yogurt—or a scoop of ice cream. You may find low-fat versions on the menu. Either way, the small or kids' size offers a

Have You Ever Wondered

... about herbal mix-ins in smoothies? Bee pollen, ginseng, and other herbal mix-ins may cost extra in smoothies, yet not offer the benefits you think. *See "Herbals and Botanicals: Help or Harm?" in chapter 23.*

taste without indulging. For fewer calories, go easy on fudge sauce, candy pieces or mix-ins, or syrup toppings. A little of these toppings goes a long way. Ask for cut-up or dried fruit, nuts, or granola instead.

Pizza—as You Like It!

Pizza is nutritious fast food with the nutritional benefits of three or more food groups in one or two slices. The crust supplies starches and B vitamins, the cheese is a good source of calcium and protein, and the tomato sauce and vegetable toppings add vitamins A, C, and phytonutrients. Meat or seafood toppers add protein, iron, and some vitamins, too.

The actual nutrient content depends on what you put on top—and the type of crust you order. The good news is: You can be the architect of your pizza, controlling the toppings along with the nutrient and calorie content and the flavor.

● Consider the crust. For more fiber, build your pizza on a whole-wheat crust. To trim the calories, order a thin-crust pizza rather than a thick-crust or deep-dish pizza. A stuffed-crust pizza can have considerably

PIZZA TOPPINGS

ENJOY MORE OFTEN	ENJOY SOMETIMES
Artichoke hearts	Anchovies
Bell peppers	Bacon
Broccoli florets	Extra cheese
Canadian bacon or lean ham	Olives
Crabmeat	Pepperoni
Eggplant slices	Prosciutto
Green onions, chopped	Sausage
Jalapeño peppers	
Lean ground meat	
Mushroom slices	
Onion slices	
Pineapple chunks	
Shrimp	
Spinach	
Tomato slices	
Tuna or salmon	
Zucchini slices	

more calories and fat than a thinner-crust pizza; for example, 1 slice of a large stuffed-crust pizza may have 20 fat grams or more, and 450 calories or more.

● Load up on vegetable and fruit toppings for less fat, more fiber, and more vitamins. *Check out "Pizza Toppings" in this chapter for low-fat choices.*

● Go easy on higher-fat toppings: bacon, pepperoni, prosciutto, sausage, olives, anchovies, and extra cheese. If you like higher-fat toppings, stick with just one. These foods add sodium, too. Many combination or deluxe pizzas have several high-fat toppings.

● Choose lean toppings from the Meat and Beans Group, such as lean ham, Canadian bacon, or shrimp.

● Enjoy the variety of toppings and new combinations available in some pizza parlors. Many new toppings are vegetables—artichoke hearts, broccoli florets, eggplant, red bell peppers, and asparagus spears, as well as salmon, tuna, chicken, and shrimp! Want more flavor? Sprinkle on hot pepper flakes for no calories but lots of flavor.

● Order a salad to complement your pizza. Salad not only adds nutrients and fiber, it also helps you fill up. You may be less likely to eat another pizza slice.

● Order a reasonable-size pizza. Limit yourself to two or three slices—or one slice if you're really watching calories. Calories from any pizza, even a veggie pizza, add up when you eat just one more slice. A typical slice—an eighth of a 12-inch thin-crust meat and cheese pizza—supplies about 185 calories.

● If a bigger size is the better deal, wrap up the extra for the fridge before you start eating. You'll enjoy pizza again—and save time with lunch—the next day!

● Go halfzies. Order half the pizza your way if someone else prefers toppings with more fat. In that way you both get what you want.

● For a different flavor, enjoy wood oven-baked pizza, or pizza with a regional twist: perhaps a Southwest pizza; a Cajun-style pizza; or a Hawaiian pizza with pineapple and lean ham.

Deli Sandwiches and Wraps

Sandwiches, subs, and wraps, as well as yogurt, fruit, salads, soups, bagels and muffins, milk, flavored waters, coffee, and tea—the deli bar sells an array of foods and beverages. Of the many foods, the sandwich takes center stage. The great thing is that you often can order a deli sandwich just as you want it!

● Just start with bread. Choose a whole-grain bread, roll, or pita pocket for more fiber. Or try a bagel or herbed foccacia.

● Next, the filling—2 to 3 ounces of lean meat or poultry contribute protein, iron, and other nutrients. Add a slice of cheese to boost the calcium content. For fillings with less fat, order lean roast beef, ham, chicken breast, or turkey. Some delis use meats that are 90 percent or more fat-free—just ask. Request tuna, ham, or egg salad made with less mayonnaise or with reduced-fat or fat-free dressing if available.

● Have your sandwich made to order with a spread that adds flavor, such as mustard, light mayonnaise, or fat-free dressing. To control fat and calories, ask the server to go easy on higher-fat spreads.

● Layer on vegetables: red or green peppers, jalapeños, tomatoes, sprouts, cucumbers, carrot shreds, onions, or grilled veggies. They're low in fat and supply vitamins A and C, fiber, and other nutrients.

● Choose "sides" to fit your healthful eating style. To cut down on fat, ask for carrot or green pepper sticks rather than chips or creamy slaw. For less sodium, enjoy a cucumber spear instead of a pickle.

● Look for a sandwich "wrap" in a soft tortilla. Often the fillings are low in fat, perhaps rice blended with seafood, shredded chicken, or vegetables, or grilled vegetables and chicken breast.

● When sandwiches, subs, and wraps get big, buy one to share, or keep some in the fridge for the next day.

Eating Out Ethnic Style

As a nation of immigrants, the United States has always been home to ethnic cuisine. The real interest in "foreign theme" restaurants grew in the 1960s with pizza parlors and Japanese tabletop cooking. From there, our exposure to ethnic foods became more sophisticated. We added Mexican and more Asian flavors to our restaurant repertoire. Today, ethnic restaurants appear in almost every city and town.

FFF—Fast Food Facts

The nutritional values for similar foods differ among chains; their menus differ, too. Check the chain's Web site for nutrition information about its menu.

Menu Item	Portion Size	Calories	Fat (g)	Saturated Fat (g)	Cholesterol (mg)	Sodium (mg)
Breakfast Items						
Egg and sausage biscuit	1 (180 g)	580	39	15	300	1,140
Egg and cheese croissant	1 (127 g)	370	25	14	215	550
Danish, fruit	1 (94 g)	335	16	3	20	335
English muffin with butter	1 (63 g)	190	6	2	15	385
English muffin with egg, cheese, and Canadian bacon	1 (137 g)	290	13	5	235	730
French toast sticks	5 (141 g)	515	29	5	75	500
Hash brown potatoes	½ cup	150	9	4	10	290
Pancakes with butter and syrup	2 (232 g)	520	14	6	60	1,100
Chicken						
Chicken nuggets	6 pieces (96 g)	285	18	4	55	550
Fried chicken, dark meat	drumstick and thigh	430	27	7	165	755
Fried chicken, white meat	side breast and wing	495	30	8	150	975
Chicken fillet sandwich	1 (182 g)	515	30	9	60	960
Rotisserie chicken white meat, quarter with skin	5 oz.	330	18	5	150	530
Rotisserie chicken dark meat quarter with skin	5 oz.	330	22	7	150	450
Grilled chicken breast sandwich	1 (225 g)	405	11	2	90	960
Fish						
Fish fillet, fried	3 oz. (91 g)	210	11	3	30	485
Fish sandwich with tartar sauce	1 (158 g)	430	23	5	55	615
Sandwiches						
Bacon cheeseburger, large	1 (195 g)	610	37	16	110	1,040
Cheeseburger, regular	1 (113 g)	295	14	6	35	615
Hamburger, regular	1 (90 g)	275	12	4	35	385
Hamburger, large, with lettuce and tomato	1 (218 g)	510	27	10	85	830
Hamburger, double meat patty	1 (226 g)	540	27	10	120	790
Submarine sandwich	1 (228 g)	455	19	7	35	1,650
Roast beef sandwich	1 (139 g)	345	14	4	50	790
Hot dog	1 (98 g)	240	15	5	45	670
Chili dog	1 (114 g)	295	14	5	50	480
Mexican						
Taco, small	1 (171 g)	370	21	11	55	800
Taco salad, large with shell	21 oz.	905	49	16	100	1,935
Burrito, bean and cheese	2 (186 g)	380	12	7	30	1,170
Burrito, beans and meat	2 (231 g)	510	18	8	50	1,335
Enchilada, beef and cheese	1 (192 g)	325	18	9	40	1,320
Refried beans with cheese	1 cup (167 g)	225	8	4	35	880
Nachos with cheese	6–8 nachos (113 g)	345	19	8	20	815
Nachos with cheese, beans, beef, and peppers	6–8 nachos (255 g)	570	31	12	20	1,800

FFF—Fast Food Facts *(continued)*

Menu Item	Portion Size	Calories	Fat (g)	Saturated Fat (g)	Cholesterol (mg)	Sodium (mg)
Other						
Pizza, cheese	1/12 of 14-in. pie (75 g)	200	7	3	15	405
Pizza, meat and vegetables	1/12 of 14-in. pie (97 g)	235	11	4	25	575
Pizza, pepperoni	1/12 of 14-in. pie (79 g)	220	9	4	20	505
Chili con carne	1 cup (253 g)	255	8	3	135	1,010
Sides						
Coleslaw	¾ cup (99 g)	145	11	2	5	265
French fries, fried in vegetable oil	30–40 fries (114 g)	350	18	3	0	220
	20–25 fries (74 g)	225	12	2	0	145
Onion rings	8–9 rings (83 g)	275	16	7	15	430
Potatoes, mashed, with gravy	½ cup (136 g)	120	6	1	0	440
Potato, large, baked, plain	1 (299 g)	280	<1	Trace	0	30
Potato, large, baked, with cheese and broccoli	1 (339 g)	405	21	9	20	485
Potato, large, baked, with cheese and chili	1 (395 g)	480	23	13	30	700
Salad, vegetables without dressing*	1½ cups (207 g)	35	<1	Trace	0	55
Salad with egg and cheese, without dressing*	1½ cups (217 g)	100	6	3	100	120
Salad with chicken without dressing*	1½ cups (218 g)	105	2	<1	70	210
Vegetables, steamed	1 cup (3.7 oz.)	30	<1	Trace	0	10
BBQ baked beans	¾ cup(156 g)	130	3	1	5	760
Pasta salad, tortellini	1½ cups (417 g)	380	21	3	50	1,570
Fruit, cut-up	½ cup (113 g)	65	0	0	0	15
Applesauce	4 ounces (127 g)	95	<1	Trace	0	5
Carrots, baby	4 ounces (113 g)	40	<1	Trace	0	90
Desserts						
Cookies, animal crackers	1 box	300	9	4	10	270
Cookies, chocolate chip	1 box	235	12	5	10	190
Sundae, hot fudge	1 (158 g)	285	9	5	20	180
Ice milk, soft serve	1 cone (103 g)	165	6	4	30	90
Fruit pie, fried	1 pie (128 g)	405	21	3	0	480
Fruit-yogurt parfait	5 ounces (149 g)	155	2	<1	5	85
Beverages						
Milk, 1% low-fat	8 oz.	100	2	1.5	10	105
Soft drink, cola, regular	12 oz.	150	0	0	0	15
Soft drink, cola, calorie-free	12 oz.	5	0	0	0	15
Iced tea, sweetened, store bought	12 oz.	135	0	0	0	75
Iced tea, unsweetened	12 oz.	5	0	0	0	10
Orange juice	8 oz.	105	<1	0	0	5
Shake, chocolate	12 oz.	360	10	7	35	270
Coffee with 1 tbsp. half-and-half cream	6 oz.	25	2	1	5	10

*See "Build a Healthful Salad" in this chapter for nutrition information about salad dressings, and see "Milk: A Good Calcium Source" in chapter 10 for nutrition information for flavored and unflavored milk.

Source: U.S. Department of Agriculture, Agricultural Research Service, 2005. *USDA National Nutrient Database for Standard Reference,* Release 18.

What ethnic cuisines are most popular? Italian, Mexican, and Chinese (Cantonese), say trend-trackers. They're so mainstream today that they're no longer considered ethnic. French and fine Italian cuisines have been upscale restaurant cuisine for years. According to the National Restaurant Association, appreciation for ethnic flavors is growing, with more restaurants featuring Japanese (sushi), Thai, Vietnamese, Caribbean, Indo-Pakistani, Nuevo Latino, and Middle Eastern cuisines. From every corner of the globe, urban areas offer even more ethnic flavors to try!

For fun, find the restaurant pages of your phone book. Now count—how many different ethnic cuisines could you enjoy? To expand the variety in your eating style, try a new cuisine the next time you eat out!

Italian . . . Not Just Pizza and Pasta!

Italian cuisine is the most popular restaurant food in the United States. Two-thirds of all restaurants feature Italian dishes—and not just pizza and pasta. With foods from every region, Italian foods are simple, flavorful, and nourishing.

Italian food is one of several Mediterranean cuisines receiving attention from both food and nutrition experts. Featuring pasta, risotto (rice dish), and polenta (cornmeal dish), Italian food is high in starches. The cuisine relies on smaller meat portions, and cheese is used to flavor many dishes.

Particularly with the foods of southern Italy, olive oil is the primary cooking fat, in contrast to butter, used in many northern Italian dishes. High in heart-healthier monounsaturated fatty acids, olive oil has some nutritional benefits. Regardless, go easy; any oil is still fat, with the same number of calories per ounce as margarine and butter. *For more about this cuisine, see "Take Your Taste Buds to the Mediterranean" in chapter 9.* Consider these tips for Italian foods:

● Enjoy crusty Italian bread—a slice or two, but not the whole basket! For less fat, go easy on butter or on olive oil for dipping, or enjoy the flavor of fresh bread as it is, without a spread. *Hint:* Garlic bread usually is lathered in high-fat spreads, Parmesan cheese, and garlic before it arrives at your table. Plain bread is a lower-calorie, lower-fat choice.

Have You Ever Wondered

. . . what "primavera" and "fresco" on menus mean? Translated from Italian, "primavera" means "spring style." In cooking terms it refers to dishes prepared with raw or lightly cooked fresh vegetables. "Fresco" means fresh.

● Go easy on antipasto. "Antipasto" means "before the pasta," and it usually refers to a variety of hot or cold appetizers. In the Mediterranean tradition, they include cheese, olives, smoked meats, and marinated vegetables and fish. While they're nutritious, some may be high in fat and sodium. Nibbling appetizers, followed by a heavy meal, may add up to more calories than you expect.

● Order a fresh garden salad, or "insalata," to round out your meal, with salad dressing, perhaps herbed vinegar and olive oil, served on the side. Salads in Italian restaurants often are tossed with a variety of raw vegetables and mixed greens, including arugula, radicchio, bell peppers, tomatoes, and onions. As an entrée, salad with bread makes a nice, light meal.

● Look for traditional bean and vegetable dishes on many Italian menus. Minestrone is a hearty, tomato-based soup with beans, vegetables, and pasta. White beans, called "fagioli," are featured in soups and risotto (rice dishes). "Florentine" dishes are prepared with spinach.

● Know menu lingo. For example, dishes described as "fritto" (fried) or "crema" (creamed) are higher in fat. "Primavera" refers to dishes prepared with fresh vegetables and herbs. Sometimes primavera dishes are served with a creamy sauce; ask your server.

● For enjoyment, order different types of pasta dishes—in shapes and sizes you may not find on supermarket shelves. Made of flour and water, pasta is a carbohydrate-rich food. Fat comes from the sauces and other ingredients tossed with pasta. Did you know that a tomato-based sauce usually has fewer calories than a creamy white pasta sauce or a pesto sauce? Look for marinara and other tomato-based sauces that usually have more vegetables and less fat, too, than creamy white sauces such as alfredo and carbonara. *See "Gourmet's Guide to Sauces" earlier in this chapter.*

● For polenta, gnocchi, or risotto, ask how these are made before ordering.

● *Polenta,* similar to a cornmeal mush, typically is served with sauce, vegetables, and meat; some ingredients may have more fat.

● *Gnocchi,* usually made from potatoes or flour, means dumplings; sometimes eggs, cheese, or chopped vegetables are mixed into the dough. After they're cooked in boiling water they may be baked or fried, then served with a flavorful sauce.

● *Risotto,* typically made from arborio rice, usually is cooked in broth and perhaps butter, often with meat, seafood, cheese, and vegetables. Be aware that the broth may be salty.

● As another option, order ravioli, which are square "pillows" of pasta filled with meat, seafood, cheese, or vegetables. Usually they're served with a sauce. Ask about preparation before you order; as appetizers, they may be fried.

● Watch portion size. If you know the restaurant offers generous servings, order an appetizer portion, or share with someone else.

● If you need to watch fat carefully, go easy on veal scaloppini, and chicken or veal parmigiana, which are sautéed or pan-fried. Parmigiana entrées—made with Parmesan cheese—also are breaded, so they absorb more fat. As an alternative and a lower-fat option, order chicken or veal cacciatore, marsala, or piccata. Cacciatore is a tomato-based sauce; marsala is broth-based and cooked with wine; and piccata is pan drippings, lemon juice, and chopped parsley.

From the Italian Menu

Enjoy more often:

● Minestrone soup
● Garden salad
● Bread sticks
● Vinegar and oil dressing
● Pasta with red sauce, such as marinara
● Chicken cacciatore
● Cappuccino (Ask your server to have it made with fat-free or low-fat milk.)
● Italian fruit ice or fruit

POPULAR ITALIAN FARE: FITTING WITHIN THE FOOD GROUPS

MyPyramid.gov
STEPS TO A HEALTHIER YOU

Grains
Bread sticks
Gnocchi (dumpling)
Italian bread
Polenta (cornmeal mush)
Risotto (rice specialty)
Spaghetti, linguini, other pasta

Vegetables
Artichokes
Beans (white kidney, fava, garbanzo)*
Bell peppers
Eggplants
Grape leaves
Greens
Mushrooms
Tomatoes, tomato sauces
Spinach

Fruits
Dates
Figs
Grapefruit
Grapes
Olives
Oranges
Pomegranates
Dried fruits

Milk
Cheese: mozzarella, pecorino, ricotta, others
Gelato
Milk
Yogurt

Meat and Beans
Beef
Chicken
Fish (anchovies, tuna, others)
Beans (white kidney, fava, garbanzo)*
Nuts (pine nuts, almonds)
Sausage, proscuitto, ham
Shellfish (clams, shrimp, calamari)
Veal

Oils
Olive oil
Oils in nuts, olives, anchovies, tuna, other fatty fish

*Legumes (dry beans) fit in either food group.

Enjoy sometimes:

- Antipasto plates
- Buttered garlic bread
- Creamy Italian dressing
- Pasta with white sauce such as alfredo or carbonara
- Italian sausage and prosciutto
- Fried dishes such as eggplant Parmesan
- Cannoli (Cannoli, cannelloni, and cannellini often get mixed up. Cannoli are deep-fried pastry shells filled with ricotta cheese or whipped cream and perhaps chocolate bits, nuts, and candied fruit. Cannelloni are pasta tubes filled with meat and cheese and topped with sauce. Cannellini are white kidney beans.)

It's Greek Food to Me!

Another Mediterranean cuisine is popular: Greek food. For many consumers, experience with Greek restaurants comes from fast-food courts in shopping malls. The popular gyro sandwich, souvlaki, Greek salad, rice pilaf, moussaka, and baklava are best known. But like other cuisines, full-service restaurants offer far more variety. To order smarter, consider these menu tips:

- For a creamy dressing on salads, or a sauce on pita sandwiches, enjoy tzatziki. It's made with yogurt, garlic, and cucumbers. Sometimes tzatziki is listed on the menu as a salad. Try tzatziki as an appetizer dip with pita bread, too.

- Enjoy smaller amounts of baba ghanouj, a higher-fat dip made with eggplant and olive oil, and of hummus, made with mashed chickpeas and sesame seed paste.

- Flavorful olive oil for dipping is often served with a basket of pita bread. Again, go easy. Although high in monounsaturated fat, low in saturated fat, and cholesterol-free, olive oil contains just as much fat as butter or margarine. Bread often can soak up a lot of oil!

- Ordering saganaki as an appetizer? Saganaki is thick kasseri cheese that's fried and sometimes flamed in brandy. To trim the fat, share with someone else.

- For nutritious fast food order pita bread stuffed with Greek salad, lean meat, tabouli, or other ingredients. Tabouli is bulgur wheat mixed with chopped tomatoes, parsley, mint, olive oil, and lemon juice. For more fiber ask for whole-wheat pita. Another popular use of the pita is the gyro, which is minced lamb molded and roasted vertically. When cooked, the lamb is sliced and tucked into pita bread with grilled onions, bell peppers, and tzatziki sauce.

- As a main dish, look for broiled and grilled meat, poultry, and seafood: perhaps shish kebob, which is skewered and broiled meat and vegetables; souvlaki, which is lamb marinated in lemon juice, olive oil, and herbs, then skewered and grilled; or plaki, which is fish broiled with tomato sauce and garlic.

- As another menu option, try dolmas, or stuffed vegetables. Grape leaves are most commonly stuffed with ground meat; other vegetables, such as bell peppers, cabbage leaves, eggplant, and squash, are stuffed with mixtures of ground meat, rice, dried fruit, and pine nuts. Because they're steamed or baked, fat usually isn't added with cooking.

- To boost fiber, order dishes made with legumes. In a full-service restaurant you'll likely find mixed dishes and soups made with fava beans and other legumes.

- Order a Greek salad to go with meals. Ask for dressing on the side. And go easy on the higher-fat, higher-sodium ingredients: anchovies, kalamata olives, and feta cheese.

- Go easy also on rich Greek desserts such as baklava. Made with phyllo and plenty of butter, honey or sugar, and nuts, this sweet, compact pastry is very high in calories. It's wonderful-tasting, but a small serving is enough to satisfy a sweet tooth!

From the Greek Menu

Enjoy more often:

- Broiled, grilled, simmered, or stewed dishes
- Greek salad
- Tabouli
- Dolmas
- Tzatziki
- Fresh fruit
- Pita bread

Enjoy sometimes:

- Pan-fried dishes
- Vegetable pies such as spanakopita and tyropita
- Baba ghanouj (a Middle Eastern dish that appears on some Greek menus)
- Baklava and phyllo pastry dishes
- Deep-fried falafel and calamari
- Moussaka and other creamy casseroles

Mexican Food: Tacos, Tamales, and More

From fast-food establishments to full-service restaurants, Mexican food and its Tex-Mex offspring are among America's favorite ethnic foods. And Mexican flavors now appear in pizzas, entrée salads, wraps, and stir-fries. The staples—tortillas, beans, and rice—are great sources of starches, and pinto or black beans supply fiber as well. Moderate portions of meat and poultry contribute adequate, but not lavish, amounts of protein. And beans and rice, or beans and tortillas when eaten together, also supply high-quality protein.

Depending on the choices, Mexican or Tex-Mex cuisine can be high in fat—and sodium, too. In most restaurants, vegetable oil (no longer lard) is the fat used in cooking (except perhaps in refried beans). Cooked with vegetable oil, the saturated fat may be lower, but not the calories or the total fat. As with foods of every culture, enjoy variety, but go easy on foods with more total fat, especially saturated fats, and *trans* fats, cholesterol, and sodium.

- Order guacamole and sour cream on the side to control the amount. Or ask for low-fat or fat-free sour cream. For more vitamins A and C, use a heavy hand with tomato-based salsa. Made with tomatoes, onions, chiles, and herbs, it's virtually fat-free, yet bursting with flavor. So are the cilantro, hot sauce, and peppers!

- Ask for soft tacos. Crispy tacos and tostadas are deep-fried. Corn tortillas have a little less calories and fat than flour tortillas.

- Ordering a taco salad? Enjoy, but go easy on the big, crisp tortilla shell it's served in—or the taco chips on top—to trim fat and calories. Enjoy warmed, soft tortillas on the side. And dress it with salsa!

- Go easy on nachos and cheese, or chile con queso, especially if it's just the appetizer before the meal. To cut in half the fat and the calories from cheese, ask for half a ladle of cheese sauce, or half as much cheese shreds. For the starter of chips and salsa, enjoy one basket or less, then have it taken away if you can't resist, or skip the nacho basket altogether.

- Order a low-fat appetizer: gazpacho (chilled tomato soup), jicama and salsa, tortilla soup, or black bean soup.

- Since portions in Mexican meals tend to be large, choose the regular plate, not the "deluxe combo" plate. For most people, the regular plate is plenty! Ask for more shredded lettuce and tomato instead.

- Choose mostly baked or stir-fried entrées such as enchiladas or fajitas on a soft tortilla. Go easy on fried dishes such as chiles relleños, chimichangas, or flautas.

Although tacos, tamales, enchiladas, and burritos are among the most popular items, especially in Tex-Mex restaurants, Mexican and Southwest restaurants offer a far broader menu, especially in authentic restaurants. Next time, check the menu further. You may find salads with nopales, or cactus pads; chayote and jicama, which are starchy vegetables; and tomatillos, or green tomatoes. For prepared foods look for Veracruz-style seafood dishes, which are cooked in a herbed tomato sauce; or chile verde, which is pork simmered with vegetables and green chiles.

- Want a margarita? "On the rocks" has fewer calories than "frozen." Skip the salt if you have high blood pressure.

From the Mexican Menu

Enjoy more often:

- Jicama with fresh lime juice
- Salsa
- Soft tacos
- Burritos, enchiladas, tamales, fajitas
- Red beans and rice*
- Spanish rice*
- Refried beans (no lard)
- Steamed vegetables
- Black bean soup, menudo (spicy soup made with tripe and hominy), gazpacho
- Arroz con pollo (chicken with rice)

- Fruit for dessert such as guava, papaya, or mango
- Flan or pudding
- Grilled meat, poultry, fish

* The fat and calorie content varies depending on the ingredients and the preparation method.

Enjoy less often:

- Guacamole dip with taco chips
- Sour cream and extra cheese
- Crispy, fried tortillas
- Crispy tacos, taco salad
- Tostadas, chiles relleños, quesadillas, chimi-changas, chalupas
- Refried beans (cooked in lard)
- Honey-sweetened pastry and sopapillas
- Chicharonnes (fried pork rinds)
- Fried ice cream
- Chorizo

Mexican Menu Language

Learn to speak Mexican menu talk. Look for descriptions that offer clues to the fat content.

Menu clues—less fat and perhaps calories:

- Asada (grilled)
- Mole sauce (chile-chocolate sauce)
- Served with salsa verde (green chile sauce)
- Simmered
- Tomato sauce, picante
- Topped with lettuce and tomato
- Veracruz-style (tomato sauce)
- With chiles
- Wrapped in a soft tortilla

Menu clues—more fat and perhaps calories:

- Crispy
- Fried
- Layered with refried beans
- Mixed with chorizo (Mexican sausage)
- Served in a crisp tortilla basket
- Smothered in cheese sauce
- Topped with guacamole and sour cream
- Chile con queso

POPULAR MEXICAN FARE: FITTING WITHIN THE FOOD GROUPS

MyPyramid.gov
STEPS TO A HEALTHIER YOU

Grains
Posole (soup made with corn kernels)
Rice
Sopa (thick rice soup)
Taco shells
Tortillas, flour and corn

Fruits
Avocado
Mango
Papaya
Platano (cooking banana)
Zapote (sweet yellow fruit)

Vegetables
Beans and peas (pigeon peas, garbanzos, black, kidney, red beans)*
Chayote
Corn
Jicama
Nopales
Peppers
Refried beans*
Salsa
Tomatoes
Tomatillos

Milk
Coffee con leche (with milk)
Flan (custard)
Jack cheese

Leche (milk)
Queso blanco (cheese)

Meat and Beans
Beans and peas (pigeon peas, garbanzos, black, kidney, red beans)*
Beef
Chicken
Chorizo sausage
Eggs
Fish
Shrimp
Refried beans*

Oils
Corn oil
Vegetable oil

*Legumes (dry beans) fit in either food group.

Chinese Fare

Chinese cuisine is complex and highly developed, offering significant contributions to the world's food experiences. With its focus on vegetables, rice, and noodles, Asian-style cooking also has earned its place as a nutritious option in a healthful eating pattern.

Chinese cuisine reflects the different cooking styles, ingredients, and flavorings of China's many regions. Restaurants may specialize in foods from Canton, Hunan, Peking (Beijing), Shanghai, or Szechuan, for example. Cantonese-style cooking is the most popular in the United States, largely due to the number of Cantonese immigrants in the mid-1800s who brought their cooking styles with them. Cantonese cuisine of southeastern China features roasted and grilled meat, steamed dishes, stir-fried dishes, and mild flavors. Szechuan and Hunan foods tend to be hot and spicy, and perhaps higher in fat. Peking cuisine of northeastern China is noted for skillful, subtle uses of seasonings. Shanghai-style has more seafood. The term "Mandarin" on menus usually refers to aristocratic cuisine, featuring the finest aspects of all regional cuisines.

Chinese meals emphasize rice or noodles, and vegetables, with their contribution of starches. Vegetables are good sources of fiber, beta carotene (which forms vitamin A) and vitamin C, and phytonutrients, too. Meat, poultry, and seafood are served in small portions, often sliced and cooked with vegetables. Tofu, or soybean curd, is a common, high-protein, low-fat, cholesterol-free ingredient, too. Many Chinese dishes are roasted, simmered, steamed, or stir-fried, so they're likely to be low in fat.

From a nutritional standpoint, the areas of caution in Chinese dining are the fat and the sodium content. Deep-fat frying is a common cooking technique for many menu items. Sometimes foods are stir-fried in large amounts of oil. For those who are sodium-sensitive, know that two ingredients with more sodium—monosodium glutamate (MSG) and soy sauce—often are used to flavor foods. MSG, however, has a third the sodium of table salt. *See "MSG— Another Flavor Enhancer" in chapter 7.*

Calcium-rich foods are limited on Chinese menus since milk, cheese, and yogurt aren't part of the traditional cuisine. Most calcium comes from fish with edible bones and from vegetables such as broccoli and greens, although the amount of calcium per half cup portion is much lower than in eight ounces of milk.

Whether you eat in or carry out, keep these ordering tips in mind at a Chinese restaurant:

● Enjoy the flavorful soups as a starter or a main dish. Many are made with clear broth with small amounts of meat and vegetables. Made by cooking eggs in the broth, egg drop soup and hot-and-sour soup are higher in cholesterol; the amount, however, is small since there's not much egg in a single serving.

● Go easy on fried appetizers. Fried wontons, crab rangoon, and many egg rolls are deep-fat fried. As an option, order steamed spring rolls or egg rolls.

● Enjoy the vegetable variety in Chinese dishes! Besides the familiar bell peppers, broccoli, cabbage, carrots, chile peppers, green onions, mushrooms, and bean sprouts, Chinese dishes feature bamboo shoots, bok choy, lily pods, napa, snow peas, and other vegetables. Flip to the vegetarian section of the menu, for dishes featuring tofu and legumes.

● For less fat look for dishes that are braised, roasted, simmered, steamed, and stir-fried. Ask that stir-fried dishes be cooked in just a small amount of oil.

● Order plain rice and noodles rather than fried versions. Plain rice and noodles usually are lower in sodium, too, than fried versions, which are flavored with soy sauce. Crispy skin on poultry dishes such as Peking duck is high in fat.

● Be aware that the meat, poultry, or fish in sweet-and-sour dishes is typically breaded and deep-fat fried. Instead, ask for roasted or grilled meat with sweet-and-sour sauce to cut down on fat.

● For less sodium, go easy on foods prepared with MSG, soy sauce, or high-sodium sauces such as black bean, Hoisin, and oyster sauce. Ask to have your dish prepared to order without high-sodium seasonings or sauces. You might ask for light or reduced-sodium soy sauce to add yourself. Or instead, choose dishes prepared with hot-mustard, sweet-and-sour, plum, or "duck" sauce, which have less sodium.

● For a small bite, enjoy dim sum. Translated as "little heart," these small portions include steamed dumplings and steamed spring rolls. Go easy on fried dim sum dishes. To order dim sum, you choose your dishes from a server, who passes your table with one dish after another. As a result, you can easily overeat!

● Enjoy your fortune cookie—and the fortune inside! A single cookie has just 15 calories and 0 fat gram. Typically, Chinese meals don't give much attention to sweet desserts. Usually you'll have ice cream, fresh fruit, or almond cookies.

● Control the urge to overeat. In Chinese restaurants portions are often quite ample. For a sit-down meal order the amount you need, not necessarily a meal special with several courses. Ask for half a portion if you can. Plan to share a dish; perhaps order two or three dishes to serve four people. Or take leftovers home with you. Skip popular Chinese buffets, or go easy.

From the Chinese Menu

Enjoy more often:

● Wonton soup

● Hot-and-sour soup

● Steamed spring rolls

● Chicken, scallops, or shrimp with vegetables

● Whole steamed fish

● Steamed rice

● Steamed dumplings and other dim sum

● Soft noodles

● Stir-fried dishes*

● Steamed and simmered dishes

● Tofu

● Fortune cookies

POPULAR CHINESE FARE: FITTING WITHIN THE FOOD GROUPS

MyPyramid.gov
STEPS TO A HEALTHIER YOU

Grains:
Fortune cookies
Dumplings (potstickers, others)
Noodles
Rice
Rice noodles, rice sticks
Rice congee (rice soup)
Wonton or eggroll wrappers

Fruits
Guava
Kumquat
Lychee
Orange, mandarin oranges
Persimmon
Pineapple
Pummelo (large citrus fruit)

Vegetables
Asparagus
Baby corn
Bamboo shoots
Bean sprouts
Bell peppers
Bok choy
Broccoli
Carrots
Chives
Long beans
Mushrooms (straw, wood ear, others)
Napa cabbage
Pea pods
Tofu*
Water chestnuts

Milk
Milk
Soy cheese (calcium-fortified)
Soy beverage (calcium-fortified)

Meat and Beans
Beef
Cashews
Chicken
Eggs
Fish
Mung beans
Pork
Tofu*
Shellfish (shrimp, crab, lobster, scallops, octopus)

Oils
Peanut oil
Sesame oil
Vegetable (soybean) oil
Healthy oils from cashews, fatty fish

Legumes (dry beans) fit in either food group.

Enjoy less often:

- Fried wontons
- Fried egg rolls or spring rolls
- Peking duck
- Fried fish with lobster sauce
- Fried rice
- Fried dim sum
- Fried noodles
- Fried "crispy" dishes, sweet-and sour dishes with breaded, deep-fried ingredients

* If cooked in just small amounts of oil, they can be quite low in fat. Stir-fry dishes, however, can be quite oily (e.g., lo mein).

Thai and Vietnamese Cuisine

For restaurant patrons who enjoy an Asian kitchen, "spicy hot" defines many Thai dishes. Similar to Thai dishes in many ways, Vietnamese dishes are not known for their spiciness. Both cuisines also are noted for plenty of fruits, vegetables, rice, and noodles. The fresh, unique flavor of these cuisines comes from the contrasting seasonings, unique herbs and spices, and fresh ingredients.

Rice is a staple that's simply cooked or enjoyed as an ingredient in rice noodles, rice flour, and rice "paper." Enjoy it plain: long-grained jasmine rice with its perfumelike flavor; or sticky, plump rice. Try a dish in moistened rice "paper," used to wrap chopped, cooked vegetables; meat, seafood, and poultry; and fresh herbs. Or order translucent rice noodles, tossed in salads and stir-fried dishes. You'll find wheat flour noodles on the menu, too.

Vegetables and fruits add flavor, nutrients, and interest to Thai salads, soups, and mixed dishes. Look for dishes made with less familiar fruits and vegetables such as bamboo shoots, banana blossoms, bananas, bitter melons, green mangoes, pomelos, or straw mushrooms, as well as the familiar: cucumbers, bean sprouts, eggplant, green peppers, or snow peas. Thai restaurants are unique for Asian cuisine because you can order a salad! (Often the salad is cooked.)

In this mixed style of cooking, the portions of meat, poultry, and seafood are reasonable. Look for all kinds of seafood, including shrimp, mussels, and scallops, as well as beef, pork, chicken, and duck.

If you choose to go meatless, look for dishes made with tofu or egg, or combinations of noodles or rice, and vegetables. The popular pad Thai (with noodles, sprouts, tofu, eggs, scallions, and peanuts) may be a good choice; just leave off the eggs and some shrimp on top to cut the cholesterol.

What's the special flavor in Thai cooking? In menu descriptions you'll find a unique variety of herbs native to Thailand that add flavor but no sodium: coriander, ginger, galangal, kaffir lime leaves (citrus leaf), lemongrass, and Thai basil. Look for spices in curry dishes. Peanuts and cashews, common to Thai cooking, may add texture and flavor as well as protein.

The small, green or red bird's eye chiles (prik kii noo suan) are viciously hot and distinctively Thai. But they aren't the only chiles used in Thai cooking. Check the menu for clues to the "heat." If you can't take the heat, ask for "toned-down Thai." Many dishes can be prepared to suit your taste.

Consider the nutritional bounty in Thai cuisine—especially because it has less fat and sodium—and great flavor! Keep these points in mind:

- If you enjoy Thai food often, go easy on soups, curries, desserts, and other dishes made with a Thai staple: coconut milk or cream. The fat in regular coconut milk is highly saturated and high in calories. The popular satay (grilled chicken or meat skewers) usually is marinated in curried coconut milk and served with a sauce of peanuts and coconut milk. To control the amount, ask for the peanut sauce on the side.

- Find out what type of oil the kitchen uses. If it's lard or coconut oil, ask to have vegetable oil substituted.

- Look for stir-fried, sautéed, braised, grilled, and steamed dishes. In Thai cooking you'll also find deep-fried foods and ingredients. Go easy.

- Ask for a light touch with nam bla (Thai fish sauce), a high-sodium sauce, and with soy sauce. Or see if they can use light soy sauce in place of either one. The distinctive flavors of Thai curries come from a blend of nam bla with chiles, garlic, and other unique seasonings: coriander, cumin, and turmeric in Indian-type curries, and gingerroot, lemongrass, and shrimp paste. Go easy on dishes made with salty condiments such as salty eggs, dried shrimp, and fish paste, too.

If you pick a Vietnamese restaurant, the cuisine is similar, also based on rice, noodles, similar vegetables, seafood, and meat, so order with the same mind-set. Vietnamese cuisine also is flavored with fish sauce but contains more fresh coriander root and leaf (cilantro) and less garlic and chile pepper.

From the Thai and Vietnamese Menu

Enjoy more often:

- Broth-based soups such as tom yum koong
- Spring rolls in moistened rice paper
- Stir-fried noodle dishes such as pad Thai
- Stir-fried or sautéed vegetables with meat, poultry, fish, or tofu
- Broiled or steamed dishes
- Steamed rice
- Tropical fruits and juices
- Grilled or charbroiled meat, chicken, or seafood

Enjoy less often:

- Soups made with coconut milk such as tom ka gai
- Fried spring rolls
- Peanut-coconut milk sauce
- Dishes (including curries) made with coconut milk
- Deep-fried tofu or eggplant
- Dishes with deep-fried fish, duck, or meat
- Fried rice and fried noodles
- Fried banana
- Desserts made with coconut milk

Japanese Cuisine

Interest in Japanese-style restaurants has grown in recent years. It started with the Japanese steak house. There, Americans experienced the flair of tabletop, stir-fry cooking, seated around the grill. In either full-service or fast-food restaurants, today's Japanese menu offers more variety.

With its use of rice, noodles, tofu, vegetables, seafood, and small meat portions as staples, and limited use of oils, Japanese cooking is noted for being low in fat. Glazes and sauces are typically made with ingredients that are low in fat: broth, soy sauce, rice vinegar, and sake (rice wine). While some foods are fried, the more common cooking methods are low in fat and include braising, broiling, grilling, simmering, and steaming. Rice, noodles, and vegetables contribute starches (complex carbohydrates), and vegetables supply fiber, beta carotene, and vitamin C. Meat, poultry, seafood, and tofu are high-protein ingredients, usually served in moderate-size portions. Calcium-rich foods are limited. For those whose blood pressure is sodium-sensitive, the use of high-sodium flavoring is a nutrition concern.

To the Japanese cook, artistry ranks as important as nourishment. Edible garnishes of ginger or vegetables, or seaweed carefully wrapped around raw fish and rice, or an artful food arrangement on a plate are among the aesthetic touches that make Japanese food beautiful. Enjoyment of food has always been an important dietary guideline for the Japanese diet!

The language of a Japanese menu might be new to you. Use these guidelines to sharpen your menu savvy:

- Know that tempura is a popular battered, fried dish. Agemono and katsu dishes are also breaded and fried. To control fat and calories, go easy on fried dishes, but don't avoid them altogether or you'll miss some outstanding taste treats! Just balance these foods with other, lower-fat choices.

- Look for menu terms that suggest less fat, such as *nimono* (simmered), *yaki* (broiled), and *yaki-mono* (grilled). Two examples of this for meat, poultry, or fish: yakitori, which is skewered, then grilled or broiled; and teriyaki, which is marinated in soy sauce and mirin (rice wine), then grilled.

- Looking for another low-fat choice? Try sashimi (raw fish) or sushi (vinegared rice, prepared with seaweed, raw fish, and/or vegetables). If sodium is a concern, go easy on the soy sauce for dipping. *See "Is Raw Seafood Safe to Eat?" in chapter 12 for choosing a sushi restaurant and for those who need to avoid raw fish.*

- As another bowl meal, try domburi, or rice covered with vegetables, meat, or poultry, and perhaps egg. For less cholesterol, ask for it without the egg.

- To cut back on sodium, go easy on high-sodium sauces such as soy sauce, miso sauce, or teriyaki sauce, as well as broth and pickled vegetables. Many dishes, such as soup, noodle dishes, and stir-fried dishes, also are flavored with soy sauce. As an alternative, ask for dishes prepared without soy sauce, such as shabu shabu, foods that are not marinated, or steamed seafood; then dip them in a low-sodium soy sauce. For flavor without sodium, use a bit of the shredded or mashed green wasabi, which is a very strong and hot horseradish. Beware—a very little wasabi goes a long way!

● For more vegetables, order a salad as a side dish. Try edamame (fresh, steamed soybeans, often in the pod). For less sodium, ask for a lemon slice to squeeze on your salad, rather than miso dressing. Miso, a common flavoring in Japanese cooking, is derived from fermented soybean paste and is high in sodium.

● Enjoy Japanese noodles—udon (wheat noodles) or soba (buckwheat noodles). Noodles are often served under cooked dishes such as sukiyaki or in soups.

● Order fresh fruit for dessert. You won't find rich pastries on Japanese menus.

● Take time to enjoy the aesthetics of a Japanese meal in a full-service restaurant. Learn to use chopsticks. They may slow down your eating, and that can be a good part of the dining experience!

From the Japanese Menu

Enjoy more often:
- Stir-fried dishes such as sukiyaki
- Simmered dishes such as shabu shabu
- Grilled dishes such as yakitori
- Stir-fried tofu
- Clear soups such as miso and suimono
- Steamed rice
- Sashimi and sushi

Enjoy less often:
- Deep-fried dishes such as tempura
- Breaded and fried dishes such as tonkatsu
- Fried tofu

Eating for Travelers

Does eating on the road challenge your waistline and good nutrition sense? Overdoing is all too easy—especially when portions are big; the desserts are rich;

and the menus, tantalizing. Dehydration and food safety also demand thought and action for travelers.

Dining at 35,000 Feet!

What's to eat at 35,000 feet? Food service depends on the carrier, where you sit on the plane, and the length and time of your flight. As airlines cut back to control costs, food service is often just a light snack, a pack of pretzels or peanuts, or no food—and a beverage.

Whether you're a frequent flier or an occasional passenger, plan ahead so the plane "fare" fits into your eating style—and promotes your health.

● Except for long (often international) flights, don't count on an airline meal. Instead, check with your travel agent or the airline before the flight to verify the type of food service.

● If there's no meal served and you want to eat, take your own food on board, especially if you travel with small children. Dried fruit such as apricots, an apple or a banana, raw vegetables, packaged crackers and sliced cheese, muffins, bagels, pretzels, and peanuts are among portable foods that travel well. For safety's sake, don't keep a sandwich with meat or other perishable food for too long at cabin temperature—no more than two hours. That includes transit time from your kitchen, if it's packed there.

● Want a special meal on a long flight? If you or your travel agent call at least twenty-four hours before your flight, you can arrange for special meals on major carriers—vegetarian, kosher, low-calorie, low-fat, low-sodium, diabetic, and fruit plate, among others—for no extra cost if the flight has meal service. Often special meals are available for infants and children. Some carriers offer Hindu, Muslim, or Asian meals. In fact, the most efficient time to place your request is when you make your reservation.

● Remember: It's okay to say "no." You don't need to eat airline food just because it's offered. If you just ate or plan a nice meal on the ground, let the serving cart roll by. Today there may be a cost, too!

● To avoid dehydration, drink plenty of fluids (even if you're not thirsty)—8 ounces every hour of your flight. Juice and water are great choices. For the same reason, go easy on alcoholic drinks. With the low humidity and recirculating air within the pressurized

PASSPORT TO FLAVOR: SIX MORE ETHNIC CUISINES

Add variety and adventure to eating out. Try these cuisines, too! Enjoy menu items with fewer calories and less fat more often. Go ahead and enjoy a higher-fat food if you prefer; share or have a smaller portion. This are just a few menu items to whet your appetite:

ENJOY MORE OFTEN	ENJOY LESS OFTEN

Caribbean

• Beans and rice dishes	• Fried fish
• Chicken and rice	• Fritters (conch fritters)
• Grilled meat and chicken (jerk chicken or goat)	• Fried plantain
• Vegetable stews (callaloo)	

Middle Eastern

• Bean and bulgur salad	• Baba ghanouj
• Cold yogurt soup	• Fried chickpea cakes (falafel)
• Couscous (perhaps whole wheat)	• Fried meat-bulgur patties (kibbeh)
• Fatoosh (bread salad)	• Rich pastries, often with honey (baklava)
• Lamb and vegetable stew	
• Rice and lentil/bean dishes	

German

• Cooked cabbage	• Breaded and fried meat and poultry (schnitzel)
• Dumplings	• Creamy soup
• Potato salad with a sweet-sour dressing	• Noodle and cheese dishes
• Roast pork (lean) with gravy on the side	• Sausages
	• Thick, creamy gravy

French

• Broth-based fish soup (bouillabaisse)	• Cheese
• Demiglace sauces	• Cream soups
• Poached fruit	• Creamy sauces
• Roasted or braised meat, poultry, or fish	• Croissants
• Salad greens with vinaigrette	• Goose or duck liver (foie gras), paté
• Steamed or sautéed vegetables	• French fries (pommes frites)
• Vegetable casserole (ratatouille)	• Rich desserts (mousse, Napoleon)
• Provençal dishes (with tomatoes)	• Soups with gratinée (cheese)

Russian

• Boiled or baked dumplings (pelmeni)	• Blini
• Broiled meat skewers (shaslyk)	• Dishes made with sour cream gravy (stroganoff)
• Kasha	• Fried dumplings
• Meat-stuffed cabbage	• Salads with mayonnaise or sour cream
• Whole-grain breads	• Soups made with cream or sour cream (borscht)

Indian

• Baked roti (bread, such as naan), chapati	• Dishes, such as curry dishes, made with coconut milk
• Dishes prepared with yogurt	• Fried bread (poori, paratha, pakora)
• Lentil dishes, curries with vegetable sauce	• Fried dishes (samosa, shami)
• Roasted chicken or fish dishes with vegetable sauces; grilled kebobs	• Ghee (clarified butter)
• Tandoori cooked chicken	• Korma (meat dish with rich cream sauce)
• Papadum (lentil wafers)	

cabin, airline travel can be dehydrating; you lose body fluids through evaporation on your skin. Dehydration causes fatigue. Pack bottled water in your carry-on luggage as an extra supply. Especially on a long trip, drink plenty of liquids before, during, and after flying.

● Want to relax or sleep on the flight? If you're sensitive to caffeine, avoid caffeinated beverages: coffee, tea, and colas. For some people, too much caffeine can promote sleeplessness, anxiety, and overstimulation . . . especially for those anxious about flying anyway!

● If you drink alcoholic beverages, go easy—even if you have free drink coupons or you're in first class, where they're free. It's wise to stop after one or two drinks. On a long flight, wine or cocktails may not help you sleep—and may not relax you, either. Instead, larger amounts may have the opposite effect, making you more restless.

● When the beverage cart rolls by, make your choice count for overall nutrition, not just calories—especially if you may come up short during the day. Ask for fruit juice, tomato juice, or milk.

● Especially on a long flight, get out of your seat and move around as allowed by the flight attendants. Even a little exercise, such as walking the aisles, will help you feel better than just sinking into the seat with your headset on or with a good book.

● If you buy airport food to take onboard or eat as you wait, try to order sensibly—even if choices are limited. Rather than sit as you wait for a flight, exercise: walk the concourses, skip people movers!

Travel Fare—on the Ground

For the businessperson, eating on the road can be an "occupational hazard." For the leisure traveler, calories add up, too, especially when food is the main event. Eating just 500 extra calories a day can add up to 3,500 extra calories a week. Unless you compensate with more physical activity, those 3,500 extra calories can turn into a pound of body fat!

● Whether traveling on business or leisure, be a wise restaurant consumer. *As with any meal out, the "Restaurant Eater's Tip List" and "Fast Food, Healthful Food" in this chapter apply.*

● On an expense account? Avoid the urge to overeat just because you aren't paying the bill. Promising to "cut down when I get back home" may not be enough to keep trim, especially if you're a frequent traveler.

● Schedule your wake-up call to allow time for breakfast. An early morning meal is, after all, a smart way to start any day. If you're in a hotel with room service, order breakfast the night before.

● When you work during a meal or a cocktail hour, be as attuned to your food and drinks as you are to business issues. Overordering is easy when you're not paying attention to your body's hunger and satiety signals. A second round of drinks or another basket of chips can appear without much notice.

Drinking is often part of the social side of business travel, or viewed by the traveler as a way to relax. However, calories in a cocktail or two, and perhaps

Your Anti-Jet Lag Plan

The best advice: Organize yourself so you're well rested and relaxed before you travel. Avoid skipping meals as you rush to prepare for your trip; stick to a healthful meal pattern.

When flying, being dehydrated actually promotes jet lag. To minimize the effects, drink a glass of water or juice before your airline flight, then each hour in flight. Alcoholic beverages also can promote dehydration and may increase jet lag. Go easy if you drink them. During long flights, get up, stretch, and walk around the cabin.

On the ground, keep drinking fluids. After a long flight, drink extra fluids for several days. Immediately adjust your meals and sleep to the new time if you've traveled over several time zones. If your body clock skips from late afternoon to early morning and you lose the night (as you often do with overseas flights), take a short nap when you arrive, then continue with a normal day—lunch, dinner, and an early evening. If you leave in the morning and arrive at night, have dinner and go to bed—even if your body clock says it's midday.

No evidence shows anti-jet lag formulas or diets are effective. You may have heard anti-jet lag claims about a dietary supplement called melatonin. While this claim may be partially true, the amount of melatonin that promotes sleep is far less than the amount in over-the-counter products. *For more information on melatonin and other supplements, see chapter 23.*

wine with dinner, add up fast. Depending on the size, a single drink can supply 10 percent of your day's calorie needs—so go easy. Moreover, be careful that cocktails and salty snacks don't replace a nutritious meal.

Too often people complain that travel upsets their physical activity routine. As a leisure or business traveler, make time to move: explore museums, historic spots, parks, and shops on foot. Take time to use athletic facilities at the hotel or local park. *For tips on fitting physical activity into our travel schedule, see "When You're on the Road" in chapter 19.*

Breakfast on the Road

A 2-egg omelet, 3 strips of bacon, 1/2 cup hash browns, 1 slice of toast with 2 teaspoons of butter or margarine, 3/4 cup of fruit juice, and coffee: this hearty restaurant breakfast can total up to 685 calories and 40 fat grams. For a quick, nutritious start, order one of the following breakfasts instead for 400 calories or less:

- Fresh fruit, bagel with jam, low-fat milk

- Cereal (hot or cold) with low-fat milk, fresh berries or banana, coffee or tea

- Low-fat yogurt, whole-wheat English muffin with spread served on the side, fruit juice or fresh fruit, coffee or tea

- Whole-wheat pancakes topped with fruit; hot cocoa made with milk

- One poached egg, whole-wheat toast with jam, 1/2 grapefruit, fat-free milk

Ordering just a Continental breakfast (bread, juice, and coffee)? For breads with less fat, ask for a bagel, toast (perhaps whole-wheat or rye), or an English muffin with jam or with butter or margarine served on the side. Skip doughnuts, sweet rolls, croissants, and other pastries to cut down on fat.

Have Food, Will Travel

If your job, vacation, or weekend outings take you on the road, brown-bag it—or fill a cooler—so you don't need to rely on vending machines, convenience stores, fast-food chains, or snack bars.

- Fill sealable plastic bags with vegetable finger foods: raw vegetables (broccoli and cauliflower florets,

Have You Ever Wondered

... how to enjoy the floating feast on a cruise ship without overdoing or feeling guilty? Use the ship's outer deck as a running or walking track, or take advantage of the ship's fitness center, pool, or workout classes so you can indulge a little more. Check the menu; many of today's cruise ships offer lighter or spa fare. Take advantage of the built-in variety on cruise ship menus. If you stay up to enjoy the midnight buffet, balance it by going easy at other meals. If you can't resist the urge to order another course, ask for a small portion; just because your meals are prepaid doesn't mean you must order everything on the menu. Don't feel forced to order a beverage when you sit down to an evening show or sit around the pool.

Problem with seasickness? Skipping food entirely isn't the answer. Instead, ask the passenger desk for motion sickness medication, and eat something light, perhaps crackers, to keep something in your stomach.

To control infectious disease, use the hand sanitizer often available to passengers near dining areas.

jicama and carrot sticks, zucchini and bell pepper circles, or snow peas). Take seasonal fruit. Besides taking the edge off hunger, fruit can be a thirst quencher.

- Tuck in single-portion beverages: canned or boxed fruit juice, canned tomato juice, boxed milk, and bottled water. Take other portable, nonperishable foods—for example, crackers, peanut butter, raisins, small boxes of ready-to-eat cereal, single-serving cans of tuna or fruit, other dried fruit, pretzels, or plain popcorn. Tuck in packages of instant oatmeal for a quick, easy, hot breakfast in your hotel.

- Stock an insulated cooler with perishable foods: deli sandwiches, yogurt, and cheese, among others. Keep fresh fruit and raw vegetables in the cooler, too, to keep them crisp. *For more tips, see "Carry It Safe" in chapter 12.*

- When you're hungry, stop to eat. Get out of the car. Stretch. Take a short walk. You'll enjoy your meal more—and feel more relaxed as you continue driving. To help prevent constipation—a frequent complaint on long-distance car trips—stop every hour or two for a brisk walk and drink of water.

Food in Faraway Places

From cozy cafés, small food stores, and open-air markets . . . to rice paddies, hillsides with tropical fruit trees, and fishermen hauling in their nets . . . food offers a unique cultural experience for the curious traveler. Americans' growing enjoyment of ethnic foods comes in part from their travel experiences. Savvy travelers take the opportunity to try the adventure of new foods and flavors.

As the world grows smaller and as adventure travel grows in popularity, more business and pleasure travelers (adults and youth) venture to places where sanitation standards are not as high as in the United States. In certain environments, bacteria, parasites, and viruses can transfer to food from poor sanitation or agricultural practices. To help control the spread of disease, immigration forms for entering the United States ask if you've visited a farm; travelers and their baggage also go through an agricultural inspection.

No matter what you call it—Montezuma's Revenge, *turista,* or something else—travelers' diarrhea most often is caused by contaminated food and/or water. Typically, it lasts no more than three to four days, but that's enough to upset or even ruin an otherwise wonderful vacation—and certainly puts a business trip into a tailspin. The first bout won't "immunize" you from the next. But the good news is that you can reduce your risk by being cautious and careful. Pay attention to everything you eat and drink, remembering the same food safety rules you follow at home.

Food Safety: Ounces of Precaution

Like other types of foodborne illness, travelers' diarrhea is most commonly caused by bacteria—probably 80 percent of the cases. For travelers, improperly handled, contaminated food and drink also can cause *E. coli* infections, hepatitis, giardiasis, shigellosis, and other contagious diseases. *To avoid foodborne illness, the guidelines in "Eating Out Safely!" in this chapter apply no matter where you eat away from home.* In less developed areas, you need to take added precautions: "boil it, cook it, peel it, or forget it." *For more about foodborne illness, see chapter 12.*

● If you're traveling to developing or rural areas, ask your physician and county health department about immunizations and preventive medication suggested for your travel destination. The Centers for Disease Control and Prevention (*www.cdc.gov/travel*) provides food, water, and immunization alerts and advice for travelers in many regions of the world. That includes advice about diseases such as bird flu. If you're traveling with an infant, child, or someone at high risk *(see chapter 12),* immunizations are a must, as are pre-travel precautions for foodborne and other infectious illness. Even if you're visiting friends and relatives abroad and perhaps staying in their homes, you need pre-travel preventive care.

● Avoid buffets if food is just rewarmed after sitting for a while, or if it's been kept at room temperature for longer than 1 to 2 hours.

TRAVELING ABROAD? EATING FOR SAFETY'S SAKE

BE CAUTIOUS—SKIP THESE FOODS . . .	EAT THESE FOODS INSTEAD . . .
Salads, fruit with peels, raw vegetables (in uncertain areas)	Fruit peeled by you, cooked vegetables
Raw, rare, or partly cooked meat, poultry, or fish	Well-cooked meat, poultry, or fish
Softly scrambled or sunny-side up eggs (unless the egg is well cooked)	Well-cooked scrambled eggs or hard-cooked eggs
Unpasteurized milk	Canned or ultrapasteurized (UHT) boxed milk, or pasteurized milk from a large commercial dairy (ask to be sure)
Cheese made from unpasteurized milk	Cheese made from pasteurized milk
Food and drinks sold by street vendors	Only commercially bottled drinks and commercially packaged foods from vendors

● Be aware: A few fish and shellfish contain toxins even when they're cooked; avoid barracuda and puffer fish. Especially in tropical waters of the West Indies, Pacific, and Indian Oceans, a few other fish are occasionally toxic, such as tropical reef fish, red snapper, amber jack, grouper, and sea bass.

● Like at home, always wash your hands before eating! Remember: Your hands can transfer diarrhea-causing bacteria to your mouth. Carry an antibacterial hand wash, wet wipes, and maybe a small bar of soap.

● When you aren't sure what you may encounter, carry packable, nonperishable foods. Single-serve foods, sold for lunch boxes, are great for travelers.

● Check travel guides and talk to staff in the better hotels, or to your tour guide, to find restaurants with high sanitation standards. Restaurants in better hotels usually have high standards. Food and drinks eaten from street vendors increase the chance of illness.

● If you travel with a baby, breast milk guarantees food safety. If your infant takes formula, prepare it from commercial powder, and boiled or commercially bottled water. *For more about infant formula, see "Another Healthful Option: Bottle-Feeding" in chapter 15.*

What's Safe to Drink?

You're always smart to play it safe. In developed countries, tap water should be fine.

Better hotels in lesser-developed areas also may filter and chlorinate their tap water to make it safe. Before you use water from the faucet, find out if the hotel has a water purification system. When you're not sure, don't drink or brush your teeth with tap water. Instead, use commercially bottled or canned water with the seal or cap intact. Keep a bottle or can of water in your carry-on bag.

Soft drinks, canned or bottled juices, beer, and wine are safe to drink. Coffee, tea, and other hot beverages are usually safe because the long heating time destroys most and perhaps all of the bacteria, viruses, and parasites that might be present in the water. You also can boil or chemically treat water you drink. The Centers for Disease Control also advise you to dry any wet cans or bottles before opening them, then wiping clean any surfaces where your mouth contacts the can or

bottle. *For guidelines on treating water to make it safe for drinking, see "Safe Enough to Drink" in chapter 8.*

In less-developed areas, avoid beverages made with water or ice cubes—unless you know that commercially bottled water was used. Also avoid bottled water served to you without an intact seal or cap; it may have been refilled with local tap water. Be cautious of locally bottled water because the standards may not be high for bottling. Even crystal-clear water in wilderness areas anywhere, including the United States and Canada, should be treated before drinking it.

If You Do Get Sick . . .

● For most cases of travelers' diarrhea, dehydration is the biggest concern. If it strikes you, increase your fluid intake—with plenty of safe water, canned juice, and soup. Canned soft drinks (preferably without caffeine) are okay, too.

● If the problem persists (more than three or four days) or if your symptoms are severe, seek qualified medical care. Your hotel or tour guide should be able to suggest a physician.

● Prepare before you travel; talk with your physician at home, and take any precautionary medication recommended. *For more about dealing with diarrhea, see "Gastrointestinal Conditions" in chapter 22.*

Flavor on the Menu

For healthful eating, you don't need to give up flavor in today's restaurants! More than ever, chefs use culinary techniques to enhance foods' natural flavors, while retaining their nourishing qualities. This phenomenon isn't reserved for table-service or upscale

---

Need more tips on eating out? Check here for "how-tos":

● Eat out with kids and deal with their "fussy" restaurant eating—see chapter 16.

● Eat out vegetarian-style—see chapter 20.

● Handle allergies when eating out—see chapter 21.

restaurants. Gradually it's happening in many fast-food, deli, and family restaurants.

What flavor techniques do chefs use? Their culinary secrets can work in your kitchen.

● Poaching fish, poultry, or meat in flavorful broth, rather than cooking them in oil . . . or poaching fruit in juice, rather than cooking in sugary syrup

● Intensifying flavors with high-heat cooking, such as pan-searing, grilling, or broiling, to brown the meat and seal in the juices

● Grilling or roasting vegetables, then featuring them center stage as an entrée

● Adding fuller flavors with more whole grains, including brown rice, amaranth, and quinoa, as well as wild rice

● Flavoring and adding volume and color to plates with more creative fruit and vegetable sides and garnishes, often with exotic fruits and vegetables

● Serving bean purees or tapenade (anchovy-olive spread) instead of butter or margarine as table condiments

● Using salsa, chutney, or vinaigrette in place of rich sauces

● Adding nuts: hazelnuts, pecans, almonds

● Flavoring creatively with herbs and spices: perhaps a sweet spice, such as cinnamon, with meat, or a savory herb, such as rosemary, with fruit

● Using big, bold flavor ingredients, but perhaps small amounts, such as feta or blue cheese, pomegranate seeds, chipotle pepper (with a smoky taste), cilantro, or bitter broccoli rabe

● Layering flavors, with a variety of ingredients of contrasting flavors—as easy as a mixture of many greens, citrus fruit, and nuts in a salad

● Varying and balancing flavors in a dish or meal, for example, a fruit sauce for fish with mango

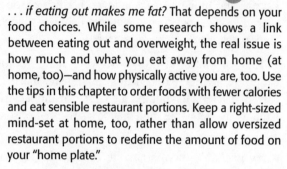

Have You Ever Wondered

. . . if eating out makes me fat? That depends on your food choices. While some research shows a link between eating out and overweight, the real issue is how much and what you eat away from home (at home, too)—and how physically active you are, too. Use the tips in this chapter to order foods with fewer calories and eat sensible restaurant portions. Keep a right-sized mind-set at home, too, rather than allow oversized restaurant portions to redefine the amount of food on your "home plate."

. . . how to encourage your kids to eat healthfully from the kids' menu? Many restaurants feature more vegetables and fruits on children's menus these days. To go with the common grilled cheese sandwiches, chicken nuggets, hot dogs, and burgers, encourage an order of steamed broccoli, a fruit cup, carrot sticks, other fruit and vegetable side dishes, and milk to go with it. Or offer something from the adult menu, perhaps to share.

. . . about nutritional information for restaurant foods? It's happening! Restaurants all over the country are finding more ways to provide nutrition information to customers at point of purchase—on packaging, kiosks, posters, brochures, and tray liners. Since different information formats are currently used, check the chain's Web site or ask the restaurant manager for tips on using this consumer information.

(sweet), tarragon (bitter), vinegar (sour), broth (umami), and a touch of salt

● Experimenting with unique ingredients, including flavorful local or ethnic foods and seasonings.

For more about food and flavor, refer to "'Flavor' the Difference" in chapter 13.

PART IV

Food for Health

Every Age, Every Stage of Life

CHAPTER 15

Off to a Healthy Start

Should our baby be breast-fed or bottle-fed?" "Can solid foods be given too soon?" "How do I know if my baby has eaten enough?" "Do I give my baby juice from a cup or a bottle?" "Should solid foods be warmed?"

New and experienced parents ask so many questions! Wouldn't it be great for parents and other caregivers if newborns were delivered into their parents' arms with a "how-to" manual filled with feeding instructions? Still, it's amazing how fast infant feeding becomes routine. However, as soon as babies and parents master one feeding stage, they're both ready to move on and learn the next.

As you feed your baby, keep two main goals in mind: provide enough food energy (or calories) and nutrients to support your baby's optimal growth and development . . . and nourish the emotional bonds between you and your baby.

Learning baby feeding basics takes the guesswork out of infant feeding. Practical guidance from your pediatrician, pediatric nurse, registered dietitian, and other parents is a blessing. Your own patience, time—and creativity—build warm, memorable feeding experiences for your baby, your family, and you.

Breast-Feeding Your Baby

Nature provides ideal nourishment for babies: breast milk. Medical and nutrition experts highly recommend breast-feeding at least for an infant's first year of life. Breast milk alone can provide enough nourishment to support your baby's optimal growth and development during the first six months of life. Then when solid foods are introduced, they complement breast milk. Breast milk continues to be important for your baby for the first year—and even longer.

The decision to breast-feed is a personal one. It takes into account the family's lifestyle, economic situation, and cultural beliefs, along with the mother's physical ability to do so.

For Good Reasons . . .

Breast-feeding offers a host of physical, emotional, and practical benefits for both baby and mother. The benefits of breast-feeding are greatest when mother's milk is your baby's exclusive source of nourishment

Breast-Feed or Bottle-Feed?

If you're a new parent, either approach—*breast- or bottle-feeding*—can provide adequate nourishment and the strong emotional bond that your growing baby needs. Whenever possible, though, breast milk is best for baby during the first year of life. If you're not sure which approach to use, start with breast-feeding. If it isn't right for you, switch to bottle-feeding. Starting with a bottle, then trying later to breast-feed is difficult. *If you choose to breast-feed, you'll find guidance in "Breast-Feeding Your Baby" on this page. For bottle-feeding, see "Another Healthful Option: Bottle Feeding," also in this chapter.*

for the first six months, and continue when solids are introduced at about six months. The longer a baby breast-feeds, the greater the benefits. However, your baby benefits even when breast-feeding lasts for only a short time, perhaps only during your six- to eight-week maternity leave.

Breast milk has the right amount of fat, sugar, water, protein, and other nutrients to meet the growth, development, and energy needs of infants. And as a baby matures and grows, the composition and amount of breast milk that a mother produces naturally changes.

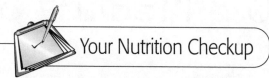

Your Nutrition Checkup

Do You Baby Your Baby?

There's a lot to know about feeding an infant and a toddler—and about ensuring a positive eating experience from day one.

Check yourself out on these baby-feeding basics. Which infant-feeding practices do you follow (or have you followed) when feeding your baby—or perhaps when helping a new parent?

YES **No**

☐ ☐ 1. Count the number of wet diapers (six or more every twenty-four hours) to make sure your breast- or formula-fed baby is getting enough to eat.

☐ ☐ 2. Offer breast milk or formula, not cow milk, to your baby up to twelve months of age.

☐ ☐ 3. If your baby is bottle-fed, choose an iron-fortified formula—unless your baby's doctor advises otherwise.

☐ ☐ 4. Discard unused expressed breast milk or infant formula after a bottle feeding.

☐ ☐ 5. Wait to start solid foods, as directed by your doctor—perhaps until six months if your baby is exclusively breast-fed.

☐ ☐ 6. Always wash your hands before feeding your baby.

☐ ☐ 7. Clean all baby-feeding equipment with hot, soapy water, and rinse well.

☐ ☐ 8. Avoid putting your baby to bed with a bottle.

☐ ☐ 9. Offer infant cereal that's iron fortified.

☐ ☐ 10. Start with single foods—one new food at a time.

☐ ☐ 11. Monitor your baby's reaction to a new food, in case of a reaction.

☐ ☐ 12. Offer your baby enough to eat, rather than trying to restrict calories or fat.

☐ ☐ 13. Check the temperature of food or bottles that are heated so they're evenly warmed, not hot!

☐ ☐ 14. Try new foods several times, rather than giving up after one or two tries.

☐ ☐ 15. Let your baby—not you—set the feeding pace.

☐ ☐ 16. Remain patient as your baby learns to feed himself or herself.

☐ ☐ 17. Offer smooth foods until your baby is ready for mashed or finely chopped foods.

☐ ☐ 18. Always stay with your baby while he or she is eating.

☐ ☐ 19. Discard unused food after a feeding.

☐ ☐ 20. Make infant feeding a special time to nurture and enjoy your baby—these days don't last!

Now Score Yourself:

Give yourself—and your baby—a big hug if you said "yes" to all twenty items. If you said "no" to any item, read on. Then practice what you learn. Your baby's health depends on it!

For most nutrients, what a mother eats has little if any effect on the nutritional content of breast milk. If the mother's nutrient intake is low, her body's own stored nutrients may be used for breast milk, putting her at potential nutritional risk. That's especially true for calcium and folate. For overall health, a nutritious diet during breast-feeding is important, as it was during pregnancy. *See "For Those Who Breast-Feed" in chapter 17.*

Breast-fed babies get protection from both allergies and common illnesses. Unlike formula, breast milk is rich in antibodies and other substances that help protect an infant from illnesses such as ear infections, diarrhea, respiratory illnesses, allergies, intestinal infections, and perhaps sudden infant death syndrome (SIDS). Breast-fed babies aren't sick as often and have fewer doctor's visits. In fact, human milk contains at least a hundred ingredients that infant formula doesn't have!

Colostrum, the clear or yellow fluid secreted for two to four days after delivery, is rich in protein and vitamin A, with more antibodies than the mature milk that follows. It helps protect a newborn's intestines from infection during the first few months. Think of colostrum as a newborn's first immunization. Colostrum also helps a baby pass his or her first stool.

Breast milk changes with baby's changing needs. From about the third to the tenth day after delivery, the body produces transition milk—a mix of colostrum and mature milk. And then mature milk, bluish in color and thinner in consistency, comes in. As your baby needs to eat more and more often, your breasts produce more milk.

Breast milk is easy for babies to digest. It's clean and safe. Babies may react to something their mothers eat, but they're rarely allergic to their mother's milk. Breast-feeding requires more sucking than bottle-feeding. This helps strengthen and develop the baby's jaw and so helps teeth and speech patterns.

Later on, those who were breast-fed may be less likely to develop certain chronic diseases, including heart disease, diabetes, asthma, some types of cancer, and certain stomach and intestinal diseases. Research in this area is not conclusive, but it is promising.

Have You Ever Wondered

. . . if breast size affects the success of breast-feeding? No, and it doesn't affect the volume of milk production, either. When a woman isn't breast-feeding, glands that produce milk are very small, regardless of breast size. The amounts of fat and fibrous tissue a woman has, not the glands that produce breast milk, determine breast size.

. . . if premature babies can breast-feed successfully? Many premature babies can. But if your baby is born prematurely, get help from a lactation counselor, pediatric nurse, or your doctor. You may need to express milk at first; you'll still feed your milk to your baby, perhaps mixed with a nutrient supplement for preterm infants. For premature babies, breast milk offers benefits that help them grow and stay free from illness. There's another reason to start right away: you need to establish your milk supply if you plan to nurse.

. . . if the foods you eat during pregnancy or breast-feeding increase your baby's risk for food allergies? Plenty of research indicates that breast-feeding reduces the risk for food allergies, particularly if there's a family history of allergies. In fact, food allergies are less common in breast-fed babies than in formula-fed babies.

No conclusive evidence shows that all pregnant or nursing mothers should avoid certain foods to protect against allergies. However, as a precaution against potential allergens in breast milk, the American Academy of Pediatrics suggests that nursing mothers of susceptible infants (with a family history of allergies) are wise to skip peanuts and peanut-containing foods.

. . . what to do if your baby reacts to something you eat? Be watchful. If your baby seems to react poorly after you eat certain foods, including those with known allergens, stop eating them for a while. Any allergic reaction usually comes from a protein in a food that a mother consumes, not from breast milk itself. If your pediatrician identifies an allergy, eliminate that food or ingredient in your diet until your baby is weaned. *See "Food Allergies: Commonly Uncommon" in chapter 21.*

Other areas of research: breast-fed babies tend to gain less unnecessary weight and tend to be leaner, perhaps with less chance for obesity later. Breast-feeding also increases mental function; breast-fed babies score higher on childhood IQ tests, especially those born prematurely.

How about Mom?

Besides knowing that your baby is well fed, you as a nursing mom get many benefits from breast-feeding, too. The longer a woman breast-feeds, the greater the benefits to both baby and mother.

Breast-feeding nurtures a close bond between mother and baby. That's often a gratifying, emotionally fulfilling extension of pregnancy and a chance to build self-esteem as a parent.

Always ready-to-feed, breast milk doesn't need measuring, mixing, or warming. So it's easy, especially in the wee hours of the night. With no bottles to prepare or wash and no infant formula to shop for, nursing moms have more time to relax with the baby, or to catch a nap as baby sleeps.

Breast-feeding also may help a new mother regain her prepregnancy figure and reduce postpartum bleeding. Because nursing stimulates the release of oxytocin, a hormone that helps the uterus to contract and shrink, a mother's abdomen trims down more quickly. Her body also uses the fat pad that was deposited on her hips and thighs during pregnancy as some fuel for milk production. Gradual weight loss during breast-feeding doesn't affect milk production.

Breast-feeding is economical, too—even when you account for the extra food a mother eats. The average cost of infant formula is about $700 a year, or more depending on the brand, for families who don't breast-feed. And since breast-fed babies often aren't sick as much, there's less cost for doctor visits and lost work income when babies are breast-fed. Women who breast-feed do need to add about 500 calories a day to their normal diet to cover the energy required for milk production. These calories are best added with nutrient-rich food-group foods. *See "Planning to Eat," chapter 10.*

There's less odor involved with breast-feeding. Diaper-changing odor is less offensive, and if a breast-

Do Babies Need Extra Water?

Newborns need little or no extra water. Except for periods of hot weather when your baby perspires, breast milk or infant formula usually supply enough fluid. If water is needed, offer 1 to 2 ounces of plain water after a feeding; water shouldn't take the place of breast milk or formula. For safety's sake when your baby is less than four months of age, boil water first, then chill it, or offer sterilized bottled water. When babies begin eating solid food, offer plain water.

Your child needs water to replace fluids lost through diarrhea or vomiting. Diarrhea and vomiting can lead to dehydration—and its complications—if fluids aren't replaced. Rather than water or juice, your doctor or pediatric nurse may recommend an oral electrolyte maintenance solution, sold near baby foods in your grocery store, to prevent dehydration. Besides fluid, the solution contains glucose (a form of sugar) and minerals (sodium, chloride, and potassium) called electrolytes. Electrolytes help maintain fluid balance in your baby's body cells. These minerals are lost through body fluids.

Consult your doctor or pediatric nurse before feeding an oral electrolyte maintenance solution to children under two years of age (or older children, too). Besides the risk of dehydration, diarrhea and vomiting signal possible illness that may require medical attention! If diarrhea, vomiting, or fever persist longer than twenty-four hours, consult your doctor or pediatric nurse. An electrolyte maintenance solution won't stop diarrhea or vomiting, but it does prevent dehydration.

fed infant spits up, there's very little smell, and it doesn't stain clothing.

An added benefit: with nursing, a mother takes time to relax every few hours. That's often a welcome and needed change of pace from the added demands of being a new parent.

What about long-term benefits? Women who have breast-fed have a lower risk of developing premenopausal breast cancer, ovarian cancer, and osteoporosis and hip fractures. Breast-feeding also helps with blood glucose levels for women with gestational diabetes.

To learn more about eating while breast-feeding, see "For Those Who Breast-Feed" in chapter 17.

Perfecting the Breast-Feeding Technique

While breast-feeding is nature's way of providing ideal nutrition for infants, the "art" of breast-feeding might not come as naturally! Like learning any new skill, the keys to success are knowledge, practice, and the support of family, friends, and perhaps coworkers and employers. Discuss your decision to breast-feed with your doctor before delivery, and remind hospital staff when you arrive at the hospital.

Getting Started

● To build confidence and to help ensure an adequate milk supply, start nursing as soon after delivery as possible. The best time to start is within twenty to thirty minutes after your baby is born, perhaps right in the delivery room. The first feeding will be short, about ten minutes. "Rooming in" at the hospital may make your first days with nursing more successful.

● Relax and make yourself comfortable. Find a comfortable chair with good arm and back support. Or lie down with pillows strategically positioned to help you support your baby. If you are comfortable and well supported, it's easy to hold your baby, and you won't feel much tension in your neck, back, and shoulders.

● Plan to nurse on demand—that is, whenever your baby says it's time to eat. Increased alertness or activity, rooting toward your breast, or mouthing are all signs that your baby is hungry. Typically, crying is a late signal of hunger. Trying to establish a schedule early on may frustrate you both. As reassurance, you can't "spoil" your baby by feeding on demand. Most babies fall into a schedule with time.

● Be prepared to nurse very frequently during the first months—about eight to twelve times every twenty-four hours. That's because a newborn's stomach is small and because nutrient needs are exceptional now during rapid growth and development.

Frequent nursing helps establish your milk supply and keeps your breasts from becoming hard and swollen. Full and heavy breasts signal that it's time to nurse. As milk "lets down," or moves from the inner breast to the nipple, you may feel a tingling feeling.

Latching On

Some newborns instinctively suck when they're first put to their mother's breast. (Maybe they practiced sucking their thumb before birth.) Others nuzzle first, just to get used to the warmth, security, and softness from their mother. Either way is normal.

● Help your baby by stroking baby's cheek nearest your breast. As your baby turns toward your nipple, guide your baby's mouth so that he or she can take in as much of the areola (dark area of the nipple) as possible, not just the nipple. Newborns have a "rooting reflex" at the breast; they open their mouths naturally.

● Try to offer both breasts at each feeding. Let your baby nurse as long as he or she wants (about ten to twenty minutes on each breast). The last portion from each breast is "hind milk." This milk is higher in fat and helps the baby feel full and satisfied after feeding.

● Release your baby from the breast by gently putting your finger into the corner of his or her mouth. (Wash your hands before nursing.) This will ease the baby's grip and break the suction without discomfort. Wait until you feel the suction release before pulling away.

Latching on correctly helps your baby get enough milk and protects you from sore nipples. Ask about breast compression if latching on is a problem.

Breast-Feeding: About Your Baby

● Burp your baby when you change breasts and at the end of the feeding. This relieves any discomfort from air swallowed while nursing. Hold him or her upright on your shoulder, or lay your baby "tummy-side down" across your lap. Then gently rub or pat your baby's back. It's normal for a baby to spit up a bit of milk.

● Trust your baby to let you know when he or she has had enough to eat. When your baby feels full, he or she may close his or her lips, turn away, or even fall asleep. Sometimes babies rest during a feeding, too, making it hard to know when one feeding stops and the next begins! Is your baby getting enough milk? *See "Nursing: Reassuring Signs of Success" in this chapter.*

● Don't worry about your baby's loose stools. It's normal for a breast-fed baby to have loose, yellowish stools, which may resemble watery "mustard seeds."

● Try to skip a pacifier or bottle nipple, at least for the first month. It can interfere with your baby's ability to learn to breast-feed.

Breast-Feeding: About You

● Because babies nurse more vigorously when they start feeding, alternate the breast you offer first. Clip a safety pin to your bra as a reminder. Alternating ensures that both breasts are emptied regularly, and helps prevent breast tenderness. Vary the nursing position and allow your nipples to "air dry" after feedings to avoid breast tenderness and cracking.

● If your breasts are tender or reddened, or if you feel achy and feverish, contact your doctor. You may have a plugged duct or breast infection (mastitis). An antibiotic might be prescribed. Usually you can keep on nursing while an infection clears up.

● If your breasts feel tight and full, soften them with a warm shower, or express a small amount of milk. To express milk means to stimulate milk flow by hand or with a breast pump. Fullness and discomfort are signs of engorgement and may happen when your milk supply first comes in or if you've gone too long between feedings. Feed your baby often. Wearing undergarments with proper support helps, too. When breasts become too full, your baby won't be able to latch on correctly, which can cause nipple soreness.

● Don't be surprised if your milk "lets down" and leaks a bit when you hear your baby cry, or even when you think about him or her. It's natural. You might wear pads (without plastic liners) to protect from any leaking.

● Pour yourself some water or juice before nursing.

Breast-Feeding Cautions

Use caution if you smoke, drink alcoholic beverages, use some herbal supplements, or take medication. These substances may affect milk production and the

---

Some Steps in Breast-Feeding

1. *Snuggle "tummy to tummy."*
Cradle baby in your arms with his or her tummy against your tummy. Baby's head should rest in the bend of your elbow. Your forearm should support the baby's back, with your hand on his bottom.

2. *Place nipple directly in front of your baby's mouth.*
Your baby's head should be in a straight line with his or her body. If his or her head is tilted back or your baby has to turn to reach your nipple, your baby is in the wrong position.

3. *Keep a good position.*
Keep your baby well supported. Make sure your baby is facing straight on to the nipple and does not have his or her head back or neck turned. Make sure your back is straight and you are not leaning over your baby.

4. *Nurse as long as your baby wants.*
Try to use both breasts at each feeding. To take your baby off the breast, release the suction by putting your little finger in the corner of his or her mouth. Wait until you feel the suction release before removing your baby.

let-down reflex. But some pass into the mother's milk, too, at the same levels as in her bloodstream.

When you're nursing, avoid smoking and drinking alcoholic beverages. The Dietary Guidelines advise: *Alcoholic beverages should not be consumed by lactating women.* Alcohol concentrates in breast milk; drinking alcoholic beverages can inhibit milk production. An occasional drink to celebrate is okay—consumed at least two hours before nursing. When mothers smoke, babies are more likely to get sinus infections, colic, or become fussy. Even secondhand smoke is harmful, so dads and other caregivers are wise to avoid smoking, too. Smoking around babies increases the risk for Sudden Infant Death Syndrome (SIDS).

Talk to your doctor about taking medications, including over-the-counter medications, and herbal supplements during breast-feeding. Take your own medications, even if they're safe for babies, after nursing, not before.

In a few circumstances, breast-feeding isn't advised. Mothers who test positive for HIV can pass the virus on through breast milk. Women with untreated tuberculosis or on chemotherapy should not breast-feed. And babies born with galactosemia, who can't tolerate breast milk, need a special diet free of lactose and galactose. Some illegal drugs can also pass to the baby and cause serious side effects.

Getting Help for Breast-Feeding

You and your baby are learning about breast-feeding together. It's okay to ask for help. Besides the delivery room nurse, certified lactation consultants in many hospitals teach breast-feeding techniques and answer parents' questions. Some may visit at home later to help you perfect your skills.

Within the first one to two weeks, nursing mothers and their newborns should see their pediatrician or healthcare professional. That's another chance to check your feeding techniques. If you're discharged from the hospital less than forty-eight hours after delivery, your first checkup should be within two to four days after birth.

You can also seek help and get support and reassurance from the La Leche League, a registered dietitian (RD), a nurse midwife, or another health professional with experience in lactation counseling. Women who have been successful at breast-feeding, such as La Leche League volunteers, offer great support and practical advice to new mothers. The government's National Women's Health Information can also help: 800-994-9662. *To find sound, reliable advice on infant feeding and breast-feeding, see "How to Find Nutrition Help . . ." in chapter 24.*

Nursing: Reassuring Signs of Success

Not knowing how much milk their infant consumes, some parents feel uncomfortable about breast-feeding. You probably don't need to worry about having enough milk. Your body is miraculous. If your baby needs and demands more, your body probably will make more milk to satisfy the demands of nursing—even when you try to lose extra pounds gained during pregnancy. Even mothers of twins and triplets can produce enough milk to nurse successfully.

Look for these signs that nursing is going well:

● Following the third or fourth day after birth, your baby has six or more wet diapers, soiled with light-colored urine, every twenty-four hours. Most newborns wet fewer diapers with only colostrum.

● Your baby nurses at least eight times every twenty-four hours, and maybe up to twelve times daily, in the first month. If your baby sleeps longer than a four-hour stretch, you may need to awaken him or her for a feeding. While nursing, you should feel sucking and hear the infant swallowing.

Have You Ever Wondered

. . . if you can breast-feed if you're sick? Yes—usually it's safe to continue breast-feeding. It even offers added protection for your baby, who already has been exposed to any "bug" before you experienced any symptoms. In breast milk you pass on some immunity through the antibodies your own body produces to fight the infection. If you're taking any medications to treat an illness, talk to your pediatrician to make sure they're compatible with breast-feeding. Severe illness may require weaning; again consult your doctor.

Breast-Feeding Positions

If you're a nursing mom, you may want to experiment with these positions as you feed your baby:

Cradle position. Sit up straight with your baby cradled in your arm. His or her head should be slightly elevated and resting in the crux of your elbow. You and your baby should be comfortably positioned "tummy to tummy," with baby's mouth level with your nipple. Be sure that your baby is facing straight toward you, without having his or her head, back, or neck turned.

Lying down. Lie on your side with the baby on his or her side, too. Place pillows under your head and behind your back for comfort. Position your baby "tummy to tummy" so his or her mouth is next to your nipple. Use a folded towel or a pillow to elevate your baby to the correct height. This position is especially comfortable for women who've had a cesarean delivery. You can feed your baby from both breasts on one side, or turn onto your other side to nurse from your second breast.

"Football" position. Hold your baby with the head facing your breast, and his or her body tucked under your arm at your side. Your forearm supports the baby's back, and his or her legs and feet should point toward your back. Rest the baby on a pillow near your elbow to give support and slightly raise his or her head.

Whatever the position, enjoy eye contact with your baby. This helps build the mother-baby bond and helps your baby feel secure.

● The baby's weight steadily increases. Make certain your baby is weighed at the doctor's office within a week or two after delivery to monitor weight gain, and regularly thereafter. During checkups, your baby's weight and length will be assessed. Doctors check a baby's measurements against reference growth curves. If your child doesn't gain weight properly, there may be a feeding or a medical problem.

Initially babies may lose a little weight right after their birth. That's normal. However, if your baby doesn't regain his or her birthweight by three weeks of age, your doctor or pediatric nurse will need to monitor him or her frequently. From birth to six months, babies typically gain 4 to 8 ounces per week.

Other signs of breast-feeding success: your baby's urine will be pale yellow urine, not deep yellow or orange, and he or she will sleep well, yet be alert and healthy when awake.

A Few Words for Dad . . .

A father can play a very important role in the success of breast-feeding. He can offer support, encouragement, and confidence to a new mother. Ways that fathers can get involved include attending prenatal breast-feeding classes with an expectant mother, reading a book on breast-feeding, arranging pillows, and bringing a snack or a beverage for mom when breast-feeding. A father also can burp the baby, change diapers, massage mom's neck and shoulders to encourage relaxation, and give baby a supplemental bottle. By sharing household responsibilities, caring for other children, shopping, and doing other tasks, he takes other pressures and interruptions away from mom.

What about Supplemental Bottles?

Breast-feeding abides by the law of supply and demand. Nursing stimulates the flow of milk—and increases its production as baby demands more to meet his or her needs. So supplemental bottles usually aren't needed—unless your pediatrician advises it, perhaps if your baby loses weight and doesn't regain it.

Although nursing may temporarily limit your independence, offering a supplemental bottle too soon may discourage your baby from nursing. Until your milk supply is established, stay close at hand for feeding.

If you choose to offer a supplemental bottle or a pacifier, wait about four weeks after birth, or until breast-feeding is well established. Because the nipple on a bottle or a pacifier is different from the breast, it can confuse a baby who is just learning to breast-feed.

Once the milk supply is constant—and both you and your baby are comfortable with nursing—a supplemental bottle lets dad, siblings, and other caregivers share in feeding. Expressed breast milk or commercially prepared infant formula may be offered in a supplemental bottle. *Note:* When nursing sessions are replaced regularly with supplemental bottles—without expressing milk—a mother's breasts will compensate by producing less milk.

For guidance on storing breast milk, see "Breast Milk: Safe Handling and Storage" in this chapter. For more about infant formula and bottle feeding, see "Another Healthful Option: Bottle-Feeding," also in this chapter.

Breast-Feeding for a Back-to-Work Schedule

To continue breast-feeding, changing from maternity leave to a back-to-work schedule takes adjustment. Some moms express milk during their workday. In that way, their baby can have bottles of mother's milk when mom's away. Other moms breast-feed when they can be with their baby; caregivers offer infant formula when mom can't. And some babies take both— bottles of expressed breast milk and of formula. Choose the option that works best for you and your baby.

If you're a back-to-work nursing mom (or need to be away from home regularly), consider these guidelines for breast-feeding success:

● Before you take maternity leave, work out a plan with your employer. Perhaps work at home for a while, or plan your schedule for short days, flextime, or longer breaks. Check your state law for breastfeeding at your job.

● Select a caregiver for your baby who is supportive of breast-feeding.

● Plan to nurse before you leave for work, soon after you return from work, and during the evening to keep your milk supply strong. A routine helps.

● If you plan to express milk during the workday, try to make your plans before your maternity leave. If necessary, arrange for a private area to relax, free from interruptions. (You'll need fifteen to thirty minutes, usually twice a day.) Unoccupied offices or women's lounges may be options. And you'll need access to a refrigerator, or a small cooler with ice packs, to store breast milk, and an outlet if you use an electric pump. *For tips on safe handing of expressed milk, see "Breast Milk: Safe Handling and Storage" in this chapter.*

● Before you go back to work, help your baby learn to take expressed breast milk or infant formula from a bottle. Wait at least four weeks after delivery so your own milk supply is well established. If you wait too long, your baby may be less willing to take a bottle. Experiment with different types of bottle nipples to find one your baby likes. This may be the perfect chance to involve dad in feeding! *For more about the different types of bottle nipples, see "Bottles and Nipples: Baby Feeding Supplies" later in this chapter.*

● If your work schedule and the travel distance from work allow, schedule feeding visits with your baby during your breaks. Let the caregiver know when you'll arrive. In that way, your baby won't be fed too soon before your visits. To make it easier, choose a caregiver near your workplace.

● For the same reason, let the caregiver know when you'll pick up your baby after work. Together, schedule feedings so your baby won't eat too close to the end of your workday.

Vitamin and Mineral Supplements for Breast-Fed Babies

Until solid foods are introduced—preferably at about six months—breast milk can be a complete source of nutrition for infants. However, three nutrients may warrant additional consideration. Ask your doctor for advice.

Iron. Iron is important for the manufacture of hemoglobin, the part of red blood cells that carry oxygen throughout the body. Iron also is essential for your baby's brain development and growth.

In the last trimester before birth, babies accumulate enough iron stores to last through their first four to six months of life. Breast milk also contains easily absorbed iron. After four to six months, however, most babies need more iron. Breast-fed babies may be at risk for being iron-deficient if another source of iron—usually iron-fortified cereal—isn't introduced. Talk to your dietitian or health professional about what is best for your baby.

Premature infants who breast-feed may need iron supplementation earlier. They had less time to build adequate iron reserves before birth.

Fluoride. Your baby's teeth started to develop even before you could see them. Fluoride, a mineral often found in tap water, helps develop strong teeth and prevent cavities later.

Breast milk contains little fluoride—even if the mother's drinking water is fluoridated. If your breast-fed infant takes supplemental formula made with fluoridated water—at least 0.3 ppm (parts per million) of fluoride—your baby may get enough fluoride. If your child is breast-fed only or drinks formula made with well water, distilled water, unfluoridated bottled water, or city unfluoridated water, your doctor may advise a fluoride supplement starting at about six months. Breast-fed infants who take supplemental ready-to-use formula also may need a fluoride supplement; these formulas usually are prepared with water low in fluoride.

If fluoride supplementation is needed, about six months of age usually is a good time to start. At your baby's six-month checkup, ask your doctor. A fluoride supplement may be prescribed.

Vitamin D. This vitamin helps your baby use calcium from breast milk (and infant formula) to help bones grow and develop. When skin is exposed to sunlight,

Breast Milk: Safe Handling and Storage

● Wash your hands before expressing milk.

● If you use a breast pump, review the operation and cleaning instructions.

● Glass or plastic? Store refrigerated breast milk in plastic (made specifically for storing breast milk) or clean collection bottles. Plastic retains the protective properties of refrigerated breast milk better. You also can freeze breast milk in either plastic or glass containers.

● Use expressed breast milk stored in the refrigerator. Use refrigerated breast milk within 24 hours. Otherwise freeze it.

● If you work outside your home, or need to be away, consider stocking a milk supply in your freezer during maternity leave. Breast milk can be frozen:
  ● In a freezer compartment inside the refrigerator, not the freezer door, for up to two weeks
  ● In a refrigerator-freezer with a separate freezer door for three to four months
  ● In a separate freezer at temperatures below 0° F for six months or longer.

Date expressed milk kept in the refrigerator or freezer. Then rotate the milk—first in, first out.

● Store expressed milk in 2- to 4-ounce portions to avoid wasting unused milk after a feeding. Because bacteria from the baby's mouth can contaminate milk in the bottle, always discard milk that's left in the bottle after feeding.

● Thaw breast milk in the refrigerator, under warm, running water, or in a pan of water on the stove. Do not thaw or heat breast milk in a microwave oven. Before feeding thawed breast milk, gently shake the container to mix layers that may have become separated. Once thawed, use breast milk within 24 hours; avoid refreezing it.

the body can make vitamin D—but a baby's skin should be protected from sunlight with sunscreen or clothing.

Unlike infant formula and fortified cow milk, breast milk doesn't contain much vitamin D. A vitamin D supplement is advised for all breast-fed babies and babies consuming less than 16 ounces of formula daily.

Other vitamins. Babies of strict vegetarian mothers may need a vitamin B_{12} supplement. *See "The Vegetarian Mom" in chapter 20 for more advice for vegetarian moms who breast-feed.*

Always get advice from your baby's healthcare provider or a registered dietitian before giving nutrient supplements to a baby, child, or teen of any age!

Weaning . . . When and How?

Weaning is the slow, gradual process that helps your baby eat and enjoy your family's foods. The time for weaning is an individual matter for mother and baby. Experts encourage moms to breast-feed for at least twelve months. Babies benefit from breast-feeding for as long as it's mutually right for mother and baby.

No matter how long you choose to nurse, start complementary foods, too, when your baby's ready. If your baby is exclusively breast-fed, that's about at six months of age. Talk to your pediatrician about timing. When your baby eats other foods, too, you'll probably nurse less often: typically first thing in the morning, naptimes, and bedtime.

When you choose to wean your baby, introduce either infant formula or cow milk, depending on your baby's age. If your baby is under twelve months of age, wean from breast milk to iron-fortified infant formula. If your baby is twelve months or older, whole cow milk is appropriate.

Should you wean your baby to a bottle or a cup? That depends on his or her developmental readiness. Between four and six months, most infants will drink or suck small amounts of liquid from a cup or a glass when someone else holds it. Older babies and toddlers usually have the coordination to drink fluids from a cup or a straw. However, for infants under six months of age, a bottle is probably the best choice.

Another Healthful Option: Bottle-Feeding

Breast-feeding may or may not be right for you. In rare cases, a woman may not be able to breast-feed for physical or health reasons. Some may feel uncomfortable. Others may take medications that wouldn't be safe if passed through their breast milk to the baby. Still others have cultural or work-related reasons. In all of these cases, parents can feel reassured that bottle-feeding is a healthful option.

Infant formula also is a good supplement for nursing moms when a mother chooses to skip a breast-feeding, or when the mother doesn't make enough breast milk for her baby.

If you choose bottle-feeding, feel assured: commercially prepared infant formulas are as similar to mother's milk as currently possible. Infant formulas have enough nutrients and food energy (calories) for your baby until you introduce solid foods—usually at about four to six months of age. And infant formulas supply the right balance of fats, carbohydrates, and proteins. Unlike breast milk, formulas lack protective factors such as antibodies to promote immunity.

Even after babies take solids, continue infant formula until your baby's first birthday. Similar to breast-feeding, cuddling a baby while he or she takes a bottle also builds a close, nurturing relationship with all those who share the responsibility of feeding: dad, siblings, grandparents, and other caregivers.

Formula: What Type?

Commercially prepared infant formulas are powdered, liquid concentrate, or ready-to-feed. Before feeding, dilute powdered and liquid-concentrate formulas with boiled or sterile water. Ready-to-feed formulas don't need to be diluted. They're ready "as is"—packaged in cans or in bottles.

What's in a name? Regardless of which formula you use, commercially prepared infant formulas are usually cow milk–based or soy-based. Formulas based on modified cow milk are appropriate for most babies. A soy-based or specialty formula might be best for the small number of babies who are sensitive to protein in cow milk. Vegetarian moms who don't choose to breast-feed may prefer a soy-based formula, too. For premature or low-birthweight babies, a soy-based formula probably won't be recommended. Ask your baby's healthcare provider.

Old-fashioned homemade formulas from canned evaporated milk and corn syrup may have nourished you or your mother, but they're nutritionally inferior to today's commercial formulas. And corn syrup may contain botulinum spores, which can produce a deadly toxin. Your baby's better off with commercially prepared, iron-fortified infant formula.

Consider this when choosing a formula:

Iron. Many infant formulas are fortified with iron. Iron is a key mineral in forming hemoglobin, the part of red blood cells that carries oxygen to cells to make energy. Your baby also needs iron for brain development; an iron deficiency may cause irreversible delays in your baby's development. Full-term babies are born with enough iron stores to last four to six months. An iron-fortified formula right from the start helps keep a baby's iron stores adequate.

Cow Milk: When? What Type?

As a great source of calcium and other nutrients, cow milk is an ideal food for toddlers, children, and adults. However, it isn't appropriate for infants younger than twelve months of age. While some infant formulas are made from cow milk, it's been modified for infants.

Unmodified cow milk isn't the best food for young infants for several reasons. Its high protein content is hard for a baby's immature system to digest and process. The potassium and sodium contents also are higher than recommended for babies. Cow milk is low in iron; the iron it does contain isn't absorbed well. And it doesn't provide enough zinc, vitamins C and E, copper, and essential fatty acids—nutrients that babies need to grow and develop.

Goat milk isn't a suitable alternative either, for many of the same reasons as cow milk. If you choose to offer goat milk after age one, make sure it's vitamin D fortified. To clear up a misconception, babies who are allergic to the protein in cow milk are probably allergic to the protein in goat milk, too.

Knowing When Your Baby's Had Enough

There's no exact science to bottle-feeding, but these are some signs that suggest that your baby's had enough:

- Your baby may close his or her mouth or turn away from the bottle.
- Your baby may fall asleep.
- Your baby may get fussy with your repeated attempts to offer the bottle.
- Your baby may bite or play with the bottle nipple.

With Baby . . . That's More Than One!

Are you an experienced parent—with one or more other children? If so, feeding a newborn isn't new to you. Yet, every baby is different—so be prepared to learn new parenting skills. One child may be a fussy eater; another, ready and eager to eat. One may be ready for solid foods at four months; another, at six months. Observe, respect, and enjoy their unique differences.

Do you wish that you had handled infant or child feeding differently with your first child? That's normal, too, especially for a first-time parent. You were learning! It's okay to change your feeding approach with your next child.

Perhaps the biggest change is trying to do several things at once: trying to feed a baby, older children, and others in your family—including you. Enlist help from your preschooler or school-age child, without expecting too much. An older child can be your helper, but shouldn't be responsible for your baby. Tasks as simple as wiping baby's sticky hands, getting a bib, or picking up a bottle that falls to the floor make your older child feel helpful, "grown up," and important.

Remember, too: A new baby competes for your attention, which may lead to fussy eating from another child. Give your older child personal time at the table, too; include him or her in table talk. And try to keep mealtime calm and pleasant—despite all that's happening around the table.

Choose an iron-fortified formula, or ask your baby's doctor, pediatric nurse, or a registered dietitian to recommend one. If your baby starts on a formula without iron, switch to an iron-fortified formula by four months. To clear up a common misperception, iron added to infant formula won't cause constipation or other feeding problems. Continue an iron-fortified formula until twelve months, when your baby is already eating a variety of foods, and starts cow milk.

Fluoride. The mineral fluoride helps your baby develop strong teeth and protects teeth from cavities. Use fluoridated water if available. When you mix powdered or liquid concentrate formulas with water, you add fluoride, too—if your water supply is fluoridated. Ready-to-feed formulas aren't prepared with fluoridated water. If you regularly offer ready-to-feed formula or if your water supply isn't fluoridated, ask your baby's doctor about fluoride supplementation. After six months a fluoride supplement may be advised.

Have You Ever Wondered

. . . if you can substitute vegetarian milk, such as soy or rice beverages, for breast milk or formula? No, even if they're fortified with vitamins and minerals, they don't have enough proteins (except soy beverage) and fats. Wait until after two years of age, but even then talk to your doctor, pediatric nurse, or registered dietitian first.

. . . if your baby needs formula fortified with DHA and ARA? Infant formulas with two fatty acids—docosahexaenoic acid (DHA) and arachidonic acid (ARA)—now are sold in the United States.

Found naturally in breast milk, DHA and ARA are important components of cell membranes in the brain and the retina. Infants also produce these fatty acids inside the body when adequate amounts of essential fatty acids—alpha-linolenic acid and linoleic acid—are present in infant formula. *See chapter 3, "Fat Facts."*

DHA and ARA added to infant formula may provide developmental benefits (brain and vision), especially for premature infants. As of 2002, these nutrients have been reviewed and are generally recognized as safe (GRAS) for full-term infants by the U.S. Food and Drug Administration (FDA), but not yet for preterm infants. The benefits of these formulas are still inconclusive. For more current information, check www.FDA.gov. Ask your physician before choosing these formulas for your infant. The formula label will indicate the presence of DHA and ARA.

Recipe for Success

For mixing infant formula, careful measuring, cleanliness, and refrigeration constitute the "recipe for success." When properly mixed, powdered, concentrated, and ready-to-feed infant formulas are identical in their nutritional composition. The primary differences are price and how much time you need to prepare formula. Pay attention to "use by" dates on the label.

Whatever type of formula you choose, follow these guidelines:

● Wash your hands first. With an immature immune system, your baby is highly susceptible to foodborne illness.

● Pay careful attention to mixing instructions on the formula label. Adding too much water dilutes it. Then your baby may not get enough nutrients or food energy. Conversely, adding too little water concentrates the formula too much. Then it's hard for a baby to digest, and it supplies too much food energy at one feeding and not enough fluids to prevent dehydration.

Powdered and concentrated formulas are best mixed with water that's been brought to a rolling boil for at least one minute, and then allowed to cool. Bottled water that's labeled as "sterile" is also an option, unless otherwise advised by your baby's doctor. *See "What about Bottled Water?" in chapter 8.*

● If your baby does well with one type and brand of infant formula, stick with it unless your baby's doctor advises otherwise. If you switch, check the label. The "recipe" for mixing the new formula may differ from the brand you used first.

● Always use clean bottles and baby-bottle nipples. *See the following "Bottles and Nipples: Baby Feeding Supplies" for cleaning tips.*

● For convenience, prepare a supply of bottles— enough for the day ahead. Date and refrigerate the prepared infant formula. Once opened, ready-to-feed formula and liquid concentrates must be refrigerated and used within forty-eight hours.

● Infant formula can be fed to a baby at a cold temperature, room temperature, or slightly warm. Always test the temperature of the formula to avoid burning the baby. *To bring chilled bottles to room temperature or to slightly warm, see "Play It Safe: Warming Baby's Bottle and Food" later in this chapter.*

● Make only as much as your baby needs. Discard formula left in the bottle after feeding. Bacteria from your baby's mouth can contaminate formula and cause spoilage. To avoid too much leftover, fill the bottle with less. Make more as your baby's appetite dictates.

Bottles and Nipples: Baby Feeding Supplies

Baby bottles. Plastic or glass bottles, or disposable bottle bags? The choice is yours. Some parents keep a variety of baby-bottle sizes and styles on hand for different purposes. For example, disposable bottle bags are handy when you're on the go and when washing facilities are limited. For convenience, bottles with disposable liners let you toss away the used liner when the feeding is done. Small-size bottles are perfect for holding 2- or 3-ounce feedings during the first weeks after delivery. Be cautious of bottles with cute shapes; they're often hard to clean.

Baby-bottle nipples come in a variety of shapes and sizes, too. Choose nipples that correspond to your baby's mouth size and developmental needs. A baby's comfort and ease of sucking are the criteria to use when choosing a nipple.

There are four basic baby-bottle nipple types: a regular nipple with slow, medium, or fast flow (the number and size of the holes will determine flow); a nipple for very small or premature babies; an orthodontic nipple, which imitates the shape of a human nipple during breast-feeding; and a cleft-palate nipple. A cleft-palate nipple is meant for babies who have a lip or palate problem that keeps them from sucking properly.

Keep bottle-feeding equipment in good working order:

● Discard cracked or chipped bottles that could break and spill formula onto your baby.

● Replace nipples regularly as they can become "gummy" or cracked with age. Check them by pulling the tip before each use.

● Check the size of the opening on new nipples and then periodically as you use them. Formula should

How Much Formula?

Your baby's appetite is a good guide to the amount of infant formula he or she needs—and how often. That depends in part on the stage of development. In addition, some babies drink a little more or less depending on when solid food is introduced. Use this chart *only* as a guide.

AGE	NUMBER OF BOTTLE FEEDINGS PER DAY	TOTAL AMOUNT OF FORMULA PER DAY (OZ.)
Birth to 4 months	6–8	18–32
4 to 6 months	4–6	28–45
6 to 9 months	3–5	24–32
9 to 12 months	2–4	24–32

flow from the nipple in even drops—not a steady stream. If the milk flows too quickly, your baby could choke, so discard the nipple. If the milk flows too slowly for your baby, consider trying a nipple with more holes, designed for older babies.

When it comes to preparing infant formula and washing bottles, cleanliness is essential! Your baby's immune system isn't fully developed, so he or she is very susceptible to foodborne illness from improperly cleaned feeding equipment.

● Use plenty of hot, soapy water to wash your hands, work area, measuring utensils, bottles, and nipples. If possible, wash bottles right away when they're easier to clean.

● Thoroughly clean bottles and nipples by washing them with hot, soapy water and rinsing well. Sanitize nipples and bottles by placing them in boiling water for two minutes. Then let them air-dry. Or wash bottles, rings, and caps in the top rack of the dishwasher. Look for special dishwasher baskets designed to hold bottle parts, and keep them from falling to the bottom of the dishwasher.

● Remember that the outer "shell" of bottles with disposable bottle bags needs regular washing to destroy bacteria.

Bottle-Feeding Techniques: All in the Family!

Bottle-feeding gives the whole family warm, cozy moments with the baby. Nestled in the arms of a parent, sibling, grandparent, or other caregiver, babies feel safe and comfortable. Consider these tips for your bottle-feeding techniques:

● Find a comfortable place, perhaps a chair with an armrest. Hold your baby with his or her head slightly raised, resting on your elbow. That allows a baby to suck from the bottle and to swallow easily.

● Avoid propping your baby in bed or in an infant seat with a bottle. Babies can choke! And if they fall asleep with a bottle in their mouth, formula that bathes the teeth can promote baby-bottle tooth decay. Remove the bottle promptly if your baby falls asleep while eating.

● Angle the bottle to help prevent your baby from swallowing too much air. The nipple should stay full with formula when your baby is eating.

● To ease discomfort from air bubbles swallowed during feeding, burp your baby in the middle and at the end of feedings. Hold him or her upright at your shoulder, or lie your baby tummy down across your lap. Then gently pat or rub your baby's back.

● Keep a clean, damp washcloth handy. It's normal for babies to spit up some formula during burping.

● When your baby's done, take the nipple out of his or her mouth. Sucking on an empty bottle causes air bubbles in your baby's tummy.

● If your baby doesn't finish a bottle, don't refrigerate it for later. Don't keep formula at room temperature for more than two hours, either.

Baby's Bottle-Feeding Routine

Newborns eat frequently in the first months after birth—perhaps every two hours! Since their stomachs are small, just 2 ounces, or as many as 4 ounces of infant formula, may be enough for the early feedings. *See "How Much Formula?" on page 386 for guidelines during the first twelve months.*

Formula-fed babies usually need twenty to thirty minutes to finish a bottle. If it takes less than fifteen minutes for a newborn to finish a bottle, use a nipple with smaller holes. If it takes longer and if the baby

Need more parenting tips for feeding your baby? Check here for "how-tos":

● Look ahead to toddler and preschool feeding—see chapter 16.

● Eat smart during pregnancy and breast-feeding—see chapter 17.

● Know signs of food allergies or intolerances—see chapter 21.

● Find a nutrition expert experienced in infant feeding—see chapter 24.

Physical Activity: Guidelines for Infants

Physical activity is important from the beginning of life! Activity can encourage rolling over, crawling, and walking as well as cognitive development, and can lead to a preference for active play. Conversely, inactivity may set the stage for childhood obesity. Rather than confine your baby to a stroller or playpen too much, start a habit of active living now. During this first year of life:

● Spend part of each day with active baby games such as peekaboo and pat-a-cake.

● Find ways to help your infant safely and actively explore his or her surroundings. Floor play is great!

● Avoid restricting your infant's movements for prolonged periods of time.

● Choose activities that encourage your infant to move large muscles (arms, legs, hands, and feet).

● Play when your baby's awake; don't interrupt sleep to play.

is sucking actively, make sure the holes aren't clogged. Or try a nipple with more holes.

As with a breast-fed baby, plan to bottle-feed on demand—when a baby signals hunger. Trying to impose a feeding routine will frustrate you both. You can't spoil your baby by feeding on demand. A formula-fed baby may not eat as often; formula digests more slowly than breast milk.

Should formula be warm, cool, or at room temperature? That's up to you. Your baby will become accustomed to whatever temperature you usually provide. If you warm it, just be careful so your baby doesn't get burned. *For tips, see "Play It Safe: Warming Baby's Bottle and Food" later in this chapter.*

Let your baby decide how much to drink. Pay attention to his or her appetite; your baby doesn't need to finish a bottle. In fact, forcing your baby to finish it focuses too much on eating—which may lead to over- or underfeeding. To learn good eating habits, babies need to learn hunger and fullness cues.

If your baby has six or more wet diapers a day, seems content between feedings, and if his or her weight increases steadily, your baby's probably getting enough. If not, check with your doctor or pediatric nurse. *For more hunger and fullness cues, see "Knowing When Your Baby's Had Enough" earlier in this chapter.*

Solid Advice on Solid Foods

Just when parents master breast-feeding routines or formula mixing, babies show that they're ready to join the high-chair crowd! Starting solid foods is just one more adventure in the journey of child feeding.

Throughout the first year, breast milk or iron-fortified infant formula continues to be your baby's most important source of nutrients and energy. (Wait until after twelve months for cow milk.) Around the middle of your baby's first year, he or she will be ready to start solid foods to complement the nutrition from breast milk or formula. Typically they're added in this order:

● Iron-fortified, single-grain infant cereal (mixed with breast milk or formula), single strained fruits and vegetables—six months or somewhat sooner.

● Strained meats/poultry, unsweetened 100 percent fruit juices (vitamin C fortified) in a cup, plain toast, and teething biscuits—seven to nine months.

● Chopped soft fruits and vegetables; meats; unsweetened dry cereals; plain, soft bread; and pasta—ten to twelve months.

The order isn't important—as long as solids provide your baby with an iron source.

For more detailed guidelines, see "Infant Feeding Plan: A Basic Guideline" later in this chapter.

Ready, Willing, and Able

Although most babies are ready to start solid foods about six months of age or perhaps somewhat earlier, don't rely solely on the calendar! Babies must be physically and developmentally ready for solid foods. Remember: Each baby is different. Age is just a point of reference. If babies aren't ready to eat solid food, it will likely end up on their laps—not in their tummies. Offering solids too soon only frustrates baby, parents, and other caregivers.

Until about four months, babies are unable to effectively coordinate their tongue to push food to the back of their mouth for swallowing. Well-meaning friends and family may tell you to start solid foods earlier to help your baby sleep. However, babies sleep through the night only after their nervous system

Have You Ever Wondered

... if it's okay to offer solid foods in a bottle? No, not for most babies. One problem? Possible delay in learning feeding skills. Cereal or other foods from a bottle also can cause choking. This practice may encourage your baby to overeat (too much food energy, or calories). With spoon-feeding, resting between bites gives your baby time to feel full and so learn self-regulation. Cereal in a bottle also may take the place of breast milk or formula, along with the nutrients they supply. To clarify a misconception, offering cereal in a bottle won't help baby sleep or stop crying.

... what you can do to relieve the discomfort of teething? You might rub your baby's tender gums gently with your clean finger, perhaps with a little teething gel along the gumline. A chilled teething ring—kept in the refrigerator, not in the freezer—also can help. Chewing on textured solid foods, such as teething biscuits or bagel pieces, helps teething, too. Offer these foods when your baby is sitting up, and stay nearby. Chill baby foods, too; they may feel better than warm foods.

More drooling and swollen, tender gums signal teething. Be aware that a runny nose, diarrhea, fever, or rash probably are symptoms of illness, not teething.

Caring for Baby Teeth

Good dental care begins at birth—even before baby teeth appear! Healthy teeth let children chew food easier, learn to talk clearly, and smile with self-assurance.

Make cleaning your baby's teeth and gums part of the daily bathtub routine. Starting at birth, clean your baby's gums with a soft infant toothbrush and water, or use a clean, wet washcloth or gauze pad. Do this after every feeding. Skip toothpaste, which babies often swallow.

Schedule your baby's first visit to a pediatric dentist after the first tooth appears (at about six to twelve months).

Fluoride is a mineral that helps teeth develop and resist decay. In many places, fluoride is naturally present in local water supplies at various levels. If you live in an area that doesn't have fluoridated water, ask your baby's doctor if your baby or child needs a fluoride supplement. Unless your child's dentist advises otherwise, wait until after age two or three years to start with fluoridated toothpaste. *For more information on fluoride, see "Vitamin and Mineral Supplements for Breast-Fed Babies" and "Formula: What Type?" earlier in this chapter. For more about fluoridated water, see "The Fluoride Connection" in chapter 8.*

To avoid tooth decay, do not put your infant, toddler, or young child to bed with a bottle of juice, formula, or milk. The liquid that bathes the teeth and gums from sucking on the bottle stays on teeth and can cause tooth decay. That happens even if a baby's teeth haven't yet erupted through the gums. If your child won't nap or go to bed without a bottle, fill it with plain water instead.

For more about dental care, see "Your Smile: Sugar and Oral Health" in chapter 5.

---

develops more fully. In fact, solid foods offered too soon stress a baby's immature digestive system, and most passes right through to the diaper.

When is the right time to start solid foods? Usually, no sooner than six months of age. Then, if your baby weighs at least 13 pounds and has doubled his or her birthweight, it might be time. Let your baby be the judge. There's no one calendar date that's right for all babies. Research on timing for introducing solid foods doesn't show an effect on childhood obesity. Watch for these milestones that suggest that he or she may be ready to join the league of solid-food eaters:

● *Baby can sit with little support.* Your baby can control his or her head and may be able to lift up his or her chest, shoulders, and head when lying tummy down. By now your baby can turn away to signal "enough."

● *Baby has an appetite for more.* If your baby is hungry after eight to ten breast-feedings or drinks more than 32 ounces of formula, it may be time for solids.

● *Baby shows interest in foods you're eating.* As the baby watches, he or she leans forward and may even open his or her mouth in anticipation. Take a trial run with appropriate solid foods. If your baby doesn't seem interested, wait a few weeks, then try again. Avoid forcing a child to eat solid foods.

● *Baby can move foods from the front to the back of the mouth.* Up to about four months of age, babies will try to push food out with their tongue. As they develop, the tongue becomes more coordinated and moves back and forth. This allows your baby to swallow foods from a spoon.

Something New: Eating from a Spoon!

Learning to eat the first solid food—usually iron-fortified cereal—from a spoon is a big transition in infant feeding. It's a step toward independence. And it encourages chewing and swallowing skills.

Spoon feeding has challenges. It's messier. At first, more food may end up on the bib and face than in the mouth. Try this to make the transition pleasant:

● Relax. This is a new eating adventure for both of you! Pick a time when your baby is relaxed and not ravenously hungry. Smile, and talk as you feed your baby. Your soothing voice will make new food experiences more pleasant—and talking helps with language development, too.

● Of course, wash your hands first. And keep baby food safe and clean.

● Use a small spoon with a long handle—and just a little bit of food on the tip of the spoon.

● Start with a teaspoon or two of food. Then work up to one to two tablespoons, two to three times a day.

● Let your baby set the pace for feeding. Don't try to go faster or slower.

● Seat your baby straight or propped upright, facing forward. This makes swallowing easier and helps prevent choking.

● Introduce new foods at the start of the meal. Once satisfied, your baby may be less willing to try a new taste. If he or she refuses a new food, that's okay; try it again in a few days or weeks.

Infant Cereal: Timing Is Everything

Your baby's first solid food should be a source of iron, such as iron-fortified infant cereal, which is often the most convenient iron source. With cereals, opt for ones developed for babies. They digest easier than varieties for older children and adults. Iron-fortified infant cereals help babies maintain their iron stores.

● Although there's no strict order, you might start with rice cereal. It's often best as the first cereal because it's least likely to cause allergic reactions. *To determine if a food may be causing a reaction, see "Food Sensitivities and Your Baby."* Hold off on wheat cereal until after your baby's first birthday. Some infants are sensitive to wheat before one year of age.

● When it comes to your baby's first cereal feedings, keep the cereal mixture thin. Start with just one part cereal to four parts of breast milk or infant formula. Once your baby develops eating skills—and a taste for cereal—mix in less liquid so it's thicker. Don't mix in honey or corn syrup, which may contain small amounts of bacteria *(Clostridium botulinum)* spores that can be harmful to infants.

● Be prepared if your baby refuses cereal at first. Try again in a few days. Infant cereal tastes different from the familiar breast milk or formula. The texture is different, too—not to mention the difference between a nipple and a spoon!

● Once your baby starts eating more cereal, he or she will take less breast milk or infant formula. Breast milk or iron-fortified formula still should be the mainstay of the diet during the first year.

Solid Foods: What Comes Next?

Once your baby accepts cereal, try strained vegetables and fruits; after that, meats and breads. It doesn't matter which you offer first: vegetables or fruits. Some parents opt for vegetables first.

Food Sensitivities and Your Baby

Some babies are sensitive to certain foods. You know by their reaction—perhaps a rash, wheezing, diarrhea, or vomiting. Most babies outgrow these reactions once their digestive and immune systems mature. (To reassure you . . . a baby's stool often changes color and consistency when new foods are eaten. These changes don't necessarily indicate a food sensitivity.) To best monitor your baby for food-induced reactions:

● Keep track of foods your baby eats. Choose single-grain infant cereals and plain fruits, vegetables, and meats instead of mixed varieties or "dinners" until you know what your baby can handle. If your baby has a reaction, stop that food for a while.

● As you introduce new foods, offer one new food at a time. Wait three to five days before offering the next new food. If your baby has trouble with a certain food, you'll more likely know what food causes the reaction.

● Save egg whites until after your baby's first birthday. Young babies may be sensitive to the protein in egg whites. Cooked egg yolks are okay.

● Be watchful of foods that contain common allergens, including peanuts, tree nuts, soy, eggs, fish, shellfish, wheat, and milk. Use the ingredient list and allergen labeling on food labels to identify these ingredients.

● If any food causes a significant and ongoing reaction, talk to your baby's doctor, pediatric nurse, or registered dietitian about it. Together, you can establish an eating plan that's best for your baby.

For babies with a family history of food allergies, the American Academy of Pediatrics advises waiting to introduce some foods: citrus, cow milk, soy, and wheat until after the first year, and eggs, fish, and peanuts until after two to three years.

For more about food intolerances and allergies, see chapter 21, "Sensitive about Food."

● One by one, offer a variety of foods to your baby. This lays the groundwork for a healthful diet throughout life. *For more about the importance of variety, see "Variety: Good for You, Good for Baby!" on page 392.*

● Try single foods first: for example, fruits—applesauce, pears, peaches, prunes (dried plums), bananas; vegetables—sweet potato, carrots, squash, peas, green beans; meat—beef, chicken, turkey, ham; legumes or tofu (for vegetarian infants); and egg yolks.

● Start with smooth foods that are easy to swallow. Babies can eat mashed or finely-chopped foods when their teeth start to appear and when they start to make chewing motions.

● If you offer juice, offer from a cup, not a bottle. Sucking juice too long from a bottle exposes a baby's teeth to natural sugars in fruit juice. Prolonged contact with sugars can promote tooth decay.

● At about six to nine months of age, most babies enjoy drinking from a cup—or at least trying to! Offer formula, breast milk, or water in a child-size unbreakable cup. A cup without handles may be easier for a young child to hold. Covered cups with a spout also are helpful at this stage. Babies are clumsy with a cup at first but usually catch on quickly.

● As your baby gets more teeth and gets interested in self-feeding—at about nine to twelve months of age—introduce finger foods. Soft, ripe fruit without peels or seeds and cooked vegetables are good for tiny fingers. Avoid foods a baby can choke on. *See "For Babies, Toddlers, and Preschoolers: How to Avoid Choking" in this chapter.*

● Teething biscuits, bread sticks, and rice cakes are good natural "teethers." Chewing on these foods eases a baby's sore gums while offering a healthful snack—eaten "all by myself"! *For more on self-feeding, see "'Feeding Myself'" in this chapter.*

● Babies need the opportunity to develop a taste for the natural flavor of foods without added sugar, salt, or other flavorings. Seasonings are not added to many varieties of commercially prepared baby foods. Read the product label to find out.

● Gradually expose your baby to foods with herbs and spices, including flavors that are part of your

Have You Ever Wondered

. . . if it's okay to sweeten baby foods with honey or to dip a pacifier in honey? No. Until after a baby's first birthday, avoid giving honey or corn syrup in any form. Very occasionally, honey can harbor spores of a toxic bacterium called *Clostridium botulinum.* For adults and older children, these spores are harmless. But for babies younger than twelve months, they can cause botulism, a severe foodborne illness that can be fatal. *Note:* Sucking on a sweetened pacifier promotes cavities.

. . . when your baby can have fruit juice? Before six months fruit juice offers no nutritional benefits, advises the American Academy of Pediatrics. After six months pasteurized 100 percent fruit juice (not fruit drinks) is an option, as long as your baby doesn't drink too much of it. Four to 6 ounces of juice a day are more than enough.

Offer juice in a small cup at mealtime or snacktime—not from a bottle, covered cup, or juice box, which promotes sipping juice throughout the day. Juice shouldn't be given in a bedtime bottle, or to manage diarrhea. Except that fruit has more fiber, fruit juice and fruit offer the same nutritional benefits for older babies.

. . . if a chubby baby is more likely to become an overweight adult? Relax if you're concerned. Chubbiness during infancy generally doesn't lead to adult overweight. Rather than worry or restrict food, respect your baby's appetite. That helps your baby learn to eat the right amount of food, not over- or undereat. Restricting food may keep your baby from getting nutrients and energy needed to grow and develop, and may cause a failure to thrive.

. . . if your baby needs a vitamin supplement when he or she starts solid foods? Ask your pediatrician. A specially formulated infant supplement may be recommended if you're not sure if foods supply enough, if your family is vegetarian, or if your baby needs to restrict food for any reason.

Feeding Myself

As babies master spoon feeding, they're gradually ready to feed themselves. Watch for signals that suggest your baby is ready: perhaps trying to help you, or taking a cup away, or putting his or her hand on yours.

● Start with finger foods. It's easy because eating by hand is utensil-free.

● Give your baby a spoon to hold in one hand while you use another for feeding. This gives your baby practice grasping a utensil.

● Offer baby-friendly utensils: a small, rounded spoon with a straight, wide handle, and a dish with high, straight sides.

● Use the two-spoon approach. Give an empty one to your baby, and fill the other with baby food. Then switch so baby has a filled spoon for self-feeding.

● Be patient—and relaxed. Food will end up on the floor. Your baby will need lots of practice before being able to eat a whole meal without your help.

● Always stay with your baby when he or she is self-feeding. In that way you'll be around if he or she starts to choke.

Tip: Start a lifelong habit of family mealtime. Bring your baby's high chair to the family table, even if you need to feed your baby first.

family's food culture. There's no need to keep food plain.

● As you choose foods for your baby, don't restrict fat. Growing babies need the energy and essential fatty acids that fat provides. *See "Fat Facts for Kids" in chapter 16.*

● As your baby grows and develops a bigger appetite, offer more solid foods. *The chart "Infant Feeding Plan: A Basic Guideline" in this chapter suggests when.*

Variety: Good for You, Good for Baby!

Variety certainly is the spice of life—especially when it comes to forming good eating habits for your baby. Offering your baby a wide variety of foods with different flavors, colors, shapes, and textures helps ensure that his or her nutrition needs are met. Variety makes mealtime more fun, too! As an aside, babies perceive sweet tastes first; both amniotic fluid and breast milk are sweet. Other taste perceptions develop during a baby's first year.

Like you, your baby may like some foods better than others. That's normal. Likes and dislikes may change from week to week. Continue to offer food variety. You may offer a new food or flavor eight to ten times before a child accepts it—so keep trying. If not now, try again in a few days. Don't let your own food biases limit your baby's preferences. Your baby or toddler may like those foods!

Learning to enjoy a variety of solid foods helps establish a lifetime of good eating habits. This is why variety is so important, even in the early years.

Fruits and Vegetables

They're good sources of vitamin C, beta carotene, other nutrients, and phytonutrients. By offering these foods frequently at mealtime, children become familiar with fruit and vegetable flavors. That helps set the stage for accepting and enjoying them throughout life.

Consider these tips for encouraging your baby to eat and enjoy vegetables and fruits. Introduce them in any order. If you want to start with applesauce, bananas, and carrots, that's fine. Offer new flavors along with familiar vegetables and fruit. Respect what your baby likes and may not like. No one fruit or vegetable is essential for health, so relax. Start now by encouraging a rainbow of colorful vegetables and fruits. The goal? Learning to like as many vegetables and fruits as possible.

Breads, Cereals, and Other Grain Foods

Offer iron-fortified cereal to babies and toddlers. To enhance iron absorption, serve those that contain iron along with foods that contain vitamin C, such as fruits and fortified infant juices. Other grain products include soft, cooked pasta or rice, soft breads, dry cereals, crackers, and teething biscuits.

Caution with high-fiber foods: Some high-fiber cereals, such as bran, are low in calories yet high in bulk. Avoid offering large amounts of them to infants; they fill a small stomach without providing many nutrients or calories. Infants and young children can get enough fiber from a variety of foods.

Have You Ever Wondered

... what foods help your baby avoid constipation? Offer a combination of foods to keep stools a consistency that's easier to pass. Some foods produce softer stools: for example, apricots, peas, peaches, pears, and prunes (dried plums). Drinking enough fluid helps soften stools.

If your baby gets constipated, offer apple juice twice a day, or prune juice for something stronger. Get advice from your pediatrician if this doesn't work.

... how to tell if your older baby is hungry or full? Older babies might signal hunger by opening and moving their mouth toward a spoon, by trying to swipe food toward their mouth, or by pointing, nodding, or grabbing a spoon. Fullness signals might be turning their head away from the spoon, spitting out or pushing familiar foods away, or being distracted. Learn your baby's hunger and fullness cues, as you help him or her learn to avoid overeating later in life.

... whether lead poisoning is an issue for your infant? You need to check! The American Academy of Pediatrics and the Centers for Disease Control and Prevention advise lead screening at ages one and two. Talk to your doctor. *Refer to chapter 8 for more about lead poisoning.*

Meats, Milk Products, and Other Protein Sources

These foods are valuable sources of protein, calcium, iron, zinc, and other minerals that your baby needs to develop bones and muscles, as well as for his or her blood supply and brain development.

Offer a variety of soft, pureed, or finely chopped meats such as chicken, turkey, or beef. By age seven to eight months, well-cooked, pureed legumes (perhaps strained) or mashed tofu are options for vegetarian infants; since tofu is made of soy, be watchful for potential food allergies. (Wait until after one year of age to offer smooth nut and seed butters, spread on bread or crackers.) After twelve months, if children no longer take breast milk or infant formula, whole milk is an important source of energy, calcium, proteins, essential fatty acids, and some other nutrients. Growing bones need an adequate supply of calcium

from food. Good sources include cheese, milk, and calcium-fortified cottage cheese. Health experts don't advise feeding lower-fat dairy foods, such as low-fat or fat-free milk, to children under two years of age. If you offer yogurt (often sold as low-fat), make sure your child also consumes whole-milk dairy foods.

Play It Safe: Warming Baby's Bottle and Food

Babies enjoy breast milk, infant formula, and baby foods either warm or cool. Unlike most adults, babies have no physical or emotional need for warmed liquids and warmed foods.

● If you want to serve foods at warm temperatures, play it safe so your baby won't get burned. Warm bottles of formula or breast milk in a pan of warm water that's removed from the stovetop, or under a stream of warm tap water. You can do the same with frozen breast milk, or defrost it overnight in the refrigerator.

● Avoid heating milk to a boiling temperature. Boiling temperatures destroy some nutrients, and for breast milk, some protective properties.

● Shake the bottle during and after warming to evenly distribute the heat. And always test a few drops on the back of your hand, not your wrist; the back of your hand is more sensitive. The formula or milk should be tepid, or just slightly warm to the touch.

Microwave Warming: Be Very Cautious

Be very cautious if you heat formula or baby food in a microwave oven. Microwaving creates uneven heating, or "hot spots," that can burn a baby's mouth, throat, and skin. A bottle or food may feel cool on the outside while the inner contents reach scorching temperatures. And since food doesn't heat evenly, microwaving may not destroy bacteria that cause foodborne illness. Another problem: sometimes plastic bottle liners explode if their contents become too hot.

Better yet, avoid using the microwave oven to warm breast milk or infant formula. Besides the chance of burning your baby, microwave heating produces high temperatures quickly; some vitamins and protective factors in breast milk may be destroyed.

INFANT FEEDING PLAN: A BASIC GUIDELINE

Babies differ in their size, appetite, and readiness for solid food. This guide offers a general time frame for introducing baby foods and table foods into an infant's eating pattern.

However, some babies may be ready for certain foods a little sooner; others, somewhat later. Your baby's doctor, pediatric nurse, or a registered dietitian will recommend an eating pattern to meet your baby's individual needs.

What Are Your Baby's Developmental Signs?

	NEWBORN/HEAD UP	SUPPORTED SITTER	INDEPENDENT SITTER
Physical Skills	—*Newborn:* need head support —*Head Up:* has more skillful head control	—Sits with help or support —On tummy, pushes up on arms with straight elbow	—Sits independently —Can pick up and hold small objects in hand —Leans toward food or spoon
Eating Skills	—*Newborn:* establishes a suck-swallow breathing pattern —*Head Up:* tongue moves forward and back to suck	—May push food out of mouth with tongue —Moves pureed food forward with tongue to swallow —Recognizes spoon and holds mouth open as spoon approaches	—Able to keep thick purees in mouth —Pulls head downward and presses upper lip to draw food from spoon —Rakes food toward self in fist —Can transfer food from one hand to another —Can drink from a cup with help
Appropriate Foods and Textures	—*Newborn & Head Up:* breast milk or formula	—Breast milk or formula —Infant cereals —Thin pureed foods, such as single-ingredient baby foods	—Breast milk or formula —Infant cereals —Thin pureed foods, such as single-ingredient baby foods —Thicker pureed foods, such as more advanced pureed baby foods —Soft, mashed foods without lumps, such as cooked potatoes and carrots, 100% juice
What You Do to Help	—If breast-feeding, eat a wide variety of healthy foods to teach your baby flavors, tastes, and aromas through your breast milk	—Enhance baby's acceptance of cereal by mixing it with breast milk or formula —Respect baby's hunger and fullness cues—stop feeding when he/she indicates he/she is full	—Introduce one new food 2 to 4 days in a row before starting a new one —Give baby a variety of thin and thick textures to help develop the skills needed

Source: Copyright 2005 Gerber Products Company. Reprinted with permission.

For solid foods . . . warm foods in the microwave oven until only just lukewarm.

● Warm food in a microwave-safe dish. As in baby bottles, food heated in jars can develop hot spots.

● Heat only the amount you'll need. Less food heats faster than more food, and some ovens heat faster than others. Fifteen seconds on high (100 percent power) for 4 ounces of baby food are enough. Heat higher-fat foods such as meat and eggs on the stove, not in the microwave oven. They heat faster and splatter or overheat more.

● Read warming guidelines on baby food labels. And remember that baby foods can be served cold, at room temperature, or slightly warm.

● After microwaving, allow food to "rest"; food will continue to heat through. Stir the food to distribute the heat. Let it stand for at least 30 seconds.

● Test the temperature of the food before feeding it to your baby; the food should be just lukewarm. Use a clean spoon to feed the baby.

For more about the safe use of a microwave oven, see "Play It Microwave-Safe" in chapter 12.

Baby Food—Make It Yourself?

In spite of the added work, some parents get satisfaction from preparing baby food themselves. However, that requires extra care to keep baby's food safe and to retain the nutrients from fresh foods.

Commercial baby foods are nutritious options for feeding baby, too. Today's commercial baby foods provide balance and variety with carefully controlled and consistent nutrient content.

Follow these guidelines if you choose to prepare homemade baby food:

● Wash your hands before preparing baby food.

● Always use clean cutting boards, utensils, and containers to cook, puree, and store homemade baby food.

● Wash, peel, and remove seeds or pits from produce. Take special care with fruits and vegetables that are grown close to the ground; they may contain spores for *Clostridium botulinum* or contain other harmful bacteria that can cause foodborne illness.

● Start with fresh or frozen vegetables. Cook them until tender by steaming or microwaving, then puree or mash. There's no need to add salt, other seasonings, or sweeteners. Remember: A baby's tastes aren't the same as yours.

● Puree or mash fresh fruit or fruit canned in its own juice. Never add honey or corn syrup.

● Avoid putting egg whites in homemade baby food until the baby's first birthday. Egg whites, more likely than egg yolks, may cause an allergic reaction. Cook any egg whites you feed your toddler.

● Cook meats, poultry, and egg yolks until well done. Babies are especially susceptible to foodborne illnesses caused by eating undercooked meats, poultry, and eggs. Again, there's no need for added flavorings.

● Prepare foods with a texture appropriate for the baby's feeding stage. Puree foods in a food processor, blender, or baby food grinder, or mash them with a fork; or chop them well, so your baby won't choke.

● Cover, and refrigerate or freeze homemade baby food immediately after it's prepared. If refrigerated, keep homemade baby food in a covered container for one to two days in the refrigerator or three to four months in the freezer. Label and date homemade baby food.

● For convenience, freeze prepared baby food for later use. Freeze it in small portions in a clean ice cube tray. Once frozen, put the cubes into clean, airtight, plastic bags for single-serve portions. As another method, use the "plop and freeze" technique: plop meal-size spoonfuls of pureed food onto a cookie sheet, freeze, then transfer the frozen baby food to clean plastic bags for continued freezing.

For Babies, Toddlers, and Preschoolers: How to Avoid Choking

Having teeth doesn't mean children can handle all foods. Small, hard foods . . . slippery foods . . . and sticky foods can block the air passage, cutting off a child's supply of oxygen.

● Don't offer these foods to children younger than three or four years of age:

Avoid Feeding from the Baby Food Jar

Feeding directly from the jar introduces bacteria from your baby's mouth to the spoon and into the food. If you save the uneaten food, bacteria in leftovers can grow and may cause diarrhea, vomiting, and other symptoms of foodborne illness if used at a later feeding.

- Instead, spoon small amounts of baby food from the jar into a feeding dish, and feed from there. Toss what's uneaten from the dish. If your baby needs a second helping, just take more from the jar with a clean spoon.

- As soon as you finish feeding your baby, cap opened jars of baby food that haven't come in contact with your baby's saliva. You may then safely refrigerate them: opened strained fruits for two to three days; strained meats and eggs, one day; and meat and vegetable combinations, one to two days.

Unopened jars of baby food have the same shelf life as other canned foods. Check the product dating on the label or lid, then use the baby food while it's still at its peak quality. *To learn how to read product dating, see "More Reading on the Food Label" in chapter 11.* Most jars of baby food have a safety button on top. If the button's down, the food should be safe. As the vacuum seal releases, you'll hear a "pop" when you open the jar. Discard jars with chipped glass or rusty lids.

- *Small, hard foods*—nuts, seeds, popcorn, snack chips, pretzels, raw carrots, raw celery, raw peas, whole olives, cherry tomatoes, snack puffs, raisins. For toddlers and preschoolers, cut foods cut into slightly larger pieces that they can bite and chew, but not put whole into their mouths.

- *Slippery foods*—whole grapes; large pieces of meats, poultry, and frankfurter; and hard candy, lollipops, and cough drops, which may be swallowed before they're adequately chewed. Chop grapes, meat, poultry, hot dogs, and other foods in small pieces. Avoid offering chewing gum.

- Be careful with sticky foods, too, such as peanut butter. Spread only a thin layer on bread. Avoid giving your baby peanut butter from a spoon or finger. If it gets stuck in your baby's throat, he or she may have trouble breathing.

- Watch out for these foods: taffy, soft candies with a firm texture such as gel or gummi candies, caramels, marshmallows, jelly beans, raw peeled apple and pear slices, cherries with pits, and dried fruits.

- Avoid propping your baby's bottle. Refrain from feeding your baby in the car, too; helping a choking baby is harder when the car's moving.

- Offer appropriate foods. Finger foods for older babies and toddlers are pieces of banana, graham crackers, strips of cheese, or bagels.

- Watch young children while they eat. That includes watching older brothers and sisters who may offer foods that younger children can't handle yet.

- Insist that children sit to eat or drink, not when they're lying down, walking, or running. As they develop eating skills, encourage them to take time to chew well.

Tips for Travel, Tips for Day Care

- Pack unopened jars of commercial baby food. Even cereal comes in jars. Ready-to-feed formula in a prepackaged bottle is handy, especially since it doesn't require refrigeration. Or use powdered formula. Just premeasure water and powder into separate containers, then mix when it's needed.

- Keep perishable food, such as bottles of prepared infant formula or breast milk, well chilled. Pack them in an insulated container with frozen cold packs or buried in ice in a plastic bag. When you arrive at your destination, refrigerate.

  Bottles, already cold from your refrigerator, can stay safe for up to eight hours in sterile sealed bottles in an insulated bottle bag, or for about four hours if they're stored in ice cubes in a plastic bag.

- Have everything handy: food, utensils, bib, and baby wipes or a clean, damp washcloth. If someone else is feeding your baby, provide feeding instructions, too, including the time and approximate amount to feed.

- Keep food separate from soiled diapers. And don't put food and bottles in a diaper bag that's frequently exposed to soiled diapers.

Food Labels: For Childen under Four Years

The Dietary Guidelines for Americans don't apply to children under age two—and neither do the Nutrition Facts on food labels, which are for adults and children ages four years and above.

Although they use the Nutrition Facts format, infant and toddler food labels are different from adult food labels—and supply different information. *This page shows two typical Nutrition Facts panels: for a toddler food (less than two years) and for food for children under age four years.* The label gives information that helps parents choose food with the kinds and amounts of nutrients that infants, toddlers, and young children need.

Serving size. For infant foods, serving sizes are based on average amounts that infants and toddlers under four or two years of age usually eat at one time. For example, for oatmeal, that's ¼ cup. On adult food labels, serving sizes are based on average amounts adults typically eat at one time; again for oatmeal, that may be given as ½ cup or 1 ounce of uncooked oatmeal.

Total fat. Infant food labels (foods for children under two years and four years) list the total fat and *trans* fat content in a single serving of food. But unlike adult food labels, they don't give the calories from fat or from saturated fat. The saturated fat and cholesterol content are listed only on labels for foods for children ages two to under four years. These details aren't included on foods for babies and toddlers under two years of age who need fat as a concentrated energy source to fuel their rapid growth. Parents and other caregivers shouldn't try to limit an infant's fat intake.

% Daily Values (DVs). The % Daily Values for protein and some vitamins and minerals are listed on food labels for infants and children under four years of age. You won't find % DVs for fat, cholesterol, sodium, potassium, carbohydrates, and fiber, however; no Daily Values for them are set for children under age four.

For more about food labels, see "Today's Food Labels" in chapter 11, which includes more detail on the Nutrition Facts panel on adult food labels.

Check the required use-by date on a food label for infant formula and baby food, too, so you don't offer baby food with an off-flavor or texture. That date is for quality, as well as for nutrient retention.

Nutrition Label Format, Food for Children under 2

Nutrition Label Format, Food for Children under 4

Source: 2004 Food Products Association, *Food Labeling Manual,* 2nd ed.; pp. 169–170.

● Be prepared to use the Heimlich maneuver quickly to dislodge solid foods that obstruct the air passage. Do this when a child is choking and can't breathe, cough, talk, or cry. The technique for infants and toddlers differs somewhat from that for adults. *See the illustrated description. For the Heimlich maneuver for older children, teens, and adults, see chapter 12.*

● Always have your doctor see your child after a serious choking incident to be sure that the lungs and airway are clear.

Another Food Safety Reminder for Feeding Infants

Infants and young children are very vulnerable to foodborne illness! Their immune systems aren't developed enough to fend off foodborne infections. Safe food handling and preparation is very important. The Dietary Guidelines offer advice for feeding infants: *Do not eat or drink raw (unpasteurized) milk or any products made from unpasteurized milk, raw or partially cooked eggs or foods containing raw eggs, raw or undercooked meat and poultry, raw or undercooked fish or shellfish, unpasteurized juices, and raw sprouts.*

Have You Ever Wondered

. . . if a human milk bank is an option if you can't breast-feed? Perhaps—but generally only as a medical emergency. Human milk banks require a prescription. Currently supplies are limited, and the cost is high.

. . . if breast-feeding affects fertility? Ovaries may stop releasing eggs, but it's still possible to get pregnant. If you don't want to get pregnant while you're nursing, talk to your doctor about a birth control method that's right for you.

. . . how to successfully breast-feed twins? Wonder if you'll produce enough milk? Remember: Your milk supply operates on the principle of supply and demand; with more breast-feeding, your body produces more breast milk. In the early weeks, you may be able to feed both infants simultaneously—an efficient use of time.

Talk to your pediatrician about the need for a supplemental bottle. If your babies are growing normally, it's probably not needed unless you need help from other caregivers. Seek help from a lactation counselor for any special guidance for successfully nursing "multiples," such as help with positioning for two infants.

When an Infant Is Choking . . .

Lay the child down, face up, on a firm surface and kneel or stand at victim's feet, or hold infant on your lap facing away from you. Place the middle and index fingers of both your hands below his rib cage and above his navel. Press into the victim's abdomen with a quick upward thrust. Be very gentle. Repeat until object is expelled.

If your baby isn't breathing: Clear any obstructions from the mouth. If there is no pulse, start CPR (two breaths followed by five gentle chest thrusts). Continue CPR until baby starts breathing or help arrives.

Source: Courtesy of the Heimlich Institute, Cincinnati, Ohio.

Heart Health Starts In Infancy!

The American Heart Association advises developing heart-healthy eating habits from the start. Breast-feed for the first year and transition to other nutrient sources between four to six months. Wait until a baby is at least six months old to offer juice, then limit it to 4 to 6 ounces per day. Avoid overfeeding or forcing a baby to finish meals if he or she isn't hungry. Repeatedly give healthful foods, even if he or she initially won't eat them. And avoid introducing foods without overall nutritional value, just to provide calories.

CHAPTER 16

Food to Grow On

Food nourishes at every age and stage in a child's life: infancy, the toddler and preschool years, school-age years, and adolescence. Careful food choices not only help ensure the physical nourishment of a child's growing body but also nourish his or her social, mental, and psychological development. Childhood is also a time to establish patterns of healthful eating and active living that lead to health and wellness—from childhood on.

Whatever the age, children and teens need the same nutrients as adults. Only the amounts differ. Like you, they need energy from food—but more relative to their body weight. They enjoy many of the same foods you like, but the form and combinations may differ.

Your challenge as a parent or a caregiver? First, be a good role model for healthful eating and active living for kids. After all, parents and other caregivers are a child's first and most influential teachers. Second, support your child's chances to make wise food choices and enjoy food. It's up to you to recognize and respect his or her unique needs, to make a variety of nourishing, appropriate foods available, and to set a routine (time and place) for eating. Your child has responsibilities: learning skills to make sound food choices, listening to body cues to learn to eat the right amount, and making active play part of daily living!

You have more influence on your child or teen's food choices and daily living patterns than you may think. When you take care of yourself (eat smart and move more), you care for your child and family!

Toddlers and Preschoolers: Food and Play for the Early Years

Do young children seem like sponges, absorbing all the sights, sounds, and tastes around them? Young children are impressionable, ready and eager to learn. That makes the preschool years a great time to nurture positive attitudes toward eating and help children learn to eat and enjoy a variety of foods. Establishing good eating habits and active lifestyles now starts a lifelong pattern.

While toddlers and preschoolers grow at a slower rate than infants, they need enough energy from food to fuel active play, learning, and the next stages of growth. They also need enough nutrients to promote their growth and health. Starting in the early years, good nutrition and healthful lifestyle habits can reduce the risks for overweight and obesity, diabetes, heart disease, cancer, and other chronic diseases later in life.

Food for Hungry Tummies

What's healthful eating for young children? A variety of foods with different textures, tastes, and colors—in adequate amounts—provides the nutrients and the food energy children need to thrive. Nourishment comes from a wide array of food.

What about nutrients? Carbohydrates should be children's main energy source. How much? Their

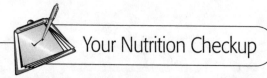

Your Nutrition Checkup

Eating and Activity: Family Matters

Family styles influence a child's eating and physical activity patterns and attitudes for life. What children eat and how much they move—and their attitude toward both—have lifelong implications.

Take a moment to assess your own family's eating and physical activity practices. As a parent, family member, or caregiver:

Do You . . .	ALWAYS	USUALLY	SOMETIMES	NEVER
Eat your meals together as a family at least once a day?	___	___	___	___
Serve meals and snacks on a regular schedule?	___	___	___	___
Give your youngster freedom to choose the foods he or she eats?	___	___	___	___
Respect a child's appetite and offer only child-sized portions?	___	___	___	___
Involve children in planning and preparing family food?	___	___	___	___
Make an effort to keep mealtimes pleasant?	___	___	___	___
Include snacks as part of the day's eating plan?	___	___	___	___
Attempt to keep eating to the kitchen, dining room, or another designated place?	___	___	___	___
Set a good role model with your food decisions?	___	___	___	___
Avoid rewarding or punishing a child with food?	___	___	___	___
Give kids enough time to eat—make meals last at least fifteen minutes?	___	___	___	___
Turn off the TV while you eat together?	___	___	___	___
Offer foods that appeal to children?	___	___	___	___
Serve a variety of foods for meals and snacks?	___	___	___	___
Offer new foods and new food combinations?	___	___	___	___
Avoid forcing a child to eat everything on the plate?	___	___	___	___
Set a good role model by being physically active?	___	___	___	___
Limit TV time to one to two hours daily?	___	___	___	___
Encourage children to play actively?	___	___	___	___
Enjoy physical activity regularly as a family (at least once or twice weekly)?	___	___	___	___
Subtotal	___	___	___	___

Now score yourself:

Count the number of check marks in each column. Then multiply by these scores.

What's your total?

"Always":   3 points

"Usually":   2 points

"Sometimes": 1 points

"Never":   0 point

Your total score _____

What does your score suggest?

If you scored 40 to 60 points, you already apply what you know about nurturing positive eating and physical activity patterns. Read on for more ideas.

A score of 20 to 39 suggests you're on the right track for feeding and exercising with kids. But you still have room to make positive changes in your family's lifestyle. Check this chapter for more practical tips.

Less than 20, try to incorporate a few changes in your family's approach to food and physical activity. Read on for some steps to get you started.

energy needs depend on their growth rate, body size, and level of physical activity. Most moderately active to active children, ages three to five, likely need 1,200 to 1,600 calories a day, depending on their age, gender, size, and level of physical activity. Younger children need somewhat less. They need enough protein (5 to 20 percent of their total calories) for growth and for substances (hormones and enzymes) that stimulate body processes. Children need moderate amounts of fat, too, again for growth and to meet their energy needs; see *"Fat Facts for Kids" later in this chapter.* Food variety can supply the vitamins and minerals that young children need to thrive, although calcium and iron are among the nutrients that may need your attention. Fiber is important, too! For children ages one to three years, the Institute of Medicine advises 19 grams of total fiber a day; for children ages four to eight years, the advice is 25 grams a day. A variety of foods provides all these important nutrients. *See the Dietary Reference Intakes in the Appendices.*

Variety for young children includes enough calcium-rich dairy foods and iron-rich protein foods, as well as enough nutrient-rich, fiber-rich vegetables, fruits, and whole-grain foods. For overall good nutrition, offer foods with less added sugars, and from age two years on, lower-fat dairy choices. For preschoolers ages two years on up, use MyPyramid to guide and plan a day's worth of healthful meals and snacks— with enough food variety in the right amounts. For food-group amounts, *find your child's age and gender with his or her activity level on the "MyPyramid Food Intake Pattern Calorie Levels" chart in the Appendices*, then the food group plan to match the recommended calories.

For every nutrient, children have many choices. If your children won't touch sweet potatoes, offer a wedge of cantaloupe; both are good sources of vitamin A. Is milk rejected? Try chocolate or another flavored milk or offer other calcium-rich foods—such as cheese or yogurt. If you offer different kinds of healthful foods regularly, your child will learn to enjoy many of them—and reap their benefits. Children often refuse foods the first time. Keep trying!

Whole milk, rather than low-fat varieties, is recommended for children twelve to twenty-four months of age. Whole milk supplies more fat and calories than low-fat or fat-free milk. As a concentrated source of

Have You Ever Wondered

... what to do if your preschooler seems overweight? First discuss your concerns with your child's doctor. Your child's size may be normal. A growth chart, recorded in regular health exams, will track your child's height and weight and show how he or she fits within a healthy range. Some kids gain a little extra weight to support an upcoming growth spurt.

If your child is overweight, withholding food isn't healthful. Low-calorie diets often don't supply the food energy and nutrients he or she needs to grow, develop, and learn properly. Healthful eating habits, combined with plenty of active play, can help most overweight kids grow into their healthy weight—without a special diet. *See "Weighty Problems for Children—Overweight" in this chapter.*

... if a vegetarian diet is okay for kids? A well-planned vegetarian diet—even a vegan diet—can supply all the nutrients that children need for their growth and energy needs. Calcium and iron need special attention. If your child doesn't eat any meat, poultry, fish, eggs, and dairy foods, be especially cautious about good sources of protein, vitamin B_{12}, vitamin D, and zinc. *For more guidance, see chapter 20, "The Vegetarian Way."* A nutrient supplement might be a good idea; ask your healthcare provider.

... how to find out if your child is getting enough iron? For young children, iron deficiency anemia is the most common nutrition problem. That's why children are screened for anemia in regular checkups. Children need enough iron to support growth, replace normal iron loss, and produce energy for learning and play. *See chapter 4 for ways to include iron-rich foods in family meals.*

energy, fat helps fuel this period of fairly rapid growth. And the extra cholesterol in whole milk helps a young child's brain develop properly. After the second birthday, any type of milk is okay to drink. Choose the type that matches your child's energy needs.

Enough to Eat, without Overfeeding

You can lead a young child to the table, but you can't make a child eat—nor should you! Let your child's appetite guide how much food is enough. A pattern of overeating can lead to overweight, starting in these early years. Of concern: even among two- to five-year-

"Do as I Do": Are You a Good Role Model?

Did *you* eat *your* vegetables today? Did *you* drink milk? Did *you* take a walk or do something physically active, not just sit by the TV or the computer? Did *you* eat just a handful of chips, or the whole bagful?

Children learn their habits, attitudes, and beliefs about eating and physical activity as they watch and interact with you: parent, older sibling, other caregiver. By mimicking you, they explore their world, try "grown-up" behavior, and hope to please you. Whether you intend to or not, role modeling probably is the most powerful, effective way to help your child eat smart and move more.

Most kids want to do what others do! So the next time you order a drink to go with a fast-food meal, eat when you're stressed or bored, or decide how you'll spend a leisurely afternoon, think about the messages you send. The best way to help your child eat healthier and be physically active is for you to do so!

olds, more than 10 percent are considered overweight. Underfeeding also can lead to weight gain if your child sneaks food to satisfy hunger when you're not looking.

How much do toddlers and preschoolers need to eat? Although they're no longer babies, young children aren't ready for adult-size portions. Adult servings can overwhelm small appetites and lead to overeating and too many calories. Children's stomachs aren't big enough to handle large portions, and they don't need as much as you do! Judge how much your child needs to eat:

● Serve a toddler or a preschooler small helpings—smaller than yours. Let the child ask for more. As a guide, some experts advise one tablespoon of every food served for every year in age.

● Respect your child's hunger and satiety cues. When he or she starts to play with food, becomes restless, or sends signals of "no more," remove the food. Knowing what it feels like to be full—and when to stop eating—helps children learn to eat enough, but not to overeat.

● Do away with the "clean plate" club. This practice may encourage overeating or a food aversion—habits that could set up a child for weight or eating problems

later. If your child always leaves food on his or her plate, you may be offering too much food. Offer smaller portions to smaller people!

Day-to-day and meal-to-meal appetite fluctuations are normal. Children's appetites often decrease after their first birthday as their growth slows. In fact, expect a child to pick at meals on occasion. Chances are that he or she will make up for it later. If your child is growing normally, seems healthy, and has energy to play, he or she probably is eating enough. Unsure? Talk to your child's doctor.

How often should young children eat? Most children do best with a routine—when meals and snacks are served at about the same time each day. "Pacifier snacks" eaten while standing in line at the supermarket—or snacks just a half hour before a meal—may interfere with a child's eating routine.

Younger children may need to eat five to six times a day because their small stomachs don't hold much. Plan food-group snacks as part of the day's meal schedule, and space them between meals. It's never too early to help youngsters learn to make healthful snack choices. *See "Snacks Equal Good Nutrition" in this chapter.*

For menus that meet the nutrient and energy needs of most young children, see "For Starters: Sample Menus for Preschoolers" in this chapter.

Have You Ever Wondered

. . . how to make sure food is safe for your young child? Infants and young children are less able to fight infection than you can. As for everyone in your family, handle food properly to avoid foodborne illness; *chapter 12 offers plenty of advice.* The Dietary Guidelines also advise: *Do not eat or drink raw (unpasteurized) milk, raw or partially cooked eggs or foods containing raw eggs, raw or undercooked meat and poultry, raw or undercooked fish or shellfish, unpasteurized juices, and raw sprouts.* Among the many lessons: teach kids about proper handwashing and skip the raw cookie dough!

Another food safety issue: avoid offering foods your child could choke on. *Refer to page 395 for advice.*

Mealtime Tactics

Parents and caregivers supply the three *w*'s of meals and snacks: *what* foods are offered, and *when* and *where* they're eaten. The child fills in the other *w* and *h*: *which* offered foods to eat and *how* much.

- While physical activity promotes a healthy appetite, plan a quiet time before meals and snacks. Kids eat best when they're more relaxed.

- Remember that your child learns by watching you and older siblings. Eat together as a family. Set a good example by eating a variety of foods—including vegetables—yourself. Eating together also is a good chance to talk and to practice appropriate table manners.

- Even if you can't eat together, be there! Young children need supervision in case they start to choke. Someone who's choking may not be able to make sounds you can hear easily. *For foods that may cause choking or ways to safely handle a choking incident, see "For Babies, Toddlers, and Preschoolers: How to Avoid Choking" in chapter 15.*

- Encourage kids to sit while they eat. Give youngsters a booster seat so they can reach their food easily. Discourage eating while standing, walking, or lying down.

- Reward children with affection and attention—not food. Using food as a reward or a punishment only promotes unhealthy attitudes about food and perhaps emotional overeating.

- Respect food preferences. Give young children the freedom to choose and reject foods, just as older children and adults do. Just encourage young children to politely say "No, thank you." Making food choices is a competency children need to master.

- Avoid the notion of "forbidden" foods. That may cause your child to want them more. All foods can be part of your child's healthful eating plan.

- Serve "designer dinners," featuring a variety of colors and textures. Cut food into interesting shapes, and arrange it attractively on the plate. Kids react to inviting foods just as you do!

- Get kids involved in preparing meals. Even young children can tear apart lettuce leaves for a salad or break up green beans into smaller pieces. Children are more likely to try foods that they have helped prepare.

- Offer foods with kid appeal. Many younger children prefer unmixed foods. Foods with funny names—such as Monster Mash potatoes (mashed sweet potatoes) or Bugs on a Log (raisins and peanut butter on celery)—may help kids to try new foods. Kids often like finger foods, too. Offer raw vegetables to easily nibble in hand; be careful with foods that may cause choking. *For vegetables that taste good raw, see "Produce 'Package'" in the Appendices.*

- Encourage children to practice serving themselves—for example, pouring milk from a pitcher, spreading peanut butter on bread, or spooning food from a serving bowl to their plate. Even though spills are messy, they're part of becoming independent.

- Make eating and family time the focus of meal and snack time—not TV watching. Use this chance to talk together and reinforce their good eating habits.

- Focus on the whole meal, not just on desserts. Avoid making desserts a reward.

- Stock your kitchen with child-size dishes and utensils that children can use with ease: cups they can get their hands around; broad, straight, short-handled utensils; spoons with a wide mouth; forks with blunt tines; and plates with a curved lip.

- Even in this fast-paced world, give kids enough time to eat. Remember: They're just learning to feed themselves. Time pressure puts stress on eating and takes the pleasure away.

- Toddlers and preschoolers live to play! Encourage a sense of fun and adventure by making family meals pleasant. Recall the day's events, share each other's company, and talk about the food: its colors, flavors, and textures.

Feeding Choosy Eaters

Does your child refuse to eat green foods? Does he or she suddenly react to an all-time favorite food with an "I don't like this," or simply "no"? Are you concerned because your youngster won't eat vegetables?

Bouts of independence are part of being a toddler or a young child. "Choosy" eating may be your child's early attempts to make decisions and be assertive—a natural part of growing up. It may reflect a smaller appetite as his or her growth rate slows a bit, too. Or "no" may really mean "I want your attention."

Relax; be patient. Arm yourself with practical solutions to handle the "downs and ups" of child feeding:

● Avoid the "short order cook" routine. At mealtime, serve at least one food you know your child likes. But expect your tot to at least try foods that the rest of the family enjoys.

FOR STARTERS: SAMPLE MENUS FOR PRESCHOOLERS

SAMPLE MENU	AMOUNT FOR A MODERATELY ACTIVE CHILD, AGE TWO (ABOUT 1,000 CALORIES)	AMOUNT FOR A MODERATELY ACTIVE CHILD, AGE THREE TO FIVE (ABOUT 1,400 CALORIES)
Breakfast		
Cream of wheat made with milk	¼ cup	½ cup
Hard-cooked egg, medium	½	1
Banana, medium	½	½
1% milk*	½ cup	½ cup
Midmorning snack		
Cheese, Cheddar	½ ounce	½ ounce
Whole-wheat crackers	3	3
Orange juice	½ cup (4 ounces)	¾ cup (6 ounces)
Lunch		
Vegetable-bean soup	½ cup	¾ cup
Peanut butter	1 tablespoon	2 tablespoons
Whole-wheat bread	1 regular slice	1 regular slice
Cooked carrots	¼ cup	¼ cup
Bell pepper sticks	¼ cup	¼ cup
1% milk*	½ cup	½ cup
Midafternoon Snack		
Canned peaches in juice	¼ cup	½ cup
Vanilla wafers	2 small	2 small
Dinner		
Meat loaf	2 ounces	2½ ounces
Cooked spaghetti noodles	¼ cup	½ cup
Broccoli	¼ cup	½ cup
Shredded lettuce salad	¼ cup	½ cup
Soft margarine	1 teaspoon	1 teaspoon
Whole-wheat dinner roll	1 small	1 small
1% milk*	½ cup	¾ cup

*Children older than two years can be given milk with less fat content.

- Offer choices, but not too many, rather than asking open-ended questions such as, "What do you want to eat?" Deciding between or among two or three foods gives your child a feeling of control. It's also good practice for learning to make food decisions.

- Make food simple and recognizable. "Unmix" the food if it's an issue; put aside some ingredients for mixed dishes before assembling the recipe, even a salad or a sandwich. Then let your child put food together as he or she likes.

- Involve kids. Even choosy eaters eat foods they help plan, buy, or make. Together, plan a meal around foods your child likes. When you shop, ask your child to pick a new food for the family to try. Ask for a kitchen helper; even small children can wash fresh fruit or put meat between bread slices for a sandwich.

- Allow hot food to cool down and cold food to warm up a little before serving it. Many children dislike extreme temperatures.

- If your child won't eat certain foods, perhaps spinach, don't worry. Just offer a similar food-group food, maybe broccoli. Or try carrots. Foods from the same food group supply similar nutrients.

- Moisten dry foods such as meat if they're hard to chew. A little cheese sauce or fruit or vegetable juice might help. Serve drier foods alongside naturally moist foods such as mashed potatoes or cottage cheese. Or offer "dipping" sauces with finger foods— kids love to dip!

- Trust your child's appetite. Forcing children to eat can start a lifelong habit of overeating. Instead,

Fat Facts for Kids

For a young child's eating plan, put away some adult notions about fat. A low-fat eating plan isn't advised for children under two years of age—and cutting way back on fat for older children isn't recommended either.

Fat is an important source of the energy, or calories, that support a young child's rapid growth, learning, and play. Two fatty acids—linoleic and alpha-linolenic acid— are essential for growing and brain development. Food must supply them because the body can't make them. Kids also need some fat from food to help their bodies use vitamins A, D, E, and K and to add flavor to food.

Starting at age two, advice for children and teens is similar to the advice for their parents: eat a diet moderate in total fat and low in saturated fat and *trans* fat. More specifically, the Dietary Guidelines offer this advice for children and adolescents: *Keep total fat intake between 30 to 35 percent of calories for children two to three years of age and between 25 to 35 percent of calories for children and adolescents four to eighteen years of age, with most fats coming from sources of polyunsaturated and monounsaturated fatty acids, such as fish, nuts, and vegetable oils.*

Grain products, fruits, vegetables, low-fat dairy foods, and other protein-rich foods (lean meat, poultry, fish, beans, and nuts) should supply most of a child's food energy. Remember that this guideline refers to your child's overall eating plan *and yours* for several days— not to one food, one meal, or even one day's intake.

If that's true, can your child eat French fries, chicken nuggets, cheese, and ice cream occasionally? Sure. Reasonable amounts of higher-fat foods can fit in a child's healthful eating plan. Just be sure his or her overall choices are moderate in fat and low in "sat fats" and *trans* fats.

Going easy on fat is good family advice, too. Family meals and snacks, prepared with less fat, teach a lifelong habit of lower-fat eating. Later in life that habit reduces your child's risk for many health problems. Another benefit: eating too much fat may add excess calories and result in weight gain, even at an early age.

For more about fat in a healthful diet, see chapter 3, "Fat Facts"; chapter 13 offers ways to prepare family foods with less fat.

Food Jags

What do you do when youngsters get "stuck" on a food? If he or she keeps asking for the same food meal after meal, the child is on a "food jag." Food jags are common in the toddler years.

More frustrating for you than harmful for kids, you're smart to remain low key about food jags. The more you focus on them, the longer they may last.

Actually, it's okay to offer the food they want again and again and again! Just include other foods alongside to encourage variety. Most "monotonous diners" soon tire of eating the same food so often.

If your child rejects whole categories of food for more than two weeks, talk to your child's doctor or a registered dietitian.

following hunger and satiety cues is part of learning to eat the right amount.

● Limit table time. Sitting at the table without eating for a long time doesn't teach good food habits. At the end of mealtime, quietly remove the plate.

● Most of all, relax. And be a good role model (eat your veggies, drink your milk) yourself.

● Avoid conflict and criticism at mealtime; otherwise your child may use food for "table control." Focus your attention on the positives in your child's eating behavior, not on your child's food. And unless you're prepared for a self-fulfilling prophecy, skip labeling your child as a "picky eater."

● Remember: What your child eats over several days—not just one meal—is what really counts!

Tasting Something New!

Babies try one new food after another as they start solids, each time adding more food variety to their diet. The tasting adventure continues throughout childhood—and on into adulthood. More variety increases the chance for good nutrition and adds interest and fun to eating. And more variety can mean more vitamins, minerals, and phytonutrients.

Help children be willing food "tryers." It's part of the challenge and pleasure of learning about food. Be aware: young children typically have more tastebuds and may be more sensitive to flavors than you are.

● Offer new foods at the start of meals. That's when children are the most hungry. But make the rest of the meal familiar.

● Encourage children to taste at least one bite of a new food—or a food prepared in a different way. Don't force them. Just be matter-of-fact.

● Keep quiet about foods you don't like. Try not to let your food dislikes keep your child from trying new foods.

● Before offering the new food, talk about it: color, texture, size, shape, aroma, not whether it tastes "good" or "bad." Let kids help you prepare it. They'll be more willing to taste!

● Serve the same food in different forms—for example, raw carrot sticks and cooked carrot coins.

Hand-Washing Basics

Kids can't see them—but germs that cause illness are everywhere! For children, who have less immunity, proper hand washing and food safety are especially important.

Teach children good hand-washing habits—always before and after handling food and eating, and after using the bathroom, touching a pet, combing hair, blowing their nose, or coughing or sneezing into their hands:

● Wash hands with soap and warm water, rubbing hands for twenty seconds. (It's good counting practice, too.) And dry hands well.

● Get a safe stool so your child can reach the sink, the faucet, the soap, and a towel.

● Practice with your child. Rub a little cinnamon and oil on your child's hands. Watch what happens if he or she doesn't wash hands well. Cinnamon that stays on hands represents germs.

● Be a good role model. *Always* wash and dry your hands properly, too.

● Keep trying! Kids may need to taste a food at least eight to ten times before they learn to like it. Accept a fact of life: it's okay not to like every food.

Whenever you expose children to some foods but limit others, you also limit the variety of foods they learn to eat and enjoy. That has an impact on the overall nutritional quality of their food pattern for life!

Snacks Equal Good Nutrition

Young children like to snack. That's good news! With their small stomachs, they may not meet their nutrition needs with just three meals a day. Snacks can fill in the nutrient and food-energy gaps from their meals.

If snacks conjure up images of high-calorie, low-nutrient foods—think again! Wise snack foods for people of all ages, including young children, come *mostly* from nutrient-rich foods in MyPyramid's five food groups. Milk (flavored or not) is a good snack drink; go easy on fruit juice. Make snacks a healthful part of your child's day:

● Let snacks supplement regular meals, not replace them. Plan for two to three food-group snacks plus three meals a day. Children age two to five usually need to eat every two to three hours. Younger children may need to eat more often.

● Plan ahead by keeping food-group snacks handy. *Check "Child-Friendly Snacks" on this page.* An occasional piece of candy is okay, but avoid labeling it as a "special treat" to avoid undue emphasis. Just be matter-of-fact about it.

● Offer snacks two hours or more before meals. In that way youngsters are hungry at mealtime.

● Offer snacks when kids are hungry, not to calm tears or reward behavior. Otherwise you teach a pattern of emotional overeating. Maybe your child just needs attention, not food.

● Choose snacks to fill in the gaps from meals. If your child's meals come up short on vegetables or grain products, offer them at snacktime.

● Offer small snack portions. Let your child ask for more if he or she is still hungry.

● Think "fun" at snacktime. Children enjoy foods with sensory appeal: brightly colored fruits and vegetables; the aroma of baking bread or freshly cut watermelon; the texture differences of soft, creamy cheese with crisp, crunchy crackers.

● Encourage tooth brushing after snacks of any kind, not only after sweets.

Exploring More about Food

Food offers a world of experiences well suited to how children learn. Because food can become a "hands-on" activity, everyday tasks can get kids involved in food—and so promote healthful eating. Try these simple ways to explore food with young children:

● As you walk the store aisles, encourage children to name the fruits and vegetables in the produce aisle or the canned food aisle, or to say the colors of foods they know. Find foods that are new to them; talk about their color, shape, size, and feel.

● At home, as you take vegetables out of grocery bags, talk about the part of the plant each one grows on: leaf (cabbage, lettuce, greens), roots (carrot, potato), stalk (celery, asparagus), flower (broccoli, cauliflower, artichoke), and seed (peas, corn).

Child-Friendly Snacks

For children under age four, avoid popcorn, nuts, seeds, and other hard, small, whole foods to avoid choking. Chop raw carrots and grapes and cooked hot dogs in small pieces.

Grains Group
Animal crackers; cereal (dry or with milk); bagel; English muffin; graham crackers; pita (pocket) bread; rice cake; toast; tortilla; air-popped popcorn; pretzels. Go for whole-grain varieties whenever possible.

Milk Group
Cheese; cottage cheese; pudding; milk (including flavored milk); string cheese; yogurt; frozen yogurt

Vegetable Group
Any raw vegetable (cut in strips or circles); vegetable soup

Fruit Group
Any fresh fruit (sliced for finger food); canned or frozen fruit; fruit juice*; fruit leather; dried fruit

Meat and Beans Group
Bean soup; peanut butter; hard-cooked egg; turkey or meat cubes; tuna salad

* See advice about fruit juice in "Have You Ever Wondered . . . are fruit juices and fruit drinks good choices for kids?" in this chapter.

● Grow foods from seed in your backyard garden. Perhaps start the seeds in paper cups on your windowsill. Kids enjoy eating foods they grow themselves—and it's a great science lesson!

● Have children help decide what foods to serve. Perhaps show them pictures of vegetables and fruits. Have them pick the ones to make for family meals.

● As preschoolers are ready, give them simple tasks to help with family meals. They might wash fruit, arrange bread in a basket, put ready-to-eat cereal in bowls, or help set the table. Most children like to help. They feel good about themselves when they can say, for example, "I poured it!" Working together in the kitchen offers many chances to nurture children. *"Kids' Kitchen" later in this chapter provides more ideas.*

● Expand their world by reading books about food to children. Ask a librarian, preschool teacher, or head

Have You Ever Wondered

... what to do if you think your child can't drink milk? Before you say "can't," know that milk sensitivity is often a matter of degree. Lactose intolerance, or difficulty digesting the sugar in milk, is more common than a milk allergy. And it's easy to manage—often by giving the child smaller, more frequent portions of milk. Also easier to digest: chocolate milk; cheese, which has milk's nutrients; and milk itself enjoyed with an oatmeal cookie, banana, or other snack.

If you suspect a milk sensitivity, seek advice from your child's doctor, pediatric nurse, or a registered dietitian. Don't simply give up milk! Your child depends on you for calcium and other nutrients that milk provides for proper growth. For tips on handling a child's sensitivity to milk, *see "Lactose Intolerance: A Matter of Degree" in chapter 21.*

... what to do if your child has a phobia, or a fear, of trying new foods? Just relax, and give your child time to outgrow it. Even kids who resist trying new foods can eat in a healthful way, according to studies of kids' eating behavior. In the meantime, offer a variety of foods, and enjoy them yourself.

of the children's book department in a store to suggest titles. Prepare some foods from the stories.

For more about cooking with kids, including kitchen safety tips, see "Kids' Kitchen" later in this chapter.

Food in Child Care: Check It Out!

Warm and caring staff, a safe environment, opportunities for development and self-expression—that's what most parents look for when they choose child care. If you look for child care, rank good nutrition, food-safety standards, and active play high on your checklist, too. If your child has a food allergy or needs to avoid any food for religious or other reasons, find out how that's handled.

Consider the importance of the food served. A child may eat two or more meals and snacks in a child-care facility, so the nutritional quality must be high. Since a young child is developing eating skills and food attitudes that will affect long-term health, the overall eating environment is important, too.

A child-care setting offers many opportunities for spreading illness: food service, diapering, toileting, and close contact with others. For this reason, cleanliness and safe food handling are "musts." Infants and young children have immature immune systems; they're more vulnerable to catching a cold, flu, or other illness from others.

To help establish a lifelong habit of active living, children regularly involved in child care need a program with safe, fun, and developmentally appropriate ways to move more and sit less. Choose a program that makes active play a priority. Besides health, active living teaches social skills and helps develop body skills.

As you choose child care, these factors suggest high standards of cleanliness, nutrition, and active play:

Food preparation and storage areas ...

- Neat and very clean
- Properly labeled and well-covered foods
- Adequate refrigeration and heating equipment
- Perishable foods stored in the refrigerator

Hand-washing area ...

- Child-size sinks, or safe stepping stools for adult-size sinks
- Soap and paper towels

Mealtimes and snacktimes ...

- Meals and snacks with a variety of foods from the five food groups of MyPyramid. (Most child-care settings have specific guidelines and menus; ask to see them.)
- Tables and chairs appropriately sized for children's comfort, or high chairs, or booster seats
- Child-size utensils and covered cups with spouts to help young children master their feeding skills
- Adult supervision at snacktimes and mealtimes and adequate staffing for feeding infants and children with special needs

Diaper-changing and toilet areas ...

- Very clean
- Located away from food, eating, and play areas
- Closed containers for soiled diapers, tissues, and wipes
- Daily removal of soiled items

Other areas . . .

- Separate storage for each child's toothbrush, comb, and clothing

- Ample space between cots, nap rugs, or cribs

Observe what goes on in the child-care setting. You should be able to answer "yes" to these questions:

- Do children, staff, and volunteers wash and dry their hands before and after eating or participating in food activities?

- Do children wash and dry their hands after outdoor play, toileting, touching animals, sneezing, or wiping their nose?

- Does each child have his or her own washcloth?

- Are child-care providers practicing appropriate sanitation and food-handling techniques?

- Are bottles and foods brought from home refrigerated, and if necessary, heated safely? (*Hint:* When you send food, always label it with your child's name. Transport perishable foods in an insulated sack with a cold pack.)

Active Play
for Toddlers and Preschoolers

Run, jump, throw, and kick! Active living helps your child learn a variety of body skills, mental skills, and social skills, and begins a habit of lifelong active living and a healthy weight. And it's fun! Those skills develop when children have opportunities to move in their daily life. As a parent, it's up to you to encourage active play:

- Balance quiet play (such as reading together) with plenty of active play.

- Choose day care that makes safe, active play a priority.

- Set aside time each day to play together, perhaps tossing a ball, playing tag, or taking a family walk.

- Designate an inside and an outside area that's safe, where your child can freely jump, roll, and tumble.

- Pick toys that "move"—perhaps a ball or a tricycle.

- Join a play group together.

  Inactive TV watching is discouraged for kids under two years. Videos that encourage active "follow me" games can encourage moving for older children.

Have You Ever Wondered

. . . are fruit juices and fruit drinks good choices for kids? Actually, that takes a two-part answer.

Fruit juices: You know that kids are urged to eat fruit every day. Fruit juice is one option, but be aware that too much juice can add up to a lot of calories, or crowd out other nourishing foods and beverages such as milk, and can spoil appetites. An excessive amount also can lead to diarrhea and intestinal discomfort. Sipping a lot of juice even promotes tooth decay. For children and teens, the American Academy of Pediatrics advises:

- *ages 1 to 6 years:* ½ to ¾ cup (4 to 6 ounces) of fruit juice daily, maximum

- *ages 7 to 18 years:* 1 to 1½ cup (8 to 12 ounces) of fruit juice daily, maximum

For food safety sake, avoid unpasteurized juice.

Fruit drinks: They have some juice and perhaps added vitamin C or calcium, but offer fewer nutrients than 100% fruit juice or milk. Read the Nutrition Facts and ingredient list to compare. *See "Juicy Story: Fruit Juice, Juice Drink, Fruit Drink . . . or Just Plain Water?" in chapter 8.*

. . . about iron poisoning—how does it happen? Iron poisoning from adult iron capsules or tablets—or from vitamin pills with iron—occurs when children accidentally swallow them. This can happen, too, if iron tablets meant for children aren't taken as directed, but instead at a higher dosage in a short period. If your doctor prescribes extra iron for your child, give it *only* as directed.

Iron poisoning can cause serious injury, even death. Call your doctor or a poison control center immediately if your child accidentally swallows a supplement with iron. Keep all pills in child-safe containers where your child can't reach them. *Note:* A healthful diet with iron-fortified foods won't cause iron poisoning!

- Is food that's left on a child's plate discarded properly?

- Do children each have their own dish, cup, and utensils, rather than share?

- Does an adult eat with the children, serving as a good role model? Can you volunteer from time to time?

- Are menus posted, or are they sent home with the children?

Need more practical, easy ways to help your kids eat healthy? Check here for "how-tos":

- Help your child with proper dental care—see chapter 5.

- Help your child or teenager eat smart for sports—see chapter 19.

- Feed a vegetarian child or teen—see chapter 20.

- Deal with food allergies or intolerances at home, at day care, in school, or in a restaurant—see chapter 21.

- Find a nutrition expert experienced in issues for feeding kids—see chapter 24.

- Are the foods appropriate for the age of the children (e.g., no foods that may be choking hazards)?

- Are plates, cups, and utensils washed and sanitized after each use?

- Are toys that go into a child's mouth sanitized regularly?

- Do child-care providers and parents wash their hands thoroughly after every diaper check and change?

- Are food activities such as tasting parties, food preparation, growing food from seed, field trips, and circle time activities part of the child-care program? Can you be a parent volunteer?

- Is safe, physically active play part of the daily routine? Is it well supervised? Does it match the abilities of children?

Parents as Partners

For the many children in child care, feeding is a shared responsibility. Together, parents and child-care providers offer foods that nourish kids. And together they help children develop skills and a positive attitude about eating. Here's what you can do:

- If your child has a feeding problem—perhaps a food sensitivity—address it with your child and the caregivers.

- Ask for a meal and snack menu. Identify new foods. Talk about and prepare them at home. Reinforce tasting by serving foods your child tries first in day care.

- Practice hand washing before kids start child care.

- If schedules allow, volunteer in a child-care setting to support the center's nutrition program. Offer to help with meal planning. Prepare a family food as a group activity for your child to share with classmates. Occasionally eat with children or help chaperone a food-related field trip. Or gather empty food packages and other kitchen supplies for play areas or for food activities. Early childhood educators appreciate this help!

School-Age Kids: Eat Smart, Move More

School-age youngsters—no longer preschoolers, not yet teens—are establishing habits that last a lifetime. For their good health and healthy weight, nutrition *and* physical activity should rank high as priorities.

During these years, children gain control of the world around them. They push for independence, associate more with their peers, and make more choices of their own. Because they're away from home more often, people other than family have a growing role in shaping their food decisions. A recent study showed that school-age children acknowledge teachers and schools, then parents as their main sources of nutrition information; television, books, then health professionals ranked next. Another "info" source: some nutrition Web sites for kids.

Nutrition for Active, Growing Kids!

Help your school-age child develop healthful eating and active living habits that last a lifetime!

Nutrients and Calories. Children don't need any special foods for their growth, energy, and health, just enough food energy (but not too much) and nutrients. In fact, they need the same nutrients as their parents do, only in different amounts.

For children, what nutrients may need special attention? The Dietary Guidelines identify calcium, potas-

BMIs for Kids: Tracking Their Growth

Growth charts—using the Body Mass Index (BMI) designed for children ages two and over, and teens—track growth, and a child's or a teen's weight in relation to height. These charts are used to assess whether a child *may be* underweight, at risk for overweight, or overweight. As importantly, the BMI charts assure parents and kids that there's a wide range of "normal." A muscular kid isn't necessarily fat, and a slim kid isn't necessarily underweight. They're simply different.

As children mature, it's normal for their body fat to change. Each child's growth clock, body size, and shape are individual; girls and boys differ, too. Some kids plump up before puberty to prepare for their next rapid growth spurt. Remember: Your child will likely grow as one of his or her parents did at the same age.

As a parent, you, with your healthcare provider, can use these charts to help track your child's growth. Be aware that even the extremes—5th percentile or 95th percentile—don't necessarily mean your child is underweight or overweight. Let your physician make that determination, using additional measures. *See the Appendices for the Growth Charts with Body Mass Index for Age Percentiles for Boys and for Girls, 2 to 20 Years.*

sium, magnesium, vitamin E, and fiber as nutrients that may be low enough among children for concern. Zinc, important for growth, and iron may be issues for some children, too.

With a day's worth of meals and snacks that follow MyPyramid guidelines, they can consume enough of these nutrients. For example, consuming two to three cups of milk or an equivalent supplies enough calcium, and eating more whole fruit, vegetables, and whole-grain foods helps kids eat more fiber. *See Pyramid Power for Kids in this chapter.*

Many children consume more calories than their bodies use—especially inactive kids. What foods deliver their excess calories? Perhaps too many energy-dense foods, "too big" portions, or poorly chosen snack and snack drinks. *"Weighty Problems for Children" on page 418 addresses this issue.*

The calorie sources are an issue, too. Regarding carbohydrates, children need to avoid too many foods and drinks with added sugars. The more foods eaten with a lot of added sugars, the harder it is to consume enough nutrients without gaining weight. Another "carb" issue: preventing cavities. *Refer to "Your Smile: Carbohydrates and Oral Health" in chapter 5. For advice about fat intake for children, refer to "Fat Facts for Kids" on page 405.*

Growth. Children age six to twelve years grow about 2 inches per year. This represents a weight gain of about 5 pounds yearly. To look at it another way, children grow 1 to 2 feet and almost double their weight during these years.

Before you compare your child with another, remember that even in this period of steady growth, children's body sizes, shapes, and growth patterns vary. Most children grow in a pattern that's more like a parent than an unrelated friend. (Get out your family photo album for a visual memory.) *"BMIs for Kids: Tracking Their Growth" in this chapter helps you look at your child's growth pattern.*

Empower Your Kids: Seven How-tos for Smart Snacking

Here's the key to healthful food choices: very visible, convenient, effortless—great taste.

1. Ask your kids what food-group foods they'd like to have on hand. Buy them!

2. "Walk" your kids through the kitchen so they know where these foods are kept.

3. Keep fresh fruit on the counter where kids see it.

4. Wash and cut up veggies ahead, so they're ready to eat.

5. Use see-through containers, clear plastic bags, or containers covered with plastic wrap so kids can see what's inside.

6. Put nutrient-rich food where kids can reach it, perhaps on lower shelves in your refrigerator, pantry, or cabinet. Keep "sometimes" foods such as cookies and chips away in cabinets where they're less convenient to reach, especially for impulse eaters.

7. Buy food in single-serve containers for grab-and-go eating—for example, milk, raisins, juice, fruit cups, pudding, baby carrots. "Single serve" are sensible portions.

A school-age child's appetite gradually increases; most eat more just before a growth spurt. During childhood, growth is gradual, accelerating most just prior to and during early adolescence: for girls, from ages ten through fourteen, and for boys, from ages twelve through sixteen. As long as a child is growing normally, he or she is getting enough calories. By tracking a child's weight and height, your child's healthcare professional will advise if your child is consuming adequate calories for healthy growth.

Food Preferences and Habits. Children's appetites and food preferences are changeable. Eating small amounts or not eating certain foods simply may mean that your child is testing his or her tastes, or perhaps exerting independence.

Children learn their food habits by watching others—not just parents, but also siblings, friends, teachers, and media. For parents and caregivers, your food choices and lifestyle habits help set their food decisions and behavior. How big are your portions? Do you eat a variety of foods including vegetables? Try new foods? Skip the urge to eat to relieve stress? Fit in physical activity each day? Set up chances for your child to make healthful choices and establish good eating habits. Early influence from parents is linked to the way children relate to food later in life.

Healthy Eating for Growing Up

School-age children love to measure their progress from year to year on a growth chart. They want energy to run and play—and the energy to do well in school. Parents, teachers, and other caregivers have the same priorities: helping children grow up healthy—and have the energy to experience their world.

Pyramid Power for Kids

MyPyramid is a healthy eating guide for all members of the family. That said, a kid-friendly version—MyPyramid for Kids—motivates children, ages six to eleven, to "Eat Right. Exercise. Have Fun." Among its goals: it's meant to help combat obesity, starting at a young age. What does MyPyramid for Kids on page 413 say to active, growing children?

● *Be physically active every day.* The child climbing the steps reminds kids to be physically active every

day: 60 minutes of moderate activity on most days! *Read "Get Up and Move!" in this chapter.*

● *Eat foods from every food group every day.* With a stripe for each food group, MyPyramid for Kids reminds children to eat a variety of foods from all five food groups—Grains, Vegetables, Fruit, Milk, and Meat and Beans Groups—plus healthy oils. Encourage many colorful vegetables, not just fries; fruit as a sweet snack, not just ice cream; and chicken or fish sandwiches.

● *Choose healthier foods from each group.* Every food group has foods that kids should eat more often—more nutrient-rich foods. Offer mostly whole-grain crackers instead of cookies; yogurt rather than ice cream; raw veggies instead of chips; fruit in place of fruit pies. *See "Foods to 'Chews'" on page 414 for more ideas.*

● *Eat more from some food groups than others.* The stripes of MyPyramid are different sizes, suggesting how much from each group. Most children need more vegetables and fruits than they eat now. *"Vegetables for Kids: The Challenge," on page 413, offers tips.* Most children need more whole-grain foods, too; choose whole grains for crackers, breakfast cereals, and sandwich bread.

● *Make the right choices for you.* For help in making personal choices for eating better and moving, check the Web site (www.MyPyramid.gov).

● *Take it one step at a time.* For kids and parents, learning to eat smart and move more is sensible. Start with one new, good thing a day. Add another new one every day.

The Dietary Guidelines advise everyone ages two on up to consume enough fruits and vegetables, yet stay within their calorie needs. For school-aged kids, there's more food-group advice: *Consume whole-grain products often; at least half the grains should be whole grains. Children two to eight years should consume two cups per day of fat-free or low-fat milk or equivalent milk products. Children nine years of age and older should consume three cups per day of fat-free or low-fat milk or equivalent milk products.*

For more about the nutrients, foods, and amounts from the food groups and healthy oils, refer to chapter 10.

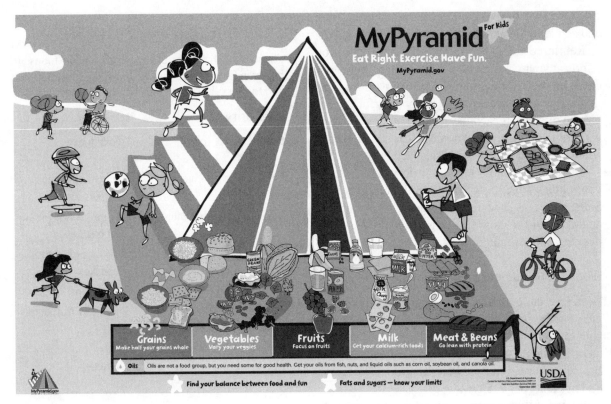

Vegetables for Kids: The Challenge

Kids—and adults, too—are urged to eat a variety of colorful, nutrient-rich vegetables for plenty of health reasons! American kids typically eat more than half their vegetable intake as potatoes (most often high-fat fries) or tomatoes. Snacks are often cookies, chips, other salty snacks, candy, and dessert foods rather than fruit or veggies.

What's a parent to do when vegetables are greeted with a chorus of "yuck"?

● Add veggies to kid favorites. Mix peas into macaroni and cheese. Add carrot shreds to spaghetti sauce, chili, lasagna, even peanut butter. Put zucchini shreds into burgers or mashed potatoes.

● "Fortify" ready-to-eat soup with extra vegetables or canned beans.

● Offer raw finger-food veggies. Kids may prefer uncooked vegetables. They like to "dip," too. So offer salsa, bean dip, or herb-flavored plain yogurt.

● Kids like the bright colors and crisp textures of vegetables. To keep them appealing, steam or microwave veggies in small amounts of water, or stir-fry.

● Start a "veggie club." Try to taste vegetables from A to Z, and check off letters of the alphabet as you go! As you shop, let kids pick a new vegetable as a family "adventure." Post a tasting chart on the refrigerator door to recognize family tasters.

● Grow veggies together. If you don't have a garden, plant a container garden. Most kids eat vegetables they grow!

● From your library, check out children's books about vegetables. Read the story, then taste the veggies together!

● Nothing works? Offer more fruit, another source of vitamins A and C, and phytonutrients.

Source: "Healthy Start: Food to Grow On," volume IV (Food Marketing Institute, American Dietetic Association, and American Academy of Pediatrics, 1995). Reprinted with permission by the Food Marketing Institute, ©1995.

Learning about Healthful Eating

Depending on their age, many children know the basics of healthful eating. And most know they need to eat smart and move their bodies to stay healthy. But it usually doesn't just happen. As a parent or caregiver, take time to help your child practice healthful eating and active living until they become everyday habits.

Reinforce the nutrition and physical education efforts at your child's school. For example, help your child: use MyPyramid to choose or help plan a family meal or snacks; count how many colorful vegetables he or she eats each day; prepare foods (perhaps with fruit or vegetables) at home that he or she learned about at school; and track physical activities.

Encourage healthful snacks and physical activity in your child's after-school program or activities, too. Some programs and clubs offer "junior chef" or gardening activities. Pick one that gives your child experiences with healthful food choices.

What about Nutrient Supplements?

Does your child eat a variety of foods? Do his or her meals and snacks follow MyPyramid advice? If so, your child probably doesn't need a nutrient supplement. Meals and snacks likely supply enough vitamins and other nutrients for growth and health. Food is the best nutrient source, anyway.

If your child has a feeding problem that lasts for several weeks or if you're unsure about your child's nutrient intake, get expert advice. Before you give your child a supplement, talk to your child's doctor or a registered dietitian.

Beware of claims for supplements targeted to help children get over colds, depression, or attention deficit disorder, among others. These claims aren't supported by sound science; such supplements may be harmful. An appropriate supplement may be recommended if your child avoids an entire food group due to a food dislike, allergy, or intolerance; or if your child is a vegetarian. If your water supply isn't fluoridated, a fluoride supplement may be advised by your dentist.

Have You Ever Wondered

... if herbal supplements are good for kids? Although touted as "natural" remedies or "healthy" alternatives, herbal supplements should be used only under the guidance of a qualified healthcare provider. Their effects can be powerful, potentially harmful to your child, and perhaps ineffective for the advertised benefit.

Foods to "Chews"

Chances are that some of your child's favorite foods are higher in fat and food energy. To get the most nutrition and to trim calories and fat, offer these foods:

MORE OFTEN . . .	LESS OFTEN . . .
Baked potato, colorful veggies	French fries
Baked or grilled chicken	Fried chicken strips and nuggets
Bagels or English muffins	Doughnuts and breakfast pastries
Graham crackers, animal crackers, fig bars	Chocolate-chip cookies, cupcakes
Pretzels, plain popcorn	Potato chips
Low-fat or fat-free milk, 100% fruit juice	Soft drinks, fruit drinks
Raw vegetable snacks, fruit	Candy
Frozen yogurt	Ice cream

If your health provider recommends a nutrient supplement for your child:

● Buy what's advised, perhaps a children's supplement. Check with the pharmacist if you need help. It should have no more than 100 percent of the Daily Values (DV). Unless stated otherwise, the % Daily Values stated on the Supplement Facts panel are meant for children age four or older, as well as for adults. On supplements meant for younger children, look for the % DV for children under age four. *Beware:* An adult iron supplement can be dangerous for children!

● Choose a supplement with a childproof cap. Store it out of your child's reach.

● Give a supplement only in the safe, recommended dose. Too much can be harmful.

● Remember: Supplements are just that—supplements—not an excuse to forgo smart eating.

● Remind children that supplements aren't candy, even if they come in fun names, colors, shapes, and package designs.

● Remember that enriched and fortified foods may

have the same added nutrients that the supplement has. Read labels so your child doesn't get too much.

For more about supplements, see chapter 23.

Eating Strategies for Children

How can you help your school-age child eat well? Many feeding strategies you used during the preschool years apply now, too. *See "Mealtime Tactics" earlier in this chapter.* Keep these ideas top-of-mind, too:

Most school-age children do best with a regular meal schedule. Like preschoolers, they can't compensate for hunger as adults can. When meals aren't regular or when meals are missed, children tend to snack more heavily throughout the day, so they're less hungry at mealtime. Space snacks at least one hour before a meal. Two to three snacks per day are enough for most children; make their calories count for good nutrition!

Breakfast skipping is a concern. Breakfast is a healthful, important start for a day of learning and active play. *See "Nutrition and Learning" and "Easy Breakfasts for Kids to Make" in this chapter.*

The family table offers nutrition benefits—and more! According to recent research, kids who eat frequent family dinners also eat more calcium, iron, fiber, and several vitamins, and less saturated fat and *trans* fats. They also eat more fruit or vegetables daily. Family mealtime offers more than nutrition to school-aged kids: some studies link frequent family meals to healthier weight, better school performance, and language development from family "talk time" at the table—and for teens, less risk for substance abuse. So the family table matters!

Telling kids to eat nutritious foods and have good table manners is one thing; showing them is better! The family table promotes family bonding—a time to talk, listen, and create family memories.

● Eat as a family—if possible, at least once a day. If it's breakfast, set the table the night before for less effort in the morning.

● If your family is always "on the go," designate family dinner nights. Planning ahead makes it easier to fit family meals in.

● Cook fast, eat slowly. Spend your kitchen time together at the table rather than on making a fancy meal. *See "Quick-to-Fix-Meal Tips" in chapter 10.*

● Turn off the TV, and put the phone answering system on to make food and family important.

● Eat around a table, not side by side at the counter. That's better for conversation and eye contact.

● Keep family mealtime positive: pleasant talk, a chance for everyone (including your child) to share and get attention, a mealtime that's neither rushed nor prolonged.

Children need to make their own food decisions. They usually eat better when they feel in control of their choices. As an adult, provide a variety of nutrient-rich foods—new and familiar—from which your child can choose.

● Let your child choose what and how much to eat from what you offer. Respect his or her food preferences and appetite. Help your child learn to eat slowly and pay attention to feeling full. By learning hunger and fullness cues, your child will learn to eat enough, but not overeat. Give your child the freedom to politely refuse foods he or she doesn't want.

● Involve kids in planning meals and snacks. It's a chance to practice making food decisions. Children often eat foods that they help plan and prepare.

● Encourage your child to try new foods—without forcing or bribing them. Trying new foods is like a new hobby; it expands his or her food knowledge, experience, and skills. Include foods from cultures other than your own. Acknowledge that your child will like some, but not all, of those foods. That's okay.

Kids learn to like foods they eat often. If you offer fruits and vegetables regularly—and if they see you eating them—your child likely will learn to like them.

Snacks help children eat for health. Chosen carefully, they supply nutrient-rich food-group foods—and nutrients—that may be missing from the day's meals. Snacks can help supply food energy that growing, active children need. Kids who use more energy in active play, organized sports, or after-school activities need more food energy—and more snacks—than kids who watch a lot of TV, play video games, spend time on a computer, or have a sedentary after-school routine. *For snacks kids can make, see "Kitchen Nutrition: Healthful, No-Cook Snacks for Kids" later in this chapter. See "Challenge Three: That Snack Attack!" in chapter 10.*

What children eat over several days counts—not what they eat for one meal or one day. There's no need for concern if your child occasionally skips food-group foods or doesn't eat much at a meal.

Children develop good eating habits when mealtimes and snacktimes are pleasant. Mealtime stress can lead to emotional overeating or undereating, so try to avoid fussing, nagging, arguing, or complaining at the table.

Nutrition and Learning

Why do kids need breakfast? Among other reasons, a well-nourished child is ready to learn. Fit kids more likely have the energy, stamina, and self-esteem that enhance their ability to learn. Healthful eating, along with regular physical activity, helps kids get and stay fit.

Nutrition experts, other health professionals, and educators recognize that severe nutrient deficiencies—which may be linked to improper growth, retarded mental development, and very low energy levels—hinder learning. Iron deficiency among children leads to poor behavior, difficulty concentrating, and poor performance.

Mild undernutrition isn't easily recognized. But it may affect how children learn—for example, a mild iron deficiency can affect brain function. Mild undernutrition may not be an economic issue, but instead come from poor food choices or meal skipping.

Regular breakfast skipping is linked to lower school achievement and performance. Conversely, a morning meal may help children succeed with learning and provide energy to learn. Studies show that breakfast eaters tend to have higher school attendance, less tardiness, and fewer hunger-induced stomach aches in the morning. Their overall test scores tend to be better. And they may concentrate better, solve problems more easily, and have better muscle coordination. Kids who eat breakfast are less likely to be overweight and more likely to get enough calcium, too. *For more about breakfast, see "Why Breakfast?" in chapter 10 and "Easy Breakfasts for Kids to Make" in this chapter.*

For Kids Only—Today's School Meals

What's for school lunch? What's for school breakfast? For parents, school meals offer an inexpensive, convenient, and nutritious solution for one or two meals daily for their kids. For many, school meals contribute significantly to their overall nutrient and energy intake. For kids who aren't hungry first thing in the morning, school breakfast may offer the perfect solution.

In most school districts—probably yours—school meals are regulated through the U.S. Department of Agriculture (USDA). The USDA meal patterns are designed carefully to supply about one-quarter of a child's need for key nutrients and energy from School Breakfast, and about one-third of them from School Lunch, at different age or grade groups.

The USDA's National School Food Service Program (NSFSP) helps children and teens make healthful food choices. The challenge? Serving meals that appeal to kids and support advice from the Recommended Dietary Allowances, calorie goals, and the Dietary Guidelines for Americans. School breakfast and lunch menus must meet nutrient standards for adequate calories and nutrients for specific age groups, with fat and saturated fat reduced to advised levels. Local school meal programs are charged with planning and serving meals that help children expand the variety of foods in their diet; add more fruits, vegetables, and grains, preferably whole grains, to the foods they already eat; and construct a diet lower in fat.

Many schools have modified their menus—for example, serving leaner beef, oven-baked fries, more vegetable and fruit variety, sandwiches served on whole-grain bread, dried and fresh fruit, salad bars, and fat-free milk.

Because most school meals have federal financial support, children and teens of all income levels have access to nutritious meals during school at a low cost. Some kids qualify for free or reduced-price meals.

If your child buys school meals, he or she may have choices on the cafeteria line, perhaps more than one vegetable or several types of milk. In many schools, students can select three to five items from the school lunch menu for the same price. Other schools provide up to seven items, including more fruits and vegetables. Having choices helps students build smart eating skills—and it helps ensure that children eat healthful meals. It's part of "eating right" education!

As a parent volunteer, you can be involved in and support school meals in your community—and help your child or teen choose healthful meals at school:

● Get familiar with the menu. Keep a current school lunch menu and perhaps a breakfast menu in your kitchen. Find menus in school mailings or in your local newspaper. You can ask for nutrition information about the menus from the school food service director.

● Go over the menu with your child. Talk about making choices on the cafeteria line; practice at home.

● If your child has a food allergy, restricts food for any reason (perhaps for religious, cultural, or health reasons), or chooses to be a vegetarian, talk to a school administrator and school food service staff. Most schools can prepare meals that match your child's unique needs—if they know ahead. *For dealing with food allergies, refer to chapter 21.*

● Join or set up a parent advisory committee for the school food service program. In 2006, schools involved in the NSFSP were required to have Local Wellness Policies. Parents can be involved!

● Have lunch—or breakfast—with kids occasionally. Parents usually are welcome to eat a school meal to become familiar with the school food program, the foods served, and the atmosphere in the cafeteria.

● Get to know the school food service staff. Volunteer to help with meal events, with food tastings, or at regular meal hours. Help in a school garden. Express your support. As you build relationships, pass along constructive suggestions.

● Support school nutrition education. Find out what your children are learning about food, nutrition, and active play, and help them practice at home. There's plenty of sound, often interactive, nutrition education for kids and families on Web sites. *See www.kids.gov. Refer to chapter 24 for judging "Nutrition in Cyberspace."*

● When school menus offer burgers, pizza, and tacos, encourage your child to choose a salad, fruit, yogurt, and/or milk to go with them.

● Encourage school clubs and parent associations to serve nutrient-rich snacks and drinks for fund-raising events, school parties, and in school vending machines. Advocate for school policies that ensure that the foods available at school help children make healthful food and beverage choices.

Another school-related tip: Be an advocate for moderate to vigorous physical activity as part of every school day. Encourage your child to play actively during recess. Balancing stringent academic standards with physical activity during the school day is chal-

---

Easy Breakfasts for Kids to Make

Breakfast—with food from the Milk, Grains, Vegetable, Fruit, and/or Meat and Beans Groups—can set your child or teen in a healthful nutrition direction for the day. What's for breakfast? Even if kids are on their own in the morning, most can make these easy breakfasts. And they go down even "healthier" with juice or milk!

G = Grains , **V** = Vegetable, **F** = Fruit, **M** = Milk, **MB** = Meat and Beans

● Cheese slices served with—or melted on—whole-wheat toast, fruit juice   **M** **G** **F**
● Iron-fortified cereal and milk, with banana slices   **G** **M** **F**
● Peanut butter spread on toasted whole grain bread or a waffle, or rolled inside a wheat tortilla, tangerine   **MB** **G** **F**
● Fruit—bananas, strawberries, raisins—and milk on instant oatmeal   **F** **M** **G**
● Cold pizza   **G** **M** **V**
● Leftover spaghetti or macaroni and cheese, banana   **G** **M** **F**
● Apple and cheese slices between whole-wheat or graham crackers   **F** **M** **G**
● Breakfast cereal topped with fresh fruit and a scoop of frozen yogurt   **G** **F** **M**

lenging for schools. Encourage your school to make physical education part of the curriculum. Being active helps children learn and stay healthy.

Brown-Bagging It!

Often, the older the children are, the more they want to join classmates in the cafeteria line. But some children prefer to carry a bag lunch. If that's true for your child, pack easy-to-prepare and fun meals that are healthful, safe, and nutritious.

● What tote will your child choose: brown bag, insulated bag, or lunch box? Ask what your child prefers. For some kids, having the "right" tote is important. A lunch box is easier to clean; it may keep food cool longer. Wash it after every use! Always use a clean, new brown bag.

● If you send perishable foods, such as a sandwich with meat, include a small, frozen cold pack. And remind the child to bring it back home! A frozen pouch or box of juice also keeps food cool.

● Plan easy-to-eat foods—for example, sandwiches, raw vegetable pieces (carrots, red or green bell peppers, cucumbers, cherry tomatoes), crackers, cheese slices or cubes, string cheese, whole fruit, individual containers of pudding, or an oatmeal cookie. If you pack an orange, score the rind so it's easy to peel—or tuck in a tangerine instead! It's okay to pack a brownie or a small bag of chips as part of a healthful bag lunch. Kids may need the extra energy they supply.

● Expect children to help plan and prepare their school lunches. When they're involved, they'll probably eat every morsel—rather than trade their raw veggies for someone else's cookie.

● Remind kids to store their carried meals at school in a clean, safe place—away from sunlight and the heat vent in the classroom and not in a dirty gym bag!

● *Hint:* Add extra pleasure to a carried meal with an occasional surprise tucked inside—a riddle, a comic, or a note that says, "You're somebody special!" Knowing that someone cares is "nourishing" in its own way.

See "Carry It Safe" in chapter 12.

Weighty Problems for Children

Over the past thirty years, the number of overweight children in the United States has more than tripled, with about 15 percent of kids ages six to eleven considered overweight, and 15 percent of teens ages twelve to nineteen overweight, according to 2002 data from the Centers for Disease Control and Prevention. Obesity rates have risen, too. In fact, overweight has been described as the most common nutrition problem among American children today.

Excess weight during these early years can have long-term physical and psychological consequences. Compared with normal-weight peers, overweight children more likely become obese adults, and so more prone to health problems later in life—for example, diabetes, heart disease, high blood pressure, stroke, osteoarthritis, gallbladder disease, and some forms of cancer. Research shows that about 60 percent of overweight children, ages five to ten, have at least one heart disease risk factor besides being overweight, such as elevated total cholesterol, triglycerides, insulin, or blood pressure; 25 percent had two or more risk factors for heart disease. They also may have sleep apnea (short cessation of breathing while sleeping), problems with balance or ease of moving, and early puberty. With early puberty girls have more estrogen

---

Have You Ever Wondered

... how you know if your child is eating right? Start by asking: Is my child growing well? Does he or she have energy to play and learn? If so, he or she probably is eating enough. Your child's doctor, pediatric nurse, or a registered dietitian can help you monitor your child's growth and development by plotting his or her progress on a growth chart. The other question to ask: Is your child eating a variety of foods and enough from the five food groups of MyPyramid? If so, he or she probably is getting enough nutrients to grow well.

... if your child gets enough to drink? Active children need eight or more cups of water during the day, as you do. Children perspire with active play, even outside in cold weather when they're bundled up. Just plain water is great for replenishing fluids; bring some along if you plan to be out for longer than an hour, or go on an extended car trip. Kids may drink more water if it's offered in appealing "sports bottles." *Check chapter 19 if your child is involved in sports.*

over a lifetime, and perhaps greater risk for breast and ovarian cancer later on.

Of concern, children who may be overweight are more likely to develop insulin resistance, which often precedes adult-onset type 2 diabetes. Type 2 diabetes, usually seen in overweight adults, now is being seen in children and teens as well! Complications from diabetes are appearing sooner, too. *See "Children and Diabetes" in chapter 22.*

There are psychological prices, too: overweight children may lose their self-esteem, have a poor body image, or feel emotionally stressed. Another consequence: overweight children may be teased or bullied, feel stigmatized, or isolate themselves from their peers, teachers, and family.

Why do children become overweight? There's no one reason. Family history, inactivity, and poor food habits all contribute to childhood weight problems. A child with one or two overweight parents has a higher risk; the reasons may be genetic, behavioral, or both. It's probably not limited to genetic factors. It's true, however, that children often mimic the food and lifestyle habits they observe at home. Heavy snacking, irregular meals, inactivity, and eating more calories than they use in daily physical activity results in weight problems, too. It's highly unlikely that a child's weight problem is caused by a hormone imbalance.

A family history doesn't destine children to being overweight adults. Often children shed extra "kid" fat during the rapid growth spurt of puberty. Overweight kids won't necessarily be overweight adults, either. However, the risk goes up as children get older if they still carry excess weight. Increased physical activity and balanced, healthful eating are key to helping prevent a child from becoming overweight. Addressing weight problems early is important.

How do you know if your child is overweight? Adults should never assess a child's body weight by their own standards. BMI charts for adults aren't meant for kids! *Instead see "BMIs for Kids: Tracking Their Growth" earlier in this chapter.* At each stage of development, children have different amounts of body fat. Children of the same age aren't necessarily the same shape either. Your child's doctor should make the assessment.

How can adults help overweight children achieve a healthy weight—while supporting good nutrition?

Because their bodies are growing and developing, weight loss isn't the best approach for most children. Instead, for most kids, slowing or stopping weight gain so a child grows into his or her weight is usually best. In other words, let a child's height catch up with his or her weight. A diet that's too restrictive—with too few calories—may not supply the food energy and nutrients a child needs for normal growth and development and can trigger unhealthy binge eating if the child feels too deprived.

For overweight children, the Dietary Guidelines advise: *Reduce the rate of body weight gain while allowing growth and development. Consult a healthcare provider before placing a child on a weight reduction diet.* For overweight kids with chronic disease and/or who are on medication: *Consult a healthcare provider about weight loss strategies prior to starting a weight-reduction program to ensure appropriate management of other health conditions.*

Weight problems aren't just about food. Many factors, such as emotions, family problems, lifestyle, and self-image, intertwine with eating behavior. Address the whole child—emotionally, socially, mentally, and physically—as you address weight management.

Lifestyle changes—often for the whole family—offer a good approach for helping an overweight child manage his or her weight. *"Eating Strategies for Children" earlier in this chapter apply to every child—overweight, normal weight, or underweight.*

If Your Child or Teen Has a Weight Problem . . .

● Seek professional advice. Your child needs a medical evaluation first. A registered dietitian, your doctor, or the school nurse can help you find an approach that's right for the nutritional and developmental needs of your child. Keep in mind that weight loss approaches for adults aren't right for children. *See "How to Find Nutrition Help . . ." in chapter 24.*

● Encourage physical activities your child enjoys. Besides burning calories, physical activity indirectly affects eating—for example, appetite control, stress release, and mental diversion from eating. Make physical activity a family affair. When parents are physically active, their kids are often active, too.

● Overweight children are often self-conscious in

organized or competitive games. Instead, encourage activities such as walking the dog or biking, where skill and an audience are less important. *For more about physical activity, see "Get Up and Move" on page 422.*

● Give your child more control over how much to eat. That may seem counterintuitive; however, when parents pressure or restrict food choices too much, kids don't learn self-regulation. They may overeat if they can't read their body signals for hunger and satiety.

● Consider other reasons to avoid restricting food. An overly restricted eating approach may keep your child from getting nutrients he or she needs. Restrictions also may lead to sneaking food elsewhere, then feeling guilty or bad about themselves.

● Involve your whole family in healthful eating so your overweight child won't feel singled out.

● Tailor portion sizes for your child. Large portions encourage overeating. Use smaller plates so less looks like more. A hungry child can ask for more.

● Avoid undue attention to eating. For example, for-

Have You Ever Wondered

... if foods grown with pesticides are safe for kids? With more than a hundred required tests directly relevant to children and infants, there's no evidence that children are being harmed from pesticide residues in food, water, or the environment. Any residue is hundreds to thousands of times lower than what might potentially pose a health risk. The safety evaluation takes children's diets, body weight, and rapid growth into account. And the Food Quality Assurance Act of 1996 includes additional provisions aimed at protecting children from pesticides. The health benefits of eating fruits and vegetables far outweigh any potential risk.

As a precaution, rinse vegetables to remove any residues. *For more about foods grown with pesticides, see "Pesticides: Carefully Controlled" in chapter 9.*

... if lead in drinking water is harmful to children? Infants and children are at higher risk for lead poisoning than others. Among other problems, lead that builds up in the body over time can cause brain damage. Health experts advise that children get screened at ages one and two, perhaps more often if there's a risk. *For more about screening and addressing lead in drinking water, see "Get the Lead Out!" in chapter 8.*

get rewarding or punishing a child with food. In that way you won't reinforce an emotional link to eating.

● Stock your kitchen with lower-calorie snack choices such as raw vegetables, fruit, milk, or vanilla wafers. Instead of heavy snacking, meals should provide most of your child's nutrients and food energy.

● Avoid labeling food as "good" or "bad." Instead, help your child see how any food can fit in a healthful eating pattern. Even kids who need to reduce body fat can have an occasional cookie or a piece of candy. In fact, they probably need a high-calorie snack from time to time to meet their energy needs. Anyway, the body doesn't see food in black-and-white terms. It's the whole eating plan that counts.

● Store food out of sight; be careful about bringing a lot of higher-calorie foods into the house. When food sits on the kitchen counter, grabbing a cookie or chips may be more habit than hunger. For many people—kids, too—just seeing food stimulates the appetite.

● Set time limits on watching television—no more than one or two hours daily of total media time, advises the American Academy of Pediatrics. Limit video games and computer time, too. All three keep kids away from active play. Children who watch four or more hours of television a day are twice as likely to be overweight as youngsters who don't.

● For everyone: eat only in the kitchen or dining room. Kids probably won't eat as much—and they'll be more conscious about eating. High-calorie snacks may go along with TV watching or homework.

● Refrain from eating meals in front of the TV. It's easy to eat more when attention is shifted away from the meal and satiety cues, and instead to a TV show.

● Talk to your child about his or her feelings. Observe emotions and subsequent behavior. Together look for ways other than eating to address emotions. Help your child understand: even though eating may feel good for a while, food can't solve problems!

● Be aware: kids may say they're hungry when they're bored or want attention. Probe a little. Offer a snack, perhaps a cracker or an apple. If neither appeals, the child is probably bored, not hungry.

Consider this advice about childhood weight issues, even if your child's weight seems healthy: *see "Obesity and Kids: A Heavy Burden" in chapter 2.*

Should You Have Your Child's Cholesterol Level Checked?

Perhaps. It's not routinely recommended for all children. The American Heart Association advises screening for children with a family history of risk factors: blood-related parents, grandparents, aunts, and uncles with high cholesterol levels, high triglyceride levels, or cardiovascular disease before age fifty-five for men and age sixty-five for women.

If your child has a higher than normal blood cholesterol level, don't panic. High cholesterol levels among children don't necessarily predict high levels in adulthood. But when children come from high-risk families, it's prudent to check with a doctor and work with a registered dietitian to bring the levels down: good advice for the whole family!

For cardiovascular health, young people, ages two through nineteen years, should maintain acceptable blood cholesterol levels:

LEVELS	TOTAL CHOLESTEROL (MG/DL)	LDL CHOLESTEROL (MG/DL)
High:	200 or greater	130 or greater
Borderline:	170 to 199	110 to 129
Acceptable:	Less than 170	Less than 110

HDL levels should be greater than or equal to 35 mg/dL; triglycerides should be less than or equal to 150 mg/dL.

Compelling research suggests that fatty buildup in arteries begins in childhood and is more likely with higher blood cholesterol levels. For that reason, the American Heart Association offers advice for children and teens about these related health risks:

● Cigarette smoking: discourage it.

● High blood pressure: identify and treat it.

● Obesity: prevent it or reduce weight.

● Diabetes: diagnose and treat it.

● Inactivity: encourage regular aerobic exercise (30 to 60 minutes), on most days of the week. At the same time, kids need to eat enough fruits and vegetables each day, and choose foods that are low in saturated fats, *trans* fats, and cholesterol.

For more about blood cholesterol levels, refer to "Your Healthy Heart" chapter 22. For the American Heart Association guidelines for cardiovascular health for infants, children, and adolescents, go to www .americanheart.org.

Fear of Weight Gain

A desire to be overly thin, prompted by media messages and by what parents say and do, is reaching down to school-age children. Children, mostly girls, as young as age six express concerns about their body image and gaining weight. Inappropriate weight loss can interfere with growth—and may lead to eating disorders down the road.

Parents may play an even bigger role than media in shaping a child's body image. Even before your child hits adolescence:

● Quit worrying about your child's weight. Instead, strive for a positive eating relationship with your child. Teach healthful eating habits.

● Refrain from negative comments about your own weight or anyone else's weight. Avoid pressuring your child to conform to any body size or shape.

● Set a good example in the way you manage your own weight and feel about your own body image. Skip the lure of fad dieting yourself.

● Encourage physical activity to build muscles and coordination. And work to develop your child's social skills, self-confidence, and self-esteem.

See "Disordered Eating: Problems, Signs, and Help" in chapter 2 and "Mainly for Girls: Pressure to Be Thin" later in this chapter.

On another note: Whether or not your child has a weight problem, he or she can be a thoughtful classmate, friend, or sibling to those who are overweight or underweight. Remind your child that dealing with weight problems isn't easy. Yet all children have the same basic needs and lots to offer, no matter what their body size. Teasing or bullying isn't caring, respectful, or fair.

Eating Out with Kids

Eating out with kids? A necessity in your busy lifestyle—or a special treat for your family? To make restaurant meals a healthful and pleasant experience for the whole family, and a chance to teach kids how to make healthful choices and behave away from home:

● Choose a restaurant that caters to children, perhaps with healthier children's menus. A place that serves food quickly probably is best; waiting too long at the table is hard for kids. If you have a young child, ask for a high chair or a booster seat. Save upscale table service for older children, teens, and adults.

● Match your eating-out schedule to a child's needs. When meals are delayed, kids can't compensate for hunger pangs as adults can. You'll only end up with a cranky meal companion! Offer a small snack ahead.

● Look beyond the children's menu for foods on the regular menu. Skip the urge to just order fries or fried chicken nuggets for your child. A good alternative: take home half the order; order other foods, too.

● Before ordering, ask about the preparation. Most children like plain foods with the sauce or the dressing on the side. In that way they have a choice. Substitute "sides": perhaps carrot sticks in place of fries.

● Choose two or three suitable menu items. Then let your child pick—and even place the order if he or she wants to. (Avoid pressuring your child.) Making choices encourages independence and gives kids control over their eating.

● Let kids order familiar favorites when they eat out. For new foods offer a bite or two from your order.

● If regular portions are too big for children, ask for appetizer portions. Or share an order . . . perhaps between two kids or with you. Kids shouldn't be urged or expected to "polish" their plate. Instead, consider bringing leftovers home safely.

● Curb your child's appetite while you wait. Ask for a small portion of raw vegetables or bread—just enough to take the edge off hunger, not enough to interfere with a meal. Ask for drinks *with* the meal, not before, so your child doesn't fill up on liquids.

● Make eating out a pleasant experience for kids. Engage them in table talk as you wait for your meal.

For more about restaurant ordering, see chapter 14.

Get Up and Move!

Smart eating is just part of a healthy start on life. Kids need to be physically active, too. Inactivity is linked to the dramatic rise in childhood overweight!

What if . . . Your Child Gets Fussy in a Restaurant?

● Excuse yourselves from the table. Take a short walk.

● Talk in a calm, quiet, and positive way. This isn't the place for loud discipline.

● Avoid forcing your child to eat. Instead, have the meal packed to take home.

● Ask if the restaurant has a paper place mat to color or draw on. Bring your own crayons—just in case.

● Bring along a stuffed animal to "share" the fun.

Source: Duyff, R. L. *Nibbles for Health* (Washington, D.C.: U.S. Department of Agriculture, 2002).

Today's children often watch TV during their "prime time" for play. In fact, by first grade, many kids have watched five thousand hours of TV. According to health experts, children who watch too much TV may not get enough physical exercise or time for creative activity. Besides spending too much leisure time at the computer, TV, or video games, there's concern about safe outdoor play. Kids often ride instead of walk to school and have less chance at school for noncompetitive play. To prevent your "tater tots" from becoming the next generation of "couch potatoes," make physical activity fun and part of your family's routine.

Active Play: Good Moves for Children

What makes physical activity so important for kids? Good physical health and fitness are obvious. Through active, safe play, children can develop social skills, build a positive self-image, enhance their ability to learn, and even help protect themselves from danger. An active child is also more likely be an active adult!

● Regular physical activity helps with a child's physical development. It builds muscular strength, including a strong heart muscle. Strong muscles promote good posture, which, in turn, affects a child's health and self-image. Weight-bearing activities such as running and skating help strengthen growing bones. Being active also helps build stamina, a quality that promotes learning and play.

● Can children quickly run in case of danger? Although each circumstance has different physical demands, strong, physically fit children deal better with many emergencies. Regular physical activity offers better protection from danger!

● Active kids are more likely to keep their bodies lean and avoid the growing problem of overweight. Health experts recommend increased physical activity as one of the best ways for kids to trim extra body fat.

● Regular physical activity supports learning. Many activities develop coordination. Playing catch develops eye-hand coordination. Jumping rope or hopscotch helps teach spatial relationships, while soccer helps develop manipulative skills.

● As children play actively with others, they also develop and practice social skills. With games of all kinds, they can share, cooperate, communicate, support each other, and act as a team.

● Being on a winning team isn't the only way to build self-esteem. Succeeding at any physical activity—riding a bike, swimming a lap, or catching a ball—helps build self-confidence and a positive self-image.

● Active play is part of the joy of childhood! Physical activity that's pleasant more likely becomes a lifelong habit. A lifestyle that includes regular physical activity lowers the risk of many chronic diseases.

Kids, Go for It!

For good health, children need to move! For children, the Dietary Guidelines advise: *Engage in at least sixty minutes of physical activity on most, preferably all, days of the week.* Kids don't need a structured activity program to meet this goal. And competitive sports may not be appropriate for some kids; they can create unnecessary pressure and take the fun away.

Active play—biking, in-line skating, playing tag, jump-roping, swimming, or tossing a Frisbee, among others—can offer enough exercise for most children. Besides, it can be fun! *Hint:* Be sure that children have appropriate safety gear such as helmets, knee pads, or life jackets, as well as sunscreen (even in cold weather) and appropriate clothing.

Next time your kids say they don't know what to do, suggest something active. *See "Ten Things for Kids to Do Instead of Watching TV" on this page.*

To promote an active lifestyle you need to make

your moves, too. Be a role model. Join kids in active play—perhaps hike together as a weekend outing, ride bikes after dinner, play a quick game of catch or hopscotch after work, clean up a local nature trail, knead a loaf of bread, or take an active vacation (perhaps with hiking, swimming, or skiing). Plan for family activities, perhaps after dinner or every Saturday morning so that exercise happens! Party time? Make fun activities the main event: backyard "Olympics" with relay races, bowling, or skating. Going to a party? Give gifts that encourage physical activity, such as sporting equipment or physically active games.

Ten Things for Kids to Do Instead of Watching TV

1. Encourage kids to set up a jump rope contest. If they're older, go "double dutch" with two ropes. (A Hula Hoop contest is fun, too.)
2. Take the dog for a brisk walk together. Don't have a dog? Have kids take their teddy bears for a stroll instead. Walking as a family is good talking time!
3. Give kids colored chalk to create a sidewalk mural. Or draw a hopscotch game—fun to play alone or with friends.
4. Don't let rainy days put a damper on fun! Turn up the radio and dance inside.
5. Start a "hundred" walking club. Who's first in your family to walk a hundred times up and down the sidewalk or the stairs in your house?
6. Play a game of tag or kickball in the playground, park, or backyard.
7. If there's snow, make a snowman or go sledding. Or take the family ice skating at any time of year at an ice rink—even in July!
8. On warm days, go in-line skating or ride bikes (remember the helmet and pads), or run through sprinkler "rain."
9. Enjoy a hike together in a nearby park or forest preserve. Have kids find ten points of natural interest to enjoy as you hike.
10. Host a neighborhood bicycle wash outside—or a dog wash instead!

Source: Adapted from *"Healthy Start: Food to Grow On,"* vol. IV (Food Marketing Institute, American Dietetic Association, and American Academy of Pediatrics, 1995). Reprinted with permission by the Food Marketing Institute, ©1995.

Healthful, No-Cook Snacks for Kids

Kids have a case of the after-school munchies? Try these healthful, no-cook snacks. They're easy and fun to make—and depending on your child's age, require little or no adult supervision.

G = Grains, **F** = Fruit, **V** = Vegetable, **MB** = Meat and Beans, **M** = Milk

- *Snack Kebobs.* Cut raw vegetables and fruit into chunks. Skewer them onto thin pretzel sticks. **V** **F** **G**
(*Note:* To prevent discoloration, dip cut apples, bananas, or pears in orange juice.)

- *Veggies with Dip.* Cut celery, zucchini, cucumbers, or carrots into sticks or coins. Then dip them **V** into prepared salsa.

- *Banana Pops.* Peel a banana. Dip it in yogurt, then roll in crushed breakfast cereal; freeze. **F** **M** **G**

- *Fruit Slices and PB.* Spread peanut butter on apple or banana slices. **F** **MB**

- *Fruit Shake-ups.* Put ½ cup low-fat fruit yogurt and ½ cup cold fruit juice in a nonbreakable, **M** **F** covered container. Make sure the lid is tight. Then shake it up, and pour into a cup.

- *Sandwich Cutouts.* Using cookie cutters with fun shapes like dinosaurs, stars, and hearts, cut slices **M** **MB** **G** of cheese, meat, and whole-grain bread. Then put them together to make fun sandwiches. Eat the edges, too.

- *Peanut Butter Balls.* Mix peanut butter and bran or cornflakes in a bowl. Shape the mixture into **M** **G** balls with clean hands. Then roll them in crushed graham crackers.

- *Salsa Quesadillas.* Fill a soft tortilla with cheese and salsa, fold over, and grill. **G** **M** **V**

- *Ice Cream–Wiches.* Put a small scoop of ice cream or frozen yogurt between two oatmeal cook- **M** **G** ies or frozen whole-wheat waffles. Make a batch of these sandwiches ahead, and freeze them.

- *Ants on a Log.* Fill celery with peanut butter. Arrange raisins along the top. **V** **MB** **F**

Until the teen years, avoid the urge to compete with your kids in organized games such as tennis; usually a child is no match for adult strength and skill. Physical activity needs to feel good to the body and the mind. Encourage "personal best."

Encourage active play so exercise doesn't seem like punishment. If your child feels embarrassed about not being good enough in a sport, find something active your child likes or feels good about. It doesn't need to be a team or group activity. Do it together to build confidence.

Do you need after-school care for your kids? Look for programs that include physical activity: perhaps in Scout groups, outdoor centers, recreational and community centers, or your child's school. Or sign them up for gymnastics, dance, or swim classes.

For more ideas, see "Twenty Everyday Ways to Get Moving" in chapter 2.

Kids' Kitchen

Your kitchen is a learning laboratory! Just like learning to read and write, becoming self-sufficient with food preparation is a life skill your child or teen needs to accomplish. In the kitchen kids learn about food and become health-wise consumers of food.

If you're a single parent or in a dual-career household, your child also may share responsibility for family nutrition and be expected to feed himself or herself sometimes. Depending on age, your child may help with food shopping, preparation, and cleanup. Kitchen skills are more than fun. They may be a necessity!

Let's Cook!

Prepare food with your child—and explore a wide variety of foods. At the same time, your child can learn how to handle and prepare foods in a safe, healthful way.

When kids cook, they practice many skills—besides how to handle and prepare foods to nourish themselves and keep food safe to eat. By reading a recipe, children learn new words and practice reading. They identify foods and learn their qualities as they gather ingredients. By preparing a recipe, they practice measuring, counting, timing, sequencing, and following directions. Slicing, pouring, rolling dough, and shaping meat patties are among the food preparation activities that develop small-muscle movement and eye-hand coordination. Food preparation is practical science. Children might watch dough rise, see eggs coagulate, or observe how sugar dissolves in water.

Preparing food also promotes your child's social and emotional development. Children feel good about themselves when they successfully prepare foods to eat—and share with others. It's an opportunity to explore foods of other cultures and respect the similarities and the differences. Most important, preparing food together is a chance to be together.

Consider these guidelines for kitchen success:

● Choose foods and recipes that match your child's abilities. With foods a child might prepare alone, first make them together.

● For young cooks, choose illustrated children's cookbooks that show the foods, measurements, and steps along the way. Go over the safety and sanitation tips at the front of a child's cookbook.

● Ask your child to suggest foods he or she would like to make. Make it a total experience by shopping for ingredients together, too.

● Start with hand washing! And review safety precautions. Supervise children as they learn to work with knives, the stove, and other potentially dangerous equipment. Follow good cleanliness habits. *See "Kitchen Safety Alert" below.*

● Besides cooking together, have your child help you store food properly for food safety.

● Use this chance to show your child how to handle food to keep it clean and safe from spoilage and foodborne illness. Among the things to learn and practice: hand washing, using clean utensils for different foods, and using a meat thermometer. *For more guidance, see chapter 12.*

For easy recipes that children can prepare for snacks—or any meal of the day—see "Kitchen Nutrition: Healthful, No-Cook Snacks for Kids" on page 424.

Microwave Oven Safety for Kids

Because burns are a common hazard related to microwave oven use, make sure children know how to use a microwave oven safely.

● Make sure the microwave oven is on a sturdy stand—one that's low enough for kids. If children need to reach too high, they may pull a hot dish down on themselves.

● Teach children to read the controls on the microwave oven—the time, the power level, and the "start" and "stop" controls. If kids can't read them, they're too young to operate a microwave oven alone.

● Keep microwave-safe containers in one place—within a child's reach.

● Always have a child use potholders to remove heated food from the microwave oven—whether the food is hot or not. In that way it becomes a habit. Keep potholders handy for kids.

● Teach children to stir heated food before tasting. That distributes the heat and avoids hot spots that can cause burns.

● Show them how to open containers so that steam escapes away from their face. That includes packages of popped microwave popcorn.

● Until you're sure that children have mastered the art of microwaving, provide supervision.

For more tips on using a microwave oven safely, see "Play It Microwave-Safe" in chapter 12.

Kitchen Safety Alert

With all that goes on in a kitchen, food preparation sends some "red flags" for kids' safety. Cooking is safe—if your child learns to be careful. Make the kitchen a fun, rewarding place for kids; teach the basics of kitchen safety.

● Remind children to always wash their hands with soap and water before and after they handle food, and dry them well.

● Supervise your child around food, especially when he or she handles hot liquids, knives, appliances, and other potentially dangerous equipment.

● As your child is ready, teach kitchen safety tips: to use potholders when handling hot pans, pots, and dishes . . . to handle knives safely . . . to be very careful with hot liquids . . . and to use appliances safely. *See "Microwave Oven Safety for Kids" on page 425.*

● Set limits on what your child can—and can't—do without proper supervision. For example, your child can't use the oven if he or she is home alone.

● Remind your child to be aware of his or her hair and clothes before using the stove. Large, loose-fitting garments and long hair can catch fire.

● Practice what you preach. Your child will take his or her kitchen-safety cues from you.

● Practice what to do in case of fire. That includes "drop and roll" to smother the flames in case his or her clothes catch fire. Keep a fire extinguisher in view and teach your child how to use it.

● Try to keep food and utensils your child will use within easy reach. Keep a sturdy stool handy if he or she needs to reach higher. Remind your child not to climb on the counters or on a wobbling stool!

● Teach kids—even preschoolers—to call 911 (or emergency numbers such as those for the fire department, poison control center, or police in your area). Post the phone numbers in your kitchen where children can see them easily. Include the phone numbers of your doctor, a neighbor, and a relative.

● Practice the Heimlich maneuver with children. Like you, they can save the life of someone who's choking—if they know how. *See "How to Avoid Choking" in chapter 12. For infants, see "For Babies, Toddlers, and Preschoolers: How to Avoid Choking" in chapter 15.*

● Keep a first-aid kit handy and stocked. Teach your child how to use it for a minor cooking injury.

For more on preventing injuries, see "Quick Tips for Injury Prevention" in chapter 12.

Feeding the Teen Machine

By adolescence, many kids make most of their own decisions about food. Other than filling the refrigerator and kitchen shelves with food and preparing family meals, parents have far less control over what their adolescent child eats. Teenagers themselves exert stronger influence over family eating than before, perhaps sharing the shopping and food preparation. Compared with their childhood years, they probably consume more food and beverages away from home.

Chances are that teenagers know the basics of nutrition and healthful eating. However, peer pressure, school and work schedules, a sense of independence, lack of personal discipline, unrealistic notions about body weight, and a poor self-image are among the barriers to healthful eating. Food choices may not reflect what teens know about eating for fitness—much to their parents' dismay!

The same holds true for physical activity. Kids know why they should move more, but doing so has barriers, too.

Sound familiar? In a nutshell, adolescents often don't connect their immediate food and physical activity patterns to their long- or short-term health. Many teens live in a wonderful world of invulnerability. Others follow misguided advice: supplements for muscle building, unsafe dieting for weight loss, energy drinks—for energy! Read on for a few "teen-friendly" fitness strategies.

Many nutrition issues for adults also apply to your teenager: for example, calorie-dense snacking, meal skipping, fad diets, eating too few fruits and vegetables, smart vegetarian eating, smart fast-food choices, sports nutrition. Throughout the book, you'll find strategies your teen can use to address these issues.

Food, Nutrients, and the Teen Years

Second only to infancy, adolescence is the fastest growth stage in life! Even when teens reach their adult height (for girls sooner than for boys), their bodies are still growing and developing.

Puberty marks the start of the teenage growth spurt. That time differs for each child. For girls, puberty typically begins at about age twelve or thirteen, about two years younger than for boys. From the school-age years through the teens, the average youngster grows to be 20 percent taller and 50 percent heavier. Body changes that happen as children mature are stressful for some, and may affect their self-image and perhaps the choices they make about eating and physical activity. (Some overweight children may start puberty

Teens, Did You Know

... unhealthy dieting can stop you from growing to your full height? Your body needs calories and other nutrients to grow and develop fully. Most teens shouldn't "diet."

... your bones take in the most calcium during your teen years and early twenties? The best sources are milk, yogurt, and cheese, and most teens need the equivalent of three cups of milk daily.

... if you don't eat breakfast, your body is like a computer without power?

... eating cookies, candy, or other sweet foods before an athletic event won't give you an energy boost?

... for girls, when you have a menstrual period you lose iron? If you don't eat iron-rich foods to replace this loss, you may feel weak and tired.

... pizza and hamburgers are healthful food choices, especially if you know which toppings to choose (veggies, fruit, beans, lean protein)—and you eat sensible amounts?

... eating smart and moving more help you feel good, look good, and do your best!

sooner, but for now, there are too many unanswered questions to know why.)

How your teenage child grows—when, how, and how much—has more to do with genes than with food choices. However, smart eating does help determine if your child grows to his or her maximum height potential—with strong bones and a fit body.

All teens need enough calcium for bone growth and strength, protein for every body cell including muscles, carbohydrates and fats for energy, vitamins and minerals for the "sparks" that make it all happen, and enough water. Energy and nutrient needs increase to meet the growth demands of adolescence. Teens need understanding parents who appreciate that their adolescent's growth pattern, although different from a friend's, is perfectly normal.

Food Energy: How Much?

Teens need somewhat more calories than when they were a bit younger. Teenage boys on average need 1,800 to 2,600 calories a day if they're eleven to thirteen years, and 2,200 to 3,200 calories a day if they're fourteen to eighteen years of age. Teenage girls need

more, too: 1,800 to 2,200 calories a day if they're ages eleven to thirteen, and 1,800 to 2,400 calories a day if they're age fourteen to eighteen. Their gender, body size, growth rate, and activity level specifically determine how many calories they need. Those involved in strenuous physical activity such as soccer, basketball, football, or other sports may need 3,500 calories (more or less) daily.

Nutrients: For Some, An All-Time High

Many nutrient recommendations go up during adolescence. *Check the Dietary Reference Intakes in the Appendices to see how much.* As teens consume more food-group foods, they also get a nutrient and food energy boost to meet the demands of growth, health, and perhaps more physical activity. Typically, teens need to eat more fiber-rich foods, too.

Several nutrients may need attention in a teenager's food choices: calcium, iron, and perhaps zinc. That's usually due to poor food choices, or for girls especially, simply not eating enough. Dairy foods and lean protein foods provide these nutrients. Potassium, magnesium, vitamin E, and fiber likely need attention, too; eating enough fruit, vegetables, whole-grain foods, and healthy oils can provide enough of these. Read on to learn more.

Pregnancy affects a teenage girl's nutrition needs. Like any pregnancy, the need for nutrients and energy goes up; for teens, the recommendations are higher than for adult women, for their own growth and development, and for the developing fetus. *For more on the nutrition needs of a teenage pregnancy, see "For Pregnant Teens: Good Nutrition" in chapter 17.*

Calcium: A Growing Issue. "I'm sixteen, and I've stopped growing. So why do I need milk?" Actually, bones keep on growing into the adult years. Even when teenagers reach their adult height, bones continue to grow stronger as they become more dense. In fact, almost half of an adult's bone mass forms during the teen years. The stronger bones become during adolescence, the lower the risk of osteoporosis later on. Yet, only about 14 percent of girls and about 36 percent of boys ages twelve to nineteen in the United States consume the recommended amount of calcium!

Osteoporosis is really an adolescent health problem that manifests itself in later years. Teenagers—

children, too—who don't consume enough calcium put their bones at risk for the long term. They may start their adult years with a calcium deficit in their bones. With bone loss that comes as a natural part of aging, they have less to draw on, and their risk for osteoporosis, or brittle bone disease, goes up.

Teens are advised to consume enough calcium-rich foods so their bones become as strong as they can be. For children and teens ages nine through eighteen, the equivalent of three cups of calcium-rich dairy foods each day provide enough calcium for growing bones. According to the Dietary Reference Intakes, 1,300 milligrams of calcium daily is considered an Adequate Intake (AI). An 8-ounce glass of milk has about 300 milligrams of calcium.

What foods are teens' best calcium sources? Milk Group foods including milk, yogurt, and cheese—although a variety of foods have smaller amounts of calcium. Milk also contains other nutrients essential to healthy bone and tooth development: vitamins D, A, and B_{12}, potassium, magnesium, and protein. Canned salmon and sardines with bones, as well as some vegetables (such as mustard greens, collard greens, okra, broccoli, and bok choy), supply calcium. And some prepared foods are calcium-fortified, including some juice, soy drinks, breads, and breakfast cereal. *For more on calcium and a list of calcium-rich foods, see "Calcium: A Closer Look" in chapter 4.*

Why don't many teens consume enough calcium-rich dairy foods? Perhaps there's no milk on hand at home, or perhaps they don't like it. Maybe kids haven't made a habit of drinking milk with fast food. Or perhaps soft drinks compete. If milk is cold, convenient, and "cool," your teen more likely will drink it. *Tip:* Fill the fridge with flavored milk or yogurt drinks sold in "cool," single-serving containers.

Many teenage girls misguidedly link milk drinking to their fear of getting fat, including teens on fad diets or those with eating disorders. Yet those who watch calories can consume low-fat or fat-free dairy foods. Eight ounces of fat-free milk supplies fewer calories than 8 ounces of a soft drink or juice: only 86 calories and almost no fat, yet fat-free milk has as much calcium as whole milk!

Vegan eating patterns and lactose intolerance may be barriers, too. In either case, teens have plenty of practical ways to get enough calcium. *See chapter 20 for more about vegetarian eating, and chapter 21 for more about lactose intolerance.*

For more about bone health during adulthood, see "Osteoporosis: Reduce the Risks" in chapter 22.

Iron: The Fatigue Connection. Does your teenager seem chronically tired? Fatigue may come from too little sleep, an exhausting schedule, strenuous activity (a good kind of fatigue), or the emotional ups and downs of adolescence. Feeling tired also may be a symptom of a health problem or low iron levels in blood.

Iron is part of blood's hemoglobin, which carries oxygen to body cells. Once there, oxygen helps cells produce energy. When iron is in short supply, there's less oxygen available to produce energy—hence fatigue.

Iron needs go up dramatically in the teen years. During childhood (ages nine to thirteen) both boys and girls need about 8 milligrams of iron daily, according to the Dietary Reference Intakes. For adolescence, more muscle mass and a greater blood supply demand more iron, so the recommendation jumps to 15 milligrams of iron daily for girls ages fourteen to eighteen, and 11 milligrams daily for boys that age. Girls need more to replace iron losses from their menstrual flow. *See "Menstrual Cycle: More Iron for Women" in chapter 17.*

Many teens—girls especially—don't consume enough iron. Poor food choices or restricting food to lose weight are two common reasons. Kids who don't

Have You Ever Wondered

. . . besides drinking milk, how can teens keep their bones healthy? Like milk, yogurt, cheese, and pudding are all calcium-rich, bone-building foods. In addition, calcium-fortified soy beverage and tofu, as well as calcium-fortified juice and dark green vegetables, provide calcium, too. Regular weight-bearing activities such as dancing, soccer, running, weight lifting, tennis, and volleyball are important since they trigger bone tissue to form. Going easy on soft drinks if they edge out calcium-rich milk is smart advice. Smoking also may have a negative effect on bone formation; teens who smoke are smart to kick the habit for many reasons!

eat meat regularly may not consume enough either. Unlike calcium, the effects of low iron intake can be apparent during the teenage years.

Iron comes from a variety of foods: meat, poultry, and seafood as well as legumes, enriched grain products, and some vegetables. For example, the iron in some common foods is:

- 3-ounce hamburger—2.5 milligrams
- ½ cup of cooked, baked, or refried beans—2 to 3 milligrams
- 1 slice of enriched bread—1 milligram
- 1 cup of iron-fortified breakfast cereal—4 milligrams (more or less). For cereal, check the Nutrition Facts on food labels for the specific amount. *For information on reading labels, see "What's on the Label?" in chapter 11.*

Teens who drink orange juice with their morning toast or cereal get an iron boost, too. Its vitamin C content makes iron from plant sources and eggs more usable by the body. Kids who just grab toast to eat at the bus stop, but skip the juice, don't get the full benefit of the iron in bread. For some teens, vitamin C is a problem nutrient, too.

For more on iron in a healthful diet, see "Iron: A Closer Look" in chapter 4.

Zinc: Also Essential. Although it gets less attention, zinc often comes up short for teens. Besides other functions, zinc is essential for growth and sexual maturation. For teens who don't eat meat and other animal-based foods, a lack of zinc may affect development.

MyPyramid for Teens

MyPyramid, with its five food groups and healthy oils, is meant for teens, too! How much from the food groups for teens? That depends on how many calories they need. The more active they are, the more calories they need—and the more they can eat. *Check the Appendices to estimate calorie needs and find a food-group pattern that matches.*

Here's top-line food group advice for teens. *For more guidance, refer to chapter 10, "Planning to Eat."*

- Grains Group—*make their calories count.* "Carbs" should provide most food energy for teens. The best choices have more fiber, and less saturated fats, *trans*

Have You Ever Wondered

. . . if you should be concerned if your teenager skips meals? No, if meal skipping is just occasional. But if your teen skips meals regularly, nutrients needed for growth, development, and health may come up short.

Teenage girls often skip breakfast or lunch to save on calories, then perhaps miss out on nutrient-rich foods of special concern: high-calcium foods such as milk, iron-fortified cereals, fiber-rich whole grains, and fruits and vegetables. Later teens may satisfy their hunger with high-calorie, high-fat snack foods. The net result: more calories, fewer nutrients. *See "Meal Skipping: Poor Option!" in chapter 10.*

fats, and added sugars. The Dietary Guidelines advise: *Consume whole-grain products often; at least half the grains should be whole.* Order pizza on whole-grain crust; sandwiches on whole-wheat bread; plain popcorn or whole-wheat crackers.

- Vegetable and Fruit Groups—*eat more* fruits and veggies than you're used to. They deliver vitamins, minerals, fiber, and more, generally with fewer calories.

Choose with variety in mind, less fat, and without added sugar. Go for color! Ease up on fries!

- Milk Group—*eat enough* low-fat or fat-free dairy foods for calcium and its nutrient partners for a lifetime of healthy bones. The Dietary Guidelines advise for teens: *Consume 3 cups per day of fat-free or low-fat milk or equivalent milk products.*

- Meat and Beans Group—*eat enough* lean meat and beans to get the iron your body needs. These foods, along with poultry, fish, eggs, and nuts, provide protein, too. Go easy on chicken and fish that's fried!

- Healthy Oils—*choose an amount within your energy budget* from vegetable oils, fatty fish, and nuts, in place of foods with more saturated and *trans* fats.

Healthy eating at school makes a difference. For school lunch, encourage teens to eat the full variety of foods on the menu, preferably not a burger, pizza, or fries every day—and to make lunch a chance to drink milk. *For more about school meals, see "For Kids Only—Today's School Meals" earlier in this chapter.*

Great Snacking!

With their high energy and nutrient needs, especially during their growth spurt, teens often need snacks as a "refueling stop." Boys especially may need snacks to fill their bottomless pit. Snacks help to fill in nutrient gaps that meal choices miss: yogurt as a snack, for example, if a teen doesn't drink milk for lunch. Snacking is part of a social pattern and something to do when teenagers get together!

The real issue with teen snacking isn't whether they do—or don't. Instead, these are among the nutrition issues: (1) high-calorie snacks replacing nutrient-rich meals; (2) mindless or emotional snacking that adds to excess calories; (3) large, even oversized, portions that add up on calories, and perhaps total fat, saturated and *trans* fats, and cholesterol and added sugars; and (4) overdoing on drinks and snacks that are high in total fat, including "sat fat," *trans* fats, and cholesterol, and high in added sugars; for example, regular soft drinks, sweetened tea, candy, chips, cookies, and fruit pies.

Teens snack! Support their ability to snack smart: water, milk, or juice from a vending machine; a small burger with milk at a fast-food restaurant; or fruit, raw vegetables, yogurt, or cereal with milk from the kitchen at home. *For easy, nutritious snack ideas, see "Challenge Three: That Snack Attack!" in chapter 10.*

Your Teen's Food Choices: What You Can Do

Bigger appetites, busy lifestyles, emotional swings, struggles for independence, peer pressure: they challenge how and what teens eat. As a parent you can influence your teen's eating habits—subtly, of course!

● Stock the kitchen with easy-to-grab nutrition. Foods that take little or no effort—for example, whole fruit, yogurt, hummus, cut-up veggie sticks, string cheese, and bagels—are most likely eaten. (Ease is one reason why kids reach for chips.) *See "Empower Your Kids: Seven How-tos for Smart Eating" earlier in this chapter for more ideas.*

● Still . . . make time for family meals, even if you need to schedule around after-school activities and jobs, and put family meals on the calendar days in advance. It's a good time to get connected. (Save stressful conversations for later.) What's more, research suggests nutritional benefits! For teens, eating family meals is linked to eating more fruit and vegetables and less soft drinks and less fried, high-fat, and sugar-laden foods. Another link: Some research also links family meals with better emotional health; fewer risk-taking behaviors, such as alcohol and drug abuse; and better school performance.

● Encourage an elective class in foods, nutrition and wellness, or consumer health. That's a great way for teens to learn practical basics of sound nutrition and healthful eating. These classes are also full of applied science, math, and social studies!

● Help teens build skills. Your teen can plan, shop for, and cook family meals. The kitchen is a place to practice what's learned in a foods class. *Some tips in "Kids' Kitchen" in this chapter might help younger teens.*

● Check out the options together at fast-food restaurants, vending machines, and convenience stores. Your teen may be clueless about all the choices out there. There's more than burgers, fries, chips, and soft drinks.

● Help kids tune into portion size. A small bag of chips can be as much fun to eat as a bigger bag, with far fewer calories! The same goes for soft drinks. *See "Portion Distortion?" in chapter 10.*

● Set a good example for wellness and lifestyle—for example, with regular physical activity, lower-fat eating, sensible portions, and not smoking. Kids notice when adults "walk their talk." Not surprisingly, research suggests that boys tend to follow their dad's lifestyles; girls, their mother's.

● Help your teen deal with peer pressure. In that way he or she will have strategies to follow personal goals for smart eating, rather than going with the crowd.

● In your talk, tie smart eating and active living to what matters to your teen—growing normally; feeling good; looking good; and doing well in school, sports, or a personal interest (music, drama, art, whatever). Even when teens seem to disregard what you suggest, they likely "hear" your encouragement, concern, and example.

If Your Teen Decides to Become a Vegetarian. Support the decision by helping him or her make food choices that continue to promote growth and health. It's not uncommon for teenagers to opt for an eating style that reflects their independence and emerging beliefs. Regardless, a vegetarian eating style can supply all the

Move It!

Choose your FUN!

Your body counts on you to be active to help strengthen your bones and heart, and build muscles.

How much physical activity do kids need?

- **GET AT LEAST** 60 minutes a day of moderate activity, most days of the week.

United States
Department of
Agriculture

Food and
Nutrition
Service

September 2000

Do...

LESS
Spend less time sitting around watching TV or using the computer.

ENOUGH
Do enough strengthening activities to keep your muscles firm.

MORE
Do more intense activities that warm you up and make you glow!

PLENTY
Walk, wiggle, dance, climb the stairs. Just keep moving whenever you can.

nutrients and energy teenagers need if they know how.

A strict vegetarian diet with no animal foods, if not planned properly, may not supply all the nutrients an adolescent needs to grow. It's easiest to meet teens' nutrient needs with an eating plan that includes dairy foods and eggs, plenty of legumes, and small amounts of meat, seafood, and chicken. *See chapter 20, "The Vegetarian Way."*

Move Your "Bod"

Does your teen move in high gear on a "24/7" schedule—school to after-school activities and perhaps to a job? Do homework, time with friends, and hours on the phone or the Internet fit in between? Remember: A busy schedule may not be an active lifestyle!

Moving more promotes benefits that are dear to teenage hearts: looking good, being in shape, being strong, feeling energetic, being self-confident, doing well in school, and having a good outlook on life.

There's more. Being active now helps reduce the risk for some chronic health problems later,

including diabetes, heart disease, obesity, and osteoporosis—especially if teens make active living a lifelong habit.

The physical activity guideline for teens? For adolescents, the Dietary Guidelines advise: *Engage in at least sixty minutes of physical activity on most, preferably all, days of the week.* Research shows that physical activity drops dramatically when kids hit the teen years. Kids and parents: *use the Activity Pyramid here* to get a good balance of activities that stretch, strengthen, and give your heart a workout. Kids of every ability, shape, and size benefit with regular physical activity. *For more about guidelines and benefits of physical activity, see "Get Physical!" in chapter 2.*

Kids on the Move: Overcoming the Barriers

Why are more and more teenagers less and less active? Perhaps it's the family pattern they "inherited." But for every reason teens give, there's an easy, often fun solution. Offer these tips as starters to teens:

Reason: "I'd rather watch TV." In fact, about 50

percent of children and youth watch more than three hours of television a day!

Solution: Get some self-discipline: limit your TV time to fit in other types of fun. Or multitask: watch TV while you do something active, perhaps lift weights, do push-ups or sit-ups, or dance in front of the TV. (Kids: it's not weird to move more.)

Reason: "It's too far to walk there." So kids ride in or drive cars to school, the store, friends' homes, the library, or work.

Solution: Skip the school bus or car if you can. Walk or use a bike, scooter, or in-line skates. (Remember a helmet and perhaps knee pads, for safety.)

Reason: "I'd rather play video games or get on the computer."

Solution: Mental exercise is great, but—take an active break from sitting. It's good for your eyes and your head. In fact, your brain's synapses may work faster with some physical activity!

Get Fit with a Friend

Is your teenager looking for something to do? Suggest these active ways to get fit with a friend—and have fun!

- Do something active: play tennis, go in-line skating, go hiking, or enjoy dancing at a school function. *Hint:* You don't need a partner for line dancing.

- Instead of talking on the phone, walk and talk with your friends.

- Sign up for a school or community sports team. You don't need to "play varsity" for health benefits.

- Join the marching band if you play a musical instrument. Try out for cheerleading, majorettes, or the pom-pom squad.

- Volunteer as a stagehand for school plays. You'll get plenty of activity doing stage chores.

- Do community service—perhaps at a community garden, home-building project, children's day camp, community clean-up, or animal center.

- Baby-sit! Play actively with children.

- Get a neighborhood job: mow lawns, shovel snow, wash cars, do yardwork.

    For more physical activity ideas for teens, see "Twenty Everyday Ways to Get Moving" in chapter 2.

Have You Ever Wondered

. . . what to eat to control acne? Although all kinds of foods get blamed, teenage acne is linked to hormonal changes, rarely to food choices. The best approach to healthy skin is to eat an overall varied and balanced diet, keep skin clean, get enough rest—and wait. After the body matures, most acne clears up. If problems are severe or persist, talk to a dermatologist. Sometimes a skin application that contains a derivative of vitamin A is prescribed; simply taking a vitamin A tablet won't clear the skin.

Caution: If the doctor prescribes Accutane (isotretinoin) to treat severe acne, avoid supplements with vitamin A. Together, Accutane and vitamin A have toxic effects. Taking Accutane can also raise cholesterol and blood lipid (fat) levels until the treatment stops. Because of the many potential psychological (depression, lack of concentration, irritability, and suicidal thoughts, among others) and physical (including unusual fatigue and appetite loss) side effects of Accutane, make sure your teen follows dosage directions carefully, *under close supervision of a physician.*

. . . if kids who wear braces should avoid eating raw vegetables and fruits? No! It's true that hard, crunchy, or sticky foods can damage braces. But kids don't need to give up vegetables and fruits. Instead they might choose softer types: perhaps a ripe peach or a banana rather than a crisp apple, or cucumber sticks rather than a whole, raw carrot. Or they might cut these foods into bite-size pieces instead of eating them whole. Consult your child's orthodontist for a list of foods that might damage braces.

Reason: "I don't have time." Perhaps leisure time for active fun is limited.

Solution: Fit physical activity into what you need to do anyway. Perhaps wash the family car. Volunteer for your share of the household chores—the ones that make you move more, like raking leaves or sweeping sidewalks.

Reason: "My school doesn't require PE."

Solution: Sign up for PE at school anyway, not as a summer course. (For parents, support efforts for more physical education at school.) Or take a community aerobics, dance, or martial arts class.

Reason: "I'm self-conscious." Some kids feel that way, perhaps if they're less adept at sports or overweight.

Solution: Focus on individual sports such as biking and in-line skating, where the emphasis is on fun, not performance.

Reason: "I don't want to sweat or mess up my hair." "Exercising isn't 'cool.'" That's probably more true for teenage girls than boys.

Solution: Do everyday activities, such as walking to school or household tasks, that don't work up a sweat. Even if you do sweat, fitness is more important.

Weight: Right-Sized?

Eager for acceptance, yet self-conscious about body changes, most teens view their body image as a big issue. Even though their bodies come in different sizes, shapes, and stages of growth, many weigh in within a healthy range. In growing numbers, some deal with overweight. Others use misguided approaches for trying to achieve an unrealistic weight or body size. Still others are victims of disordered eating. Remember: The right weight is a range, not a single number; and it's about health, not just looks.

If Your Teen Is Overweight

Teens who truly are overweight—or at risk for it—need a healthful, realistic, safe way to manage their weight. That includes both physical activity and smart eating, not "dieting." Adult diets aren't meant for teens. Unless a doctor advises it, the teen years aren't a time for a weight loss diet. For many, growing into an appropriate weight is healthier; dieting may deprive a growing teen of needed nutrients.

Weight is a sensitive issue for everyone, especially kids. The best approach is positive—no nagging, forbidden foods, or criticism; a negative approach is sure-fire defeat. Instead, understanding, love, and support go a long way in helping teens and children cope with and address weight issues.

- Help eliminate eating triggers, such as the sight of high-calorie snacks on the kitchen counter.
- Reassess the family's eating style. Make gradual improvements together. Gradual changes often become permanent ones.

- Do fun, active things together. You both benefit!
- Talk, listen, and offer support and alternatives for emotional issues that trigger eating.
- Gather the resources your teen needs. Keep nutritious, lower-calorie foods, including vegetables and fruits, on hand. Prepare family meals that support your teen's strategies for managing weight.
- Most of all, be accepting. Your love doesn't depend on your teen's weight loss. Unconditional acceptance goes a long way in promoting a positive self-image, which helps promote a healthy weight.

For more about weight issues, see "Weighty Problems for Children" earlier in this chapter.

Pressure to Be Thin

To many teens, looks are almost everything! As their bodies develop and take on adult curves, it's normal to focus on body image. Often, however, teens have unrealistic notions about their own weight. Many girls especially—about 50 percent of nine- to fifteen-year-olds—see themselves as overweight. And about 23 percent of boys in the same age group do, too. In reality, about 15 percent of twelve- to nineteen-year-olds are overweight.

Pressure to be thin is closely linked to pressure to fit in and to be accepted by peers. Thin people are viewed as successful, popular, and attractive. This message gets reinforced by media images and celebrities—and often by parents and friends. However, even celebrities they try to emulate may not have a "perfect look" in reality; computers can manipulate photo images.

Teenage girls tend to diet, often poorly, as their main approach to an attractive body, while boys often put more emphasis on exercise. For girls, the pursuit of thinness often leads to fad dieting—usually ineffective, often dangerous. These diets are especially risky during adolescence, when teenagers' nutrient needs for growth and energy are high. Trying to lose weight fast to "look good" for a dance or a swim party is neither realistic nor healthful. *For more on fad diets, see "'Diets' That Don't Work!" in chapter 2.*

Teens who truly are overweight—or at risk for overweight—need a realistic, safe way to manage their weight. That includes both physical activity and a smart eating plan, not "dieting."

Disordered Eating. Sometimes a teen's pursuit of thinness leads to obsession, perhaps caused by trauma or a life change. Although not overweight, and perhaps even underweight, some teenagers see themselves as fat. Sometimes a distorted body image begins as teens develop sexual characteristics.

A distorted body image may lead to disordered eating. Teens, whose nutrient needs are high, instead may eat very little, or purge with self-induced vomiting or laxative abuse. Disordered eating can result in extreme undernourishment and weight loss—even death. Because eating disorders are linked to psychological problems, attention from a mental health professional, as well as your child's physician, is essential.

Most victims of eating disorders are teenage girls and young women. For example, 1 percent of girls age twelve to eighteen have anorexia nervosa. Although less common, teenage boys, in increasing numbers, have eating disorders, too. Other eating disorders, such as bulimia and binge eating disorder, also afflict adolescents. *To learn more, see "Disordered Eating: Problems, Signs, and Help" in chapter 2.*

Bodybuilding

Most teenage boys want to build muscle (have great "abs"), not lose weight, to look good. Many know the value of weight training for bodybuilding. But for some, the size and shape of their muscles become obsessions that lead to seemingly constant weight lifting and workouts. They may also have the misguided notion that eating more protein builds muscle mass, too. Some opt for more meat portions, perhaps at the expense of whole-grain starchy foods; others take protein supplements and "bulk-up" drugs such as steroids. Muscle-building steroids are dangerous; *see "Ergogenic Aids: No Substitute for Training" in chapter 19.*

Although protein needs go up from childhood, an extra amount has no bodybuilding benefits. Following the recommendations of MyPyramid supplies the protein that most teens need—whether they're involved in weight training or not. Like extra carbohydrate or dietary fat, extra protein calories are deposited in the body as fat, not muscle.

A high-protein diet may contribute a high percentage of calories from fat. That's especially true when teens opt for fewer foods high in starches, such as bread, pasta, rice, and cereal. The best advice for teenage bodybuilders? Follow MyPyramid guidelines and be sensible with a weight-training program.

The key to building muscle is a good exercise program and plenty of carbohydrates to fuel longer workouts. Through exercise, which creates a demand for more muscle, protein enters the muscles and makes them larger. *See "Muscle Myths" in chapter 19.*

What about making weight for wrestling or football—or for a lean strong body for gymnastics, figure skating, or cheerleading? Unhealthy weight management—either to gain or to lose weight—can be dangerous for anyone, including young athletes. Cutting down on food and beverages, along with overexercising and sweating off water weight, can lead to dehydration, heat stress, and other health problems—and certainly does not enhance performance. Instead, muscles may get weaker and smaller, even if you consume protein. If you don't eat enough calories, your body burns some protein in your muscles for energy. Crash dieting for sports and body image, along with a poor self-image, are factors that can lead to disordered eating and decreased performance.

For more on food for sports and making weight, see "Making Weight" in chapter 19.

Have You Ever Wondered

. . . if kids can turn computer time into physically active fun? Sure—if they find the right Web site! VERB (www.VerbNow.com) from the Centers for Disease Control gets kids moving while they're online.

. . . about soft drinks and other foods and drinks that compete with school meals? More and more schools are eliminating foods that compete with the school lunch program and with nutrient-rich à la carte foods. It's too soon to know how this will affect the eating habits of children and teens. That said, being an advocate for healthy food choices in your child's or teen's school can support school nutrition policies.

For Women Only

Women—this chapter is meant especially for you and your unique nutrition needs! Only in the past fifteen to twenty years have women's unique health needs received much attention in medical research. Until then, women's health needs were projected in studies done mostly with men! Except for pregnancy and breast-feeding, health concerns for women were largely ignored. Today medical research, health promotion, and healthcare address gender differences. And nutrition often is center stage in initiatives for women's health.

Consider briefly a few gender-related nutrition differences. Of course, you need the same nutrients that men do—perhaps more of some, depending on your age. Yet, if you're physically smaller, you likely need fewer calories to deliver those nutrients.

Unless men shift their physical activity level, the nutrition needs of healthy males don't change much over a lifetime. That's not true for women. Complexities of the reproductive system, the ups and downs of female hormones, and the physical demands of childbearing affect nutrition needs and healthcare. Menstruation, pregnancy, breast-feeding, and menopause all have nutrition implications.

● *If you're in your reproductive years,* check the beginning of the chapter for healthful eating advice specific to women's health.

● *For nutrition advice during pregnancy and breast-feeding,* go to the middle of the chapter.

● *If you're near or dealing with menopause,* turn to the chapter end, where you'll find nutrition guidance for your continued health and well-being.

Childbearing Years: Nutrition, Menstruation, and Prepregnancy

The choice is yours! Healthful eating, active living, and hormones are intertwined in the unique and complex issues of women's health. Whether or not you choose to have children, the choices you make now, during your childbearing years, affect the quality and length of your life for the long run. Many of those choices are uniquely female.

Menstrual Cycle: More Iron for Women

In your childbearing years you need more iron than men do. Why? To replace iron loss from menstrual flow. On average, women lose about ¼ cup of blood with each menstrual period. Those with a heavy flow may lose more. For women who don't replace that iron, menstrual loss—combined with low iron intake, frequent dieting, and a low vitamin C intake—contribute to iron deficiency and perhaps to anemia.

The Dietary Guidelines advise women of childbearing age: *Eat foods high in heme-iron and/or consume iron-rich plant foods or iron-fortified foods with an enhancer of iron absorption, such as vitamin C-rich foods.* For women ages nineteen to fifty, the Recommended Dietary Allowance (RDA) for iron is 18 milligrams of iron daily. During pregnancy, the recommendation increases to 27 milligrams daily. To compare, adult men need only 8 milligrams of iron daily. With menopause, a woman's need for iron drops and equals that of men.

To get enough iron from food, eat iron-rich foods such as meat, poultry, fortified cereal, enriched rice, and legumes. Remember that iron from grain products, legumes, and eggs isn't absorbed as well. So enjoy these foods with vitamin C-rich foods: perhaps citrus fruit with your morning cereal or scrambled egg. Consult your healthcare provider about an iron supplement, too. *For more about iron and food sources, see "Iron: A Closer Look" in chapter 4. See chapter 22 for "Anemia: 'Tired Blood'" and "Iron Supplements: Enhancing the Benefit" in chapter 23.*

Food Choices: Control for PMS?

Do you experience uncomfortable symptoms of premenstrual syndrome (PMS)? Women describe as many as two hundred symptoms: physical, such as acne, backaches, bloating, tender breasts, and headaches; food cravings; and psychological, such as anxiety, irritability, and insomnia.

PMS—a condition, not a disease—starts as many as fourteen days before a woman's period, then stops when menstrual flow starts. Shifts in hormone levels are the likely cause. Because body water fluctuates during the menstrual cycle, your body may retain fluids prior to your period. Fluid retention usually disappears soon after it's over.

PMS gets plenty of attention in women's media, yet there's little consensus on its causes or treatment, and little conclusive research on links between nutrition and its symptoms. Despite claims, no evidence links PMS and nutritional deficiencies. Here's what's known—and unknown—about PMS "headlines."

● *Calcium* may help reduce fluid retention and regulate mood-related brain chemicals, but research isn't conclusive. Regardless, there's good reason to boost your calcium intake. Calcium is essential for lifelong bone health, yet most women don't get enough!

● *Phytoestrogens* are weak, naturally occurring plant estrogens that may help relieve some PMS symptoms. Science hasn't yet determined how much is adequate, or the interaction between phytoestrogens and other hormones. Still, foods with phytoestrogens such as tofu, tempeh, soy beverage, and many other soy foods are worth enjoying for their potential health benefits.

● *Salt.* If you retain a lot of water (five pounds or more) before your period, try cutting down on salt for a week to ten days before your period, or ask your doctor about a diuretic. Research suggests that higher progesterone levels before your period cause your body to excrete sodium naturally. Limit sodium intake to 2,300 milligrams per day; for most women there's no need for further limits. Do not limit fluids!

● What about dietary supplements? Despite anecdotal claims, no conclusive research indicates that vitamin B_6, vitamin E, or magnesium alleviate PMS symptoms—and megadoses of vitamin B_6 can cause nerve damage. Except for the psychological effect, large doses of other vitamins, herbals, or botanicals such as evening primrose oil don't alleviate the symptoms either, and they may be harmful. *For more about supplements, see chapter 23.*

Until more is known, general guidelines for good health may help you cope with PMS, if it's a problem. Eat an overall healthful diet. Live an active lifestyle. Relax, learn to alleviate stress, and cope with mood swings. And get plenty of rest.

Physical activity may offer benefits! First, a good workout stimulates the release of brain endorphins, which can help relieve PMS moodiness. Just before your period, endorphin levels are low. Second, if you tend to eat more before your period, exercise can help you keep your weight stable. And third, sweating may help reduce bloating if you retain less fluid.

Consult your doctor if PMS symptoms incapacitate you. Before you attribute ongoing symptoms to PMS, talk to your healthcare provider. Diabetes, pelvic infections, depression, and other health problems may be misdiagnosed as PMS.

Other Health Issues: A Nutrition Link?

Vaginal Yeast Infections

Do food choices either promote or prevent vaginal "yeast infections," or *Candida vulvovaginitis*?

Have You Ever Wondered?

. . . if you need extra vitamins if you use oral contraceptives? No. An overall eating plan that's varied and balanced can supply enough nutrients if you're on the pill. However, taking an oral contraceptive over a period of time may exacerbate symptoms of a nutrient deficiency. For example, vitamin B_6—found in whole grains, legumes, meat, poultry, and fish—helps the body produce serotonin, which helps regulate mood and pain. A vitamin B_6 deficiency may trigger mood-related side effects related to oral contraceptives.

. . . if drinking cranberry juice helps protect you from urinary tract infections? Maybe. It appears that substances in cranberries and blueberries (same berry family) may help prevent certain bacteria that cause infection from sticking to the urinary tract wall. Many women suffer from urinary tract infections sometime in their lives. Although urine is normally bacteria-free, bacteria can travel from the rectum, across the skin surface, and into the bladder and cause infection. Studies are investigating the role of drinking cranberry juice in reducing urinary tract bacteria.

If you feel the symptoms—frequent and urgent need to urinate, painful urination, cloudy or bloody urine, or lower back or abdominal pain—seek advice for proper treatment from your doctor.

. . . can food choices reduce the symptoms of fibromyalgia? A syndrome more common in women in their twenties and thirties than in men, fibromyalgia results in chronic pain in fibrous tissues, muscles, tendons, and other connective tissues, and often sleeplessness. Although there's no known cure, a healthy weight helps keep pain in check by putting less pressure on muscles and tissues around joints. Relieving stress, staying physically active, and avoiding caffeine six to eight hours before sleeptime helps. *For more sleep-promoting tips, see "Drink Smart—and Get Your Zzzzzzzs!" in chapter 8.* Some herbal supplements are touted for relief, but research isn't conclusive; some may be harmful.

("Vulvo" means the external female genitals.) *Candida* is a fungus that commonly lives in the mouth, intestinal tract, vagina, and other moist, warm, and dark body areas. For teenage girls and women, *Candida* may cause vaginal "yeast infections" with several symptoms: vaginal itching, redness, or pain; a thick, white, "cheesy" vaginal discharge; discomfort during urination; and perhaps white or yellow skin patches around the vaginal area. Recent use of antibiotics, uncontrolled diabetes, pregnancy, high-estrogen contraceptives, immunosuppression, thyroid or endocrine disorders, and corticosteroid therapy are among the risk factors linked to yeast infections.

Does eating yogurt prevent it? Eating a cup of yogurt with *active cultures* each day may offer some protection from vaginal "yeast infections." However, the evidence isn't conclusive. Regardless, that same cup of yogurt does supply 300 to 450 milligrams of calcium, which is good for bone health!

To refute a commonly heard myth, there's no scientific evidence that eating sugary foods contributes to "yeast infections." Neither do processed foods, fruit, or milk. Avoiding these foods or taking certain dietary supplements or antifungal drugs doesn't appear to prevent it.

Be aware that *Candida* isn't the only cause of vaginitis. Bacteria, viruses, and chemical irritants are among other causes. The best way to proper treatment is accurate diagnosis from your healthcare provider. If you're prone to "yeast infections," lower your risk with good hygiene, avoiding vaginal sprays and douches, and wearing cotton garments that don't hold in moisture and heat.

Fibrocystic Breast Disease

Between 10 and 20 percent of women experience fibrocystic breast disease (FBD), benign but often painful breast lumps. Despite anecdotal claims, no carefully controlled research evidence links noncancerous breast lumps to caffeine intake. In fact, both the National Cancer Institute and the American Medical Association's Council on Scientific Affairs report that FBD isn't associated with caffeine intake. The use of vitamin E as a treatment is controversial.

Because fibrocystic breast disease is linked to hormone levels, it usually subsides with menopause—

unless a woman receives hormone replacement therapy.

As a safety check for breast health, examine your breasts carefully each month. Get regular mammograms and professional examinations yearly after age forty. And consult your doctor about any breast lumps.

Polycystic Ovary Syndrome

Are you aware of polycystic ovary syndrome (PCOS)? It's an often undiagnosed hormonal problem with a cluster of symptoms, including obesity (one of the most common clues), ovarian cysts, irregular menstrual cycles, acne, excess facial hair, fertility problems, and male pattern hair thinning. The concerns extend even farther. PCOS increases other health risks: diabetes, heart disease, high blood pressure, and uterine and breast cancer.

Although the causes of PCOS aren't known, it's a lifelong problem that may run in families and begin in adolescence. Insulin resistance (which affects the way your body uses blood sugar), obesity, and a high level of male hormones such as testosterone may explain some symptoms. PCOS isn't easy to diagnose; however, blood tests for hormone levels and ultrasound exams for ovarian cysts reveal clues.

Because of the short- and long-term health implications, talk to your healthcare provider if you suspect PCOS or have its symptoms. Some women with PCOS have no signs. Treatment may include weight loss and hormone therapy. Some women also need treatment for diabetes or high blood pressure.

Before Pregnancy

Thinking about pregnancy? If so, inventory your health and nutrition habits now. Initiating good health and nutrition habits before pregnancy—or simply nudging healthful eating and active living back into your lifestyle—promotes your health and establishes the healthy environment your baby needs to develop normally during pregnancy. And you'll be fit and ready! Your baby develops rapidly during the first weeks of pregnancy, perhaps before you even know you're expecting.

Whether you're preparing for pregnancy or not, advice for all healthy women is the same: To get enough of the forty or so nutrients essential for your good health—and your baby's health, too—*customize MyPyramid, explained in chapter 10, as your "before, during, and after" pregnancy guide to healthful eating.*

Fertility: Nutrition Links

Healthful eating not only prepares your body for pregnancy but also can affect fertility in ways that aren't yet clear. If you're trying to get pregnant:

● Aim for your healthy weight. Either extreme underweight or extreme overweight may affect the menstrual cycle and ovulation and so reduce fertility. How? The body produces estrogen in the ovaries and in fat cells. Being very thin, the body won't produce as much estrogen in fat cells. With obesity, the body's fat cells produce too much. Either way throws off the delicate hormonal balance that promotes fertility.

● Take caution with dietary supplements touted to enhance fertility. Not enough is known about the risks or the benefits of extra vitamins, minerals, or herbals and how they might affect the unborn baby.

● If you're having difficulty getting pregnant, explore the reasons and a sound approach to infertility with your doctor. In that way you'll also eliminate any health problems that you or your spouse may have. *See "Polycystic Ovary Syndrome" on this page.*

Folic Acid: Take Note!

To prepare for pregnancy, all nutrients are essential. One merits special consideration: folate, or folic acid (a B vitamin). Folic acid is the form of folate in fortified foods and supplements. Folate is essential to good health, and your body needs it to manufacture new cells and genetic material. Soon after conception, folate helps develop the neural tube, which becomes your baby's spinal cord and brain.

Women who consume enough folate, particularly in the weeks prior to conception and during the first three months of pregnancy, may reduce the risk of neural tube defects, which occur when the neural tube does not close completely. In fact, as many as 75 percent of serious birth defects in the spine and neural tube (spina bifida) and brain (anencephaly) might be prevented if women consumed enough folic acid in the critical time before and in the early weeks of pregnancy.

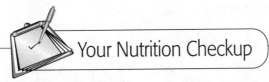

Your Nutrition Checkup

Ironing Out the Differences, for Calcium and Folate, Too!

How do your food choices stack up for three nutrients of concern to women: calcium, iron, and folate? In each pair, which food would you choose?

For more calcium . . .

COLUMN A

_____ ½ cup frozen yogurt
_____ 1 oz. Cheddar cheese
_____ 3 oz. canned tuna
_____ 1 cup milk
_____ 1 slice cheesecake
_____ 2 tbsp. yogurt cheese*
_____ ½ cup lettuce
_____ ½ cup tofu (with calcium sulfate)

COLUMN B

_____ ½ cup ice cream
_____ ½ cup cottage cheese
_____ 3 oz. canned salmon with bones
_____ 1 cup apple juice
_____ ½ cup pudding
_____ 2 tbsp. cream cheese
_____ ½ cup turnip greens
_____ ½ cup pinto beans

See "Kitchen Nutrition: Yogurt Cheese" in chapter 3 for a recipe.

For more iron . . .

COLUMN A

_____ 1 cup fortified breakfast cereal
_____ 3 oz. broiled sirloin steak
_____ ½ cup cooked green beans
_____ ½ cup cooked zucchini
_____ 1 egg yolk
_____ ⅓ cup grapes
_____ 2 tbsp. peanut butter
_____ 1 oz. pumpkin seeds

COLUMN B

_____ 1 slice whole-wheat toast
_____ 3 oz. broiled cod
_____ ½ cup cooked kidney beans
_____ ½ cup boiled spinach
_____ 1 egg white
_____ ⅓ cup raisins
_____ 3 oz. broiled chicken breast
_____ 1 oz. pretzels

For more folate . . .

COLUMN A

_____ 1 cup fortified breakfast cereal
_____ ½ cup mashed potatoes
_____ 6 oz. apple juice
_____ 1 cup raw spinach

COLUMN B

_____ 1 bread slice
_____ ½ cup pasta
_____ 6 oz. orange juice
_____ 1 cup iceberg lettuce

Now score yourself:

For each pair, these foods contain:

● *More calcium*—frozen yogurt, Cheddar cheese, canned salmon with bones, milk, pudding, yogurt cheese, turnip greens, tofu (with calcium sulfate)

● *More iron*—fortified breakfast cereal, sirloin steak, kidney beans, spinach, egg yolk, raisins, chicken breast, pumpkin seeds

● *More folate*—fortified breakfast cereal, pasta,* orange juice, spinach

*Most enriched grain products are fortified with folic acid by law; whole-grain products may or may not be.

Give yourself 5 points for each selection you got right—perfect score, 40 points for calcium, 40 points for iron, and 20 points for folate. The higher your score, the more calcium, iron, and folate you likely consume—*if* these foods really are your "picks" for the day. *Tip:* Partner eggs and plant sources of iron with meat, poultry, or fish, or with a vitamin C-rich food to enhance its absorption.

To check specific calcium and iron content in these food pairs, see "Counting Up Calcium" and "Counting Up Iron" in chapter 4. Fruits and vegetables are among your best folate sources; *assess your fruit and vegetable intake using "How Do Your Fruits and Veggies Stack Up?" in chapter 4.* Fortified grain products, some whole-grain products, nuts, legumes, and liver are good folate sources, too.

About twenty-five hundred newborns in the United States are born each year with neural tube defects. Since 1998, when grain products became fortified by law with folic acid (a form of folate), the incidence has gone down significantly. A diet with insufficient folic acid is one cause of neural tube defects.

Even a varied, well-balanced eating plan may not supply enough folate to protect against birth defects. So nutrition experts advise that all women of child-bearing age consume 400 micrograms of folic acid daily from fortified foods, vitamin supplements, or both, in addition to the folate naturally found in food.

● Eat a variety of foods with naturally occurring folate—for example, citrus fruits and juices; dark-green leafy vegetables; nuts; legumes; and liver.

● Read food labels to identify foods fortified with folic acid—for example, in most refined grains, such as breads, flour, crackers, cornmeal, farina, pasta and rice. If folic acid is added to breakfast cereals, it's listed on the Nutrition Facts. For fortified foods, the label may carry a health claim—that adequate folate intake may decrease the risk for neural tube defects. If most of your grains are "whole," your food choices may not provide much folate; some whole-grain products are voluntarily folic acid fortified.

● Consult your doctor or a registered dietitian (RD) about appropriate levels of supplements with folic acid. Taking too much folate (more than 1,000 micrograms a day) can mask the symptoms of pernicious anemia, which can cause nerve damage. (Pernicious

---

EVERY AGE AND STAGE OF LIFE: WHY A HEALTHY WEIGHT?

For girls . . . A healthy weight—not overweight—during childhood offers protection for the long term: protecting them from adult obesity and type 2 diabetes, and helping blood cholesterol and triglyceride levels stay at healthy levels. During the growing-up years, a healthy weight boosts self-esteem, important for emotional, mental, and social development. Overweight increases the chance of early puberty.

For teen and young-adult women . . . As with girls, a healthy weight—not overweight—reduces the chances of adult obesity later and helps ensure a healthy pregnancy and nursing. Beyond that, maintaining a healthy weight promotes physical health in other ways: lower risk for high blood cholesterol levels, for type 2 diabetes, and for high blood pressure; less arthritis risk in later life; and perhaps easier breast cancer detection. On the flip side, a healthy weight—not underweight—helps teens and young women develop and maintain strong bones for peak bone mass. For emotional health, a healthy weight feels good and boosts self-esteem.

For women in their child-bearing years . . . The benefits of a healthy weight mirror those of the teen and young-adult years. In addition, a healthy weight promotes fertility and helps reduce the risk for gallbladder disease.

For pregnant and breast-feeding women . . . Most important, healthy weight gain (not dieting) helps ensure a healthy pregnancy: promotes normal fetal development and improves the chances of a healthy, full-term birth. When maternal weight is healthy, childbirth is easier and safer. Obesity increases the risk for high blood pressure, gestational diabetes, induced labor, and caesarean sections. Maternal obesity may affect a child's health in other ways, too, including increased risk for childhood obesity. During breast-feeding, a healthy weight helps maintain the quality and volume of breast milk. A healthy weight during pregnancy and breast-feeding lowers a woman's risk for obesity later.

For women after menopause . . . As before, a healthy weight protects against some health problems, including breast cancer, some other cancers, heart disease, and diabetes. Among other benefits, helping to prevent risky abdominal weight gain, as weight shifts after menopause. As always, a healthy weight feels good!

For older women . . . A healthy weight continues to protect against some cancers, heart disease, and type 2 diabetes. A healthy weight—not underweight—helps bones remain strong, cushions bones and organs from fracture and other injury (in case of a fall), and protects against wasting related to serious illness.

See "Weighing the Risks" in chapter 2 for more reasons!

anemia may result from a vitamin B_{12} deficiency.) Taking large doses from vitamin pills, not food sources, is the usual reason why symptoms are masked.

Even if pregnant women do consume enough folate, obesity increases the chance of neural tube defects. *For more on folate, see chapter 4.*

More Prepregnancy Advice

● Even before pregnancy, refrain from practices that may harm your developing baby: cigarette smoking, drinking alcoholic beverages, and inappropriate drug use. Important stages in your baby's development start right after conception. Before you know you're pregnant, potentially harmful substances may have effects.

● Discuss over-the-counter and prescription medications you take with your doctor. They may be harmful to your developing baby.

● Stay physically active or initiate moderate physical activity in your daily lifestyle. That will help prepare you to be "fit" for a healthy pregnancy.

● Two foodborne risks can affect your baby, even before you conceive: methylmercury and toxoplasmosis. *Refer to chapter 12 to learn how to protect yourself now!*

You're Expecting!

Being a nurturing parent begins at the moment of conception and even before. Although you can't change your age or genetic traits, there's plenty you can do during the nine months of pregnancy to ensure your well-being and that of your unborn baby: eat wisely, stay physically active, get plenty of rest. More good advice: see your doctor regularly, stop smoking (if that's a habit), and avoid alcoholic drinks and inappropriate drugs. The likely outcome: fewer complications during pregnancy, labor, and delivery, and a healthier baby.

"Weighting" for Your New Arrival

"How much weight should I gain?" That's one of the top questions expectant mothers ask. In the last twenty-six weeks of pregnancy, your baby will grow fast, gaining about 1 ounce every day. Besides "baby weight," the weight you gain supports changes in your body and helps prepare you for breast-feeding.

Appropriate weight gain helps ensure a healthy outcome. In fact, your baby's birthweight depends on your weight gain during pregnancy. If you don't gain enough, your chance for delivering a low-birthweight infant goes up. Babies who weigh less than $5\frac{1}{2}$ pounds at birth are at greater risk for developmental difficulties and health problems. Gain too much? Both delivery and returning to your prepregnancy weight may be more difficult. Excessive weight gain during pregnancy has been linked to rising obesity rates among women. And for women with a BMI >26 for pregnancy, excessive weight gain increases an infant's risk for being large-for-gestational-age, which is linked to excess body fat during childhood.

If you were dieting for weight loss before pregnancy, put that regimen aside for these nine months. Pregnancy is *not* a good time to skimp on calories, follow a weight-loss diet, or restrict weight gain!

How much should you expect to gain during pregnancy? Because every woman is unique, your doctor will advise you about the weight-gain range that's right for you. That advice depends on:

● *Your weight before pregnancy.* For a healthy pregnancy outcome, here's the general guideline for weight gain for prepregnancy BMIs:

- ● BMI <19.8: 28 to 40 pounds
- ● BMI 19.8 to 26: 25 to 35 pounds
- ● BMI >26 to 29: 15 to 25 pounds
- ● BMI >29: 15 pounds

Talk to your doctor about what's right for you. A healthcare professional can help calculate your Body Mass Index. *For more about healthy prepregnancy weight see chapter 2.*

● *Your height.* Because all women are different, a range of weight gain is recommended—not just one targeted weight. For instance, very short women (62 inches or less) should aim for the lower end of the range for weight gain.

● *Your age.* Young teens (until age eighteen), who are at greater risk for delivering low-birthweight babies, are encouraged to gain at the higher end of the weight-gain range. Pregnancy puts greater demands on their own growing, developing bodies. *For more on teenage pregnancy, see "For Pregnant Teens: Good Nutrition" in this chapter.*

● *Expecting multiples?* Regardless of your BMI, your doctor may recommend a 35- to 45-pound weight gain for twins, and a 50-pound weight gain for triplets.

Weight Gain and Loss: Slow and Steady

Your rate of weight gain during pregnancy is as important as the amount. Expect 2 to 4 pounds of weight gain during your first three months; for teens, 4 to 6 pounds. (More weight than that is likely body fat without added benefit to mother or baby.) After that, you'll probably gain ¾ to 1 pound per week. From month to month, you may gain a little more or a little less.

If you gain weight faster, you can cut calories without depriving yourself or your baby of nutrients:

● Substitute fat-free or lower-fat milk, yogurt, and cheese for whole-milk products. And choose lean meats, poultry, and fish.

● Broil, bake, grill, or stir-fry foods instead of frying them.

Where Does Weight Gain Go?

Your baby may weigh about 7 to 8 pounds at birth—but you'll gain more. Why? Many parts of your body support pregnancy. For example, your blood volume expands by about 50 percent. Your breasts increase in size. Your body stores fat to sustain the baby's rapid growth and to provide energy for labor, delivery, and breast-feeding.

	AVERAGE WEIGHT GAIN (POUNDS)
Baby	7 to 8
Placenta	1 to 2
Amniotic fluid	2
Mother	
Breasts	1
Uterus	2
Increase in blood volume	3
Body fat	5 or more
Increased muscle tissue and fluid	4 to 7
Total	At least 25 pounds

● Eat smaller portions. *See chapter 10 for advice and tips on the right amounts.*

● Cut down on foods high in fat and calories and low in nutrients, such as candy, cake, pastries, and rich desserts. Eat more fruit and vegetables instead.

● Increase your physical activity within your doctor's guidelines.

Excessive weight gain during pregnancy can lead to a difficult delivery, back and joint problems, gestational diabetes, and postpartum weight gain. The Dietary Guidelines for pregnancy advises: *Ensure appropriate weight gain as specified by a healthcare provider.*

Delivering your baby may be the fastest weight you ever lose! Between the baby and fluid loss, some moms lose up to 10 pounds right after delivery, and another 5 pounds within the first month or so. For others, weight comes off gradually, over a longer period. Most women continue to lose weight slowly and steadily for six to twelve months after delivery. How fast you shed "baby weight" depends on how physically active you are, your calorie intake, and if you breast-feed.

Return to your prepregnancy weight—slowly and steadily—for continued health. That may mean a shift in your lifestyle. In fact, studies suggest that lifestyle changes, not physical changes related to pregnancy, are likely reasons for postpregnancy weight gain. *For guidance on healthy weight loss, see "Weight Management: Strategies That Work!" in chapter 2.*

Nutrients: For You and Baby, Too!

During pregnancy, your need for most nutrients and food energy goes up somewhat. Eating a variety of foods from all five food groups is the best way to get what you need. An inadequate diet may impair your baby's development, and he or she may be underweight at birth. *See "MyPyramid: Your Healthful Eating Guide" in chapter 10.*

Caution: If you've been pregnant recently, or if you've breast-fed within the past year, your body's nutritional reserves may be low. Problems during a previous pregnancy are another reason to make a special effort to eat wisely for a healthy pregnancy.

For specific nutrient recommendations during pregnancy, see the Appendices. If you're vegetarian, see "The Vegetarian Mom" in chapter 20.

Pregnancy: A Meal Ticket for Two

Did you know that it takes about 75,000 calories (about 340 to 450 extra calories a day after the first trimester) over nine months for a healthy baby to develop? Eating for two doesn't need to be much different than eating for one. The key is to "choose your calories by the company they keep"—in other words, choose nutrient-rich foods for extra calories.

MyPyramid provides the guidelines for the nutrients and the energy needed for your "meal ticket for two." A few more nutrient-rich food-group foods can supply all you need. *See chapter 10 for more about MyPyramid.*

How do 340 calories translate into "real food"? Try these nutrient-rich "combos" for about that amount:

- 1 ounce of cold cereal, a banana, and 1 cup of fat-free milk, *or*
- 1 baked potato with skin, topped with ½ cup each of broccoli and cauliflower, and 1 ounce of low-fat cheese, *or*
- 2 ounces of turkey on 2 slices of whole-grain or enriched bread, topped with lettuce and tomato.

Baby-Building Protein

The structural components of body cells—your baby's and yours—are mostly protein. Changes in your own body, particularly the placenta, also require protein. An eating plan that matches MyPyramid advice provides enough protein for a healthy pregnancy.

Pregnancy requires somewhat more protein. The Institute of Medicine advises 71 grams of protein (compared with 46 grams before) daily for pregnant teens and adult pregnant women. Most nonpregnant women easily consume that much. To put the extra in perspective, a 3-ounce meat patty has about 20 grams of protein; 8 ounces of milk, about 8 grams of protein.

Eggs and dairy foods can provide enough protein for lacto-ovo-vegetarians. Vegans who consume plenty of legumes, grain products, vegetables, and nuts can get enough, too. *See "Protein Power" in chapter 20.*

Fuel for Your Unborn Baby

Your baby needs a constant supply of energy . . . every minute for about 280 days . . . to grow! For protein to build body cells, your body also needs an adequate energy supply. Otherwise your body uses protein for energy instead of cell building.

Eating for two (or more!) doesn't mean your calorie need doubles. Calorie needs increase during the course of pregnancy. For the first trimester you don't need more. However, the Institute of Medicine advises an additional 340 calories a day during the second trimester and 450 calories more than when you're not pregnant during the third trimester. Your individual calorie needs may differ—certainly if you're pregnant with twins or triplets. If you're physically active, you may need more. Talk with your doctor.

Most of your food energy should come from carbohydrates. How much? The Recommended Dietary Allowance advises at least 175 grams of carbohydrate a day, just for enough glucose for both mother and baby. For overall nourishment during pregnancy, you need more: 45 to 65 percent of total calories from carbohydrates. Let "carbs" come from nutrient-rich fruits, vegetables, legumes (dry beans), and grain products (including whole grains).

Dietary fat? For your baby's central nervous system, including brain cells, you need enough essential fatty acids. During pregnancy, the Institute of Medicine advises an Adequate Intake of 13 grams of omega-6 fatty acids and 1.4 grams of omega-3s daily. The percentage of calories advised from fat doesn't change during pregnancy. Restricting fat too much isn't advised. *Refer to chapter 3 for more about fat, including essential fatty acids.*

To fuel a healthy pregnancy, make your extra calories count! Choose mostly nutrient-rich foods from MyPyramid's five food groups. They provide you and your baby with a healthful dose of nutrients, too. *For ways to "spend" extra calories for pregnancy, see "Pregnancy: A Meal Ticket for Two" in this chapter.*

Vital Vitamins

If carbohydrates are the fuel of human life, vitamins are sparks that make body processes happen! Although all vitamins are important during pregnancy, some need special attention, including those important for cell division and the formation of new life.

A varied and balanced approach to eating is the best way to get the vitamins you and your unborn baby need. Your doctor may prescribe a prenatal vitamin/

mineral supplement, too. *See "Vitamin/Mineral Supplements: Benefits and Risks" in chapter 23.*

Vitamin A. Vitamin A, for example, promotes the growth and the health of cells and tissues throughout the body—yours and your baby's. There's no need for any extra from a supplement. Your everyday food choices can provide enough vitamin A for pregnancy.

What about supplements? Research suggests that excessive amounts from supplements (10,000 IU of vitamin A, or 3,000 mcg preformed vitamin A, daily) increase the risk of birth defects. Take supplements only in amounts recommended by your doctor. Check the Supplement Facts panel on the label, and choose one with no more than 100 percent of the Daily Value for vitamin A.

Eating plenty of fruits and vegetables high in beta carotene (which forms vitamin A) isn't a problem. Beta carotene does not convert to vitamin A when blood levels of vitamin A are normal.

Have You Ever Wondered

... if intense sweeteners are safe to consume during pregnancy? Current research shows no reason to avoid foods and beverages with very-low-calorie, or intense sweeteners: such as aspartame, saccharin, acesulfame potassium, sucralose, tagatose, or neotame. Instead of calorie-free soft drinks and candies, more nutritious foods and beverages may be better choices. Drink milk, juice, and water.

Exception: Pregnant women with the rare genetic disorder called phenylketonuria (PKU) should avoid foods sweetened with aspartame starting before pregnancy. People with PKU cannot break down phenylalanine, which is an amino acid in aspartame. Then phenylalanine can reach high levels in the mother's blood and may affect the developing baby. Studies show that women with the PKU gene, but not the disease, metabolize aspartame well enough to protect their unborn baby from abnormal phenylalanine levels. If you have PKU or carry the gene, talk to your doctor.

Nonnutritive sweeteners can be useful to pregnant women with diabetes, or to pregnant women who enjoy sweet flavors. Since most women need more energy during pregnancy, calorie restriction usually is discouraged. *For more about intense sweeteners and about aspartame and PKU, see "Intense Sweeteners: Flavor without Calories" in chapter 5.*

Folate and Other B Vitamins. By consuming an extra 340 to 450 calories a day, you'll likely consume enough extra of most B vitamins. During pregnancy you need more thiamin, riboflavin, and niacin to use the extra energy from food. And you need more vitamin B_6 to help protein make new body cells.

The Dietary Guidelines for women of childbearing age who may become pregnant and those in the first trimester of pregnancy: *Consume adequate synthetic folic acid daily (from fortified foods or supplements) in addition to food forms of folate from a varied diet.* The amount increases to 600 micrograms daily. Get 400 micrograms from fortified foods or supplements, and the remaining 200 micrograms from foods with naturally occurring folate. Consuming enough during the first three months is especially critical for lowering a newborn's risk for neural tube, or spinal cord, damage. *For more about folate prior to and during pregnancy, see "Before Pregnancy" in this chapter.*

The need for vitamin B_{12} also goes up during pregnancy. This vitamin is found in foods of animal origin such as milk, eggs, cheese, and meats. Vegetarian women who don't consume any foods of animal origin need a reliable source of vitamin B_{12}—perhaps a fortified breakfast cereal or a vitamin B_{12} supplement.

Vitamin C. The need for vitamin C goes up a bit, too. But ¾ cup of orange juice supplies enough for a day! Besides its other functions, vitamin C helps your body absorb iron from plant sources of food. That's important because your iron needs increase by about 50 percent during pregnancy.

Vitamin D. To help your body absorb the calcium needed for pregnancy, consume enough vitamin D. Vitamin D-fortified milk is a good source. Calcium-fortified foods with vitamin D, too, are other options. If you're a vegetarian who doesn't consume dairy foods, you may need a vitamin D supplement—especially if you aren't exposed to direct sunlight. Your body produces vitamin D when your skin comes in contact with sunlight.

See "Vitamins: The Basics" in chapter 4.

Minerals—Giving Body Structure

Minerals are part of a baby's bones and teeth. Along with protein and vitamins, minerals help make blood cells and other body tissues, too. Minerals also take part in many body processes that support pregnancy. A few minerals require special attention during pregnancy: calcium, iron, and sometimes zinc.

Calcium. You need enough calcium now for two reasons: your baby's developing bones, and preserving your own bone mass. Without enough calcium, your body will withdraw calcium from your bones to build your baby's bones. You can't afford the loss! Research suggests that you also may reduce the chances of developing toxemia and high blood pressure if you consume enough calcium.

The calcium recommendation doesn't change for pregnancy. The body absorbs calcium more efficiently during pregnancy: 1,000 milligrams of calcium daily for adult women; 1,300 milligrams daily for pregnant teens. Yet before, during, and after pregnancy, many women don't get enough—often not enough calcium to protect against osteoporosis later in life. *See "Osteoporosis: Reduce the Risks" in chapter 22.*

The equivalent of three cups of milk from the Milk Group supply nearly all the calcium adult women need daily. An 8-ounce serving of milk or yogurt provides about 300 milligrams of calcium. *For more about calcium and calcium-rich foods, see "Calcium: A Closer Look" in chapter 4 and "Calcium Supplements: A Bone-Builder" in chapter 23.*

Doctors may prescribe a supplement for women who don't consume enough calcium-rich foods.

Iron. Why do you need so much more iron during pregnancy—up from 18 to 27 milligrams daily for adult women? Iron is essential for making hemoglobin, a component of blood. During pregnancy your blood volume increases by about 50 percent. Hemoglobin carries oxygen throughout your body, including to the placenta for your unborn baby.

For enough iron, consume good iron sources every day: lean meat; poultry; legumes; eggs; iron-fortified grain products; and green, leafy vegetables. Eat good sources of vitamin C such as citrus fruits and juices, broccoli, tomatoes, and kiwifruit, with iron-rich foods since vitamin C helps your body absorb iron.

Besides an iron-rich diet your doctor probably will prescribe a low-dose (30 milligrams per day) iron supplement or a prenatal vitamin supplement with iron. Why? Iron deficiency, the most common nutri-

Have You Ever Wondered

... if you need a multivitamin/mineral supplement during pregnancy? Check with your doctor. A balanced diet with a variety of foods can provide healthy women with enough nutrients for pregnancy. Your doctor or registered dietitian may recommend a prenatal multivitamin/mineral supplement to help ensure that you get enough iron, folic acid, and other nutrients.

If you follow a vegan diet (no foods of animal origin), if you're pregnant with more than one baby, if your diet lacks critical nutrients, or for those who have abused alcohol or drugs, a doctor may prescribe a supplement, too. *See chapter 23, "Supplements: Use and Abuse."*

tional deficiency during pregnancy, increases the risk for a premature or a low-birthweight delivery. Although widely available in food, iron isn't always well absorbed. Many women start pregnancy with marginal iron stores, which increases the chance for anemia. If you have iron-deficiency anemia, your doctor may prescribe a higher dosage.

Your body absorbs iron from a supplement best on an empty stomach or with vitamin C-rich juice but not with meals. Conversely, taking an iron supplement with coffee or tea may decrease its absorption.

Iron can interfere with the absorption of some other minerals. An iron supplement with 15 milligrams of zinc and 2 milligrams of copper is recommended.

Iron supplements during pregnancy may cause side effects such as nausea, constipation, and appetite loss. If that happens, try taking the supplement with meals even though the iron may not be absorbed as well. Then make sure you eat more food sources of iron. A lower dosage might help, too; talk to your doctor.

For more about iron, see "Iron: A Closer Look" in chapter 4 and "Iron Supplements: Enhancing the Benefit" in chapter 23.

Zinc. The need for zinc, essential for cell growth and brain development, increases by 50 percent during pregnancy. Zinc comes in a variety of foods, but it's most available from foods of animal origin such as meat, seafood, and poultry. Whole-grain products have zinc, too, but it's not absorbed as well. Most women, except perhaps some vegetarian women, get enough zinc during pregnancy from their everyday food choices, especially from protein-rich foods. **Caution:** Take an iron supplement according to the recommended dosage; too much iron can interfere with zinc absorption.

Sodium. You don't need to restrict sodium during pregnancy—unless your doctor advises you to do so. And if you limited your sodium intake before pregnancy, continue to do so as your doctor recommends. Pregnant or not, choosing and preparing food with little salt—and more potassium-rich fruits and vegetables—still is good advice. *See chapter 7, "Sodium and Potassium: A Salty Subject."*

For more about minerals in a healthful eating plan, see *"Minerals—Not 'Heavy Metal'" in chapter 4.*

Fiber

Getting enough fiber—from whole-grain foods, bran, vegetables, legumes, fruits, nuts, and seeds—is important during pregnancy. The Adequate Intake for total fiber for pregnant women, regardless of age, is 28 grams per day—likely more than normally consumed.

And Water, Too

Remember: Water is a nutrient. As part of your body's transportation system, it carries nutrients to body cells and carries waste products away. That includes nourishment that passes through the placenta to your baby. You need fluids—about 3 liters (12 cups) daily—for your own and your baby's increased blood volume. When you feel thirsty, drink more!

For Pregnant Teens: Good Nutrition

School, activities, and social schedules often take good nutrition off a teen's "top ten" list. Still growing, pregnant teens may need more food energy, protein, and some vitamins and minerals than an adult woman. What a pregnant teen eats affects her own short- and long-term health and her baby's future.

Figure-conscious teens may be reluctant to gain weight during pregnancy. However, teens need to understand that pregnancy isn't the time to restrict calories or follow a weight-control diet! Pregnancy is just a temporary body change, and extra pounds aren't just the fetus or mother's body fat.

Until age eighteen, pregnant teens need to gain more weight than adult women do. Most healthy young mothers gain about 35 pounds by the end of their pregnancy. Gaining at the upper end of the suggested range helps the teen mother deliver a healthier, normal-birthweight baby.

A baby grows "around the clock." Yet, typical teen food habits—meal-skipping, high-calorie/low-nutrient foods and drinks—often don't provide the ongoing nutrient supply an unborn baby needs. A pattern of three meals and three nutritious snacks daily, which follow MyPyramid guidelines, can provide enough nourishment for a teenage pregnancy. *Use MyPyramid, explained in chapter 10, as a guide.*

A varied, balanced eating plan is the only way to provide enough nutrients and food energy during pregnancy and to "feed" an unborn baby! A multivitamin/mineral supplement for pregnant teens is meant to supplement, not replace, meals or snacks.

Adolescent pregnancy is high risk. A teenager's body is still growing, perhaps competing with the unborn baby for nutrients. With poor food choices and an inadequate nutrient intake, a teenage mom more likely delivers a low-birthweight baby. The chances of anemia and pre-eclampsia (or toxemia) are higher, too. Untreated pre-eclampsia is dangerous and potentially life-threatening for the mother and the baby. Symptoms include sudden weight gain, abdominal pain, and high blood pressure. Prenatal care with nutrition counseling is essential

For more about nutrition during adolescence, see *"Feeding the Teen Machine" in chapter 16.*

Discomforts of Pregnancy

With so many changes taking place in your body, occasional discomforts during pregnancy really aren't surprising. A few changes in what—and how—you eat may relieve vomiting and nausea, constipation, heartburn, and swelling.

Dealing with Nausea and Vomiting

Often referred to as "morning sickness," nausea or vomiting is experienced by many moms-to-be. Hormonal changes, particularly rising estrogen levels, are likely responsible. Somewhat of a misnomer, "morning sickness" may occur at any time—day or night.

. . . if vegetarian eating can promote a healthy pregnancy? Yes, *if* you plan your food choices carefully. Getting enough nutrients and food energy during pregnancy is often easier for women who have already mastered vegetarian eating skills. If you decide to become a vegetarian during pregnancy, *first* consult a registered dietitian for guidance.

What about nutrient supplements? The same advice applies to all pregnant women, vegetarian or not. In addition, a vitamin B$_{12}$ supplement—and perhaps a vitamin D supplement if sunlight exposure is limited—are advised for vegan women. Some vegetarian women also may need zinc or calcium supplements if their food choices come up short. Vegetarian women usually consume more folate than nonvegetarian women; still, a folic acid supplement or folic-acid-fortified foods are advised. *For more guidance, see "The Vegetarian 'Mom'" in chapter 20.*

. . . if caffeinated drinks are okay during pregnancy? There's no conclusive evidence about the effects of caffeine on fetal development. However, moderation is best when you're expecting: one or two servings of coffee, tea, or other caffeine-containing drinks a day are enough. Prudent advice: Keep caffeine intake below 300 milligrams a day. *Refer to chapter 8 for more about caffeinated drinks.* For some pregnant women, caffeine can cause nausea and heartburn. *For more about caffeine, see chapter 8.*

And it may continue past the first three months of pregnancy.

Some women complain about just minor queasiness. Persistent, severe nausea with spells of vomiting can leave other pregnant women at risk for dehydration and weight loss. If these discomforts continue beyond the first trimester, get advice and support from your healthcare provider. These suggestions might keep nausea at bay:

● Skip foods with strong flavors (perhaps spicy foods) or aromas if they trigger nausea. Pregnant women often have an exaggerated sense of smell, making a common aroma seem unappealing.

● Before getting out of bed, eat starchy foods such as crackers, plain toast, or dry cereal. That helps remove stomach acid. Get out of bed slowly.

● Enjoy small meals every two to three hours to prevent an empty stomach. Drink beverages between, not with, meals, and stay well hydrated!

● Eat easy-to-digest carbohydrate foods, such as plain pasta, crackers, potatoes, rice, fruits, and vegetables, and low-fat protein foods such as lean meat, fish, poultry, and eggs. Limit fried and other high-fat foods if they cause discomfort.

● Savor every bite! Eat meals slowly. In fact, try to make your surroundings stress-free.

● Before bedtime eat a small snack such as peanut butter on crackers and milk, or cereal and milk.

● Experiment with beverages that may calm a queasy stomach: lemon or ginger tea, lemonade, ginger ale, or water flavored with lemon or ginger.

● Choose those foods that appeal and that "stay down." Even if your food choices aren't "nutritionally perfect," that's okay if queasiness doesn't last longer than a few days. If the problem persists, talk to your doctor or a registered dietitian.

● Consult your doctor, especially if severe nausea and vomiting continue after fourteen weeks.

Constipation during Pregnancy

Since becoming pregnant, do you occasionally feel constipated? Many women do. Hormonal changes relax muscles to accommodate your expanding uterus, and that slows the action in your intestine. Taking an iron supplement can aggravate constipation, too.

For some women, constipation, along with pressure from the baby, leads to hemorrhoids. Hemorrhoids are large, swollen veins in the rectum.

Try these ways to prevent or ease constipation and the discomfort of hemorrhoids:

● Consume about 12 cups of fluid daily. Besides water, include milk, fruit juice, and perhaps broth in your fluid allowance. *For more about fluids in a healthful eating plan, including food sources of water, see chapter 8.*

● Eat high-fiber foods: whole-grain foods, bran, vegetables, fruits, and legumes.

● Enjoy the natural laxative effect of dried plums (prunes), prune juice, and figs.

● Be physically active every day. Like swimming

and prenatal exercise classes, walking is good exercise during pregnancy. Regular activity stimulates normal bowel function.

● Unless your doctor prescribes them, don't take laxatives. For hemorrhoids, ask your doctor to recommend a safe suppository or ointment.

Just Heartburn

Especially during the last three months, you may complain about heartburn. That may happen as a result of hormonal changes that slow the movement of food through the digestive tract. To relieve your discomfort:

● Eat small meals often, every two to three hours.

● Cut down on caffeinated and carbonated beverages, chocolate, and highly seasoned food.

● Eat slowly in relaxed surroundings.

● Walk after you eat to help gastric, or stomach, juices go down, not up. Or at least remain seated for an hour or two after eating, rather than lie down.

● Avoid large meals before bedtime.

● Sleep with your head elevated to avoid acid reflux.

● Wear comfortable, loose-fitting clothes.

● Consult your doctor before taking antacids. Some contain sodium bicarbonate (baking soda), which can interfere with nutrient absorption.

Swelling—Part of Pregnancy

Swelling is normal, especially in the last three months of pregnancy. Water retained in your ankles, hands, and wrists is a reservoir for your expanded blood volume. It offsets the water lost during delivery, and it's used later for breast milk. Even with swelling, drink plenty of water!

Unless your doctor advises otherwise, avoid diuretics that increase water loss through urination. There's no need to limit salt to prevent swelling; use iodized salt—just enough to match your taste. Iodine is a mineral essential for you and your baby.

To relieve the discomfort of moderate swelling:

● Put your feet up. When you sit, get up to stretch to improve your circulation. Try not to stand for a long time. Rest on your left side to aid circulation.

Pregnancy and Alcoholic Beverages Don't Mix!

Your blood passes through every organ in your body, through the placenta, and into the circulatory system of your unborn baby. Your baby will be exposed to any alcohol or drugs in your blood.

Even at moderate levels (one drink a day), women who regularly consume alcohol during pregnancy may increase their risk for miscarriage or delivering low-birthweight babies. Fetal alcohol syndrome (FAS) is associated with excessive drinking. Infants with FAS may be born with birth defects: retarded growth, mental impairment, or physical malformations.

If you're trying to conceive or you're already pregnant, health experts advise to avoid beer, wine, or other alcoholic beverages completely. A safe level for alcohol intake during pregnancy is unknown. Health experts don't know if babies differ in their sensitivity to alcohol. As a reminder, alcoholic beverages carry a label warning about the dangers of drinking during pregnancy and its relation to birth defects.

> GOVERNMENT WARNING:
>
> (1) ACCORDING TO THE SURGEON GENERAL, WOMEN SHOULD NOT DRINK ALCOHOLIC BEVERAGES DURING PREGNANCY BECAUSE OF THE RISK OF BIRTH DEFECTS. (2) CONSUMPTION OF ALCOHOLIC BEVERAGES IMPAIRS YOUR ABILITY TO DRIVE A CAR OR OPERATE MACHINERY, AND MAY CAUSE HEALTH PROBLEMS.

● Wear comfortable shoes, perhaps a larger size. Avoid tight clothes, tight stockings, tight-fitting rings, and anything else that restricts circulation.

Excessive swelling may signal pre-eclampsia, or toxemia. Other signs include high blood pressure, a sudden weight gain, headaches, and abdominal pain. Advise your doctor right away if you develop these symptoms. Untreated, pre-eclampsia can be dangerous later in pregnancy, even life-threatening for mother and baby. Pre-eclampsia is linked to low calcium and low protein intake during pregnancy.

Pregnancy and Diabetes

Gestational diabetes—which may start around the middle of pregnancy and end after delivery—is a health problem for some pregnant women. Who's at risk? Women with a family history of diabetes, obese women, those with a problem pregnancy, and women over age forty. Most women are routinely tested for gestational diabetes at about twenty-four to twenty-eight weeks.

Whether it's preexisting or gestational, diabetes during pregnancy increases the risk for high blood pressure and toxemia. Toxemia, accompanied by swelling, high blood pressure, and excess protein in urine, is dangerous. Women with gestational diabetes often have big babies, who may be difficult to deliver, and they may need a cesarean delivery. The risk for getting diabetes later in life is higher among women who develop gestational diabetes.

If you have diabetes, you can deliver a healthy baby. However, it's important for your doctor to monitor it carefully and prescribe treatment, typically a combination of diet and physical activity. A registered dietitian can help you develop an eating plan to control your blood sugar levels. *See "Diabetes: A Growing Health Concern" in chapter 22.* Controlling existing diabetes before pregnancy is important.

Pregnancy: More Reasons for Food Safety

Handling food properly to avoid foodborne illness is always essential. Pregnancy is no exception. Besides general cautions, some issues are of special concern:

● *Listeria,* a bacterium that may contaminate soft cheese, unpasteurized milk, hot dogs, and deli meats, can cause miscarriage in the first trimester and serious illness, premature birth, or stillbirth later.

● *Toxoplasmosis,* a parasite linked to undercooked meat or poultry, can be passed from mother to unborn baby, causing severe symptoms including infant death or mental retardation. Because cat feces carry this parasite, avoid cat litter, always wash your hands with soap and water after handling a cat, and keep your cat indoors.

● *E. coli O157:H7,* a bacterium associated with raw and undercooked meat and unpasteurized milk, is highly toxic. This life-threatening strain, which can cause severe kidney, intestinal, and brain damage, can pass to your unborn baby.

● *Lead* exposure during pregnancy is linked to miscarriage and stillbirth, low-birthweight babies, and damage to a baby's nervous system. Among the sources of lead: water from lead pipes or pipes with lead solder, food served on ceramic plates with improperly applied lead glaze, and beverages kept and served in lead crystal decanters or glasses.

● *Methyl mercury and PCBs (polychlorinated biphenyls),* chemical pollutants found in some fish, are especially harmful to unborn babies and young children, whose bodies are just developing. Mercury poisoning, for example, may damage the nervous system. No matter how you prepare or cook fish, you can't get rid of the methyl mercury! Since you may pass these contaminants on, pregnancy and breast-feeding are not the time to eat large, long-lived fish (shark, swordfish, king mackerel, and tilefish), which contain the highest levels of methyl mercury.

Especially during pregnancy, avoid raw fish and seafood to reduce viral and bacterial infection risks. Enjoy shellfish, canned light tuna, smaller ocean fish, or farm-raised fish, such as catfish or salmon. You can safely eat 12 ounces of these varieties of cooked fish weekly. For locally caught fish, check advisories; limit to 6 ounces if an advisory isn't posted.

See chapter 12 for specific precautions for these foodborne illnesses and for general food safety guidance. Chapter 8 addresses lead poisoning and water.

Stay Active!

For most pregnancies, mild to moderate physical activity benefits the mom—and won't affect the unborn child. Consider the unique benefits!

● Helps you look and feel good as your body changes

● Promotes muscle tone, stamina, and strength

● Helps reduce leg and back pain, constipation, swelling, and bloating

● Promotes blood circulation and may help prevent varicose veins

Have You Ever Wondered ?

. . . if herbal supplements or botanicals are safe during pregnancy and nursing? There's not enough scientific evidence yet to recommend safe levels for herbal supplements for pregnant or nursing moms. However, some are known to be harmful to a baby—for example, comfrey may cause liver damage, blue cohosh may cause heart defects, and pennyroyal may cause spontaneous abortions. Other herbs identified as potentially harmful include aloe, buckthorn, burdock, cascara, chamomile, coltsfoot, cornsilk, devil's claw root, Dong Quai, ephedra, feverfew, ginseng, goldenseal, hawthorne, horseradish, licorice, lobelia, mate, rue, sassafras, senna, St. John's wort, uva ursi, and yarrow.

. . . if herbal teas are okay to drink during pregnancy? Some are considered safe if you enjoy no more than two to three cups a day. Blackberry, citrus peel, ginger, lemon balm, orange peel, and rosehip teas are among those considered safe if they've been processed according to government safety standards.

During pregnancy the Dietary Guidelines also advise: *Do not eat or drink raw (unpasteurized) milk or any products made from unpasteurized milk, raw or partially cooked eggs or foods containing raw eggs, raw or undercooked meat and poultry, raw or undercooked fish or shellfish, unpasteurized juices, and raw sprouts. Only eat certain deli meats and frankfurters that have been reheated to steaming hot.*

● Helps your posture and balance—important as your center of gravity shifts

● Helps you sleep better

● Prepares your body for labor and childbirth

● After delivery, helps your body get in shape!

During pregnancy, the Dietary Guidelines advise: *In the absence of medical or obstetric complications, incorporate 30 minutes or more of moderate-intensity physical activity on most, if not all, days of the week. Avoid activities with a high risk of falling or abdominal trauma.*

Caution: Pregnancy isn't the time to exercise to lose or keep from gaining weight.

Healthcare professionals advise moderate activity for most pregnant women: perhaps walking, swim-

ming, modified low-impact aerobics, or stationary cycling. The right level of physical activity depends on your health and how active you've always been. If you haven't been physically active, talk to your doctor before starting.

Caution: Avoid strenuous activity during your first trimester. Overexertion, which may cause your unborn baby to become overheated at a critical time of development, increases the risk for birth defects.

With minor changes you may be able to continue your regular physical activity routine. Just remember: As your body shape changes and you gain weight, your center of gravity shifts, too. That puts more stress on your muscles and joints, particularly in your lower back and pelvis. Some activities get harder to do, especially during the last three months. Injury is more likely, too, as changes in your hormones cause ligaments in your joints to stretch. Exercise with care. Avoid jerky, bouncy movements—and don't overdo. Keep these pointers in mind:

● Talk with your doctor about physical activity during pregnancy—including any new activities you plan to do. Doctors may advise against exercise for a high-risk pregnancy: high blood pressure induced by pregnancy, symptoms or a history of early contractions (preterm labor), vaginal bleeding, or early rupture of membranes. Other health conditions, such as heart or lung disease, may limit physical activity.

● With your doctor, choose an activity plan that keeps you fit, matches your health needs and lifestyle, and prepares you for delivery. Your hospital, clinic, or health club may offer an exercise program for pregnant women with exercises to help with labor.

● Start slowly. If you haven't been active, start with low-intensity activity, as your doctor advises.

● Stick with a routine—every day for 30 minutes if you can. This isn't the time to stop and start with spurts of heavy exercise.

● Enjoy activities that build strength and condition your heart and lungs. Stretch your muscles before and afterward.

● After the first twenty weeks, avoid any exercises you do while lying on your back. In that position it may be harder for your blood to circulate.

● Drink plenty of water—before, during, and after physical activity—and wear appropriate clothing to avoid getting overheated and dehydrated. Avoid brisk exercise in hot, humid temperatures.

● Wear a supportive bra to protect your breasts.

● If you feel tired, stop before you feel exhausted. If you can talk as you move, your level of physical activity is right. Talk with your doctor about the right target heart rate for you. *See "Your Physical Activity: How Intense?" in chapter 19.*

● If you experience any problems, stop your activity and consult your doctor right away. These are warning signs: breast pain, headaches, pain (in general, or in your back or pubic area), dizziness or feeling faint, vaginal bleeding, shortness of breath, rapid or irregular heartbeat, discomfort when you walk, uterine contractions and chest pain, edema, nausea, and fluid leaking from your vagina.

● After delivery, resume your prepregnancy routine gradually, as you're physically able. Start with walking; use a stroller or a front/back carrier so you and your baby can walk together. Another option: Check in your community for a postpartum exercise class.

For Those Who Breast-Feed

The decision to breast-feed is personal. If you decide it's right for you and your baby, make smart eating a priority. Your needs for energy and some nutrients are higher now than during pregnancy.

If you're able, breast-feeding is good for your baby—and for you. Besides the physical benefits to your baby and the emotional nurturing you share, breast-feeding can help you return to your prepregnancy shape and weight, and reduce blood loss after pregnancy. While inconclusive, research suggests that breast-feeding may offer health benefits later: reduced risks of breast cancer, ovarian cancer, and osteoporosis. *See "Breast-Feeding Your Baby" in chapter 15.*

Your Energy Sources

Your fuel supply for milk production comes from two sources: energy stored as body fat during pregnancy, and extra energy from food choices. To produce breast milk, your body uses about 100 to 150 calories a day from the fat you stored during pregnancy. That's why breast-feeding helps many new mothers lose pregnancy weight —often without trying!

While breast-feeding, you also need to eat more calories daily than you would if you weren't breast-feeding: an extra 330 calories during the first six months, an extra 400 calories for the second six months.

Get those added calories by enjoying more nutrient-rich foods from MyPyramid's five food groups. Adding a little nutrient-dense food-group foods during the day provides enough extra energy and nutrients for breast-feeding. *See "How Many Servings a Day for You?" in chapter 10.*

After you've established your breast-feeding routine, evaluate your energy intake. Consider your activity level, your weight gain during pregnancy, and your weight loss since delivery. Do you need more or less than 500 extra calories a day? Ask your lactation counselor or a registered dietitian for guidance.

For breast-feeding women, the Dietary Guidelines advise: *Moderate weight reduction is safe and*

Pass the Pickles: Cravings and Food Aversions

Whether it's pickles and ice cream or other foods, cravings, as well as food aversions, are common during pregnancy. Although the exact cause is unknown, taste perceptions may change with hormonal changes. Usually taste buds "realign" after the first trimester, or sometimes not until after the baby's birth.

If you avoid an entire food group, food aversions are harmless unless foods you crave replace more nutritious foods. Instead substitute nutritionally similar foods. For instance, if broccoli loses its appeal, substitute another vegetable that you enjoy and tolerate.

Caution: Cravings for nonfood substances, a condition called pica, can be dangerous. The cultural practice of craving cornstarch, ashes, laundry starch, clay, or other odd substances comes from folklore that started hundreds of years ago. It was believed that eating a particular substance might decrease nausea, promote a healthy baby, or ease delivery. There's no evidence that this practice works—and it can be harmful for you and your baby. Some substances contain lead or other toxicants.

does not compromise weight gain of the nursing infant.

While nursing, steer away from restrictive weight-loss regimens. Dipping below 1,800 calories daily may decrease your milk volume and compromise your nutritional status. Losing 2 to 4 pounds a month, probably won't affect your milk supply; gradual weight loss is healthier anyway. Losing more than 4 to 5 pounds a month after the first month isn't advised.

Now about Nutrients

The need for most nutrients increases during breast-feeding. A few need special attention, especially if you breast-feed longer than two or three months:

Macronutrients. When you breast-feed, the advice for protein, essential fatty acids, and carbohydrate (from glucose) is higher than if you didn't breast-feed. Everyday food choices can supply enough if choosen wisely. *Refer to the Appendices for amounts.*

Calcium. Your calcium needs don't change when you're breast-feeding. Still, make sure you consume enough. If you come up short, your body may draw from calcium in your bones so the calcium content in breast milk remains adequate. Calcium losses in your bones may put you at greater risk for osteoporosis later in life. Periodontal problems also may crop up after pregnancy and nursing, perhaps related to calcium drain. Enjoy the equivalent of 3 cups of milk daily. And eat leafy-green vegetables, and fish with edible bones; they're both good calcium sources. *See "Osteoporosis: Reduce the Risks" in chapter 22.*

Have You Ever Wondered

... if your food choices affect the flavor of breast milk? Eating strongly flavored foods such as onions, garlic, broccoli, cabbage, cauliflower, garlic, "hot" spicy food, or beans may give breast milk an unfamiliar flavor. These flavors make some babies fussy; other babies don't notice. If some foods seem to upset your baby, eat less of them, less often. What you eat may cause a harmless color change. Breast milk usually is white or bluish-white.

Zinc. Nursing increases the need for zinc. Zinc easily comes from foods of animal origin. Pay special attention to zinc, especially if you're a vegetarian.

Vitamin B_{12} and Vitamin D. Make sure you consume enough to ensure an optimal amount of these vitamins in breast milk. Because vitamin B_{12} is found only in foods of animal origin, some vegetarians may need a vitamin B_{12} supplement. If you eat meat, poultry, fish, eggs, and dairy products, you're likely getting enough.

Breast milk doesn't have much vitamin D. If your diet is low in vitamin D or if you aren't exposed to sunlight, your breast milk may have less. Milk is fortified with vitamin D; sunlight helps your body produce it. Some vegetarians may need a vitamin D supplement.

Folate. Especially if you're considering another pregnancy soon, consume the recommended 500 micrograms daily of folate—from fortified grain products and supplements as well as from fruits and vegetables—while breast-feeding. *For more about folate, see "Before Pregnancy" earlier in this chapter.*

Vitamin B_6. The need for this B vitamin goes up, yet nursing mothers often don't consume enough. Chicken, fish, and pork are the best sources, followed by whole-grain products and legumes.

Multivitamin/mineral Supplement. If you took a prenatal vitamin/mineral supplement during pregnancy, your doctor may recommend that you continue. You probably can get enough nutrients from food—if you choose wisely. If your own food choices come up short on calories or nutrients, in most cases your breast milk still will be sufficient to support your baby's growth and development—but at the expense of your own nutrient reserves! *See "Vitamin/Mineral Supplements: Benefits and Risks" in chapter 23.*

For more about vitamins and minerals, see chapter 4; for specific Dietary Reference Intakes during breast-feeding, see the Appendices.

Remember Fluids!

To ensure an adequate milk supply and to prevent dehydration, drink enough fluids to satisfy your thirst. That's the amount to keep your urine pale yellow or nearly colorless. During breast-feeding, you need about 15 cups of fluids daily—more if you're thirsty.

That includes water from food sources. If you're constipated or if your urine is concentrated, drink more! *Tip:* Keep water, milk, or juice handy to sip as you nurse. Milk and juice supply other nutrients you need in extra amounts for nursing: calcium from milk and vitamin C from most fruit juices.

Nonfoods: Effect on Breast Milk?

While you breast-feed, take the same precautions you did during pregnancy. Food, beverages, or other substances: what you consume may be passed to your baby.

Alcoholic Beverages

The alcohol you drink passes into breast milk, so steer away from wine or beer for relaxation. Contrary to popular belief, no scientific evidence suggests that an alcoholic drink promotes the "letdown" reflex.

An occasional alcoholic drink probably won't affect your baby or interfere with nursing, but heavy drinking may inhibit your "letdown" reflex. Alcohol in breast milk may cause your baby to be less alert. In excess, it may affect brain development.

The Dietary Guidelines advise: *Alcoholic beverages should not be consumed by lactating women.* Alcohol passes into breast milk; drinking alcoholic beverages can decrease milk production. For a celebration drink, do so after breast-feeding, or postpone nursing for at least two hours.

Smoking

Nicotine passes into breast milk. If you're a smoker and quit during pregnancy, breast-feeding isn't the time to start again. Nicotine can reduce your milk supply, and increase your baby's chance for colic, a sinus infection, or fussiness. Smoking near your baby is risky, exposing him or her to secondhand smoke and possibly getting burned. Too close to a nursing session, smoking may inhibit your "letdown" reflex. Smoking is also linked to the increased rate of lung cancer.

If you choose to smoke, don't smoke near your baby—not even in the same room. Try to avoid smoking for 2½ hours before nursing: never smoke as you nurse!

Have You Ever Wondered

. . . if you can drink caffeinated beverages while you're nursing? Yes, enjoy your morning coffee, or a soft drink for a snack, in moderation. Caffeine does pass into breast milk. However, caffeine in 1 or 2 cups a day probably won't bother your baby.

. . . if vegetarian eating supplies adequate nutrition for breast-feeding? A vegetarian mom who consumes dairy products, and perhaps eggs, can easily get enough nutrients. For vegans, who avoid all foods of animal origin, calcium, vitamin D, iron, and vitamin B_{12} need special attention. *See "The Vegetarian Mom" in chapter 20.*

. . . if you can pass food allergens through breast milk to your baby? For starters, it's highly unlikely that your baby can't tolerate breast milk; allergic reactions from human milk are extremely rare. While uncommon, some babies react to allergens passed through breast milk—for example, cow milk protein or protein in peanuts. If your family has a history of food allergies, the American Academy of Pediatrics advises avoiding peanuts during the nursing period to lower your baby's peanut allergy risk. If you suspect an allergy, never make the diagnosis yourself! Talk to your doctor. Then get help from a registered dietitian to help you manage any allergy and continue breast-feeding. *See "Food Allergies: Commonly Uncommon" in chapter 21.*

Food Safety Issues

Food safety precautions are advised during nursing: *refer to page 449.*

Medications

Consult your doctor about any prescription and over-the-counter medication you're taking, even an aspirin! Most pass into breast milk in concentrations that pose no harm to your infant. But there are some exceptions.

Recreational drugs—which pass into breast milk—are never considered safe for you or your baby!

See "Breast-Feeding Your Baby" in chapter 15.

Stay Active!

Being physically active now helps shed "baby weight." It's good for your health and mental outlook. During breast-feeding, the Dietary Guidelines advise: *Be aware that neither acute nor regular exercise adversely affects the mother's ability to successfully breast-feed.*

Being active likely won't affect the amount or the composition of breast milk. If you're highly active, your milk may have more lactic acid right after exercise, which may affect flavor, but doesn't appear harmful to infants.

Show yourself as a role model. Walk with your baby in a stroller. Play actively together. Be active for you.

Now for Menopause

Menopause, when hormone levels slowly drop, is a natural passage in a woman's life cycle—not a health problem. So relax. Accept the changes as normal and very individual. Once symptoms such as hot flashes, mood swings, and sleeplessness disappear, post-menopausal women are free of discomforts from a monthly menstrual cycle.

The menopausal years are gradual. Menopausal changes are linked closely to hormone levels, most specifically to estrogen. As reproductive hormones

Breast Cancer: Do Food Choices Make a Difference?

Breast cancer: it's a common fear for good reason. Breast cancer is the most common cancer among North American women, striking nearly two hundred thousand women annually. It's the second most common cause of cancer death for women, killing nearly fifty thousand women a year.

All women are vulnerable to breast cancer—eventually. What's your risk? Among the probable risk factors: family history of breast cancer, early menstruation, late menopause (after age fifty-five), older-age pregnancy of a first child, some forms of benign breast disease, obesity after menopause, ovarian and endometrial cancer, exposure to ionizing radiation, and simply getting older.

The causes of breast cancer aren't understood. Yet, healthful eating and lifestyles, maintaining healthy weight throughout life, being physically active, and reducing alcoholic-beverage consumption may help protect you from breast lesions and cancer.

Are you a "pear" or an "apple"? The place where extra pounds of body fat settle on your body may make a difference. Early research suggests that women who carry excess body fat around the abdomen (apple shape) may have an increased breast cancer risk. After menopause, more excess weight accumulates there. After menopause, weight gain is linked with increased cancer risk, perhaps related to estrogens formed in the body's fat tissues. Being physically active helps you keep your healthy weight, so move more, too!

Another possible link: excessive alcoholic beverage consumption may increase breast cancer risk. A daily limit of 5 ounces of wine, 12 ounces of beer, or 1½ ounces of 80-proof distilled spirits is recommended. If you're at high risk for breast cancer, you may be better off enjoying non-alcoholic drinks instead.

If you are considering hormone therapy, weigh the benefits and the risks. Although it may reduce discomforts of menopause and the risk of osteoporosis, hormone therapy is linked to increased breast cancer risk. Talk to your doctor about the best approach for you. *Refer to "Menopausal Symptoms: Nutrition and Lifestyle Strategies" later in this chapter.*

Are foods with phytoestrogens—for example, soy with the isoflavone genistein—an appropriate alternative to hormone therapy if you're at high risk for breast cancer? On one hand, the estrogenlike effects in isoflavones may be harmful for women already at high risk for breast cancer. New research also suggests that phytoestrogens in soy are selective and don't have much effect on breast tissue. Since the jury's still out, talk to your physician before adding soy to your meals and snacks if you have breast cancer, if you're at high risk for breast cancer, or if you're taking tamoxifen, a hormone-blocking drug related to estrogen. Dietary soy supplements aren't advised, either. Research is under way to explore another food that may protect against hormone-sensitive cancers: flaxseed, which contains a type of phytoestrogen called lignan.

Aim for your healthy weight. And make early detection a habit: monthly self-examination, yearly mammograms, and routine breast examination. *See chapter 22 for more about nutrition and cancer.*

Have You Ever Wondered

. . . if foods designed for women are worth it? "Feminine foods," or those nutritionally designed for women's needs, may offer health benefits—for example, soy beverage products, cereals fully fortified with folic acid, and juice with added calcium. Read food labels, then decide if you need what they provide. These foods often cost more. If you already consume enough from other foods, you may not need them.

. . . if feeling tired could be a thyroid problem? Perhaps. Symptoms of hypothyroidism include fatigue and mood swings. However, with mild hypothyroidism, you may feel fine. Cold intolerance; dry, brittle hair and skin; hoarseness; difficulty swallowing; and forgetfulness are other symptoms, usually associated with more severe hypothyroidism. Of the eleven million people in the United States with hypothryroidism, most are women and elderly people. *For more about a thyroid problem and its potential consequences, see chapter 22.*

diminish, every body cell—particularly in the cardiovascular, skeletal, and reproductive systems—is affected. Perimenopause typically starts in a woman's midforties and lasts for four to six years as the body gradually produces less estrogen and progesterone. Menopause is twelve months after the last period, on average—at age fifty-one; postmenopause follows.

As always, an overall healthful diet—with enough from MyPyramid—is important advice for menopause. Healthful eating and active living promote good health, and good health minimizes the discomforts of menopause. *See "MyPyramid: Your Healthful Eating Guide" in chapter 10.*

Physical activity remains a priority, with benefits to weight management; to heart and bone health; and to lower risks for heart disease, diabetes, and cancer. An active lifestyle also can reduce the discomforts of menopause. *See "Get Physical!" in chapter 2.*

Iron Needs Drop

Your iron need drops with menopause—from 18 to 8 milligrams of iron a day. Since you no longer have menstrual loss, your risk for iron deficiency goes down. Unless your doctor advises otherwise, stop taking iron supplements. Consuming too much iron, typically from a supplement, can be harmful—especially if you have a genetic disorder called hemochromatosis.

Weight Gain: A New Problem?

On the "down" side, some menopausal women gain weight—some having weight problems for the first time in their life! Why? It's partly age. Metabolic rate, or the speed at which the body uses energy, often slows as hormone levels change. There's often another reason. In midlife, many women shift to more sedentary living, using less food energy. That promotes weight problems if eating habits remain unchanged. As an aside, research doesn't support the perception that hormone therapy causes weight gain.

Besides going up in dress size, what are the risks? Being overweight increases the chances for many health problems that start to appear after menopause. Changing hormone levels affect body fat distribution as more fat gets stored around the abdomen. Central body fat appears to be riskier for heart disease, higher cholesterol levels, high blood pressure, and insulin resistance than lower body fat.

You don't need be resigned to weight gain after menopause! To maintain your weight or to drop a few pounds if you need to, adjust your food choices. Follow MyPyramid guidelines and choose mostly lean and lower-fat foods, also with fewer added sugars. Balance the calories you take in with those you burn. Move more, too—that includes strength training to maintain muscle and to keep your bones healthy! *See chapter 2, "Your Healthy Weight."*

Bone Health: Calcium and Vitamin D Needs Go Up

Bone loss is part of aging. With a drop in estrogen levels during menopause, women lose bone faster, so calcium needs increase. In the first years after menopause women lose 3 to 5 percent of bone mass per year and 1 percent bone loss per year after age sixty-five.

Boosting your calcium and vitamin D intake and regular weight-bearing exercise helps slow bone loss and reduce risks for osteoporosis and fractures. After age fifty, the Adequate Intake for women, set by the Institute of Medicine, is 1,200 milligrams of calcium daily, and for vitamin D, 10 micrograms a day. As a reference, 8 ounces of milk supplies about 300 milligrams of calcium and 2.5 micrograms (or 100 International Units) vitamin D. *For more about calcium and bone health, see "Calcium: A Closer Look" in chapter 4.*

Taking a calcium supplement does make a difference in bone health—as noted in further investigation of the Women's Health Initiative Study. This was questioned when this study was first published.

For bone health, phytoestrogens (*see chapter 4*) haven't been shown to prevent osteoporosis or lower fracture risk. While hormone therapy may reduce bone loss, any benefit—from estrogen only—must be balanced against increased heart disease risk. *Refer to "Osteoporosis: Reducing the Risks" in chapter 22.*

Heart Disease: A Woman's Issue, Too!

As estrogen levels drop with menopause, women no longer have the same protection that estrogen gives from heart disease and high blood pressure. HDL levels drop; triglyceride levels increase. That's true whether menopause is natural or surgical. As a result, women's heart-disease risks parallel those of men—seven to ten years later in life! Their death rate is higher, perhaps due to increased age or more risk factors. In fact, heart disease (not breast cancer) is the top killer and disabler of American women; a woman is three times more likely to get cardiovascular disease than breast cancer. About two-thirds of women who die of heart disease had no previous symptoms.

The signs of heart disease for women often differ from those of men—and may go unrecognized or ignored. Women often have angina first, rather than a heart attack. A woman's symptoms may be intermittent: unexplained heartburn, profound fatigue, nausea, shortness of breath, and pain that comes and goes. Treadmill stress tests for diagnosis are less reliable for women than for men, too. Also less reliable: taking a lose-dose aspirin.

Women—if you haven't done so already, make heart-healthy choices. Start with small steps, then work up. This book is full of practical advice:

● Eat a colorful variety of fruits and vegetables, grains (including whole grains), low-fat or fat-free dairy foods, fatty fish, legumes, and other lean protein foods. Make overall choices that are low in sat-urated fat, *trans* fat, and cholesterol.

● Stay physically active, or start. Fit in at least 30 minutes of moderate physical activity daily, or on most days.

● Keep a healthy weight. Your risk for heart disease is higher if most body fat is around your abdomen, rather than your hips and thighs.

● Control diabetes if you have it. A healthy weight lowers your risk of type 2 diabetes. Diabetes increases heart disease risk, for women even more than for men. Aim for a normal blood glucose level.

● Prevent high blood pressure, or lower your blood pressure to optimal levels. Choose and prepare foods with little salt; consume potassium-rich foods to blunt sodium's effects on blood pressure.

● Control stress in your daily life, especially if it leads to overeating, smoking, or other risky behaviors.

● If you drink alcoholic beverages, do so in moderation.

● If you smoke, quit. If you don't, don't start. And stay away from secondhand smoke.

Refer to chapter 22 for more on heart disease, high blood pressure, and diabetes.

Menopausal Symptoms: Nutrition and Lifestyle Strategies

Menopause sets the stage for two conditions: osteoporosis and heart disease. Many women deal with uncomfortable menopausal symptoms, too. Instead of hormone therapy, nutrition and lifestyle strategies may help. If you're approaching or experiencing menopause, talk with your healthcare provider about the best approach for you. Nonhormonal medications may be prescribed.

Hot Flashes

What about phytoestrogens? Foods with estrogenlike compounds called isoflavones (genistein and daidzein) in soy are getting research attention. Under study, these substances, found in many soy foods (tofu, tempeh, soy beverages—not soy oil) may help offset the effects of reduced estrogen production by the ovaries for some women. Currently there's no solid evidence that they reduce hot flashes, but more soy from food likely can't hurt. *See "What's 'Soy' Good?" in chapter 11.*

Lifestyle changes can help you cope: sleeping in a cool room, wearing clothes that don't make you too warm, and reducing stress. Avoiding caffeine and spicy foods, according to the National Institutes of Health, may help.

Insomnia

Trouble sleeping? Try consuming milk or yogurt (low-fat or fat-free) at bedtime, and perhaps taking a hot shower or bath. Keep physical activity, preferably early in the day, in your daily routine; physical activity later may keep you awake at night.

Other Symptoms

Many women experience mood swings and memory problems, too. Getting enough sleep and staying physically active help—yet another reason to fit in at least 30 minutes of moderate physical activity every day!

Need more tips specific to women's health? Check here for "how-tos":

- Help an adolescent girl address some nutrition issues that start during puberty—see chapter 16.
- Follow a safe, effective strategy for reaching and keeping your healthy weight after pregnancy, menopause, or at any other time of life—see chapter 2.
- Protect yourself from—or deal with—chronic health problems that afflict women: heart disease, diabetes, cancer (including breast cancer), osteoporosis, and anemia—see chapter 22.
- Choose a supplement ("multi," calcium, iron) if you need it—see chapter 23.
- Find a nutrition expert experienced in women's health issues—see chapter 24.

Have You Ever Wondered

. . . if supplements are safe, effective treatments for menopause symptoms? Even though they're "natural," herbal and botanical supplements may not be safe or effective. The American College of Obstetricians and Gynecologists advises:

- *Soy foods and their isoflavones* in amounts in food are safe and perhaps helpful. Because soy products have some estrogenlike qualities they may have some risks.
- *Black cohosh* may act like estrogen. It may offer some relief of hot flashes and night sweats. But side effects may include nausea and low blood pressure.
- *Dong quai* doesn't appear effective when used alone. Of concern, it may increase sensitivity to sunlight and perhaps affect blood clotting time, which can be risky.
- *Wild or Mexican yam* doesn't appear to reduce menopause symptoms, unless perhaps large amounts are consumed.
- Other products without proof of effectiveness: *evening primrose, valerian root, ginseng, and chasteberry.* Again, probably not worth the money.

Before you take supplements to reduce menopause symptoms, talk to your doctor. They may interfere with other medications you're taking. *Refer to chapter 23 for more about dietary supplements.*

Hormone Therapy

Hormone therapy may ease menopausal discomforts for some women, bothered by moderate or severe symptoms, and it may help reduce osteoporosis risk. However, although low for many women, there's an increased risk for heart disease, stroke, or breast cancer with its use. Discuss with your doctor whether hormone therapy outweighs your personal risks. If you choose to use it, see your healthcare professional regularly. If you already use hormone therapy, reconsider your options.

CHAPTER 18

For Mature Adults

Healthful Eating!

Are you catching the age wave—or how about an older relative or a friend? Are you in the "sandwich generation"—in between caring for kids and older parents?

Due to better healthcare, longer life expectancy, and the aging of the baby boom generation, the number of mature American adults is on the rise. By 2010 ninety million Americans may be "fifty plus" mature adults, according to projections, with only seventy-four million age eighteen or under. And by 2030, people aged sixty-five or older are expected to make up 20 percent (compared to 12 percent in the mid-1990s) of the U.S. population, with the eighty-five-plus group projected to grow the fastest!

What is a "mature adult"? Actually, there's no one concise category to describe the diversity of "mature adults" whose ages span a half century—from their fifties into their hundreds. Many live a full, active lifestyle that differs little from life in their thirties or forties. Others are limited by health and lifestyle challenges that began at a younger age. Except for a few shifts in nutrient needs, overall health and attitude define aging more than calendar age does.

So, with what you know now, do you wish you were sixteen again? If so, would you make smarter food choices? Fit more physical activity into your life? Deal with stress better? Try to sleep more?

You can't change the past—or stop the clock. "Anti-aging" is impossible, but the choices made now or at any age and health condition can slow the changes and the challenges that come with getting older, and perhaps even extend youth. The results? Feeling good longer, and enjoying life now and in years to come. Sound good? Start now—to eat smarter and move more! Good lifestyle choices can be powerful influences on healthy aging!

Aged to Perfection!

It's no secret: how you eat—and how active you are—have plenty to do with your biological age. *For healthy, mature adults, the Dietary Guidelines, described in chapter 1, and MyPyramid, described in chapter 10, serve as sound, credible advice for healthful eating.* Thirty minutes of moderate physical activity each day are now recommended as a smart lifestyle choice.

Smart food choices and active living today may help you feel younger, stay healthier, more productive and self-sufficient, enjoy a higher quality of life—and even prevent, or at least delay, health problems that often come with aging. *See "How 'Old' Are You? Biomarkers of Age" on page 459.*

Of course, life and health change gradually as the years go by. Yet for each of us, getting older differs. And diversity describes every decade of the mature years: "fifty plus," "seventy plus," even "ninety plus"!

Eating for Healthy Aging

Whether you're over fifty or seventy, you (or an older relative or friend) need the same nutrients—proteins,

How "Old" Are You? Biomarkers of Age

Eager to slow the physical changes of aging? Want to feel as young as you are? Rather than wait until you notice signs of aging, a fitness routine—healthful eating and regular physical activity—can help slow or reverse "biomarkers," or changes, that come with getting older.

● *Your muscle mass and strength.* Stamina, ease of movement, ability to handle heavy objects, feeling energetic, and even physical appearance depend on muscle strength and flexibility. Yet, with age, muscle size and strength decrease naturally; for each decade of adult life, people lose about six to seven pounds of muscle. That rate hastens after age forty-five. Regular physical activity helps you maintain muscle size, strength, and other qualities of youth.

● *The rate your body uses energy.* The rate your body uses energy declines with age: about 2 percent for every decade. Body composition, along with hormone changes, is part of the reason. You can't fool Mother Nature entirely. But if you're physically active and keep your muscle mass, your body burns energy a little faster; muscle burns more energy than body fat.

● *Your percentage of body fat.* With age, body fat gradually replaces muscle—even if your eating and activity patterns stay the same. Besides losing that firm, muscular shape of youth, any extra body fat increases your risk for high blood pressure, heart disease, stroke, some cancers, diabetes, arthritis, and breathing problems. "Midriff bulge" is a sure sign that you're probably not twenty-five anymore! The bottom line: try to keep lean.

● *Your bone density.* Healthy bones let you enjoy physical activity as you age with less risk of fractures. Yet bone loss is a natural part of aging. If you keep your bones strong, you may avoid a "dowager's hump," which often appears with osteoporosis. *See "Osteoporosis: Reduce the Risks" in chapter 22 for ways to slow bone loss.*

● *Your cholesterol/HDL levels.* Age is one reason why total and LDL cholesterol rise. As a heart-healthy strategy, losing weight, regular physical activity, and smart eating can help bring down your total and your LDL blood cholesterol levels, lower your triglycerides, and raise your "good" HDL blood cholesterol levels. *See "Heart Disease: The Blood Lipid Connection" in chapter 22.*

● *Your blood sugar tolerance.* With age, blood sugar levels may rise for several reasons. In part, your body may not produce as much insulin with age. Physical activity, along with keeping a healthy weight, can help keep blood sugar levels within normal range and help you avoid type 2 diabetes.

● *Your body's "thermostat."* Fluids are your body's natural cooling system. As you get older, your sense of thirst may diminish, putting you at greater risk for dehydration. Still, your body needs at least 9 to 12½ cups of fluid daily from water, juice, milk, other beverages, and food. Physical activity helps your body regulate its internal temperature.

● *Your aerobic capacity.* With age, your body's ability to use the oxygen you breathe efficiently declines. With continued vigorous physical activity, your body pumps more oxygen to your muscles.

---

carbohydrates, fats, vitamins, minerals, and water—but perhaps in slightly different amounts. When health or lifestyles limit food choices, or when meals and medications need careful coordination, consuming enough may be a challenge!

After age fifty, a few nutrients may need special attention: protein, calcium, vitamin D, vitamin C, iron, vitamin A, folate, vitamin B$_6$, vitamin B$_{12}$, zinc, and water. Among the reasons? Physical changes with aging affect how your body digests food, absorbs its nutrients, and excretes wastes. Eating enough fiber-rich foods aids digestion and helps prevent the discomfort of constipation—two problems that may come with aging. To ease this discomfort, the Adequate Intake for total fiber after age fifty is 30 grams for men and 21 grams for women daily.

For nutrients, the DRIs provide guidance for two groups of mature, healthy adults: those age fifty-one or over, and those age seventy-one or over. *For specific amounts, see the chart in the Appendices. Advice may differ with health problems; see chapter 22.*

Nutrient-Rich: Spending Calories Wisely

As people get older, most use less energy, or calories, than they did in their younger years. In fact, calorie needs may decrease by as much as 25 percent for two reasons. First, basic body processes use energy at a slower rate. Most adults lose about 2 to 3 percent of their lean body mass, or muscle, each decade of their adult life; the body uses less energy to maintain body fat than to maintain muscle. Second, many mature adults need fewer calories for their less physically active lifestyles. Yet nutrient needs don't change much; in some cases they're somewhat higher.

How many calories? Although calorie needs vary for activity level, gender, health status, and age, as well as height and weight, many women over age fifty need 1,600 to 1,800 calories daily. Many older men need about 2,000 calories each day. Doesn't seem like many calories? Chosen carefully, those calories can—*and should*—be nutrient-rich! The problem for many older adults is: as calorie intake declines, vitamin and mineral intake often does, too. That's why nutrient-rich foods are so important! *Use "MyPyramid Food Intake Calorie Pattern Levels" in the Appendices to estimate your calorie needs.*

The challenge for healthy, older adults: Get about the same amount of nutrients as before, but likely with fewer calories! To do that:

● Make smart choices with plenty of variety from all five food groups to get the nutrients you need—including those of special concern for older adults. Make the most of your discretionary calories with more healthful oils in place of saturated and *trans* fats.

● Get the most nutrition from your food and beverage choices—and your calories. Pick foods such as fruits, vegetables, whole-grain products, fat-free or low-fat milk and milk products, lean meat, poultry, fish, and eggs. Go nutrient-rich!

● Find a balance between food and physical activity. That includes paying attention to your food and drink portions—and being physically active in ways that match your lifestyle and health.

Use MyPyramid, *described in chapter 10*, to help you make and monitor your healthful eating plan. If you're computer savvy, the Food Tracker on www.MyPyramid.gov can help.

Eat Your Fruits and Vegetables!

The advice you've likely given kids applies to you, too: Eat your fruits and vegetables! Colorful and nourishing, they're mostly nutrient rich and provide plenty of phytonutrients. Along with their many health-promoting benefits, their fiber can help overcome constipation. Their potassium may help counter the effects of sodium on blood pressure, and their antioxidants may provide anti-aging properties that may reduce disease risk.

Chewing problems? That's no reason to give up fruits or vegetables. Make "softer" choices: perhaps ripe bananas, baked or steamed squash, cooked peas, sliced peaches, baked sweet or baking potatoes, cooked spinach, stewed tomatoes, or steamed cauliflower.

Concerned that fresh produce might take a bite out of your pocketbook? Buy seasonal fruits and vegetables, when they typically cost less. And stock up on canned and frozen fruits and vegetables, and dried fruits, when they're specially priced. Canned and frozen fruits and vegetables offer convenience, especially for housebound adults. If you or someone you're caring for needs a special diet, talk to a registered dietitian about buying these foods. Use the Nutrition Facts on food labels, too. Some canned vegetables and frozen vegetables with sauces contain added salt and added sugars. Plain, frozen vegetables and no-salt-added canned vegetables may be better choices for a low-sodium diet. Canned fruit in natural juices and frozen fruit without added sugars may be better choices for "carb"-controlled eating.

As in younger years, mature, healthy adults are urged to keep their overall food choices low in saturated fats, *trans* fats, and cholesterol, and to moderate total fat intake. Remember that a gram of fat supplies more than twice the calories that a gram of either carbohydrate or protein does, so watching your fat intake is one approach to eating more nutrient-rich foods and balancing your calories for weight control. Limiting fat, *trans* fat, saturated fat, and cholesterol may also be part of managing risk factors for heart disease and other chronic health problems.

MyPyramid is meant for healthy people. If you have diabetes, high blood pressure, or other health problems (or if you're at risk for them), your food and nutrient needs may differ. Get advice from a registered dietitian or your doctor. *Refer to chapter 22, "Smart Eating to Prevent and Manage Disease."*

Protein: An Issue for Some

Protein: you still need it! If you follow advice from the Meat and Beans Group of MyPyramid, you're likely consuming enough protein. So what's the issue?

Some older adults don't consume enough protein-rich foods. Sometimes meat or poultry are hard to chew and swallow, so they may be left on the plate. Other people may have trouble digesting milk, another good protein source. Those with limited finances might avoid meat, poultry, or fish because they often cost more than many other foods.

Emerging research suggests: Eating somewhat more protein as you age may help you retain muscle mass as you become more sedentary. How can you get enough high-quality protein?

● Choose lean meat, poultry, and fish. Combine them with other ingredients in casserole dishes so a small amount goes farther. Consider less-expensive protein sources, such as eggs, legumes, and peanut butter.

● Chop your meat or poultry well if you need to.

● Trouble chewing? Have your teeth and gums (perhaps dentures) checked. *See "Chewing Problems?" on page 474.*

● Include dairy products. Milk, cheese, and yogurt—and foods made with these ingredients—supply protein. If milk disagrees with you, try cheese or yogurt. *See chapter 21 if you're lactose-sensitive.*

● Consult a registered dietitian for other ways to ensure enough high-quality protein in your food choices.

See "Protein Power" in chapter 20.

Calcium: As Important as Ever

Why is calcium still so important? Calcium plays a primary role in keeping your bones healthy and so

Have You Ever Wondered

. . . why milk doesn't seem to agree with you anymore? Some older adults have trouble digesting milk, even though they had no problem in younger years. The reason? The small intestine may no longer produce as much lactase. Lactase, an enzyme, digests the natural sugar, called lactose, in milk and some milk products.

To continue to enjoy milk and reap its calcium and vitamin D benefits, try this. Drink milk in small amounts; usually your body can handle a little at a time. Try buttermilk, yogurt, cheese, or a special lactose-reduced milk. Custard, pudding, and cream soup may be tolerated better, too. Try other foods that supply calcium, including some dark-green leafy vegetables and canned fish (sardines and salmon) with bones. *For more tips, see "Lactose Intolerance: A Matter of Degree" in chapter 21.*

. . . if you should avoid animal-based foods (meat, eggs, milk, cheese) with fat and cholesterol to protect yourself from heart disease? There's no reason for "fat phobia." Thinking that you need to avoid meat, dairy foods, and eggs to protect against heart disease is unfounded—especially if that means missing out on these nutrient-rich foods. They supply other nutrients that often end up short in the diets of older adults: calcium, iron, zinc, and vitamins B_6 and B_{12}.

If you don't have heart disease, and if your blood cholesterol levels are within a healthful range, be sensible—and enjoy these foods in moderation, using guidelines from MyPyramid.

. . . if extra vitamin E will keep you young? We all dream of the fountain of youth. Many claims made for vitamin E are really distortions of research done with animals that shouldn't be applied to humans. Taking vitamin E supplements won't stop or reverse the aging process. And in the bigger picture, they won't cure sterility, premenstrual syndrome for younger women, or ulcers, to name a few.

Research is being done to explore the potential benefits of taking extra amounts of vitamin E, however. As an antioxidant it may play a protective role against some health problems including building immunity, cataract formation, and Alzheimer's and Parkinson's diseases. It's too soon to advise levels higher than the Recommended Dietary Allowance of 15 milligrams of alpha-tocopherol a day; *see chapter 4 for more about vitamin E.*

Until more is known, make food choices that supply enough vitamin E. If you take a supplement, choose one with no more than 100 percent of the Daily Value for vitamin E. And talk to a registered dietitian to help you sort through the current facts about vitamin E.

helps reduce the risks of osteoporosis, or brittle-bone disease. That's true for both men and women!

For mature adults, calcium needs are higher. To help maintain bone mass, calcium recommendations increase by 20 percent. For both men and women over age fifty, the Adequate Intake level is 1,200 milligrams of calcium daily. That's almost as much as growing children and teens need daily.

The risk for osteoporosis goes up with age. By age seventy, between 30 and 40 percent of all women have had at least one fracture linked to osteoporosis. The percent continues to climb, even for men, who may develop bone disease later in life. *See "Osteoporosis: Reduce the Risks" in chapter 22.*

Age is only one reason why older adults have a higher risk for bone disease. Many don't consume enough calcium-rich foods, especially if dairy foods aren't a regular part of their meals or snacks. With age, the body doesn't absorb calcium from food as well. In addition, many older adults don't get enough weight-bearing exercise, which helps to keep bones stronger. Vitamin D, which helps the body use calcium, may be limited in food choices, too, and it isn't absorbed as well as it once was.

There's good news if you're an older adult: even if you haven't been consuming enough calcium all along, it's not too late to consume more now. You still can reduce your risk of bone fractures as you get older. At the same time, consume enough vitamin D and do some weight-bearing exercise, such as walking. Aim for thirty minutes of moderate physical activity each day, taken all at once or split into shorter segments.

Which foods supply calcium? Milk, yogurt, and cheese are the best sources. For example, an 8-ounce glass of milk supplies about 300 milligrams of calcium, so two or three cups put you well on your way. Milk is a good source of vitamin D and potassium, too, which might come up short for many mature adults. In addition, some dark-green leafy vegetables, fish with edible bones (such as canned salmon), calcium-fortified soy beverages, tofu made with calcium sulfate, and other fortified foods also have significant amounts of calcium.

Hint: Calcium in food is more bioavailable than from a supplement. But if you do take a calcium supplement, choose one with vitamin D, and take it between meals. Calcium can hinder the absorption of iron from your meals. *See "Calcium Supplements: A Bone Builder?" in chapter 23.*

Calcium and vitamin D aren't the only nutrients important for bone health. Others, including protein, vitamins A and K, magnesium, as well as phytoestrogens, play a role—another reason why overall healthful eating is so important to reducing disease risk!

Vitamin D: The Sunshine Vitamin

To keep bones strong as you age, your body needs calcium—along with its partner vitamin D. Vitamin D helps deposit calcium in your bones and together they help protect you from bone disease.

Vitamin D is unique. It's known as the "sunshine vitamin" because your body makes it after sunlight, or ultraviolet light, hits your skin. If you stay indoors, your body may lack vitamin D, especially if you don't drink milk fortified with vitamin D.

With age, the body doesn't make vitamin D from sunlight as easily; by age seventy, 50 to 75 percent less vitamin D is made than for someone age twenty. The body doesn't absorb as much vitamin D from food in later years either. Adding to the risk, many older adults are housebound or covered outside, especially in northern climates, so sun exposure is limited.

Like calcium, the need for vitamin D goes up after age fifty. In fact, it doubles to 400 International Units (IUs), or 10 micrograms, daily. And after age seventy, the recommended daily intake level goes up again, to 600 IUs for both men and women.

Vitamin D is added to most milk and other fortified foods such as cereals. You'll find vitamin D listed on the Nutrition Facts on food packages if it's been added. Even if you drink milk regularly, though, you may need a vitamin D supplement; consult your doctor or registered dietitian. Taking high doses from a dietary supplement can be harmful. Kidney damage, weak bones or muscles, and excessive bleeding are all associated with taking too much over time.

For older adults, the Dietary Guidelines advise: *Consume extra vitamin D from vitamin D-fortified foods and/or supplements.*

The Iron–Vitamin C Connection

Most people who follow guidelines of MyPyramid consume enough iron and vitamin C. Yet, for mature adults, a poor diet may lead to a deficiency in one or both. Iron deficiency causes anemia, which can make you feel weak, tired, and irritable, or lose concentration. *See "Anemia: 'Tired Blood'" in chapter 22.* Iron deficiency may have other causes: reduced iron absorption as the body secretes less digestive juices or when antacids interfere; blood loss from ulcers, hemorrhoids, or other health problems; and medications (perhaps too many aspirins) that cause blood loss.

Although iron and vitamin C come from very different foods, their health roles are connected. Vitamin C helps your body absorb iron from eggs and from plant sources of food. Vitamin C is especially important if you rely heavily on beans, whole-grain foods, and iron-enriched cereals as iron sources.

Choose economical sources of iron, including iron-enriched cereals; legumes (dry beans); whole-grain foods; lean, ground meat; eggs; and liver. Partner eggs, beans, and whole-grain and iron-enriched breads, pasta, and cereals with either vitamin C-rich foods or with some meat, poultry, or fish. *Refer to "Iron: A Closer Look" in chapter 4.*

Vitamin C (in citrus, fruit, melon, and berries) may offer some other health-promoting benefits. As an antioxidant, it may help lower the risk for cataracts and some cancers, for example. For any nutrient, including vitamin C, try to get enough from food first, not a supplement. Besides, vitamin C-rich foods have other nutrients, such as potassium, and phytonutrients that promote health. Insufficient intake of vitamin C is linked to memory loss. Excessively high amounts from supplements can be harmful, especially if you have hemochromatosis, recurring kidney stones, or kidney disease.

For iron, the advice for adults ages fifty-one on is 8 milligrams a day; that's less than half of what women need before menopause. Consult with your doctor before taking an iron supplement. A supplement with too much iron for you can be harmful. For some people with a genetic illness called hemochromatosis, iron is absorbed more readily and can build up in body organs, causing irreparable damage.

Other Nutrients and Phytonutrients

Besides those just mentioned, a few others may need attention in the eating patterns of mature Americans. Not getting enough of any single nutrient on one day

or even for several days isn't a cause for concern. But for those who don't consume a balanced diet with enough nutrients over a longer period—several weeks or months—a nutrient supplement may be prescribed, especially for elderly people.

Vitamin A and Carotenoids (forms vitamin A). Vitamin A helps your eyes adjust to darkness, a safety precaution. Carotenoids also may help reduce the risk of age-related macular degeneration and cataracts. Colorful vegetables and fruits are good food sources. Consult with a registered dietitian or your healthcare provider before taking vitamin A supplements regularly. With age, the liver can't handle excess vitamin A as well; too much from supplements can be especially harmful.

Folate. Folate, a B vitamin, helps your body make red blood cells. Not consuming enough over time may

Miracles? Dream On!

Charlatans prey on mature adults with promises of easy cures or ways to stay young. Many products they peddle are foods, substances from food, or supplements. No substantial evidence is provided for many claims that their products offer benefits for treating arthritis, cancer, Alzheimer's disease, or other maladies—or for helping people live longer.

Many "miracle" products are costly. Money used to buy them is better spent on healthful, flavorful foods.

Their harm may go farther than the pocketbook. These remedies may mask symptoms, offer false hope, or worse yet, keep people from seeking reliable healthcare. These products also may interfere with the action of prescribed medications—or perhaps with the absorption of nutrients in food.

Always be cautious of promises that seem too good to be true. *To learn how to judge what you read and hear about nutrition and health, see chapter 24.* Always consult your doctor or a registered dietitian before trying these products—or any alternative healthcare. *Chapter 23 explores what's known and unknown about many supplements, some promoted as "antiaging."* Many people claim to be nutrition experts, but some aren't qualified. *To find a registered dietitian, other qualified health expert, or resources in your community, see chapter 24.*

lead to anemia and age-related hearing loss. Along with other B vitamins, folate from food may play a role in heart health, by removing homocysteine from the bloodstream; high homocysteine levels are a potential risk factor for heart disease. Good sources: leafy green vegetables, some fruits, legumes, liver, fortified cereals, other grain foods, and wheat germ.

Vitamin B$_{12}$. Vitamin B$_{12}$, or cobalamin, works with folate to make red blood cells. Not getting enough

---

A Day of Good Nutrition

Here's an easy-to-make, easy-to-digest, low-cost menu for a whole day of good nutrition. If you count up the servings, you'll see it supplies enough from all five food groups of MyPyramid. It's a menu that adds up to about 1,700 to 1,800 calories. *Note:* Choose mostly foods with little added salt.

Breakfast:

½ medium grapefruit
½ cup fortified oat flakes with ½ cup low-fat or fat-
    free milk
Coffee, tea, or water

Snack:

2 squares graham crackers
1 cup low-fat fruit yogurt
½ cup orange juice (perhaps calcium fortified)

Lunch:

1 cup split-pea or lentil soup, low sodium
½ cup coleslaw
1 small corn muffin
½ cup canned, juice-packed peaches
½ cup low-sodium tomato juice

Dinner:

3 ounces skinless chicken breast, baked with Italian
    seasoning
1 medium baked sweet potato
½ cup green beans, frozen or canned, no-salt-added
1 small dinner roll
½ cup low-fat ice cream
Coffee, tea, or water

Snack:

½ whole-wheat English muffin with 1 tablespoon
    apple butter
1 cup low-fat or fat-free milk

---

vitamin B$_{12}$ also can lead to anemia and high levels of homocysteine. Among mature adults, low levels of vitamins B$_{12}$ and B$_6$ are linked to memory loss, and low levels of B$_{12}$, to age-related hearing loss. With coexisting conditions, other symptoms of vitamin B$_{12}$ deficiency may go unrecognized. Meat, poultry, fish, eggs, and dairy foods are all good sources. To avoid deficiency, mature adults are urged to eat vitamin B$_{12}$-fortified foods and to take a supplement with vitamin B$_{12}$. Some health problems impair the body's ability to absorb naturally occurring vitamin B$_{12}$. If you're over age fifty, the Dietary Guidelines advise: *Consume vitamin B$_{12}$ in its crystalline form (from fortified foods or supplements)*—and meet the recommendation of 2.4 micrograms per day.

Vitamin B$_6$. Vitamin B$_6$ often comes up short for older adults, too. The recommendation for vitamin B$_6$ goes up slightly after age fifty, from 1.3 milligrams per day for men and women to 1.5 milligrams daily for women and 1.7 milligrams daily for men. Among the good sources: chicken, fish, and pork, and to a lesser degree, whole grains, nuts, and legumes.

Sodium and Potassium. The risk rising with age, many mature adults develop high blood pressure. Older adults are more salt-sensitive, yet potassium blunts sodium's effects on blood pressure. To balance these nutrients, the Dietary Guidelines advise older adults: *Aim to consume no more than 1,500 milligrams of sodium per day, and meet the potassium recommendation (4,700 milligrams per day) with food.*

Zinc. Zinc from foods such as beef, whole grains, and milk helps your body fight infections and repair body tissue. Yet absorption decreases with age. Even a marginal deficiency may affect the ability to taste, heal wounds, and provide immunity.

For more about these nutrients, see chapter 4.

Thirst Quenchers: Drink Fluids

Thirsty? The average healthy adult uses about 3 quarts or more of fluid daily by urinating, perspiring, breathing, and eliminating other body wastes. To keep from getting dehydrated, your body needs its fluids replaced. Thirst is a signal to drink more.

With age come changes that affect fluid intake. The sense of thirst often diminishes, so mature adults may not be able to count on thirst as their primary reminder to drink fluids. Kidneys may not conserve fluids as they once did either, so the body holds on to less water. Those who have trouble getting around may deliberately limit fluid intake to avoid bathroom trips. Fear of incontinence also keeps some people from drinking enough.

Dehydration is a health concern during the mature years, especially in warmer weather and for those who don't drink enough fluid. And adequate fluid intake is linked to other health issues:

● Everyone needs enough water to help rid the body of wastes. With less fluid, the chances of constipation rise.

● While fluid helps keep kidneys healthy, dehydration can cause kidney problems.

● Many older adults have less saliva to help with chewing and swallowing. Drinking water or other liquids at meals makes eating easier.

● Some medications need to be taken with water. Some, such as diuretics, cause the body to lose water. Understand how medications affect fluid status!

● In older adults, dehydration may cause symptoms that seem like dementia, or impaired mental function, or might worsen existing dementia.

● In extreme cases dehydration can lead to death.

Mature adults need plenty of fluids. Food provides some water, but drinking at least 9 to 12½ cups daily depending on your gender is important. Any beverage—juice, milk, soup, tea, coffee, soft drinks—supplies water. Plain water is great! Juice, milk, and soup offer nutrients as well.

Caffeinated beverages such as regular coffee, tea, and colas are best consumed in moderation. Caffeine can have a mild diuretic effect, perhaps increasing the need to urinate. The beverage itself usually cancels out any fluid loss.

The Dietary Guidelines also advise: *Don't consume alcoholic beverages if you take medications that can interact with alcohol or have certain medical problems.*

If you have trouble remembering how much water you drank, try this: fill a jug (or two) or a jar with at least 9 cups (72 ounces) of water each morning. Place it in your refrigerator. Use that water for drinking and for making juice, lemonade, soup, tea, and coffee. When the water is gone, you've probably met your day's fluid goal.

For more about water as a nutrient and the risks of dehydration, see "A Fluid Asset" in chapter 8.

Never Too Late for Exercise

No matter what your age, it's never too late to get moving. Whether you're pushing sixty, seventy, eighty, or perhaps even ninety, you can strengthen your muscles, improve agility and balance, and get other benefits, even if you haven't been physically active for a while. Regardless of overall health, most people can participate in some form of enjoyable physical activity.

For older adults, the Dietary Guidelines advise: *Participate in regular physical activity to reduce functional declines associated with aging and to achieve the other benefits of physical activity identified for all adults.*

The Reasons Are Many

What are the benefits of physical activity for mature adults? They're about the same as for anyone.

● Moving your body burns energy. That's an aid to keeping a healthy weight and important for energy balance!

● Activities that put weight on your bones, such as walking, help preserve bone density. The benefit? Helping to reduce your bone disease risk.

● Regular physical activity of all kinds helps keep your heart and lungs healthier. Aim for a total of thirty minutes of moderate activity each day. Do aerobic activity if you can; ask your doctor first.

● Being active helps keep your blood pressure, blood cholesterol, and blood sugar normal. That reduces the risks related to health problems, such as high blood pressure, heart disease, and diabetes.

● Many activities help minimize muscle loss and keep muscles strong. With strength you often have better balance and may be able to remain independent. You're less likely to fall and fracture your bones.

● Being active often helps your digestion and appetite—a benefit if food seems to lose its appeal.

● For those with trouble sleeping, a problem that often comes with getting older, physical activity helps promote sleep.

● If you feel depressed, being active—especially if you enjoy group activities—can be the antidote! Being active has a way of boosting your outlook on life.

You Can Do It!

For healthy older adults, like their younger counterparts, health experts advise a total of thirty minutes of moderate activity every day, if possible. If you walk, that's about two miles. You don't need to do all your activity at one time. Instead try three ten-minute spurts of activities that you enjoy. Even low-intensity activity can make a difference.

The key to fitting physical activity into your everyday routine is to make it fun! Choose activities that improve endurance, strength, and flexibility.

● Try walking—around the block or around the mall. Walk a dog or invite a friend if you'd like companionship. If you don't have a sidewalk, mall walking is safe—especially in bad weather.

● Do some gardening without electric tools.

● Go swimming. Or try aqua exercises, such as stretching, walking, dancing, or doing aerobics in the water. These are great activities, especially if you're not steady on your feet. They may help relieve some joint pain that accompanies arthritis.

● If you golf, "go the course"—without the cart.

● Go dancing. Even a moderate two-step is good exercise—and a great way to be with other people.

● Take a class in Tai Chi, a series of slow, controlled movements.

Health Alert: Foodborne Illness

Keep food safe! Mature adults are at greater risk for foodborne illness. The reason? The immune system can't always fight back as easily with age, especially for those battling other health problems, such as diabetes or kidney disease, or for those dealing with some cancer treatments. With age, stomach acids, which help reduce intestinal bacteria, decrease. Even mild foodborne illness can have a serious health effect.

Although the kitchen seems clean, poor eyesight or inadequate lighting may keep people from noticing food spills or visual signs of food spoilage. And for those with less energy, proper cleaning may be hard to do.

For anyone, especially older adults:

● If you need glasses, wear them as you handle food.

● Turn up the lights. Mature adults may have more trouble with glare from one light source.

● Label perishable food with a date. Use a dark marker that's easy to read. Don't count on memory alone to know your own "use by" date.

● Don't rely on your senses of sight, smell, or taste to determine if food is safe to eat. Contaminated food may not have an off-flavor or off-smell. With impaired vision, cross-contamination of salad vegetables and raw meat juices may not be obvious.

● Cook simply to save your energy for cleanup, too. Frozen and canned foods are quick, nutritious, and easy to cook.

● Feeling short on energy? Feel comfortable about asking a younger family member or a friend to help occasionally with kitchen tasks.

● Portions too big when you eat out? If you bring food home in a "doggie bag," refrigerate it right away, and reheat it to steaming or boiling before you eat it—within a few days.

Follow the general steps for food safety described in chapter 12, "The Safe Kitchen."

To reduce health risks from foodborne bacteria, *the Dietary Guidelines for Americans advise older adults to avoid raw (unpasteurized) milk or any products made from unpasteurized milk; raw or partially cooked eggs or foods containing raw eggs; raw or undercooked meat and poultry; raw or undercooked fish or shellfish; unpasteurized juices; and raw sprouts. The guidelines also advise: Only eat certain deli meats and frankfurters that have been reheated to steaming hot.*

● To keep your arms strong, lift "weights." Use canned foods from your kitchen shelves, bean bags, or 1- to 5-pound hand or ankle weights.

● Learn some chair exercises—good for people who aren't steady on their feet or who have degenerative joint disease. You can "sit and be fit" even if you're confined to a wheelchair or need a walker.

● Want to keep up with everyday tasks such as bending for a newspaper, reaching an upper shelf, or making a bed? Fit in some stretching activities that increase the range of motion in your ankles, knees, hips, shoulders, neck, and back.

● Sign up for an exercise class or an individual fitness program especially designed for mature adults. If needed, check with your community center or area hospital for special classes.

For more ideas, see "Twenty Everyday Ways to Get Moving" in chapter 2.

If you haven't been physically active, talk to your doctor before getting started. Together plan activities and a sensible approach that's safe, effective, and right for you. Most important, start slowly, work toward your goal gradually, and enjoy!

Tip: No matter what activity you're involved in, drink plenty of water before, during, and afterward.

When Lifestyles Change

Lifestyle changes accompany each stage in life. Think about the independence that came with becoming an adult, the responsibility with parenthood, or the freedom of having kids finally leave the "nest." At some point the mature years also bring new lifestyles and health conditions that impact what, where, when, and even with whom you eat. And losing a spouse, moving away from a lifelong community, even retiring can change social interaction that includes food.

Eating Alone—Special, Too!

For many, eating provides a time to enjoy others. That's especially true for those who've spent their time cooking for a family. However, the pleasure of preparing food, even eating, may diminish when eating alone. Eating alone can feel boring or depressing. If you're

in that position, or know someone who is, you can help spark a tired appetite. Eating together may enhance nutrition!

Making Meals Special: Solo or Not

If you're a "single," you don't need to always dine alone. Eat with friends occasionally:

● Set a standing date with a friend, a relative, or a grandchild for lunch or dinner at your home.

● If you're "into cooking" but need someone to cook for, organize a dining club of like-minded friends.

● Cut down on the effort. Get together with other mature adults for weekly or monthly potluck suppers. Take turns acting as host.

● Take advantage of meals offered at senior citizens' centers. Many serve full midday meals on weekdays. Usually the price is right. In some communities, religious centers and schools serve meals for older adults.

Added benefits: Senior citizen meals offer a place to meet old and new friends. You can enjoy a meal that takes more work to prepare than you may do for yourself. Take advantage of an exercise class when you go!

● When eating out, enjoy early-bird specials, when the portions are usually smaller and the prices are lower. Consider splitting an order or take home half for another meal if restaurant portions seem too large. Eat out for breakfast or lunch, when portions are smaller and prices are lower. Some restaurants also have senior citizen prices—just ask. *For more tips on eating out, see chapter 14, "Your Food Away from Home."*

When you do dine solo, make eating a special event. Looking forward to mealtime can offer a boost to both your appetite and your morale!

● Set your place at the table, perhaps with a place mat, napkin, and centerpiece. You'll feel more like you've had a meal—and with more enjoyment—than if you had eaten right from the cooking pot!

● For a change of pace, enjoy eating in different places: the kitchen, patio or deck, dining room, or perhaps on a tray by the fireplace.

● Create some atmosphere or interest. Turn on the radio. Play a favorite music tape or CD. Or watch your favorite television show as you eat.

● Make food preparation easy—and healthful!

See "Have You Ever Wondered . . . how to feel comfortable when you dine alone?" in chapter 14.

Meals–Fast, Simple, Nutritious

Some mature adults say they have no time to cook. They're too busy living life to its fullest. For others, lack of inclination or energy or perhaps less mobility require quick and easy solutions for nutritious eating.

Whatever the reason, try these tasty "meals in minutes" for starters:

● For a quick breakfast, add milk to instant hot cereal. It's as fast to prepare as ready-to-eat cereals.

● Keep frozen dinners and entrées (perhaps a low-

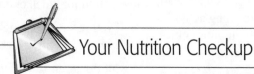

Your Nutrition Checkup

Mature Adults: Nutritionally Healthy?

If you're a mature adult, use this checklist for insight into your nutritional health. If you care for an older adult, perhaps a parent, use it to be a better caregiver.

Read each statement. If a statement applies to you or someone you know, circle the number in the "yes" column. Then tally up the nutritional score of "yes" answers.

	YES
I have an illness or a condition that made me change the kind and/or amount of food I eat.	2 points
I eat fewer than two meals per day.	3 points
I eat few fruits or vegetables, or milk products.	2 points
I have three or more drinks of beer, wine, or spirits almost every day.	2 points
I have tooth or mouth problems that make it hard for me to eat.	2 points
I don't always have enough money to buy the food I need.	4 points
I eat alone most of the time.	1 point
I take three or more different prescribed or over-the-counter drugs a day.	1 point
Without wanting to, I have lost or gained 10 pounds in the past six months.	2 points
I am not always physically able to shop, cook, and/or feed myself.	2 points
Total	_____ points

What's your nutritional score? If it's . . .

0–2 . . . Good! But check again in six months.

3–5 . . . You're at moderate nutritional risk. Try to make some changes—suggested here—that improve your eating habits and lifestyle. Get advice from a registered dietitian or another qualified nutrition professional . . . or from an office on aging, a senior citizens' center, health department, or senior nutrition program. And check again in three months.

6 or more . . . You're at high nutritional risk. The next time you see your doctor, registered dietitian, or other qualified health or social service professional, bring this checklist. Talk about any problems, and ask for help to improve your nutritional health. Read on for practical ways to follow their advice.

Source: Reprinted with permission by the Nutrition Screening Initiative, a project of the American Academy of Family Physicians, the American Dietetic Association, and the National Council on Aging, Inc., and funded in part by a grant from Ross Products Division, Abbott Laboratories Inc. Go to *www.aafp.org/nsi.xml* for a print or interactive copy of this checklist.

calorie version) on hand for quick cooking and easy cleanup. For the most nutrition, buy frozen meals with meat, poultry, or fish; a starchy food (such as rice, pasta, or potato); and a vegetable. Team them with a salad, a roll, a piece of fruit, and milk for a hearty meal that takes little effort.

● Watching your salt intake? Check the sodium on frozen meals and canned foods (stews, soups, and chili). Many have more sodium; look for those with less. Use other seasonings instead of salt. Enhance flavor with MSG, with only one third of the sodium that the same amount of salt has. One-half teaspoon is enough for a pound of meat or 2 to 3 cups of cooked vegetables. Before using MSG, know if you or your guests are sensitive to it.

● Prepare food ahead, or to freeze as leftovers. Perhaps make lower-fat meatballs with lean, ground turkey or beef. Brown, drain any grease, then com-

DETERMINE the Warning Signs of Poor Nutrition

If you're a mature adult, or if you care for someone older, be alert for these warning signs of poor nutrition. They spell the word "determine." Anyone with three or more of these risk factors should consult a doctor, a registered dietitian (RD), or other healthcare professional:

Disease

Eating poorly

Tooth loss or mouth pain

Economic hardship

Reduced social contact

Multiple medicines

Involuntary weight loss or gain

Needs assistance in self-care

Elder years above age eighty

Source: Reprinted with permission by the Nutrition Screening Initiative, a project of the American Academy of Family Physicians, the American Dietetic Association, and the National Council on Aging, Inc., and funded in part by a grant from Ross Products Division, Abbott Laboratories Inc.

These warning signs suggest risk but don't diagnose any health condition.

Meals in Minutes

Check the clock. You can prepare this nutritious, flavorful supper without much effort!

● Place a sliced red or white potato and sliced carrots into a small baking dish sprayed with vegetable oil spray. Toss with 2 teaspoons of olive oil and ½ teaspoon of crushed rosemary or basil, or your favorite herbs. Bake at 350° F for about thirty minutes, until tender.

● In another small baking dish, place a chicken breast or two smaller pieces of chicken. Sprinkle with lemon juice or Italian salad dressing before placing it into the oven. Check the internal temperature; the chicken's done when it reaches 170° F.

● Set the table. Relax with a book or television for about twenty minutes.

● Spoon canned apricot halves into a dish.

● Take out a whole-wheat dinner roll.

● Pour a tall glass of refreshing milk.

● Enjoy your dinner!

bine with tomato sauce. Serve over pasta on one day, over rice the next, and freeze the rest for later.

● Freeze homemade soups, stews, lasagna, and other casserole dishes in single-serving containers. Then thaw enough for one or two meals at a time. Label and date your packages to track what's in the freezer.

● For easy-to-prepare salads, wash, tear, and dry salad greens. Then store them in a plastic container for three or four days. Or purchase pre-washed and cut salad greens in a bag. So when you want a salad, just top greens with sliced tomatoes, grated carrots, sliced deli meat, cheese, or canned kidney beans. Serve with milk, whole-wheat bread, and canned fruit.

● Visit the supermarket salad bar for single servings of washed and chopped fruits and vegetables.

"Maxing Out" Your Food Dollar

Another adjustment may affect food decisions: learning to live and eat on a fixed income. If medical and prescription costs go up at the same time, there may not be much money to spare. For many older adults, economic challenges can get in the way of healthful eating. By shopping wisely, you can maximize your food dollar and get the most nutrition for your money.

Depending on income, many older adults qualify for food stamps, a program of the U.S. Department of Health and Human Services. Food stamps are used like cash in food stores, giving people access to a healthful diet and nutrient-rich foods. Usually food stamps aren't meant for dining out, although for older adults, some restaurants are authorized to accept them in exchange for low-cost meals; check before you order.

Another program, the Senior Farmers' Market Nutrition Program, gives some people ages sixty years and older more access to fresh fruits and vegetables. Other government programs also provide food and nutrition assistance for older adults who qualify. *Refer to chapter 24 for more information.*

To find out if you—or someone you know—qualifies for food stamps or other food assistance, talk to a registered dietitian, social worker, or your local senior center. Or check the government pages in your phone book for your local food stamp office. *See "Nutrition $ense" in chapter 11 for more ways to maximize your food dollar.*

Hassle-Free Shopping

As people get a little older, popping in and out of the supermarket may take more effort. Learn to shop without the hassles:

● Start your shopping trip before you get to the store. Plan ahead. Make a grocery list, then you won't need to repeat your steps through the store.

● Shop at quiet times, such as weekday mornings, when stores aren't crowded. Daytime shopping, when it's easier to see curbs and potholes, is safer anyway. If you must shop at night, pick a store with a well-lit parking lot, or ask someone to go with you.

● Ask for help with your groceries. It's also extra security for you in the parking lot.

● Feeling less stable? Use the shopping cart for balance—even to buy just a few items.

● If you're less mobile, shop in stores with a battery-powered, sit-down grocery cart. It's a courtesy service that your supermarket may offer.

● If you have trouble with night vision, shop during daylight hours.

● Don't drive or use public transportation? Check with your local area Agency on Aging for shopping assistance. Your community may offer shopping transportation for senior citizens.

● Keep an emergency supply of nonperishable foods on the shelf: nonfat dry milk or boxed milk, dried fruit, canned foods (fruit, vegetables, juice, tuna, soup, stew, beans), peanut butter, and cereal. Then you won't need to head to the store when it's raining or snowing.

● If you have ideas to make shopping more convenient for older shoppers, talk with the store manager. With the growing numbers of older customers, they'll likely listen.

● If you qualify, get a sticker for your car that lets you park in spots for the handicapped.

● Ask about special services from your supermarket: home delivery or phone orders. If you're computer savvy, you might order online.

When Cooking Is Too Much

Can't cook anymore? That doesn't necessarily mean giving up living on your own. Many communities offer services for older adults to assure access to nutritious meals. Look for these services:

● Meals on Wheels brings food to housebound people.

● Home healthcare aides help by shopping and preparing meals for older disabled people.

● Community centers offer hot meals. Some are part of adult day programs. Minivans may be available to transfer people to the center. *See "Food in Adult Day and Residential Care: Questions to Ask!" on page 471.*

● Many churches, synagogues, mosques, and other community groups provide volunteers who help older adults with shopping and food preparation.

For assistance, talk to a registered dietitian, a social worker, or call your local Agency on Aging. *See "How to Find Nutrition Help . . ." in chapter 24.*

Food in Adult Day and Residential Care: Questions to Ask!

Meals offer more than nourishment to daily life. That's especially true for many older adults, who look forward to meals as a time to be with others.

As you look for adult day or residential care for yourself, or for a friend or family member, find out about the food service. Look for "yes" answers to these questions:

Sandwiched In?

Are you among the many adults who fit in the "sandwich generation," with children or teens yet to raise and an elderly parent to care for? If so, learn to cope without becoming overly stressed:

- Start by taking care of you: eat smart, fit regular physical activity in, and try to stay rested. Overcome stress or lack of time so they don't become barriers! You'll be more effective in all your family roles as parent, son or daughter, or perhaps spouse—and perhaps in the workforce or your volunteer work.

- Plan openly with your whole family, including kids and an elder parent(s), so that goals, responsibilities, and expectations are clear. That includes activities that surround eating: shopping, food preparation and cleanup, eating schedules, and family meals.

- Share responsibilities as a family rather than attempt to do everything yourself. Try to avoid neglecting one family member to care for another.

- Gather a support network that may include adult day programs, home-delivered meals if you work all day, and other senior citizen services for your parent. Ask for help, and accept when it's offered.

- Accept the fact that you'll be tired and perhaps angry sometimes. That's okay, so discard any feelings of guilt. Instead, get help so you can have a break, even if it's just for a few hours. Maybe it's a good time to do something physically active. If negative feelings trigger eating, find another emotional outlet.

- Respect privacy, dignity, and independence.

Facilities:

- Is the dining area clean and attractive?

- Are menus printed with lettering that's big enough for older people to read?

- Is the dining area well lit throughout, not just with "mood" lighting or single lights that cause glare?

- Does the dining area encourage socializing?

Food:

- Are people given choices from a variety of foods?

- Are plenty of beverages and snacks available throughout the day?

- Is the menu changed often, so the menu cycle doesn't get monotonous?

- Are fresh fruits and vegetables served often?

- Is food served attractively?

- Are religious and cultural food restrictions honored and respected? How about special food preferences?

- Are holidays and special events celebrated with special menus or appropriate foods?

- Are special meals, such as low-sodium or soft meals, provided to those who need them?

- Are people offered a chance to make food requests that aren't on the menu?

Staff:

- Is mealtime viewed as important to daily life at the facility?

- Is a registered dietitian on staff?

- Are people encouraged to eat in a common dining room? Are they offered assistance to get there?

- Do staff or volunteers help those with eating difficulties, perhaps cutting food or helping them eat?

- Do staff or volunteers wear sanitary gloves when they're helping people eat so they don't spread infection?

- Are people given enough time to eat, and not rushed?

- For those who can't leave their rooms, is food brought to them on attractive trays?

● If they need help, is it given promptly so food doesn't get cold? Are trays also removed promptly?

● For a nursing home, does the staff track each person's weight, and how much they eat and drink?

● Are special food and nutrition needs given individual attention? Are special utensils offered if needed?

Changes That Challenge

What's changed? That depends. If you've inherited a great set of genes, and taken care of yourself throughout life, you have a better chance of living a long, vital life. You may feel "fit as a fiddle" without many apparent physical signs of aging. Wrinkles and gray hairs hardly seem to count. In fact, they make you look wise and distinguished.

In the long run, some physical changes are inevitable. The reasons that the human body ages—and the rate of change—are still scientific speculation. But genetics, nutrition, lifestyle, disease, and environment are among the reasons. Many physical and lifestyle changes affect food choices and nutrition.

Have You Ever Wondered

... if taking lecithin or gingko biloba can help prevent memory loss? No, but it's a common wish, especially for those who constantly misplace eyeglasses or shoes! In fact, no conclusive studies show that taking lecithin (a type of fat) or gingko biloba improves memory, thinking, or learning. Under a doctor's supervision, gingko biloba may be used to help treat the symptoms of age-related memory loss and dementia.

... if taking a multivitamin/mineral supplement is a good idea? Consuming a wide variety of food, in sufficient amounts, is the best approach to adequate nutrition, no matter what your age, if you're healthy. However, your physician may suggest a multivitamin/mineral supplement meant for older adults, especially if you limit your food choices. For older adults, supplements with vitamin B_{12}, vitamin D, and perhaps calcium are recommended. Talk to your doctor about any supplement before you take it.

Medications may have side effects related to food or nutrition. *To learn about interactions among food, nutrients, and medications, see "Food and Medicine" in chapter 22.*

Aging with "Taste"

"That recipe just doesn't taste the way I remember!" You might hear that comment from an older adult. Maybe you've said it yourself! The truth is that the senses of smell, taste, and touch decline gradually, with acuity loss starting at about age sixty; some people notice the effects more than others. Medications or health conditions also may alter your flavor perceptions. Fortunately, there are ways to boost the flavor and the appeal of food.

Less Sense-Able

You've probably given it little thought, but throughout your life, smell and taste have affected the quality of your life, your overall health, and your personal safety. Think about simple pleasures: the variety of flavors in a holiday meal, the aromas of bread baking or turkey roasting in the oven, the sounds of popping popcorn, or the sizzle of food on the grill. Food's wonderful flavors encourage a healthy appetite and help stimulate digestion.

Your senses also provide clues to the off-flavor or appearance of deteriorating food, or perhaps to a kitchen fire or a gas leak in the kitchen stove. All these sensory experiences may change, with age and health problems posing potential health risks.

Consider this. Flavor is really several perceptions: the senses of smell and taste, as well as touch (temperature and mouth feel). With aging, taste buds and smell receptors may not be quite as sensitive or as numerous. Loss of smell is often greater than loss of taste. When the flavors change, people often mistakenly think they can't taste as well; loss of smell may be the issue. The ability to sense sweet and salty tastes may wane sooner than bitter and sour tastes. That's why many foods may seem bitter, and why some older people reach for the salt shaker or the sugar bowl. Differences in saliva—composition and amount—may affect flavor, too. *For more about food and flavor, see "'Flavor' the Difference" in chapter 13.*

Age isn't the only reason for changes in taste and

smell. Medications and health problems may interfere. Some medicines leave a bitter flavor that affects saliva and, as a result, flavor. Some cause nausea, resulting in appetite loss, or dry mouth. Medicines may suppress taste and smell. And health problems such as diabetes, high blood pressure, cancer, and liver disease, common among older people, may alter taste and smell.

Fortunately, you can overcome, or at least accommodate to, many sensory changes that affect your food experiences and your personal nutrition.

● Can't easily read food labels, an oven thermometer, or medication instructions? Get glasses for the first time, change your eyeglasses or contact lens prescription, or keep a magnifying glass handy. Large-print cookbooks are useful, too.

● Have trouble hearing a kitchen timer, food bubbling over on the stove, or a faucet you forgot to turn off? Find out from a doctor if you need a hearing aid.

● Pay attention to smell and taste losses—and their effects on nutrition and the pleasure of eating. When food "just doesn't taste as good as it used to," some older adults lose interest in eating. Small appetites and skipped meals can result in poor nutrition.

"Sage" Advice for a Flavor Boost

Compensating for diminished taste or smell is within your control. One approach: intensify the taste and the aroma of food. Vary the temperature and the texture—-and make it more visually appealing. Despite a common myth, older adults can tolerate spicy foods.

● Perk up flavors by using more herbs, spices, and lemon juice—not with more salt or sugar! To compensate for age-related taste loss, you might need two or three times as much herb or spice and twice the flavor extract. For example, accent roasted poultry, poultry stew, or stuffing with sage. Carrots and creamed spinach taste good with a dash of nutmeg. Simmer a bay leaf in soups and stews. Add a pinch of thyme or cumin to peas or legumes. Or try dill weed in potato soup or coleslaw. *See "A Pinch of Flavor: How to Cook with Herbs and Spices" in chapter 13.* Hint: If any spices cause stomach irritation, stick with herbs.

● Add crunch to lunch—and dinner, too! Texture adds to the mouth feel and flavor of food. A variety of textures helps make up for a loss of taste and smell. What's easy? Crushed crackers on soup, chopped nuts on vegetables or in rice dishes, coleslaw as a salad, or crushed cornflakes on ice cream or pudding.

● Use strong-flavored ingredients: garlic, onion, sharp cheese, flavored vinegars and oils, concentrated fruit sauce, and jam. Use fats that add flavor: olive oil, nut oils, peanut butter, and a little butter.

● For less fat, impart flavor with herb rubs instead of gravy or sauces. Use a little healthy oil for health benefits. Fat carries flavor, too. A little dribble will do!

● Enjoy food variety with different flavors, colors, and textures.

● Include foods of different temperatures at each meal to perk up your sensations of flavor. Serve hot foods hot, not lukewarm, to enhance flavor. Extreme hot or cold temperatures, however, tend to lessen flavors.

● Serve yourself colorful, attractive food. A simple parsley sprig or a tomato slice on the plate adds appeal.

● Chew well to enjoy the foods' full flavors.

● If you smoke, stop. Smoking reduces the ability to perceive flavors.

● Avoid overexposing your taste buds to strong or bitter flavors, such as coffee, which can temporarily deaden sensitivity to other flavors.

● If you've lost interest in eating, talk to your doctor, and consult a registered dietitian about other ways to make food more appealing. Be aware: sensory loss may signal serious health problems; tell your doctor!

For more about flavor, see " 'Resetting' Your Table . . . for Taste and Health" in chapter 13.

A Few Words about Constipation

Constipation is a persistent problem for many people as they get older. The reason? The digestive system may get a little sluggish. Not getting enough fluid or fiber and being inactive may compound the problem. With constipation, stools get hard and can't be passed out of the body without straining. And the body's normal elimination schedule may change.

Have You Ever Wondered

. . . if taking mineral oil helps keep you regular? Taking mineral oil isn't recommended. It can promote the loss of fat-soluble vitamins (A, D, E, and K).

Being physically active, drinking enough fluids, and eating enough fiber are ways to stay regular—and avoid constipation. If these remedies don't work, ask a registered dietitian or your doctor for more advice.

● Drink enough water or other fluids daily. Fluids help your stools stay softer, bulkier, and easier to eliminate. *See page 464.*

● Consume plenty of fiber-rich foods: legumes, whole-grain breads and cereals, vegetables, and fruits. Fiber gives bulk to stools, making them easier to pass through the colon. *For more about fiber for health, including fiber pills and powders, see chapter 6, "Fiber: Your Body's Broom."*

● Listen to nature's call! The longer waste remains in your large intestine, the more difficult it is to eliminate. The body continues to draw out water, so stools get harder.

● Keep physically active and get enough rest. Both help keep your body regular.

● Avoid taking laxatives, as well as fiber pills and powders, unless your doctor recommends them. Food may pass through your intestinal tract faster than vitamins and minerals can be absorbed. And some may cause your body to lose fluids and potassium. A cup of tea or warm water with lemon, taken first thing in the morning, can act as a gentle, natural laxative.

For more about dealing with constipation, see "Gastrointestinal Conditions" in chapter 22.

Not Hungry?

While many older adults say they just don't have an appetite, there's no single cause for that complaint. As noted, sensory loss plays a role. Some have digestive problems that cause appetite loss. And medication or health problems also may be a cause. For some, the problem is psychological: loneliness, depression, or anxiety, among others.

Regardless, people who don't eat adequately increase their chances for poor nutrition and its negative consequences. To perk up a tired appetite:

● Try to identify the problem. If certain foods cause heartburn or gas, find alternatives. Talk to your doctor about your medication; if it's the cause, something else might be prescribed.

● Eat four to six smaller meals; keep portions small. You may take seconds if you're hungry for more. And smaller meals may be easier to digest.

● Give yourself enough time to eat. Rushing through a meal can cause discomfort.

● To get your digestive juices flowing, serve foods hot. Heat brings out the aroma of food, usually making it more enticing.

● Make your overall meal look appealing. Food that's attractively arranged and served may help bring your appetite back!

● If possible, increase your physical activity. That may promote a healthier appetite.

● If you're confined to bed, ask someone to help keep your room pleasant. Remove bedpans and other unpleasant things. Enjoy a plant, and turn on some music!

Chewing Problems?

For many mature adults, poor appetite isn't much of a nutrition problem. Instead, tooth loss or mouth pain may be. An astounding number lose all their teeth by age sixty-five. Many also have poorly fitting dentures that cause chewing problems and mouth sores.

What's at the root of oral health problems? Cavities may come to mind first. Yet gum, or periodontal, disease is the most common cause of tooth loss among older adults. As a result, many have missing, loose, or diseased teeth and sore, diseased gums. People with dentures may be able to eat all the foods they've always enjoyed if dentures fit right. If not, the resulting discomfort and mouth pain may keep them from eating a well-balanced diet. Osteoarthritis also can hinder chewing if it affects the lower jaw.

A dry mouth is another problem that may cause

Need more practical, easy ways to eat smart as the years go by? Check here for "how-tos":

- Boost your appetite if you don't feel hungry—see chapter 2.

- Find smart ways to lose, gain, or maintain your weight—see chapter 2.

- Make a personal plan for healthful eating—see chapter 10.

- Make quick, simple meals if you don't have a lot of energy—see chapter 10.

- Get more for your food dollar on a fixed income—see chapter 11.

- Protect yourself from foodborne illness—see chapter 12.

- Get more nutrition for fewer calories—see chapter 13.

- Perk up food's flavor with herbs and spices if food no longer tastes as good. Improve food's look, too—see chapter 13.

- Eat out, yet still match your health needs—see chapter 14.

- Eat to manage health problems—see chapter 22.

- Get easy, personalized tips from a nutrition expert—see chapter 24.

chewing and swallowing difficulties, especially if food is dry and hard to chew. As people get older, they may not have as much saliva flow to help soften food and wash it down. Medications, some health problems, and treatment such as chemotherapy also may decrease saliva flow or cause chewing and swallowing problems. *See "Cancer Treatment: Handling Side Effects" in chapter 22.*

If you have chewing problems, make sure oral problems don't become a barrier to good nutrition.

- See your dentist, or go to a dentist who specializes in care for older adults. Many oral health problems can be treated. And dentures that don't fit properly should be adjusted.

- Choose softer foods that are easier to chew. Chop foods well to reduce your risk of choking. All five food groups of MyPyramid have foods that are softer and easier to eat. *See "MyPyramid: Your Healthful Eating Guide" in chapter 10.*

- *Grains Group:* cooked cereal, cooked rice, cooked pasta, soft bread or rolls, softer crackers
- *Fruit Group:* fruit juice, cooked or canned fruit, avocados, bananas, grapefruit and orange sections, soft fruit
- *Vegetable Group:* vegetable juice, cooked vegetables, mashed potatoes, salads with soft vegetables, chopped lettuce
- *Milk Group:* milk, cheese, yogurt, pudding, ice cream, milk shakes
- *Meat and Beans Group:* chopped, lean meat, chopped chicken or turkey, canned fish, tender cooked fish, eggs, tofu, hummus, peanut butter

- Drink water or other fluids with meals and snacks to make swallowing easier.

- Consult a registered dietitian. Together you can plan for foods that you can eat comfortably without compromising your nutrient intake.

There's good news! Tooth loss and chewing difficulty aren't inevitable parts of aging. Good oral care—starting now, whatever your age—can help you keep the teeth you were born with. *See "Keep Teeth and Gums Healthy" in chapter 5.*

Gum disease is highly preventable. Proper brushing, daily flossing, and regular cleaning by a dentist or a hygienist can keep gum disease at bay. If you can, have your teeth cleaned twice a year, and perhaps more often if you have gum disease. *For more about gum disease, see "Keep Smiling: Prevent Gum Disease" in chapter 22.*

Weight Loss—or Gain?

Have you lost weight as a result of a poor appetite or health problems? Or have extra pounds crept on? Maintaining or improving your weight may be a health step you need to take. Talk to your doctor or a registered dietitian about the weight that's healthy for you.

Whether you need to keep weight on, or take it off, eat in a healthful way and remain as physically active as you can. *See "Never Too Late for Exercise" earlier in this chapter.*

Weight Loss: A Concern

Weight loss may be a health problem, especially if you haven't tried to lose weight. If that happens, first and foremost, find out why! Perhaps the reason is poor oral health or immobility that makes grocery shopping or food preparation difficult. Weight loss may signal an emotional problem, perhaps depression and/or bereavement, or social isolation. Unexpected weight loss also is a symptom for some serious health problems, including cancer. Talk to your doctor!

Besides other health implications, weight loss may be linked to physical weakness when muscle mass, not just body fat, is lost. Loss of physical strength increases the risk for falls, and as a result, bone fractures. Being underweight also may slow recovery from sickness or surgery.

To gain or to maintain weight:

● Eat enough. Use MyPyramid as your guide for consuming enough total amount, and enough variety among and within its five food groups.

● Eat five or six small meals a day if you fill up quickly at meals.

● Stick to a regular meal schedule so you don't forget to eat.

● Keep healthful, easy snack foods handy: milk, yogurt, fruit, vegetables, crackers, whole-wheat bread, cereal, and peanut butter.

● Eat with someone else to spark your appetite.

● Instead of coffee or tea, which supplies few calories, drink cocoa, milk, soup, or juice.

● Make casseroles, soups, stews, and side dishes heartier. Add whole milk, cheese, beans, rice, or pasta.

● Talk to a registered dietitian (RD) or your doctor about ways to boost calories and nutrients in your meals and snacks. An RD can provide ideas for high-calorie meals and drinks, and if necessary, can help you select the right canned nutrition supplement drink or dietary supplement. Find an appropriate way to stay physically active so you maintain your body's muscle mass—and your strength. Again talk to your doctor, and perhaps a trained physical therapist.

Be aware that some medications, including low-dose antidepressant drugs, may enhance appetite.

Weight Gain: An Issue, Too

As you get older, you need fewer calories to maintain your weight. It's not surprising, then, to gain a few pounds—especially if you're more sedentary and still eat as you always have. The concern is that being overweight increases the risks for high blood pressure, heart disease, diabetes, and certain cancers. If you have one of these problems already, dropping just a few pounds may lower your blood pressure, total blood cholesterol level, or blood sugar level. Extra body weight affects how easily you move and intensifies the discomfort of arthritis. It also can contribute to disabilities, which may lead to an earlier death.

Before you start trying to lose weight, talk to your physician about an effective, safe approach that matches your health needs. These strategies may help you:

To lose weight:

● Use MyPyramid as your daily eating guide. Choose mostly lean and low-fat or fat-free foods and those without much added sugars. Eat the recommended amount of nutrient-rich foods from the five food groups and healthy oils, taking your budget for discretionary calories into account.

● Eat regular meals. Meal-skipping often leads to snacking and possibly overeating.

● Choose snacks carefully: fruits, vegetables, low-fat yogurt, fat-free or low-fat milk, breakfast cereal, and frozen yogurt.

● Trim fat and added sugars from food choices to cut calories. Remove skin from turkey or chicken before eating it. Choose lean meats and trim visible fat. Bake, broil, microwave, or steam foods instead of frying them. Use low-fat or fat-free milk, yogurt, and cheese. Go easy on butter, margarine, cream, and sour cream and sugary desserts. *For more ways to trim fat and added sugars in food preparation, see chapter 13.*

● Eat smaller portions—and still meet MyPyramid guidelines for your calorie needs.

● If you drink alcoholic beverages, do so in moderation: no more than one drink a day for women, and two for men. If you take medication, you might need to avoid alcoholic drinks altogether.

● Keep physically active and busy to prevent eating

from boredom or loneliness. And learn to recognize signals for hunger and satiety (fullness).

● Find safe and appropriate ways to move more and sit less. You'll get more health-promoting benefits than weight control alone!

● Beware of weight-loss plans with unrealistic promises. *See "'Diets' That Don't Work!" in chapter 2.*

"Moving Ideas" for Physical Limitations

Some older adults move with the same grace, stamina, and dexterity of their earlier years. For others, health problems limit physical abilities: for example, arthritis, diabetes, osteoporosis, Parkinson's disease, respiratory diseases, and strokes. Even healthy, mature adults may become gradually less active, so they have less strength and stamina for everyday tasks.

For those who enjoy independent living, some general tips can make food preparation and eating easier:

● Does your tile or wooden floor seem slippery? Wear flat, rubber-soled shoes in the kitchen. And wipe up spills immediately so you don't slip!

● Be careful of loose rugs by the sink or other places in your kitchen. They may feel good underfoot, but they're easy to trip or slip on.

● If you're unsteady or need a cane, use a rolling tea cart to move food, dishes, and kitchen equipment from place to place.

● A wheelchair or a walker with a flat seat can be used to move things, too; check with a medical supply store to find them.

● Sit while you work. Use the kitchen table for food preparation, or get a stable chair or stool that's high enough for working at the counter or the stove.

● Give yourself time. Things may take a little longer to do as you get older.

● Get a loud kitchen timer if you have trouble hearing. Especially if you're forgetful, using a timer when you cook can avoid burned food and kitchen fires.

● Cooking for just one? Use a microwave or toaster oven rather than the conventional oven.

● Organize your kitchen for efficiency—everything within easy reach. Keep mixers, blenders, and other heavy, small appliances on the counter. Keep heavy pots and pans on lower shelves, too.

● If you have vision problems, keep a magnifying glass handy, and have your eyes checked and fitted for glasses. That makes it easier to read expiration dates and small type on food labels.

● Use a cutting board with contrasting colors if you have trouble with vision; for example, it may be hard to safely cut an onion on a white plastic cutting board.

● Have trouble with manual tasks such as opening jars and cans, or perhaps cutting? Kitchen devices are sold to make food preparation easier for people with arthritis or other problems, and for those partly paralyzed by a stroke. Again, check a medical supply store. Place a wet paper towel under the cutting board so it doesn't move around. *See "Have You Ever Wondered . . . if you can eat anything to relieve arthritis?" in chapter 22.*

● Get a cordless or cell phone and keep it charged. You won't need to dash to the phone while you're cooking. Just keep it near you. It's a good safety measure, too, in case you fall.

● If you use a walker or a wheelchair, talk to a registered dietitian or a physical therapist about ways to change your kitchen for independent living.

● Another kitchen safety tip: avoid using your oven as a room heater. It can be dangerous! If heating is a problem where you live, let someone know—a relative, landlord, building manager, or social worker, among others. *For other kitchen safety tips, see "Quick Tips for Injury Prevention" in chapter 12.*

● Use an all-in-one fork and spoon if you have trouble with one hand. Check with a medical supply store or catalog to find one.

● Drink soup from a mug. It's easier than using a soup spoon—and there's one less utensil to wash.

● Get dishes with a high rim and a rubber, no-slip back. The rim helps you push food onto your spoon or fork.

● Set your table with plastic placemats. They're easy to clean. And dishes won't slide on them, as they might on the table surface.

● Shaky with a cup? Get a covered cup with a drinking spout or place for a straw.

● If you use a wheelchair, buy an oven with front controls and a side-hinged door. Install it next to the sink or your work area, not across the kitchen. Put in low countertops and "pull-outs," such as cutting boards, in your kitchen. Talk to a physical therapist or a registered dietitian about other kitchen solutions.

● Rather than avoid certain categories of foods, accept help if you need it. You need nourishment from a variety of foods.

Meals and Snacks: When You Need a Special Diet

Many health problems—physical and emotional— that arise with aging require major changes in what and how people eat. Discuss that with your doctor during your regular checkups—annually or more often as your doctor advises. Never self-diagnose an ongoing disease, or prescribe your own special diet or dietary supplement to treat it. And be careful of so-called miracle cures. *See "Miracles? Dream On!" earlier in this chapter.*

For any health condition, there's no one recommended diet. Each person needs individual nutrition advice because needs differ so much. And sometimes more than one health problem needs to be treated at the same time. If a special (therapeutic) diet is prescribed for you, consult your doctor or a registered dietitian for guidance. Have your progress monitored, as advised. *For more tips, see "If Your Doctor Prescribes a Special Eating Plan . . . " in chapter 22.*

To manage your health, your food choices may need as much of your attention as following directions for medications. It's all for your good health! To find a registered dietitian, ask your doctor. *See "How to Find Nutrition Help" in chapter 24.*

Give a Helping Hand!

To people who are sick, weak, or injured, good nutrition is often the best medicine! Regardless of age, those with difficulty feeding themselves may need a caring, helping hand.

If you offer help, make mealtime pleasant:

● Help with hand washing before and after eating. Use a wet, soapy washcloth or premoistened towels or a hand sanitizer if the person can't get to the sink. Offer a towel for drying.

● Make sure that the food is the right consistency. You might need to chop or puree it if chewing is difficult.

● Let the person decide what foods to eat first, next, and so on. Even when people can't feed themselves, most want to feel in control of their lives.

● For dignity's sake, provide a napkin or an apron to help him or her keep clean.

● Offer some finger foods to eat independently. For example, try banana slices, orange sections, bread (cut in quarters), a soft roll, cheese sticks, or meat (sliced in strips).

● Offer a drink between bites to help with chewing and swallowing. Provide a straw and a cup that's not too big. You can always pour more.

● Consider how far the person can reach for a cup or a dish. Arrange the place setting for easy reach.

● Sit together at the same level as you offer food. Share pleasant conversation in a normal tone, even if you need to do all the talking. To be sure you understand a response, repeat or rephrase it.

● Relax and be patient. Encourage self-expression of any kind. The meal should not feel rushed, especially if the person has trouble chewing or swallowing.

● Offer small bites, and suggest a spoon rather than a fork. It's easier for holding food and less likely to jab his or her mouth.

● If you can, eat your meal at the same time to continue the joy and the normalcy of social interaction at mealtime.

● Clean any spills right away. You might keep a clean cloth handy.

● Most important, respect the person's needs and desires. Expect frustration, and handle it without a negative reaction. Counting on others for personal care can be emotionally difficult.

● Let the nurse or other caregivers know what and how much the person has eaten. In that way other meals and snacks can be adjusted accordingly.

PART V

Healthful Eating
Special Issues

CHAPTER 19

Athlete's Guide
Winning Nutrition

On your mark . . . get set . . . go! Whether you train for competitive sports, or work out for your own good health or just for fun, what you eat and drink—and when—is part of your formula for athletic success. Good nutrition can't replace training, effort, talent, and personal drive. But there's no question that what you eat and drink over time makes a difference when your goal is peak performance or your personal best.

Whether competitive or recreational, physical activity puts extra demands on your body. As an athlete, you use more energy, lose more body fluids, and put extra stress on your muscles, joints, and bones. Fortunately, your "training table" can increase your endurance and help prevent dehydration and injury. Most important, healthful eating helps you feel good and stay fit overall: the positive "mental edge!"

Nutrients for Active Living

Nutrition is fundamental to your peak physical performance. To put in your best effort, you need the same nutrients as nonathletes: carbohydrates, proteins, fats, vitamins, minerals, and water. If you're highly active, you may need slightly more of some nutrients.

What are the major differences in your nutrient needs? To replace fluid losses, athletes need more fluids to stay hydrated during high activity. And working muscles need more energy-supplying nutrients, especially carbohydrates.

Thirst for Success!

Do you drink plenty of water without overdrinking? Your physical endurance and strength depend on it!

When you're physically active, you lose fluids as sweat evaporates from your skin. As you breathe, often heavily, you exhale moisture, too. A 150-pound athlete can lose 1½ quarts, or 3 pounds, of fluid in just one hour. That equals six 8-ounce glasses of water. With heavy training, fluid loss can be higher. To avoid dehydration you need to replace the fluids you lose.

Fluids for Peak Performance

What's the risk if you begin physical activity even slightly dehydrated, or lose too much fluid while you're active? Even small losses of 1 percent of your body weight may hinder your physical performance, particularly during warm weather. Losing more than 1 percent is a known detriment. (That's about 2 or 3 pounds for a 150-pound person.) Dehydration can

Did You Know

. . . heat stroke, caused by severe dehydration, ranks second among the reported cases of death among high school athletes?

. . . taking extra vitamins or minerals (beyond the Recommended Dietary Allowances) offers no added advantage to athletic performance?

. . . a high-carbohydrate diet can boost your endurance?

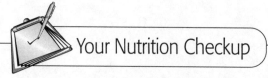

Eat to Compete

Sports nutrition is filled with misconceptions—all based on the drive for top performance. As an athlete, are you tuned into the facts or the myths?

TRUE OR FALSE?

T	F	
___	___	**1.** If you train properly for sports, you don't need to worry as much about replacing fluids.
___	___	**2.** Vitamin supplements supply extra energy for heavy workouts.
___	___	**3.** A steak dinner is the best precompetition meal.
___	___	**4.** Fasting is a good approach for "making weight."
___	___	**5.** Except for football and other contact sports, the leaner you are, the better.
___	___	**6.** Drinking milk before a heavy workout causes stomach cramps.
___	___	**7.** Salt tablets prevent muscle cramps.
___	___	**8.** If you eat a lot of protein, you'll build a lot of muscle.
___	___	**9.** Creatine supplements are necessary to build muscle and give you energy to train.

Now score yourself:

Do you eat smart to compete? Be aware that *every statement above is false.* These are the facts:

1. *Fact:* To avoid dehydration, everyone—even well-trained athletes—needs to stay hydrated before, during, and after physical activity. Besides water, sports drinks are an option. Training won't protect you from dehydration!

2. *Fact:* Vitamins don't supply energy; carbohydrates, fats, and proteins do. If you're already following the advice of MyPyramid and eating enough to meet your energy needs, there's no reason for vitamin supplements. The small amount of extra vitamins—for example, B vitamins—you need to produce extra energy from carbohydrates, fats, and proteins comes from extra amounts of nutrient-rich food-group foods.

3. *Fact:* A high-carbohydrate meal is the best precompetition meal. It supplies the primary fuel for working muscles. Although a steak dinner may taste great, the fats and proteins in steak take longer to digest than carbohydrates do.

   If steak gives you a "mental edge," enjoy a small portion. And eat plenty of carbohydrate-rich foods with it: perhaps baked potato, pasta, or rice; carrots; a dinner roll; a fruit salad; and frozen yogurt for dessert. Allow several hours for the meal to digest.

4. *Fact:* Fasting is never advised for athletes! It often causes fatigue, reduced glycogen stores (storage form of carbohydrate in muscles and the liver), the potential for muscle loss, dehydration, and decreased performance. For young athletes, fasting keeps them from consuming nutrients essential to their growth and development.

5. *Fact:* Although a lean, muscular body may enhance health and athletic performance, you can be too lean. Among its many functions, fat cushions body organs, providing protection from injury. During endurance sports (running, cycling, swimming), both carbohydrate and fat provide energy for working muscles. If you're too lean, you may tire too quickly. And restricting energy intake too much to avoid body fat may create a nutrient deficiency.

6. *Fact:* Contrary to popular myth, drinking milk before physical exertion doesn't cause stomach discomfort or digestive problems. Besides its role in bone health, calcium is needed for muscle contraction. Whether you choose to drink milk before a heavy workout is a personal matter.

   If you have trouble digesting milk, the problem might be lactose intolerance. If so, you can still drink milk in your training diet. *For guidance, see "Lactose Intolerance: A Matter of Degree" in chapter 21.*

7. *Fact:* Sodium loss is only one factor that contributes

to muscle cramping during exercise, especially during hot weather. Muscle fatigue and dehydration also increase the chance of muscle cramps. You don't need salt tablets to replace the small amount of sodium you lose in sweat. Your normal diet supplies enough.

8. *Fact:* Exercise, not a lot of extra protein, builds muscle mass. To build muscles, you need to work them more and gradually increase their workload. You may think of muscles as all protein. But actually 15 to 20 percent is protein; 70 to 75 percent is water; and 5 to 7 percent is fat, glycogen, and minerals.

9. *Fact:* Creatine supplements are not needed to build muscle. Smart food choices, hard work in the weight room, and adequate rest are the main factors that build muscle. Some college and professional athletes use creatine to help store this energy source in their muscles, but creatine use is not recommended for athletes under age eighteen.

Read on for more facts about eating for peak physical performance.

affect your strength, endurance, and aerobic capacity. How does fluid promote performance?

For energy production. Fluids are part of the energy-production cycle. As part of blood, water helps carry oxygen and glucose to muscle cells. There, oxygen and glucose help produce energy. Blood removes waste by-products as muscle cells generate energy and passes them to urine. Fluid losses decrease blood volume; your heart must work harder to deliver enough oxygen to cells.

For cooling down. Exercise generates heat as a by-product of energy production. Evaporation of sweat helps cool you down.

As you move your body, your body's overall temperature goes up, and you sweat. As sweat evaporates, your skin and the blood just under your skin cool. Cooler blood that flows throughout your body helps protect you from overheating. If you don't replace fluids lost through perspiration, your body's fluid balance is thrown off—a bigger problem as working muscles continue to generate more heat.

For transporting nutrients. Water in your bloodstream carries other nutrients for performance, including electrolytes, which help maintain body fluid balance.

As a cushion. The water around your body's tissues and organs offers protection from all the jostles and jolts that go along with exercise.

Protection from dehydration. Fluid loss—beyond the early stages of dehydration—increases your chances of heat injury, such as heat cramps, heat exhaustion, and heat stroke. *Severe dehydration can be life-threatening. See "Dehydration Alert!" in this chapter. See "A Fluid Asset" in chapter 8.*

Fluids: Tips to Drink Enough

No matter what your sport—running, bicycling, swimming, tennis, even walking and golfing—or rigorous activity, drink enough fluid to avoid dehydration. Getting enough isn't always easy.

● Drink plenty of fluids—before, during, and after physical activity. Carry a water bottle in a bottle belt or fluid pack, especially if you have no available water source. Or find out where you can get fluids: store, water fountain, others; bring money. Rehydrating yourself after activity helps you recover faster, both physically and mentally.

● Drink early and often—but don't drink too much. Drink fluids on schedule (every fifteen minutes during activity)—even when you don't feel thirsty. Your thirst mechanism may not send thirst signals when you're exercising. Thirst is a symptom of dehydration; drink fluids before that happens. *Follow the schedule in this chapter, "For Physical Activity: How Much Fluid?"*

● Stop to drink if you need fluids. You'll more than make up for any lost time with better performance.

● Wear lightweight, loose-fitting clothing that wicks moisture, especially in warm weather. Be aware that fabrics that hold heat—such as tights, body suits, heavy gear—as well as helmets and other protective gear, won't let sweat evaporate.

● Replace water weight. Weigh yourself before and after a heavy workout. Your nude weight is best. Wear the same clothing when you weigh yourself—before and after. Replace each pound of weight you lose with 3 cups of water, carbohydrate drink, or other fluid to bring your fluid balance back to normal. And plan to drink more before your active workout next time. If

For Physical Activity: How Much Fluid?

Make a point of drinking fluids at all times during the day—not just after your workout or competition. How much fluid is enough? Here's a schedule that can keep you from becoming dehydrated:

When to Drink	About How Much (One medium mouthful of fluid = about 1 ounce; 1 cup = 8 ounces.)
2 hours before activity	2 cups (and drink plenty with meals)
15 minutes before activity	1 to 2 cups
Every 15 minutes during activity	½ to 2 cups, enough to minimize body weight loss, without overdrinking
After activity	3 cups for each pound of body weight lost

Adapted from: Marie Dunford, ed., *Sports Nutrition: A Practice Manual for Professionals* (Chicago: American Dietetic Association, 2006).

you weigh more after exercise, you drank too much during activity; drink less while exercising next time.

● Check the color of your urine. Dark-colored urine indicates dehydration. Drink more fluids, so your urine is pale and nearly colorless before exercising again.

● Be especially careful if you exercise intensely in warm, humid weather. Consider how much hotter you feel on humid days. Sweat doesn't evaporate from your skin quickly, so you don't get the cooling benefits. That's why on humid days it's easier to get hyperthermia, or overheated, as you exercise. Hyperthermia can lead to heat stroke, which can be fatal!

● Know the signs of dehydration. Some early signs are flushed skin, fatigue, increased body temperature, and faster breathing and pulse rate. Later signs are dizziness, weakness, and labored breathing with exercise. Replace fluids before symptoms get serious. *See "Dehydration: Look for Body Signals!" in chapter 8.*

● Drink, rather than simply pour water over your head. Drinking is the *only* way to rehydrate and cool your body from the inside out.

For more about fluids and active children, see "Fluids: Caution for Kids" later in this chapter.

Be cautious about overdrinking, especially during intense exercise when your kidneys can't excrete the excess. Called hyponatremia, or abnormally low blood sodium levels, extra water moves instead into body cells, including brain cells. The extra pressure affects vital functions, with potentially fatal outcomes.

Which Fluids?

What should you drink before, during, and after rigorous activity? Try water, fruit juices, sports drinks, or other beverages. For workouts of less than thirty minutes of continuous activity and recreational walking, sports drinks, juices, and water are good choices. For fluid replacers for other sports, read on.

Water: A Good Choice. Water helps lower and normalize your body's core temperature from inside when you're hot, and it moves quickly from your digestive tract to your tissues.

Cold water is a fine choice. Contrary to popular myth, drinking cold water during exercise doesn't cause stomach cramps for most athletes; stomach cramps may be caused by dehydration, not by drinking cold water. For outside activity in cold weather, drink water that's warm or at room temperature to help protect you from hypothermia, or low body temperature. Cool water, preferred by many exercisers, can enhance performance.

Have You Ever Wondered

. . . if swimmers need to worry about dehydration? Like any athlete, swimmers perspire to keep from overheating. However, swimmers probably don't notice their sweat—at least not while they're in the water. Like other athletes, they need to drink plenty of fluids before, during, and after rigorous swimming.

. . . if dehydration is a concern with cold-weather sports such as ice skating or skiing? Even in a cool or cold environment, you sweat. Attire for cold weather sports such as downhill skiing, snowmobiling, and ice hockey doesn't "breathe" or allow the body to cool down, either.

Sports Drinks. Sports drinks can benefit some athletes, especially in hot, humid conditions. Sports drinks with 6 to 8 percent carbohydrate (14 to 19 grams of carbohydrate per 8 ounces) may be better than water or diluted fruit juice for fluid replacement. More than 8 percent carbohydrate solution may decrease the rate of fluid absorption and gastric (stomach) emptying.

For activities lasting longer than an hour, try sports drinks. If you're a long-distance runner or long-distance bicyclist, or involved in other endurance events (longer than ninety minutes), sports drinks may offer some performance benefits. New research shows

Have You Ever Wondered ?

. . . if caffeine can boost your physical performance? Maybe—and maybe not. People react to caffeine in different ways. Caffeine does stimulate the central nervous system, so it may help you feel more alert and attentive. And it may enhance your performance.

For caffeine-sensitive athletes, caffeine may exacerbate pre-event anxiety and its symptoms. Although caffeine may have a mild diuretic effect that may not last long, noncaffeinated beverages are advised when rapid rehydration is needed, perhaps between tournament events. That's also an issue in hot weather and for endurance athletes.

If you enjoy coffee, tea, or soft drinks with caffeine, experiment during training, not competition. A single cup may help—or at least not hinder—your performance. But avoid caffeine tablets or several cups of caffeinated drinks. The National Collegiate Athletic Association (NCAA) limits caffeine concentration to no more than 15 micrograms per milliliter of urine. You likely won't reach this level from caffeine in food (equivalent to seventeen caffeinated, 12-ounce sodas). But athletes who consume three 200-mg caffeine tablets may exceed this limit. Beginning in 2004 the International Olympic Committee no longer prohibited caffeine but monitors caffeine content in urine instead.

If you drink caffeinated beverages, drink enough other fluids, too. Despite any mild, short-term diuretic effects of caffeine, caffeinated beverages contribute to total fluid intake. Caffeine doesn't cause dehydration or electrolyte imbalance. *For more about caffeine, see "Drinks: With or without Caffeine?" in chapter 8.*

a benefit for high-intensity activity (perhaps sprinting or playing hockey) lasting thirty minutes or more.

Glucose (simple form of carbohydrate), in sports drinks is a more immediate fuel, or energy, source for working muscles. It may help prevent muscle glycogen from depleting too fast and so help lengthen performance time. (Muscle glycogen is carbohydrate stored in muscle.) Glucose in sports drinks also helps fluid get out of the gut and into the bloodstream.

Compared to juice or soft drinks, sports drinks are more diluted. This means that the fluid and glucose in a sports drink can be absorbed and used more readily by the body. If you'd like to see if a drink has about 6 percent carbohydrate, use this formula:

● Find the carbohydrate grams and serving size (in milliliters—mL) on the label (8 ounces is about 240 mL).

● Divide the carbohydrate grams by the serving size (in mL) and multiply by 100 to determine the percent of carbohydrate.

● Example: 14 grams carbohydrate/240 mL × 100 = 6%

Besides fluid and energy, sports drinks supply electrolytes. As you perspire, your body loses very small amounts of sodium and other electrolytes. For most athletes, a normal diet replaces what's lost. But endurance athletes perspire much more, so they're at greater risk for sodium depletion. Sodium and other electrolytes in sports drinks may be beneficial. During exercise that's longer than 60 minutes, or for exercise performed in high heat or humidity, drinks with electrolytes help to enhance fluid absorption. *See "Electrolytes: Sweat 'Em!" later in this chapter.*

You don't lose vitamins when you sweat, so you don't need sports drinks with extra vitamins. The extra food you eat for more food energy also provides any extra B vitamins you need for energy production.

If you're an endurance athlete, experiment with sports drinks and other fluids during practices and low-key competition. If the flavor of sports drinks encourages you to drink more fluids—or if they give you a psychological boost—enjoy them, but don't overdo. Watching your weight? Remember: They supply calories.

"Energy" Drinks? These drinks typically contain more carbohydrates than commercial sport drinks.

They're also usually higher in caffeine. Since they aren't formulated for athletes' needs, they aren't advised for use during exercise.

Fruit Juice or Soft Drinks? Compared with sports drinks, sugars in soft drinks and fruit juice are more concentrated: 10 to 15 percent carbohydrate. They aren't recommended during exercise because of their high sugar content and, for soft drinks, their carbonation. Drinks with a lot of sugar take longer to be absorbed, and they may cause cramps, diarrhea, or nausea. Carbonation can make you feel full and make your throat burn, so you drink less fluid.

You can dilute fruit juice—if you like the flavor. Unlike sports drinks, diluted fruit juice doesn't provide sodium; depending on how much it's diluted, it may not contain enough "carbs" to help the athlete.

Alcoholic Drinks: Not Now! Alcoholic beverages can impair, not enhance, your physical performance. Consider the reasons to skip alcoholic drinks—at least until *after* you replenish the fluids lost in your workout:

● If you're looking for a carbohydrate source, look elsewhere. A 12-ounce can of beer has less than a third of the "carbs" provided by a 12-ounce serving of orange juice. Calories from alcohol don't fuel muscles.

● Alcohol may have a short-term diuretic effect. It works as a depressant, affecting your brain's ability to reason and make judgments and perhaps your reaction time. And it may impair your coordination, balance, muscle reflexes, and visual perception.

● For the endurance athlete it has another effect: When you drink a beer, wine, or mixed drink, your liver works to detoxify and metabolize the alcohol. This process can interfere with the liver's job of forming extra blood glucose for prolonged physical activity. The possible result? Early fatigue.

Energy to Burn

Athletes: The only way to have enough energy for physical activity is to consume enough energy. How much energy, or calories, should you consume per day? That's a very individual matter. A 200-pound body builder has very different needs than an 80-pound gymnast. A physical training program may use 500 to 3,000 or more calories daily—a huge range.

Dehydration Alert!

As you exercise, be alert for conditions that increase your fluid loss through sweat. With more perspiration, your body dehydrates faster.

● *Temperature.* The higher the temperature, the greater your sweat losses.

● *Intensity.* The harder you work out, the greater your sweat losses.

● *Body size.* The larger the athlete, the greater the sweat losses. Males generally sweat more than females.

● *Duration.* The longer the workout, the greater your fluid losses.

● *Fitness.* Well-trained athletes sweat more, starting to sweat at a lower body temperature. Why? Sweating cools the body. The well-trained athlete cools his or her body more efficiently than an untrained person.

Source: Debbi Sowell Jennings and Suzanne Nelson Steen, *Play Hard, Eat Right* (Minneapolis: American Dietetic Association, Chronimed Publishing, 1995).

● The amount of energy for sports depends partly on your body composition, body weight, and level of fitness. Body size (consider a male football player and a female gymnast) also makes a big difference. When two people ski together at the same intensity, the person weighing more likely burns more calories.

● The harder, the longer, and the more often you work out, the more energy required for muscle work. Any activity such as cycling, power walking, or swimming is a bigger energy burner if done more vigorously.

● Not surprisingly, some sports burn more energy than others. That's simply because they're more intense or their duration is longer. Both a golf game and downhill skiing may last several hours. But skiing uses more energy since it's more physically demanding for larger muscle groups.

Carbohydrates supply energy for activities that take high-intensity, short bursts of energy, and both carbohydrates and fats supply energy for longer activity.

For the energy costs of several sports, see chapter 2. To estimate your energy needs, see "Your 'Weigh': Figuring Your Energy Needs" in chapter 2. Or have a registered dietitian (RD) help you.

Carbohydrate Power

For sports and everyday living, carbohydrates are your body's foremost energy source—and the main fuel for working muscles. Nutrition experts advise athletes to consume 5 to 10 grams of carbohydrate a day for every kilogram of body weight depending on their sport. For an athlete who weighs 120 pounds (55 kilograms), that's 275 to 550 grams of carbohydrate; for a 175-pound (80-kilogram) athlete, that's 400 to 800 grams of "carbs." While 5 to 7 grams of carbohydrate per kilogram of weight daily is good for general training, some athletes, especially male endurance athletes, need 7 to 10 grams per kilogram body weight daily. Some elite athletes may need more. (One pound equals 2.2 kilograms.)

Along with training, a high-carbohydrate eating plan promotes overall fitness and offers a competitive edge. With "carbs" (not fats or proteins) as the main fuel, you can maintain rigorous activity longer. Training helps your body use carbohydrates efficiently and store more as muscle glycogen. Stored in muscles, glycogen is fuel ready to power your physical activity.

For Working Muscles

To power working muscles, stored energy comes mostly from glycogen in muscle or the liver, and from blood sugar (or blood glucose). Glycogen is your body's storage form of carbohydrate. Depending on the intensity and the duration of exercise, fat and, for endurance athletes, even a small amount of protein supplies energy, too.

Carbohydrates are broken down during digestion and changed to blood sugar, or glucose. Some blood sugar, which is circulated in your bloodstream, is used immediately for energy. The rest is stored as muscle and liver glycogen, or it's converted to fat if excess calories are consumed. The more muscle glycogen you can store, the more you have to power physical activity.

Your body's glycogen stores are continually used and replenished. For more energy, your body fuels muscles with a mix of both carbohydrate (glycogen) and fat. The higher the immediate intensity of an activity, the more glycogen used. Lower-intensity and longer activities use more fat and less glycogen.

● For sports that require short, intense energy spurts (anaerobic activities), muscle glycogen is the main energy source used. That includes tennis, volleyball, baseball, weight lifting, sprinting, and even bowling.

● Sports requiring both intensity and endurance use mostly muscle glycogen. Basketball and football are two examples.

● For endurance activities (aerobic activities) such as long-distance running or bicycling, your body uses glucose, glycogen, and fat for fuel; the proportion depends mainly on the activity's intensity and duration.

See "Carbohydrates: Your 'Power' Source" in chapter 5.

Fuel Up!

"Carbs" are an athlete's best energy source. (Eat enough every day to keep your muscle and liver glycogen stores up.) Both starches and sugars supply energy and replenish your muscle glycogen.

What foods contain carbohydrates? Starches come from cereals, breads, rice, pasta, vegetables, and legumes (beans and peas). Sugars (naturally occurring and added) are in fruit, fruit juice, milk, cookies, cakes, candy, and soft drinks, among other foods.

Get "carbs" from mixed dishes:

YOUR DAILY CARBOHYDRATE GOAL IS ABOUT . . .*

IF YOU WEIGH . . .	5 GRAMS	7 GRAMS	10 GRAMS
	PER KILOGRAM OF YOUR BODY WEIGHT		
100 pounds (45 kg)	225	320	455
125 pounds (56 kg)	280	400	570
150 pounds (68 kg)	340	475	680
175 pounds (80 kg)	400	560	800
200 pounds (91 kg)	455	640	910
225 pounds (102 kg)	510	715	1,020
250 pounds (114 kg)	570	800	1,140

Energy needs vary among athletes. For your target amount check with a registered dietitian.

*Amounts are rounded.

How does that translate to food? *See the chart "Carbohydrates in Food: Quick Rule of Thumb" in this chapter.*

● *Made with breads, grains, cereals, and pastas:* wild rice pilaf; pasta salads; whole-wheat or buckwheat pancakes; sandwiches made with bread, including a bagel or pita bread; animal crackers, gingersnaps, graham crackers, or oatmeal-raisin cookies; homemade fruit and nut breads.

● *Made with fruits or vegetables:* dried fruit; stuffed spuds such as a baked potato with broccoli; fresh fruit salad; and raw vegetables with yogurt dip.

● *Made with legumes* (chickpeas, kidney beans, black beans, lentils, and other dried peas and beans): bean enchiladas; split pea soups; vegetarian baked beans; and chili.

For the specific carbohydrate content of many foods, see "'Carbo' Foods" in the Appendices.

Carbohydrate Loading

Your muscles and liver store glycogen—only a limited amount—which must be replaced after each bout of exercise. Endurance athletes worry that they may "hit the wall," or feel extremely fatigued, before finishing. When this happens, they're out of glycogen.

The more glycogen you store, the longer it lasts. Carbohydrate loading (or glycogen loading) may help you "stockpile" two to three times more glycogen in your muscles for extended activity. Carbohydrate loading won't make you pedal harder or run faster. But it may help you perform longer before getting tired.

How do you "load up" your muscles if you're an endurance athlete? Combine training, rest, and eating extra carbohydrates.

Have You Ever Wondered

. . . how you can avoid "hitting the wall"? When endurance athletes run out of glucose, they're too tired to continue exerting themselves. To maintain your supply for as long as possible for endurance sports, follow an eating regimen that's high in carbohydrates. Have a sports drink if your workout lasts an hour or more. Eat a carbohydrate-rich snack right afterward when your body can store glycogen at a faster rate. Regular physical training also helps; your muscles adapt, gradually storing more glycogen for intense workouts.

"Carbohydrates" in Food: Quick Rule of Thumb

Food	Carbohydrates
Breads and cereals: 1 slice bread, or ½ cup rice or pasta, or 1 ounce dry cereal	About 15 grams
Starchy vegetables: ½ cup	About 15 grams
Fruits: ½ cup, or 1 small to medium whole fruit	About 10 to 15 grams
Vegetables: ½ cup cooked or raw	About 5 grams
Milk: 1 cup	About 12 grams

● Start a week before the endurance event. On the first day (six days before), train at a normal level to deplete the glycogen in your working muscles. For the next two days (four and five days ahead) taper off on training to rest your muscles so they can "re-stock" muscle glycogen. During those four to six days ahead, consume a normal mixed diet with 5 grams of carbohydrate per kilogram of your weight. (2.2 lb. = 1 kg)

● For three days before the event, cut back on training and gradually increase your carbohydrate calories to 10 grams of carbohydrate daily per kilogram of body weight—without increasing your total calories. Make most of those "carbs" complex, or starches. Rest (no exercise) the day before competition.

Recently researchers have tried to simulate carbohydrate loading with a short bout of high-intensity exercise, then one to two days of 'high-carb' eating. More research is needed to see if this works for storing extra muscle glycogen.

Reminders: In your normal training diet, most of your energy should come from carbohydrates. Whole grains, cereal, legumes, and starchy vegetables are good sources of starches (complex "carbs").

"Carbohydrate loading is most effective for trained endurance athletes. Generally having more muscle, their bodies have more capacity to store extra glycogen. "Occasional" or "weekend" athletes, and those involved in sports that don't require prolonged endurance, shouldn't expect the same results.

What sports should you "carb load" for? If you're a trained athlete, try it for either endurance events such as marathons and triathlons that last longer than ninety minutes, or for all-day events such as swim meets, a series of tennis matches, distance bicycling, or soccer games. For shorter events, a normal, carbohydrate-rich approach to eating supplies enough glycogen.

Caution: Carbohydrate loading is not advised for school-age children or teens. If you have diabetes or high blood triglycerides, talk to your doctor and a registered dietitian before trying this regimen.

Smart About Fat, Still Best!

Fat also fuels working muscles. In fact, it's a more concentrated energy source. And it performs other body functions, such as transporting fat-soluble vitamins and providing essential fatty acids. For good health, consume fat as one source of fuel. Rather than try to eat almost "fat-free," be smart: low in saturated fat and *trans* fat, and moderate in your fat intake.

Fat as Fuel

For energy, fat helps power activities of longer duration such as hiking or marathon running. Because fat doesn't convert to energy as fast as carbohydrates, fat doesn't power quick energy spurts such as returning a tennis serve or running a 100-yard dash.

Unlike glycogen, fat needs oxygen for energy metabolism. That's why endurance sports, fueled in part by fat, are called aerobic activities. "Aerobic" means with oxygen, and aerobic activities require a continuous intake of oxygen. The more you train, the more easily you breathe during longer activity; the oxygen you take in helps convert fat to energy.

No matter where it comes from—carbohydrates, proteins, or fats—your body stores extra energy as body fat. These fat stores supply energy for aerobic activity. Even if you're lean, you likely have enough fat stores to fuel prolonged or endurance activity. You don't need to eat more fat!

For Athletes: How Much Fat?

Advice for athletes is the same as that for all healthy people: eat a diet low in saturated fat, *trans* fat, and cholesterol and moderate in total fat. To get enough calories for sports, yet not too much fat, 20 to 35

percent of your total calories from fat is a good guideline. Most of your food energy should come from carbohydrates. With a high-fat diet your carbohydrate or protein intake may come up short. Less than 15 percent of calories from fat doesn't provide enough calories or enough fat for other health roles, especially for those involved in endurance sports. Getting enough essential fatty acids is also important for health and peak performance.

Athletes who consume too little fat, often to keep weight and body fat down, may risk a shortfall in food energy; young athletes on a very low-fat diet may not consume enough essential fatty acids for normal growth and development. For female athletes—often dancers, gymnasts, and skaters—a very-low-fat diet may interfere with menstrual cycles, with lifelong health implications.

Do you burn a lot of energy? Since your calorie needs are higher, your total fat intake is probably higher, too. That's often true for football linemen and weight lifters, who may use 4,000 calories or more a day. Still, fats shouldn't contribute more than 35 percent of total energy.

Action plan. Do you need to cut back on fat? If so, get more food energy from carbohydrates. Remember that

Have You Ever Wondered

. . . if eating a candy bar right before rigorous activity supercharges your body? No; even though carbohydrates supply energy, a candy bar won't supply extra energy right away.

For endurance activities of ninety minutes or longer, a sugary snack food (energy) bar or drink before exercise (or even during an event) may enhance your stamina. It slowly makes its way to your muscles as your glycogen stores get used up. Fig bars, graham crackers, bananas, and raisins work, too. Drink water along with these snacks.

Keep your snack or drink small: no more than 200 to 300 calories. Too much sugar may slow the time it takes water to leave your stomach, so your body won't replace fluids as quickly. Your best approach? Enjoy a sports drink. You'll consume a little sugar to fuel your muscles—but not too much to impair rehydration.

fat isn't stored as muscle glycogen; "carbs" are. Here's one strategy for cutting fat and boosting carbohydrates: Eat a baked potato more often than fries. Replace the fat calories you didn't eat from fries with a slice of whole-grain bread, a nutirent-rich source of "carbs."

For more about fat in a healthful eating plan, and for ways to moderate fat in your food choices, see chapter 3, "Fat Facts."

Protein—More Is Not Necessarily Better

Athlete or not, you need protein. But what's enough? Is more protein better? This nutrient needs no special attention just because you're physically active or building muscle. For overall fitness or strength building, extra protein—beyond the amount recommended—offers no added performance benefits.

Your body uses protein for many purposes: to build and repair tissues; to make enzymes, hormones, and other body chemicals; to transport nutrients; to make your muscles contract; and to regulate body processes such as water balance. If you don't consume enough carbohydrates for your high-energy demands, your body uses protein for energy instead. That's counterproductive to your physical goals!

Although protein supplies energy, extra amounts aren't your best fuel. The extra calories from excess protein is stored as fat, and not used for energy—if you've already consumed enough food energy. For anyone, protein should supply 10 to 35 percent of overall energy intake.

Most athletes need just slightly more protein than nonathletes do. Because athletes usually eat more, they easily get what they need.

How Much Protein?

How much protein do you need for sports? Base the amount on your body weight, not your energy need.

● For most recreational exercisers, 0.5 to 0.75 gram of protein per pound of body weight is enough. (The upper end of the range is recommended for athletes involved in strength or speed training.) For a 150-pound athlete that's about 75 to 115 grams of protein each day . . . and just 2 to 4 ounces more meat, chicken, or fish a day than recommended for nonathletes. As a point of reference, 3 ounces of lean beef supply about

30 grams of protein, 8 ounces of milk supply 8 grams of protein, and a slice of bread has 2 grams of protein or more.

● Adult endurance athletes need 0.6 to 0.7 gram of protein per pound of body weight. Adults building muscle mass, including weight lifters and football players, may need 0.7 to 0.8 gram of protein daily per pound. Teen athletes need enough for growth and muscle building: 0.7 to 0.9 gram of protein per pound.

Source for protein needs: N. Clark, *Nancy Clark's Sport Nutrition Guidebook*, 3rd ed. (Champaign, Ill.: Human Kinetics, 2003).

Muscle Myths

You've likely heard the long-held myth that extra protein builds more muscle. In truth, only athletic training builds muscle strength and size. Consuming more protein—from food or dietary supplements—won't make any difference. You've got to work your muscles!

Can amino acid supplements build muscle? Despite claims, amino acid supplements won't increase your muscle size or strength. By definition, amino acids are the building blocks of protein. Twenty different amino acids link together to make proteins in food and in body tissue. Food supplies amino acids in proportions your body needs. To your body, amino acids in supplements are no different from those in foods. In food they "taste" better and likely cost much less.

Most athletes get enough protein—and enough amino acids—from food. Protein-rich foods supply other nutrients, too; amino acid supplements supply only amino acids.

Caution about excess protein: Extra protein is *not* stored in your body for future use as protein. Instead, it's either used as energy or stored as body fat. A high-protein diet also may be high in fat.

Excessive protein or amino acids can be harmful. Side effects include metabolic imbalance, toxicity, nervous system disorders, and perhaps kidney problems. No research supports any benefits from the amino acids arginine or lysine for muscle growth.

When you consume excess protein, you need more water to excrete the urea, a waste product formed when protein is broken down. So excess protein increases the chances of dehydration—and increases the need to urinate. That's an inconvenience during a workout.

Bottom line: To build muscle, consume enough

calories from "carbs," follow advice for protein from food (no need for extra), and train regularly.

See "Ergogenic Aids: No Substitute for Training" at the end of this chapter.

Protein-Rich Foods: How Much?

The average American diet supplies more than enough protein. Just 6 to 7 ounces total of lean meat, poultry, or fish, or the equivalent from eggs, beans, nuts, or seeds daily, along with protein from dairy foods and grain products, supply enough for most athletes. Athletes involved in endurance sports and weight lifters need somewhat more.

Good protein sources include lean meat, poultry, and fish; milk, cheese, and yogurt; eggs; beans and tofu; and nuts, seeds, and peanut butter. Cereal, breads, and vegetables also contain smaller amounts of protein. If you're a vegetarian, you can consume enough protein for rigorous activity; just choose a variety of protein-containing foods carefully.

For more about protein and amino acids, see "Protein Power" in chapter 20.

Vitamins and Minerals: Sense and Nonsense

Vitamins and minerals trigger body processes for physical performance. Although not energy sources, some help produce energy from carbohydrates, fats, and proteins. Some help your muscles relax and contract. Others are part of hemoglobin in blood that carries oxygen to cells to power aerobic activity. *For more about their role in health, see chapter 4, "Vitamins, Minerals, and Phytonutrients: Variety on Your Plate!"*

If you burn more energy, you need more of some vitamins and minerals. By following advice from MyPyramid and so eating enough from each food group, you likely consume enough vitamins and minerals. For those who might need slightly more, eating more food probably provides the extra. In fact, an athlete with a hearty appetite has a better chance of consuming enough vitamins and minerals than someone who's less active and so eats less. However, athletes who try to lose weight by consuming too few calories or eliminating whole food groups are at greater risk for vitamin and mineral deficiencies.

For enough vitamins and minerals, eat recommended amounts from all five food groups; see chapter 10.

Electrolytes? Sweat 'Em!

Your sweat is made of water along with three minerals known as electrolytes: sodium, chloride, and potassium. Among their many functions, electrolytes help maintain your body's water balance—a critical function for athletes. They also help your muscles, including your heart muscle, contract and relax. And they help transmit nerve impulses.

Taste the sweat on your upper lip. How salty it can be! As you perspire during a physical workout, your body loses small amounts of electrolytes, mostly sodium. Most athletes replace sodium and other electrolytes through foods they normally eat. The average American consumes more than enough sodium to replace losses from perspiration—no need for extra sodium or salt tablets. When you perspire heavily, focus your attention on extra fluids instead.

Endurance athletes, who sweat heavily for long periods, may need to replace sodium and other electrolytes. Again, salt tablets aren't advised; they may cause stomach irritation, promote dehydration, and impair exercise performance. Instead, a sports drink with electrolytes, or salty foods, such as crackers and cheese, probably offer enough. Sodium from those

Have You Ever Wondered

. . . if athletes benefit from extra chromium? No, but misleading claims about chromium picolinate, which is a dietary supplement, have raised the question. No scientific evidence shows that taking a chromium supplement improves physical performance, builds muscle, burns body fat, or prolongs youth. For that matter, the role of chromium in your overall health isn't well understood, although early research suggests benefits to some people with diabetes or glucose intolerance.

Whole-grain foods, ready-to-eat cereals, beans, apples, and peanuts are some sources of chromium; most people get enough from their normal diet. Supplements aren't advised; chromium supplements may interfere with the work of iron in the blood.

sources helps speed rehydration. *See "Sports Drinks?" earlier in this chapter.*

For more about electrolytes, see "Sodium: You Need Some!" in chapter 7.

About Iron

Athletes: your muscle cells need iron to produce energy! Iron is part of hemoglobin, the part of red blood cells that carries oxygen to your body cells. Oxygen is used in energy metabolism, specifically for aerobic activities where fat converts to energy. An iron shortfall, even if it's small, can affect your physical performance. Women who engage in vigorous, prolonged activity may be at special risk for iron depletion.

The Recommended Dietary Allowance (RDA) for iron is 18 milligrams daily for premenopausal women and 8 milligrams daily for men. Premenopausal women have a higher iron need because of iron losses in monthly menstrual periods. For teens it's 15 milligrams of iron a day for females and 11 milligrams of iron for males. How much is too much? The Tolerable Upper Intake Level (UL) is 45 milligrams of iron per day for ages fourteen and over.

Getting enough iron may be an issue—especially if you're female, or if most of your iron comes from foods of plant origin such as legumes and grains. Plant sources of iron aren't absorbed as efficiently as from animal sources. To improve iron absorption, eat these foods with a vitamin C-rich food such as citrus. Good sources include lean red meat, dark poultry meat, iron-fortified cereals, and legumes.

Even if you consume enough iron, you may be iron-depleted if you're involved in endurance sports. Prolonged exercise such as marathon running and long-distance bicycling promotes iron loss. With more exercise you sweat more, losing some iron through perspiration. Endurance athletes may lose iron through urine, feces, and intestinal bleeding. If you're an endurance athlete, have your iron status checked periodically by your doctor.

Unless prescribed by your doctor, don't take an iron supplement. Be aware that iron supplementation is harmful to those with a genetic disorder called hemochromatosis; *see "Iron" in chapter 4.*

For more about iron and its food sources, see "Iron: A Closer Look" in chapter 4 and "Menstrual Cycle: More Iron for Women" in chapter 17.

Calcium and Weight-Bearing Exercise: Bone-Building Duo

Calcium and weight-bearing exercise: they're a winning combination for building and maintaining strong, healthy bones. Your goal? To maximize your calcium stores early in life, then maintain that level to later minimize the loss that comes with age.

Consuming enough calcium, at least 1,000 to 1,300 milligrams a day, depending on your age, offers protection against bone loss. Weight-bearing activity such as running, cross-country skiing, tennis, and soccer promotes the deposit of calcium into the matrix, or structure, of bones. While swimming and cycling offer many benefits of physical activity, they aren't weight-bearing, so they don't help to build bone.

Calcium and Female Athletes. Calcium is an issue. Why? To start with, many (including teens) don't consume enough calcium for bone health.

Active women who repeatedly consume too few calories—perhaps due to disordered eating—to meet their training needs risk having their menstrual periods stop. For teens and young women this hinders the deposit of calcium into bones at a time when bones should be developing at their maximum rate. Female athletes who've stopped menstruating are at special

Have You Ever Wondered

. . . if heavy training causes "sports anemia"? Perhaps, in the early stages of training. However, "sports anemia" isn't really anemia. Because blood volume increases in the early weeks of endurance training, iron concentration in blood dilutes slightly as your body adapts to more physical activity.

If you develop sports anemia, that's normal. It will disappear once your training program is off and running. With endurance training your blood's capacity to carry oxygen and your athletic performance will improve. Taking iron supplements isn't helpful or advised.

Feeling tired may result from other aspects of training. If fatigue persists, or if you think you're at risk for other types of anemia, including iron-deficiency anemia, check with your doctor. *See "Anemia: 'Tired Blood'" in chapter 22.*

risk for developing stress fractures, decreased bone mineral density, and other bone problems.

Women: For your bones' sake, pay attention if your periods stop. Talk to your doctor. This is *not* a normal outcome of physical activity. Stress fractures caused by weakened bones may seriously affect your physical performance. And the long-range impact on bone health: increased osteoporosis risk. For bone health, your doctor may recommend a higher calcium intake, or perhaps a calcium supplement. *See "Osteoporosis: Reduce the Risks" in chapter 22.*

Supplements: Not "Energy-Charged"

Contrary to unscientific claims, there's likely no need for vitamin or mineral supplements for sports if you're already well nourished. The "extra" won't offer an energy boost or added physical benefits—immediately or over the long run. Even if you're deficient in one or more nutrients, popping a supplement pill right before physical activity has no immediate effect.

Although B vitamins help your body use energy from food, no vitamin supplies energy. Since you likely eat more when you're physically active, you'll get the extra B vitamins you need from food—if your food choices are nutrient-rich. Just choose from MyPyramid's five food groups.

If you decide to take a supplement, choose a "multi" with no more than 100 percent of the Daily Values (DVs) for vitamins and minerals—unless your doctor prescribes more for special health reasons. *See "Dietary Supplements: What Are They?" in chapter 23.*

A High-Performance Diet

Training that includes healthful eating prepares you to achieve and maintain your strength, flexibility, and endurance. What's the best training diet? One that's varied, moderate, and balanced. Sound familiar? It's high in carbohydrates, with enough proteins, vitamins, minerals, and moderate in fat. High-performance eating is appropriate for all physically active people, not just those training for sports.

MyPyramid for Athletes

Except for food energy, healthful eating for athletics and for rigorous active living doesn't differ much

Have You Ever Wondered

. . . how to eat after you're no longer in training? Many athletes never address that! Whether you're a college athlete who stops training or an elite athlete who retires, "retrain" for healthful eating. Less physical activity; loss of muscle mass; and for some, increased food intake can contribute to weight gain. You'll likely need fewer calories, even though your nutrient needs remain about the same. *For guidance see chapter 10, "Planning to Eat Smart." A registered dietitian can help you, too. See "How to Find Nutrition Help . . ." in chapter 24.*

from advice for nonathletes. Both on- and off-season, MyPyramid offers good eating guidelines. Because it's flexible, it works, no matter how much food energy you need or what sport you choose. There's no single eating plan for sports. You can customize!

From chapter 10, you're well aware that MyPyramid categorizes foods into five groups and healthy oils. How much you need from the variety of foods in the five food groups and the healthy oils category depends on your energy needs. *The charts, "MyPyramid Food Intake Pattern Calorie Levels," in the Appendices help you determine the amount. Refer to chapter 10 for more on using MyPyramid.*

For many athletes, energy needs are higher—as many as 6,000 calories a day, for example, for some football players. To meet higher energy demands, choose more servings of nutrient-rich, carbohydrate-rich foods, mostly from the Grains Group and the Vegetable and Fruit Groups of MyPyramid. In contrast, although a high-fat diet offers plenty of concentrated energy (from fat), it carries risks for heart disease—even for highly active people. *For more about MyPyramid, food-group amounts, and serving sizes, see "MyPyramid: Your Healthful Eating Guide" in chapter 10.*

An added reminder: Drink enough fluids during training. It's a good time to practice drinking "on schedule," not just for thirst.

Especially for Children and Teens

You've heard that today's kids don't move enough. Yet many do enjoy vigorous play or competitive sports.

And their food and beverage choices power all they do: first and foremost, for growth and development, and second, for the added demands of physical activity.

Many situations, often unplanned, affect what kids eat and, as a result, their physical performance: early lunch hours and after-school competition; practice that goes into family meal hours; two-sport athletes with little time to recover before competing again; sports fatigue that preempts homework and meals; and nervousness so kids don't eat planned precompetition carried food. These challenges need smart, practical snack and meal solutions.

Nutrients for Active Kids. Healthy eating guidelines from MyPyramid apply to young athletes. Except for calories and fluids, the nutrients for young athletes and nonathletes are about the same. For serious young athletes who train intensely, talk to your doctor or a registered dietitian for guidance; getting enough iron, calcium, and vitamin D, for example, may be issues. Also be aware that growing bones are more susceptible to sports injury from impact and excessive use.

Food Energy for Active Kids. Energy needs depend on age, developmental stage, body size, and sport. *For active kids, check the estimated energy needs in the "MyPyramid Food Intake Pattern Calorie Levels" in the Appendices.* Some very active kids may need more energy to fuel activity.

Does your highly active child consume enough food energy? Here's a clue: Watch his or her performance. Children who tire easily may not be eating enough. Another clue: Monitor your child's growth with your physician. If your child is growing normally, his or her energy (caloric) intake is likely okay. If you're still unsure, ask your doctor to refer you to a registered dietitian who can help you create an eating plan that matches your child's energy needs.

Fluids: Caution for Kids. Children are more likely to get overheated from strenuous activity. As a result, they're at greater risk for dehydration than teens and adults. Even when children play actively in the backyard, they need plenty of fluids.

Why is the risk for dehydration higher? Because kids don't perspire as much as teens and adults, a kid's body's "air conditioning" system is less effective. Kids generate more body heat with exercise, too. A child's "thermostat" doesn't adjust as quickly during

Weight: For Young Athletes

For all children, normal growth and development should be the top priority. Their weight should never be manipulated to meet goals required for sports!

Remember: Child athletes aren't the same as teen and adult athletes. Because they're growing and because their growth spurts aren't always predictable, their body composition can't be judged in the same way. At certain times—for example, before puberty—a child's body naturally stores more body fat to prepare for the next growth spurt. And each child matures at his or her own time and rate.

An eating approach for sports can't change the genetic "body clock" and so speed up physical changes that enhance athletic performance. Supplements and ergogenic aids that are promoted to build muscle, prevent fat gain, or improve performance are never appropriate for children and teens! *For more about healthful eating during the childhood years, see "Eating ABCs for School-Age Children" in chapter 16.*

For young athletes, weight goals should be healthy ones. A distorted body image that drives overexercising and undereating can lead to serious developmental and health problems. That includes the "female athlete triad": a problem of disordered eating, low bone density, and amenorrhea (cessation of menstruation).

Always talk to your doctor about the best weight for your child. An inaccurate assessment may result in a weight goal that isn't healthy.

For more information about body weight, see "Compete in a Weight Category?" later in this chapter.

exercise in hot weather. Protective gear used in many sports, such as hockey and football, hinders their bodies' ability to cool off, too.

To protect children from becoming dehydrated:

● Encourage them to drink plenty of cool fluids before, during, and after physical activities.

● Offer regular fluid breaks (every fifteen minutes) and ensure that fluids are readily available. Perhaps give them a water bottle. Once they're thirsty, they're already on the way to dehydration.

● Weigh them before and after exercise, then replace fluids: 3 cups per pound of weight loss.

● Supervise them carefully, especially on hot days, when fluid needs are even greater.

Refer to chapter 16, "Food to Grow On," for more about food for active kids.

During Pregnancy and Breast-feeding

Pregnancy. With their doctor's approval, active women may continue their sport—at least in the earlier part of pregnancy. Less active women may initiate low-level activities gradually—again with their doctor's approval. Being physically active during pregnancy offers many benefits, among them a psychological lift, optimal weight gain, better aerobic fitness, and an easier labor and delivery

If you're a pregnant woman, or planning to be, ask your doctor about precautions. Overheating your body from exercise, a sauna, or steam room early in pregnancy can affect the development of your unborn baby. If you have anemia, hypertension, diabetes, and other health problems, rigorous activity during pregnancy may not be advised.

All the nutritional issues that relate to a healthy pregnancy apply to female athletes, too. The guidelines? Eat a varied and balanced diet—with enough energy to support your pregnancy, your own needs, and the demands of physical activity. If your energy intake is too low, you may not gain enough weight and your baby may not grow adequately.

Fluid replacement, always important, has even more health implications now. During pregnancy you need more fluids as your own and your baby's blood volume increases. If you don't drink enough, you're at greater risk for dehydration and overheating.

Breast-feeding. With a doctor's guidance, most women can engage in sports or some other form of regular physically activity if they're breast-feeding.

Breast-feeding requires an additional 330 to 400 calories a day for milk production. With more physical activity, you need more; the actual amount depends on the duration and the intensity of your workout.

MyPyramid offers guidance for planning a varied, balanced, and moderate eating plan during breast-feeding—whether you're an athlete or not. Your fluid needs increase during breast-feeding, too. Without exercise, you need about 4 cups more, or at least 15 cups daily from food, beverages, and drinking water. When you work out, drink even more to avoid dehydration.

For more about healthful eating and physical activity during pregnancy and breast-feeding, see "You're Expecting!" and "For Those Who Breast-feed" in chapter 17.

For Vegetarians

Are you among the athletes and physically active people who choose a vegetarian eating style? Vegetarian eating can provide enough fuel and nutrients for peak athletic performance—if you choose meals and snacks carefully with a variety of plant-based foods.

As with any high-performance diet, carbohydrate-rich foods should provide the most food energy—usually not a problem for vegetarians. Follow the advice from MyPyramid (vegetarian-style). And focus on a varied and balanced diet.

If you're a vegetarian who consumes dairy foods and perhaps eggs, getting enough of most nutrients, including protein, poses little challenge. If you're a vegan who eats no foods of animal origin, choose carefully to ensure adequate intake of protein, vitamin B_{12}, iron, zinc, calcium, and perhaps energy (for muscular athletes, who use more energy).

For some vegetarian athletes, consuming enough energy—from an eating plan of bulky, plant-based foods—is a challenge. Eating six to eight meals or snacks a day might be a practical solution.

See chapter 20, "The Vegetarian Way."

Different Sports, Different Approaches to Eating?

No matter what sport you choose, MyPyramid is a basic guide for high-performance eating. Choose enough nutrient-rich food-group foods for the food energy you need.

The most significant nutrition difference from sport to sport relates to energy. The duration and intensity of activity, as well as body size, make the difference.

● A 200-pound football player uses more energy than a 90-pound gymnast.

● A baseball player uses less energy than a soccer player, who's almost constantly in motion.

● An endurance cross-country skier or a long-distance runner likely uses more energy overall than a tennis player or a golfer, who uses spurts of energy for a shorter time.

Every sport demands adequate fluids to replace perspiration and breathing losses, too. In sports with prolonged, intense activity, athletes may perspire more—especially during hot weather.

Endurance Sports

Both in training and in competition, endurance sports—cross-country and marathon running, cross-country skiing, distance bicycling, field hockey, long-distance swimming, and soccer—require more energy. Activity that lasts longer than several hours depletes glycogen stores. Carbohydrate consumed during exercise helps endurance athletes maintain a fast pace; fat is used more efficiently for fuel as exercise continues. Also, protein is a minor fuel source during endurance exercise. Endurance athletes do not need to consume more protein than strength-training athletes; adult endurance athletes should aim for 0.6 to 0.7 gram of protein per pound of body weight.

Energy needed for endurance sports depends on body size, duration of activity, and overall effort. For the elite athlete that may be as high as 4,000 to 6,000 calories daily, chosen from a high-carbohydrate diet. Best sources: nutrient-rich foods from all groups of MyPyramid.

Nonendurance Sports

Nonendurance sports—baseball, bowling, golf, martial arts, softball, speed skating, sprint swimming, tennis, track and field, volleyball, and weight lifting—are fueled by short bursts of energy, perhaps just for two or three minutes or even several seconds. While these sports take an intense, all-out effort, they don't use as much energy overall because their duration is shorter.

Still, nonendurance sports might be of high or moderate intensity. The overall energy demand depends not only on the duration but also on the intensity and the athlete's body size.

Except for calories, nutrient needs for athletes involved in endurance and nonendurance sports are about the same. Again, MyPyramid offers a healthful eating guideline, with an emphasis on nutrient-rich, carbohydrate-rich foods.

Food for Your Training Table

For meals that are high in carbohydrates, adequate in protein, and moderate in fat, try these meal combos:

- Chili made with kidney beans and lean beef.
- Stir-fry with vegetables and lean pork, chicken, shrimp, or tofu served over rice (easy on the oil).
- Soft corn tortillas filled with vegetarian refried beans and topped with tomato sauce or salsa, and cheese. (On a can of refried beans, check the fat content on the label's Nutrition Facts.)
- Grilled fish kebobs (chunks of fresh fish alternating with cherry tomatoes, green peppers, and pineapple on a skewer) served on brown rice.
- Lentils (alone or mixed with lean ground beef) in spaghetti sauce on whole-wheat pasta.
- Green peppers stuffed with a mixture of lean ground turkey and brown rice. Add a mixed green salad, and finish the meal with angel food cake topped with strawberries.
- Lean roast sirloin strips with a baked potato, steamed carrots and cauliflower, and whole-wheat rolls.
- Chicken salad (made with reduced-calorie mayonnaise, grated lemon peel, and tarragon) on rye bread with tomato slices and sprouts. Serve with vegetable soup, whole-wheat crackers, and cantaloupe slices.

Making Weight

Most athletes are concerned about their weight. For football, extra weight may be an advantage for a defensive lineman. For swimmers, some body fat may offer buoyancy. For gymnasts and skaters, a slim body may add to the aesthetics of performance.

For some athletes, weight cycling is an issue. Those who weigh more during their off-season may need to drop a few pounds for training and competition. Others need to "bulk up," perhaps to train and compete in contact sports. Either way, what's the healthful, most effective approach to your best competitive weight?

Whatever your sport, for your peak performance,

enter the competitive season at your best weight. Instead of trying to "make weight" quickly to train and compete, stay at your best weight year-'round.

Body Composition: Fit, Not Fat

For athletic performance (strength, speed, endurance), your body composition is more important than your weight—even if you compete in a weight category. (That's true for nonathletes, too.) Health risks go up as the proportion of body fat increases beyond "healthy." A lean, muscular body has benefits beyond athletics and good looks: overall fitness for life!

What's healthy for athletes? There's no single body fat percentage to aim for, even for the same sport. For your own best performance, the percent body fat for you depends on the body type you were born with. *Refer to the chart, "Body Fat for Adults: Leaner with Physical Training," on this page for a range.* Too little body fat not only jeopardizes athletic performance but also health. In general, less than 5 percent body fat for men, and less than 12 percent body fat for women, has been defined as risky; the percent body fat that's considered risky for you may differ.

You can't measure your body fat or composition accurately on your own. Instead, seek a trained health expert who uses professional methods for measurement, such as skinfold measurements, underwater weighing, and bioelectrical impedance (done with a computer). A registered dietitian or an exercise physiologist can help you target goals for a healthy weight and body composition (percent body fat) for your best physical performance. *See "How to Find Nutrition Help" in chapter 24. For more about body composition, see "Body Weight, Body Fat" in chapter 2.*

Lose Fat, Not Muscle

Do you need to lose weight? Choose an approach that helps you lose fat, not muscle. Start your weight loss strategies ahead—well before training and competition. Then maintain your healthy weight so you have energy and strength when you need them most.

Getting the Lean Advantage

Most important, set a weight goal that's realistic and healthy for you—one that considers your body com-

---

Body Fat for Adults: Leaner with Physical Training

What's the right body composition for sports? For people involved in substantial physical training, the percent of body fat is less than that considered healthy for most people.

Body fat ranges vary from athlete to athlete, sport to sport, and even for a specific position or event on a team. If you're a serious, perhaps an elite, athlete, talk to your physician, qualified trainer, or registered dietitian to set your goal for body fat composition.

		PERCENT BODY FAT	
AGE (YEARS)		WOMEN	MEN
For overall health	<55	20 – 35	8 – 22
	>55	25 – 38	10 – 25
For people in substantial	<55	16 – 28	5 – 15
physical training	>55	20 – 33	7 – 18

Source: Marie Dunford, editor, *Sports Nutrition: A Practice Manual for Professionals* (Chicago: American Dietetic Association, 2006).

---

position and that offers the best competitive edge for your sport. If you need to drop a few pounds, make your weight loss gradual: ½ to 1 pound a week. To lose about 1 pound a week, cut back on your day's energy intake by about 250 calories and boost your training to burn 250 calories more. (*Hint:* 1 pound of body fat equals 3,500 calories.) To cut back on calories, follow guidelines of MyPyramid at a calorie level that's lower for you than usual, and somewhat lower in calories than what your body uses. *See "MyPyramid for Athletes" earlier in this chapter.*

Remember that carbohydrates are the fuel that your working muscles need. Get most of your energy from starches (complex carbohydrates): grain products, including whole grains, legumes, vegetables, and fruits. Cut back on higher-fat foods.

For weight loss, physical activity does more than burn calories. Exercise boosts your metabolic rate, or the rate at which your body uses energy. Muscles use more energy than body fat does.

Be aware that a quick weight-loss regimen that's

low in calories may interfere with your physical performance, first by shorting your energy supply. With many quick regimens you may lose muscle, along with body fat, and deplete your stores of muscle glycogen. Weight loss may be partly water loss—a problem for athletes, who need to keep adequately hydrated.

In your off-season training program, learn to maintain weight so you stay at the best weight for your sport. *To lose weight in a healthful way, see "Weight Management: Strategies That Work!" in chapter 2.*

"Leanest" Isn't Always Better!

The notion that you can never be too thin or too lean may compromise your physical performance! Athletes obsessed with a lean, thin body risk eating disorders and all the dangers (some life-threatening) that accompany severe weight loss. Among the other concerns, for athletes, a body that's too lean may not sweat and cool down properly. The chance for dehydration goes up, and physical endurance is reduced.

If you, someone you train with, or your child or teen show signs of an eating disorder, seek help. Talk to the person about your concern, as well as the family, friends, or the coach. A registered dietitian can offer an expert perspective on eating disorders. *See "Disordered Eating: Problems, Signs, and Help" in chapter 2.*

Compete in a Weight Category?

If you're a wrestler, weight lifter, oarsman, boxer, or body builder who competes in a weight category, body weight may be critically important. Being the heaviest competitor in a lower weight class often is believed to provide a competitive edge. Even an extra pound or two may affect weight class or performance.

For good health, endurance, strength, and best performance, the better advice is to compete in a weight class that's realistic for your body composition and to maintain your optimal weight throughout the competitive season, rather than cycle to "make weight" in unhealthful ways for competition.

Water weight is *not* unnecessary body weight, so sweating off pounds to make weight for wrestling—or any other sport—only hinders performance. Because it leads to dehydration, losing as little as 2 to 3 percent of body weight from sweat (e.g., 3 or 4 pounds, or 6 to 8 cups of fluid, in a 150-pound ath-

lete) can be very dangerous. Even a 1 percent weight loss from fluid loss makes a difference!

Fasting, or drastically cutting back on food, isn't healthy or performance-enhancing, either! And feeling hungry is distracting. More importantly, with fasting, your body won't store the muscle glycogen you need as energy for training and competition. A careful healthful eating plan—that starts well before "weigh in"—is the smartest way to reach and stay in your weight class. Without ongoing, sensible weight management you might continue with the same weight dilemma and "weight cycle" for the next competition—and the next and the next!

Gain Muscle, Not Fat

Hockey and football are among the sports where extra body weight aids performance. Trying to "bulk up" too fast, however, may put more fat on than muscle—especially if you eat extra calories without enough exercise. If you're already in strenuous training, gaining weight may not be as easy as it sounds. You may use energy faster than you consume it!

To build muscle, engage in strength-building activity and consume enough energy from food. Contrary to popular myth, you need only a little extra protein to help build muscle, from a variety of nutritious foods. *See "Muscle Myths" earlier in this chapter.*

As with weight loss, the key to weight gain is "gradual and steady": about ½ to 1 pound a week. To get the extra energy to fuel exercise and build muscle:

- Eat frequent minimeals.
- Increase portions at mealtime.
- Snack between meals.
- Get most of your extra energy from nutrient-rich, high-carbohydrate foods—for example, granola or muesli topped with nuts or dried fruit.
- As an extra meal or snack, try liquid meal supplements for convenient, high-carbohydrate nourishment.

For guidance on healthy weight gain, see "When You Want to Gain" in chapter 2.

The Game Plan

It's the day of the big event. You're excited and perhaps a bit anxious. You've trained hard. What should you eat to maximize your performance? Your game plan now—what you eat before, during, and after competition or a heavy workout—makes a difference.

For endurance events, think further ahead—before your pre-event meal. Several days beforehand, you might eat more carbohydrates and gradually rest your muscles. In that way, you'll store extra muscle glycogen and won't tire as quickly during the event. *See "Carbohydrate Loading" earlier in this chapter.*

For any sport, eat for peak performance well ahead. Most energy for competition comes from foods you ate earlier, not from your pre-event meal. For training, eat plenty of carbohydrates, moderate amounts of protein, not much fat, and drink plenty of fluids.

On competition day, even carefully planned meals can't make up for a poor training diet. Eat for fitness all along.

Read on for general advice. For sports-specific nutrition guidelines, talk with a sports dietitian, a registered dietitian with a specialty in sports nutrition.

Before You Compete

Before competition? Choose a pre-event meal or snack—light, easy to digest, high-carbohydrate—that matches your physical performance goals. In that way you can perform to your ability without tiring too soon. Eating helps prevent the distraction of hunger pangs. Although eating won't provide immediate energy, it can supply energy for exercise that lasts an hour or more. Drink enough, too, to fully hydrate your body before strenuous exercise.

The "right" pre-event meal or snack differs from athlete to athlete, event to event, and time of day. During your training, experiment with different foods, food combinations, amounts, and timing.

Timing. Finish eating one to four hours before your workout or competition. That allows enough time for food to digest so you don't feel full or uncomfortable.

What about morning competition? Eat a hearty, high-carbohydrate dinner and bedtime snack the night before. Then in the morning, eat a light, high-carbohydrate meal or snack. Eating two hours before exercise helps replenish your liver glycogen and satisfy hunger.

Small meals. Choose a small meal or snack. The amount depends on what makes you feel comfortable.

High "carbs." Enjoy a high-"carb" meal or snack that's moderate in protein and low in fat. It gets digested and absorbed faster. (About $\frac{1}{2}$ gram to 2 grams of carbohydrate per pound of body weight is about right.)

Make pasta, rice, potatoes, or bread the "center" of your plate. A high-fat meal may cause indigestion

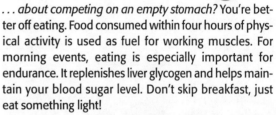

Have You Ever Wondered

... about competing on an empty stomach? You're better off eating. Food consumed within four hours of physical activity is used as fuel for working muscles. For morning events, eating is especially important for endurance. It replenishes liver glycogen and helps maintain your blood sugar level. Don't skip breakfast, just eat something light!

... what to eat before competition if you feel too nervous to eat? Drinking a liquid meal supplement or a fruit milk shake might help. It provides nutrients and fluids needed for competition. And it might be more easily digested and absorbed than a full meal. Liquid meals also contribute fluids.

... if fructose tablets during prolonged exercise are a good energy source? Fructose isn't converted to energy as fast as glucose is; fructose converts to liver glycogen first. You're better off with a drink that offers glucose or sucrose. Fructose also can cause gastrointestinal distress (bloating, cramping, or diarrhea).

... if a "complete nutrition supplement," perhaps an energy bar or drink, or a power gel, aids performance? Not "complete nutrition," energy bars and drinks may be an energy source, but not a meal replacement, for physical activity. Power gels supply "carbs," too, but usually few vitamins or minerals. A quick check of the Nutrition Facts reveals their calorie and nutrient contribution. Although energy bars, drinks, or gels may be convenient during an endurance event, eat fruit or a starchy snack such as a bagel afterward instead.

... where to get nutrition advice for athletic performance—or to find out if your food choices help or hinder your training? Talk to a sports dietitian, a registered dietitian with a specialty in sports nutrition, or other qualified expert for help in determining your energy needs, evaluating your eating plan, and strategizing ways to eat for peak performance. Be aware: "personal trainer" isn't a regulated professional specialty. Some trainers are highly qualified exercise specialists; others aren't.

Pre-Event Meals–for Starters

There's no single menu prescribed for pre-event eating, but these three high-carbohydrate menus show what you might eat before you compete:

MEAL 1	MEAL 2	MEAL 3
● 1 cup cereal	● 2 cups beef noodle soup	● 2 pancakes with 2 tbsp. syrup
● 1 banana	● 6 crackers	● 1 cup fat-free yogurt
● 8 oz. fat-free milk	● 1 medium baked potato	● ½ cup strawberries
● 1 bagel with 1 tbsp. jelly	● 1 cup vegetable juice	● 1 cup apple juice
● ¾ cup cranberry juice drink		
Calories 630	*Calories* 620	*Calories* 625
Carbohydrates 136 g	*Carbohydrates* 116 g	*Carbohydrates* 110 g

or nausea with heavy exercise. *See "Pre-Event Meals—for Starters" on this page.*

Contrary to common belief, eating small amounts of fat won't keep your body from storing muscle glycogen. A little fat adds flavor and helps you meet your overall energy needs.

No discomfort. Skip foods that may cause intestinal discomfort during competition: gas-causing foods such as beans, cabbage, onions, cauliflower, and turnips, and bulky, high-fiber foods such as raw fruits and vegetables with seeds and tough skin, bran, nuts, and seeds.

Familiar foods. Enjoy familiar foods and beverages. This isn't the time to try something new that may disagree with you.

Enough fluids. About two hours ahead, drink at least 2 cups of fluid. Then about fifteen minutes ahead, drink another 1 to 2 cups of fluids. Milk's okay. Stress and loss of body fluids—not milk—often slow saliva flow, causing "cotton mouth," or a dry mouth.

"Feel-good" foods. If a certain food or meal seems to enhance your performance, enjoy it—if you can fit it into your pre-event eating strategy.

During Competition

Nourishment now depends on your sport.

● *During most activities,* drinking plenty of fluids is the only real issue. Every fifteen or so minutes, you're wise to drink enough to minimize loss of body weight, without overdrinking: ½ to 2 cups every 15 minutes.

● *During endurance sports of sixty minutes or more,* a slightly sweetened carbohydrate drink (sports drink) or snack may help maintain your blood sugar levels, boost your stamina, and enhance your performance. Figure about 0.5 gram of carbohydrate per pound of your body weight per hour.

Sports drinks are easy to digest, especially if you're involved in intense activity. And they count as fluids. Their flavor may encourage their consumption, especially among children. Remember to also drink fluids every fifteen or so minutes!

● *During day-long events or regional tournaments,* snack on high-carbohydrate, low-fat foods. Between matches, sets, or other competitive events, these foods are good choices: crackers, bagels, rice cakes, orange slices, apples, bananas, and fruit bars. Bring snacks so you don't need to rely on a concession stand. Consuming fluids all day long remains important.

After You Compete

Your cool-down routine is just as important as your warm-up. And what you eat and drink after a workout is as important as your pre-event eating routine.

Make fluids your first priority! First and foremost, after competition or a heavy workout, replace your fluid loss. The amount depends on how much weight you lose through exercise. Simply weigh yourself before and afterward; the difference is your water weight. For every pound you lose, drink 3 cups of fluid. And continue to drink fluids throughout the day or several days until you return to your pre-exercise weight if you lost weight.

What fluids are best? Drink fluids with carbohydrates, such as juice or sports drinks. They replace fluids and help your body replenish muscle glycogen. Sports drinks may have sodium, as well; juice has potassium. Plain water and watery foods, such as soup, watermelon, and grapes, are good fluid recovery foods, too. *See "Food: A Water Source" in chapter 8.*

Refuel your muscles with carbohydrates. Within the first several hours after competition or a heavy workout, eat a carbohydrate-rich meal or snack. For muscle recovery, the sooner, the better. For strength training, include a high-quality protein source, such as milk, lean meat, fish, or poultry.

For every pound of body weight, strive for about 0.5 gram of carbohydrates. For example, if you weigh 150 pounds, eat at least 75 grams of carbohydrates. That's easy to do with a high-carbohydrate snack or meal. For strenuous exercise that lasts ninety minutes or longer, consume that much in carbohydrates within thirty minutes after exercise, then again about two hours later. A little protein eaten with carbohydrate foods, perhaps milk with cereal, aids recovery. *See "'Carbo' Foods" in the Appendices.*

If you aren't hungry right away, drink juice or a sports drink for fluids and "carbs." Because sports drinks are a diluted source of "carbs," you need to double the amount of sports drink to get the same amount of carbohydrates—for example, 32 ounces of a sports drink and 16 ounces of juice each supply about 50 grams of carbohydrates. When your hunger returns, enjoy a carbohydrate-rich meal or snack.

How about electrolytes? Through perspiration, you lose electrolytes such as sodium. Because the average American diet supplies more than enough, enjoy your meal—and perhaps a sports drink—after endurance sports. You'll likely get enough sodium and other electrolytes to replace your losses.

You don't need a salt tablet. It may cause cramping, dehydration, and stomach irritation. Concentrated amounts of salt cause the stomach to draw fluids from other parts of the body as they dilute the salt. For some athletes a little salt may aid rehydration.

Ergogenic Aids: No Substitute for Training

"Blast your body with energy!". . . "Best muscle volumizers!" . . . "Guaranteed for muscle growth!". . . "For faster muscle recovery and longer endurance!"

Of course, you want to make the most of every workout and increase your competitive edge. But do you take supplements without questioning their merits? It's easy to be lured by advertising claims that ergogenic aids (dietary and hormonal supplements) improve strength, endurance, or recovery time, especially when anatomical graphics and charts make claims appear credible. Adding confusion, valid and invalid advice often appear side by side in fitness magazines.

"Ergogenic" means the potential to increase work output. Despite slick advertising and marketing, only proper training and nutrition can do that.

What about "proven results"? Perceived performance benefits of ergogenic aids often come from individual reports, a misunderstanding of physiology, or from claims taken out of scientific context. Their purported claims may be more psychological than physical. It's well documented that the side effects of many ergogenic aids may hinder performance and may cause harm, especially in the long run!

Dietary Supplements

A slew of dietary supplements—amino acid supplements, bee pollen, carnitine, chromium picolinate, ephedra, glutamine, HMB (beta-hydroxy beta methylbutyrate), and whey protein, among others, as well as many herbs—are promoted for better physical performance. Yet, their effectiveness and safety are undetermined. (*Note:* Ephedra is now banned by the U.S. FDA for sale as a supplement although the ruling has been challenged; some over-the-counter medications may contain ephedrine.) And they're costly!

● *Amino acids.* Amino acid supplements such as arginine, branched-chain amino acids (BCAAs), and ornithine are often promoted to build muscle and increase fat loss among athletes. But most athletes consume more than enough amino acids from food, so these products are an unnecessary expense. *See "Muscle Myths" in this chapter.*

● *Carnitine.* Carnitine is a body chemical composed of two essential amino acids, lysine and methionine. As an ergogenic aid, carnitine has been promoted for more energy, aerobic power, and body fat reduction. However, the human body produces adequate amounts, and foods of animal origin are good sources. There's no need to take extra. For improved athletic performance, it's ineffective.

● *Chromium picolinate.* Chromium picolinate is promoted as an ergogenic aid for athletes, and an aid

When You're on the Road

Planes, trains, and automobiles get you where you're going. But to keep physically active—or perhaps keep up a training regimen—when you travel, plan ahead!

● Pack comfortable workout clothes and footwear. Take a jump rope, running or walking shoes, or plastic dumbbells to fill with water. You won't need work-out facilities.

● Choose a hotel with exercise equipment, then make time to use it. Before you make your reservation, ask about the facilities: an indoor or outdoor pool; tennis courts; bicycle rentals; and gym equipment such as a treadmill, step machine, or rowing machine.

● If you belong to a health club at home, check ahead for membership benefits elsewhere.

● At the airport, wait for your flight by walking the concourse; skip people movers. On a long train or plane trip, walk up and down the aisle several times if allowed. Ask for an aisle seat so you won't have to climb over your fellow passengers. Do simple stretching exercises to avoid feeling stiff.

● Ask for an early wake-up call so you can get a jump start on your day with a thirty-minute walk or jog. Get a guidebook to map out your way—or the hotel's front desk may have a walking map.

● Skip the taxicab. If it's a safe, reasonable distance, walk to your business meeting, museums, shops, or restaurants in comfortable walking shoes.

● If you're driving, take regular breaks. You'll ride more comfortably after some physical activity.

● Check the television guide for a workout or yoga program. Or take an exercise DVD and a player.

to weight loss. Because chromium works with insulin, it plays a role in energy production. Deficiencies of chromium from food choices are rare, however. When chromium levels are normal, there doesn't appear to be any benefit from taking a supplement. In supplements, chromium levels are significantly higher than the Recommended Dietary Allowance (RDA). Excess levels may have adverse effects—and offer no benefits.

● *Creatine monohydrate.* This ergogenic aid is promoted to increase muscle mass and strength, enhance energy, and delay fatigue. In fact, creatine is a nitrogen-containing compound that's found naturally in meat and fish and in the human brain and in muscle. Research suggests that creatine supplements may promote muscle strength, help increase body weight, and aid recovery after strength training or short bouts of high-intensity activity; yet there's only limited research on its long-term effects. In addition, athletes tend to take larger doses than manufacturers recommend. Creatine supplements aren't advised for teenage athletes; safety and effectiveness are unknown.

● *Pangamic acid.* Touted as vitamin B_{15}, it's not a vitamin at all. Instead it's an inconsistent mixture of substances, including some that are potentially hazardous. Although extolled as an energy enhancer for athletes, it has no proven benefits.

● *Spirulina.* Spirulina, a blue-green alga, is often touted as a high-energy food. It can offer nutrients to the diet, but it has no energy-producing qualities. Spirulina is high in protein and contains small amounts of vitamin B_{12}. However, much of its vitamin B_{12} is inactive and cannot be absorbed by humans.

● *Wheat germ and wheat germ oil.* Both products are promoted as ergogenic aids. Although no proven benefits exist, there are no known side effects or adverse reactions from ingesting them. Wheat germ supplies nutrients such as proteins, B vitamins, and vitamin E.

See chapter 23 for more about dietary supplements.

Hormone Supplements

Hormone supplements, or steroids, are another type of dietary supplement that may increase muscle mass—but at a price to health. An ergogenic aid, they're powerful yet dangerous drugs!

Teens should *never* use steroids. Contrary to many a young adolescent boy's wish, steroids won't bulk up muscles before puberty. Adolescents who use them may not grow to their normal height.

● *Androstenedione*, or "andro," is an anabolic steroid that acts like testosterone, a male sex hormone. "Anabolic" refers to the metabolic processes of synthesizing body tissue. Steroids can help build bigger muscles, as well as increase strength, alter mood, and decrease body fat, but don't ensure better physical performance.

Of concern, their use can have dangerous and often permanent side effects. For example, in men, steroids may cause acne, testicular damage, enlarged breasts, and a lower sperm count. Used by women, steroids may cause masculine qualities: a lower voice, facial hair, smaller breasts, and loss of (or irregular) menstrual cycle. Other potential risks: increased risk for injury, blood clots, and gastrointestinal problems as well as liver damage, heart disease, and cancer. Steroid use is banned by the International Olympic Committee (IOC) and most other sports governing bodies, and condemned by the American Academy of Pediatrics and the American College of Sports Medicine. In the Anabolic Steroid Control Act androstenedione is a controlled substance, listed as a banned anabolic steroid and an illegal performance-enhancing drug.

Need more tips specific to eating for active living? Check here for "how-tos":

● Manage weight for sports sensibly—see chapter 2.

● Spot the signs of eating disorders in athletes—see chapter 2.

● Exercise safely during pregnancy—see chapter 17.

● Sort through claims for ergogenic dietary supplements—see chapter 23.

● Seek advice from a sports dietitian, especially if you're an athlete who aspires to peak performance, an elite or professional athlete, or a physically active person with a health condition—see chapter 24.

● *Dehydroepiandrosterone (DHEA),* sold as a safe alternative to anabolic steroids, is androgenic steroid, banned by the IOC and the National Collegiate Athletic Association. "Androgenic" refers to the development of male characteristics. Evidence doesn't back up these claims: to increase energy, decrease body fat, counteract stress, and slow aging. In the short run, DHEA can have unpleasant side effects, including facial hair growth, acne, enlarged liver, rapid heartbeat, and testicular damage. With its potential effect on testosterone and estradiol (a female steroid produced in the ovaries) levels, its use may be risky for people with a family history of prostate or breast cancer.

Building muscle gradually through physical activity is still the healthful, time-honored, most effective, and fair approach! *See "Muscle Myths" in this chapter.*

Your Physical Activity: How Intense?

Light, moderate, or intense? Estimate your activity level: determine if your heart rate is within your target zone.

1. *Decide on your goal:*
   ● *Moderate intensity:* Your target heart rate should be 50 to 70 percent of your maximum heart rate.
   ● *Vigorous intensity:* Your target heart rate should be 70 to 85 percent of your maximum heart rate.

2. *Figure your maximum heart rate.* It's 220 minus your age. So, if you're 50 years old, your maximum heart rate is 220 minus 50 to equal 170 beats per minute (bpm).

3. *Determine your target zone.* Multiply your maximum heart rate by your workout intensity. For example, for moderate intensity, multiply 170 bpm by 50 percent to equal 85 bpm, or by 70 percent to equal 119 bpm.

4. *Take your heart rate.* Stop exercising. With your index and middle fingers, take your pulse at your neck, wrist, or chest. Count the beats for 60 seconds; the first beat is zero. (Or count for 30 seconds, then double it for bpm.) In this example, between 85 and 119 beats is moderate activity.

The talk-sing test, *described in chapter 1,* is another quick way to assess your workout intensity.

CHAPTER 20

The Vegetarian Way

Pasta salad with vegetables. Polenta topped with homemade tomato sauce and freshly grated Parmesan cheese. Bean burritos. Portobello mushroom sandwich layered with stir-fried onions and peppers. Split-pea soup with rye bread. Veggie-cheese pizza. Barley-cheese stuffed peppers. Lentil curry. Bean curd lo mein.

Today's cookbooks, magazines, and restaurant menus are full of vegetarian dishes with nutritious, flavorful food combinations. Whether you choose a vegetarian eating style or not, these dishes add food variety, interest, and flavor to smart eating.

A plant-based diet isn't new. Yet today vegetarian eating styles and dishes are capturing more attention among consumers, health professionals, fast-food and sit-down restaurants, and the food industry. Have you noticed how many vegetarian products have hit the market, including tofu burgers, veggie cheese, soy-burgers, frozen dinners, and bowl entrées?

Being Vegetarian

What does it mean to be a vegetarian? For some, it's a way of eating; for others, a whole lifestyle. And non-vegetarians simply may enjoy the flavors and get the health benefits from plant-based dishes—regularly or as an occasional switch from their everyday fare.

Why Vegetarian?

Vegetarian eating styles differ, as do the many reasons why people choose to become vegetarians. With today's focus on wellness, many cite health reasons. Others express concerns about the environment, compassion for animals, or their belief in nonviolence. For some, religious, spiritual, or ethical reasons define their strict vegetarian lifestyle. Several religions advocate vegetarian eating—for example, Hinduism and the Seventh-Day Adventist Church. For some, being a vegetarian reflects their ethical approach to addressing world hunger. Still others simply prefer the flavors and food mixtures of vegetarian dishes, and may recognize that a plant-based diet often costs less.

Health Benefits

Either choice—vegetarian or nonvegetarian eating—can supply enough nutrients and food substances to nourish you, promote your health, and help prevent health problems. No matter what your approach, the nutrition bottom line depends on your food choices over time. In fact, eating a vegetarian diet can be an easy way to follow the advice of the Dietary Guidelines for Americans and MyPyramid.

Studies show a positive link between vegetarian eating and health. In general, the incidence of, or the death rate from, some health problems—heart disease, high blood pressure, type 2 diabetes, and some forms of cancer—tends to be lower among vegetarians. Body Mass Index, an indication of overweight and obesity, is typically less, too. Among vegetarians, total blood cholesterol and LDL ("bad") cholesterol are usually lower; however, HDL ("good") cholesterol and triglyceride levels may or may not be affected.

Potential health-promoting benefits of vegetarian eating may come from the nutrients and phytonutrients (or plant substances) in the overall food choices. A vegetarian approach to eating tends to be lower in saturated fat, cholesterol, and animal protein, and higher in carbohydrates, fiber, folate, carotenoids, vitamins A and C, magnesium, and other phytonutrients. Those same qualities can come from a carefully chosen nonvegetarian diet.

Food choices may not be the only reason for the health benefits, however. Vegetarians often make other lifestyle choices that promote health, such as regular physical exercise, not smoking, and moderating ingestion of or avoiding alcoholic beverages.

Being vegetarian doesn't ensure a healthful eating style. Poorly planned, the chance for some nutritional deficiencies can go up. Like any way of eating, a vegetarian eating style also can be high in fat and cholesterol, low in fiber, or both. The nutritional content of a vegetarian style of eating depends on overall food choices over several days—and on focusing on the bounty of plant-based foods!

What Type?

In its broadest definition, being "vegetarian" means avoiding foods from animal sources. Instead, plant sources of food—grains, legumes (dry beans and peas), nuts, vegetables, and fruits—form the basis of the diet. That's what vegetarians have in common.

As a matter of choice, many vegetarians eat dairy products, and perhaps eggs. Among today's vegetarians, nearly half avoid foods of animal origin. If you're a vegetarian, you may describe yourself in one of these ways:

● *Lacto-ovo-vegetarian,* who chooses an eating approach with eggs and dairy products but no meat, poultry, and fish. The prefix "lacto" refers to milk; "ovo" refers to eggs. Most vegetarians in the United States fit within this category.

● *Lacto-vegetarian,* who avoids meat, poultry, fish, and eggs (and egg derivatives such as albumin or egg whites) but eats dairy products.

● *Strict vegetarian, or vegan* (VEE-gahn or VEHJ-ahn), who eats no animal products: no meat, poultry, fish, eggs, milk, cheese, or other dairy products.

Vegans frequently avoid foods with animal products as ingredients, too: for example, *no* refried beans made with lard; *no* fries cooked in beef tallow; baked goods made *without* butter, eggs, or albumin (from eggs); *no* margarine made with whey or casein (from milk); *no* foods flavored with meat extracts; and *no* foods with gelatin (from animal bones and hooves). Some avoid honey, which is made by bees.

● *Semivegetarian,* who usually follows a vegetarian eating plan but sometimes eats meat, poultry, or fish, perhaps as a condiment or side dish.

Vegetarian Diets: Nutritionally Speaking

Can vegetarian eating supply your body with enough nutrients? Yes. As with any eating style, you need to

Have You Ever Wondered

. . . if "vegetarian" on a food label means "low-fat," too? No, it doesn't. Foods labeled as "vegetarian" on their package labeling—and on restaurant menus—may contain high-fat ingredients. Foods that can be higher in fat include textured soy patties, soy hot dogs, soy cheese, refried beans, and snack bars. Even tofu may have more fat than you'd think: 4 ounces (about ½ cup) has about 95 calories and 6 fat grams, mostly from polyunsaturated fats, compared with about 145 calories and 4 fat grams in 3 ounces of cooked lean beef round steak. Read the Nutrition Facts panel on food labels to compare the calories and the nutrients in food.

. . . if a macrobiotic diet is nourishing? Like any approach to eating, the answer lies in how the overall eating plan stacks up to today's healthful eating guidelines. *(See page 519.)* A macrobiotic diet has been described as predominantly vegetarian, emphasizing minimally processed foods. Food choices are mostly grains, legumes, and vegetables, with fruits, nuts, and seeds eaten to a lesser extent. Some who follow a macrobiotic diet consume limited amounts of fish. For the record, the Zen macrobiotic diet, followed several decades ago typically for spiritual reasons, is different and highly restrictive.

Not Just for Vegetarians: Quick and Healthful Snacks

Popcorn, plain

Dairy or soy yogurt, low-fat or fat-free

Pretzels

Cottage cheese

Crackers*

Muffins*

Oatmeal cookies*

Sunflower and pumpkin seeds

Fresh or canned fruit

Dried fruit

Peanuts, soy nuts, or tree nuts

Fruit shakes

Fruit juice

Raw vegetables (carrots, broccoli, zucchini)

Dried fruit rolls (fruit leather)

Tomato juice

Crackers* and cheese

Trail mix

Bean tacos or burritos

Cheese and veggie pizza (or cheeseless pizza)

Bagels and peanut butter

Focaccia bread (with or without cheese)

Hummus (mashed chickpea dip) with pita points

Nut butter and crackers

Fruit/cereal bars, calcium fortified

Milk or calcium-fortified soy beverages or rice beverages

Fig cookies

Tofu dip

Smoothies made with milk, or with soy or rice beverages

*Choose those with less *trans* fat.

choose foods carefully—and consume enough food energy, or calories, yet not too many.

For vegetarians who consume dairy products and perhaps eggs, nutrition issues don't differ much from those of nonvegetarians. Balance the calories you eat with those you burn—smart advice. Go easy on saturated fats, *trans* fats, and cholesterol—as well as added sugars and salt. If you choose mostly lower-fat or fat-free dairy products, plenty of grains (especially whole grains), vegetables, and fruits, as well as nuts and healthy oils, a typical lacto-ovo-vegetarian diet can be high in fiber, low in saturated fat, *trans* fats, and cholesterol, and moderate in total fat: nutrition goals for all healthy people!

For vegans, the nutrition issues differ somewhat. Without any foods of animal origin, getting enough calories to maintain a healthy weight can be a challenge, especially for growing children and teens. And nutrients that may come up short need special attention: vitamin B_{12}, vitamin D, calcium, iron, and zinc. Nonetheless, planned wisely, a vegan diet can provide enough nutrients for overall good health, too.

Protein Power

With vegetarian eating, the issue of protein often arises. Why? Because vegetarians eat less—or perhaps no—foods of animal origin; lean meat, poultry, fish, eggs, and dairy foods are all sources of concentrated protein. For most vegetarians, adequate protein isn't a concern, however. Except for fruit, almost every food of plant origin contains protein—at least a small amount. Legumes, nuts, and seeds are good sources.

Is the protein sufficient? Probably yes—even though a vegetarian diet may be slightly lower in total protein than a nonvegetarian diet. If protein quality is lower, vegetarians may need somewhat more protein overall. Yet a plant-based diet, chosen wisely with plenty of food variety and sufficient food energy, likely provides more than enough protein for most vegetarians. Here's why—and how!

More about Proteins

We often think of protein as a single nutrient. Yet, proteins in both food and your body cells are made up of building blocks, or amino acids, each with a somewhat different structure. Although many more appear in nature, your body uses about twenty amino acids to make body proteins. Like carbohydrates and fats, amino acids are unique combinations of carbon, hydrogen, and oxygen. However, amino acids also have nitrogen, which makes their physiological structure and functions uniquely their own.

How proteins are made. Of the twenty or so amino acids your body uses, nine are considered essential.

Because your body can't make them, your food choices must supply them. Their names may sound familiar: histidine, isoleucine, leucine, lysine, methionine, phenylalanine, threonine, tryptophan, and valine. You might see some—perhaps phenylalanine and tryptophan—on food labels.

Other amino acids are nonessential. Your body makes them—if you consume enough essential amino acids and enough calories during the day from other amino acids. Just eat many different foods with protein during the day for the full variety of amino acids.

Amino acids are described as protein's "building blocks." Like notes in a music scale or letters of the alphabet, they're arranged in countless ways. The same music notes create symphonies, jazz, and pop hits. And the same twenty-six letters of the alphabet form thousands of words in many languages, each word with its own meaning. It's the same for amino acids. In a single cell in your body, ten thousand different proteins may exist—each with a different arrangement of amino acids.

For their meaning, words must be spelled correctly. Amino acids in proteins must be arranged in a precise order to function normally. The genetic code in every cell—called DNA, or deoxyribonucleic acid—carries "spelling" instructions for each protein.

What proteins do. As nutrients, proteins perform many functions. For one, proteins are part of every body cell. Your body's different tissues—skin, muscles, bone, and organs, for example—are unique because the amino acid patterns in their proteins differ. Your body needs a constant supply of proteins to repair body cells as they wear out. During times of growth—infancy, childhood, adolescence, and pregnancy—the body also needs proteins to make new body tissues.

Beyond that, proteins help regulate body processes. As enzymes and hormones, they make various chemical reactions happen—for example, a nonessential amino acid, L-arginine, may play a role in heart health by helping to keep blood vessels open. As antibodies, amino acids help protect you from disease-carrying bacteria and viruses. Proteins are also in membranes, working as transport carriers.

Proteins also supply your body with energy if you don't consume enough from carbohydrates and fats. If you do consume enough calories from "carbs" and fats, proteins can be saved for their unique function:

to build and repair body tissue. When you consume more protein than you need, it's broken down and stored as body fat, not as a protein reserve.

How much protein. For vegetarians and nonvegetarians, the Recommended Dietary Allowance (RDA) for protein per day set by the Institute of Medicine is based on body weight (*see Appendices*): for children ages 4 to 8, 19 grams; for kids ages 9 to 13, 34 grams; for teen boys 14 to 18, 52 grams; for teen girls ages 14 to 18, 46 grams; for adult men ages 19 or over, 56 grams; and for adult women ages 19 or over, 46 grams. For pregnancy and breast-feeding, the RDA is 71 grams of protein. And the Acceptable Macronutrient Distribution Range (AMDR) for protein: for children and teens, ages 4 to 18 years, 10 to 30 percent of total calories, and for adults ages 19 or over, 10 to 35 percent of total calories. The RDA falls at the lower end of the AMDR. The lower your calorie needs, the higher percent of calories you need from protein to meet your RDA.

Where proteins come from. Meat, poultry, fish, eggs, milk, cheese, yogurt, and soy provide all nine essential amino acids. For that reason they're often referred to as high-quality "complete" proteins.

Almost all plant-based foods supply the indispensable amino acids, but not the same amounts as "high-quality" protein foods do; for some amino acids, the amounts are quite small. Legumes (beans and peas), seeds, and nuts supply plenty of proteins. Grain products and most vegetables supply proteins, too, with smaller amounts of some essential amino acids. Even fruit provides small amounts.

Consider this: a 1-cup serving of rice and beans (half rice, half beans) supplies about 10 grams of protein. Add 1 cup of milk or soy beverage for, respectively, 8 or 6 grams of protein; a green vegetable side dish for 1 gram or 2 grams of protein; one whole-wheat roll, about 4 more grams of protein. That adds up to at least 21 grams of protein.

Completing the Equation

For the body to make its many proteins, your food choices must supply essential amino acids—in sufficient amounts. Animal proteins supply them all, in proportions needed to make new body proteins. Except for soybeans, foods with plant proteins lack significant amounts of one or more of them. That's why their protein is often called "incomplete." When your meals and snacks provide a variety of plant-based foods and your food energy needs are met, you get all the amino acids your body needs.

For complete protein, there's no need to combine specific foods at each meal, as once thought. Your body makes its own complete proteins if you eat a variety of plant foods—legumes, nuts, seeds, grains, vegetables, and fruits—and enough calories throughout the day. Whatever amino acid one food lacks can come from other foods you eat. For vegetarians, protein is an issue only when calories are overly limited or when they come mostly from energy-dense, nutrient-poor food and drink choices.

Vitamin B$_{12}$: A Challenge for Vegans

Like other B vitamins, vitamin B$_{12}$, also called cobalamin, fulfills many functions in health. For one, it helps your body make red blood cells and use fats and amino acids, and it's part of every body cell. A deficiency of vitamin B$_{12}$ isn't likely in the short run. Vitamin B$_{12}$ needs are small, and it's a nutrient that's stored and recycled in your body. Over time, however, a vitamin B$_{12}$ deficiency can result in anemia and severe, irreversible nerve damage. That said, suboptimal intakes of vitamin B$_{12}$ may be linked to higher levels of homocysteine, a risk factor for heart disease.

Unlike some nutrients, vitamin B$_{12}$ doesn't make the health news much, perhaps because it's so widely available in foods of animal origin. With some exceptions, getting enough isn't a concern for most vegetarians—at least those who consume dairy products or eggs.

For vegans, vitamin B$_{12}$ is a nutrition concern. Plants only supply this nutrient when soil with vitamin B$_{12}$-producing microorganisms clings to fruits and vegetables and isn't removed completely before eating. In the United States, fruits and vegetables are scrubbed clean; they usually have no soil with these microorganisms on them. Most vegans need to look elsewhere for a reliable source of vitamin B$_{12}$.

For those who limit or avoid foods from animal sources, a vitamin B$_{12}$ supplement or foods fortified with vitamin B$_{12}$ are advised. Since vitamin B$_{12}$ isn't absorbed as well with age, even older vegetarians who consume dairy foods or eggs benefit by taking a supplement as well.

● Look for vitamin B$_{12}$-fortified breakfast cereals, soy or rice beverages, or vegetarian burger patties. Or consider a vitamin B$_{12}$ supplement. Read the Nutrition Facts panel on food and supplement labels to check the vitamin B$_{12}$ content. Know that "cyanocobalamin" is its most bioavailable form. In other words, it's the form the body absorbs most easily.

● If you choose a supplement, look for one that provides 100 percent of the Daily Value (DV) for vitamin B$_{12}$. Check the Supplement Facts. Vitamin B$_{12}$ in fortified foods and supplements is produced synthetically from bacteria, not from animal sources.

● Be aware that seaweed, algae, spirulina, and fermented plant foods such as tempeh and miso aren't good sources of vitamin B$_{12}$—even if the package says so. The vitamin B$_{12}$ is inactive, so it's not in a form that the human body can use. Vitamin B$_{12}$ in beer and other fermented foods isn't reliable, either.

● Nutritional yeast can be a source of vitamin B$_{12}$ if grown on a medium that's enriched with vitamin B$_{12}$—for example, Red Star Vegetarian Support Formula Nutritional Yeast. Yeast typically used in baking doesn't supply any. Check the label. Don't count on yeast to supply vitamin B$_{12}$ unless you've checked it out.

For more about vitamin B$_{12}$, see chapter 4.

Fatty Acid: An Essential

Somewhat like the amino acids that make up proteins, fats are made up of fatty acids. Among them, alpha-linolenic acid (ALA) and linoleic acid (omega-6s) are considered essential since your body can't make them. In your body, alpha-linolenic acid converts to omega-3 fatty acids (DHA, or docosahexaenoic acid and EPA or eicosapentaeoic acid), which keeps your brain, central nervous system, and membranes throughout your body healthy. Omega-3s also may offer protection against some ongoing health problems such as heart disease.

Vegetarians are urged to consume alpha-linolenic acids from plant-based ingredients—for example, canola oil, soy oil, walnuts, ground flaxseed, and soybeans—since they convert to omega-3s. Fatty fish and some eggs supply omega-3 fatty acids for some vegetarians. Choosing these sources of fats, instead of those that add up to a lot of saturated fats and *trans* fats, is a good strategy. Check the label's Nutrition Facts.

Vegetarian diets tend to be low in omega-3s, but often high in omega-6 fatty acids. The imbalance can inhibit production of important omega-3s from alpha-linolenic acid (ALA). *(Refer to page 53 for more about ALA.)* Omega-6s come from corn, safflower, and sunflower oils.

The Institute of Medicine set Adequate Intake levels (AI) for omega-3s; *see chapter 3*. The recommended amount supplies about 15 calories or a little less from omega-3s daily.

Vitamin D: Not Just from Sunshine!

Vitamin D works as a nutrient partner, helping your body absorb calcium and phosphorus, then depositing them in bones and teeth.

Your body also makes its own vitamin D when your skin is exposed to sunlight. About ten to fifteen minutes on your hands, arms, and face without sunscreen twice weekly is ample time for your body to produce enough vitamin D. If you're darker-skinned or live in a cloudy or smoggy area, you may need more sun exposure; just don't overdo! For lighter skin, less.

Few foods are naturally high in vitamin D, so in the United States, most milk is vitamin D fortified; some flavored milks are not vitamin D fortified. Egg yolks also supply smaller amounts.

Vitamin D isn't an issue if you drink enough milk or if you're regularly exposed to sunlight. Just 8 ounces of milk provide 100 International Units of vitamin D, or about half the amount that adults age fifty or under need daily.

However, vegans—or anyone who doesn't drink milk or eat fatty fish—need to be careful to get enough vitamin D, especially during the winter in northern climates and if housebound. That's true, too, for older adults, who don't synthesize vitamin D as efficiently.

● If you're a vegan, check the Nutrition Facts on food labels—some breakfast cereals, some soy and rice beverages, some cereal bars, and some calcium-fortified juices are fortified with vitamin D.

● If you're in doubt, talk to your doctor or a registered dietitian (RD) about taking a vitamin D supplement. Choose one with no more than 100 percent of the

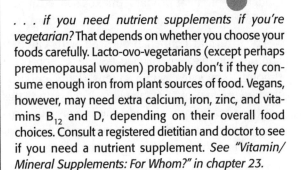

Have You Ever Wondered

. . . if you need nutrient supplements if you're vegetarian? That depends on whether you choose your foods carefully. Lacto-ovo-vegetarians (except perhaps premenopausal women) probably don't if they consume enough iron from plant sources of food. Vegans, however, may need extra calcium, iron, zinc, and vitamins B_{12} and D, depending on their overall food choices. Consult a registered dietitian and doctor to see if you need a nutrient supplement. See *"Vitamin/ Mineral Supplements: For Whom?" in chapter 23.*

Daily Values (DVs) per day. Larger doses can be dangerous and should be avoided.

For more about vitamin D, see chapter 4. For more about vitamin D and older adults, see "Vitamin D: The Sunshine Vitamin" in chapter 18.

Calcium: Getting Enough

Calcium—you know it best as a bone builder. Calcium also helps muscles contract; transfers nerve impulses; helps your blood clot; helps your heart beat; and for kids, builds healthy teeth, among its many tasks. If you're a vegetarian, how can you consume enough?

Vegetarians who consume dairy products have excellent calcium sources in their daily eating plan: milk, cheese, and yogurt. The equivalent of 3 cups of milk daily contributes much of the calcium advised by the Dietary Reference Intakes—for many people.

Vegans can get enough calcium from plant foods and calcium-fortified foods. But it may take more planning. Vegans may not need quite as much calcium, as some studies suggest. The typically high-protein diet of nonvegetarians actually may increase calcium's excretion through urine; in contrast, soy protein may decrease calcium excretion, perhaps due to its lower sulfur amino acid content.

If you're a vegan, what's the calcium advice? Currently, consume the level established in the DRI for your age group—for example, 1,000 milligrams of calcium per day is an Adequate Intake if you're age nineteen to fifty (more if you're a teenager or over age fifty). You'll need enough vitamin D to help your body absorb and use the calcium you consume effectively. If you can't consume enough calcium from food, a supplement probably makes sense for you.

Which foods of plant origin supply calcium?

● Try tofu and tempeh processed with calcium, calcium-fortified soy or rice beverages, broccoli, almonds, soybeans, some greens (kale, collards, mustard greens), okra, rutabaga, bok choy, dried figs, tortillas (made from slaked lime-processed corn), and calcium-fortified juice, bread, cereal bars, and cereal. These grain products may not be vegan.

● Beet greens, rhubarb, spinach, Swiss chard, and a grain called amaranth supply calcium, but your body cannot use it. These foods contain oxalates that bind calcium, blocking its absorption. Some grain products also contain small amounts of calcium, but they may contain phytates that block calcium absorption.

See "Calcium: A Closer Look" in chapter 4. For food "prep," see "Calcium Boosters" in chapter 13.

Iron—Make the Most of It!

Because it often comes up short, iron needs special attention, especially by growing children and women of childbearing age. That's true whether you're a vegetarian or not. Among other reasons, your body needs iron as part of the complex process of energy production. It carries oxygen in the blood to cells. Not consuming enough may result in fatigue and perhaps iron-deficiency anemia.

What are the iron-related issues for vegetarians? Foods of plant origin contain iron, called nonheme iron, which isn't absorbed as well as heme iron in meat and other foods of animal origin. The challenge for vegetarians is this: Improve the absorption of nonheme iron from food—easy, if you know how.

● Start by consuming plant sources of food that contain nonheme iron: legumes; iron-fortified cereals and breads, especially whole-wheat breads; whole-grain products; tofu; some dark-green leafy vegetables (such as spinach or beet greens); seeds; tempeh; prune juice; some dried fruits (dried apricots, prunes, raisins); and blackstrap molasses. For lacto-ovo-vegetarians, eggs also supply nonheme iron.

● Include a vitamin C-rich food at every meal. Vitamin C-rich foods (citrus fruits or juices, broccoli,

tomatoes, and bell peppers) help your body absorb iron from plant sources of food and from eggs. *For vitamin C-rich fruits and vegetables see chapter 4.*

● If you're a semivegetarian, eating a little meat, poultry, and fish helps your body absorb nonheme iron from plant sources of food, and perhaps from eggs.

● If you cook foods in iron pots or skillets, some iron from the pots or skillets may pass into food—a good thing! That's especially true when ingredients being cooked are high in acid, such as tomatoes, and when you simmer foods (such as soups and stews) for a while.

See "Iron: A Closer Look" in chapter 4.

Zinc: Not to Overlook

Zinc, a mineral, is essential for growth, repairing body cells, and energy production. And it's associated with more than two hundred enzymes that control your body processes and that help the immune system function normally. Without meat, poultry, and seafood, zinc may come up short in a vegetarian diet.

For lacto-ovo-vegetarians, milk, cheese, yogurt, and eggs all supply zinc. In addition, many foods of plant origin contain zinc—but its bioavailability (availability to your body) is less than from animal foods. Most vegetarian diets supply enough zinc to keep blood levels within a normal range.

Science hasn't yet clarified the effect of marginal zinc status. Yet even mild deficiencies may impair mental performance; that's an issue not only for adults but for children and teens as well.

To make sure you consume enough zinc:

● Eat a variety of foods with zinc: whole-wheat bread; whole grains, especially the germ and bran; many legumes (white beans, kidney beans, chickpeas); tofu; seeds; and nuts in amounts recommended for health. Be aware that grains lose zinc when they're processed to make refined flour. And substances in plant sources such as fiber and phytates can inhibit zinc absorption. Phytates, however, are broken down during the process of yeast fermentation called leavening in baking yeast breads.

● Be cautious of zinc supplements, which can have harmful side effects in high dosages. If your doctor or registered dietitian recommends a supplement, stick with a vitamin-mineral combination with 100 percent or less of the Daily Value (DV) for zinc.

For more about zinc, see chapter 4.

Throughout the Life Cycle

People at any age can eat vegetarian style—and get the nourishment they need. Nutrition issues differ somewhat, depending on their stage in life.

If you or someone in your family becomes a vegetarian, consult a registered dietitian for help in planning a nutritious vegetarian eating plan. Some dietitians specialize in vegetarian nutrition. Getting sound nutrition advice is especially important during pregnancy, breast-feeding, recovery from illness, and for times of growth (infancy, childhood, and adolescence). *See "How to Find Nutrition Help . . ." in chapter 24.*

The Vegetarian Mom

For pregnancy and breast-feeding: either a lacto-ovo-vegetarian eating plan or a vegan eating plan can supply the nutrients and the food energy needed to support the increased needs of both mother and baby.

If you've already mastered the skills of vegetarian eating, adjusting your food choices for pregnancy and breast-feeding won't require much extra effort. However, if vegetarian eating is new to you, seek nutrition advice from a registered dietitian to make sure your diet is healthful for you and your baby.

You know that good nutrition during pregnancy and breast-feeding is important for both mother and baby. When a mom puts herself at nutritional risk, her baby's development may be affected, too.

If you're pregnant or nursing, follow these tips if you choose a vegetarian approach to eating:

● Keep tabs on your weight gain during pregnancy. For vegetarian and nonvegetarian women, pregnancy requires about 340 to 450 extra calories a day in the second and third trimesters; breast-feeding, about 330 to 400 calories more than needed before pregnancy. Healthy weight gain for a full-term pregnancy is 25 to 35 pounds for most women. *See " 'Weighting' for Your New Arrival" in chapter 17.*

Research shows that babies born to vegetarian moms are similar in birthweight to babies born to nonvegetarian women—as long as the mother is well nourished during pregnancy. That's good news. **Caution:** If you don't consume enough food energy (calories) during pregnancy, your weight gain may be too low to sustain the normal development of the fetus. As a result, your baby may be born with a low birthweight. And if your calorie intake is less than needed while nursing, your body may not produce enough breast milk.

● For enough calcium during pregnancy and breast-feeding, you need 1,000 milligrams daily if you're age 19 or over, and 1,300 milligrams daily for teens. If you consume dairy products, getting enough calcium for pregnancy and breast-feeding is easy. Just follow the guidelines from MyPyramid. *If you're a vegan, see "Calcium: Getting Enough" earlier in this chapter for more about plant sources of calcium.* A calcium supplement may be advised for you, too; check with your healthcare provider.

Babies need calcium for developing bones and teeth. If you don't consume enough calcium during pregnancy and breast-feeding, your body will give up some calcium stores in your bones. That may put you at greater risk for bone disease as you get older.

● During pregnancy and breast-feeding, your need for vitamin D is the same as before—but you still need enough to help absorb calcium. If you're lacto-vegetarian, drink milk fortified with vitamin D. If you're a vegan, you may need a vitamin D supplement, especially if your exposure to sunlight is limited.

● Most pregnant women—vegetarians and nonvegetarians—are advised to take an iron supplement. Consult your doctor or a registered dietitian. If you take one, follow the recommended dosage. Too much iron can interfere with zinc absorption, putting your newborn at risk for a zinc deficiency.

● For vegetarians, vegans especially, getting enough vitamin B_{12} during pregnancy and lactation is of special concern. For vegans, consume a reliable source of vitamin B_{12}—perhaps fortified breakfast cereals or a vitamin B_{12} supplement. During pregnancy, you need more for the developing fetus and your own increased blood supply. Without enough vitamin B_{12} during pregnancy and nursing, your baby may be at risk for anemia and nerve damage.

● With a vegetarian diet you probably consume enough folate. Still, as a precaution, get enough folate prior to and during pregnancy to avoid neural tube (spinal cord) defects in the fetus. Many plant-based foods are good sources: leafy vegetables, legumes, some fruits, wheat germ, and grains products fortified with folic acid. Be aware that whole-grain foods may not be folic-acid fortified. A folate (folic acid) supplement still may be advised. Consult your doctor or a registered dietitian.

● During pregnancy and breast-feeding, consuming enough essential fatty acids is essential for the infant's brain and neurological development. If you're a vegan, make sure you consume sources of linolenic acid (ground flaxseed and flaxseed, canola, or soy oil) to help increase the linolenic acid in breast milk. Or perhaps get more from a supplement. Limit corn, safflower, and sunflower oils, as well as *trans* fats to increase the essential fats in breast milk.

● The need for zinc increases by 50 percent during pregnancy. Vegetarian women may need a zinc supplement if they don't consume enough from food.

For more about nutrition during pregnancy and breast-feeding, see chapter 17.

Feeding Vegetarian Kids

Are your kids vegetarians? That's okay—as long as their overall food choices are healthful. Chosen carefully, either a lacto-ovo-vegetarian or a vegan eating style can provide for the nutrient and energy needs of growing kids. They also need skills for making smart choices from the array of foods that fit in their vegetarian diets.

For vegetarian children on very restricted eating plans, not getting enough calories may result in poor growth. Vegetarian meals can be low in fat and high in fiber ("bulky"), so they fill kids up without supplying enough calories.

To meet the nutrient and calorie demands of growth, offer frequent meals and snacks. Provide some foods with more unsaturated fats such as nuts, seeds, and nut butters. Foods with some added sugars, such as oatmeal cookies and ice cream, may provide food energy, but go easy. These nutrient-rich

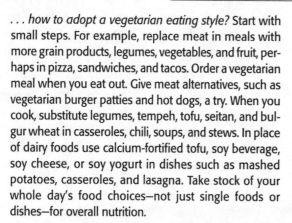

Have You Ever Wondered

. . . how to adopt a vegetarian eating style? Start with small steps. For example, replace meat in meals with more grain products, legumes, vegetables, and fruit, perhaps in pizza, sandwiches, and tacos. Order a vegetarian meal when you eat out. Give meat alternatives, such as vegetarian burger patties and hot dogs, a try. When you cook, substitute legumes, tempeh, tofu, seitan, and bulgur wheat in casseroles, chili, soups, and stews. In place of dairy foods use calcium-fortified tofu, soy beverage, soy cheese, or soy yogurt in dishes such as mashed potatoes, casseroles, and lasagna. Take stock of your whole day's food choices—not just single foods or dishes—for overall nutrition.

. . . if soy beverage is a good substitute for cow milk for children and adults? Check the Nutrition Facts. The calcium content of soy beverages varies. Some are fortified with calcium and vitamin D, but not all. If the cost of fluid soy beverage is an issue, look for powdered soy beverage. Cow milk also supplies other nutrients, including vitamin A, riboflavin (vitamin B$_2$), vitamin B$_{12}$, and

phosphorus—nutrients needed by adults and growing children alike. Fortified soy beverage commonly has many of these nutrients, too; check the label. Make sure other food choices supply enough of these nutrients.

As an aside, fortified rice beverage is another option, but it doesn't provide as much protein as soy beverage does. It doesn't offer all the nutrients that cow milk does.

. . . if it's okay for your teenager to control weight with a vegetarian diet? Yes, if your teen's food choices are varied and balanced—and if your teen keeps a healthy weight. Vegetarian eating doesn't lead to eating disorders, but may be used to camouflage one. However, if a vegetarian teen loses too much weight or shows other signs of disordered eating, it's time to be concerned. Eating disorders can be harmful, even life-threatening. If that happens, seek professional help. And help your teen understand that vegetarian eating isn't always low-calorie; energy, or calorie, content depends on your teen's overall food choices. *See "Eating Disorders: Problems, Signs, and Help" in chapter 2.*

snacks provide food energy too: a peanut butter sandwich and milk, raw vegetables with hummus or tofu dip, ready-to-eat breakfast cereal, fruit, or finger-food veggies. *See "Not Just for Vegetarians . . . Quick and Healthful Snacks" earlier in this chapter.*

Lacto-ovo-vegetarian kids generally can get enough nutrients from well-chosen foods alone. In fact, vegetarian eating may encourage more fiber, folate, vitamins A and C, fruits and vegetables, and perhaps fewer sweets, fast foods, and salty snacks, than nonvegetarian eating. For vegan infants, children, and teens, some nutrients may need special attention: calcium, iron, zinc, vitamin B_{12}, and vitamin D. If your child is a vegan, offer a variety of foods with adequate amounts of these nutrients. Poor choices can put vegetarian kids at greater risk for nutrient inadequacies and their health consequences.

Especially for Babies

Breast milk is the best "first food" for babies. When breast-feeding isn't chosen, commercial infant formulas, including soy formulas, are a healthful option. **Caution:** Cow or goat milk, regular soy beverage or rice beverage, or homemade formula are not suitable substitutes for commercial infant formula!

Infants exclusively breast-fed for longer than six months are at risk for iron and vitamin D deficiencies. That's true whether the mom is a vegetarian or not. As a guideline for all infants at this time: Healthcare providers may advise an iron-fortified cereal or an iron supplement, and perhaps a vitamin D supplement if the baby's exposure to sunlight is limited. Vegetarian or not, the American Academy of Pediatrics advises a vitamin D supplement for breast-fed babies starting at two months of age; infant formula contains vitamin D. For breast-fed vegan infants a vitamin B_{12} supplement may be recommended, too, if the mother doesn't consume vitamin B_{12}-fortified foods.

Time to introduce protein-rich solid foods? Offer pureed tofu, cottage cheese, cooked egg yolk, soy or dairy yogurt, and pureed or strained legumes to vegetarian babies. Later start tofu cubes, cheese or soy cheese, and soyburger pieces. At age one year or older, it's okay to start full-fat commercial, fortified soy beverage or cow milk. When infants are weaned, provide energy-rich, nutrient-rich foods, such as mashed avocado, bean spreads, and tofu. Before age two, babies

need enough fat to develop a healthy nervous system; this isn't the time to restrict fat in food! If your family has a food-allergy history, you may be advised to be especially cautious of some foods; *see page 390.*

Health advice. If your infant, child, or teen follows a vegetarian eating style, consult a registered dietitian, your doctor, or a pediatric nurse for support and nutrition counseling. For vegans, ask about nutrient supplements. *For more about feeding infants, children, and teens, see chapters 15 and 16.*

Vegetarian Fare for Older Adults

Are you an older vegetarian? If so, your overall nutrition needs and concerns are similar to those of other older adults and other vegetarians. With age, your energy need is likely less, but your calcium, vitamin D, vitamin B_6 and perhaps protein needs are higher.

If Your Teen Decides to Become a Vegetarian

Many teens today equate being vegetarian with being "cool." Support a smart approach:

- Make a shopping list together of food group foods that fit your teen's vegetarian "style"—and keep those foods on hand: perhaps hummus, cheese, and crackers; cow milk; calcium-fortified soy beverage; trail mix with nuts; fruit; raw veggies; yogurt; and other quick, portable vegetarian snacks.

- Plan vegetarian dishes that your whole family can enjoy, such as chili with beans, vegetarian pizza, or bean tacos, so you aren't a short-order cook.

- For some dishes, prepare them two ways with just a simple substitution: a veggieburger for your teen and beefburgers for the rest of the family.

- Prepare vegetarian foods that can be the main dish for your teen and a side dish for others—for example, rice and beans, or pasta primavera. Offer milk.

- Encourage your teen to help prepare food to practice the basics of healthful vegetarian eating.

- Talk about eating-out options so your teen is prepared to make wise choices with peers.

- Whether you're a vegetarian or not, be a role model for healthful eating and healthful living.

- Most of all, be supportive and learn about smart vegetarian eating together.

For older vegetarians, vitamin D and vitamin B_{12} need special attention. Those confined to the house without exposure to sunlight may be deficient in vitamin D unless they drink milk. With age, the body may not absorb vitamin B_{12} efficiently, either. Eating foods fortified with vitamin B_{12} or taking a supplement can prevent a deficiency.

Good news: Fiber in a vegetarian eating plan may help older adults with constipation.

In later years, people are at greater risk for some health problems if they don't get the variety of nutrients they need, especially those recovering from illness. *Use the "MyPyramid for Vegetarians" in this chapter as a healthful eating guide. See chapter 18, "For Mature Adults: Healthful Eating!"*

"Vegging Out" the Healthful Way!

Planned carefully, a vegetarian eating style can provide what is needed for growth and for good health. That takes commitment. But once you understand it, being a smart vegetarian takes no more effort than any other approach to smart eating. Start here:

● For food variety and the right amounts, follow MyPyramid advice (*see page 519*) for your age, gender, and activity level. Consume enough protein, calcium, iron, zinc, vitamins B_{12} and D, and essential fatty acids.

● Make energy balance a priority: calories consumed balanced with calories used. Vegetarian eating isn't necessarily lower in calories. *Refer to chapter 2 on energy balance.*

● Build meals around protein sources that are naturally nutrient-rich, such as beans and lentils. Avoid overloading on high-fat cheeses to replace meat. Make meat or poultry dishes vegetarian: pasta primavera, veggie pizza, vegetable lasagna, tofu-vegetable stir-fry, vegetable lo mein, vegetable kabobs, and bean burritos or tacos.

What's on the Menu?

To make food preparation fast and easy, choose dishes that everyone—vegetarians and non-vegetarians—around your table will enjoy! This vegetarian menu was planned for a 2,000-calorie-a-day eating plan, using the Food Tracker from www.MyPyramid.gov.

Breakfast

1 cup oatmeal* (made with milk or calcium- and vitamin D-fortified soy beverage) with 2 tablespoons sliced almonds and 2 tablespoons raisins

1 slice whole-wheat toast with 1 tablespoon jelly

½ cup orange juice

Coffee or tea

*or ready-to-eat breakfast cereal fortified with vitamins B_{12} and D

Lunch

1½ cups hearty lentil soup

¼ cup carrot and ¼ cup green pepper sticks with ¼ cup salsa

1 small whole-grain muffin

1 cup fat-free milk or calcium- and vitamin D-fortified soy beverage

Snack

½ small bagel with 1 tablespoon peanut butter

Iced tea with fresh lemon

Dinner

Rice and beans made with ¾ cup kidney beans, ½ cup herb-seasoned rice, and ¼ cup tomatoes

¾ cup steamed broccoli with lemon juice and 1 tablespoon sesame seeds

½ cup fresh fruit salad

1 small slice Italian herb bread

1 cup fat-free milk or calcium- and vitamin D-fortified soy beverage

½ cup fruit sorbet beverage

Snack

Fruit smoothie made with ½ cup plain, fat-free yogurt or soy yogurt, and ½ cup sliced strawberries

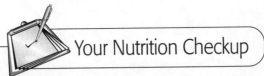

Your Nutrition Checkup

Your Nutrition Checkup: For Vegetarians

You've chosen to follow a vegetarian diet—perhaps with health in mind. But are you making smart choices? Take this survey as a quick check. This is based on a 2,000-calorie-a-day eating plan. *To see how many calories you need, check "MyPyramid Food Intake Pattern Calorie Level," in the Appendices.*

Do you eat:

Yes   **No**

1. A wide variety of grain products (including whole grains), legumes, nuts, vegetables, and fruits?

2. About six ounces of bread, rice, pasta, and other grain products daily, of which at least three are whole grain?

3. About 2½ cups of vegetables daily?

4. About 2 cups of fruit daily?

5. A vitamin C-rich food with meals whenever you can?

6. A day's meals and snacks that balance the calories you consume with those you use—in a lifestyle that's physically active?

7. Mostly nutrient-rich foods, go easy on solid fats and added sugars, and eat just moderate amounts of total fat?

8. About 6 ounces or an equivalent of legumes and other meat alternates each day?

Just for lacto- and lacto-ovo-vegetarians (if you're a vegan, skip ahead):

9. The equivalent of three cups of milk, yogurt, or cheese daily?

10. Eggs occasionally (so you stay under 300 milligrams of cholesterol a day)? *(Skip this question if you're a lacto-vegetarian.)*

Just for vegans (if you're a lacto- or lacto-ovo-vegetarian, skip these two questions):

9. Plant-based foods that are high in calcium such as calcium-fortified juice or soy beverage?

10. Foods that are fortified with vitamins B_{12} and D (or take a supplement that provides no more than 100 percent of the Daily Value)?

Now score yourself. Give yourself a point for every "yes."

If you scored a perfect "10," your food choices do promote your good health. If you scored "9" and only answered nine questions, the same applies—your food choices probably supply enough nutrients and perhaps offer other health benefits.

If you said "no" to any item, read on, then make changes to eat healthier—the vegetarian way!

● For vegans, consume reliable sources of vitamin B_{12} such as fortified breakfast cereal or soy beverage and vitamin D, especially if your exposure to sunlight is limited.

● Enjoy variety: plenty of vegetables (as well as beans), fruits, grain foods (especially whole grains), nuts, and seeds for their nutrient, fiber, and other phytonutrient benefits. You may choose to eat eggs and dairy foods, too.

● Choose mostly nutrient-rich foods. Go easy on foods and drinks high in fat, especially saturated fat and *trans* fat, and/or added sugars. Stick within your budget for discretionary calories; *see chapter 10.* Being plant-based doesn't mean low in fat, added sugars, or calories!

Follow the Food Guide

For good health, follow the advice of the Dietary Guidelines for Americans and MyPyramid, meant for vegetarians and nonvegetarians alike. *Refer to page 519 for recommended food group amounts.*

Vegetarian Way: Grains

Make at least half your grains whole—equal to at least 3 ounces of whole-grain foods a day: whole-wheat bread, breakfast cereal, and pasta; brown rice; and other whole grains. *See "What Is a Whole Grain?" in chapter 6.* Besides the starches (complex carbohydrates), iron, fiber, and phytonutrients they provide, whole grains supply zinc, which may come up short for vegetarians.

● Make grain dishes the centerpiece of your menu—perhaps tabouli, barley, rice pilaf, risotto, rice or noodle dishes, gnocchi, or polenta. Add interest to vegetarian meals with a greater variety of breads, including focaccia, bagels, tortillas, pita, chapatis, and naan. (Pay attention to portion size.) Try breads with a variety of grains: oats, rye, and cornmeal, to name a few. *Tip:* Because of their processing method, some corn tortillas supply calcium. Check the label.

● Add cooked grains to many foods. Stuff vegetables (eggplant, bell peppers, cabbage, zucchini) with cooked grain mixtures: rice, oats, and barley, among others. Blend cooked grains with shredded vegetables and perhaps tofu for vegetable patties or croquettes.

Toss cooked grains (not just rice or noodles) with stir-fried vegetables. And add bulgur, barley, and other cooked grains to soups, stews, and chili.

● Choose fortified breakfast cereals. Read the Nutrition Facts panel on food labels for added nutrients, including iron, vitamin B_{12}, and zinc.

Vegetarian Way: Vegetables

Vary your veggies! For everyone—especially vegans—choose vegetables that are good sources of calcium: dark-green leafy vegetables (such as kale, mustard, collard, or turnip greens), bok choy, and broccoli. Dark-green leafy vegetables also supply iron.

● Choose vegetables that are high in vitamin C—for example, broccoli, tomatoes, and green and red peppers. Vitamin C helps your body absorb iron in eggs and in plant sources of food. *See "Vitamin C: More than Citrus" in chapter 4.*

● Plan meals with different vegetables, not just garden salads, baked potatoes, and fries. That way you get the nutrient and phytonutrient benefits of variety.

Vegetarian Way: Fruits

Focus on fruit!

● Enjoy a variety of fruits, including a good food source of vitamin C, such as citrus fruits, melons, and berries. Among the other benefits, vitamin C-rich fruit is an important partner for iron from eggs and plant-based foods. *For vitamin C in various fruits, see "Vitamin C: More than Citrus" in chapter 4.*

● To get enough fruit, enjoy it for dessert and snacks—whole or sliced; prepared in cobblers; ice cream toppers; or in thick, fruity smoothies.

● Look for calcium-fortified juice as an added source of calcium, especially if you're a vegan.

Vegetarian Way: Legumes and Other Meat Alternates

Build your meals around legumes, lentils, and other meat alternates every day. These foods supply protein and iron, as meat, poultry, and fish do for nonvegetarians. Except for eggs, most meat alternates are low in total fat and saturated fat, and they have no cholesterol.

Stocking the Vegetarian Kitchen

Today's supermarkets sell all the foods you need for a healthful, vegetarian diet—even vegetarian convenience foods. You don't need to shop elsewhere, but specialty stores may carry less common items (such as textured soy protein, quinoa, kosher gelatin, and wheat gluten).

No matter where you shop, plan ahead. Shop with a list. Read food labels to find foods with ingredients that match your needs. The ingredient list helps identify animal-derived ingredients. Check the grocery aisle for shelf-stable foods such as boxed soy beverage. For your vegetarian kitchen, stock up on foods such as these:

Grain Products

- Ready-to-eat, fortified, and whole-grain breakfast cereals
- Quick-cooking whole-grain and enriched cereals such as oatmeal and muesli
- Whole-grain and enriched breads,* bagels,* rolls,* and crackers such as rye and whole wheat, and mixed grain rice such as brown, wild, basmati, and white.
- Pastas such as macaroni, spaghetti, fettuccini, couscous (perhaps made without eggs), and whole-grain pasta
- Corn or flour tortillas
- Popcorn
- Wheat germ, bran, and wheat gluten (seitan)
- Other grains such as barley, bulgur, millet, and quinoa
- Flour—whole wheat, rye, cornmeal

*Read labels if you're vegan; some breads have ingredients derived from eggs, or they're brushed with eggs to make them shine.

Legumes and Meat Alternates

- Canned, frozen, and fresh legumes such as pintos, black beans, split peas, soybeans, and garbanzos
- Dried legumes (beans) and lentils
- Vegetarian refried beans
- Dried legume mixes such as refried beans, falafel, and hummus (mashed chickpeas)
- Tofu and tempeh
- Miso
- Soy-protein patties, soy bacon, soy sausages
- Lentil or "veggie" burgers
- Falafel mix (for chickpea patties)

- Soy beverage, soy cheese, soy yogurt
- Soy nuts
- Soy flour, soy grits
- Textured soy protein
- Myco-protein (Quorn) meat alternatives sold as patties, sausages, and cold cuts
- Peanut butter
- Nut and seed spreads such as almond butter and tahini (sesame seed spread)
- Nuts such as pecans, almonds, walnuts, hazelnuts, and cashews
- Seeds such as sesame, pumpkin, and sunflower
- Eggs or egg substitute*

*For vegans, egg replacer powder, made from tapioca starch and leavenings (not a meat alternative)

Fruits and Vegetables

- Frozen and canned fruit, vegetables, and juice
- Fresh fruits and vegetables
- Tomato sauce
- Frozen and boxed (shelf-stable) fruit juice concentrate
- Dried fruits such as raisins, dried plums (prunes), dried cranberries, dates, and dried apricots

Dairy and Dairy Alternatives

- Vitamin D-fortified milk, reduced-fat or fat-free
- Calcium-fortified soy beverage
- Cheese (dairy or soy-based)
- Yogurt (dairy or soy-based)
- Dry milk powder
- Ice cream, frozen yogurt, or nondairy ice cream

Combination Foods

- Canned and frozen vegetarian soups
- Frozen vegetarian entrées such as bean burritos or vegetable potstickers
- Canned vegetarian dishes such as meatless chili
- Vegetable pizza

Fats and Sugars

- Vegetable oil, plain and flavor-infused
- Margarine (perhaps soy margarine or soft, tub, or liquid margarine for less *trans* fat) and butter

Stocking the Vegetarian Kitchen *(continued)*

- Salad dressing (perhaps made without eggs), tofu-based mayonnaise
- Vegetarian gravy and sauce mixes
- Syrup, jam, jelly, and molasses
- Refined sugar, brown sugar, honey, and other sweeteners

Condiments, Seasonings, and Other Flavorings
- Herbs and spices
- Vinegar, plain and flavored
- Sauces such as chutney, salsa, soy sauce, teriyaki sauce
- Canned vegetable broth and broth mix, bouillon

● Make legumes a mealtime regular—eat them most days of the week. They contribute proteins and are good sources of starches (complex carbohydrates), fiber, and phytonutrients. *For a description of the variety of legumes and tips for cooking them, see chapter 6.*

● Use soybean products—tofu, tempeh, textured soy protein, and soy beverage. Try them in stir-fry dishes, casseroles, lasagna, soups, and burger patties. *See "What's 'Soy' Good?" in chapter 11.*

● If you eat eggs, watch how much. For cardiovascular health, try to limit your cholesterol intake to less than 300 milligrams a day; one large egg yolk has about 215 milligrams of cholesterol. Make egg-based dishes lower in cholesterol by substituting egg whites for some whole eggs. Examples of egg-based dishes include quiche, omelettes, frittata, scrambled eggs, French toast, egg salad, and egg foo yung.

● Include nuts, nut butters (almond butter, cashew butter, peanut butter), seeds, and seed spread (tahini, or sesame seed spread). They, too, supply protein and an array of phytonutrients. Since they're fairly high in fat, go easy; most fat from nuts is unsaturated.

Vegetarian Way: Milk, Yogurt, and Cheese

Lacto-vegetarians can enjoy milk, yogurt, and cheese—choose mostly lower-fat and fat-free dairy products for less fat.

For vegans—in fact, all vegetarians—calcium-fortified soy beverage offers an alternative; look for soy beverage that's also fortified with vitamin D. Read the Nutrition Facts on food labels to compare soy beverages. Milk supplies about 300 milligrams of calcium per serving; choose soy beverage with at least this much. If soy-based products aren't calcium fortified,

they can't count as an alternative to milk. Especially if you're vegan, look for other calcium-rich foods in other food groups, too. Find adequate sources of cow milk's other nutrients.

Vegetarian Way: Healthy Oils

As with any approach to eating, choose healthy oils since their fats are less saturated. For vegetarians, oils from nuts, seeds, avocadoes, and olives are among the sources, along with vegetable oils. Sources of omega-3s include flaxseed, soybean, and canola oils, as well as walnuts and ground flaxseed. *Another tip:* Choose vegetable oil and tub margarine more often than stick margarine, which is higher in *trans* fats.

Adapting Your Recipes

Looking for vegetarian recipes? Check the bookstore and magazine racks for many flavor-filled dishes from vegetarian cookbooks and publications. Go online! Or with just a few changes, adapt recipes from almost any cookbook or magazine for vegetarian-style eating—even if you choose to avoid eggs and dairy products. Try these recipe hints for adjusting recipes.

Instead of meat, poultry, or fish . . .

● *In casseroles, stews, soups, lasagna, and chili,* substitute cooked or canned legumes for meat: perhaps kidney beans in chili or stew, or red lentils in spaghetti sauce or stuffed cabbage rolls, or refried beans in burritos, tacos, and enchiladas. Or add textured soy protein, often sold in granular form.

● *In stir-fry dishes,* use firm tofu, tempeh, soyburgers, or sausage, cooked beans, nuts, or sesame seeds in place of meat, poultry, or seafood. *Hint:* For more flavor, marinate tofu before adding it to dishes.

MyPyramid for Vegetarians

Here's the daily advice for a 2,000-calorie-a-day eating plan. If you need more or less calories, adjust the amount from each food group. *Refer to "MyPyramid Food Intake Patterns" in the Appendices for how much from each food group.*

GRAINS GROUP
6 ounces or the equivalent (Make at least half whole grains.) One ounce is: *

1 slice bread

1 cup ready-to-eat cereal

½ cup cooked rice or pasta

½ cup cooked cereal

FRUIT GROUP
2 cups or the equivalent
One cup is:*

1 cup cut-up or canned fruit

1 cup fruit juice

MILK GROUP
3 cups or the equivalent
One cup is:*

1 cup milk

1 cup yogurt

1½ ounces natural cheese

2 ounces processed cheese

ESPECIALLY FOR VEGANS:

● Calcium-fortified juices, cereals, breads, soy beverages, rice beverages

● Soybeans and other soy products (soy-based beverages, soy yogurt, tempeh), some other dried beans, and some leafy greens (collard and turnip greens, kale, bok choy). The amount of calcium that can be absorbed from these foods varies. Check www.MyPyramid.gov for specifics on nondairy sources of calcium.

VEGETABLE GROUP
2½ cups or the equivalent
One cup is:*

1 cup raw or cooked vegetables

2 cups raw leafy greens

1 cup vegetable juice

1 cup cooked beans (legumes)

1 cup (8 ounces) tofu

MEAT AND BEANS GROUP
6 ounces or the equivalent
One ounce is:*

1 egg

½ ounce nuts (12 almonds, 24 pistachios, 7 walnut halves)

½ ounce seeds (pumpkin, sunflower, squash seeds), hulled

1 tablespoon peanut butter or almond butter

¼ cup cooked dry beans

¼ cup cooked dry peas (chickpeas, lentils, split peas)

¼ cup baked beans or refried beans

¼ cup (about 2 ounces) tofu

1 ounce tempeh, cooked

¼ cup roasted soybeans

1 4-ounce falafel patty

2 tablespoons hummus

Note: ½ cup split pea, lentil, or bean soup counts as about 1 ounce.

Refer to chapter 10 for more foods (and amounts) for this food group.

Some foods can count in more than one food group, for example legumes (beans) in the Vegetable Group and the Meat and Beans Group. Choose one.

Other essentials for those who consume little or no animal-based foods:

Vitamin B$_{12}$—fortified foods or a supplement

Vitamin D—fortified foods or a supplement

Omega-3 fats—ground flaxseed; canola, flaxseed, and soybean oils

● *For grilling,* cube and skewer firm tofu and tempeh with vegetables.

● On pizza, hot sandwiches, sloppy joes, and other dishes that typically call for meat, use soy-protein patties, bacon, or sausages.

● Prepare pasta sauces, pizza, soups, stews, and other mixed dishes as always—but skip meat. Add more chopped vegetables and beans. If you eat dairy products, top with cheese for more protein and calcium.

Instead of eggs . . .

Eggs offer functional qualities to recipes—for example, thickening, binding ingredients together, clarifying stock, coating breaded foods, and leavening. A leavener lightens the texture and increases the volume of baked goods. Without eggs, the qualities of food often change. So experiment!

● Try these ingredients in place of eggs—but know that the results may differ from the original recipe. In place of one egg:
  ● ½ mashed banana (in breads, muffins, or pancakes)
  ● 2 tablespoons of cornstarch or arrowroot
  ● ¼ cup of tofu (Blend it with liquid ingredients until smooth; then add it to dry ingredients.)
  ● ¼ cup of pureed fruit, applesauce, or canned pumpkin
  ● Egg replacer powder, or vegetarian egg replacement (often sold in specialty stores)
  ● ¼ cup of cooked oatmeal, mashed potatoes, mashed beans, or tofu (in vegetarian burgers or loaves)
● Try scrambled tofu with herbs for breakfast!

Instead of dairy foods . . .

● For vegans, use soy margarine in place of butter or other margarines. Most margarine contains some ingredients derived from milk, such as whey or casein. Cookies, pastries, and other baked goods made with margarine may have a different texture than those made with butter. Remember that lard is another fat of animal origin and that stick margarine contains *trans* fatty acids; use mostly soft or liquid margarine.

● Enjoy thick, creamy fruit shakes? If you're a lacto-vegetarian, make them with milk, ice cream, or frozen yogurt. If you're a vegan, blend fruit instead with soft tofu, soy beverage, soy yogurt, or nondairy ice cream—or make all-fruit smoothies!

● Use tofu, soy beverage, soy cheese, and soy yogurt in recipes that call for dairy products. Crumbled tofu, for example, can take the place of ricotta cheese in lasagna. Soft tofu makes a great dip or sauce; blend it with other ingredients. And in baked foods, 1 cup of soy beverage plus 1 tablespoon of vinegar may take the place of 1 cup of buttermilk.

● Enjoy fruit sorbet in place of sherbet and ice cream.

Instead of gelatin . . .

● Use kosher gelatin, made from a sea vegetable. Find it in a specialty food shop.

Now for Eating Out

What choices do you have when you eat out? Plenty! More and more traditional restaurants and cafeterias cater to "all the time" or "sometime" vegetarians. Fast-food restaurants offer meatless salads that are big enough to enjoy as an entrée—as well as vegetarian deli sandwiches, pita pockets, pizzas, and tacos. In many ethnic restaurants—for example, Indo-

---

Need more strategies for healthful vegetarian eating? Check here for "how-tos":

● Get a great list of interesting fruits, vegetables, and grains—see chapter 9.

● Check vegetarian options from MyPyramid—see chapter 10.

● Scout for soy and other plant-based foods when you shop—see chapter 11.

● Lock vitamins in and boost calcium when you prepare food—see chapter 13.

● Ask questions about vegetarian options when you eat out—see chapter 14.

● Follow a vegetarian eating plan as an athlete—see chapter 19.

● Use dietary supplements appropriately to fill in any nutrient gaps—see chapter 23.

Pakistani, other Asian, and Middle Eastern—vegetarian dishes are among their specialties.

Whether you're a vegetarian or simply enjoy an occasional vegetarian meal, be savvy.

● Before you order, talk to your server about the dish. Even ask about ingredients in vegetarian dishes prepared without eggs and dairy products if you're vegan. For chain restaurants, contact the company to ask about ingredients if you frequently dine there.

● If the menu doesn't offer a vegetarian entrée, order a salad with vegetable soup and perhaps bread, or several vegetable appetizers. A fruit plate—with or without cheese or yogurt—can make a great entrée. Ask for meatless sauces. Omit meat from stir-fries; add vegetables or pasta in its place. It's easier to substitute at restaurants that make food to order.

● If you choose the salad bar, "toss" your salad with kidney beans, chickpeas, and a few sunflower seeds . . . as well as vegetables that have more vitamin C. (Remember that vitamin C helps your body absorb iron from plant sources of food.) If you're a lacto-ovo-vegetarian, spoon on cottage cheese, shredded cheese, and chopped or sliced hard-cooked eggs. (*Hint:* If you're vegan, find out if the dressing has ingredients derived from egg; if so, vinegar and oil is great!)

● Choose an ethnic restaurant that's likely to have vegetarian options. Perhaps try cuisines of the Middle East, Greece, India, China, Mexico, or parts of Africa. (*Tip for vegans:* Ghee, used in many dishes from India, is melted, clarified butter.) *Also see "Vegetarian Dishes in the Global Kitchen" on this page.*

● Ask for a vegetarian meal when you book long airline flights. If you need to, find out ahead if the meal is egg- and dairy-free. For airlines that don't offer vegetarian meals, request a fruit plate or pack snacks. *See "Dining at 35,000 Feet!" in chapter 14.*

● For organized meal functions, request a vegetarian meal ahead.

School Meals for Vegetarian Kids

● Review school menus with your child, and practice what he or she might order. If the school doesn't provide menus to parents, ask the school staff.

● Suggest the salad bar as a nutritious option—if it's available. A salad bar can be a good place to go for fresh vegetables and possibly for other nutrient-packed choices, including fruits, beans, sunflower seeds, cheese, or hard-cooked eggs.

● When the school menu doesn't offer an option for your child, pack a lunch. A peanut butter sandwich is always popular (if your child doesn't have a peanut allergy). For the child who doesn't want to appear different, it's the food that almost all kids eat—vegetarian or not!

Vegetarian Dishes in the Global Kitchen

Delicious and nutritious—vegetarian dishes are typical fare in many parts of the world. As you flip the pages of ethnic cookbooks or glance through the menu of an ethnic restaurant, try to build your meal around dishes like these. They're typically made without meat, poultry, or fish—but check to be sure. Internationally, rice and beans—a high-protein food combination—also comes to the table nearly everywhere uniquely prepared and seasoned.

Caribbean

   Callaloo: one-pot meal (stew) made with dark-green leafy vegetables, a variety of other vegetables, peppers, and seasonings

   Black-eyed pea patties: black-eyed peas mashed with eggs and seasonings, then quickly pan-fried in a small amount of oil

   Pois et ris: kidney beans and rice flavored with smoked meat and seasonings

   Gunga: pigeon peas and rice

China

   Vegetable-tofu stir-fry: variety of thinly sliced vegetables and cubed bean curd stir-fried with soy sauce and perhaps vegetable broth

   Egg foo yung: frittatalike dish made by combining slightly whipped eggs with sliced vegetables, then frying in a skillet until browned; also may be prepared with meat or poultry

   Hot and sour soup: hot soup with tofu

   Vegetable potstickers: steamed vegetable dumplings

   Soybean cakes: stir-fried tofu with steamed rice

Vegetarian Dishes in the Global Kitchen *(continued)*

East Africa

Kunde (bean and groundnut stew): stew made of black-eyed peas, peanuts (groundnuts), tomatoes, and onions; a similar stew is made in West Africa, often without peanuts

Injera and lentil stew: flat bread served with cooked lentils; this is an Ethiopian dish

France

Vegetable quiche: pie with a custard of egg and cheese mixed with chopped vegetables such as leeks, spinach, asparagus, and mushrooms

Ratatouille: soup or stew made of eggplant, tomatoes, onions, green peppers, and other vegetables; enjoy with crusty French bread

Greece

Tzatziki (cucumber-yogurt salad): plain yogurt mixed with shredded cucumber, garlic, and perhaps black olives; served with crusty bread

Vegetable-stuffed eggplant: eggplants hollowed and filled with chopped vegetables, cooked grains, and sometimes nuts

Spanakopita (spinach pie): pita made with a phyllo-dough crust and filled with a mixture of spinach, feta cheese, and eggs

India

Dohkla: steamed cakes made of rice and beans

Vegetable curry dishes: combination of chopped vegetables and lentils flavored with a curry mix and perhaps served with basmati rice

Idli or dhoka: steamed bean and rice cakes

Indonesia

Gado-gado: cooked vegetable salad with a peanut sauce; often seasoned with chiles

Italy

Pasta primavera: cooked pasta tossed with lightly cooked vegetables, with or without Parmesan cheese

Vegetable risotto: arborio rice, cooked in vegetable broth and combined with cooked vegetables and perhaps cooked beans or nuts, with or without grated cheese

Eggplant parmesan: sliced eggplant prepared by dipping it into a mixture of eggs and milk, coating it with breadcrumbs and Parmesan cheese, and sautéeing it; serve, with tomato sauce

Pasta e fagioli: pasta and white bean "stew" seasoned with herbs; usually prepared without meat

Mexico

Bean burrito: vegetarian refried beans wrapped in a soft tortilla, with or without cheese topping

Chiles relleños: poblano peppers stuffed with cheese, dipped in an egg batter, and baked or fried; if they're fried, they're high in fat

Huevos rancheros (Mexican eggs): scrambled eggs prepared with onions, and served with tomato salsa, vegetarian refried beans, and tortillas

Vegetable fajitas: stir-fried vegetables and perhaps tofu rolled in a soft tortilla; often served with guacamole

Middle East

Falafel sandwich: ground chickpea patties (fried), tucked in pita bread with lettuce shreds and chopped tomato, topped with tahini (sesame seed spread)

Tabouli: salad made with bulgur, tomatoes, parsley, mint or chives, lemon juice, and perhaps cooked white beans

Ful: brown bean casserole made with tomatoes, lemons, parsley, and eggs

Mujadarah: lentils and rice seasoned with cumin, onions, and lemon

Native American Southwest

Maricopa bean stew: stew made of corn, beans, and cholla buds

South America

Ochos rios: kidney beans and rice flavored with shredded coconut

Spain

Tortilla à la española (Spanish omelette): egg omelette, made with potatoes, onions, and other vegetables

Vegetable paella: saffron-flavored rice dish with tomatoes and other vegetables

Switzerland

Cheese fondue: cheese melted with wine and served with chunks of crusty bread

Raclette: cheese "scraped" from a melted piece of hard cheese, then spread on a boiled potato or dark bread

Sensitive about Food

Sensitive to certain foods? Maybe and maybe not. A queasy stomach, itchy skin, or diarrhea might be a reaction to something you ate. But it may or may not be what you think. So avoid the urge to give foods a bum rap without exploring the cause!

A food sensitivity, or adverse reaction to food, can't be overlooked as a health issue. It can seriously affect and disrupt the quality of life and may even be life-threatening. The causes of discomfort are more numerous, and perhaps more complex, than you may think. Among the types of food sensitivities:

● *Food intolerances.* For metabolic reasons, people with a food intolerance can't digest part of certain foods or a food component. Food intolerances have other causes as well.

● *Food allergies.* A food allergy rallies the body's disease-fighting (immune) system to action, creating unpleasant, sometimes serious, symptoms. In other words, the immune system starts to work even though the person isn't sick. That's why symptoms appear.

● *Other adverse reactions to food.* Infectious organisms such as bacteria, parasites, or viruses, which cause foodborne illness, or contaminants such as chemicals in water where seafood is harvested, can cause an adverse body reaction.

● *Psychological reasons.* Feelings of discomfort after eating can also be wrapped up with emotion. Even though there's no physical reason, just thinking about

a certain food that may be associated with an unpleasant experience can make some people feel sick!

If a certain food seems to bother you, skip the temptation to self-diagnose. Instead, check with your physician. For example, a reaction to milk could be an intolerance rather than a food allergy; let your doctor diagnose your symptoms. This chapter can help you get familiar with possible causes. Be aware that an adverse reaction may be a foodborne illness; *see chapter 12, "The Safe Kitchen," for a closer look at identifying and preventing foodborne illnesses.*

Food Intolerances and Other Adverse Food Reactions

If your body reacts to food or a food component, you may have a food intolerance, not an allergy. Unlike food allergies, food intolerances don't involve the immune system. Because they prompt many of the same symptoms (nausea, diarrhea, abdominal cramps) food intolerances are often mislabeled as "allergies."

With a food intolerance, physical reactions to a food often result from faulty metabolism. The body can't adequately digest a certain component of a particular food—perhaps because a digestive enzyme is deficient. Substances that are part of a food's natural chemistry—such as theobromine in coffee or tea, or serotonin in bananas or tomatoes—may cause reactions, too.

Depending on the type of food intolerance, most people can eat small servings of the problem food without unpleasant side effects. (People with gluten intolerance and those with sulfite sensitivity are exceptions.) In contrast, people with food allergies usually need to *eliminate* the problem food from their diet.

Lactose Intolerance: A Matter of Degree

Do you like milk but think that milk doesn't like you? Then you may be lactose-intolerant—and not allergic to milk. The good news is: A serving of milk may be "friendlier" than you think!

Lactose is a natural sugar in milk and milk products. During digestion, an intestinal enzyme called lactase breaks down lactose into smaller, more easily digested sugars. People with lactose intolerance produce too little lactase to adequately digest the amount of lactose in foods and beverages containing milk. Left undigested, lactose is fermented by "healthy" bacteria in the intestinal tract. This fermentation produces uncomfortable symptoms—for example, nausea, cramping, bloating, abdominal pain, gas, and diarrhea.

For people with lactose intolerance, symptoms may begin from fifteen minutes to several hours after consuming foods or drinks containing lactose. Their severity varies from person to person—and how much and when lactose is consumed in relation to other foods.

A milk allergy is quite different. It's an allergic reaction to the protein components, such as casein, in milk. People who have a milk allergy usually must avoid all milk products. People with lactose intolerance can eat dairy products in varying amounts; that's because lactose intolerance is a matter of degree. If you suspect lactose intolerance, avoid self-diagnosis. Instead, see your doctor for a medical diagnosis; the symptoms might be caused by another condition. Lactose intolerance is diagnosed with several tests: a blood test, a hydrogen breath test, or a stool acidity test for infants and young children.

Who's Likely to Be Lactose-Intolerant?

Anyone can be lactose-intolerant. From birth, most infants produce the lactase enzyme. With age, however, the body may produce less lactase.

How many people have low levels of lactase? Between thirty to fifty million Americans; however, a large proportion of them have few if any symptoms. And many people who think they're lactose-intolerant really aren't. Certain ethnic and racial populations are more widely affected than others. In the United States as many as 80 percent of African Americans and 75 percent of American Indians, 90 percent of Asian Americans and 60 percent of Hispanics are lactose-

HOW MUCH LACTOSE?

PRODUCT	SERVING SIZE (APPROXIMATE)	LACTOSE (GM)
Milk: whole, reduced-fat, low-fat, fat-free, sweet acidophilus milk, or buttermilk	1 cup	10–12
Goat milk	1 cup	9
Lactose-treated milk	1 cup	1
Nonfat dry milk	⅓ cup	12
Half-and-half	½ cup	5
Whipping cream	½ cup	3
Sour cream	½ cup	4
Sweetened condensed milk	1 cup	30
Evaporated milk	1 cup	24
Butter, margarine	1 tsp.	Trace
Cottage cheese	½ cup	2–3
Yogurt, low-fat	1 cup	5
Cheese: American, Swiss, blue, Cheddar, Parmesan, or cream cheese	1 oz.	1–2
Ice cream, regular and low-fat	½ cup	6–9
Sherbet, orange	½ cup	2

Lactose-free foods include:
- Broth-based soups
- Plain meat, fish, and poultry
- Fruits and vegetables, plain
- Tofu and tofu products
- Soy and rice beverages
- Breads, cereal, crackers, and desserts made without milk, dry milk, or whey

intolerant to some degree. The condition is least common among persons of northern European descent who tend to maintain adequate lactose levels throughout their lives. Researchers have identified a genetic link with lactose intolerance.

Lactose intolerance is sometimes linked to other issues. For example, some medications lower lactase production in the body. Lactose intolerance can be a side effect of certain medical conditions, such as intestinal disease or gastric (stomach) surgery. Depending on the cause, lactose intolerance may be short-term.

Lactose in Food: Which "Whey"?

Lactose usually comes from foods containing milk or milk solids. *The chart "How Much Lactose?" on page 524 suggests how much.* Prepared foods, even those labeled "nondairy," may contain lactose. If you're *very* lactose-intolerant, check labels carefully.

● Look for label ingredient terms that suggest lactose: milk, dry milk solids (including nonfat milk solids), buttermilk, lactose, malted milk, sour or sweet cream, margarine, whey, whey protein concentrate, and cheese.

● Spot baked and processed foods that often contain small amounts of lactose: bread, pancake or baking mixes, candy and cookies, cold cuts and hot dogs (other than kosher), drink mixes, commercial sauces and gravies, cream soups, dry cereals, prepared foods (such as frozen pizza, lasagna, waffles), salad dressings made with milk or cheese, margarine, sugar substitutes, and powdered meal-replacement supplements.

● Be aware: some medications contain lactose. If you're lactose-intolerant, consult with your doctor or pharmacist about appropriate medications.

Dairy Foods: Don't Give 'Em Up!

So you've been diagnosed as lactose-intolerant. That's not a reason to give up dairy foods! Lactose intolerance isn't an "all or nothing" condition. Instead, it's a matter of degree. Most people with difficulty digesting lactose can still consume foods with lactose. It's just a matter of knowing which foods contain lactose—and knowing your personal tolerance level.

Needlessly avoiding milk and other dairy foods may pose nutritional risks. They're important sources of calcium, protein, riboflavin, vitamins A and D,

For Those with Lactose Intolerance: Another Option

As another option, food products have been developed for people with lactose intolerance. Some products are lactose-reduced. Others contain lactase, the enzyme that digests milk sugar and that's deficient to some degree in people with lactose intolerance. *If you're lactose-intolerant and if "Lactose: Tips for Tolerance" in this chapter aren't enough:*

● Look for lactose-treated milk and other dairy foods at the store. Lactose-reduced milk has 70 percent less lactose than regular milk; lactose-free milk is virtually free of any lactose.

● Add lactase enzyme, available in tablets or in drops, to fluid milk before drinking it. You'll find instructions on the package. Your milk will taste slightly sweeter because added lactase breaks down the lactose in milk into simpler, sweeter sugars.

● As another option, look for a lactase supplement to chew or swallow before eating lactose-rich foods. With a supplemental supply of lactase, you can eat without discomfort. Read the timing and dosage instructions on the package label.

magnesium, phosphorus, and many other nutrients.

Calcium is especially important because of its role in growing and maintaining strong bones. An adequate amount of calcium helps children and teens grow strong, healthy bones and helps prevent the bone-thinning disease called osteoporosis. Milk and other dairy foods supply about 72 percent of the calcium in the American food supply. Without these foods, meeting your calcium requirement can be challenging. *For more about calcium in a healthful diet, see "Calcium: A Closer Look" in chapter 4.*

If you're lactose-intolerant, consult a registered dietitian (RD) to help you plan a diet, adequate in calcium and vitamin D, while controlling the lactose in your meals and snacks. In extreme cases or for children or pregnant women with lactose intolerance, a physician or a registered dietitian also may recommend a calcium supplement. Most older children and adults can eat some foods with lactose, in some amount. For infants and young children, talk to your doctor about lactose-containing foods.

Lactose: Tips for Tolerance

Lactose intolerance is easy to manage. Most people with difficulty digesting lactose can include some dairy and other lactose-containing foods in their meals and snacks. In fact, most people with lower levels of lactase can drink a cup of milk without discomfort.

If you—or someone in your family—has trouble digesting lactose, try these tips to comfortably include lactose-containing foods in meals and snacks:

● Experiment! Start with small amounts of lactose-containing foods. Then gradually increase the portion size to determine your personal tolerance level.

● Enjoy lactose-containing foods as part of a meal or a snack, rather than alone. Try a milk-fruit smoothie, or milk and fruit on your morning cereal. The mix of foods slows release of lactose into the digestive system, making it easier to digest. Think of this as "diluting" the lactose.

● Eat smaller, more frequent portions of lactose-rich foods. For example, drink ½- or ¾-cup servings of milk several times throughout the day instead of 1-cup servings one, two, or three times daily.

Have You Ever Wondered

... if goat milk is a good substitute for cow milk for someone with lactose intolerance or with a milk allergy? Goat milk has slightly less lactose: 9 grams of lactose per cup, compared with 11 grams of lactose in one cup of cow milk. For a milk allergy, the protein in goat milk is similar to that of cow milk; it's not a safe alternative.

... if a nondairy creamer can replace milk for someone who's lactose-intolerant? How about nonfat dry milk? No. Nondairy creamers may contain lactose. Check the label. The nutrient content of the creamer and the milk is different. In a nondairy creamer, the protein quality and the amounts of calcium and vitamins A and C are lower than in milk. Regarding nonfat dry milk, remember that fat, not lactose, has been removed from milk.

... if a/B milk offers unique health benefits? Milk with added a/B cultures (acidophilus and bifidobacteria cultures) is similar to the milk it's made from. Although research isn't conclusive, these cultures may help improve lactose digestion, promote healthy bacteria in the GI tract, and help lower blood pressure.

● Choose calcium-rich foods that are naturally lower in lactose, such as aged cheese. When cheese is made, curds (or solids) are separated from the whey (or watery liquid); most lactose is in the whey. Aged cheeses such as Swiss, colby, Parmesan, and Cheddar lose most of their lactose during processing and aging. Much of the lactose is removed with the whey.

● Try yogurt and buttermilk with active cultures. Their "friendly" bacteria help digest the lactose. Not all cultured dairy foods contain live cultures. Look for the National Yogurt Association's seal "Live and Active Cultures" on the yogurt carton.

● Opt for whole-milk dairy products. Their higher fat content may help to slow the rate of digestion, allowing a gradual release of lactose. Then in your overall food choices, choose other foods with less fat.

● Even if you're sensitive to lactose, include a variety of calcium-rich foods in your diet every day. In addition to dairy foods, enjoy these other calcium sources: dark-green leafy vegetables; calcium-fortified products such as juice, bread, and cereal; and canned sardines and salmon with bones. For canned fish you need to eat the bones to get the calcium!

● Check labels for ingredients that may indicate lactose. *See "Lactose in Food: Which 'Whey'?"*

● Don't be fooled by lactobacillus or sweet acidophilus milks. Most are no lower in lactose. They're tolerated about the same as other forms of milk.

Gluten Intolerance: Often a Lifelong Condition

Pasta, tortillas, bagels, whole-wheat bread: great sources of starches, other nutrients, and perhaps fiber. Yet, those with gluten intolerance need to build their healthful eating plan with other grain products.

Gluten intolerance—also referred to as gluten-sensitive enteropathy or celiac disease—is an intestinal disorder and not a true food intolerance. For those who have it, the body can't tolerate gluten (a form of protein) in wheat, rye, barley, and perhaps oats.

For people with gluten intolerance, consuming gluten damages the small intestine lining, and the damaged intestine can't absorb nutrients as well. For those with gluten intolerance, the risk for malnutrition, especially among children, is high. Other potential risks: premature osteoporosis, colon cancer, autoimmune

Label Lingo

Words That Indicate Gluten

For people with gluten intolerance, label reading is very important! These are among the ingredients to watch out for:

Grains and ingredients derived from grains that contain gluten:

- Barley
- Rye
- Triticale
- Wheat (durum, graham, semolina, kamut, spelt, emmer, faro)
- Malt or malt flavoring (can be made from barley)
- Malt vinegar (made from barley)

Food components that often contain gluten:

- Breading, coating mixes, Panko*
- Broth, soup bases
- Brown rice syrup
- Candy—e.g., licorice, some chocolates
- Croutons
- Flour or cereal products
- Imitation bacon
- Imitation seafood
- Marinades
- Pastas
- Processed luncheon meats
- Sauces, gravies
- Self-basting poultry
- Soy sauce or soy sauce solids
- Stuffing, dressing
- Thickeners (roux)
- Communion wafers
- Herbal supplements
- Drugs & over-the-counter medications
- Nutritional supplements, vitamins, & mineral supplements
- Playdough: A potential problem if hands are put on or in the mouth while playing with playdough or are not washed after use.

Source: Gluten Intolerance Group of North America.

*Bread crumbs used in Japanese cooking.

disorders (including thyroid disease and type 1 diabetes), arthritis, miscarriage, and birth defects.

Who's at risk? As a genetic disorder, gluten intolerance is more common among people with European roots. The actual incidence in the United States is unknown but may run as high as 1 in every 133 Americans. The challenge is: Gluten intolerance is often misdiagnosed, and its varying symptoms often imitate other health problems. Often it goes undetected until triggered by other body stresses: perhaps surgery, a viral infection, or pregnancy.

The symptoms? They vary. Weakness, appetite loss, weight loss, chronic diarrhea, and abdominal cramps and bloating are common; some experience a painful rash, muscle cramps, or joint pain. Among women, gluten intolerance may interfere with the menstrual cycle. For children, gluten intolerance is especially risky. Unless well managed, gluten intolerance can affect a child's behavior and ability to grow and learn. Chronic irritability is a warning sign. For growth and development, a child's high energy and nutrient needs require adequate nourishment.

Gluten intolerance can occur at any age. Symptoms may appear first during infancy when cereal is started. Most cases are diagnosed in adulthood, often ten years after the first symptoms. Temporary lactose intolerance may accompany gluten intolerance, at least until the condition is under control and the small intestine heals. Healing may take months or years.

Primary treatment for gluten intolerance is a lifelong, strict eating regimen; *a gluten-free diet is a "must."* Once gluten is eliminated, the small intestine can heal. Nutrient absorption then improves; symptoms disappear. Those with gluten intolerance can live a long, healthy life. If you think you have gluten intolerance, ask your physician for a diagnosis.

Which Foods for Gluten Intolerance?

Gluten in wheat, rye, barley, and perhaps oats is damaging. To manage gluten intolerance, these four grains, and any food or food component made from them, must be avoided. Even trace amounts of gluten in the diet can damage the small intestine.

Avoiding wheat is probably the biggest challenge for people with gluten intolerance. That's because wheat is the main ingredient in so many foods: baked foods, bread, breakfast cereal, breaded foods, crackers, pretzels, and pasta, among others. Gluten-containing ingredients show up as additives (thickeners, fillers, and stabilizers) in many other products, too, including batter-dipped vegetables, scalloped potatoes, canned soup, lunch meat, pudding, beer, salad dressing, canned tuna—and even some medications, toothpastes, and mouthwashes.

Gluten-containing ingredients may be hard to detect because they may appear under a different name or as part of another ingredient. *See "Label Lingo: Words That May Indicate Gluten" in this chapter.* The U.S. Food and Drug Administration is working on labeling regulations to help consumers more easily identify gluten-free products. Knowing how to identify gluten is important for using ingredients' information from food manufacturers. Technically, "gluten" describes the protein component of grain. Although rice and corn contain gluten, it's in a different form, so it's not harmful. Avoid gluten from barley, rye, wheat, and perhaps oats.

Eating Gluten-Free!

Coping with gluten intolerance requires a strict eating regimen. While it's hard to follow at first, this condition can be managed with food choices, not medication. If you—or someone you know—deals with gluten intolerance, these are some guidelines to follow:

● Consult a registered dietitian who can help you learn how to live with gluten intolerance—and enjoy eating! *See "How to Find Nutrition Help . . ." in chapter 24 for tips on finding a qualified nutrition expert.*

● Use grains and other starchy foods *without* gluten: amaranth, arrowroot, beans (legumes), buckwheat, corn, garfava, millet, Montina, nut flours, potato, quinoa, rice, sorghum, soy, tapioca, and tef. Skip oats since they may be produced and harvested in equipment used for handling wheat. As a result, cross-contamination may be a problem.

● Look for gluten-free grains, flour, and food products in stores. Today more gluten-free food products are available than ever before. Can't find them in your grocery store? Check specialty or health food stores. Mail-order outlets also can be a source of alternate flours for baking, as well as prepared foods, mixes, grains, and specialty ingredients.

● Read food labels carefully! Many commercially prepared foods—baked, frozen, and canned—have gluten-containing ingredients. These are among the many foods that may or may not be a problem: flavored and frozen yogurt, rice crackers, luncheon meats, egg substitutes, French fries (especially in restaurants), salad dressings, pudding mixes, canned soups, flavored teas, candies, seasoning mixes, tortilla chips, and Worcestershire sauce. Spotting ingredients and additives with gluten *must* become second nature. *Check the ingredient list in "Label Lingo: Words That May Indicate Gluten" in this chapter.*

● Know the origin, composition, and production of ingredients. For example, flavored chips may be dusted with an ingredient made with wheat. Since the amount is less than 2 percent by weight, the ingredient may not be listed on the label. Another example: vinegars, distilled from grain, are okay except for malt vinegar in the United States. Malt vinegar is a problem because malt by definition in the United States is barley; it may be added to or used as the starting mash to produce malt vinegar. Ingredients used in prepared foods, such as marinades and barbecue sauce, may have malt vinegar, too.

● Substitute gluten-free flour for wheat flour in food prep. Use corn, rice, soy, arrowroot, tapioca, or potato flours, or perhaps a mixture, instead of wheat flour. These flours are gluten-free. Because they give a dif-

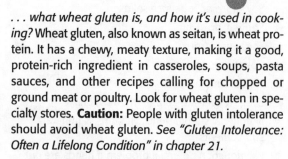

Have You Ever Wondered

. . . what wheat gluten is, and how it's used in cooking? Wheat gluten, also known as seitan, is wheat protein. It has a chewy, meaty texture, making it a good, protein-rich ingredient in casseroles, soups, pasta sauces, and other recipes calling for chopped or ground meat or poultry. Look for wheat gluten in specialty stores. **Caution:** People with gluten intolerance should avoid wheat gluten. *See "Gluten Intolerance: Often a Lifelong Condition" in chapter 21.*

. . . if carrageenan is a problem if you're allergic to fish or shellfish? No, it's a seaweed extract, not a fish. An additive in many foods, it appears safe for most people with allergies to fish and seafood.

Have You Ever Wondered

... if a wheat allergy is the same as gluten intolerance (celiac disease or gluten-sensitive enteropathy)? No, they're two different conditions: different physiological responses, treated in different ways. With a wheat allergy, wheat products and foods made with wheat products must be avoided. If you're allergic to wheat, you can consume wheat substitutes, including oats, rye, and barley. *See "Gluten Intolerance: Often a Lifelong Condition" in this chapter for ways to cope.*

ferent flavor and texture to baked foods, using these flours takes practice and experimentation.

● Keep up-to-date with food products so you can choose gluten-free foods. Contact food manufacturers for their current ingredient lists. As you know, recipes for prepared foods change. You'll find the company name, address, and perhaps a toll-free consumer information service number on the food label.

● Eating away from home? Pack gluten-free foods. Read restaurant menus carefully, and ask questions. If you're a guest in someone's home, tell him or her about your special food needs ahead, and offer to bring food. *For more tips on ordering from a menu, see "Restaurant Eater's Tip List" in chapter 14.*

● Find local and national support groups to share information and recipes with others with the same condition. Many support groups publish lists of acceptable food products by brand name. That makes shopping and following a gluten-free diet easier. A registered dietitian can help you find a support group.

Sensitive to Additives? Maybe, Maybe Not

Do you wonder what hard-to-pronounce ingredients listed on the food label do? You probably know most are additives, but you may not know exactly why they're used.

Additives serve important functions in food. *(See the chart in the Appendices.)* For instance, they may improve the nutritional value of food if B vitamins and iron are added to flour. Some additives, such as spices and colors, enhance a food's taste and the appearance. Others prevent spoilage or give foods the

consistency you expect. Without them our food supply likely would be far more limited. *See "Additives: Safe at the Plate" in chapter 9 for more on food additives.*

Except on rare occasions, we consume many food additives without side effects. For those who do experience adverse reactions, the response is commonly an intolerance—not a true allergy—to the additive.

The U.S. Food and Drug Administration (FDA) regulates food additives; food intolerances and allergies are considered in the approval process. Certain food additives—preservatives, colors, and flavors— are linked more commonly to food sensitivities than others. How strong is the link? Read on.

For the Sulfite-Sensitive

Have you ever wondered why dried apricots and dehydrated potatoes list "sulfites" on the ingredient list of a food label? Sulfites help prevent certain foods from browning, such as light-colored fruits, dried fruits, and vegetables. In beer, wine, and other fermented foods, sulfites slow the growth of bacteria.

The term "sulfites" is a catchall, referring to a variety of additives commonly used in food. Usually they have "sulf" in their names. Sulfites may be listed on food labels as sulfur dioxide, sodium sulfite, sodium or potassium bisulfite, sodium or potassium metabisulfite sulfurous acid, and sodium dithionite.

Sulfites, as part of a varied diet, pose no risk of side effects for most of us. However, the U.S. Food and Drug Administration (FDA) estimates that one out of 100 people is sensitive to sulfites. Asthmatics more often react to sulfites, and the reaction may be severe.

For those who are sulfite-sensitive, reactions may

Where Might You Find Sulfites?

● A variety of cooked, processed, and baked foods
● Dried fruits, canned vegetables, guacamole, maraschino cherries
● Condiments, jams, gravies, dehydrated or precut or peeled potatoes, molasses, shrimp, soup mixes
● Beverages such as wine, beer, hard cider, fruit and vegetable juices, tea

Source: American Academy of Allergy, Asthma & Immunology.

include wheezing, diarrhea, stomach ache, hives, or swelling. Fortunately, side effects are mild for most people. However, reactions may become life-threatening for those who are very sensitive to sulfite. *In rare cases these individuals may experience anaphylactic shock.* As with other food intolerances and allergies, consult a doctor if you think you're sulfite-sensitive. Don't self-diagnose.

Because sulfites can trigger intense reactions in sulfite-sensitive asthmatics, the U.S. FDA prohibits the use of sulfites on fruits and vegetables (except potatoes) intended to be served or sold raw. In the past, sulfites were sometimes used to keep fruits and vegetables fresh longer on restaurant salad bars, but that's no longer allowed.

Sulfites also can destroy the B vitamin called thiamin. For that reason they're not allowed in foods such as enriched bread and flour. These foods are major sources of thiamin in the American diet.

If you're among those rare individuals who are sulfite-sensitive, follow these guidelines:

● Check food labels. Choose foods without sulfite-containing additives. Be aware that they're used in varying amounts in many packaged foods—not just dried fruit, dehydrated potatoes, and fruit juices. By law, when sulfites are present in detectable amounts, the label must say so. *See "Where Might You Find Sulfites?" in this chapter.*

● Check alcoholic beverages. Labels on beer and wine must state "Contains Sulfites" if applicable. De-alcoholized beer and wine may contain sulfites.

● Ask questions in restaurants before you order. For example, ask if dried or canned foods, vegetables, or potato products contain—or were treated with—sulfites.

People sensitive to *sulfites* can consume foods with *sulfates*. Sulfates don't cause the same adverse reaction in sulfite-sensitive people.

Coloring . . . by Any Other Name!

Although the incidence is rare, a very small number of people are sensitive to a coloring added to food. FD&C Yellow No. 5, also called tartrazine, is a dye used to color foods, beverages, and medications. Research indicates that FD&C Yellow No. 5 may trigger hives, itching, and nasal congestion but not

Does Food Cause Hyperactivity?

The commonly held notion linking sugar or other food additives to hyperactive behavior or attention deficit hyperactivity disorder (ADHD) in children has never been scientifically proven. Although the exact cause of ADHD isn't known, factors such as genetics and environmental influences have been suggested.

The Feingold diet, popularized for its claimed ability to manage ADHD, has been touted as an approach for treating hyperactive children. The eating plan restricts foods containing salicylates, which are present in almonds, certain fruits and vegetables, artificial flavors and colors, and preservatives. However, the reported success is based on anecdotal data, not scientifically proven research methods. Extra attention given to children on the Feingold diet may explain why the child's behavior changes; it's not the change in food choices. Although many other studies have been conducted attempting to link eating with hyperactivity, the Feingold results haven't been replicated.

Until researchers learn more, the best management of ADHD includes behavioral modification and medication, if warranted by a doctor.

For more about the misconceptions between sugar and behavior, see "Sugar Myths" in chapter 5.

asthma attacks. But the incidence is limited to just one or two of every ten thousand people. Yellow No. 5 is the only food coloring known to cause such reactions.

Whenever added to a food or a medication, FD&C Yellow No. 5 must be listed on the label or package insert. If you're sensitive to this coloring, read labels carefully. Foods and beverages likely to contain tartrazine include soft drinks; ice cream and sherbets; gelatins; salad dressings; cheese dishes; seasoned salts; candies; flavor extracts; and pudding, cake, and frosting mixes.

Aspartame: PKU Warning

Since their discovery, intense or low-calorie sweeteners—aspartame, saccharin, acesulfame K, sucralose, and tagatose—have been thoroughly investigated by regulatory agencies around the globe as well as by leading scientific organizations. Evidence indicates that their long-term intake is safe and not associated with adverse health effects. *"Sextet of Sweet*

Have You Ever Wondered

... if you can be sensitive to MSG? Perhaps, but not likely. Some people describe varying symptoms, including body tingling or warmth, and chest pain after eating foods containing monosodium glutamate (MSG). The symptoms, usually mild, often last less than an hour. Collectively the symptoms have been referred to as "Chinese restaurant syndrome" because MSG was once so common in Chinese cuisine.

Actually, research hasn't found a definitive link between MSG or Chinese food, and any adverse side effects. Other components in those foods, perhaps a common allergen such as soy, could be the culprits if you have an adverse reaction.

If you want to moderate your MSG intake—or if you seem sensitive to it—see if you can order food without added MSG in Asian restaurants. If the menu says "No MSG," it likely means no added MSG. MSG is likely in other ingredients, such as soy sauce; glutamate itself is naturally in virtually all protein-containing foods. Check food labels to guide your food selection, too. Glutamate that naturally occurs in food won't be on the ingredient list, so you may want to consult a registered dietitian for guidance. *To learn more, see "MSG—Another Flavor Enhancer" in chapter 7.*

Options" in chapter 5 looks at these sweeteners. With one exception, low-calorie sweeteners do not cause symptoms of food sensitivity. *However, people with the rare genetic disorder phenylketonuria (PKU) should avoid foods sweetened with aspartame.*

Aspartame is made from two amino acids (aspartic acid and phenylalanine) and methanol. The same amino acids are found naturally in foods such as meat, milk, fruit, and vegetables. Regardless of the source, people with PKU cannot metabolize phenylalanine properly, so they can consume only limited amounts. Unmanaged, PKU can cause tissue damage, and in infants, brain damage. As a precaution, all babies are screened for PKU at birth.

For those who suffer from this disorder, foods and beverages containing aspartame carry a label warning stating "Phenylketonurics: Contains Phenylalanine." One of the most widely accepted food additives, aspartame is found in many products, including carbonated and powdered soft drinks, yogurt, pudding

and gelatins, frozen desserts, hot beverage mixes, and candy. You'll find aspartame listed in the label's ingredient list. The PKU warning is a signal, too.

Food Allergies: Less Common

Have you ever heard parents say that their child is allergic to milk, then remark that he or she has no adverse reactions to chocolate milk? Or maybe you avoid a particular food yourself, believing you have an allergy to it? Although food allergies are not to be taken lightly, you may be surprised at just how infrequently true food allergies occur. Consider that:

● One in three adults believes that he or she is allergic to milk. However, reports the National Institutes of Health (NIH), only 4 percent of Americans are estimated to have food allergies. About 11 million Americans overall have food allergies: 6.5 million with seafood allergies, 3 million with peanut and tree nut allergies. In recent years the prevalence of food allergy has gone up.

My Aching Head

Two to 20 percent of Americans suffer migraines (severe head pain plus a range of other symptoms such as nausea, vomiting, or increased sensitivity to light, sound, and smells). Migraine headaches can affect anyone, but women are three times more likely than men to suffer. Certain foods are blamed, but there's little agreement about the link between foods and headaches.

The causes of migraine headaches are complicated and not well understood. Certain food components— natural or added—have been suspected, not proven, to cause headaches in some people. Tyrosine (in cheese and chocolate), histamine (in red wine), caffeine (in coffee and cola), benzoic acid (a preservative), and alcohol may be food-related triggers. Susceptible individuals may be affected by several factors, not just food.

If you experience chronic headaches, check with your doctor for a medical diagnosis. To determine which foods or drinks, if any, trigger migraine attacks, keep a diary of what you eat. Depending on how often your attacks occur, you may need to keep the diary for several weeks.

If you're diagnosed with migraine headaches and feel you're susceptible to food triggers, a registered dietitian can recommend substitutes for suspected triggers.

● An estimated 6 to 8 percent of children ages four and under have food allergies, reports the NIH.

If food allergies are so uncommon, why do millions claim they're allergic? Because food allergies are often self-diagnosed and because the symptoms can mimic other food-induced ailments such as foodborne illness and food intolerances. People often use the term "allergy" loosely to describe almost any physical reaction to food—even if it's psychological!

Who is likely to develop a food allergy? Anyone. However, most occur among people with a family history of allergies. Nonfood allergies are more common than food allergies. Food allergies are often inherited, and almost all are identified early in life. Infants are much more likely to have food allergies than adults, and many allergies are outgrown. A milk allergy, for example, is usually outgrown by age three. To clarify, scientific evidence does not show that strictly avoiding a specific allergen increases the likelihood of outgrowing that allergy.

Food Allergies: What Are They?

A true food allergy, sometimes called food hypersensitivity, causes the body's immune system to react even though the person isn't sick. The body reacts to a usually harmless food substance, thinking it's harmful. An allergen, usually a protein in the troublesome food, sets off a chain of immune system reactions. When an allergy-prone person eats a food that causes an allergic reaction, his or her body scrambles to protect itself by making immunoglubulin E (IgE) antibodies. These antibodies trigger the release of body chemicals such as histamine. In turn, these body chemicals cause uncomfortable symptoms associated with allergies, such as a runny nose, itchy skin, nausea, even a rapid heartbeat, or in severe cases, anaphylaxis.

Something You Ate?

It's lunchtime. You make your toddler his or her first peanut butter and jelly sandwich. An hour later you notice the child has broken out with an itchy rash. You've heard that peanuts can be allergenic. Is your child allergic to the peanut butter in the sandwich? Maybe . . . or maybe not! In any case, a call to the child's doctor is certainly in order.

Any food can cause an allergic reaction in a susceptible person. However, some foods are more likely than others to set off a reaction. Milk, eggs, wheat, and soy, as well as fish, crustacea (especially shrimp), peanuts, and tree nuts (such as walnuts), are the most common foods with allergens, causing 90 percent of allergic reactions. Raw soybeans and soy sprouts tend to be more allergenic than tofu, tempeh, and miso. An allergy to egg, milk, soy, or wheat often is outgrown. A peanut allergy usually lasts for life.

Symptoms? Something to Sneeze About

What are the symptoms of a food allergy? Different people react to the same allergen in different ways. Even if a food contains a common allergen, you can't predict whether you may have an allergic reaction. Symptoms may appear within seconds or up to several hours after eating the food that triggers the reaction. In exceptionally sensitive people, just the touch or the smell of the food can provoke a reaction!

What's the Sign?

The most common symptoms include swelling, sneezing, and nausea. Most symptoms affect the skin, respiratory system, stomach, or intestines:

Skin reactions:
● Swelling of the lips, tongue, and face
● Itchy eyes
● Hives
● Rash (eczema)

Respiratory tract reactions:
● Itching and/or tightness in the throat
● Shortness of breath
● Dry or raspy cough
● Runny nose
● Wheezing (asthma)

What Food Allergies Are Most Common?

● *Adults:* peanuts, crustacea (crab, crawfish, lobster, shrimp), tree nuts (almonds, Brazil nuts, hazelnuts, pecans, walnuts, others), fish, eggs

● *Children:* milk, eggs, peanuts, soybeans, tree nuts, wheat, fish, shellfish

Digestive tract reactions:

- Abdominal pain
- Nausea
- Vomiting
- Diarrhea

A severe allergic reaction also can cause a drop in blood pressure, loss of consciousness, and death.

Keep in mind that these symptoms may be caused by other food- or nonfood-related conditions. For an accurate diagnosis you need a complete medical evaluation by a board-certified allergist.

Emotions linked to food experiences, not the food itself, can even cause a reaction. Just the appearance, smell, or taste of food might trigger an emotional reaction resulting in symptoms that mimic a food allergy or food intolerance. Or someone might get these symptoms by believing the food is harmful. Even if you suspect that emotions are at the root of an adverse reaction to food, check with your physician. Symptoms may stem from a more serious physical condition.

To date there's no known scientific link between food allergies and arthritis, migraine headaches, behavioral problems, ear infections, and urinary tract infections, although research in these areas is under way. Recent studies are showing a link between food allergies and severe asthma in children.

Food Allergies: The Dangerous Side

For most people with food allergies, the reactions are more uncomfortable than dangerous. In rare cases, however, an anaphylactic reaction can occur. When many different body systems react at the same time, this allergic response to food can be severe and even life-threatening. Even a touch, whiff, or tiny bite of a food allergen can be harmful.

With an anaphylactic reaction, symptoms often develop quickly—within a few seconds or minutes after eating—and progress quickly from mild to severe. They may include extreme itching, a swelling of the throat that makes breathing difficult, sweating, rapid or irregular heartbeat, low blood pressure, nausea, diarrhea, loss of consciousness, and cardiac arrest and shock. Without immediate medical attention the affected person may die. What foods may cause a severe reaction? Although the cases are rare, any food allergen can cause anaphylaxis; of the incidences,

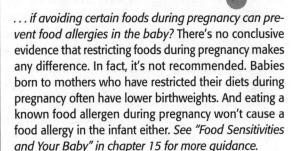

Have You Ever Wondered

... if avoiding certain foods during pregnancy can prevent food allergies in the baby? There's no conclusive evidence that restricting foods during pregnancy makes any difference. In fact, it's not recommended. Babies born to mothers who have restricted their diets during pregnancy often have lower birthweights. And eating a known food allergen during pregnancy won't cause a food allergy in the infant either. *See "Food Sensitivities and Your Baby" in chapter 15 for more guidance.*

... if breast-feeding can prevent food allergies in the baby? Perhaps so. For those with a family history of allergies, breast-fed babies are less likely to have food allergies. As a precaution against potential allergens in breast milk, the American Academy of Pediatrics suggests that nursing mothers of susceptible infants (with a family history of allergies) are wise to skip peanuts and peanut-containing foods. *See "Breast-Feeding Your Baby" in chapter 15 for more information.*

most are caused by allergens in tree nuts, eggs, peanuts, or shellfish (crustacea).

Is the reaction the same every time? Perhaps not. Its severity depends on two things: how allergic a person is and how much allergen is consumed.

Warning! If you—or a family member—experience severe food reactions, plan in advance how to handle accidental ingestion of the "trigger" allergen. The person should wear an identification bracelet or necklace to alert others, and should carry epinephrine (adrenaline) that can be injected quickly to counter the allergen. Your health care professional will give you a prescription. Because the body's responses can be life-threatening, call 911 or an ambulance immediately if someone has severe allergic reactions.

Itching for a Cause?

If you have symptoms, a doctor can help you find the cause with a medical diagnosis. A board-certified allergist (certified by the American Academy of Allergy, Asthma, and Immunology) is best equipped to diagnose food allergies. Never try to self-diagnose. Someone with a food allergy should be under a doctor's care.

True food allergies can be measured and evaluated clinically—with no need for "hunches." In that way unrelated medical conditions are eliminated. Typically the diagnosis includes a medical history, a physical exam, and possibly a food diary, elimination diet, and laboratory tests. As an initial screening your doctor may use a skin test; an allergist will confirm a food allergy with more definitive tests. *Check "Pass the Test?" later in this chapter.*

Keeping track of how your body reacts to a specific food one time after another may help you detect a food allergy or intolerance on your own. But be careful about self-diagnosis. The cause may be a more serious medical problem. Eliminating groups of foods from your eating pattern because you suspect a food allergy is not a smart idea. Sweeping dietary changes based only on a "hunch" may keep you from getting the nutrients and other food substances needed for good health!

For the Record

Suspect a food allergy? During a medical exam you'll likely need to describe your symptoms and give some medical history to unravel the mystery. Be prepared to answer such questions as:

- What are your symptoms?
- How long does it take for symptoms to appear after eating the food in question?
- How much of the food must you eat before you get a reaction?
- Do symptoms occur whenever you eat the food?
- Do other factors, such as physical activity or drinking alcoholic beverages, bring on symptoms?

Helping Kids Deal with Food Allergies

Whether your child—or his or her pal—has a food allergy, kids need to learn how to deal with food allergies. Banning allergenic foods from schools or other child-focused environments doesn't teach self-care. Instead it creates a false sense of security about the safety of food in the real world.

If your child has a food allergy, help him or her cope:

- Educate the day-care facility, school, camp director, or bus driver about your child's food allergy. Bring a signed letter from your child's healthcare provider. Together develop an approach for avoiding allergens without making your child feel "different" or isolated.

- Visit the cafeteria before school starts so your child can meet staff who can help. Choose a place to sit, perhaps an allergy-free table, to avoid cross-contact with allergen-containing foods. Arrange for a responsible "lunch buddy" to help.

- Include all the food-related events in your approach: parties, birthday treats, in-class food activities, recess, field trips, and food that children bring from home.

- With your healthcare provider, other responsible adults, and your child, make a plan for epinephrine administration (for severe reactions) or antihistamine (for milder reactions). Come up with a way your child can signal for help—fast!

- Go over the menu with your child to identify foods to avoid. Plan for substitutes—with the food service staff—or for home-prepared food.

- Teach your children why and how to avoid "food swapping" and pressure to try new foods.

For more parenting tips, see "For Kids Only—Today's School Meals" in chapter 16.

- Equip your child. When old enough to be responsible, children and teens who have severe reactions should carry an EpiPen or other form of epinephrine, a personal emergency card (perhaps in a fun backpack), a medical-alert necklace or bracelet, and a parent's phone number. An antihistamine may be enough for milder reactions.

Help your child be a friend to a food-allergic friend:

- Take friends seriously if they say they have a food allergy. Ask questions. Help them at school, with foods you offer at home, and with party foods.

- Don't swap or share food—even if you think it's safe.

- Wash your hands after you eat so you don't transfer food to other things your friend may touch.

- Get immediate help if your friend gets sick.

Label Lingo

Some Terms for Common Allergens

FOOD ALLERGY	INGREDIENTS WITH ALLERGEN	MAY CONTAIN ALLERGENS
Egg	Albumin (or albumen) Egg (dried, powdered, solids, white, yolk) Eggnog Lysozyme (used in Europe) Mayonnaise Meringue (meringue powder) Surimi	Flavoring (natural and artificial) Lecithin Macaroni Marzipan Marshmallows Nougat Pasta
Milk	Artificial butter flavor Butter, butter fat, butter oil Buttermilk Casein (casein hydrolysate) Caseinates (in all forms) Cheese Cottage cheese Cream Curds Custard Ghee Half-and-half Lactalbumin, lactalbumin phosphate Lactoglobulin Lactulose Milk (all forms: condensed, derivative, dry, evaporated, goat milk and milk from other animals, low-fat, malted, milkfat, nonfat, powder, protein, skim, solids, whole) Nisin Nougat Pudding Rennet casein Sour cream, sour cream solids Sour milk solids Whey (in all forms) Yogurt	Caramel candies Chocolate Favorings (natural and artificial) High-protein flour Lactic acid starter culture Lactose Luncheon meat, hot dogs, sausages Margarine Nondairy products
Peanuts	Artificial nuts Beer nuts Cold, pressed, expelled, or extruded peanut oil Goobers Ground nuts Mandelonas (peanuts soaked in almond flavoring) Mixed nuts Monkey nuts Nut meat Nut pieces Peanut Peanut butter Peanut flour	African, Asian (especially Chinese, Indian, Indonesian, Thai, Vietnamese) and Mexican dishes Baked goods (pastries, cookies, etc.) Candy (including chocolate candy) Chili Egg rolls Enchilada sauce Flavorings (natural and artificial) Marzipan Nougat (*Note:* Studies show that most individuals with a peanut allergy can safely eat refined peanut oil—not cold-pressed, expelled, or extruded peanut oil. Arachis oil is peanut oil. Experts advise peanut-allergic people to avoid tree nuts as well. A study showed that unlike other legumes, there is a strong possibility of a cross reaction between peanuts and lupine. Sunflower seeds are often produced on equipment shared with peanuts.)

Some Terms for Common Allergens *(continued)*

FOOD ALLERGY	INGREDIENTS WITH ALLERGEN	MAY CONTAIN ALLERGENS
Shellfish	Abalone Clams (cherrystone, littleneck, pismo, quahog) Cockle (periwinkle, sea urchin) Crab Crawfish (crayfish, ecrevisse) Lobster (langouste, langoustine, scampo, coral, tomalley) Mollusks Mussels Octopus Oysters Prawns Scallops Shrimp (crevette) Snails (escargot) Squid (calamari)	Bouillabaisse Cuttlefish ink Fish stock Flavoring (natural and artificial) Seafood flavoring (i.e., crab or clam extract) Surimi (*Note:* Any food served in a seafood restaurant may be cross contaminated with fish or shellfish. For some individuals, a reaction may occur from cooking odors or from handling fish or shellfish.)
Soy	Edamame Hydrolyzed soy protein Miso Natto Shoyu sauce Soy (soy albumin, soy fiber, soy grits, soy beverage, soy nuts, soy sprouts) Soya Soybean (curd, granules) Soy protein (concentrate, isolate) Soy sauce Tamari Tempeh Tofu TVP (textured vegetable protein)	Asian cuisine Flavoring (natural and artificial) Vegetable broth Vegetable gum Vegetable starch (*Note:* Studies show that most soy-allergic individuals may safely eat soy lecithin and soybean oil.)
Tree nuts	Almonds Artificial nuts Brazil nuts Caponata Cashews Chestnuts Filbert/hazelnuts Gianduja (nut mixture in some chocolate) Hickory nuts Macadamia nuts Mandelonas Marzipan/almond paste Nan-gai nuts Natural nut extract (i.e., almond, walnut) Nougat Nut butters (i.e., cashew butter) Nutmeal Nut meat Nut oil Nut paste (i.e., almond paste) Nut pieces Pecans (Masuga nuts)	Flavoring (natural and artificial) Mortadella (may contain pistachios) (*Note:* Mandelonas are peanuts soaked in almond flavoring. Mortadella may contain pistachios. Natural and artificial flavorings may contain tree nuts. Experts advise people allergic to tree nuts to avoid peanuts as well. Talk to your doctor if you find other nuts not listed here.)

FOOD ALLERGY	INGREDIENTS WITH ALLERGEN	MAY CONTAIN ALLERGENS
Tree nuts (continued)	Pesto Pine nuts (Indian, piñon, pinyon, pignoli, pignolia, and pignon nuts) Pistachios Pralines Walnuts	
Wheat	Bran Bread crumbs Bulgur Couscous Cracker meal Durum Farina Flour (all-purpose, bread, cake, durum, enriched, graham, high-gluten, high-protein, instant, pastry, self-rising, soft-wheat, steel-ground, stone-ground, whole-wheat) Gluten Kamut Matzoh, matzoh meal (matzo) Pasta Seitan Semolina Spelt Vital gluten Wheat (bran, germ, gluten, malt, sprouts) Whole-wheat berries	Flavoring (natural and artificial) Hydrolyzed protein Soy sauce Starch (gelatinzed starch, modified starch, modified food starch, vegetable starch, wheat starch) Surimi

Source: Adapted with permission from The Food Allergy and Anaphylaxis Network 2005.

● Does anyone in your family have allergies? Food allergies?

You may need to keep a food diary, with all the foods, beverages (including alcoholic beverages), and medications you consume over a determined period. That includes brand names of commercially prepared foods. You'll also keep track of your reactions and how soon after eating they appeared. By itself, the diary can't confirm a cause-and-effect relationship between a food and symptoms. But the information can suggest a connection to investigate.

An elimination diet offers another way to uncover a cause. Your doctor may instruct you to eliminate the suspicious food from your diet for a while. If the symptoms go away, then reappear when you eat the food again, you may be allergic to it.

Keeping a food diary or following an elimination diet on your own may seem easy. However, detecting ingredients in prepared foods that cause allergic reactions may not be so easy. A registered dietitian has the expertise to help you.

Pass the Test?

Various medical tests can help diagnose food allergies.

● The *skin-prick* test uses small amounts of diluted food extracts "pricked" into the skin. If the skin reacts to the extracts with a mosquito-bite-like bump, you may have a food allergy.

● *Blood tests* are done by checking for antibodies. Remember: The presence of antibodies, released by your immune system, signals a reaction to an allergen. For example, a test called a radioallergosorbent test (RAST) uses a sample of blood to determine the presence of IgE antibodies.

● In a *challenge test,* likely given in a doctor's office, the patient gets a sample that's either the suspected food allergen or a placebo. The placebo won't produce an allergic reaction. The response is watched carefully. If there are no symptoms, the challenge gets repeated with higher doses. This test must be done under the supervision of a physician—never on your own.

● *Tests using a food extract* are unreliable and costly.

"How-Tos" for Coping with Food Allergies

If you're diagnosed with a true food allergy, what's next? There's no cure. You'll likely need to avoid the troublesome food—and prepare and choose meals and snacks with care! If you must eliminate a food, or a category of food, plan carefully to ensure that your eating plan is nutritionally adequate and fits your food preferences and lifestyle.

Start by seeking professional help. A registered dietitian can help you learn to manage a food allergy while eating a varied and balanced diet. For example, ask about making food substitutions, reading food labels, and dining away from home. Ask about nutri-

ent supplements, too, in case you need to make up for any vitamins or minerals missed in an allergen-free diet. *See chapter 23 for more on supplements.*

Prepare for emergencies! Carry injectable epinephrine, or for less severe reactions, antihistamine and bronchodilators, in case you accidentally consume a food allergen. Be prepared to use it as directed, and to get immediate medical help if needed. Wear an identification necklace or bracelet that identifies your allergy.

Eating Allergen-Free at Home

Whether for yourself or a family member, here's how to buy, prepare, and serve food to cope with a food allergy. Simply cooking a food or scraping the allergenic food (e.g., peanuts) off the plate won't make it safe for food allergy sufferers.

● Read food labels carefully for "undercover" allergens every time you buy or use food. If, for example,

Have You Ever Wondered

. . . if peanut, soy, or nut oils can cause an allergic response? Most peanut and soy oils are highly refined, making them free of the protein allergen. Research shows that people with peanut or soy allergies don't have reactions to these commonly used oils; extremely sensitive people are still wise to be cautious. Cold-pressed peanut and tree nut oils are processed differently and may contain small amounts of protein allergens that can trigger a reaction.

. . . if chocolate really causes acne? No; chocolate doesn't cause acne or make acne worse. Hormones and hygiene, rather than a chocolate allergy, are more likely the culprits. A true food allergy to chocolate is rare. Instead, a reaction to a chocolate bar may come from other ingredients mixed in, such as nuts or milk.

. . . if foods modified by biotechnology contain allergens? It's possible. But no "biotech" foods to date have protein from known allergenic foods. The U.S. FDA policy states that any protein taken from a food causing a known allergic reaction should be considered allergenic, too. And it must be listed on the label of a food produced by biotechnology. *See "Food Biotechnology: Nutrition Opportunity!" in chapter 9.*

. . . if food allergies trigger asthma? Only in very rare cases. The usual triggers are allergens in dust, molds, pollen, and animals; pollutants in the air; respiratory infections; some medications; physical activity; and perhaps weather changes. If food appears to be a trigger, consult your doctor.

. . . if there's a cure for food allergies? At this time there's no known cure. Research is under way to find a vaccine that may reduce or eliminate the symptoms of severe food allergies. Avoiding foods with allergens is the only protective approach.

. . . if soy is a good substitute for people with other allergies? Yes, if the person isn't allergic to soy, too. Calcium-fortified soy beverage can substitute for cow milk—if you get milk's other nutrients elsewhere. Soy nuts can be used in place of peanuts or tree nuts.

. . . if foods labeled as "nondairy" are okay for people with milk allergies? You need to carefully read the label to find out. For most people with a milk allergy, a key protein in milk called casein causes a reaction. Casein or caseinates are common additives.

you're allergic to eggs, you'd need to know that eggs are common ingredients in mayonnaise, many salad dressings, and ice cream. Food labels list the ingredients in the food inside the package. The chart *"Label Lingo: Some Terms for Common Allergens" in this chapter gives some ingredients to watch for on ingredient lists of food labels if you have a food allergy.*

The Food Allergen Labeling and Consumer Protection Act, which went into effect in 2006, requires allergen labeling of U.S. FDA-regulated packaged foods sold in the United States. Under the law, all major food allergens, or ingredients with a protein derived from them, must be labeled in plain common language: milk, egg, fish (such as salmon, flounder), crustacean shellfish, tree nuts, wheat, peanuts, and soybeans. For tree nuts, fish, and shellfish, the specific types must be stated. In the new law major food allergens used in spices, flavorings, additives, and colorings must be listed, too.

For allergen labeling, the package will be labeled in one of two ways: (1) a "Contains" statement, for example, "Contains milk, egg, peanuts," at the end of the ingredient list, or (2) the common name of the allergen from which the ingredient is derived, for example "albumin (egg)," listed in parentheses after the ingredient within the ingredient list. The law doesn't apply to restaurants.

● Keep up-to-date on ingredients in food products. Periodically, food manufacturers change the ingredients; the same food from different manufacturers may have a different "recipe." So even if you're a longtime customer of a certain food, check the ingredient list on the label every time you buy it.

● If you have a milk or casein allergy, be cautious before choosing kosher foods labeled as "pareve" or "parve." For religious purposes these foods are milk-free, or perhaps have only a very small amount of milk. Although appropriate for those with lactose intolerance, it may not be milk-free from a food science perspective or for those with food allergies. However, if a "D" appears next to the kosher symbol, it does have an ingredient derived from milk. "DE" means that it was produced in equipment shared with a dairy; consider avoiding these foods, too. *See chapter 11 for kosher symbols.*

● Contact food companies for their current ingredient lists or for answers to your questions. The company name, address, and perhaps a toll-free consumer information service number are on the food label.

● Practice new ways of cooking. In time, substituting one food for another in food preparation will

Allergen-Free: Sharpen Your Cooking Skills

Preparing dishes without allergenic foods seems obvious. Just leave the ingredient out of the recipe or off the plate! However, a few other "how-tos" can help ensure a reaction-free meal or snack:

● Use *different and clean* utensils (including knives and spatulas), containers, cutting boards, and serving utensils for foods prepared *without* the food allergen.

For example, for a peanut allergy: Just wiping off a knife used to spread peanut butter isn't enough. Use a clean, separate knife for the next ingredient, perhaps jelly, you spread. The same holds true for cleaning a blender after making an ice cream shake with peanut ingredients.

● Use different oils to cook allergenic and nonallergenic foods. Frying doesn't destroy allergens.

For example, for a seafood allergy: Use different cooking oil in a clean frying pan to deep-fry shrimp rather than what you used to make French fries or other foods. Serve them on a separate plate with different utensils, too.

● Be careful to note allergenic ingredients.

For example, for a tree nut allergy: Ground nuts added to a muffin batter or a breading mix may go unnoticed. Even a bottle of gourmet barbecue sauce may have nuts!

For a fish allergy: Bottled fish sauce in a stir-fry, Worcestershire sauce, or salad dressing could be an undetected problem. Anchovies flavor some Italian foods, such as caponata.

For an egg allergy: Sometimes eggs are used to hold meatballs and fish croquettes together.

For a soy allergy: Soy flours and soy protein are used in increasingly more baked goods and other prepared foods.

For a milk allergy: Milk protein is in many brands of tuna. Currently many foods labeled as "nondairy" have casein, a milk derivative. Meat may have casein as a binder.

become second nature. Find a cookbook or online source of allergen-free recipes. You may need to experiment to find substitutions that work.

● Be careful with cooking and serving to avoid any cross-contact between the food allergen and foods prepared without the allergenic ingredient. See *"Allergen-Free: Sharpen Your Cooking Skills" on page 539.* The same rule applies elsewhere—for example, for a milk allergy, avoid deli meats since cheese and meat may be cut with the same slicer.

Eating Allergen-Free away from Home

For food allergy sufferers, eating away from home can be the greatest challenge. You're not in control of the ingredients or the food preparation:

Kitchen Nutrition

Handy Substitutions for Allergen-Free Cooking

Egg-free recipes—substitute for 1 egg:
● 1 teaspoon baking powder, 1 tablespoon liquid, 1 tablespoon vinegar
● 1 teaspoon yeast dissolved in ¼ cup warm water
● 1½ tablespoons water, 1½ tablespoons oil, 1 teaspoon baking powder
● 1 packet plain gelatin, 2 tablespoons warm water (Don't mix until ready to use.)

Wheat-free recipes—substitute for 1 cup wheat flour:
● ¾ cup rice flour plus ¼ cup cornstarch
● 1 cup fine cornmeal or corn flour
● ⅔ cup brown rice flour and ⅓ cup potato flour
● 1 cup soy flour plus ¼ cup potato starch flour
● *1 tablespoon wheat flour equals:*
    1½ teaspoons cornstarch, arrowroot, white rice flour, *or* potato starch
    2 teaspoons tapioca *or* uncooked rice

Milk-free recipes—substitute for an equal amount of milk:
● Fruit juice
● Rice or soy beverage
● Water

Need more strategies for handling food sensitivities? Check here for "how-tos":

● Sharpen up on ingredient detection as you shop—see chapter 11.

● Ask the right menu questions when you eat out—see chapter 14.

● Monitor an infant's food-induced reactions—see chapter 15.

● Get more help from a registered dietitian—see chapter 24.

● Find organizations that offer additional help—see "Resources You Can Use."

● Be "ingredient-savvy" when you eat out. Keep restaurant menus handy to review ahead.

● Make a chef card to explain your food allergy or sensitivity. Share it with your server and the chef as you order. *See page 541.*

● Explain your needs to your food server. Ask about the menu—ingredients and preparation—before you order. The same dish prepared in different restaurants may not have the same ingredients. Play it safer by ordering plain foods such as grilled meats, steamed vegetables, and fresh fruits—still ask questions!

● Ask for the chef or manager if your server seems unsure about the ingredients or preparation. It's okay to leave the restaurant if your request isn't understood.

● Skip sauces and condiments. Allergens may be present.

● Choose restaurants where you can special order.

● **Caution!** Avoid these situations:

 ● Buffet-style or family-style service—the same serving utensils may be used for different dishes.

 ● Steak—butter, which melts into meat, is often added to grilled meat for flavor, again an issue if you have a milk allergy.

 ● Coffee drinks with foam or milk topping—it may contain eggs, an issue if you have an egg allergy.

 ● Fried foods—since the same oil may be used for many different foods.

● Seafood restaurants if you have a fish allergy—since cooking utensils may contact fish protein.

● Many Chinese, Indonesian, Malaysian, Thai, Vietnamese, Mexican, and African foods if you have a tree nut or peanut allergy—since peanuts and nuts are common in these ethnic cuisines.

● Breaded foods—since the problem protein may transfer if the same breading mix is used for different foods.

● Scooped ice cream—since the scooper for several flavors may be kept in the same tub of water.

To the Chef:

WARNING! I am allergic to _____ .
In order to avoid a life-threatening reaction, I must avoid all foods that might contain _____, including these ingredients:

_____

_____

_____

_____

_____

_____

_____

_____

_____

_____

_____

_____

_____

Please ensure that my food does not contain any of these ingredients and that all utensils and equipment used to prepare my meal, as well as to prep surfaces, are thoroughly cleaned prior to use. Thanks for your cooperation.

Reprinted with permission from the Food Allergy & Anaphylaxis Network.

Have You Ever Wondered

. . . what is an exercise-induced food allergy? It's a reaction from eating a certain food before exercising. Allergic reactions may appear once exercising starts and the body temperature starts to rise. Anaphalaxis may even develop. The way to manage this: avoid eating that food for a couple of hours before exercising.

. . . if you should avoid coconut and water chestnuts if you have a tree nut allergy? Ask your doctor. Even though coconut is a nut, it's usually okay. Some people do react to coconut. Regarding water chestnuts, they're from a plant root, not a nut—so enjoy them!

. . . if you can outgrow allergies? Approximately 9 percent of children allergic to tree nuts will outgrow their allergy, including those who previously experienced a severe reaction, according to research reported in the *Journal of Allergy & Clinical Immunology,* 2005. Children allergic to peanuts have a 20 percent chance of outgrowing their allergy. A doctor should determine whether a person has outgrown an allergy; don't self-diagnose!

● Baked goods if you're allergic to soy or wheat. Today more breads, pizza crusts, and other doughs are made with soy flour; wheat is often added to rye bread. Tongs and other utensils are reused.

Refer to chapter 14, "Your Food Away from Home," for tips on being restaurant savvy.

● Carry your own food on airlines. Ask for the peanut-free snack if you have a peanut allergy.

● Not sure about the food when you eat out? Ask about the ingredients, or brown-bag your own food. If you're a guest in someone's home, offer to bring your own food or to help with food preparation.

● Be a sensitive host. As you invite your guests, ask about any special food needs—in case they feel uncomfortable telling you. Adjust the menu or prepare some foods differently if you need to.

For more education about managing specific food allergies, and a cookbook, newsletters, and other support, contact the Food Allergy and Anaphylaxis Network. *See "Resources You Can Use" at the back of this book for contact information.*

CHAPTER 22

Smart Eating to Prevent and Manage Disease

A healthful eating pattern and lifestyle from the start are your best approaches for staying healthy and preventing disease, or at least slowing its course. Most health problems don't start with a single event in your life. Instead, they're a combination of factors. Some you can't control, such as your family history, gender, or age; many you can.

This chapter addresses several common health problems that concern Americans: (1) their prevention and risk reduction and (2) the management of health problems or their symptoms. This overview may or may not apply to your unique needs. For advice specific to you or to someone you care for, consult with your doctor, a registered dietitian, and other members of your personal healthcare team.

Your Healthy Heart

We've all heard the statistics. Heart disease is America's number one killer. Although its onset is slightly postponed for women, it's a disease that affects both genders. More than 71 million of the nation's more than 300 million people have some form of cardiovascular disease, and it accounts for about 910,000, or about 40 percent, of deaths annually in the United States (preliminary 2003 data). The truth is, many deaths from heart attacks or strokes are preventable. The higher your blood cholesterol level, the greater your risk for developing heart disease or having a heart attack. High blood pressure is also a risk factor.

DAMAGE CONTROL

Of the thirteen leading causes of death in the United States, six are associated directly with diet, and six with excessive intake of alcoholic beverages. Paying attention to what you eat and drink can pay off in good health and longevity.

RANK AND CAUSE*	RISK FACTORS	
	DIET-RELATED	ALCOHOL-RELATED
1. Heart disease	x	x
2. Cancers	x	x
3. Strokes	x	
4. Chronic lower respiratory diseases		
5. Accidents		x
6. Diabetes	x	
7. Influenza and pneumonia		
8. Alzheimer's disease		
9. Kidney diseases	x	x
10. Septicemia (bacterial infection in the blood)		
11. Suicide		x
12. Liver disease and cirrhosis		x
13. Hypertension and hypertensive renal disease	x	

Source: National Vital Statistics Reports (reflecting 2003 data).

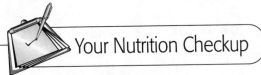

Your Nutrition Checkup

Do It for You!

Take care of you for you—and all those in your life! You can't control your age, gender, or family history, but there's plenty you can do to stay fit. For many health problems, the risk factors are the same, so the same smart living patterns may protect you from several chronic diseases.

How well are you protecting your health? If you can answer "yes" to the following questions, check to the left; fill in your own numbers in the blanks on the right.

Your Body's "Maintenance" Program . . . Your Markers of Health!

_____ Have you had a recent physical exam?

_____ Does your body mass index (BMI) fit within a range that's considered healthy?   _____ BMI*

Do you know your numbers? Are they within a normal/optimal range?

_____ Total blood cholesterol (below 200 mg/dL)   _____ mg/dL

_____ LDL blood cholesterol (below 100 mg/dL)   _____ mg/dL

_____ HDL blood cholesterol (60 mg/dL or more)   _____ mg/dL

_____ Triglycerides (below 150 mg/dL)   _____ mg/dL

_____ Blood pressure (below 120/80 mm Hg)   __/__ mm Hg

_____ Fasting blood sugar (below 100 mg/dL)   _____ mg/dL

*See "Body Mass Index: Fit or Fat?" in chapter 2 to figure your BMI.

Eat—for the Health of It!

_____ Do you try to consume the equivalent of about 6 ounces of breads, cereals, rice, pasta, and other grain products daily?* (One ounce is about 1 regular slice of bread, ½ cup of cooked rice or pasta, or 1 cup of ready-to-eat cereal.)

_____ Of these grain products, do you eat at least half as whole-grain†?*

_____ Do you try to eat at least 4½ cups or more of fruits and vegetables with a colorful variety each day?*

_____ Do you consume enough calcium-rich dairy foods daily: three cups of milk or an equivalent?*

_____ Do you try to eat protein-rich foods that add up to about 5½ ounces daily (e.g., lean meat, poultry, fish, eggs, dry beans, and nuts)?

_____ Do you choose foods low in saturated fat, _trans_ fat, and cholesterol, and moderate in total fat most of the time (e.g., lean meat, skinless poultry, fish, low-fat or fat-free dairy foods)?

_____ Do you try to eat legumes (dry beans) several times a week? (Besides being low in fat, they're high in protein, iron, and fiber.)

_____ Do you go easy on foods that deliver energy, or calories, but few nutrients (e.g., fats and sweets)? And do you try to eat foods with more nutrients and fewer calories?

_____ Do you choose and prepare food with little salt?

*For a 2,000-calorie daily diet. Check chapter 10 for more about a healthful eating pattern.
†See "What Is a Whole Grain? in chapter 6.

Do It for You! *(continued)*

Now . . . Your Lifestyle

_____ Do you get at least 30 minutes of moderate to vigorous physical activity most, if not all days, of the week?

_____ Are some of your physical activities weight-bearing (e.g., walking, dancing, tennis, basketball)?

_____ If you drink alcoholic beverages, do you do so in moderation (no more than one drink daily for women, or two for men)?

Now count up all your "yes" answers:

For each checkmark, give yourself five points. What's your total score? _____

Of course, these twenty eating and active living factors aren't the only ways to promote your good health. But the more often you said "yes," the better your chances are for a long, healthy life.

What does your score suggest? It only indicates how many different ways you already may be protecting yourself from health problems. And it suggests where you might improve.

Having a score of 50 compared with a perfect 100 doesn't mean you're twice as likely to develop heart disease, cancer, diabetes, or some other health problem. And this quick checkup is not meant for diagnosis, either. That's the role of your doctor in your regular physical checkups. However, your responses might point to risk factors that may contribute to health problems later. Read on to explore the role of nutrition in common health conditions.

What Is Heart Disease?

"Heart disease" describes several health problems that relate to the heart and blood vessels. Heart attacks and strokes may come to your mind first. However, high blood pressure, angina (chest pain), poor circulation, and abnormal heartbeats are among the other forms of heart disease.

Heart Disease: Are You at Risk?

What increases your risk for heart disease or high blood cholesterol levels? Two risk factors aren't within your control: age and genetic tendency. Yet many other risk factors are. Do any apply to you?

Risk factors you can't control:

● Family history of early heart disease (father or brother with heart disease before age fifty-five; mother or sister, before age sixty-five). African Americans, who are more likely to have high blood pressure, are at higher risk. So are Mexican Americans, Native Americans, Native Hawaiians, and some Asian Americans.

● Getting older (men over age forty-five; women over age fifty-five). Before menopause, women usually have lower cholesterol than men their age; after menopause, women's LDL cholesterol often rises.

Major risk factors that affect LDLs:

● Cigarette smoking, which is a significant risk factor for heart disease. Cigar and pipe smoking, as well as secondhand smoke, are risk factors, too.

● High blood pressure, which causes the heart to work harder and so enlarge and weaken. (High blood pressure is 140/90 mm Hg or on blood pressure medication.)

● Low HDL (less than 40 mg/dL for men, less than 50 mg/dl for women)

Other risk factors:

● Lack of physical activity.

● Overweight and obesity, especially with excess abdominal fat. The excess puts strain on the heart, raises blood pressure, raises cholesterol and triglyceride levels, and lowers the HDL cholesterol level.

● Diabetes, even if under control. People with diabetes have an especially high risk of dying from a heart attack.

● Too much alcohol intake, which can raise blood pressure, cause heart failure, and lead to a stroke. And it can contribute to high triglycerides and irregular heartbeat.

● Taking birth control pills (if you smoke or have other risk factors).

● Stress, as it often leads to overeating, smoking, and other factors that aren't heart healthy.

Having a high risk doesn't mean you're sure to have a heart attack or a stroke. That's good news! However, the more risks for heart disease you have, the greater your statistical chances. Using data from the long-term Framingham Heart Study, an interactive tool has been created to measure your ten-year statistical risk for a heart attack. Check out the Web site http://hp2010nhlbihin/atpiii/calculator.asp for your risk score. Changes in your food choices and lifestyle, and perhaps weight reduction and medication, can lower your risk score.

Insulin Resistance Syndrome, or Metabolic Syndrome

Insulin resistance syndrome, often called "syndrome X" or metabolic syndrome, is a trio of health conditions: abnormal lipid levels, high blood pressure, and obesity. When all these problems exist together, the risks for heart disease, a heart attack, and a stroke are many times higher. Several factors are among those that play a key role in the development of insulin resistance syndrome: inactivity, overeating, and insulin resistance itself.

With insulin resistance, body cells don't respond normally to insulin. The pancreas produces more insulin to overcome this insensitivity; however, insulin instead builds up in blood, contributing to high blood pressure, glucose intolerance, and abnormal levels of cholesterol and triglycerides. Upper body obesity (abdominal) adds to the problem.

The treatment? Address all conditions at the same time; the recommendations for dealing with them are consistent. This includes increased physical activity, achieving a healthy weight, and a diet that's low in saturated fat (less than 10 percent of total calories), more *moderate* in total fat content (20 to 35 percent of total calories), and *moderate* in carbohydrates. To the contrary, a high-carbohydrate, low-fat diet may aggravate the effects of this syndrome. Along with diet therapy, medications also may be prescribed to help control blood sugar, hypertension, and high blood lipids (cholesterol and triglycerides). Stop smoking if you smoke. *See "Diabetes: A Growing Health Concern" in this chapter.*

See "Heart Disease: A Woman's Issue, Too!" in chapter 17.

Heart Disease: The Blood Lipid Connection

High total and LDL cholesterol levels are major risk factors for heart disease. Conversely, lowering these cholesterol numbers and raising HDL cholesterol levels reduce the risk. What's the link?

Cholesterol, a fatlike substance produced in your liver, is found in everyone's bloodstream. As part of every body cell, it's essential to human health and cell-building. There's no Recommended Dietary Allowance for consuming enough cholesterol because your body makes it, too. The Dietary Guidelines advise eating less than 300 milligrams of cholesterol a day for adults if their LDL cholesterol is less than 130 mg/dL. As part of a therapeutic diet for adults with elevated LDL blood cholesterol ($\geq$ 130 mg/dL), less than 200 mg cholesterol per day—and less than 7 percent calories from saturated fat—are advised.

Blood cholesterol is a problem only if your total or LDL blood cholesterol gets too high and your HDL too low. When total and LDL blood cholesterol levels are elevated, deposits of cholesterol, called plaque, collect on arterial and other blood vessel walls. This condition is called atherosclerosis, or hardening of the arteries. As fatty plaques build up, arteries gradually become more narrow and may slow or block the flow of oxygen-rich blood. Chest pain may result without enough oxygen to the heart.

Plaque buildup happens silently, usually without symptoms. Warnings in the form of chest pains may not occur until vessels are about 75 percent blocked. Often a heart attack or a stroke strikes with no

Arteries

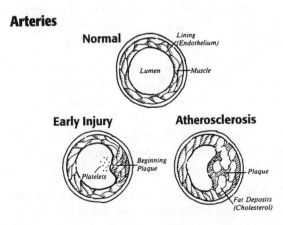

warning at all. A clot in a narrowed artery blocks blood flow to the heart, causing a heart attack. With a stroke, blood can't flow to the brain. The higher the blood cholesterol level, the greater the risk. When abnormally high total and LDL blood cholesterol levels go down, so does the risk for heart attack and stroke.

For good health, aim to fit your blood cholesterol level within a desirable range. *Check "Strive for Desirable Blood Lipid Levels" in this chapter.* High total blood cholesterol isn't the only risk factor for heart disease. Even a total of 200 or less won't automatically keep you safe.

Why Do Blood Cholesterol Levels Rise and Fall?

Usually there's no single reason. For some people, high or low blood cholesterol is an inherited tendency; in part, genetics affects how much cholesterol your body makes. Families with heart disease share more than their genetic makeup. People also grow up with similar lifestyle habits that may raise cholesterol levels—perhaps high-fat eating, excessive calories, inactivity, excessive alcohol intake, or smoking (or exposure to tobacco products).

From a nutrition standpoint, a diet high in fat, especially saturated fats and *trans* fats, is a risk factor for high blood cholesterol levels—in fact, compared to other dietary components, "sat fats" and *trans* fats have the most significant cholesterol-raising effect for most of us. Obesity, which tends to increase cholesterol levels, is a key factor. Some people are cholesterol-sensitive—that is, a high-cholesterol diet significantly boosts their total blood cholesterol level and LDL blood cholesterol level. *For more on dietary fat and cholesterol, see chapter 3.*

HDLs and LDLs: The Ups and the Downs. Lipoproteins—both HDLs and LDLs—transport "packages" of cholesterol through your blood. Here's how:

● High-density lipoproteins (HDLs), or good blood cholesterol, act like waste removal vehicles. They take cholesterol from blood and artery walls to your liver for removal from the body. According to the National Heart, Lung, and Blood Institute, an HDL level of 60 mg/dL or more protects against heart disease. *Tip:* Remember "H" stands for HDLs and "healthy."

● Low-density lipoproteins (LDLs), or bad blood cholesterol, work like delivery vehicles. They keep

blood cholesterol circulating in your bloodstream, depositing plaque on artery walls along the way. As plaque builds up, atherosclerosis risk goes up. For optimal health, keep LDLs at less than 100 mg/dL. *Tip:* Remember "L" stands for LDLs and "lousy."

With these in mind, the heart-smart goal is obvious: high levels of HDLs and low levels of LDLs (both within normal guidelines). The next questions: How do you boost your HDLs? How do you lower your LDLs?

● *To increase HDL blood cholesterol:* Stay physically active and trim any extra pounds of body fat if you're not at your healthy weight. Reduce fat intake to no more than 20 to 35 percent calories from fat in your overall diet. Replace some saturated fats with monounsaturates. Keep *trans* fats as low as you can. If you smoke, quit.

● *To decrease LDL blood cholesterol:* Substitute unsaturated fats for saturated fats, while keeping total fat and dietary cholesterol low; cut back on *trans* fatty acids (found in partly hydrogenated vegetable oils). Soluble fiber and soy protein may help lower LDL cholesterol. Keeping excess body weight off may help.

"Strive for Desirable Blood Lipid Levels" in this chapter shows target levels for HDLs and LDLs. For more about them, see "The 'Good' and the 'Bad'" in chapter 3.

Prevention: Cholesterol Countdown. A heart-healthy eating pattern—a diet low in saturated fat, *trans* fat, and dietary cholesterol—helps reduce or maintain blood cholesterol levels. *For more about fat and cholesterol in food and health, see chapter 3, "Fat Facts."*

● Be moderate in the total fat you consume—no more than 20 to 35 percent of your total calories a day advises the Dietary Guidelines for Americans, 2005 *(see chapter 3)*—rather than attempt to cut fat out of your diet entirely. You need fat to keep you healthy. And many foods with fat also contain other nutrients your body needs. *Tip:* In the Nutrition Facts on food labels, 100% Daily Value (for 2,000 calories daily) is 65 fat grams, which is 30 percent of total calories.

● Follow an eating pattern that's low in saturated fat—less than 10 percent of your total daily calories *(see chapter 3),* or not more than a third of your total fat intake advises the Dietary Guidelines. "Sat fats" boost blood cholesterol levels more than anything else you consume. You probably won't need to track "sat fats." By keeping your total fat intake moderate, you'll likely consume less saturated fat, too. Substitute foods with unsaturated fats for those higher in saturated fats and *trans* fat, without increasing your total fat intake.

● Go easy on *trans* fatty acids, too—the kind in partially hydrogenated margarines and some snack foods. They, too, are cholesterol-raising. *See chapter 3 for more on* trans *fatty acids.*

● Follow an eating plan that's low in cholesterol—less than 300 milligrams a day. Although not as significant as cutting back on saturated fat, reducing your dietary cholesterol may help lower your blood cholesterol level. You don't need to eliminate foods with cholesterol—just be prudent. Milk, cheese, eggs, poultry, fish, and meat supply nutrients your body needs.

● If you're already at your healthy weight, enjoy nutrient-rich foods with more starches and fiber as you cut back on fat. Otherwise you'll lose weight. Grain products, beans, and vegetables all contain starches (complex carbohydrates). *See "From Complex to Simple . . ." in chapter 5, and "Too Much of a Good Thing?" in chapter 3 for more guidance on fat, cholesterol, and whole-grain foods.*

● Eat more fiber. Fiber-rich foods may help lower blood cholesterol levels, especially for those with high levels, offering some protection from heart disease. Fiber also may improve the ratio between LDL and HDL cholesterol. In the intestine, fiber binds to cholesterol-rich bile acids, passing them out of the body as waste rather than reabsorbing them. Among the sources of fiber: oatmeal, oat bran, rice, wheat bran, barley, canned or cooked dried beans (such as kidney and pinto beans), and many fruits and vegetables. *For more on fiber, see "Fiber: Heart Healthy, Too!" in chapter 6.*

For the record, no long-term studies show heart-healthy benefits from fiber supplements. At least for now, they're not recommended as an approach for reducing heart disease risk.

● Eat plenty of fruits and vegetables; eat a variety daily. Besides their fiber content, emerging research also suggests a link to high intakes of antioxidant vitamins: beta carotene and vitamin C, which may be heart-protective. Prepare them with a little added saturated or *trans* fat, salt, and sugar.

On the Emerging Edge of Science. Other substances in food also may be cholesterol-lowering; hence, the interest in functional foods. *See "Functional Foods for Heart Health!" in this chapter.* For some, research evidence is strong; for others, it's preliminary but promising. Here are some new areas of scientific investigation.

● *Soybean products.* Soybeans and soy products such as soy beverage, tofu, tempeh, and soyburgers (but not soybean oil) may contain several phytonutrients that promote heart health; soy protein and isoflavones get the most consumer attention. In fact, the U.S. Food and Drug Administration has approved a health claim for labeling: 25 grams of soy protein per day, as part of a diet low in saturated fat and cholesterol, can reduce the risk of heart disease. Although research can't confirm a direct benefit between soy intake and blood cholesterol levels, there may be an indirect benefit if soy replaces foods high in saturated fats.

SOY PROTEIN: HOW MUCH?

FOODS WITH SOY PROTEIN (EXAMPLES)	AMOUNT OF SOY PROTEIN (GRAMS)
½ cup tempeh	19.5
¼ cup roasted soy nuts	19
4 oz. firm tofu	13
1 soy protein bar	14
1 soyburger patty	10 to 12
8 oz. plain soy beverage	10
1 soy sausage link	6

Source: *FDA Consumer* (May-June 2000).

● *Plant stanols and sterols.* Plant stanols and sterols, found naturally in fruits, vegetables, and plant oils, have an LDL-cholesterol-lowering effect. They work by inhibiting the absorption of cholesterol (from food and bile acids) in the intestine; instead, cholesterol passes out of the body through waste.

Some spreads, juices, yogurts, and soft gel capsules are formulated to be high in plant sterol esters or plant stanol esters. These can be effective for lowering cholesterol for those with elevated LDL cholesterol levels. To be effective, you need to consume enough: two label servings of a spread that contains plant stanol (Benecol) or sterol (Take Control) esters daily—with meals—as part of an eating plan that's low in saturated fat and cholesterol. *See "Functional Nutrition: Fatty Acids, Stanol- and Sterol-Based Ingredients" in chapter 3.*

● *Omega-3 fatty acids.* "Omega-3s" from fatty fish, such as tuna or salmon, may help reduce the risk of heart disease, although the data aren't conclusive. That's why the American Heart Association recommends eating two weekly servings (about 8 ounces total) of fatty (oily) fish. Omega-3 fatty acids from other sources—for example canola, soy, and flaxseed oil—may have a similar effect. *See "Eat Your Omega-3s and -6s" in chapter 3.*

● *Folic acid.* The fact that today's grain products are fortified with folic acid (a form of folate) to prevent neural tube defects also may benefit heart health (another reason to enjoy grain products). Here's why: A high level of homocysteine, an amino acid (a protein) in the blood, may indicate heart disease. Although the reasons aren't clear, homocysteine may promote buildup of plaque in the arteries. An area of scientific study and controversy: the role of folic acid (a B vitamin), and perhaps vitamins B_6 and B_{12}, in lowering an elevated level of homocysteine in blood, and so helping to protect against heart disease. (A doctor can order a lab test to check your homocysteine level.)

Folate comes from fortified grain products, vegetables, and fruits. Folate and B vitamin supplementation studied to reduce heart disease have not shown a benefit.

● *Antioxidant nutrients.* Antioxidant nutrients in food may benefit the heart. For example, vitamin E may offer protection from blood clots and atherosclerosis, and vitamin C may help keep blood vessels flexible. The evidence is too weak to recommend vitamin supplements; instead, enjoy a variety of nutrient-rich, plant-based foods that supply antioxidant nutrients.

● *Arginine.* The amino acid arginine may protect against atherosclerosis. However, studies haven't yet determined how much is either safe or effective. Not enough is known yet to advise any benefits from extra arginine.

Immunity ... Protecting against Infections

A strong immune system doesn't guarantee that your body can fight off every cold, sniffle, flu bug, or infectious disease. But it is your best defense! Immunity is the body's ability to use its highly complex, natural defense with highly specialized cells, organs, and a lymphatic system (a circulatory system separate from blood vessels). Even your first line of defense—your skin, hair, mucous membranes, and tears and saliva—helps protect your body from potentially harmful substances. Together they protect, defend, and clear your body from "attacks" by infectious bacteria, viruses, fungi, and parasites. A normal immune response ultimately offers protection from other health problems, too, including arthritis, allergies, abnormal cell development, and cancers.

Good nutrition, which includes handling food safely to avoid foodborne illness, is essential to a strong immune response that develops gradually from infancy on. A relatively mild deficiency of even one nutrient can make a difference in your body's ability to fight infection. Among the nutrients well recognized for their many roles in building immunity and immune response: protein, vitamins A, C, and E, and zinc. Others, including vitamin B_6, folate, selenium, iron, and copper, as well as prebiotics and probiotics, may influence immune response also.

Research is under way to investigate other nutrition-related issues that may play a role in immunity, including diabetes and hypoglycemia (low blood sugar), obesity and overnutrition, and the role of lipids (fats).

To promote your own immunity, follow a healthful eating plan. Guidelines from MyPyramid can supply plenty of immune-boosting nutrients.

American Heart Association*
for Cardiovascular Disease Risk Reduction

DIET AND LIFESTYLE GOALS

- Consume an overall healthy diet.
- Aim for a healthy body weight.
- Aim for recommended levels of low-density lipoprotein (LDL) cholesterol, high-density lipoprotein (HDL) cholesterol, and triglycerides.
- Aim for a normal blood pressure.
- Aim for a normal blood glucose level.
- Be physically active.
- Avoid use of and exposure to tobacco products.

DIET AND LIFESTYLE RECOMMENDATIONS

- Balance calorie intake and physical activity to achieve or maintain a healthy body weight.
- Consume a diet rich in vegetables and fruits.
- Consume whole-grain, high fiber foods.
- Consume fish, especially oily fish, at least twice a week.
- Limit your intake of saturated fat to <7% of energy, *trans* fat to <1% of energy, and cholesterol to <300 mg per day by:
  - Choosing lean meats and vegetable alternatives
  - Selecting fat-free (skim), 1%-fat, and low-fat dairy products
  - Minimizing intake of partially hydrogenated fats.
- Minimize your intake of beverages and foods with added sugars.
- Choose and prepare foods with little or no salt.
- If you consume alcohol, do so in moderation.
- When you eat food that is prepared outside the home, follow the AHA Diet and Lifestyle Recommendations.

Source: American Heart Association, 2006.

*The AHA's advice parallels the Dietary Guidelines for Americans, 2005, from the U.S. Department of Health and Human Services and the U.S. Department of Agriculture *(see chapter 1)*.

For more about food's functional benefits for heart health, refer to *"Phytonutrients—a 'Crop' for Good Health" in chapter 4, "Functional Foods; A New Wave" in chapter 9, and "Functional Foods: What Does Research Say?" in the Appendices.*

Triglycerides: Another Health Issue

High blood triglycerides get much less attention than cholesterol, yet they're significantly linked to heart disease. As with cholesterol, high blood triglyceride levels don't mean you'll develop heart disease, but the chance goes up if you have other risk factors.

Triglycerides are the main form of fat in foods, whether they're saturated, polyunsaturated, or monounsaturated. Once consumed, your liver processes them. Excess calories from any source—carbohydrates, proteins, or fats—change to triglycerides for storage as body fat. Alcohol also can boost the liver's production of triglycerides.

Your blood triglyceride level normally goes up after eating. Things that can increase triglyceride levels include: overweight, physical inactivity, cigarette smoking, excessive alcohol use, a very-high-carbohydrate diet, certain diseases and drugs, and genetic disorders.

Because of the risk for heart disease, the National Heart, Lung, and Blood Institute recommends treating people with borderline-high and high triglyceride levels. If your blood triglyceride level consistently exceeds normal, weight control, physical activity, and perhaps medication may bring it down. (Normal is below 150mg/dL.) In fact, the advice for lowering total blood cholesterol levels also applies to reducing triglyceride levels. Of importance:

● Maintain or improve your weight. Weight loss alone may significantly lower triglyceride levels.

● Live an active lifestyle. Regular physical activity can lower triglyceride levels and raise HDL cholesterol.

● Go easy on sugary foods.

● If you drink alcoholic beverages, consume just moderate amounts or skip them entirely. Check with your doctor and a registered dietitian.

● Eat fatty fish, such as salmon, since their omega-3 fatty acids may help lower triglycerides. *Refer to page 285 for advice on fatty fish and food safety.*

Testing, Testing: Know Your Numbers!

Numbers don't tell the whole story of heart health, but they're good predictors. Know your blood lipid numbers—total cholesterol, LDL, HDL, and triglyceride levels—whether or not you're at risk for heart disease and no matter what your adult age or gender.

Unless you're screened regularly, high lipid levels usually go unnoticed because high blood cholesterol has no symptoms. If you're age twenty or older, have your cholesterol level checked at least every five years—and more often if you're considerably older or at risk for heart disease. If your first results are high, your doctor may advise another test soon. Rather than self-diagnose, let your physician or a registered dietitian interpret your test results—and guide you to achieve and maintain your cholesterol numbers at healthy levels. *For children, see "Should You Have Your Child's Cholesterol Level Checked?" in chapter 16.*

Blood lipid levels are measured from a blood sample. What about cholesterol

screenings at a mall or a health fair? As an initial screening, these finger stick tests for cholesterol may be good indicators. If your cholesterol number is borderline high or high—or if you have other risk factors for heart disease—have it rechecked with your healthcare provider. A finger stick screening may be less accurate than a blood test done in your doctor's office or a health center.

For a complete picture, you need a blood test called a lipoprotein profile: LDL, total, and HDL cholesterol levels as well as blood triglycerides. Triglyceride levels are especially important if you have other risk factors—for example, high total blood cholesterol; two or more risk factors for heart disease, such as smoking and obesity; or health problems related to triglycerides, such as diabetes, high blood pressure, obesity,

STRIVE FOR DESIRABLE BLOOD LIPID LEVELS

To lower your heart disease risk, strive to keep your blood lipid levels at desirable levels for life. If you don't know your blood cholesterol and triglyceride numbers, check soon. Then act on the results!

LEVEL	CATEGORY
Total Cholesterol	
● Less than 200 mg/dL	Desirable
● 200-239 mg/dL	Borderline high
● 240 mg/dL and above	High
LDL Cholesterol (lower is better)	
● Less than 100 mg/dL	Optimal
● 100-129 mg/dL	Near optimal/above optimal
● 130-159 mg/dL	Borderline high
● 160-189 mg/dL	High
● 190 mg/dL and above	Very high
Triglyceride	
● Less than 150 mg/dL	Normal
● 150-199 mg/dL	Borderline high
● 200 or more	High
HDL Cholesterol	
● Less than 40 mg/dL	A major risk factor for heart disease
● 40-59 mg/dL	The higher, the better
● 60 mg/dL or more	Considered protective against heart disease

Source: National Heart, Lung, and Blood Institute, National Institutes of Health (2006).

chronic kidney disease, or circulatory disease. Before you're tested, be sure to follow the directions carefully from your doctor's office to get accurate results.

What about over-the-counter cholesterol tests? Done properly, they can be relatively accurate. However, home tests measure only total blood cholesterol levels, not HDLs, LDLs, and triglycerides. Like finger stick tests, verify the results with your healthcare provider—especially if your results are 200 mg/dL or more for total blood cholesterol and if you have other risk factors, such as a family history of heart disease. That said, you need blood tests from your healthcare provider to track your blood lipid levels!

If You're Dealing with High Lipid Levels

You can bring your numbers down. However, it takes effort and commitment, changes in your eating and lifestyle, and perhaps medication. Here's what you need to do. If you have diabetes and risk factors that affect LDLs (*see page 543*), you may need more aggressive treatment for high LDL and total cholesterol levels. Other heart-disease-related problems may require other dietary changes; get advice from your doctor or a registered dietitian.

TLC for Heart Health

If you have high cholesterol, especially high LDLs, give your heart some "TLC": Therapeutic Lifestyle Changes with guidance from the National Heart, Lung, and Blood Institute: a cholesterol-lowering eating plan, weight management, and physical activity advice.

Eating for TLC. If you're among the many Americans with high or borderline high total blood cholesterol or LDL cholesterol levels, a few changes in your food choices and lifestyle may bring your numbers down . . . and boost your HDLs. Even if your levels are normal, these guidelines make sense.

- Less than 7 percent of your calories from saturated fat. *See chapter 3 for figuring percent of calories from fat.*

- 25 to 35 percent total calories from fat.

- Less than 200 mg of cholesterol a day.

Have You Ever Wondered

. . . if high blood cholesterol could be linked to a thyroid problem? Yes, it could. Hypothyroidism—when the thyroid gland doesn't produce enough of the hormone thyroxin—has many symptoms. Among them are a sluggish feeling, poor memory, dry skin and hair, feeling cold, constipation, heavy menstrual flow, weight gain, and muscle cramps. Elevated LDL cholesterol may be another and serious side effect.

Treating hypothyroidism with medication—thyroid hormone—also helps reduce high LDL cholesterol levels associated with this condition. Untreated, hypothyroidism can damage the cardiovascular system permanently.

As part of a routine physical exam, have your physician check for thyroid problems. Hypothyroidism is much more common among women than among men.

- Limit sodium to less than 2,300 mg a day, and perhaps no more than 1,500 mg sodium daily.

- Just enough calories to achieve or maintain a healthy weight and reduce your blood cholesterol level (Ask your doctor or a registered dietitian what a reasonable calorie level is for you.)

- More soluble fiber if reducing "sat fats" and cholesterol aren't enough.

- Cholesterol-lowering, butterlike spreads, juice, and yogurt (with plant stanol or sterol esters) for more LDL-lowering benefits.

Weight Management. Maintain or improve your weight. The more excess body fat you have, the greater your risk for heart disease. If you're overweight, losing weight can help you lower LDL cholesterol, especially important if you have high triglycerides and/or low HDL cholesterol, and carry excess abdominal fat. Those who carry a "spare tire" around their abdomen have a higher cardiac risk than those with extra padding around their hips and thighs. *See chapter 2, "Your Healthy Weight."*

Keep Moving! Regular, moderate activity helps keep your blood cholesterol and triglyceride levels normal.

It helps boost your HDLs and lower your LDLs and triglycerides, helps reduce blood pressure, helps your body control stress, and helps reduce excess body weight as you burn energy. More vigorous aerobic activity gives your heart muscle a good workout and ultimately helps your whole cardiovascular and respiratory systems stay fit. *See "Ten Reasons to Make the 'Right Moves'" in chapter 1 and "Get Physical!" in chapter 2.*

Lifestyle Changes. Diet, weight management, and physical activity aren't the only ways to lower blood cholesterol levels. Lifestyle changes in support of "TLC" also can reduce your heart disease risk.

● If you have high blood pressure, get it under control. High blood pressure is a key risk factor for heart attack and stroke. *See "Blood Pressure: Under Control?" in this chapter.*

● If you smoke, give up the habit. It's a key factor in sudden death from cardiovascular disease. Smoking seems to raise blood pressure levels and heart rate. It may lower HDL cholesterol levels, too. And smoking may increase the tendency of blood to clot and so lead to a heart attack. For those who stop smoking, heart disease risk goes down over time, even for longtime smokers.

● If you have diabetes, keep it under control.

For more about "TLC" guidance, visit the Web site www.nhlbi.nih.gov/cgi-bin/chd/step2intro.cgi.

Cholesterol-Lowering Medication

Depending on your numbers, your risk factors, and if you have diabetes, your doctor may recommend cholesterol-lowering medication along with "TLC" treatment. The higher your heart disease risk, the lower your LDL cholesterol goal. By reducing your LDL and total cholesterol with eating and lifestyle choices, you may need a lower dose of medication.

For women, hormone therapy isn't an alternative for cholesterol-lowering medication. According to the National Heart, Lung, and Blood Institute, research indicates that hormone therapy doesn't reduce the risk for heart disease, stroke, or death after menopause, and it may increase the chances for gallbladder disease and the blockage of blood vessels (perhaps to the heart or brain) by a blood clot.

Talk to your doctor or healthcare provider about specific heart disease prevention guidelines for women and children.

Blood Pressure: Under Control?

Do you know your blood pressure reading? High blood pressure, or hypertension, often creeps up

---

WARNING SIGNS: HEART ATTACK AND STROKE

HEART ATTACK*

● Chest discomfort or pain: uncomfortable pressure, squeezing, fullness, or pain, usually in the center of the chest, that lasts more than a few minutes or that goes away and comes back

● Discomfort or pain in other areas of the upper body—for example, one or both arms, the back, neck, jaw, or stomach

● Shortness of breath

● Other signs: perhaps breaking out in a cold sweat, nausea, or light-headedness

STROKE

● Sudden numbness or weakness of the face, arm, or leg, especially on one side of the body

● Sudden confusion; trouble speaking; trouble understanding

● Sudden trouble seeing in one or both eyes

● Sudden trouble walking; dizziness; loss of balance or coordination

● Sudden, severe headache with no known cause

*Warning signs for men and women may differ. Women will commonly feel chest pain and discomfort. But they're more likely than men to experience other symptoms, such as jaw ache, back pain, nausea, or extreme fatigue.

Sources: American Heart Association, American Stroke Association.

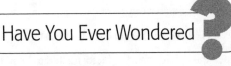

Have You Ever Wondered

. . . how many eggs you can eat for heart health? Unless your physician advises less, today's advice is more liberal than in the past—even one egg yolk daily—if you limit your overall cholesterol intake to less than 300 milligrams daily; one large egg yolk has about 215 milligrams of cholesterol. To check the cholesterol in any packaged food, check the Nutrition Facts on the label or displayed near fresh produce, meat, poultry, and seafood.

. . . if eating more olive oil will help prevent heart disease? Likely so, but not if you end up eating a diet high in total fat. An eating plan that's low in saturated fats, *trans* fats, and cholesterol and moderate in total fat is recommended for heart health. For heart-healthy eating, substitute some monounsaturated fats for some saturated fats in your food choices. Olive, canola, and safflower oils are all high in monounsaturated fats.

. . . if garlic is good for your heart? Perhaps, but the research is preliminary. The benefits of large amounts are untested. Best advice: Enjoy the flavor of garlic, but don't count on it for heart-healthy benefits. Follow accepted methods to keep your blood cholesterol under control. Stay physically active and eat a diet that's low in fat, saturated fat, *trans* fat, and cholesterol.

Although you can buy garlic pills and extracts, supplements may lack the phytonutrients that impart potential cholesterol-lowering benefits. Garlic supplements may cause stomach irritation and nausea.

. . . if fish oil supplements can protect your heart? Fish oil supplements are promoted for their omega-3 fatty acids and their potential for lowering the risk for blocked blood vessels and heart attacks. However, proper dosage has not been determined, and they can't cancel out the effects of a high-fat diet. Best guideline: Enjoy fatty fish instead, and follow an overall moderate-fat eating plan.

High-quality, contaminant-free fish oil supplements may be advised for people with high triglycerides who may benefit from consuming more omega-3s than their diet alone can provide. Some fish oils supplements are high in vitamin A; check the Supplement Facts to avoid consuming toxic levels.

. . . if fat replacers offer heart-healthy benefits? Perhaps—if you use them to replace full-fat foods and avoid consuming too many calories overall. In part because these products are relatively new, no research shows long-term benefits. Until more is known, use them to give you flexibility with fat control. *See "About Fat Replacers" in chapter 3.*

. . . what C-reactive protein testing is? It assesses inflamed arteries, caused by fatty deposits. A doctor may order this test for those with more heart disease risks.

---

slowly and quietly. Until it's advanced, there usually are no symptoms. But undetected and uncontrolled, high blood pressure may cause damage to the heart, brain, and kidneys for years without you knowing. Sometimes the first sign is a heart attack or a stroke.

Why the concern? High blood pressure is a main risk factor for heart attack, strokes, and kidney disease. In fact, more than a million heart attacks and half a million strokes yearly are caused in part by high blood pressure. By putting pressure on blood vessels in the eye, it may damage the retina, impair vision, and even cause blindness.

About one in three American adults have high blood pressure, according to 2004 data, yet only about half are being treated for it. Far fewer have their blood pressure under control. And many Americans have prehypertension. Take action to prevent and control high blood pressure. Once it develops, it usually lasts a lifetime.

What Is High Blood Pressure?

You've heard the term "high blood pressure" many times. But do you know what it really is? And how does it start? For reasons that aren't yet clear, the body system that regulates blood flow malfunctions.

Blood pressure is the force of blood against artery walls. It's normal for blood pressure to rise and fall during the day. High blood pressure, or hypertension, means consistently higher-than-normal pressure on blood vessel walls. It happens over time as blood gets pushed with more tension through arterioles, or small blood vessels, that become stiff and constricted. High blood pressure also damages artery walls and speeds

A Toast to Heart Health

Does moderate drinking reduce the risk for heart disease? Maybe, although for heart health benefits people who don't drink aren't advised to start. Moderate drinking (red or white wine, beer, or distilled spirits) may offer heart-health benefits for some people. Moderate drinking also may raise HDL levels and keep some LDL cholesterol from forming, according to recent research. Resveratrol, a phytonutrient in the skins and seeds of grapes, may function as an antioxidant, promoting heart health; it also may help keep blood platelets from sticking together. There's a fine line between how much alcohol is protective, though, and how much instead may promote heart disease, high blood pressure, and strokes. Remember, alcohol also can raise triglyceride levels. Stick to moderation.

There's reason for caution. Research linking alcoholic beverages and heart health isn't conclusive. For example, we don't yet know who may benefit. Even if a minor benefit exists, moderate drinking is only one factor related to heart health. Other lifestyle factors may play a role—for example, wine drinkers may be more physically active, and they may drink wine with meals, which may help affect blood lipid (fat) levels. *See "Red Wine: Heart-Healthy?" in chapter 8.*

Excessive and binge drinking is risky. Besides potentially leading to high blood pressure, heart failure, and excess calories, too much drinking can lead to stroke, irregular heartbeat, and sudden cardiac death. For pregnant women, drinking is the leading known cause of birth defects. Even moderate drinking isn't advised.

Alcoholic beverages also supply extra calories, so if you're trying to control weight for heart health, control calories from alcoholic beverages, too.

If you take aspirin regularly for heart health, your doctor may advise you to limit alcoholic beverages. Until we know more, moderation is advised.

For more about alcoholic beverages in a healthful eating plan and a definition of moderate drinking, see "Alcoholic Beverages: In Moderation" in chapter 8.

LIFESTYLE MODIFICATIONS TO MANAGE HIGH BLOOD PRESSURE

MODIFICATION	RECOMMENDATION	APPROXIMATE SYSTOLIC BLOOD PRESSURE REDUCTION (RANGE) *
Reduce weight	Maintain normal body weight (BMI 18.5–24.9)	5 to 20 mm Hg per10 kg (22lb) of weight loss
Adopt DASH eating plan	Consume a diet rich in fruits, vegetables, and low-fat dairy products with a reduced content of saturated and total fat.	8 to14 mm Hg
Reduce dietary sodium	Reduce dietary sodium intake to no more than 2400 milligrams of sodium** per day or 6 grams of sodium chloride.	2 to 8 mm Hg
Engage in regular aerobic physical activity	Engage in regular aerobic physical activity such as brisk walking (at least 30 minutes per day, most days of the week).	4 to 9 mm Hg
Moderate alcohol consumption	Limit consumption to no more than 2 drinks per day for men and to no more than 1 drink per day for women and light-weight persons. (One drink is 12 ounces beer, 5 ounces wine, or 1½ ounces 80-proof distilled spirits.)	2 to 4 mm Hg

For overall cardiovascular risk reduction, stop smoking.

* Blood pressure reduction is greater for some people and depends on time and dose.

Source: The Seventh Report of the Joint National Committee on Prevention, Detection, Evaluation, and Treatment of High Blood Pressure, U.S. Department of Health and Human Services, National Institutes of Health, National Heart, Lung, and Blood Institute, 2003.

** The Dietary Guidelines for Americans, 2005, advises less than 2,300 milligrams of sodium daily for most people.

plaque formation, narrowing the passage for blood. As plaque builds up in the arteries and blood flow is restricted, blood pressure goes higher.

High blood pressure causes the heart to work harder; the higher the pressure, the greater the work and the greater the risk of heart attack and stroke. High blood pressure can cause other problems: heart failure, kidney disease, and blindness. These problems result from damage that high blood pressure causes in the blood vessels of the heart, kidneys, and eyes.

Hypertension isn't emotional tension or stress, although stress may raise blood pressure temporarily. Even calm, relaxed people can have high blood pressure. For some, stress may be a factor, although the evidence isn't clear-cut. Regardless, for the overall quality of your life, learn to relieve stress.

High Blood Pressure: Are You at Risk?

High blood pressure is a complex problem, and in most cases its causes are still unknown. Only about 5 to 10 percent of cases can be attributed to known health problems, such as kidney disease. Yet health experts can identify people with increased risk.

● *Family history of high blood pressure?* There's a genetic tendency for high blood pressure. If there's been a woman under age sixty-five or a man under age fifty-five related to you in your family with hypertension or heart disease, your chances are higher.

● *Race?* African Americans have higher average blood pressure levels and tend to be more sodium-sensitive than European Americans. Typically African Americans develop hypertension earlier. As a result, they're at greater risk for kidney disease as hypertension progresses and for death from strokes and heart disease. Some Asians also are at greater risk.

● *Overweight?* Extra body fat, especially around the waist and midriff, increases the risk for high blood pressure. Excessive weight puts more strain on the heart.

● *Your age?* For many people, blood pressure goes up as they get older. For men it's sooner, perhaps starting by ages forty-five to fifty. Women often are protected through menopause; for them, high blood pressure often starts about seven to ten years later. Even if you don't have high blood pressure at age fifty-five, you have a 90 percent chance of developing it during your lifetime!

● *Sodium-sensitive?* For many in the American population, an eating plan that's high in sodium may contribute to high blood pressure. There's no way to predict whose blood pressure may be sodium-sensitive. Just in case, healthy normal adults are advised to limit sodium to less than 2,300 milligrams daily. For those with high blood pressure, African Americans, and middle-aged and older adults, the advice is: no more than 1,500 milligrams of sodium daily. For everyone, consume more potassium-rich foods to help blunt sodium's effect on blood pressure.

● *Smoker?* Smoking makes your heart work harder and raises your blood pressure.

● *Too much drinking?* Heavy drinking may increase the risk for high blood pressure, too.

● *Diabetes?* People with diabetes may develop high blood pressure if their condition isn't managed carefully—another reason to control diabetes from its first diagnosis. Up to 65 percent of people with diabetes have it. *See "Diabetes: A Growing Health Concern" in this chapter.*

● *High blood lipids?* If your blood lipids are high, they contribute to hypertension as well as to atherosclerosis. *See "Strive for Desirable Blood Lipid Levels" earlier in this chapter.*

● *Prehypertension?* Even if your blood pressure is between 120/80 to 139/89 mm Hg, be cautious. With prehypertension you'll likely develop high blood pressure later on. Take steps now to prevent it with healthful food and lifestyle choices.

Testing: Know Your Blood Pressure

A blood pressure measurement is two readings that look like a fraction. For example, an optimal reading is 120/80 mm Hg, expressed as "120 over 80" (mm Hg is millimeters of mercury). If it's less, that's okay.

● The higher number on top is systolic pressure. That's the pressure when your heart (the ventricle) contracts, pumping blood out to your arteries.

● The bottom number, diastolic pressure, is the pressure on your arteries between heartbeats, when your heart is at rest.

BLOOD PRESSURE: FOR ADULTS*

CATEGORY		SYSTOLIC†		DIASTOLIC†
Normal		<120 mm Hg	and	<80 mm Hg
Prehypertension		120-139 mm Hg	or	80-89 mm Hg
High‡	Stage 1	140-159 mm Hg	or	90-99 mm Hg
	Stage 2	≥160 mm Hg	or	≥100 mm Hg

*These categories are for people age eighteen or over. The categories are for those not on a high blood pressure medication and who have no short-term serious illness.

Source: Seventh Report of the Joint National Committee on Prevention, Detection, Evaluation, and Treatment of High Blood Pressure, U.S. Department of Health and human Services, National Institutes of Health/National Heart, Lung, and Blood Institute, National High Blood Pressure Education Program, 2003.

Whether you suspect high blood pressure or not, have your blood pressure checked at least every two years. If it's high normal (130–139 mm Hg over 85-89 mm Hg) or high, have it checked more often and take steps to bring it down. Even children should be checked as part of their regular physical exams.

If your systolic, but not diastolic, pressure is high, you can have high blood pressure. With age, systolic blood pressure goes up; diastolic pressure does too until age fifty-five or so, then often goes down. "Isolated systolic hypertension" is the most common type of high blood pressure for older Americans.

Blood pressure may fluctuate a bit during the day. Often the doctor's visit itself makes the number rise slightly; that's sometimes called "white-coat

Have You Ever Wondered?

... what to do if you have prehypertension? Even high-normal blood pressure appears to increase cardiovascular risk significantly. If you fit into this category, you're smart to monitor your blood pressure regularly—and to make lifestyle and dietary changes now to bring your blood pressure down to a healthier level. That's equally important if you have high cholesterol levels, diabetes, or other cardiovascular risk factors, or if you're an older adult.

hypertension," which refers to white medical lab coats. To diagnose high blood pressure you need two higher-than-normal readings taken one to several weeks apart.

If either your systolic or your diastolic number, or both, are consistently at or above 140/90 mm Hg, there's cause for concern. Usually high blood pressure is managed by a combination of medication, nutrition, and lifestyle changes. For those with diabetes, a still lower blood pressure goal might be advised.

Your local pharmacist may offer blood pressure readings as a free service. Or buy an electronic blood pressure measuring device to use at home. To check its accuracy, bring it to your next doctor's visit.

Not Too "Pressured"

Having a family history of high blood pressure doesn't necessarily mean you'll get it. And you can take preventive steps to lower your odds. In fact, many of the Dietary Guidelines promote blood pressure control and protect against hypertension! *See "What's Smart Eating? Guidelines for Americans" in chapter 1.*

● If you have a few pounds to shed, do so. Losing even 10 pounds, through smart eating and physical activity, may bring your blood pressure down—perhaps enough to avoid medication. As part of your weight loss plan, low-fat eating lowers blood lipid levels, too—a benefit to heart health and diabetes management. *See chapter 2, "Your Healthy Weight."*

● Fit in regular moderate to vigorous physical activity, at least 30 minutes a day, on most days. Sedentary living doesn't cause high blood pressure, but regular aerobic activity such as brisk walking, swimming, or biking may help bring it down. Moreover, physical activity can help you maintain a healthy weight.

● Eat less salt, to help limit your sodium intake to less than 2,300 milligrams a day. Put the salt shaker away. Use Nutrition Facts on food labels to find packaged foods with less sodium. Ask restaurants to go easy on the salt in the foods you order. *For more about sodium, see "Link to High Blood Pressure," "About Salt Sub-*

stitutes," and "Flavor . . . with Less Salt and Sodium" in chapter 7.

● Put dairy foods and other calcium-rich foods on the "menu." Three minerals—calcium, magnesium, and potassium—help regulate blood pressure. Calcium, and perhaps magnesium and potassium, which are all found in dairy foods, appear to be protective. *See "Counting Up Calcium" in chapter 4.* No conclusive evidence shows that calcium and magnesium supplements offer extra benefits.

● Eat plenty of fruits and vegetables. Refer to MyPyramid or the DASH eating plan. The potassium and magnesium found in many fruits and vegetables may help control your blood pressure. *For more about potassium and magnesium and their food sources, see "Minerals—Not 'Heavy Metal'" in chapter 4.*

● Follow the DASH eating plan, established by the National Heart, Lung, and Blood Institute of the National Institutes of Health. The DASH (Dietary Approaches to Stop Hypertension) eating plan emphasizes food rather than nutrients for lowering blood pressure. Similar to MyPyramid, it puts more emphasis on fruits and vegetables; like MyPyramid, it also advises low-fat and fat-free dairy foods, lean meat, poultry, and fish, and whole grains.

The DASH plan has been shown to lower blood pressure: down 2 to 8 mm Hg for systolic blood pressure. That's enough to lower hypertension risk significantly. In research studies, the DASH plan worked quickly—lowering blood pressure within two weeks. The benefits of the DASH plan were even better when combined with eating less sodium (down to 1,500 milligrams daily) in the DASH-Sodium study; blood pressure dropped even more, especially for those with hypertension. Lower in fat, abundant in phytonutrients, the DASH plan also may protect against some cancers, heart disease, and other health issues.

● Go easy on alcoholic beverages—if you drink. No more than one drink a day for women, and two for men, appear safe. Alcoholic drinks may interfere with medication for hypertension.

If You Have High Blood Pressure . . .

Relax. Although it's a lifelong condition, you can control high blood pressure and live a long, healthy life.

The key is following your doctor's advice faithfully. Treatment likely will include a shift in your eating approach, weight loss (if you're overweight), more physical activity, smoking cessation (if you smoke), and perhaps blood pressure medication.

● Make a plan of action with your healthcare provider, *following the advice in "Not Too 'Pressured'" in this chapter. Get help for adopting the DASH eating plan on the following pages.*

● If your doctor prescribes antihypertensive medication, take it faithfully. If other tactics, like weight loss, lower your blood pressure level, taking medication may not be forever. Follow directions for medications carefully. Different blood pressure medications work in different ways; some may interact with other medications—for example, for diabetes or kidney disease.

● If your doctor prescribes a sodium-modified diet, a registered dietitian can help you plan, follow through, and monitor your sodium intake.

Cancer Connection

After heart disease, cancer is the second leading cause of illness and death in the United States, currently accounting for one in four deaths. According to 2005 data, cancer will strike about one in three adults. For new cases among men, the incidence of prostate cancer is highest, followed by lung and bronchial cancer, then colorectal cancer. And for women, the prevalence of breast cancer is highest, followed by lung, then colorectal cancer. The overall death rate follows a similar order except that lung cancer for both men and women leaps to the top.

Almost half of all cancer deaths can be prevented with lifestyle changes and early detection. In fact, cancer has become a chronic disease for many, as

DASH to Health

As a way to lower blood pressure, the DASH eating plan is a taste-appealing switch from just no-salt-added eating. It may be an alternative to medication. The DASH plan has four calorie levels. Daily food-group servings vary depending on calorie needs.

FOOD GROUP	1,600 CALORIES	2,000 CALORIES	2,600 CALORIES	3,100 CALORIES	SERVING SIZES	SIGNIFICANCE FOR DASH EATING
	NUMBER OF DAILY SERVINGS					
Grains*	6	6 to 8	10 to 11	12 to 13	1 slice bread 1 oz. dry cereal ½ cup cooked rice, pasta, or cereal**	Major sources of energy and fiber
Vegetables	3 to 4	4 to 5	5 to 6	6	1 cup raw leafy vegetable ½ cup cooked vegetables 6 oz. vegetable juice	Rich sources of potassium, magnesium, and fiber
Fruits	4	4 to 5	5 to 6	6	6 oz. fruit juice 1 medium fruit ¼ cup dried fruit ½ cup fresh, frozen, or canned fruit	Important sources of potassium, magnesium, and fiber
Fat-free or low-fat milk and milk products	2 to 3	2 to 3	3	3 to 4	1 cup milk or yogurt 1½ oz. cheese	Major sources of calcium and protein
Lean meats, poultry, fish	3 to 6	6 or less	6	6 to 9	1 oz. cooked meats, poultry, or fish 1 egg***	Rich sources of protein and magnesium
Nuts, seeds, legumes	3 per week	4 to 5 per week	1	1	⅓ cup or 1½ oz. nuts 2 tbsp. peanut butter 2 tbsp. or ½ oz. seeds ½ cup cooked dry beans or peas	Rich sources of energy, magnesium, potassium, protein, and fiber
Fat and oils****	2	2 to 3	3	4	1 tsp. soft margarine 1 tbsp. mayonnaise 2 tbsp. salad dressing 1 tsp. vegetable oil	DASH has 27 percent of calories as fat, including fat in or added to foods

Food Group	1,600 Calories	2,000 Calories	2,600 Calories	3,100 Calories	Serving Sizes	Significance for DASH Eating
		Number of Daily Servings				
Sweets and added sugars	0	5 or less per week	≤2	≤2	1 tbsp. sugar 1 tbsp. jelly or jam ½ cup sorbet, gelatin 1 cup lemonade	Sweets should be low in fat

* Whole grains are recommended for most grain servings as a good source of fiber and nutrients.

** Serving sizes vary between ½ to 1¼ cups depending on cereal type. Check Nutrition Facts label.

*** Since eggs are high in cholesterol, limit egg yolk intake to no more than four a week; two egg whites have the same protein content as 1 oz. meat.

**** Fat content changes serving amounts for fats and oil: for example, 1 tbsp. of regular salad dressing equals 1 serving; 1 tbsp. of low-fat dressing equals ½ serving; 1 tbsp. of fat-free dressing equals 0 servings.

Source: U.S. Health and Human Services, 2006.
www.nhlbi.nih.gov/health/public/heart/hbp/dash

cancer survivors are living longer. At every stage of this disease—before, during, and after treatment, during remission, during recurrence, and during palliative and hospice care—good nutrition is important in dealing with cancer.

What Is Cancer?

Cancer is an assortment of diseases characterized by abnormal cell growth that can spread and destroy other organs and body tissue. Cancers are classified by the body tissues where the cancer starts, such as the colon, breast, or skin.

Cancer starts with a single cell that has divided abnormally and does not function as it should. An altered body cell multiplies at an abnormally fast rate. These abnormal cells continue to use the body's resources, including nutrients, to multiply. In the process, they disrupt and eventually destroy the normal function of the tissue or organ where they grow. These cancerous cells can metastasize, or spread through the bloodstream or the lymphatic system to other parts of the body, invading and destroying healthy body tissues and organs far from the original tumor.

The causes of cancer are varied and not always clear. Some cancers appear to be genetic and run in families. However, most cancers result from environmental and lifestyle factors. Cancer promoters, called carcinogens, include viruses, chemicals, and lifestyle and environmental factors.

Reducing Your Cancer Risk

Since some risk factors are controllable, the best prevention is to keep cancer from starting in the first place. Among the risk factors within your control: the use of tobacco; your weight; your physical activity level; your dietary intake; exposure to sunlight (ultraviolet radiation); and exposure to carcinogens, or cancer-causing agents. In fact, of all cancer cases; according to 2005 data from the American Cancer Society, one-third of cancer deaths were related to nutrition, physical inactivity, obesity, and other lifestyle factors. Taking a few small steps may be enough to significantly reduce your cancer risk.

Live Smart: Reduce Your Cancer Risk

Guidelines for cancer prevention are similar to those for preventing other health problems, including heart disease, diabetes, and high blood pressure. This same eating approach promotes overall well-being. *Throughout this book you'll find practical tips for eating to prevent cancer.* Keep in mind that no single food or nutrient causes or prevents cancer.

● Maintain a healthy weight throughout your life— and stay physically active. Obesity is linked to cancers of the uterus and breast (among postmenopausal women), and colorectal, prostate, and other cancers. The best approach to weight management is twofold: (1) stay physically active with thirty minutes or more

Nutrition and Lifestyle Advice for Cancer Prevention

For cancer prevention, the American Cancer Society (ACS) provides specific nutrition and lifestyle recommendations for individual choices. ACS also offers advice for community action—for public, private, and community organizations—to create and support environments that help people follow nutrition and lifestyle recommendations for cancer prevention. For the 2006 ACS recommendations, check the Web site www.cancer.org.

While specifically focused on cancer prevention, the ACS recommendations are similar to the advice from the Dietary Guidelines for Americans, 2005 *(see chapter 1).*

of moderate to vigorous physical activity on most if not all days of the week and (2) avoid eating more calories (food energy) than your body uses. *See chapter 2, "Your Healthy Weight."*

● Be active. Besides weight management, physical activity may help protect against cancer by affecting hormone levels and helping to stimulate your colon to eliminate waste. Regular physical activity is linked to lower risk of colon, prostate, endometrial, and breast cancers. *For more benefits of physical activity, see chapter 1.*

Adults: Engage in at least moderate activity for 30 minutes or more on 5 or more days of the week; 45 to 60 minutes may further reduce the risks of breast and colon cancers. Children and adolescents: engage in at least 60 minutes per day of moderate-to-vigorous physical activity at least 5 days per week.

● Enjoy a variety of plant-based foods: vegetables, fruits, legumes (dry beans), and whole grains. The links between fiber and cancer risk are weak, according to current research. However, fiber-rich, plant-based foods contain a complex mixture of cancer-fighting nutrients and phytonutrients. *For tips on boosting your fiber intake, see "For Fiber—Variety!" in chapter 6.*

● Eat your veggies—and fruits! Vegetables and fruits have a complex composition of vitamins, minerals, fiber, and phytonutrients, which appear to protect against various cancers—from the esophagus through the GI (gastrointestinal) tract to the rectum. What's

more, they're low in fat. These foods also may protect you from bladder, endometrial, pancreatic, lung, and larynx cancers. Following MyPyramid guidelines for fruits and vegetables may help lower your cancer risk! *See "Antioxidant Nutrients: A Closer Look" and "Phytonutrients—a 'Crop' for Good Health" in chapter 4.*

Could dietary supplements offer similar benefits? That's a question that science has not yet answered. Foods are likely more effective than supplements because they provide a full array of substances in a safe and effective mix.

● Go easy on alcoholic beverages, if you drink them. Excessive drinking increases risks for liver, mouth, throat, pharynx, larynx, and esophagus cancers—even more if you smoke. As with other health problems, moderation is the key—no more than one drink daily for women, two for men. Some studies suggest: breast cancer risk may go up even with moderate drinking. Regular consumption of even a few drinks per week is linked to increased risk of breast cancer in women—especially for those who come up short on folate. Drinking also may increase colorectal cancer risk.

● Limit saturated fat and salt. When it comes to health risks related to high-saturated-fat eating, heart disease is "top of mind" for many people. Yet this approach to eating also is linked to some types of cancer, including colon, rectum, and prostate cancers.

Why limit salt-cured, salt-pickled, and smoked foods? They may increase the risk for stomach cancer, especially among people and cultures who eat a lot of salt-preserved foods. There's no evidence that the amounts of salt used in cooking or in flavoring foods affects cancer risk.

See chapters 3 and 7 for tips on less fat and salt.

● Avoid eating charred foods. Be aware that high-temperature cooking, such as grilling, broiling, and pan-frying, of meat, poultry, and fish cause heterocyclic amines (HCAs) to form. When fat from these foods drips onto fire, smoke and flames leave another substance, polycyclic aromatic hydrocarbons (PAHs), behind. Both HCAs and PAHs are potential carcinogens. Occasional high-heat cooking and eating of darkened foods are no cause for concern. However, a lot of high-heat cooking (not vegetables or fruits) may possibly increase the chances of stomach and colorectal cancers, but that too is uncertain. For more about food's functional benefits to potentially lower cancer risk, *refer to "Phytonutrients—a 'Crop' for Good Health" in chapter 4, "Functional Foods: A New Wave" in chapter 9, and "Functional Foods: What Does Research Say?" in the Appendices. See chapter 13 for tips on smart grilling.*

Smart Living for Reducing Cancer Risk

● Make your life a "nonsmoking" zone. Smoking, chewing tobacco, and secondhand smoke are linked to most cancer deaths in the United States. Although women fear breast cancer, more die annually of lung cancer linked to cigarette smoking. Smoking also lowers blood levels of some protective nutrients. In fact, smoking increases the chances of many other cancers, including oral, throat, esophageal, stomach, liver, prostate, and colorectal cancers. By quitting, the risk gradually declines. For those who don't quit smoking, eat more fruit and vegetables. Many studies show that lung cancer risk goes down among smokers and nonsmokers when they consumed more fruits and vegetables. Be aware: Taking high doses of beta carotene and/or vitamin A supplements *increases* (not decreases) lung cancer risk. Avoid these supplements!

● Limit your exposure to the sun, as well as sunlamps and tanning booths, to reduce your skin cancer risk. As part of your daily routine, wear protective clothing and UV-absorbing sunglasses (blocking 99 to 100% UV rays), and use sunblock to protect your skin. A sunscreen with an SPF of 15 to 29 offers moderate protection; an SPF of 30 or more offers more protection, advised if you're highly sensitive to the sun. Many moisturizing creams come with built-in sunscreen. Try to avoid peak sun exposure: 10:00 A.M. to 4:00 P.M. (when your shadow is shorter than you are).

Testing, Testing: Cancer Screening for Early Detection

Cancer develops gradually. The best cure: Stop cancer as soon as possible. That's why early detection is so important! On a monthly basis, perform self-exams: breast, testicular, skin. And make sure your regular physical checkups include routine cancer screening:

● Breast cancer—mammogram for women age forty or older, every year.

● Colorectal cancer—age fifty or over, sigmoidoscopy (rectum and lower colon) and colonoscopy (entire colon and rectum) every ten years; fecal occult blood (blood in the stool) every five years; and double contrast barium enema every five years.

● Cervical cancer—annual Pap smear or as advised by your doctor for women.

● Skin cancer—a yearly all-over skin examination.

● Other screening—for prostate and testicular cancer for men, for ovarian cancer for women, and for oral and lung cancers, as advised by your doctor.

In addition to cancer screening, be alert to symptoms of cancer: thickening or a lump in the breast or elsewhere, obvious change in a wart or a mole, a sore that doesn't heal, a nagging cough or hoarseness, changes in bowel or bladder habits, indigestion or difficulty swallowing, unexplained changes in weight, and unusual bleeding or discharge. See your doctor; the symptoms can indicate other things besides cancer.

Have You Ever Wondered

. . . what medical nutrition therapy is? Often abbreviated as MNT, it's essential to comprehensive health care. For Medicare reimbursement, MNT is defined by the government as nutrition diagnoses, therapy, and counseling for the purpose of managing disease. Appropriate for many different health conditions and diseases, these services must be provided by a registered dietitian or a nutrition professional often referred by a physician, as part of safe, effective, overall care. Medical nutrition therapy is always individualized, in-depth care that's provided over time, not in a single visit, to meet very specific needs.

Most important, many people receiving care for health problems and illness can improve their health and well-being with medical nutrition therapy, and perhaps reduce their doctor visits, hospitalizations, and medication use.

Cancer Treatment: Handling Some Side Effects

Treatment and cancer itself often result in uncomfortable side effects that affect the desire and the ability to eat. If you experience these problems, these tips might make eating easier and more appealing. Remember, good nutrition is part of your treatment and your feeling of well-being.

If You . . .	You Can . . .
Have changes in your sense of taste and smell	• Try changing the temperature at which you eat certain foods. Hot foods may smell and taste stronger, so serving at a cool temperature may help. As cold foods get warmer, a sweet taste may get more pronounced, which may or may not be desirable. • Season foods with tart flavors (lemon, other citrus fruit, vinegar) or sweet flavors (sugar, honey, syrup) depending on the taste problem. • Chew sugar-free lemon drops, mints, or gum to remove bitter or metallic taste. (Avoid sugarless gums if you have diarrhea.) Use plastic, not stainless, flatware. • If a food tastes too sweet, add salt or a sour taste to counteract the sweetness. If a food is too salty, bitter, or sour, adding sugar may help. • Rinse your mouth with a water solution—1 quart water, ¾ teaspoon salt, and 1 teaspoon baking soda—before eating to clear your taste buds. Avoid mouth rinse with alcohol if your mouth is sore or irritated. • Rinse your mouth and brush your teeth frequently to help with a bad taste in your mouth.
Have a poor appetite	• Eat five or six small meals instead of three larger meals. • Make the meal more enjoyable with flowers and nice dishes. Play music or watch your favorite TV show. Eat with family or friends. • Keep nutrient-rich snacks handy to eat when you're hungry: hard-cooked eggs, peanut butter, yogurt, cereal and milk, cheese, ice cream, granola bars, nutritional drinks and puddings, crackers, pretzels, hearty soup. • Eat high-calorie, high-protein foods at meals and snacktime. • Ask your doctor about medications to help relieve constipation, nausea, or pain if these problems are causing your poor appetite. Ask about liquid meal replacements.
Feel constipated	• Try to stick to regular routines: eat at the same times each day, and try to be regular with bowel movements. This may include medications such as Metamucil or Senokot. • Drink 8 to 10 cups of liquid daily. Try water, prune juice, warm juice, decaffeinated tea, and hot lemonade. • If you feel gaseous, limit gas-producing foods such as carbonated drinks, broccoli, cabbage, cauliflower, cucumbers, legumes (beans), and onions. To keep from swallowing air, drink through a straw, limit talking while you eat, and avoid chewing gum. To avoid or get rid of gas from gas-promoting food, use a supplement like Beano, or with simethicone. • Eat high-fiber bulky foods, such as whole-grain products, fruits and vegetables (skins on), popcorn, and legumes. Make sure a high-fiber diet is advised. • Talk to your dietitian about a high-calorie, high-protein, fiber-containing liquid supplement. • Use laxatives only with your doctor's advice. Check with your doctor if you haven't had a bowel movement for three days or more.
Have diarrhea	• Drink plenty of mild, clear liquids throughout the day to prevent dehydration. Drink them at room temperature. Fluids without caffeine may be better choices. • Eat small, frequent meals and snacks during the day. • Avoid high-fiber, high-fat (greasy, fried), spicy, or very sweet foods. When diarrhea is over, gradually eat foods with more fiber. • Limit milk products to no more than 2 cups daily if you seem to have problems with milk during the period of diarrhea. • Avoid gas-producing foods. *(See tips for dealing with constipation.)* • Drink and eat foods high in sodium and potassium. *(See chapter 7.)* Some sports drinks can help replace electrolytes lost through persistent diarrhea. • Eat foods high in pectin (a type of fiber) such as applesauce and bananas. • Call your doctor if diarrhea persists or increases, or if your stools have an unusual color or odor. • Drink at least one cup of liquid after each loose bowel movement. • Limit sugar-free gums and candies with sorbitol.

If You . . .	You Can . . .
Have mouth sores or throat irritation	• Avoid tart, acidic, or salty beverages and foods (lemon, other citrus, vinegar, pickled foods). • Avoid rough-textured foods such as dry toast, crackers, granola, and raw fruits and vegetables. • Choose cool or lukewarm foods. • Avoid alcoholic and acidic drinks, carbonated beverages, commercial mouthwashes, and tobacco. • Skip irritating seasonings such as chile powder, cloves, hot sauces, nutmeg, pepper, salsa, pepper sauce, and horseradish. Season with herbs instead. • Eat soft, bland, creamy foods such as cream soups, cheese, yogurt, mashed potatoes, cooked cereals, casseroles, milk shakes, and commercial liquid supplements. Suck on fruit ices and ice chips. • Blend and moisten dry or solid foods. • Puree or liquefy foods in a blender to make them easier to swallow. • Tilt your head back and forth to help foods and liquids flow to the back of your throat for easier swallowing. • Drink through a straw to bypass mouth sores. • Eat high-protein, high-calorie foods to speed healing. • Rinse your mouth often with baking soda mouthwash (l quart of water, $3/4$ teaspoon of salt, and 1 tablespoon of baking soda) to remove food and germs.
Feel nauseous or queasy	• Eat six to eight small meals a day instead of three larger ones. • Eat dry foods such as crackers or dry cereals when you awaken and every few hours. • Choose foods that don't have a strong odor; eat foods that are cool, not icy cold or hot. • Avoid foods that are very sweet, fatty, greasy, or spicy. • Sit up or recline your head slightly for an hour after eating. • Sip clear fluids—water, juice, flat soda, sports drink—throughout the day. • Talk to your doctor about antinausea medication. • Try bland, easy-to-digest foods: perhaps chicken noodle soup with saltines. • Eat in a cool well-ventilated room without food and cooking odors or other aromas. • Rinse your mouth before and after meals, and after vomiting, with plain water. • Drink eight or more cups of fluids daily if you can, and an additional $1/2$ to 1 cup for each vomiting episode. Sip fluids 30 to 60 minutes *after* eating. Try to consume sips of apple and cranberry juice, flat soft drinks, broth, bites of frozen flavored ice.
Have a dry mouth or thick saliva	• Drink 8 to 10 cups of liquid daily to loosen mucus. Take a water bottle with you when away from home. • Eat soft, bland foods cold or at room temperature. Try blenderized fruits and vegetables; soft, cooked beef, chicken, or fish; well-thinned cereals; Popsicles; and slushies. • Moisten foods with broth, soup, sauce, gravy, butter, or margarine. Dip or soak food in what you are drinking. • Suck on sour lemon drops. Avoid chewing ice cubes that can damage your teeth. Chew sugarless gum to stimulate saliva flow. • Keep your lips moist and mouth clean with a soft-bristle toothbrush. Rinse your mouth before and after eating with plain water or a mild mouth rinse (made with 1 quart of water, $3/4$ teaspoon of salt, and 1 teaspoon of baking soda). Floss regularly. • Avoid commercial mouthwashes, alcoholic and acidic beverages, and tobacco. • Limit caffeinated drinks and foods that have a diuretic effect: coffee, tea, cola, chocolate. • Moisten room air with a cool mist humidifier. Keep it clean to avoid the spread of bacteria.
Have trouble swallowing	• Get advice from your healthcare provider on the best diet and fluid consistency for you. • Drink 6 to 8 cups of fluid daily, thickened to a consistency right for you. • Report any coughing or choking while eating to your doctor right away, especially if you have a fever. • Eat small, frequent meals. • Use liquid nutritional supplements if you can't eat enough food. • Ask a registered dietitian to recommend thickening products and help you know how to use them: gelatin, tapioca, cornstarch, or flour, commercial thickeners, pureed vegetables, instant potatoes, dry infant rice cereal.

Source: Adapted from B. Eldridge and K. K. Hamilton, *Management of Nutrition Impact Symptoms in Cancer and Educational Handouts* (Chicago: American Dietetic Association, 2004).

For more specifics on screening, check the advice of the American Cancer Society's ACS Cancer Detection Guidelines at www.cancer.org and talk to your doctor.

If You're Dealing with a Cancer Diagnosis . . .

Good nutrition is essential if you've been diagnosed with cancer. Your nutrition needs are unique to your cancer, the treatment, and your personal preferences. The goals? To maintain weight and keep up your energy level and strength. To do that, you may need high-calorie foods and more proteins. That may be a change from the way you've been eating and a challenge when you don't feel well. *For tips on boosting calories, see chapter 2.* However, some cancer treatments can cause weight gain. In that case, it is important to maintain a healthy weight.

Besides helping you feel stronger and better, good nutrition helps you handle the side effects of cancer treatment, reduce your chance of infection, and assist with your recovery from treatment or surgery.

Safe food handling takes on even more importance since your immune response may not function as well as normal. With a low white blood cell count (common during chemotherapy and radiation) your body may not be able to fight infection or harmful foodborne bacteria effectively. *For guidance on food safety, see chapter 12.*

A registered dietitian can help you with a plan for managing food choices if you're dealing with cancer. Ask your physician or healthcare professional for a referral to a registered dietitian.

Before Treatment or Surgery

Prepare—make good nutrition part of your pretreatment approach to cancer recovery. Start with a positive mind-set. Eat for health; being well nourished is a strategy for building your strength and reserves before surgery or treatment begins. Plan ahead by stocking your kitchen with foods you can eat while you're dealing with the possible side effects of treatment. Have nutritious snacks on hand; you may not have the energy to prepare food, or the appetite to eat. Gather your support team so you'll have help if and when you need it for food shopping, food preparation, and companionship. A support group dealing with

cancer also is helpful for both psychological support and practical tips. Ask your doctor, nurse, social worker, or other healthcare professional about support groups.

During "Chemo" and Radiation

Cancer treatment requires powerful medication or radiation that not only kills cancer cells but also can damage healthy body cells, resulting in possibly uncomfortable side effects. Careful food choices can help control some of the side effects that result from treatment. Most side effects go away once treatment is over.

To deal with side effects of chemotherapy or radiation that affect your ability to eat, try the strategies

Have You Ever Wondered

... how to protect against breast cancer? Scientists don't yet know, but the question is under investigation. Until we learn more, the best advice is to engage in moderate to vigorous physical activity 45 to 60 minutes five or more days per week to minimize lifetime weight gain through the combination of caloric restriction and regular physical activity and to avoid or limit intake of alcoholic beverages. Men can develop breast cancer, too. *See "Breast Cancer: Do Food Choices Make a Difference?" in chapter 17.*

... if shark cartilage is effective against cancer? Touted as an anticancer agent, the active components in shark cartilage have not been identified. Limited scientific research doesn't support its use in blocking tumor formation. Because it may affect the development of blood vessels, taking shark cartilage could be risky for pregnant women and for those recovering from wounds, surgery, or heart ailments. Beyond that, shark cartilage taken as an oral supplement may not be absorbed by the body—and it may not be pure shark cartilage.

... if laetrile is an appropriate supplement for cancer treatment? Promoted as vitamin B_{17}, laetrile (also called amygdalin) isn't a vitamin. Instead it's a substance derived from the pits of apricots and other fruits. Although proposed as a treatment for cancer, laetrile contains cyanide, which can be lethal. Laetrile is neither approved by the FDA nor legal to import into the United States.

described here to stay well nourished. Frequent minimeals, for example, might help. If you feel tired, ask your family or a friend to help you with meals—or arrange for home-delivered meals to preserve your strength. *See "Cancer Treatment: Handling Side Effects" in this chapter.* For more advice, especially if side effects persist, talk to a registered dietitian.

Caution: talk to your doctor about any alternative or complementary therapies, such as herbal products, vitamins, or minerals, before you try them to relieve symptoms or to promote the quality of your life. Although some are safe and harmless, others can interfere with the effects of radiation or chemotherapy, or with your recovery from surgery. Some may have harmful side effects.

Chemotherapy. Chemotherapy uses oral or injected medications to stop or slow the progress of cancer cell growth. Among its common side effects are fatigue, diarrhea or constipation, nausea and vomiting, mouth tenderness or sores, and changes in the way food tastes and smells. To help you cope with the unpleasant effects of chemotherapy:

- Eat before your treatment. If your treatment takes several hours, bring a light snack along unless a light snack is offered during your treatment.

- When your appetite is good between treatments, nourish yourself well.

- As important, cut yourself some slack. Some people experience changes or loss of taste and smell during "chemo." Do your best when it's challenging to eat, and know that the side effects of chemotherapy usually go away once treatment is over.

See "Cancer Treatment: Handling Side Effects" in this chapter.

Radiation. This form of therapy damages cancer cells with a series of daily treatments of radiation. Side effects depend on the area of the body being treated, the dosage, and the frequency of treatment. These can be nausea, vomiting, sore throat or mouth, loss of taste, dry mouth, difficulty swallowing, diarrhea, or loss of appetite. Many side effects contribute to eating problems, yet good nutrition is important during and after what may be several weeks of treatment. To help you cope with the side effects of radiation:

- Eat before your daily treatment.

- If it takes time to get to a treatment center, bring along food to eat before and afterward. If you need to stay overnight, make plans beforehand for convenient, easy, and nutritious meals and snacks.

- Give your body time to get over any side effects. Often they don't appear right away, but can last two or three weeks after treatments stop.

See "Cancer Treatment: Handling Some Side Effects" in this chapter.

Cancer Survival: After Treatment Ends

No special diet after cancer diagnosis and treatment can prevent the recurrence of cancer. Cancer survivors are at greater risk for other cancers. And obesity is linked to breast cancer recurrence. However, healthful eating, appropriate weight, and a physically active lifestyle can make a difference for overall health, quality of life, and longevity! Being well nourished can help you gradually rebuild your strength after treatment.

Try to follow guidance from MyPyramid. Consult with a registered dietitian about any side effects that persist. *See "Resources You Can Use" for resources for cancer treatment and cancer survival.*

Diabetes: A Growing Health Concern

Diabetes has become an epidemic, affecting about twenty-one million Americans. Yet more than six million of them—*perhaps you or someone in your family*—don't know they have it! And nearly one million more each year are predicted to get it.

In 2005 the U.S. Department of Health and Human Services and the American Diabetes Association estimated that about 41 million Americans ages 40 to 74 have pre-diabetes, which sharply raises the risk for developing type 2 diabetes and increases the risk of heart disease by 50 percent. Most people with pre-diabetes are apt to develop diabetes within a decade unless they make modest changes in both their food choices and their physical activity level.

If it's not managed properly, diabetes can have serious, even life-threatening, effects on health: eye problems including blindness, circulatory problems, nerve disease, and kidney disease and failure, among others. In fact, diabetes is the leading cause of blindness, leg and foot amputations, and kidney disease, and the sixth-leading cause of death in the United States. Diabetes also is a major risk factor for heart attacks and stroke. Damage can add up. Even during pre-diabetes, some long-term damage, especially to the heart and circulatory system, may occur. The best way to reduce the risks for these problems is to keep your blood sugar level near the normal range.

What Is Diabetes?

Simply defined, diabetes is a physiological condition that affects the way the body uses energy from sugar, starch, and other foods. Carbohydrates (sugars and starches) don't cause diabetes. Instead insulin, a hormone produced by the pancreas, isn't produced or doesn't work correctly in the body and therefore, can't be used properly for energy metabolism.

How does insulin work for healthy people? During digestion, glucose is released from carbohydrates and absorbed to circulate as blood glucose, or blood sugar, to body cells. Among healthy people, insulin regulates blood sugar levels. It allows glucose to pass from blood into body cells for energy production. Insulin also helps the body use amino acids and fatty acids from food. For people without diabetes, insulin helps blood sugar levels stay in a normal range so eating has little effect on blood sugar.

With diabetes, the body can't control blood sugar levels normally. Too little or no insulin, or the inability to use insulin properly, hinders the body's ability to use energy nutrients—carbohydrates, proteins, and fats. Instead of "feeding" cells, glucose accumulates in blood, causing blood sugar levels to rise. Since it can't be used for energy, blood glucose spills into urine and gets excreted. That makes extra work for the kidneys, causing frequent urination and excessive thirst. Over time, high blood glucose levels can cause damage to kidneys, eyes, nerves, and the heart. As a key energy source, glucose is lost.

Diabetes belongs in these main categories:

Pre-diabetes. When a person's blood glucose levels are higher than normal but not high enough for a diagnosis of type 2 diabetes, they have pre-diabetes.

Type 1 Diabetes. Type 1 diabetes, an autoimmune disease, accounts for 5 to 10 percent of diabetes cases. In this form of diabetes, the pancreas can't make insulin. Pancreatic beta cells that produce insulin have been destroyed, perhaps due to heredity or to damage prompted by a virus. The causes aren't clear. Why is it an autoimmune disease? "Auto" refers to "self"; the immune system, which normally protects the body from disease, instead attacks the beta cells that produce insulin.

The symptoms of type 1 diabetes often begin in childhood or the young adult years. However, people of any age can develop type 1 diabetes. Daily insulin injections or a continuous insulin pump, along with a careful eating and physical activity plan, are required to manage type 1 diabetes. Type 1 diabetes requires regular self-monitoring of blood glucose levels.

Type 2 Diabetes. Type 2 diabetes, a metabolic disorder, accounts for 90 to 95 percent of diabetes cases, with the incidence rising along with obesity rates, sedentary lifestyles, and an aging population, as well as better or early detection. About 80 percent of those with type 2 diabetes are overweight. With type 2 diabetes, pancreatic cells don't produce enough insulin or don't respond to insulin normally (insulin resistance), even though the pancreas produces insulin.

Type 2 diabetes develops slowly and usually becomes evident after age forty; however, obese children are increasingly at risk, too. In type 2 diabetes, blood sugar levels often can be controlled through food choices, weight control, and physical activity alone. Taking oral hypoglycemic medicines may help the body produce more insulin or better use the insulin the body makes. Sometimes insulin injections are needed, too. Type 2 diabetes also requires regular self-monitoring of blood glucose levels.

Gestational Diabetes. Gestational diabetes occurs in about 4 percent of pregnancies, resulting from changes in hormone levels. The risk is higher among obese and older women. Although it usually disappears after delivery, gestational diabetes needs careful control during pregnancy. Women with gestational diabetes often develop type 2 diabetes later in life, and usually in later pregnancies. *See "Pregnancy and Diabetes" in chapter 17 for more information on gestational diabetes.*

Early Detection

Early detection of diabetes is important. The longer the body is exposed to high blood sugar levels, the greater the damage to the nervous and circulatory systems and to the blood vessels in the eyes, kidneys, heart, and feet. The early years of diabetes offer an opportunity. If you have diabetes, that's when you can do the most to prevent or reduce its long-term consequences—and so live a longer life with fewer health problems.

According to the American Diabetes Association, many people don't know they have diabetes—despite the harmful consequences, even when diabetes goes undetected for several years.

How would you know if you have it? These are common symptoms: frequent urination, unusual thirst, extreme hunger, unusual weight loss, extreme fatigue, and irritability. In addition, those with type 2 diabetes also may experience frequent infections; cuts and bruises that heal slowly; blurred vision; numb or tingling hands or feet; or recurring skin, gum, or bladder infections. Some people with type 2 diabetes have no outward signs associated with high blood sugar levels. Keeping tabs on your blood sugar level is the way to really know.

At Risk for Type 2?

With this growing epidemic, what puts someone at risk for type 2 diabetes? The odds go up with these risk factors:

● *Being over age forty-five.* With age, the pancreas is less efficient at producing insulin.

● *Having a close family member with diabetes.* You may have an inherited tendency or share circumstances that increase your risk.

● *Being in some racial or ethnic groups.* If you're of African American, Latino, Asian American, Pacific Islander, or Native American descent, your diabetes risk is higher.

● *Being overweight or obese.* With more body fat, body cells become more insulin-resistant.

● *Being physically inactive.*

● *Having low HDL cholesterol levels or high triglycerides.*

● *Having had gestational diabetes, or delivering a baby weighing 9 pounds or more.*

Even if you're at risk for type 2 diabetes, there's good news: With regular moderate exercise and weight reduction, if you're overweight, your odds drop.

Testing, Testing: Blood Sugar Tests

Diabetes may be detected first by a urine test, given as a routine part of most physical exams. However, blood glucose readings are much more accurate. Everyone age forty-five or over should have a blood glucose test every three years. If you're at high risk, blood glucose testing should start sooner and be more frequent. Be aware that screening tests, often done at community health events, aren't diagnostic, yet they can identify those at high risk who need further testing.

Done during a checkup, a blood glucose reading is done after an eight-hour fast. A fasting plasma glucose (blood glucose) of less than 100 milligrams/deciliter (mg/dL) is considered normal. Two readings of 126 mg/dL or higher, taken on different days, are criteria for a diabetes diagnosis. A fasting blood glucose level between 100 and 125 mg/dL signals pre-diabetes. Another test, the Oral Glucose Tolerance Test (OGTT), can also be used to diagnose diabetes. It's not as fast, and it costs more.

If you're diagnosed with diabetes, you may need to self-monitor, or test your own blood glucose. Without testing you won't know your blood glucose level unless it's very high or very low. Your doctor will set realistic target blood glucose levels for you—for example, before meals and bedtime. Before meals, a blood glucose level of 90 to 130 mg/dL is considered the target; about two hours after a meal, it should be less than 180 mg/dl. Your doctor, dietitian, or certified diabetes educator will show you how to self-monitor. Be aware that target levels for young children and older adults may differ.

Checking your blood glucose is easy once you get used to pricking your finger or forearm: just a drop of blood on a test strip or a sensor, read by a blood glucose meter. Record the results, the time, and the date. Or use a blood glucose monitor that stores the readings for you. Use the information to see if your diabetes care plan (eating, exercise, and medication) is working. Share your log with your doctor.

Once you become adept at self-monitoring, you can use your blood glucose reading to know if you need to eat something or take medication. If your blood glucose is too low (perhaps below 70 mg/dL) or too high (perhaps above 240 mg/dL), you'll need to do something. Many factors determine the right blood glucose goals for someone with diabetes. While these levels have been set by the American Diabetes Association, your doctor can help you set your personal targets.

There's another blood glucose test: glycosylated hemoglobin, or hemoglobin A1c. Done every two or three months during your doctor visit, this test measures your average blood glucose over the past two to three months, and whether your blood sugar levels are under control. It may be used as a diagnostic test, too.

To control blood sugar levels and diabetes-related complications, ongoing monitoring means testing your "ABCs": A for hemoglobin A1C, B for blood pressure, and C for cholesterol levels.

If you have type 1 diabetes, your doctor also may advise you to take a urine test for ketones, which are acids that build up in urine to toxic levels. When there is no insulin available, your body cells can't use glucose for energy and so turn to burning fat, not carbohydrates, for energy. Without carbohydrates, or glucose, body cells can't burn fat completely, and ketones form as a by-product of fat burning. When ketones build up, a condition called ketoacidosis can occur and, if left untreated, can lead to a diabetic coma and even death. Talk to your doctor about the early symptoms; get immediate medical help if keto-acidosis develops.

If You Have Diabetes . . .

The goal for diabetes management is this: controlling your blood sugar levels so they stay as near to normal as possible. Like a teeter-totter, blood sugar levels go up (hyperglycemia) and down (hypoglycemia); that's part of dealing with diabetes. Those swings can be dangerous when diet, physical activity, and medication such as insulin aren't balanced properly.

● *Too much food or too little insulin?* Your blood sugar level can soar, affecting your health now and very seriously down the road.

● *Too much exercise or too much insulin?* Blood

sugar drops, and your body can't use blood glucose to produce enough energy.

To control "the ups and the downs," carefully manage what you eat, how much, and when—*no matter what type of diabetes you have.* Eating raises your blood sugar level; physical activity and medication lower it. For example, in case of low blood sugar, consume a *small amount* of a quick-acting carbohydrate, such as ½ cup juice, followed by a small amount of protein food, perhaps a cheese cube on a cracker.

Your doctor likely will advise a regular physical activity plan to help you control your blood sugar levels and prevent weight gain, too—and may advise sensible weight loss if you're overweight. For many people, smart eating, weight loss, and active living are enough to control their blood sugar level and to maintain good health. Others need diabetes medication.

Here's some general advice about managing diabetes and preventing its symptoms. For individualized guidance that matches your needs, consult your doctor and a registered dietitian (RD). Some dietitians and nurses are certified diabetes educators (CDEs).

If you've just found out that you have diabetes, you may feel healthy. Even if it's hard to remember to stick with your eating and physical activity program, the long-term benefits are well worth the effort!

Manage Your Meals and Snacks

The game plan for smart eating with diabetes follows this general strategy: *Eat about the same amount of food, in the right balance, at about the same time daily; to avoid weight gain, balance your day's food choices with regular physical activity.* In the big picture, eating with diabetes follows principles of healthful eating for anybody—in fact, for your whole family. *See the Dietary Guidelines in chapter 1.* That can make meal management simpler.

What is the "right balance"? It's *food variety* with a balance of different types of food . . . *portion savvy* to eat the right amount of food . . . and *control of energy-producing nutrients* (carbohydrates, fats, and proteins).

For diabetes, there's no single eating plan; the guidelines have built-in flexibility. The amount and proportions of carbohydrates, proteins, and fats—the energy nutrients—you consume depend on you and your weight, blood cholesterol levels, and medical

FOOD GUIDE FOR DIABETES: A GUIDE TO AMOUNTS

This food guide for diabetes can be your daily eating plan, especially for type 2 diabetes. Follow this serving guide, based on your day's calorie needs.

CATEGORIES	SERVINGS FOR 1,200 TO 1,600 CALORIES	SERVINGS FOR 1,600 TO 2,000 CALORIES	SERVINGS FOR 2,000 TO 2,400 CALORIES	A SERVING IS*
Starchy foods (bread, cereal, rice, pasta, beans, and starchy vegetables)	6	8	11	1 slice bread ⅓ cup rice ½ cup cooked cereal ¾ cup dry cereal flakes 1 small baked potato ½ cup cooked legumes (dry beans)
Vegetables (except for starchy vegetables)	3	4	4	½ cup tomato juice ½ cup cooked green or deep yellow vegetables 1 cup raw, leafy greens
Fruit	2	3	3	1 small apple ½ cup fruit juice 2 tbsp. dry fruit ½ cup canned fruit
Milk and yogurt	2	2	2	1 cup fat-free milk 8 ounces nonfat yogurt
Meat or meat substitutes	2	2	2	2 to 3 oz. cooked fish, chicken, or lean meat 2 oz. cheese ½ cup tofu
Fats	Up to 3	Up to 4	Up to 5	1 tbsp. regular salad dressing 1 tsp. regular margarine or oil 2 tbsp. light salad dressing 1 tbsp. light mayonnaise 1 bacon strip 6 whole peanuts

*Ask a registered dietitian or a certified diabetes educator where other foods fit.

Source: National Institute of Diabetes and Digestive and Kidney Diseases, 2003.

needs. Specific food choices are up to you, too, and what foods you enjoy. Your doctor, along with a registered dietitian, can help you plan what's right for you—portion sizes, types of food, and overall timing.

Portion savvy is important in diabetes management. Get out your measuring cups and spoons, and the kitchen scale. Measure your portions, as well as your cups, bowls, and dishes, until you get familiar with serving sizes.

Tip: People with diabetes often have high blood pressure and risks for heart disease, or they may acquire these conditions down the line. As precautions, eat for heart health and control your salt/sodium intake if you have diabetes. Talk to your healthcare provider for guidance. *See "Your Healthy Heart" and "Blood Pressure: Under Control?" in this chapter.*

Food Guide for Diabetes. The food guide for diabetes is a starting point to plan meals and snacks for diabetes management. *It's similar to MyPyramid shown in chapter 10,* but adjusted to help people with diabetes manage carbohydrates and other energy nutrients more easily. As you look at this guide, notice:

● The guide has "Starchy foods" with grain products, as well as starchy vegetables (potatoes, legumes, corn).

● "Meat and meat substitutes" include fish, poultry, meat, and tofu, as well as cheese. Despite their protein content, legumes (dry beans) fit with "starchy foods."

● The "Milk and yogurt" group doesn't include cheese.

It's well known that sugar doesn't cause diabetes; neither do any carbohydrates. Sugar doesn't cause blood sugar levels to rise any more than starches do. Starches (pasta, rice, bread, fruits and vegetables, and other starchy foods) and sugars have a similar effect on blood sugar levels. People with diabetes can fit small amounts of sugary foods into their eating plan as carbohydrate foods. For diabetes management, the total carbohydrates consumed counts, not just sugars. **Caution:** Many sugary foods are low in nutrients and high in fat.

If you like sweet flavors, then very-low-calorie sweeteners (acesulfame potassium, aspartame, saccharin, and sucralose) offer some choices without increasing your blood sugar level or adding calories.

For example, look for diet soft drinks, sugar-free candy, and ice cream with these sweeteners. These foods may allow you to fit other foods in. For example, by choosing yogurt sweetened with an intense sweetener instead of sugared fruit, you might fit toast, a muffin, or crackers into your eating plan, too. **Warning:** If you have the disorder phenylketonuria (PKU), avoid foods sweetened with aspartame. *See "Aspartame: PKU Warning" in chapter 21.*

Polyols (sorbitol, mannitol, and xylitol) are sweeteners with fewer calories than sugar. They affect blood sugar level, but not as much as sugar and other nutritive sweeteners do. *See "Intense Sweeteners:*

Have You Ever Wondered

. . . if going "low carb" would be a good approach for managing diabetes? Your goal should be to manage the carbohydrates in your food choices, not eliminate them. After all, you need the glucose (blood sugar) from carbohydrates as energy for your brain and other body cells. Remember: with diabetes, the issue is how insulin, which may be inadequate or not working properly, handles carbohydrates—not whether you need carbohydrates.

Whether you use exchange lists or carbohydrate counting to control energy nutrients, make the most of your "carb" choices by fitting in those foods that offer other nutrients, as well as fiber, too: whole-grain cereals, breads, crackers, and pasta; whole fruits and vegetables; soups, chili, stews, salads, and other dishes with cooked dry beans; wild rice, brown rice, and barley dishes; and vegetarian burgers. Low-fat or fat-free milk and yogurt, which contain lactose (milk sugar), are also nutrient-rich choices.

Talk to your registered dietitian or diabetes educator to help you use food labels to manage your "carb" intake. The Nutrition Facts can help you. Look at the serving number, serving size, and calories and nutrients per serving. Count the total carbohydrates, not just the sugars, in a serving. Talk to your registered dietitian or diabetes educator about adjusting for foods with fiber and sugar alcohols. Be wary of label claims, such as "net carbs," "low carb," or "low impact carbs," which aren't approved claims at this time. Consider calories, too, as you take steps to healthful eating.

Flavor without Calories" and "Sugar Alcohols: Sugar Replacers" in chapter 5.

A few more tips: As you make your choices, choose mostly lean, low-fat, and fat-free foods, not only for diabetes management but also to help keep blood lipid levels within a healthy range. Enjoy deep-yellow and orange vegetables and fruits; besides their other benefits, their beta carotene content may help reduce problems related to type 2 diabetes. *Reminder:* Sugar-free doesn't mean calorie-free. And fat-free foods can have more carbohydrates than their traditional counterparts.

How about dietary fiber? Follow the same guidelines as for those who don't have diabetes: for men up to age fifty years, the Adequate Intake (AI) is 38 grams total fiber daily; for women that age, it's 25 grams daily. After age fifty, the AI is slightly less. Besides the overall benefits, fiber slows digestion and may slow glucose absorption during digestion. And fiber helps you feel full after eating—an aid to weight control. Extra amounts, perhaps from fiber supplements, won't offer significant added benefits. *See chapter 6, "Fiber: Your Body's Broom."*

Exchanges or Carbohydrate Counting? For more control of energy nutrients (carbohydrates, fats, proteins), your dietitian or diabetes educator can help you use exchange lists or carbohydrate counting.

Exchanges are like food groups in MyPyramid. They're lists of foods grouped together because they're alike; they're similar in carbohydrate, protein, fat, and calorie content. For that reason, foods within each list can be exchanged for other foods. Exchange lists fit within three overall groups: Carbohydrate Group (starch, fruit, milk, other carbohydrates, and vegetables lists), Meat and Meat Substitutes (very lean, lean, medium-fat, and high-fat meat and substitutes lists), and Fat Group (monounsaturated, polyunsaturated, and saturated fat lists). (Alcohol counts as fat exchanges.)

With specific numbers of exchanges from each list, you plan meals and snacks to get enough food variety and to spread out calories and energy-producing nutrients throughout the day. That helps you maintain your blood sugar level near normal, and balance food with exercise and diabetes medicines. Exchanges are published in *Exchange Lists for Meal Planning* from the American Dietetic Association and the American Diabetes Association.

Carbohydrate counting is another tool for managing your food intake and for keeping your blood glucose level in check. It allows you to more precisely match your food and insulin intake. It's an approach that's good for people who need tight control and are willing to make the effort.

With this approach, you keep track of the total carbohydrate grams you eat and drink for a day, trying to eat about the same number of carbohydrates, at the same time, each day. Remember, carbohydrates have more effect on blood sugar than any other nutrient. (*Tip:* For any meal or snack, try to keep within 5 grams of your target. The more "carbs" you consume, the higher your blood glucose level.) You need to take your fat and protein intake into account, too, since they also increase your blood sugar level to some degree.

With carbohydrate counting, your "carbs" can come from any food source. Nutrient-rich foods (grain products, fruits, vegetables, legumes, and milk) are best, since together they supply vitamins, minerals, fiber, and phytonutrients. Sugary foods are often low in vitamins and nutrients, and perhaps high in fat.

Whatever approach to meal and snack planning you use:

● Get advice from a registered dietitian or a certified diabetes educator for an eating plan that's right for you—including how many exchanges from each exchange list, or how many carbohydrate grams, to strive for daily. Plan how you'll spread out your eating during the day, too.

● Choose a variety of nutrient-rich foods. Aim for 50 to 60 percent of calories from carbohydrates. In a 2,000-calorie daily plan, that's 1,000 to 1,200 calories from total "carbs," or 250 to 300 carbohydrate grams. (One carbohydrate gram supplies 4 calories.) Your calorie needs depend on your age, physical activity level, body size, and perhaps a weight-loss plan.

● Check Nutrition Facts on food labels to know total carbohydrate grams, as well as fat and protein grams, in a single serving. Serving sizes on labels also can help with meal planning, using exchange lists or *the food guide for diabetes on page 569. To learn how to use food labels, see chapter 11.*

● If you're counting "carbs" for unpackaged or restaurant foods, *check "'Carbo' Foods" in the Appendices.*

For a more extensive list, find a book or a Web site source of carbohydrate facts; ask for nutrition information for restaurant menus when you eat out. If you eat at national chains, check their Web sites. Counting "carbs" in mixed foods takes a little know-how.

● To stick to your plan, be careful about portion sizes. Even for carbohydrate counting, learn serving sizes for exchanges—for example, ⅓ cup rice, or one carbohydrate exchange, provides 15 grams of carbohydrates.

Check Your Clock. Keep to a regular meal and snack schedule—about the same amount of food, at about the same time daily—to keep your blood sugar level steady. Skipping meals or following an irregular eating pattern puts your blood sugar level out of kilter. To compound the problem, meal skipping may lead

Have You Ever Wondered

. . . if people with diabetes should make food choices based on a food's glycemic index? First the definition: Glycemic index shows a food's potential for raising blood glucose level. Eating a food with a glycemic index of less than 70 produces a lower increase in blood glucose level; above 70, it's higher. Although it may surprise you, the glycemic index for sugar (92) is less than for mashed potatoes or white bread (100).

Whether there's any health benefit to selecting foods according to their glycemic index is controversial. On one hand, some research suggests that an overall eating plan with a lower glycemic response may reduce insulin response and so help lower the chances of heart disease, diabetes, and obesity. On the other hand, a glycemic index only has been established for single foods, but not for food combinations in meals and snacks or for meal size. Having a low glycemic index doesn't mean a food is high in nutrients, either. And individual responses may differ. Plus, there isn't enough evidence yet to show that using glycemic index actually improves blood glucose levels. For now, stick to well-accepted approaches for diabetes management. *To learn more, refer to chapter 5, "Hot Topic: Glycemic Index."* For some people with diabetes, glycemic index may be used for diabetes management, with the guidance of a health care provider.

. . . if eating sugar or a carbohydrate-rich diet causes insulin resistance that results in weight gain? No, but some popular weight-loss book authors say so. Consuming carbohydrate-rich foods doesn't cause insulin resistance; excessive calories do. People who are overweight and sedentary may have symptoms of insulin resistance, a condition often diminished with moderate physical activity and weight loss.

. . . how you take insulin? Insulin needs to go directly into the bloodstream, either by injection or insulin pump. Another potential alternative: powdered insulin to take with an inhaler. Although not ready in the near future, new and easier ways to take insulin are under study: an insulin spray in the mouth; and a pill that gets past the stomach undigested, getting insulin directly to the liver.

. . . if drinking cow milk during infancy causes type 1 diabetes? There's no scientific evidence that milk protein from cow milk promotes type 1 diabetes in infants with an inherited tendency for diabetes. Regardless, the American Academy of Pediatrics (AAP) encourages breast-feeding for the first year of life, for all babies, including those with a strong family history of type 1 diabetes. Some early research suggests that breast-feeding may reduce a mother's later risk for diabetes. For children age one year or older with diabetes, AAP recommends no restriction for cow milk.

. . . if you can stop taking insulin if you take chromium supplements? No. For type 1 diabetes, chromium supplements aren't an alternative to insulin. Chromium may help control blood sugar level for type 2 diabetes, but research evidence is still preliminary. If you have type 2 diabetes, talk to your doctor before taking any supplements. Enjoy foods with chromium—meat, eggs, whole-grain products, cheese—to get what you need. *See chapter 4 for more on chromium.*

. . . if herbal products have a glucose-lowering ability? Despite claims, no conclusive research shows that herbal products offer benefits for managing diabetes. Some may interact with diabetes medication. Talk to your doctor first, if you choose to try them—and never use them in place of insulin or other prescribed medicine.

Children and Diabetes

Type 1 diabetes is the most common form of diabetes among children. With the parallel rise in childhood obesity, more and more children are at risk for or diagnosed with type 2 diabetes. Dealing with diabetes during the childhood and teenage years adds to the challenges of growing up. Most kids don't want to be different.

The first guideline—help your child maintain or grow into a healthy weight to reduce the chance of type 2 diabetes. If your child is overweight, ask your doctor about testing for diabetes at about age ten or at puberty if your child has other risk factors.

If your child is diagnosed with diabetes, accept and manage it together in a calm, careful, and positive way.

- Work closely with your child's healthcare team to manage diabetes and help your child grow normally—physically, mentally, and emotionally.

- Gradually involve your child in taking responsibility for his or her diabetes. Encourage rather than nag, even when things aren't perfect. Help your child learn when, how, and where to get help. Learning lifelong skills for diabetes management—and making them a habit—is part of growing up. Diabetes won't go away.

- Get advice from your healthcare team about handling special eating events such as birthday parties, sleepovers, field trips, and active play or sports.

- Be matter-of-fact, sensitive, and supportive as you help your child or teen learn about diabetes. A support group or diabetes camp for kids can help. Find a reliable Web site for kids about diabetes.

- Help teachers, baby-sitters, coaches, school food service staff, the school nurse, and others who supervise your child understand your child's diabetes and how they can support the diabetes care plan. Meet with them. Write instructions, list symptoms, and provide phone numbers for your doctor and other responsible adults. Provide appropriate snacks. Teach a sitter how to do blood sugar checks and give diabetes medication, if needed. Ensure that your child has the time and privacy for diabetes care without discrimination.

- Help your child or teen feel comfortable about asking to leave class or play to monitor blood sugar and take insulin.

- Make diabetes management part of your parenting responsibility, but not the sole focus. Keep the joys of growing up and a healthy family life.

For more parenting tips, see chapter 16, "Food to Grow On."

---

to overeating later and to an eating pattern that won't match your plan for managing diabetes.

- *Advice:* Stick to a regular meal and snack schedule. Carry an emergency snack in case you must change your regular eating routine. Consider several small meals, often better for blood sugar control than three big meals. A registered dietitian can help you pick the best food choices for snacking. If you need insulin or other diabetes medicine, take it on schedule, too.

Go Easy: Alcoholic Drinks. Can you enjoy alcoholic drinks now and then? That's a question to discuss with your doctor *before* you drink alcoholic beverages. Some people with diabetes are wise not to drink at all.

What are some risks? Drinking can worsen some diabetes-related health problems such as high blood pressure, nerve damage from diabetes, and high triglyceride levels. Heavy drinking causes liver damage, which makes diabetes control harder. And alcoholic drinks contribute calories when you're trying to keep your weight under control. Alcoholic beverages also interfere with some diabetes medications.

If your blood glucose levels are under control and if your doctor indicates that alcoholic beverages in moderation are okay, a registered dietitian or a certified diabetes educator can help you work them into your meal plan. Keep these guidelines in mind:

- As always, limit alcoholic drinks: no more than one serving a day for women, and two for men—the same limits as for people without diabetes. A serving of alcohol is 5 ounces of wine, 12 ounces of beer, or 1½ ounces of distilled spirits. Discuss your individual limits with your doctor and registered dietitian.

● *Always* eat when you have an alcoholic drink to reduce the chance for hypoglycemia, or low blood sugar. When your liver is detoxifying alcohol, it doesn't produce as much glucose. Blood glucose that drops too low from drinking can be dangerous.

● As an alternative, choose low-alcohol wine, beer, or distilled spirits. They have fewer calories and less alcohol and carbohydrates than regular beer or sweet wine. Ask how they fit into your plan.

● Recognize that some wine coolers and mixed drinks (made with regular soda and juice) contain sugars. Count them as part of your eating plan (as fat and carbohydrate servings/exchanges) for diabetes management. Mix drinks or spritzers with sugar-free mixers such as club soda, diet soft drinks, diet tonic, seltzer, or water. Or try "virgin" drinks without alcoholic mixers.

See *"Taking Control: Drinking Responsibly!" in chapter 8.*

Get Moving

Get moving! Active living is important in managing diabetes for several reasons. For one, regular physical activity increases insulin sensitivity, moving glucose out of blood more effectively. Second, being active can lower blood sugar as your muscles use glucose for energy. Third, physical activity burns energy, making weight management easier; your body controls your blood sugar level better at a lower body weight. And fourth, regular physical activity helps reduce your risk for heart disease and high blood pressure, both linked to diabetes.

● Before you start a physical activity plan, talk with your doctor, along with a registered dietitian or a certified diabetes educator. Balance exercise with eating to keep your blood sugar level within a target range. If you take insulin, planning for physical activity is trickier.

● Before you start your physical activity, check your blood glucose level. If it's low (below 70 mg/dL or less), eat a snack with about 15 carbohydrate grams right away (a medium apple or bread slice); wait about 15 minutes, then check again. If it's 70 to 100 mg/dL, enjoy the same snack if your next meal is at least an hour away, then get moving. If your blood sugar is 100

to 150, it's okay to start, but eat a light snack if you plan to be active for thirty minutes or more. If your blood sugar is 240 mg/dL or more, wait, and get your blood sugar level down first.

● Take a carbohydrate-rich snack along when you're physically active—just in case you start feeling lightheaded. If that happens, stop moving and eat it. Too much exercise and not enough food can lead to hypoglycemia, or low blood sugar.

● Get a partner. Besides being more fun, it's safer. Let your partner know about your diabetes, and what to do if you need help.

● Wear a tag, a necklace, or a bracelet with diabetes identification. And wear proper footwear.

● Keep well hydrated when you're active. Water is a fine choice. Check with your doctor or a registered dietitian about beverage choices if you need a fast-acting carbohydrate source; fruit juice, regular soda, or a sports drink may be advised.

Control Your Weight

Whether you're overweight or not, manage your body weight as part of your personal approach for diabetes management. If you're overweight, losing 10 to 20 pounds may make blood sugar easier to control if you have type 2 diabetes. Why? A lower weight helps lower insulin resistance, so you may no longer need diabetes medication. Other potential benefits of weight loss: lower blood lipid levels and lower blood pressure. Remember, with diabetes your risks for heart disease are higher! (Check with your doctor to see if weight loss is right for you.)

Consult a registered dietitian about losing or maintaining weight: how much you need to lose, over what time frame, and how to eat for weight loss and diabetes management. Limit weight loss to 1 pound weekly. *A few good tips for starters:* Choose mostly lean and low-fat foods. Rather than skip meals, eat smaller portions to consume fewer calories. And move more to use up calories! *See chapter 2, "Your Healthy Weight."*

Team Up for Health!

To manage diabetes properly, seek advice from your healthcare team, whose specialties help you deal with the complexities of diabetes: your physician, a registered dietitian, a certified diabetes educator, a nurse, an eye doctor, a podiatrist, and a pharmacist, among others. Follow through on your care plan.

Remember: You're the most important team member! For the team to work well:

● Set your target blood glucose levels with your doctor. For people with diabetes, near normal is generally 70 to 150 mg/dL. Be realistic; you can't avoid some "ups and downs." Numbers that are mostly within a safe range reduce your risks for complications.

● Keep all appointments for checkups, counseling, and laboratory tests. If your blood glucose levels are under control, see your doctor two to four times a year; if not under control, go in more often. Can't make it? Change your appointment—don't skip it!

● Take diabetes medications as directed, even if you're sick. Tell your doctor or pharmacist about all other medicine and supplements (including herbal products) you take, both prescriptions and over-the-counter medications. Also tell your team about any side effects or problems you have with any medicine or supplement. Plan ahead; call for prescription refills well before you run out. If you take insulin, ask about an insulin pump, which gives a constant, small dose, or other newer devices. **Caution:** Diabetes medicines can't substitute for healthful eating and physical activity.

● Learn to check your own blood glucose level. Self-monitoring, perhaps several times daily, is wise with diabetes, especially if you're taking diabetes medication, if you're pregnant, or if your blood glucose levels are low or out of control. For adults, ask about a noninvasive blood glucose monitoring device. It can check your blood glucose level every 20 minutes without puncturing your skin for a blood sample. Use it with conventional blood glucose monitoring.

● Learn how to detect and safely treat an insulin reaction, hypoglycemia, and hyperglycemia—before you get into severe danger. Immediate, appropriate treatment, perhaps medical assistance, is essential! Wear a medical alert tag or carry a card to let others know what to do in case you pass out.

● Consult a registered dietitian to create a healthful eating plan (food guide for diabetes, exchange lists,

or carbohydrate counting) specific to you, including an approach to managing weight. The dietitian also can offer specific advice on shopping, label reading, eating out, and using alcoholic beverages.

● Get help with stress control if needed. Under stress, it's harder to be diligent about diabetes care: staying active, eating smart, checking your blood sugar level, and perhaps controlling alcoholic beverages. Besides that, stress may affect your blood glucose level.

● Know that you don't need to struggle with diabetes alone. If your medications, eating plan, or physical activity program cause problems or concerns, make an appointment to explore new strategies with your health team members. Managing diabetes can be complex—but your health now and later depends on it!

Osteoporosis: Reduce the Risks

Although the signs of osteoporosis don't show up until later (usually age sixty or older), keeping your bones healthy is a lifelong process. From childhood on, your eating and lifestyle habits can protect you from this debilitating disease later. No matter what your age now, it's not too late to start caring for your bones.

Osteoporosis Is . . .

Osteoporosis is a condition of gradually weakening, brittle bones. As bones lose calcium and other minerals, they become more fragile and porous. They may break under normal use or from just a minor fall, bump, or sudden strain. Because it progresses slowly and silently, people often don't realize they have osteoporosis until they fracture a bone. The spine, hip, and wrist are the most common fracture sites.

Among older adults, a "dowager's hump" is an obvious sign of osteoporosis. Vertebrae in the spine collapse as a result of bone loss. Collapse of several vertabrae leads to a loss of height, back pain, and increasing disability.

Osteoporosis affects most Americans over age seventy, especially women. But men get it, too. In fact, even if you add up all the cases of heart disease, stroke, and diabetes in a year, osteoporosis is more common.

In the United States alone, 1.5 million bone fractures annually are attributed to this bone disease each year. About 10 million Americans over age fifty have osteoporosis; about 34 million more have low bone mass, making them at higher risk for osteoporosis. Of those with osteoporosis, about 80 percent are women. In fact, by the time women go through menopause, nearly one in three has developed osteoporosis. Osteoporosis affects men and women of all races. More people have osteoporosis than report it: four times as many men and nearly three times as many women.

Many hip fractures, common among older adults, are linked to bone disease. Besides pain, fractures cause changes in lifestyle and loss of independence. A person may no longer be able to dress alone or walk across a room. Hip fractures also can be fatal. An average of 20 percent of people with hip fractures die from complications within a year after their fracture.

Fractures have emotional consequences, too. Besides a potential loss of self-esteem and body image, there's also the worry of falling or having future fractures.

To keep your bones healthy, help them become strong and dense while you can (until your early thirties). After that, help keep them strong by slowing the natural loss that comes with age. *For more about building bones, see "Bone Up on Calcium" in chapter 4.*

You can't control some risk factors for osteoporosis: genetics, family history, gender, hormonal status, race/ethnic heritage, age, and body frame/weight. You can control other risk factors: what you eat, physical activity, cigarette smoking, alcohol intake, and using medications to help protect against osteoporosis.

Now, how bone-healthy are you?

● *Gender.* If you're female, you're about four times more likely than males to develop osteoporosis: (1) On average, most women have less bone mass to start with—and they lose it faster as they get older. (2) In young women, the hormone estrogen helps deposit calcium in bones. But as estrogen levels drop with menopause, bones are no longer protected. For the first five years after menopause, usually starting at age fifty, they lose bone faster. (3) From the teen years on, women typically eat fewer calcium-rich foods than men do. Low testosterone levels put men at greater risk.

● *Low body weight or small body frame.* If you're underweight, you likely have less bone mass than people with a healthy weight. Bone health is one of the benefits of keeping your weight within a healthy range for your height throughout your life.

Women with eating disorders and those who exercise very strenuously increase their risk, too, because they may stop menstruating. Changes in their hormone levels may speed bone loss: for example, estrogen deficiency from menopause, especially early or from a hysterectomy. Women with eating disorders may not consume enough calcium- and vitamin D-rich foods, either. *See "Disordered Eating: Problems, Signs, and Help" in chapter 2.*

● *Race/ethnic heritage.* Caucasians and Asians are at higher risk than Latinos and African Americans,

Which Bone Is Healthy?

The dense structure of healthy bone depends largely on its calcium stores. As your body withdraws calcium, bone dissolves, leaving a void where calcium was once deposited. Gradually, bones become more porous and fragile. Once the structure of bone disappears, there's no place to redeposit calcium and new bone tissue. Bone loss from osteoporosis appears to be irreversible.

Healthy bone

Osteoporotic bone

Source: Build Better Bone Now. Courtesy of National Dairy Council.

Your Nutrition Checkup

Osteoporosis: Are You at Risk?

While bone loss is a natural part of aging, osteoporosis and fractures don't need to be, according to the National Osteoporosis Foundation. As with any health problem, some women and men are at greater risk than others.

What's your risk? Check all those that apply to you.

Risk factors you can't control. Are you:

_____ **1.** Female?

_____ **2.** Thin? Or small-boned, with a slight body frame?

_____ **3.** Caucasian or Asian?

_____ **4.** Over age fifty-five?

_____ **5.** From a family with osteoporosis?

Risk factors you can control. Are you:

_____ **6.** Physically inactive?

_____ **7.** Consuming an overall eating plan that's low in calcium and vitamin D?

_____ **8.** Taking high doses of thyroid medication, or high or prolonged doses of cortisonelike medication for asthma, arthritis, or other diseases?

_____ **9.** A current smoker?

_____ **10.** A heavy drinker of alcoholic beverages?

Adapted from: National Osteoporosis Foundation.

● *Physical activity.* Being inactive—perhaps with a desk job, sedentary leisure time, driving—for a long time weakens bones. However, regular weight-bearing activities such as walking, strength training, and dancing trigger your body to deposit calcium in your bones. That makes them stronger and more dense.

● *Calcium intake.* Throughout life, calcium, along with vitamin D, is a bone builder. If your calcium and vitamin D supplies consistently have come up short before ages thirty to thirty-five, your bones may not be as dense as they could be, and less bone was built. After age thirty-five or so, adults may lose bone faster when their food choices don't supply enough calcium and vitamin D.

● *Some medications.* The use of some medications is linked significantly to increased risk for osteoporosis: ongoing use of steroids, thyroid medicine, and cortisone-like medications. Some health conditions increase risk, too.

● *Smoking.* For men and women, smoking promotes bone loss. Among women, smoking lowers estrogen levels, which further contributes to bone loss. If you smoke, that's another good reason to quit.

● *Heavy drinking.* Heavy drinking is linked to weaker bones. But reasons aren't clear—perhaps heavy drinkers make poor food choices or maybe it's a metabolic link.

Protect Your "Support System"

Good health is more than skin deep. Moisturizers and sunscreens may help keep your skin looking young. To prolong the qualities of youth, bones also need loving care.

You can't control all factors that keep your "support system," or skeleton, healthy. But regardless of age, gender, or body build, you can help reduce your osteoporosis risk with smart eating and lifestyle choices.

Never Too Young—or Too Old—to Start

Osteoporosis is often described as a disease of youth that manifests itself in the senior years. Ideally, your bone health strategies began in your childhood and have continued throughout adulthood; in fact, almost 50 percent of bone formation occurs during the adolescent growth years with 98 percent of a woman's

although people in these ethnic groups develop osteoporosis, too. Their bones usually are stronger and more dense throughout their lives, although all races and ethnic groups need the same amount of calcium.

● *Age.* Bone is dynamic with an ongoing process of bone tissue replacement called remodeling. Until your early 30s, more bone tissue is re-formed than lost. Then a few years later that equation flips. More bone is lost than is formed—up to 1 percent of bone loss per year, depending on individual differences. During the first few years of menopause, there is more rapid bone loss.

● *Family history.* Osteoporosis runs in families. Not only do people inherit a genetic tendency toward bone fractures and osteoporosis, but also families often live similar lifestyles that may increase their risk.

bone mass formed by age 20. Even in your early adult years, bones get stronger and more dense. By the early thirties, bones are as dense as they'll ever be. The denser your bones are before middle age, the better able they'll withstand bone loss that naturally goes with aging.

No matter what your age now, you're still young enough to make a difference in your bone health. Your food choices and lifestyle patterns can slow the natural process of bone loss. *For more about caring for bones in the mature adult years, see "Calcium: As Important As Ever" in chapter 18.*

The Calcium Gap

By now you're well aware of the link between calcium and bone health. So if your food choices come up short, now's the time to close the calcium gap!

As an adult you still need plenty of calcium; 1,000 milligrams daily is considered an Adequate Intake (AI) for ages nineteen to fifty; 1,200 milligrams daily for ages fifty and over. Remember, an 8-ounce serving of milk or yogurt or 1½ ounces of cheese each supply about 300 milligrams of calcium. *For calcium-rich foods, see "Calcium: A Closer Look" in chapter 4.* Teens need plenty of calcium, too; yet during this critical time of bone building, many switch from calcium-rich milk to other beverages.

Consider other links to calcium. Caffeine can increase urinary loss of calcium, but moderate caffeine intake has little influence on bone health. One cup of regular coffee prevents the absorption of the calcium found in one tablespoon of milk. If your caffeine intake is high, you may cut back on caffeinated drinks, since this effect can add up—or enjoy latte (coffee with steamed milk) or tea with milk to make up the difference. Actually, sodium has a greater effect on calcium absorption than caffeine does; however, neither is significant if calcium intake is adequate.

Alcohol and smoking can block calcium absorption. Smoking can speed bone loss; for women, a lifelong habit of smoking a pack of cigarettes a day may lower bone density by menopause an extra 5 to 10 percent. If you smoke, consider the bone-healthy benefits of quitting. Among other factors, excessive alcohol intake may inhibit some bone remodeling, increase calcium excretion, and increase the chance of falling. If you drink alcoholic beverages, drink only in moderation—for women, no more than one drink a day, and no more than two drinks daily for men.

The Vitamin D Connection

Vitamin D promotes calcium absorption. If you drink vitamin D-fortified milk, you probably consume enough to protect against bone disease. But if your calcium comes from other sources, get a little sunshine. Your body makes vitamin D when ultraviolet light touches your skin. If you can't go outdoors or if you cover up, pay special attention to getting enough vitamin D from food, or you might need a vitamin D supplement, particularly if you're over age seventy. *See "Vitamins: The Basics" in chapter 4 and "Vitamin D: The Sunshine Vitamin" in chapter 18.*

Have You Ever Wondered

... if you can get kidney stones by drinking milk? That's a common myth. Research doesn't support this misperception. In fact, drinking milk may reduce the risk. A high-calcium diet may decrease the absorption of oxalate, a substance in some plant-based foods that can form calcium oxalate kidney stones.

... if phytoestrogens in soybeans protect your bones? Maybe, since they act much like mild estrogens in the body. After menopause, as natural estrogen declines, phytoestrogens in soy products may help prevent bone some loss. *See "What's 'Soy' Good?" in chapter 11.*

Move Those Bones!

Weight-bearing and resistance training activity—at least 30 minutes daily for adults—helps maintain bone density—if you consume enough calcium. If you're swimming, bicycling, or riding a stationary bike regularly, that's great. But these activities don't promote bone health because they aren't weight-bearing.

Add activities such as these to your "activity repertoire": walking, jogging, aerobic dancing, volleyball, tennis, dancing, or weight lifting—even mowing the grass or shoveling snow. You don't need expensive equipment or a fitness club to lift weights. To build arm and shoulder strength, use things you have around your house, such as canned goods.

For anyone, including teens and young adults in their bone-growing years, eating calcium-rich foods along with regular weight-bearing activity offers a great "combo" for long-term bone health!

Hormone Therapy

Going through menopause? Consult your doctor about hormone replacement therapy. A low dose of estrogen, with or without progestin (a form of progesterone), may be prescribed to help slow bone loss and may protect against other side effects of menopause, including hot flashes. Estrogen therapy also may be advised for younger women with amenorrhea (cessation of menstrual cycles) or who've had a hysterectomy. Medical advice is to use the lowest effective dose for the shortest duration that matches a woman's treatment goals and health risks.

If you take estrogen, remember that it's just one strategy for your continued bone health. Consuming enough calcium and vitamin D and regular weight-bearing activity are important! *See "Hormone Therapy" in chapter 17.*

Calcium and Vitamin D Supplements

For many women, supplements help ensure an adequate calcium and vitamin D intake and offer protection from osteoporosis. However, the main nourishment for healthy bones should come from food, not pills. Food supplies other nutrients that your bones (and whole body) need.

If you take calcium and vitamin D pills, use them to supplement, not replace, nourishing foods. *See "Calcium Supplements: A Bone Builder" in chapter 23.*

Testing, Testing: A Bone Density Scan

For women: If you're at high risk for osteoporosis, a bone mineral density (BMD) test may be advised—especially if you've experienced early menopause, amenorrhea, a fracture from a minor strain, or if you have a family history of osteoporosis. Not at risk? Still, a BMD test at menopause offers a baseline for later, especially if you're contemplating estrogen or other drug therapy. Consult your doctor.

For women or men, BMD tests aren't invasive and take just 5 to 10 minutes. Instead, they scan your spine, hip, and wrist like other X rays do. Your bone density scans are compared to standards of people like you in gender and size: someone age-matched to you and someone younger at peak bone mass. Bone density scanning is now covered by Medicare.

If You Have Osteoporosis . . .

Preventing and treating osteoporosis has three considerations: (1) enough calcium and vitamin D, (2) weight-bearing physical activity, and (3) perhaps medication. The best guidance: protect your bones from further deterioration. *Besides the sound advice in "Protect Your 'Support System'" in this chapter, remember this:*

● Protect yourself from slips and falls, when you might easily fracture a bone, especially if you're over age sixty. Check your vision as another precaution.

● Consult with your physician about new medications that may help prevent bone loss or treat osteoporosis. Equally important, talk to your doctor about other medications and supplements you take. Thyroid hormones, oral glucocortoids (steroids), and chemotherapy, among others may promote bone loss.

● Enjoy plenty of calcium- and vitamin D-rich foods. They provide more for bone health (calcium, phosphorus, vitamin D)—and overall health—than supplements do. And a varied, well-balanced eating plan offers other nutrients that appear to promote bone density, including magnesium, potassium, and vitamin K.

● If you are not able to meet your calcium and vitamin D recommendations with foods, you may need calcium or vitamin D supplements. Ask a dietitian or your doctor about the right dosage and type. And enhance their absorption by taking them with food.

Gastrointestinal Conditions

Stomach ache? Diarrhea? Constipation? Heartburn? It's no surprise that discomfort and diseases of the gastrointestinal (GI) tract are linked to nutrition. If you don't feel like eating, or if a health problem interferes with the digestion of food or the absorption of nutrients, GI problems can affect your nutritional status.

For GI problems always see a doctor for a diagnosis if problems persist, and seek guidance from a dietetics professional for eating advice.

Gastric Reflux Disease

Is it heartburn—or gastric reflux disease? Heartburn is a main symptom of gastric reflux disease; however, gastric reflux disease is a more serious health problem. In gastric reflux disease, contents of the stomach flow backward into the esophagus. The symptoms? Besides heartburn, symptoms include pain that feels like an ulcer, difficulty swallowing, and regurgitating stomach acid. If you have these ongoing symptoms, check with your doctor.

Gastric reflux disease is associated with several health conditions, such as hiatal hernia, abdominal pressure from obesity, and probably with aging.

If You Have Gastric Reflux Disease . . .

As part of your treatment, your doctor may recommend an eating plan that eliminates or reduces foods that irritate your esophagus or that cause reflux of stomach acids. Among the common food offenders: chocolate, alcoholic drinks, carbonated drinks, citrus juice, tomato products, coffee (with and without caffeine), and mint. High-fat foods and large meals may cause problems, too. Since obesity increases the risk, your doctor may advise weight loss.

A registered dietitian can provide guidelines for meals and snack planning. These eating-related tips also can help you treat gastric reflux disease:

Have You Ever Wondered

. . . how to relieve hemorrhoids or constipation? Plenty of fiber-rich foods, plenty of fluids, and a physically active lifestyle help prevent constipation and hemorrhoids. As important, pay attention to your body's signals. Delaying a bowel movement can lead to constipation and hard, dry stools, which are difficult to pass. For travelers, lack of access to safe water, sweat loss in a hot climate, or a dry airplane cabin may contribute to fluid loss that leads to constipation.

What's the benefit of physical activity? Being active helps maintain muscle tone throughout your body, including your intestinal tract.

If constipation is a chronic or a painful problem, talk to your physician. It might signal a more serious problem or an interaction with medication.

See "Avoiding the Trio: Constipation, Hemorrhoids, and Diverticulosis" in chapter 6. For tips for easing the problems, see "Constipation during Pregnancy" in chapter 17 and the chart "Cancer Treatment: Handling Side Effects" in this chapter.

. . . how you should deal with diarrhea and vomiting? Both are symptoms of other health problems, some more serious than others. In either case, your body loses fluids that need replacing; these conditions can lead to dehydration and electrolyte imbalance.

What causes watery, loose stools, or diarrhea? Perhaps foodborne illness, infection, or medication. With diarrhea, waste passes through the intestine before fluids can be absorbed, or body fluids may pass from the cells into intestinal contents. For mild diarrhea, drink plenty of fluids and rest. For more severe or persistent diarrhea, see your physician.

Vomiting may result from motion imbalance, from a normal reaction to an irritating substance, or it may be symptomatic of many different health problems. When you vomit, the normal rhythmic movements of digestion reverse their direction, expelling your stomach, and perhaps intestinal, contents. Usually the best "medicine" is to drink fluids (in small, frequent amounts) and rest. For severe, persistent, or projectile vomiting, check with your physician immediately. You'll need proper rehydration, perhaps with electrolytes, and diagnosis and treatment of the underlying cause. *For more on dealing with diarrhea and vomiting see "Cancer Treatment: Handling Side Effects" in this chapter. For information on probiotics for gastrointestinal health, refer to page 108.*

Both diarrhea and vomiting can be especially dangerous for infants and older adults. If they persist, call your healthcare provider immediately!

- Eat small, more frequent meals.

- Sit up while you eat, and sit or stand for forty-five to sixty minutes after you eat.

- Eat at least two to three hours before bedtime. Skip late-night meals or bedtime snacks.

- Limit or avoid foods and beverages that cause discomfort, including chocolate, coffee, tea, cola, and alcoholic drinks. If other foods, such as tomatoes or oranges, give you trouble, try just small amounts, eaten with other foods.

- Wear loose-fitting clothes that don't put pressure on your abdomen.

- Achieve and keep your healthy weight.

- Sleep with your head slightly propped up on a pillow.

Your doctor also may suggest changes in your lifestyle, medication, and perhaps surgery.

Have You Ever Wondered

. . . what causes heartburn? The discomfort of heartburn, or indigestion, occurs when digestive juices (hydrochloric acid) and food from your stomach back up into your esophagus. Your stomach lining is protected from acids that form during digestion, but your esophagus lining is sensitive to the burning sensation of stomach acids. That's why you feel discomfort or pain.

Foods themselves don't cause heartburn, but they may aggravate the condition by stimulating acid production. A problem with the esophageal sphincter may be involved, too. Foods high in acids, such as citrus fruit, as well as fatty or highly seasoned foods, may also cause problems for some people.

Heartburn isn't dangerous, just uncomfortable. And it can be treated with antacids. Consult your doctor about the best type for you; antacids can interfere with other medications. The danger can come if you ignore a heart attack, thinking it's simply heartburn. *See page 552 for signs and symptoms of a heart attack.* If the pain continues or if it happens an hour or more after eating, call your doctor immediately!

Diverticular Disease

Diverticular disease is really two conditions. *Diverticulosis* is a condition in which pouches, called diverticula, develop in the weakened walls of the intestine, most often the colon. Diverticulosis is linked to an overall eating approach that's low in fiber. Constipation makes the problem worse. These pouches can become inflamed and infected from bacteria in feces that get trapped there—a health problem called *diverticulitis*. The majority (about 50 percent) of Americans ages sixty to eighty have diverticulosis; just about everybody does after age eighty.

If You Have Diverticular Disease . . .

- For diverticulosis eat plenty of high-fiber foods; keep waste moving through the intestines to avoid constipation. A high-fiber diet is likely the only treatment you need. Nuts and seeds are likely okay to eat. Studies don't support a link between inflammation of the diverticula and eating nuts and seeds. *See chapter 6 for more about dietary fiber.*

- For diverticulitis you need to clear up the infection and the inflammation. Treatment often includes antibiotics; perhaps a short-term liquid diet; bed rest; and, if the problem is severe, surgery.

Irritable Bowel Syndrome

Irritable bowel syndrome (IBS), an intestinal problem, doesn't have a clear cause; however, abnormal contractions in the intestine, stress, and food intolerance all may play a role. Symptoms might be abdominal pain or cramps as well as diarrhea, constipation, bloating, and gassiness. IBS also is known as colitis and spastic colon.

If you have these symptoms, check with your doctor. They may be a sign of other serious diseases or disorders. Several tests are used to rule out other problems: complete blood count, stool examination, and sigmoidoscopy or colonoscopy.

Irritable bowel syndrome is different from inflammatory bowel disease (IBD)—Crohn's disease and ulcerative colitis—which requires careful medical treatment. With IBD a registered dietitian helps a patient create an individualized approach to eating that

Keep Smiling: Prevent Gum Disease

From an oral health standpoint, a cavity-free mouth doesn't get you home free! Gum, or periodontal, disease, which affects about three-quarters of American adults, is the main cause of tooth loss, which, in turn, can affect food choices. As with tooth decay, bacteria in plaque (the gummy film that forms on teeth) and calculus are at the root of gum disease. In fact, these bacteria may thrive right along the gumline.

● Help prevent tooth loss by protecting your teeth from gum disease. Brush and floss regularly. By removing plaque along the gumline, bacteria in plaque are less able to irritate your gums. Plaque that isn't removed turns into calculus, or hard deposits, which you can't remove with brushing or flossing.

● Choose an overall eating plan with food variety and balance. Good nutrition makes your gums more resistant to infections caused by oral bacteria. And your gums need nutrients to stay healthy.

● Have regular dental checkups. Besides checking for gum problems and oral cancer, the dentist or dental hygienist will remove calculus buildup between teeth and along the gumline.

not only helps manage gastrointestinal (GI) symptoms but also helps to prevent malnutrition and helps the GI tract function normally.

If You Have Irritable Bowel Syndrome . . .

Many recommendations are good guidance for anyone: a high-fiber, low-fat eating approach. In addition:

● Eat small, frequent meals. Chew your food well to aid digestion. And eat slowly so you don't swallow a lot of air, which may make you feel gassy.

● To prevent constipation, eat plenty of fiber-rich foods. *See chapter 6, "Fiber: Nature's Broom," for dietary fiber advice.*

● If a food irritates or causes too much gas, avoid it.

● Limit any substance that makes symptoms

worse: perhaps caffeine; alcoholic drinks; fat; or sorbitol, a sugar alcohol. Sometimes fructose, the sugar in fruit and fruit drinks, isn't well tolerated; talk to your doctor before avoiding fruit if you suspect a problem.

● Drink more fluids to help prevent constipation. *See chapter 7, "Fluids: The Power of Water," for advice about fluids.*

● Learn to manage stress. Anxiety may affect the speed at which food residues pass through your GI tract.

● If you're lactose-intolerant, restrict lactose. *See "Lactose Intolerance: A Matter of Degree" in chapter 21.*

● Talk to your doctor about your medications. Some, such as antacids, may make symptoms worse. And some dietary supplements can have side effects that affect your GI tract—for example, aloe, black cohosh, garlic, gingko biloba, goldenseal, and saw palmetto, among others.

Ulcers

"Stress is giving me an ulcer!" In truth, it's not, although your body may secrete more stomach acid if you're under emotional strain. Most ulcers in the esophagus, stomach, and small intestine are caused by bacteria called *Heliobactor pylori;* in addition, the use of some anti-inflammatory medications and too much stomach acid, resulting from other health problems, are other causes. When the lining of the gastrointestinal tract is impaired for any number of reasons, the cells underneath can't protect themselves from stomach acids. If the damage goes deep enough, the ulcer may bleed and cause pain.

To refute another common myth, eating spicy foods doesn't cause ulcers either. In fact, no food choices cause or cure ulcers.

If You Have an Ulcer . . .

Antibiotics or antacids usually are prescribed to treat stomach ulcers: antibiotics to destroy the bacteria, or antacids to suppress stomach acids. In addition, your doctor may recommend dietary treatment. To heal an ulcer, you don't need to eat bland foods, as once thought. Instead, this advice is generally given:

... why fair-skinned people often become pale with anemia? Hemoglobin gives blood its bright red color. With less hemoglobin in circulation, skin is paler. For people with darker skin, check the lining of the eye, which may become pale with anemia.

- Follow an overall, well-balanced eating plan. Sound familiar?

- Limit foods and seasonings that stimulate the flow of gastric juices: black pepper, chile powder, cloves, garlic, and caffeinated drinks. Decaffeinated coffee or tea may be a problem, too.

- Limit frequent snacking so your body secretes less stomach acids.

- Skip alcoholic beverages, smoking, and aspirin.

- Unless a certain food causes repeated discomfort, enjoy any food you choose—as long as it fits within your healthful approach to eating.

Anemia: "Tired Blood"

Have that "run-down" feeling? Perhaps you're overworked and underrested. More sleep and relaxation may be what you need to feel energetic again. Or perhaps your fatigue is a symptom of anemia.

Actually, anemia isn't a disease, but instead a symptom of other health problems. With anemia, you may—or may not—feel fatigued. Often there's a nutrition connection.

With anemia, the body doesn't have enough red blood cells, or they're not big enough, to transport oxygen from your lungs to your body cells. Hemoglobin,

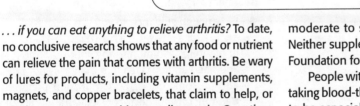

... if you can eat anything to relieve arthritis? To date, no conclusive research shows that any food or nutrient can relieve the pain that comes with arthritis. Be wary of lures for products, including vitamin supplements, magnets, and copper bracelets, that claim to help, or of taking too many aspirins to relieve pain. Over time aspirin can irritate your stomach, causing bleeding you may not be aware of. That can lead to an iron deficiency. Talk to your doctor about a safe dosage.

Can glucosamine relieve arthritis pain? That's an area of interest and study. Researchers are exploring whether glucosamine may relieve the symptoms of osteoarthritis, the form of arthritis that occurs when cartilage that cushions joints breaks down. Glucosamine is a natural component of tendons, ligaments, and cartilage.

Research suggests that, like aspirin and ibuprofen, glucosamine may help dull the pain of stiffening joints. Early findings indicate that it also may help slow the progression of osteoarthritis; however, not enough is known to confirm its safety or effectiveness. Research doesn't show that taking glucosamine and chondroitin sulfate—alone or in combination—reduces pain effectively for most people with osteoarthritis. If you have

moderate to severe knee pain, talk to your doctor. Neither supplement is recommended by the Arthritis Foundation for treating arthritis.

People with diabetes, shellfish allergies, and those taking blood-thinning medication or daily aspirin need to be especially cautious about taking glucosamine. Talk to your physician first before trying glucosamine.

The best nutritional advice for arthritis is: Follow a healthful eating plan and maintain a healthy weight. In that way you won't put too much strain on arthritic joints. The medically accepted advice also may include moderate physical activity, prescribed medication, protection of joints, and hot and cold applications.

... if antioxidants can protect your eyes from cataracts or macular degeneration? Maybe. Early research suggests that vitamins A and E, zinc, as well as lutein, zeaxanthin, and some fats may help prevent or slow (not restore) some eye changes that come with aging. Vitamin C may offer protection from cataracts. *See "Functional Nutrition: A Quick Look at Key Phytonutrients" in chapter 4 for lutein and zeaxanthin sources; chapter 4 also gives food sources of nutrients.* Talk to your eye care professional about whether an antioxidant supplement is right for you.

For other health conditions and problems, see these chapters:

- Breast cancer—chapter 17.
- Celiac disease (gluten intolerance)—chapter 21.
- Choking (Heimlich maneuver)—chapters 12 and 15 (infants and children).
- Constipation, hemorrhoids, and diverticulosis—chapters 6 and 17.
- Dehydration and heat stroke—chapter 8.
- Dental cavities—chapters 5 and 15 (infants).
- Eating disorders—chapters 2 and 16 (teens).
- Fibrocystic breast disease—chapter 17.
- Fibromylagia—chapter 17.
- Food allergies and intolerances—chapters 15 (infants) and 21.
- Foodborne illness—chapter 12.
- Lactose intolerance—chapter 21.
- Migraine headaches—chapter 21.
- Overweight and obesity—chapters 2 and 16 (children and teens).
- Polycystic ovary syndrome—chapter 17.
- Reactive hypoglycemia—chapter 5.
- Vaginal yeast infections—chapter 17.

made with iron, is the part of red blood cells that carries oxygen to other tissues. Without enough oxygen, body cells can't produce enough energy. Then fatigue, pale skin, headache, weakness, lack of concentration, or irritability, among other symptoms, may set in. To produce enough healthy red blood cells, you need enough iron in your diet, as well as enough folate and vitamin B_{12}.

Is It an Iron Deficiency?

Anemia isn't a symptom of just one health problem. A form often described as "iron-poor blood" might come to mind first. In fact, iron deficiency, with its effect on hemoglobin, is the most common form of anemia, more likely affecting adult women of childbearing age, infants and children, and teenage girls. Anemia is a health problem that develops over time. If iron intake comes up short for an extended

time, your body can't make enough hemoglobin.

Be aware that having an iron deficiency doesn't necessarily mean you're anemic. For anemia to occur you need a severe depletion of iron stored in your body, with low levels of hemoglobin in your blood.

Before menopause, women need more iron than men do, so women are at higher risk for anemia. Why?

- For starters, women need more iron due to monthly blood loss from menstruation.
- During pregnancy, women need 50 percent more

If Your Doctor Prescribes a Special Eating Plan . . .

Like your medication, a doctor-prescribed eating plan—perhaps sodium-modified, high-fiber, gluten-free, or blenderized liquid—is essential to healthcare and disease management. In the world of medicine, a special meal plan is part of medical nutrition therapy. If your doctor prescribes a special eating plan as part of your treatment for whatever conditions you might have:

- Get enough guidance so you can successfully comply. Ask for a referral to a registered dietitian for help in planning and monitoring your nutrition needs. You need an approach that matches your physical and personal needs and your food preferences. **Caution:** Let your doctor or dietitian know about any supplements you take.
- Follow the special nutrition plan faithfully. Record what you eat, your challenges, and successes to share later with your healthcare provider or dietitian. That's especially important if this is a long-term change in your eating regimen.
- Use Nutrition Facts and ingredient lists on food labels as information aids. A dietitian can help you learn to use label facts effectively.
- Get family support. Their encouragement and help in food shopping and preparation make any special eating plan easier to follow. Try to dovetail your meal plans; serve the same foods to the whole family whenever you can. For example, if you're on a DASH eating plan, almost everyone can benefit from more fruits, vegetables, and low-fat dairy foods.

For more on getting the most from nutrition counseling, see " When You Consult an Expert . . ." in chapter 24.

Have You Ever Wondered

. . . if SAM-e can help someone suffering from osteoarthritis or depression? Derived from the amino acid methionine, SAM-e (S-adenosyl-methionine) is produced in your body and sold as a dietary supplement in the United States. It may help people suffering from mild depression or joint pain—but shouldn't be used to self-medicate moderate to severe conditions. SAM-e is very costly at the doses used in research studies.

. . . if you can treat chronic fatigue with a special eating plan? Maybe. Studies are under way to determine the best treatment regimen for most sufferers. Of course, an overall healthful eating plan that provides the nutrients and the calories you need to feel energetic, combined with adequate rest, regular physical activity, and stress management, can make a difference. Other ways you might control or relieve your symptoms: improve your sleep habits, adjust your schedule to maximize when you have more energy, and join a support group. Skip unproven remedies, including dietary supplements that haven't shown effectiveness or safety. *(See chapter 23.)* Talk with your doctor about other treatment approaches.

. . . if you should heed the advice "Starve a cold and feed a fever"? Illness is no time to "starve" your body of nutrients. To fight infection, your body needs a supply of nutrients to build and maintain your natural defenses, so you still need balance and variety in your food choices. Extra rest helps, too. With a fever, drink plenty of fluids: juice, milk, soup, or water. If you don't have much appetite, eat bland, simple foods, perhaps more often. How about vitamin C? Well, it won't cure the common cold. No scientific evidence proves that a large dose, perhaps from a vitamin supplement, boosts immunity; however, it may shorten the duration of a cold and decrease the severity of cold symptoms.

. . . if lecithin can keep you healthy? Lecithin is a phospholipid, or a type of fat. Promoters make many claims for lecithin, for example, as a cure or prevention for arthritis, skin problems, gallstones, and nervous disorders, as well as memory problems and improved endurance. Others claim it dissolves cholesterol that's deposited in arteries. Because your body makes lecithin, taking it as a supplement doesn't appear to offer added benefits. Synthetic lecithin isn't well absorbed.

. . . if other healthcare treatments, such as acupuncture or herbal medicines, are safe and effective? Despite consumer attention to alternative treatments, little research backs up their safety or effectiveness. Although some have been used as traditional medicines for centuries, their success is shared mostly in individual reports, not scientific research. To gather sound research evidence to either support or dissuade their use, the National Center for Complementary and Alternative Medicine recently was established within the National Institutes of Health. Some treatments may offer promise in certain circumstances.

Until more is known, alternative approaches to healthcare shouldn't replace treatment that's known to be safe and effective. If you do choose to try alternative or complementary care, talk to your doctor first. Some alternative approaches may interfere with the effectiveness of your doctor's prescribed treatment.

---

iron: 27 milligrams a day, compared to 18 milligrams daily prior to pregnancy. The extra is needed for increased blood volume—at least three more pints of blood! Often a woman's stored iron gets used up to meet the demands of pregnancy.

● Women often don't consume enough iron-rich foods in their everyday food choices, perhaps because they restrict their food intake to their control weight.

● Vegetarian women may come up short on iron. Plant sources of iron aren't absorbed as well as iron from meat, poultry, and fish.

Infants are at risk if their mothers had low iron status during pregnancy, or, if they bottle-feed, they take formula that's not iron-fortified.

For children, teens, and adults, an iron-rich eating plan can prevent this most common type of anemia. For some, especially pregnant women, iron supplements might be recommended, too.

For more, see "Iron: A Closer Look" in chapter 4.

Anemia: More than One Cause

Although most common, iron deficiency isn't the only cause of anemia. Deficiencies in vitamin B_{12}

or folate are other nutrition-related causes. Anemia also may result from large blood loss, hereditary defects in blood cells (sickle-cell anemia), liver disease that affects body processes that use iron, infections, or congestive heart failure. "Sports anemia" isn't really anemia; *see "Have You Ever Wondered . . . if heavy training causes 'sports anemia'?" in chapter 19.*

Anemia: Linked to Vitamin B$_{12}$

Anemia from a vitamin B$_{12}$ deficiency doesn't have a single cause; it's not just poor eating, or although uncommon, a low intake of vitamin B$_{12}$. More often, it's pernicious anemia, caused by poor vitamin B$_{12}$ absorption—perhaps due to lack of intrinsic factor,

atrophic gastritis, or the surgical removal of part of the stomach or small intestine.

What's intrinsic factor? It's a body chemical, produced in the stomach, that helps your body absorb vitamin B$_{12}$ in the intestine. If gastric juices lack intrinsic factor, perhaps for genetic reasons, or if the secretion of stomach juices is impaired, vitamin B$_{12}$ can't be

Have You Ever Wondered ?

. . . if you need more potassium if you're taking a diuretic medication? That depends on the diuretic that's been prescribed for you. Talk to your doctor or a registered dietitian for advice. You probably don't need to take a potassium supplement, however. Many foods are great sources, including many fruits and vegetables, and milk. *For a list of foods high in potassium, see "Potassium: Another Reason for Fruits and Veggies!" in chapter 7.*

. . . if antacids are okay for ongoing indigestion? Although your body may produce less stomach acid with age, you may suffer from indigestion. Antacids, taken as directed, can help. However, excess amounts can deplete your body's phosphorus reserves, which may lead to softening of the bones, called osteomalacia.

Taking antacids with calcium at mealtime may prevent your body from fully absorbing iron in food. Talk to your doctor about taking antacids. Symptoms that seem like indigestion could be something more serious.

. . . what "medical foods" are? They're not functional foods. Medical foods help manage a disease or a health problem. Under a doctor's supervision, they're consumed or given in a tube feeding directly to the stomach.

. . . if Diabesity is a new disease? No, but Diabesity, a trademarked term of Shape Up America, is a growing global health issue. Because obesity and overweight are predictors of diabetes and insulin resistance, the worldwide rise in obesity parallels a rise in diabetes.

Medications: Sodium Alert

Are you on a sodium-modified eating plan? If so, talk to your doctor or pharmacist about medications. Some contain sodium, including some antacids and alkalizers, headache remedies, laxatives, sedatives, and others.

If you're taking medication prescribed for high blood pressure, eating less sodium may let your medication work more effectively. If sodium reduction helps control your blood pressure, you may be able to reduce the dosage of antihypertensive medication.

Need more tips for preventing or managing health problems? Check here for "how-tos":

- Put more physical activity in your lifestyle —see chapters 1 and 2.
- Manage your weight sensibly and effectively—see chapter 2.
- Manage alcoholic drinks for health—see chapter 8.
- Follow overall eating guidelines for health promotion—see chapter 10.
- Shop smart to match your health needs—see chapter 11.
- Prepare foods to manage your health conditions—see chapter 13.
- Stick to your eating plan when you eat out—see chapter 14.
- Use supplements appropriately to avoid or manage health problems—see chapter 23.
- Find a nutrition expert trained to help with your health problems—see chapter 24.
- Identify resources to help deal with specific health conditions—see "Resources You Can Use."

properly absorbed. With age (typically over age sixty), atrophic gastritis, a condition that causes the acid content of stomach secretions to decrease, can affect vitamin B_{12} absorption. Injury or surgical removal of part of the stomach also affects gastric juices and nutrient absorption. Your doctor will diagnose these problems and offer advice.

Because vitamin B_{12} comes only from animal sources of food (meat, fish, poultry, eggs, milk, and milk products), strict vegetarians, or vegans, can be at higher risk. They need a reliable source of vitamin B_{12}, perhaps a fortified breakfast cereal or a supplement, to protect against anemia. *See "Vitamin B_{12}: A Challenge for Vegans" in chapter 20.*

Anemia: Short on Folate

A folate deficiency can lead to anemia. Why? Folate is essential for cell growth and development. Without enough folate, red blood cells become enlarged but don't develop normally, so they can't carry oxygen to body cells as efficiently. Today most enriched grain products are folic acid-fortified in the United States, so most people consume enough to avoid anemia. Folate also comes from leafy vegetables, some fruits, legumes (dry beans), and liver. Some whole-grain foods are folic acid-fortified.

For women, a folate deficiency may show up later in pregnancy when folate needs are high. Early in pregnancy, a shortage of folate may lead to birth defects of the spinal cord. Whether or not you're at risk for anemia caused by folate deficiency, consume enough, especially if you're planning to get pregnant—or if you already are pregnant. *For more about folate and pregnancy, see "Before Pregnancy" in chapter 17.*

Testing, Testing: Do You Have Anemia?

Before you self-diagnose your fatigue as anemia and then pop a pill, consult your doctor about your symptoms. And ask for a blood test.

A hemoglobin test or a hematocrit test is a simple, inexpensive blood test to screen for the possibility of anemia; however, many conditions can affect the results. If the test results are positive, your doctor may conduct more specific tests, for example: *for iron-deficiency anemia*—serum ferritin or total iron-binding capacity (TIBC); *for folate deficiency anemia*—

serum folate; or *for vitamin B_{12} deficiency*—serum vitamin B_{12} or a Schilling test.

Proper diagnosis is essential for getting the right treatment for various types of anemia; their potentially harmful effects differ. For example, a folate supplement may "cure" blood-related symptoms of pernicious anemia but mask irreversible, potentially severe damage to the nervous system.

If You Have Anemia . . .

● Consult your doctor or a registered dietitian about appropriate treatment for the type of anemia you have. Follow prescribed treatment or professional advice, not self-prescribed supplements.

● Keep any supplements in a safe place, where children can't reach them.

● Enjoy good food sources of all three nutrients: iron, vitamin B_{12}, and folate.

● Follow up with your doctor, perhaps with appropriate blood tests to monitor your status.

● For more guidance, check here:
   ● *Iron—"Menstrual Cycle: More Iron for Women" in chapter 17, "Iron: A Closer Look" in chapter 4, and "Iron: The Fatigue Connection" for teenage girls in chapter 16.*
   ● *Vitamin B_{12}—"Vitamins: The Basics" in chapter 4.*
   ● *Folate—"Vitamins: The Basics" in chapter 4.*

Food and Medicine

Do you take over-the-counter medications, prescription medications, or both? Their safe, effective use is your responsibility—and an important part of medical treatment. Talk to your doctor, pharmacist, and perhaps a registered dietitian for the guidance you need.

Some Don't Mix

Taking medications may not seem like a nutrition issue. Yet, when food and medicines are taken together, they often interact. That's not surprising, since the chemistry of the stomach and the intestine differs before and several hours after eating. Food and the substances released in your body during digestion

COMMON INTERACTIONS BETWEEN FOOD AND SOME MEDICATIONS

MEDICINE CABINET PRESCRIPTION DRUGS AND OVER-THE-COUNTER PRODUCTS	KITCHEN CABINET: COMMON FOOD AND DRUG INTERACTIONS* (FOR SPECIFIC INFORMATION ABOUT YOUR MEDICATIONS, ASK YOUR DOCTOR OR YOUR PHARMACIST.)
Pain relievers ● Aspirin (e.g., Anacin, Bayer) ● Ibuprofen (e.g., Advil, Motrin, Nuprin)	Take these with food to avoid irritating your stomach. Also limit other stomach irritants, such as alcohol and caffeine.
Antibiotics ● Tetracycline (e.g., Achromycin, Sumycin) ● Penicillin (e.g., Pen-Vee K)	The calcium in dairy foods and in calcium and iron supplements can block the absorption of tetracycline-based products. Take these medications one hour or more before or after consuming dairy products or calcium supplements. When taken together, citrus fruits and fruit juices can destroy a type of penicillin.
Blood-thinning medication/anticoagulants ● Warfarin (e.g., Coumadin, Dicoumerol)	Eat in moderation a consistent amount of foods with vitamin K, such as dark-green leafy greens; spinach; kale; turnip greens; green tea; and some soy burgers. Too much vitamin K can make your blood clot faster.
Antidepressants ● MAO inhibitors (e.g., Marplan, Parnate)	When taken with foods high in tyramine (an amino acid found in protein foods), these medications may lead to increased blood pressure, fever, headache, vomiting, and possible death. Ask your doctor or a registered dietitian for a list of foods to avoid, such as beer, cheese, red wine, cured meats, aged cheese, avocados, sour cream, and yeast products.
Antacids containing ● Aluminum (e.g., Maalox, Amphojel) ● Calcium (e.g., Tums) ● Sodium (e.g., Alka-Seltzer)	Wait two to three hours after taking an aluminum-containing antacid before you drink or eat citrus fruits. Citrus fruits can increase the amount of aluminum your body absorbs. Antacids with aluminum also can cause a loss of bone-building calcium.
	Some antacids can weaken the absorption of heart-regulating medications such as digoxin (e.g., Lanoxin). Some antacids can weaken the effect of antiulcer medication (e.g., Tagamet) or drugs that treat high blood pressure (such as Inderal). Be sure to read all the alerts on the labels. If you have high blood pressure, read the label of antacids for the amount of sodium present.
Garlic pills	It is important for your blood to clot if you suffer a cut or undergo surgery. Substances in garlic appear to thin the blood. If you are already taking aspirin or other blood-thinning medications, taking garlic supplements may thin the blood too much.
Corticosteroids (Prednisone, Solumedrol, Hydrocortisone)	Because these medications increase sodium and water retention, which may lead to edema, go easy on foods high in sodium, such as ham and other cured meats, pickled vegetables (pickled beets, olives, pickles, sauerkraut, others), processed foods, cheese, salty snacks, and salt added in cooking and at the table.
Medications for cancer treatment (Tamoxifen, Methotrexate)	Flavonoids in citrus fruits can help tamoxifen inhibit cancer cell growth. Methotrexate promotes folate deficiency; a folate supplement may be prescribed.

*Many supplements including herbal products may interact with medications, too. See "Warning: Supplement Interactions!" in chapter 23.

Adapted from: To Your Health! Food & Activity Tips for Older Adults (National Council on Aging, National Institute on Aging, President's Council on Physical Fitness and Sports, and Food Marketing Institute). Used with permission.

may either enhance or hinder the effectiveness of some medications. Some medications alter appetite, taste, or smell, and may cause mouth sores or a dry mouth, making swallowing difficult. Others may induce nausea or irritate the GI tract. Medications also can improve or interfere with nutrient absorption or use.

Your goal? To get the full benefits of both food and medicine. To do that, all medications, even aspirin, should be taken as directed:

● Some medications should be taken with meals. With food, they're less likely to irritate the stomach. Aspirin and ibuprofen are two examples.

● Some medications should be taken on an empty stomach, perhaps an hour before or three hours after eating. Food may slow their absorption and action. That's true of some antibiotics, for example.

● Some food and medications shouldn't be consumed within several hours of each other. For example, fruit juice (including grapefruit juice) and other high-acid foods can destroy one type of penicillin. And calcium in dairy foods and calcium supplements binds with tetracycline, so it passes through the body without being absorbed.

● Some medications should be taken with plenty of water. That's true of most cholesterol-lowering medications.

● Many medications shouldn't be taken with alcoholic beverages. Alcohol can block the effects of some medications, and amplify the effects of others to potentially harmful levels. Medication also can intensify the effects of alcohol in your body.

How do you know to take medicine with a meal or on an empty stomach? Read the directions printed on the container or on an accompanying information sheet. You'll find information about when, how much per dose, and how long to take the medication. The directions also may state what to do if you miss a dose.

Ask the doctor or the pharmacist if you don't fully understand. You can ask that directions be printed in large type. *Note:* With the long-term use of some medications, your doctor also may prescribe a dietary supplement. *See chapter 23.*

You can't know about the potential interactions between all medicines and food. That's where the advice of your doctor, a pharmacist, or a registered dietitian comes in. *For a quick reference for some medications see "Common Interactions between Food and Some Medications" in this chapter.*

Medication: For Safety's Sake

● Talk to your doctor or pharmacist about all medications you're taking, including over-the-counter medications, dietary supplements such as herbal products, and oral supplements. Some medications and supplements have harmful interactions.

● Always take the medication as prescribed in the directions. If you don't take enough, or stop too soon, the medication may not work. Taking too much, too often can be dangerous. Depending on the medication, excessive amounts also may keep your body from absorbing essential nutrients or deplete your supply.

● Always take medicine in a well-lighted place. Put on your glasses if you wear them! Otherwise you might take the wrong medication or the wrong amount.

● Keep medicines in their original containers with the directions intact.

● Only take medicines prescribed for you, even if your symptoms seem similar to someone else's.

● Flush unused or expired medicines down the toilet.

● With each checkup, review your medication plan with your doctor to make sure it's still right for you.

CHAPTER 23

Supplements
Use and Abuse

Could a pill, a drink, or a supplement bar replace your dinner? For all those who enjoy the pleasure of eating, there's good news. The answer is unequivocally "no"!

Only food can provide the mixture of vitamins, minerals, phytonutrients, and other substances for health—qualities that can't be duplicated with dietary supplements alone. Fortunately for most Americans, there's plenty of quality, quantity, and variety in the food marketplace.

Despite this fact, more than half of Americans take dietary supplements, making it a business of $20.8 billion per year in 2005—and growing! Some people are prudent with their use, limiting the potency of their supplement to 100 percent or less of the Daily Values (DVs) and taking just the recommended dose. For others, supplements are part of or a complement to their medical care—as guided by their healthcare providers. Others self-prescribe high, potentially dangerous dosages of supplements, often at the advice of a friend or the media—not their healthcare provider.

Why do many consumers take dietary supplements? The reasons are varied—many times medically valid, sometimes not. In low or appropriate dosages, *some* supplements offer health benefits under *some* circumstances. Some people use supplements with good intention: perhaps in search of protection from or a remedy for health problems such as depression, aging skin, cancer, or arthritis. Still others seek added benefits: perhaps better athletic performance or sexual prowess. Too often, supplement use is based on scientifically unfounded marketing promises.

Supplement use is still largely a "world of the unknown": *unknown* benefits . . . *unknown* interactions with food, medicines, and other supplements . . . *undetermined* standards . . . *unknown* levels of safety and effectiveness, making dosages on package labels confusing. Steps are under way to gather scientific evidence for answers about their safety and effectiveness.

Regardless, no supplements provide a quick, easy road to health—a way that appears easier than making wise food choices and staying physically active. Good nutrition depends on overall healthful eating and active living, not supplements. Good health requires much more than a supplement or two, or more.

What, then, is appropriate—and inappropriate—use of dietary supplements?

Dietary Supplements: Defined

Dietary supplements are neither food nor drugs. Instead, they're products taken orally that contain a "dietary ingredient" meant to supplement the diet, not substitute for healthful foods. According to the Dietary Supplement Health and Education Act (DSHEA), approved in 1994, the term "dietary supplements" refers to a broad range of products: vitamins, minerals, herbs or other botanicals, and amino acids, as well as substances such as enzymes, hormones, concentrates, extracts, and metabolites.

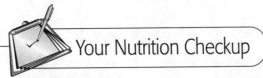

Your Nutrition Checkup

Supplements—Truth or Myth?

Many misconceptions surround dietary supplements. What do you think about using them?

....

FACT OR MYTH?

____	____	**1.** Nutrient supplements can make up for my poor food choices.
____	____	**2.** Taking supplements can prevent, treat, or cure disease.
____	____	**3.** Supplements boost my energy.
____	____	**4.** If it's herbal, it's not harmful.
____	____	**5.** "Stress" vitamins help me cope better with a lot of emotional stress.
____	____	**6.** A supplement can help me build muscle or get more from my physical performance.
____	____	**7.** A vitamin pill could protect my body from the harmful effects of smoking or alcohol.
____	____	**8.** Supplements make up for foods grown in depleted soil.
____	____	**9.** Popping a supplement pill can offer immediate benefits.

....

Here are the facts:

Misconceptions about dietary supplements are rampant. Even though consumers with these beliefs buy supplements, every statement is false!

1. *Fact:* No dietary supplement can fix an ongoing pattern of poor food choices. Supplements may supply some vitamins and minerals, but not all the substances that food supplies for your optimal health. Only a varied and balanced eating pattern provides enough nutrient variety, phytonutrients, and other substances for health. If you eat right, you probably don't need a daily supplement.

2. *Fact:* No scientific evidence in humans proves that a very high dosage of vitamin and mineral supplements prevents, treats, or cures cancer or other chronic illnesses. An extra amount of vitamin C won't prevent colds and flu, although it may reduce the symptoms. Some antioxidant nutrients, taken in higher dosages, may have protective effects, but research is still preliminary. *See "Antioxidant Vitamins: A Closer Look" in chapter 4.*

3. *Fact:* It would be great, but boosting your nutrient intake won't cause your cells to produce extra energy or more brain power. Only three nutrients—carbohydrates, fats, and proteins—supply energy or calories. Vitamins don't. Although B vitamins do *help* body cells produce energy from the three energy nutrients, they don't produce energy themselves.

4. *Fact:* Many powerful drugs and toxic chemicals are plant-based. Varieties of mushrooms can be classified as "culinary delicious" or "deadly dangerous." In the same vein, herbal supplements should be used with caution!

5. *Fact:* Emotional stress doesn't increase nutrient needs. Any claims promoting dietary supplements to "de-stress" your life are misleading, too. The best dietary advice to meet the physical demands of stress: a varied, balanced eating plan. More "de-stressing" advice: stay active, get enough rest, and take some personal time out to relax.

6. *Fact:* Athletes and other physically active people need about the same amount of nutrients as others do—just more energy, or calories, for the increased demands of exercise. The extra amount of food that active people eat supplies the very small amount of extra vitamins for energy production, too. Although protein needs are somewhat higher for some athletes, especially for those in strength-training sports, food can easily provide the extra. On another note, physical activity, not extra amino acids (protein), builds muscle. *For more on nutrition for athletes and ergogenic aids, see chapter 19, "Athlete's Guide: Winning Nutrition."*

7. *Fact:* Dietary supplements won't protect you from the harmful effects of smoking or alcohol abuse. Here's the real scoop: Smoking does increase the body's need for vitamin C; drinking excessive

Supplements—Truth or Myth? *(continued)*

amounts of alcoholic beverages can interfere with the body's use of most nutrients.

8. *Fact:* If soil can grow crops, the food produced is nutritious. When soil lacks minerals, plants don't grow properly and may not produce their potential yield. Growing area does affect a food's iodine and selenium contents.

9. *Fact:* Usually not. Supplements won't give you instant results. For vitamins and minerals to do their work, they need several hours or several days to interact and do their work in your body. For any benefits from other dietary supplements, you likely need to take them even longer.

Read on to unravel the fiction and explore the facts about dietary supplements.

Supplements are easy to spot. By law, they must be labeled "dietary supplements." About eighty thousand dietary supplements are marketed in the United States with multivitamin/mineral supplements being the biggest product category—and with an average of 500 new products launched each year. They're sold in many forms—for example, tablets, capsules, softgels, gelcaps, liquids, powders, and bars.

Vitamin/Mineral Supplements: Benefits and Risks

Do you take a vitamin and mineral supplement? Maybe you need to, maybe not. Many vitamins and minerals are sold as single supplements—for example, vitamins C and E, beta carotene, calcium, and iron. Some are sold in large doses, perhaps more than you need. Others are "combos," sold as multivitamin/mineral supplements. What's right for you?

Vitamin/Mineral Supplements: For Whom?

Do you consume a varied, balanced diet? With some exceptions, supplements usually aren't necessary—*if* you're healthy and *if* you're able *and willing* to eat a balanced, varied diet. You probably can get the vitamins and minerals you need from smart food choices. According to national studies, most Americans have enough healthful foods available to do that, yet they may not. Under some circumstances, vitamin/mineral supplements offer benefits and are advised.

Your doctor or a registered dietitian (RD) may recommend a dietary supplement. Are you . . .

● *A woman with heavy menstrual bleeding?* You may need an iron supplement to replace iron from blood loss. To enhance absorption, take iron supplements with water or juice on an empty stomach. If nausea or constipation are problems, take iron supplements with food. Absorption may be decreased by as much as 50 percent when taken with a meal or a snack.

● *A woman who's pregnant or breast-feeding?* You need more of some nutrients, especially folate and iron—and perhaps calcium if you don't consume enough calcium-rich foods. Check the label's Supplement Facts to make sure you get enough for a healthy pregnancy. Ask about a prenatal vitamin/mineral supplement. *See "Before Pregnancy" in chapter 17.*

● *A woman capable of becoming pregnant?* Consume 400 micrograms of folic acid (the synthetic form of folate) daily from fortified foods, vitamin supplements, or a combination of the two—*in addition to* folate found naturally in some fruits, vegetables, and legumes. The extra folic acid offers a safeguard against spinal cord defects in a developing fetus. Synthetic folic acid is better absorbed than food folate.

Foods fortified with folic acid include enriched grains such as flour, breads, cereals, pasta, and rice. If you take a supplement, choose one with a dosage of no more than 1,000 micrograms of folic acid daily.

● *A menopausal woman?* You'll likely benefit from a calcium supplement with vitamin D, in addition to a calcium-rich diet, to slow calcium loss from bones. *See "Calcium Supplements: A Bone Builder" in this chapter.* For some older men, a calcium supplement is advised, too.

● *Someone on a restrictive diet (<1,600 calories a day)?* You likely won't consume enough food to meet all your nutrient needs. Your doctor or a registered dietitian may recommend a multivitamin/mineral supplement. **Caution:** Unless under a doctor's supervision, very-low-calorie eating plans aren't advised. *See "'Diets' That Don't Work!" in chapter 2.*

● *A vegetarian?* You may need extra calcium, iron, zinc, and vitamins B$_{12}$ and D—if your regular eating pattern doesn't supply much, if any, meat, dairy, and other animal products. *See chapter 20, "The Vegetarian Way."*

● *Someone with limited milk intake and sunlight exposure?* If you have lactose intolerance, a milk allergy, or simply don't consume enough dairy foods, you may need a calcium supplement for bone health.

You may be advised to take a vitamin D supplement, too. (Older adults often need a vitamin D supplement.) Remember, fortified milk is the best source of vitamin D. Still, you need only a little sunlight for your body to make enough vitamin D: ten to fifteen minutes on your hands, arms, and face without sunscreen, two times a week for most people. *See "Vitamin D: The Sunshine Vitamin" in chapter 18.*

● *Someone with a health condition that affects nutrient use?* Doctors often prescribe supplements for those with health problems that affect appetite or eating, or that affect how nutrients are absorbed, used, or excreted—for example, digestive or liver problems. Surgery or injuries may increase the body's need for some nutrients. Some medications, such as antacids, antibiotics, laxatives, and diuretics, may interfere with the way the body uses nutrients. If you have a food allergy, gluten intolerance, or other health problems that restrict what you eat, a supplement may be advised; talk to your healthcare provider.

Ten to 30 percent of adults over age fifty have atrophic gastritis, a condition that causes damage to stomach cells and so reduces the body's ability to absorb vitamin B$_{12}$. For that reason, adults in this age group are urged to get extra vitamin B$_{12}$ in its crystalline form from a supplement or from fortified food.

● *Someone unable—or unwilling—to regularly consume a healthful diet?* You likely need a dietary supplement to fill in the nutrient gaps. However, eating smarter would be better if you don't have food-related health problems! Take a supplement with the advice of a doctor or a registered dietitian. For example, premenopausal women who don't consume enough calcium from food likely need a calcium supplement—unless they're willing to improve their diet.

● *Some babies* after age six months, children, and teens may need a fluoride supplement—and perhaps

iron or vitamin D. *See "Vitamin and Mineral Supplements for Breast-Fed Babies" in chapter 15.*

To know if you likely consume enough nutrients, see "How Did You Build Your Pyramid?" in chapter 10. If you have any questions about your own nutrient needs—or think you need a supplement—talk to a registered dietitian or your doctor. *See "How to Find Nutrition Help . . ." in chapter 24.*

More Isn't Always Better!

A little is good, but a lot may *not* be healthier. As with other nutrients, such as fat, added sugars, and sodium, moderation is your smart guideline for vitamins and minerals: enough, but not too much.

Supplements carry labeling, showing the amounts of vitamins and minerals in a single dosage. If you already eat a healthful diet, you probably don't need any more than a low-dose supplement. Taking a multivitamin/mineral supplement, with no more than 100 percent of the Daily Values (DVs) as a safety net, is generally considered safe. Most nutrient supplements are produced in low dosages.

Supplements that boast "high potency"—a much higher dosage than you may need—also are sold over the counter in pharmacies, grocery stores, health food stores, and through Internet and mail-order outlets. Either as single-nutrient supplements or vitamin-mineral combinations, high-potency supplements (significantly in excess of the Daily Values) can be harmful. Why can they be sold if you don't need so much? Currently no law limits supplement potency, except for potassium. Being prudent is up to you.

Risks. Consumed in excessive amounts, nutrients in some supplements can have undesirable side effects such as fatigue, diarrhea, and hair loss. Others may pose more serious risks—for example, kidney stones, liver or nerve damage, birth defects, or even death.

Because fat-soluble vitamins (A, D, E, K) are stored in the body, taking high levels of some for a prolonged time can be toxic. For example, excess amounts of vitamin D can cause kidney damage and reduced bone density. Too much vitamin A, taken over time, can cause bone and liver damage, headaches, diarrhea, and birth defects.

Supplements with water-soluble vitamins or minerals can be risky if taken in excess, over time. For

Have You Ever Wondered

. . . why a nutrient supplement label may list the percent of vitamin A from beta carotene? The supplement may contain beta carotene but not vitamin A itself. However, the body converts beta carotene to vitamin A.

. . . if ridges or white marks on your fingernails suggest a vitamin deficiency? No, but it's a common misconception. Instead, they're often caused by a slight injury to the nail. Although they may have other causes, too, a nutrient deficiency isn't one of them.

Appearance-conscious teens often hear that taking gelatin pills strengthens nails, but there's no quick nutritional cure for nails that break and split. Fingernails are mainly dead protein cells that get their strength from amino acids. Gelatin doesn't contain these amino acids.

. . . if supplements with "phytonutrients" are a good choice? From *phyto,* Greek for plant, these botanical substances are extracted from vegetables and other plant foods. There's not enough scientific evidence to know if supplement manufacturers have picked the right

active substance from plant sources for any benefit.

Plants have thousands of phytonutrients. Science hasn't yet revealed which one, if any, or what amount in a supplement might offer any health benefits. Better advice: Get "phytos" from food. Any health-promoting benefit might come from the interaction of many phytonutrients provided naturally in food.

. . . if dietary supplements can protect against biological threats? No, although some supplement promoters may make this claim. According to the Centers for Disease Control and Prevention and the U.S. Food and Drug Administration (FDA), no current and credible scientific evidence suggests that supplements on the market today offer protection from or treatment for biological contaminants such as anthrax, SARS, or bird (avian) flu.

Likewise, FDA advises against taking antibiotics for protection from foodborne illnesses caused by bacteria, unless prescribed by a doctor. Antibiotics can't protect against viruses or chemicals that contaminate food.

example, taking extra vitamin B_6 has been suggested to help relieve premenstrual tension. Yet there's limited evidence to support large vitamin B_6 doses for relief of premenstrual syndrome (PMS). Many women have viewed large vitamin B_6 doses as harmless, since they are water-soluble. Instead, they may cause irreversible nerve damage when taken in very large doses above the Tolerable Upper Intake Level (UL): 500 to 5,000 mg vitamin B_6 per day.

As other examples, very high doses of vitamin C can cause diarrhea and nausea. Liver damage may be caused by high doses of niacin (as time-released nicotinic acid); sometimes a physician will prescribe high doses of niacin to help lower an elevated blood cholesterol level. Excessive amounts of folic acid can hide symptoms of pernicious anemia, so the disease gets worse without being detected.

Children are more vulnerable to overdoses of vitamins and minerals than adults. In fact, excessive iron—perhaps from iron supplements intended for their mother—can be fatal to children.

The way your body handles large nutrient doses from dietary supplements depends on many factors. Your body size, supplement dose (amount and fre-

quency), and how long you take them influence whether a megadose will be toxic for you.

See the Appendices for the Tolerable Upper Intake Level (UL) for many nutrients. The UL is the maximum amount that appears safe for most healthy people. Consuming more may increase some health risks. *See chapter 4 for more about vitamins and minerals that may be sold in supplement form.*

Nutrient-Nutrient Interactions. High doses of some nutrients may result in deficiencies of others. For example: high calcium intake may inhibit the absorption of iron and other trace nutrients. High doses of vitamin E can interfere with the action of vitamin K and make anticoagulant drugs such as Coumadin (warfarin) more powerful.

Even low levels of dietary supplements may contribute to health problems for some people. For example, those at risk for hemochromatosis need to be careful of taking extra iron. Folic acid can mask a vitamin B_{12} deficiency, which may cause neurological damage. And zinc supplements in excess of the UL can decrease levels of "good" cholesterol (high-density lipoprotein blood cholesterol), impair immunity, and reduce copper status.

Benefits. Emerging research is exploring the link between higher levels of some antioxidant nutrients (vitamin C, vitamin E, selenium) and omega-3s with reduced risk for some health problems. However, the jury's still out. Currently available research doesn't show that levels higher than the Recommended Dietary Allowance are effective in cancer or heart disease prevention. Until more is known, be cautious about taking supplements to protect against disease. *See "Antioxidant Nutrients: Enough, or Too Much?" in this chapter.*

Except for rare medical conditions, few people need more than 100 percent of their Recommended Dietary Allowances (RDAs) of any nutrient. Large mineral or vitamin doses are prescribed only for certain medically diagnosed health problems. Even then, their use should be monitored carefully by a doctor.

That said, can you overdose on vitamins or minerals naturally occurring in food? That's highly unlikely. As we mentioned, taking very high doses of dietary supplements—or taking too many, too often—can be dangerous. The vitamin and mineral content of food is much more balanced. In amounts normally consumed, even if you enjoy extra helpings, you won't consume toxic levels of nutrients. So eat a variety of foods—and enjoy! *Note:* Nutrient amounts can add up if you consume *a lot* of highly fortified foods.

Other Cautions

You may take dietary supplements for potential health benefits. It's not uncommon for people diagnosed with cancer, AIDS, or other life-threatening health problems, who are desperate for a cure, to put their hopes and healthcare dollars in alternative treatments, including dietary supplements. However, supplements may offer a false sense of security—and a serious problem if you neglect well-proven approaches to health or delay medical attention.

If you choose to take a dietary supplement, ask your healthcare provider. *See "Guidelines for Supplement Use" in this chapter.* Seek medical attention and proven treatment for health problems first. Even if you're healthy, get regular medical checkups, eat wisely, and live a healthful lifestyle rather than rely on the "security" of supplements.

What We Know About ...

Calcium Supplements: A Bone Builder. For people of every age, food choices can supply an adequate amount of calcium. As an extra safeguard, many doctors also recommend calcium supplements, especially for menopausal and postmenopausal women and for women who simply don't consume enough calcium. The reason? To help stave off bone loss that comes with hormonal changes. If you're advised to take a calcium supplement, keep these pointers in mind:

● Read the label. Calcium in all over-the-counter supplements isn't the same. First, the calcium amount differs. Multivitamin/mineral supplements don't have as much calcium as calcium supplements do.

Calcium supplements are sold as compounds, such as calcium citrate and calcium carbonate. Their amounts and absorption of calcium differ; check the label. Aiding absorption, chewable and liquid calcium supplements dissolve even before entering the stomach. Calcium carbonate is absorbed best with food; calcium citrate can be taken any time.

● Consider a calcium supplement or a multivitamin with vitamin D if you don't get enough from food. Vitamin D is essential for calcium absorption.

● Avoid calcium supplements with dolomite, unrefined oyster shell, or bonemeal without a USP symbol. They might contain small amounts of hazardous contaminants: lead, arsenic, mercury, or cadmium. What's dolomite? A mineral compound found in marble and limestone.

● Take calcium supplements as intended—as a supplement, not as your only important calcium source. Although calcium supplements may boost calcium intake, they don't provide other nutrients your bones and body need: vitamin D, magnesium, phosphorus, and boron. Milk, for example, provides vitamin D, a nutrient that helps deposit calcium in your bones.

● If you take both calcium and iron supplements, take them at different times of the day. They'll each be better absorbed when taken on their own.

● If you take two or three low-dose tablets daily, space them throughout the day for better absorption. Calcium in supplements is absorbed best in doses of 500 milligrams or less.

- Follow the dosage advised by your healthcare provider. The Tolerable Upper Intake Level for calcium is 2,500 milligrams daily from food and supplements.

- Drink plenty of fluids with calcium supplements to avoid constipation. The lactose and vitamin D in the milk help to enhance calcium absorption.

- If you take medications or other supplements, ask your doctor or registered dietitian about interactions. For example, calcium and tetracycline bind; neither is adequately absorbed as a result. Calcium also inhibits magnesium, phosphorus, and zinc absorption.

- If you don't drink milk and want an alternative to calcium pills, consider calcium-fortified juice or soy beverage. One cup of calcium-fortified juice or soy beverage can contain about 300 milligrams of calcium, the same amount as in a cup of milk, and provides vitamin C, folate, and other nutrients. Still, you need a vitamin D source to aid absorption; some calcium-fortified juices and soy beverages are also fortified with vitamin D.

- Calcium supplements—to protect against osteoporosis (brittle-bone disease)—can't make up for your lifestyle choices or poor health habits. Regular weight-bearing physical activity is important for healthy bones. For healthy bones, avoid smoking, too.

Are calcium supplements right for everyone? For people with kidney damage or urinary tract stones, calcium supplements pose risks. If you have a history of kidney stones, take calcium supplements under your doctor's care. *See "Osteoporosis: Reduce the Risks" in chapter 22.*

Coral calcium? No evidence shows that it's better. People with shellfish allergies may react to coral calcium since it's from coral reefs. It also may contain lead, which can be dangerous. *Refer to chapter 8, "Get the Lead Out."*

Iron Supplements: Enhancing the Benefit. Physicians often advise iron supplements for premenopausal and pregnant women, and for some children and teens. If you're advised to take an iron supplement, remember:

- Pick a better-absorbed form of iron (ferrous sulfate).

- Check the dosage when choosing an iron supplement. Dosages of 15 to 30 milligrams per day are

Have You Ever Wondered

. . . if antacids are as effective as calcium supplements as an extra calcium source? That depends. Look for an antacid without aluminum hydroxides. Aluminum in antacids can interfere with calcium absorption.

. . . if vitamin nasal sprays or patches are effective? No research evidence says so, even though they're promoted for faster, more efficient absorption. In fact, they may not be absorbed at all. Here's the reality check: Fat-soluble vitamins need fat from food to aid absorption. Vitamin C in your intestine aids iron absorption—a problem if vitamin C comes from a spray. Vitamin B_{12} binds with intrinsic factor made in the stomach during digestion. That cannot happen with a spray or a patch!

likely adequate. Higher amounts should be taken only if prescribed by your healthcare provider.

- Take iron supplements on an empty stomach—between meals or before bedtime—to enhance absorption.

- Take them with water or juice—not milk, coffee, or tea, which can inhibit absorption. As an aside, drinking vitamin C-rich juice with an iron supplement isn't necessary. Unlike nonheme iron in plant-based foods, the iron in supplements is in an absorbable form.

- Drink plenty of water to help avoid constipation, a common side effect from taking iron supplements.

- Store them where children can't reach them. Adult iron supplements can be extremely toxic to children!

Herbals and Other Botanicals: Help or Harm?

Herbal and other botanical supplements may seem safe enough. After all, they're made from natural, fresh herbs or other parts of plants: flowers, leaves, roots, and seeds. And many have been used for centuries. In reality, there's nothing inherently harmless about botanical supplements, just because they're "natural." Despite the remarkable array of claims, scientific research is lacking for many herbal remedies.

Indeed, herbals and other botanicals have known medicinal qualities; 30 percent of today's drugs come from plants. Yet, herbals and other botanical supplements also are sold as dietary supplements rather than regulated as drugs. Like many plant-derived pharmaceuticals, these supplements can offer both positive health benefits and harmful side effects.

On the up side, enough scientific evidence has been collected on a handful of botanical supplements to support their limited use. For example, under a doctor's guidance, gingko biloba may be used to help treat the symptoms of age-related memory loss and dementia (including Alzheimer's disease); green tea extract may help reduce cancer risk. A growing body of research evidence is being gathered about their safety and effectiveness, as well as their limitations and dangers.

On the down side, like other supplements, herbal and other botanical supplements are regulated differently from pharmaceuticals, which are meant to cure or prevent disease. You aren't as protected from misleading claims as you might think. *See "Quality and Effectiveness: Who's in Control"? in this chapter.*

According to current law and regulations, herbal and botanical remedies and other dietary supplements can enter the marketplace without FDA approval. The burden is on the FDA to remove a dangerous dietary supplement from the marketplace. Currently dosages of herbal remedies aren't standardized, so dosages vary among products.

Although packaging claims can't say that a supplement cures or prevents disease, it may carry claims for its purported health role. Many claims have only limited scientific evidence.

Although Dietary Reference Intakes, with recommended intakes, exist for vitamins and minerals, no recommendation or safe dosage exists for herbals, other botanicals, and other nonnutrient supplements. The National Institutes of Health's Office of Dietary Supplements provides advice on many botanicals.

Herbal Ingredients: Hazardous to Health!

The FDA warns against the use of botanical supplements with these active ingredients, due to their serious, *even deadly,* side effects:

- *Aristolochic acid.* A substance in some traditional Chinese herbal products, aristolochic acid causes

ANTIOXIDANT NUTRIENTS: ENOUGH, OR TOO MUCH?

Antioxidant supplements are "hot" supplements—even though there's no conclusive evidence that taking daily amounts of antioxidant nutrients beyond their Recommended Dietary Allowance (RDA) prevents disease. If you choose to take them for their potential benefits, talk to your doctor first. Then avoid exceeding the Tolerable Upper Intake Level (UL) set for safety. To use Supplement Facts on labels, be aware that the %DVs for one serving, or dosage, are based on the Daily Values (DVs) used in labeling. *See "Antioxidants in Supplements" in chapter 4.*

ANTIOXIDANT NUTRIENT	RDA FOR WOMEN	RDA FOR MEN	DAILY VALUE (FOR LABELING)	UL FOR WOMEN AND MEN	ALSO NOTE
Vitamin C	75 mg	90 mg	60 mg	2,000 mg	Smokers need 35 mg more per day than nonsmokers.
Vitamin E	15 mg from food (equivalent to 22 IU natural sources or 33 IU synthetic form vitamin E)	15 mg from food (equivalent to 22 IU natural sources or 33 IU synthetic form vitamin E)	30 IU	1,000 mg alpha-tocopherol (equivalent to 1,500 IU natural source vitamin E or 1,100 IU synthetic form vitamin E)	
Selenium	55 mcg	55 mcg	70 mcg	400 mcg	
Beta carotene and other carotenoids	Due to conflicting evidence, no recommended level	Due to conflicting evidence, no recommended level	None identified	Due to conflicting evidence, no UL recommended	Beta carotene supplements may increase lung cancer risk among some smokers.

Adapted from: National Academy of Sciences. *Dietary Reference Intakes.* Washington, D.C.: National Academy Press, 2000. Reprinted with permission in *A Healthcare Professional's Guide for Evaluating Dietary Supplements.* Chicago: American Dietetic Association, American Pharmaceutical Association, 2000.

HERBALS AND OTHER BOTANICALS (SELECTED): CLAIMS, EFFECTIVENESS

Here's what the symbols mean:

↑ — Evidence comes from several controlled human studies.

↑? — Preliminary evidence comes from only a few controlled human studies or from laboratory studies with cell or tissue samples.

↔ — Evidence is uncertain and based on conflicting, controlled human research.

↓ — Research doesn't support the claim.

↓? — Preliminary evidence from a few controlled trials in humans does *not* support efficacy claims, but more research is needed. (Research that is negative and has only been performed in vitro is so designated in the column.)

NR — Not enough human research has been done yet, or the research quality is poor.

HERBAL OR OTHER BOTANICAL SUPPLEMENT	MEDIA OR MARKETING CLAIMS	EFFECTIVENESS	ALSO BE AWARE . . . Caution: *Dietary supplements can pose significant and serious health risks*, related to dosage, length of use, health status, age, and interactions with drugs and nutrients. *Before taking them, always* talk to your healthcare provider about their safety, risks, and interactions (*not fully listed below*), especially when treating or managing health conditions.
Echinacea	● Boosts immune function in healthy individuals	NR	● Do not take if you: — have health problems with reduced immunity (e.g,. lupus, HIV, tuberculosis, multiple sclerosis, scleroderma) — take medications that may be toxic to the liver, such as anabolic steroids ● Potential severe allergic reactions if you have asthma or sensitivity to grass pollens
	● Protects against common cold virus, upper respiratory infections	↔	
Garlic	● Reduces cholesterol levels	↑?	● May increase bleeding
	● Reduces blood pressure	↑?	● Promote undesirable body odor, even from some odor-free varieties
	● Improves circulation	↑?	● Avoid taking 7 days before surgery
	● Reduces cancer risk	↑?	● May interfere with the effectiveness of oral contraceptives and certain drugs (e.g., HIV drug saquinavir)
	● Improves immune function	↑?	● May cause stomach discomfort at high doses ● Should be monitored if taken with anticoagulant medications
Ginger	● Treats morning sickness	↑?	● Conflicting data about safety of ginger before surgery for those on anticoagulation medications
	● Treats post-surgery nausea	↔	● Should monitor closely if also taking glucose-lowering drugs for diabetes management or anticoagulant/antiplatelet drugs
	● Treats nausea associated with chemotherapy	NR	
Ginkgo biloba	● Improves memory in individuals with Alzheimer's disease or dementia	↔	● Consuming ginkgo seeds can be fatal; linked to convulsions and repetitive seizures in children
	● Improves memory in healthy individuals	↔	● Avoid taking at least 36 hours before surgery ● Avoid all fresh ginkgo plant parts
	● Improves symptoms of reduced circulation in individuals with intermittent claudication	↑?	● Can cause mild GI upset, headache, dizziness, palpitations, constipation, and allergic skin reactions ● Large doses (estimated >600 mg/day) may cause restlessness, diarrhea, nausea, vomiting, lack of muscle tone, weakness
	● Relieves tinnitus (ringing in ears)	↓	● Should be monitored if you take anticoagulant medications
	● Prevents mountain or altitude sickness	↓	
Ginseng	● Improves exercise performance	↓	● Possible hypertension, nervousness, sleeplessness, acne, edema, headache, and diarrhea linked to > 3g ginseng root/day (about 600 mg ginseng extract)
	● Improves quality of life, energy mood, cognition	↔	● Do not take:
	● Improves sexual function; aphrodisiac	NR	— during pregnancy or lactation
	● Helps control blood glucose levels in diabetes	NR	— if you are at risk or were previously treated for estrogen-related cancer (breast, ovarian, etc.)

Herbal or Other Botanical Supplement	Media or Marketing Claims	Effectiveness	Also Be Aware ...
Ginseng (continued)	• Reduces risk for cancer	NR	• Potential hypoglycemic effect; individuals with diabetes should monitor their blood glucose levels • May interfere with phenelzine, corticosteroids, digoxin (digitalis), diabetes medications, and estrogen therapy • May increase bleeding time when taken with other blood-thinning drugs or some supplements
Goldenseal (*Hydrastis canadensis*)	• Enhances immune function through antibiotic activity • Reduces risk for infectious diarrhea • Masks drug use in urine drug testing	NR NR ↓	• Safety demonstrated for short-term use • Long-term, high doses linked to cardiac spasms and death. • Oral long-term linked to gastrointestinal upset, hallucinations, delirium • Topical application results in photosensitivity to UVA exposure
Green tea extract (*Camellia sinensis*)	• Acts as an antioxidant • Reduces risk for cancer • Improves heart health • Assists in blood pressure control • Promotes weight control by increasing energy expenditure	↑ ↑? ↔ NR NR	• Moderate doses of green tea extract used for several years have been demonstrated to be safe. • Be aware that some supplements may contain caffeine • Possible nausea if consumed on an empty stomach • May interfere with iron absorption; may negatively interact with caffeine-containing medications • Discuss with your doctor if on anticoagulant medications
Kava (*Piper methysticum*)	• Reduces anxiety • Promotes restful sleep	↑? NR	• Avoid if you have: liver disease • Potentially dangerous interaction when combined with anti-anxiety medications, such as benzodiazepine, or alcohol • May affect motor reflexes and judgment; do not use while operating heavy machinery • Avoid taking with alcohol, barbiturates, or psychopharmacological agents due to possible sedative effects • Do not use for more than 3 months without medical advice • May decrease effectiveness of drugs used in Parkinson's disease, other diseases
Ma huang (*Ephedra*)	• Increases metabolism for weight loss	Do *not* use due to safety issues; products with ephedra have been banned by the FDA	• Numerous reports of adverse events after use, including heart attack, stroke, tremors, insomnia, and death in individuals otherwise in good health • Acts as a heart and central nervous system stimulant • Avoid if you have: hypertension and/or CVD disease, thyroid disease, diabetes, neurological disorders, (men) difficulty urinating due to an enlarged prostate • Do not take with any medications used to treat heart disease, hypertension, depression, Parkinson's disease, asthma, or diabetes or with stimulant herbs
Saw palmetto (*Seronoa repens*)	• Improves symptoms of enlarged prostate • Prevents prostate cancer • Prevents male-pattern baldness/hair loss	↔ NR NR	• Discontinue at least 2 weeks before surgery due to the herb's anticoagulant effects • May interfere with blood clotting and increase bleeding time if taking anticoagulant medications • May be linked to gastrointestinal discomfort in rare cases • No controlled studies testing the safety of long-term use
St. John's wort	• Alleviates depression • Promotes emotional well-being	↑? NR	• Do not take with antidepressant medications (potentially dangerous combined effects); may limit effectives of some other medications and oral contraceptives • May make skin sensitive to sunlight, especially for fair-skinned people at dosages more than 2 g/day • Discontinue before surgery • Do not take if you have: Alzheimer's disease

HERBALS AND OTHER BOTANICALS (SELECTED): CLAIMS, EFFECTIVENESS *(continued)*

HERBAL OR OTHER BOTANICAL SUPPLEMENT	MEDIA OR MARKETING CLAIMS	EFFECTIVENESS	ALSO BE AWARE ...
Valerian *(Valeriana officinalis)*	• Enhances sleep • Reduces stress and anxiety	↔ NR	• Avoid driving or operating heavy machinery while taking • Do not take if you have: liver disease (due to possible contamination); take barbiturates or other sleep medications • May cause morning drowsiness with high doses (900 mg) • Avoid if taking St John's wort, kava, L-tryptophan, or alcohol due to sedative effects • May experience serious withdrawal symptoms if abruptly discontinued; taper off slowly
Wheat grass, barley grass	• Acts as an antioxidant • Enhances immunity • Reduces cholesterol	NR NR NR	• No studies testing the safety of supplementing the diet with liquid or dried juices of wheat or barley grasses
Yohimbine *(yohimbe)*	• Increases sex drive • Aids in weight loss • Builds muscle	NR NR NR	• Potentially dangerous! • Doses of 4 to 20 mg have been associated with serious harmful effects, such abnormal heartbeat, tremors, and low blood pressure • Toxicity may be enhanced by taking phenothazines (drug used in mental disorders) • Not for people with high or low blood pressure, bipolar disorder, or liver or kidney disease • Should not be used in combination with blood pressure medications, some other drugs

Adapted from Allison Sarubin Fragakis with Cynthia A. Thomson, The Health Professional's Guide to Popular Dietary Supplements, third edition (Chicago: The American Dietetic Association, 2007).

kidney damage and is a potent carcinogen. It's known or suspected to be in many products, including those with guan mu tong, ma dou ling, birthwort, Indian ginger, wild ginger, colic root, and snakeroot.

● *Chaparral.* This Native American medicine can cause rapid, potentially irreversible liver damage.

● *Comfrey.* Supplements with comfrey (common, prickly, or Russian) pose serious health risks, notably for liver damage and as a possible carcinogen.

● *Ephedrine, ma huang* (ephedra sinica), *epitonin.* Being medicinal herbs, supplements with these ephedrine alkaloids have been touted as energy enhancers. Ephedrine also has been a component of weight-loss teas and aids. It's a stimulant closely related to methamphetamine, and is especially dangerous when combined with other stimulants. Hazards range from nervousness, dizziness, rapid heartbeat, and changes in blood pressure to muscle injury, seizures, nerve damage, heart attack, hepatitis, psychosis, stroke, and even death. People with health problems, such as high blood pressure, heart

disease, or diabetes, are at special risk. Because they are so risky, a 2004 FDA regulation prohibits the sale of dietary supplements containing ephedra; some medications, however, contain a form of it. This ruling has been challenged.

● *Kava.* An herbal ingredient promoted for relaxation, and relief of sleeplessness and menopausal symptoms, kava is linked to liver-related injuries. It's especially risky for those with liver disease or liver problems, or persons who are taking drug products that can affect the liver.

● *Lobelia.* Also called Indian tobacco, it acts like nicotine; among potential dangers: breathing problems, rapid heartbeat, sweating, low blood pressure, coma, death. It's particularly harmful to children, pregnant women, and people with heart disease.

● *Germander.* Its use may lead to liver disease, possibly to death.

● *Magnolia-stephania preparation.* Its use may lead to kidney disease and permanent kidney failure.

● *Willow bark.* Marketed as an aspirin-free product, willow bark contains an ingredient that converts to the active ingredient found in aspirin. Potential health hazards include Reye's syndrome, a potentially fatal disease that's linked to aspirin intake in children with chicken pox or flu symptoms. Adults can have an allergic reaction to willow bark.

● *Wormwood.* This herbal ingredient may cause neurological symptoms such as numbness of legs and arms, loss of intellect, delirium, and paralysis.

● *Yohimbe.* Derived from tree bark, yohimbe has several active ingredients, including yohimbine, with potentially dangerous side effects: kidney failure, seizures, nervous system disorders, paralysis, fatigue, stomach problems, and death. Because yohimbine is a MAO (monoamine oxidase) inhibitor, it is especially harmful when taken at the same time as tyramine-containing foods such as liver, cheese, or red wine, and with over-the-counter medications with phenylpropanolamine (some nasal decongestants and diet aids).

Two other ingredients, often found in herbal supplements, have potential health hazards: germanium (a nonessential mineral) may result in kidney damage, possibly death, and L-tryptophan (an amino acid) may result in a potentially fatal blood disorder that can cause high fever, muscle and joint pain, weakness, skin rash, and swelling of the arms and the legs.

Other Supplements

As supplement categories, nutrient and herbal supplements come to mind. But stores and Internet sites sell others. *Many are addressed in "Selected Other Supplements: Claims, Benefits, Risks" in this chapter.*

● Enzymes and hormones—for example, coenzyme Q10, DHEA, melatonin

● Ergogenic aids—for example, chromium picolinate, creatine

● Others—for example, bee pollen, carnitine, conjugated linoleic acid, fish oil, flaxseed, glucosamine, lecithin, royal jelly, shark cartilage.

Supplements: Safe? Effective?

Even though dietary supplements are big business, manufacturing standards for their quality, potency,

and effectiveness have lagged behind their phenomenal market growth. Product information is often misleading, despite limited government regulations. While scientific claims may be given, well-designed scientific studies for supplements are often limited.

Quality and Effectiveness: Who's in Control?

If you buy a supplement, are you getting what you think you paid for? Maybe, but maybe not, despite government regulations.

Although foods and drugs are highly regulated, supplements aren't regulated in the same way. Enacted in 1994, the FDA's Dietary Supplement Health and Education Act (DSHEA) requires that supplements be safe, unadulterated, and properly labeled, be produced with good manufacturing practices, and be promoted with label information that's truthful. The FDA proposed Good Manufacturing Practices for supplements in 2003; the rule is not yet final.

The responsibility for proof, however, lies with the manufacturer, not with the FDA. The manufacturer is expected to ensure that the supplement's label information (Supplement Facts and ingredient list) is accurate, that its ingredients are safe, and that the declared contents match what's inside the container.

The FDA doesn't currently require supplement testing—for safety, effectiveness, or interactions—before it's produced or launched into the marketplace. If, however, an ingredient is new (marketed after October 1994), manufacturers must provide the FDA with evidence that the supplement is "reasonably expected to be safe" at the labeled dosage. The FDA can take action if the supplement is either unsafe or mislabeled.

For a growing list of dietary supplements, U.S. Pharmacopeia (USP), an independent, not-for-profit organization, sets quality standards: for strength, quality, and purity of supplements. If manufacturers voluntarily comply, they may display the "USP" or "NF" (National Formulary) letters along with the lot number and expiration date of the product. This is industry-reported compliance, not third-party assessment. USP's *United States Pharmacopeia—National Formulary* manual shows supplement standards for:

● *Disintegration,* or how fast it breaks down into smaller pieces.

- *Dissolution,* or how fast and how well it dissolves in a solution similar to digestive juices.

- *Purity,* whether it has an acceptable limit of impurities.

- *Strength,* or how much of the vitamin, mineral, or active ingredient it contains.

- *Expiration,* or how long it retains its quality.

While some supplements are labeled accurately and completely, some aren't, and what's stated on the label may not be what's in the container. The potency or purity may be misrepresented or inconsistent. Herbs may be misidentified, indicating the wrong part or type of herb. The dosage's safety and effectiveness aren't regulated either. Bottom line: It's up to you to be a discriminating consumer!

Several independent organizations—e.g., NSF International, U.S. Pharmacopeia (USP), and ConsumerLab.com—have certification programs, designed to assess whether a supplement really contains what the manufacturer declares on the label. (The "USP letters" mentioned previously have a different meaning than the "USP Verified" mark.) A fee-based service to industry, each certifying organization sets its own assessment criteria—some more in-depth than others. Some audit manufacturing practices; some do ongoing surveillance.

A step in the right direction, it's hard to discern precisely what a specific certification mark on a supplement label means and how each mark's criteria differs, however. Although a certifying mark helps you know if you're getting what you paid for, it does *not* verify a supplement's overall safety or effectiveness. No certifying mark? It could mean several things: the supplement didn't meet certification criteria, or the assessment is in progress, or perhaps the supplement hasn't been submitted for review.

What about regulations for advertising supplements? The Federal Trade Commission (FTC) regulates the advertising of supplements, including media infomercials and Internet promotion. Like the FDA, its resources for monitoring are limited.

Also note, supplement recalls are voluntary. Recalling a harmful product is no guarantee that it's been removed entirely from store shelves . . . despite good intentions by reputable manufacturers.

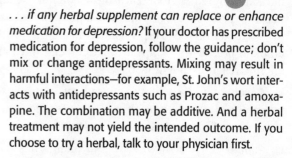

Have You Ever Wondered

. . . if any herbal supplement can replace or enhance medication for depression? If your doctor has prescribed medication for depression, follow the guidance; don't mix or change antidepressants. Mixing may result in harmful interactions—for example, St. John's wort interacts with antidepressants such as Prozac and amoxapine. The combination may be additive. And a herbal treatment may not yield the intended outcome. If you choose to try a herbal, talk to your physician first.

. . . if chromium supplements help with blood sugar levels? As a nutrient, chromium helps your body use blood sugar properly and helps break down proteins and fats. There isn't enough evidence to show that taking chromium supplements improves the way your body uses blood sugar. It may help with blood glucose control for those with diabetes.

Supplements: Marketplace Confusion

Believe it or not, many supplement manufacturers do provide reliable product information. In fact, by law, supplement labels must bear Supplement Facts and claims that cannot mislead.

However, many companies don't abide by the supplement "rules." A regulatory environment that's less restrictive than the early 1990s has allowed more products and more misinformation to enter the marketplace, and deceptive marketing tactics are present throughout the supplement industry. For well-intentioned consumers—eager to take responsibility for their health—the sea of science and fiction is often confusing and misleading, and ultimately may be costly and harmful.

What misleading tactics may be used? Supplements are often promoted with pseudoscience. *See "Ten Red Flags of Junk Science" in chapter 24.*

- *Borrowed research.* Study results that may or may not apply to the product: perhaps supplements with different potencies or formulations, or derived from different parts of the plant.

- *Distorted data.* Information that's "spun" to match the product claim. Again, the formulation or dosage may differ from the supplement used in the original study. Less reputable manufacturers may present their

OTHER SUPPLEMENTS (SELECTED) : CLAIMS, EFFECTIVENESS

Here's what the symbols mean:

↑ — Evidence comes from several controlled human studies.

↑? — Preliminary evidence comes from only a few controlled human studies or from laboratory studies with cell or tissue samples.

↔ — Evidence is uncertain and based on conflicting, controlled human research.

↓ — Research doesn't support the claim.

↓? — Preliminary evidence from a few controlled trials in humans does *not* support efficacy claims, but more research is needed. (Research that is negative and has only been performed in vitro is so designated in the column.)

NR — Not enough human research has been done yet, or the research quality is poor.

OTHER SUPPLEMENTS	MEDIA OR MARKETING CLAIMS	EFFECTIVENESS	ALSO BE AWARE . . . **Caution:** *Dietary supplements can pose significant and serious health risks,* **related to dosage, length of use, health status, age, and interactions with drugs and nutrients.** *Before taking them, always* **talk to your healthcare provider about their safety, risks, and interactions (***not fully listed below***), especially when treating or managing health conditions.**
Acidophilus/ lactobacillus acidophilus (LA)	• Reduces lactose intolerance	NR	• No reports of serious adverse effects in human studies • Some products may contain little or no LA; some may contain other strains of lactobacilli or contaminants
	• Helps control rotaviral diarrhea (LA GG)	↑	
	• Prevents antibiotic-associated diarrhea and traveler's diarrhea	↔	
	• Prevents or reduces length of vaginal yeast infections	↔ (LA yogurt) NR (LA supplements)	
	• Controls irritable bowel symptoms	↓	
	• Prevents or reduces severity of atopic disease (allergies, eczema, etc.)	NR	
	• Reduces cholesterol	↔	
	• Prevents cancer	NR	
Bee pollen	• Enhances energy, athletic performance	NR	• Evidence supports safe use of 1 teaspoon/day for up to 30 days • Anaphylactic reaction in some sensitive individuals • Not advised for people with asthma or allergies to honey or bee stings • Avoid if you have: liver disease • Avoid during pregnancy due to potential uterine stimulatory effects
	• Reduces symptoms of PMS	NR	
	• Prevents gastrointestinal upset	NR	
	• Reduces symptoms of chronic prostatitis (inflamed prostate)	NR	
	• Enhances well-being; "nature's perfect food"	↓	
Branched chain amino acids (BCAAs)	• Builds muscle; reduces abdominal fat	NR	• Doses higher than 20 g may cause gastrointestinal distress and may impair performance and induce fatigue • May stimulate insulin release and affect medications used to treat high blood glucose
	• Improves athletic performance	↓	
	• Improves appetite in the elderly	NR	
	• Helps mental function in people with liver disease	↔	
Carnitine (L-carnitine)	• Improves heart health	↑?	• No serious adverse effects reported with doses ranging from 0.5 to 6 grams a day • Larger doses associated with nausea and diarrhea
	• Improves athletic performance	↓	

OTHER SUPPLEMENTS (SELECTED) : CLAIMS, EFFECTIVENESS *(continued)*

OTHER SUPPLEMENTS	MEDIA OR MARKETING CLAIMS	EFFECTIVENESS	ALSO BE AWARE . . .
Carnitine *(continued)*	• Increases energy in people with chronic fatigue syndrome or cancer	NR	• Avoid if you have: hypothyroidism, which may inhibit thyroid hormone activity • May increase seizure frequency or severity if you have a history of seizures
	• Improves mental function in Alzheimer's disease	NR	
	• Improves thyroid function	NR	
	• Reduces male infertility	↔	
	• Improves immune function	NR	
	• Assists weight reduction	NR	
Chondroitin Sulfate	• Relieves osteoarthritis pain	↑?	• May cause epigastric pain, nausea, diarrhea, constipation • May worsen asthma symptoms • Avoid if you have: (men) prostate cancer or higher prostate cancer risk
	• Protects joints and tendons from sports injury	NR	
Coenzyme Q10 (ubiquinone)	• Improves health of people with heart disease and hypertension	↑?	• No serious adverse effects reported for 200 mg CoQ$_{10}$ daily for 1 year and 100 mg daily for up to 6 years • May cause mild gastrointestinal distress including nausea, vomiting, diarrhea, appetite suppression, and heartburn • Note: coenzyme Q10 is produced in the body and aids in energy production • May reduce effectiveness of some drugs (e.g., warfarin)
	• Improves exercise performance	↓	
	• Reduces cancer risk	NR	
	• Improves immune function in individuals with HIV	NR	
	• Helps with neurological disorders	NR	
	• Prevents migraine headache	NR	
Conjugated linoleic acid (CLA)	• Helps control weight	↓?	• No serious adverse effects found in short-term studies. • Most common side effect: gastrointestinal upset (diarrhea, nausea, loose stools, and dyspepsia); fatigue also possible • Some forms may increase insulin resistance in individuals with abdominal obesity or diabetes.
	• Stimulates immune function	↓	
	• Prevents cancer	NR	
	• Reduces risk for heart disease	↓	
	• Improves glucose tolerance	↓	
Creatine	• Increases muscle strength and mass	↑?	• Avoid exceeding a dose of 2 to 5 g/day • May cause weight gain/water retention, gastrointestinal pain, nausea, or diarrhea. • Avoid if you have: renal disease or insufficiency
	• Delays fatigue in athletes	NR	
	• Increases strength in elderly	NR	
	• Increases strength in muscular disease	↑?	
	• Increases strength in heart disease	NR	
DHEA (dehydro-epiandosterone)	• Slows aging; improves age-related memory loss	NR	• May increase breast, endometrial, or prostate cancer risks • For women, may promote masculine characteristics • With chronic use, can alter hormone levels: unknown adverse effects. • May decrease HDL cholesterol levels • Avoid if you have: breast, uterine, ovarian cancers; hormone-sensitive conditions • Banned by the National Collegiate Athletic Association and the International Olympic Committee
	• Improves immune function	↔	
	• Improves heart health	↔	
	• Helps prevent cancer	NR	
	• Reduces symptoms of lupus	↔	
	• Improves health of individuals with AIDS	NR	
	• Assists weight reduction	↔	
	• Reduces menopausal symptoms	NR	
Fish oil, contains DHA (docosa-hexaenoic acid) and EPA (eicosapent-aenoic acid)	• Reduces serum triglyceride levels	↑	• May prolong bleeding time • Should be monitored if you take anticoagulant medications or have blood clotting disorders • Avoid before surgery • During pregnancy avoid fish oil supplements high in vitamin A (halibut and shark liver oils because of vitamin A's teratogenic effects)
	• Reduces risk for athero-sclerosis/heart disease	↑?	
	• Improves glucose levels in people with diabetes	NR	

OTHER SUPPLEMENTS	MEDIA OR MARKETING CLAIMS	EFFECTIVENESS	ALSO BE AWARE . . .
Fish oil (continued)	• Improves lipid levels in people with diabetes	↑? (triglyceride levels) ↓? (LDL or HDL cholesterol levels	• May cause belching, halitosis, heartburn, or gastrointestinal upset • Up to 3 g/day considered safe; >3 g/day may suppress immune function and may increase risk of hemorrhagic stroke
	• Reduces blood pressure	↔	
	• Reduces inflammation and pain of arthritis	↑?	
	• Improves cognition in individuals with Alzheimer's disease	NR	
	• Reduces bowel inflammation in colitis or inflammatory bowel disease	↑?	
	• Helps reduce severity of symptoms of psoriasis	↓?	
	• Helps treat depression	NR	
	• Helps treat attention deficit/hyperactivity disorder	NR	
	• Prevents continued weight loss in people with cancer cachexia (wasting)	NR	
	• Reduces risk of cancer	↓?	
Flaxseed	• Improves blood lipids	↔	• Doses more than 45 g flaxseed powder linked to loose bowels • Can result in allergic and anaphylactic reactions • Not advised before surgery or for individuals with clotting disorders • Drink water when consuming whole or cracked flaxseed to prevent intestinal blockage • Fiber in ground flaxseed can interfere with the absorption of other nutrients and some medications affected by fiber • May effect antidiabetes drugs; monitor blood glucose • No specific safe intake levels for women with breast, uterine, or ovarian cancers, endometriosis, or uterine fibroids
	• Reduces risk for heart disease and stroke	NR	
	• Reduces risk of estrogen-related and other cancers	NR	
	• Reduces inflammation in individuals with arthritis	NR	
	• Improves symptoms of lupus, eczema, and other inflammatory diseases	NR	
	• Relieves constipation	↑	
Gamma-linolenic acid (evening primrose oil, black currant oil, borage seed oil)	• Reduces PMS symptoms	↔	• Not to be used with tricyclic antidepressants or anticonvulsants • Borage seed shouldn't be taken if drugs with potential liver-related side effects are being taken, too. • Potential side effects include belching, bloating, nausea, vomiting, flatulence, soft stools, and diarrhea • Avoid before surgery • Should be monitored by a physician if taking anticoagulant drugs or supplements
	• Reduces inflammation in rheumatoid arthritis	↔	
	• Reduces atopic dermatitis	↔	
	• Reduces acne	NR	
	• Improves diabetic neuropathy	NR	
	• Reduces cardiovascular disease risk NR	NR	
	• Reduces risk for breast cancer; improves response of anti-estrogen medications in breast cancer	↔	
Glucosamine	• Relieves osteoarthritis pain in knee, hip, etc.	↔	• Derived from shellfish; possible reaction for those with shellfish allergy • In three-year studies, no serious adverse effects • Some controversy regarding glucosamine and blood glucose control. To be safe, people with diabetes should have glucose levels monitored.
Lecithin/choline	• Improves exercise endurance	↓	• UL: 3.5 g choline/day for adults age 19 years and older • Mild side effects are linked to high doses (20 g): gastrointestinal symptoms, urinary incontinence, and diarrhea • Excess choline (> 20 g) may cause a fishy odor • Ongoing use may affect the nervous system
	• Improves dementia in Alzheimer's disease	↓?	
	• Improves memory, concentration	↓?	
	• Improves liver health	↓?	

OTHER SUPPLEMENTS	MEDIA OR MARKETING CLAIMS	EFFECTIVENESS	ALSO BE AWARE . . .
Lutein	• Treats age-related macular degeneration	↑?	• Not likely to have adverse effects, even with long-term use
	• Treats age-related cataracts	NR	
	• Treats retinitis pigmentosa	NR	
	• Prevents cancer	NR	
Lycopene	• Decreases risk of prostate cancer	↔	• No scientific studies specifically evaluating the safety of lycopene supplementation. Trials with supplements indicate safety at typical levels, usually at or below 30 mg/day over several weeks
	• Prevents other cancers	NR	
	• Reduces symptoms of exercise-induced asthma	NR	
	• Prevents atherosclerosis	NR	
Melatonin	• Regulates sleep-awake cycles	↔	• Long-term effects and safety have not been studied. No harmful effects reported from short-term use
	• Reduces jet lag	↑?	• Driving or using machinery for several hours after taking melatonin not advised
	• Reduces cancer risk; eases side effects of cancer treatment	NR	• Morning use may affect alertness and reflexes
	• Prevents and treats migraines	NR	• Do not take if using other sleep aids
	• Enhances sex drive	NR	• Discuss with oncologist if undergoing chemotherapy
			• Melatonin from animal pineal gland should be avoided due to potential toxin contamination
Noni juice	• Prevents cancer	NR	• Approximately the same amount of potassium as orange juice
	• Improves immunity	NR	• May reduce effectiveness of warfarin
	• Reduces blood pressure	NR	• High potassium content can cause hyperkalemia in people with kidney disease
	• Improves cholesterol levels	NR	
	• Acts as a natural pain reliever	NR	
Royal jelly	• Improves immunity	NR	• Not advised for people with asthma or a genetic predisposition to allergies
	• Contributes to a healthy heart	NR	
	• Improves stamina; reduces fatigue	NR	• *Note:* Royal jelly—exotic and expensive—isn't jelly, but instead a substance produced by worker bees to nourish future queen bees
	• Reduces PMS	NR	
	• Improves mental health, cognition	NR	
S-adenosyl-methionine (SAM-e)	• Reduces arthritis symptoms	↑?	• Mild gastrointestinal distress may occur at the beginning of use
	• Reduces symptoms of fibromyalgia	NR	• Safety well demonstrated for use as long as 2 years
	• Reduces symptoms of depression	↑?	
	• Improves liver health	↑?	
	• Promotes a healthy gallbladder	NR	
Soy protein and isoflavones	• Reduces cholesterol levels in individuals with hyper-cholesterolemia	↑?	• Avoid if you are: (women) diagnosed with breast cancer or at risk for breast cancer
	• Reduces risk of cancer	↔	• May reduce the absorption of thyroid medications
	• Reduces menopausal symptoms	↔	• Could interfere with estrogen replacement therapy
	• Reduces risk of osteoporosis	↔	
	• Improves kidney function in people with both diabetes and renal impairment	NR	
Shark cartilage	• Cures cancer	NR	• No reported adverse interactions
	• Stops cancer spread (prevents tumor from developing a blood supply)	NR	
	• Prevents blood clotting	NR	
	• Treats psoriasis	NR	

Other Supplements	Media or Marketing Claims	Effectiveness	Also Be Aware ...
Spirulina/blue-green algae	• Improves immunity • Reduces cholesterol • Reduces cancer risk • Improves intestinal health • Aids weight loss	NR NR NR NR NR	• Vegans should not rely on spirulina as their sole source of vitamin B_{12} • No long-term studies have evaluated the safety; has been consumed for centuries with few reports of adverse effects • May be contaminated with microbes or heavy metals • Patients with phenylketonuria should avoid consuming spirulina due to potential phenylalanine content
Whey protein	• Builds muscle and improves exercise performance • Improves immunity in individuals with HIV • Acts as an anticancer agent	$\leftrightarrow$ NR NR	• No long-term human studies • Should be avoided by those diagnosed with allergies or severe sensitivities to milk or milk proteins • For those with lactose intolerance, whey protein concentrate contains lactose. Whey protein isolate has insignificant quantities of lactose • Excess amounts of protein can be harmful for those with kidney disease

Adapted from Allison Sarubin Fragakis with Cynthia A. Thomson, *The Health Professional's Guide to Popular Dietary Supplements,* third edition (Chicago: The American Dietetic Association, 2007).

"proof" in a format—charts and tables, cited references—that looks like a reliable research study.

● *Claims that research is under way.* In other words, no specific data are available.

● *Unreliable studies.* Poorly designed research that hasn't been published in peer-reviewed publications.

● *Testimonials.* Statements, not based in sound science, from "satisfied" customers or celebrities.

Science behind Supplements: More Needed

To show a supplement's effectiveness and its active ingredients, more good research is needed! Good research provides data from randomized, placebo-controlled, double-blind studies—not just one study, but several that duplicate the results. In reality, current laws do not require manufacturers to conduct research. *See chapter 24 for defined research terms.*

To further complicate what's known and unknown, many supplements—for example, botanicals—have two or more active ingredients. Yet, all the bioactive substances haven't been identified, nor do we know what they do. Potencies differ when the same herbal supplement derives from different parts of a plant or different varieties. Growing conditions may affect the potency of bioactive substances. Even if sound research exists for the safety and effectiveness of one active ingredient, it may not exist for all ingredients, and usually not for the combination. Typically the potency of active ingredients in combination prod-

For up-to-date, reliable information about safe, effective supplement use, check these Web sites:

● Office of Dietary Supplement—*ods.od.nih .gov*

● U.S. Pharmacopoeia—*www.usp.org*

● National Center for Complementary and Alternative Medicine—*nccam.nih.gov*

ucts is less than the amount used in single ingredient studies. More unknowns: There's not enough scientific evidence to know how much of a supplement or its bioactive substitutes offer benefits, how much may be harmful, the health effects of dosages beyond the label dosage, or any interaction with food or medication.

In the future, sound research data may become available for more supplements from the National Institutes of Health, including the Office of Dietary Supplements (ODS) and the National Center for Complementary Medicine and Alternative Medicine. Until then, the best advice: a healthy skepticism.

See chapter 24 for more about judging nutrition information, scientific reports, and nutrition quackery.

If You Take a Supplement . . .

Before you head down your store's supplement aisle, order online, or pick up a product at your fitness center, get supplement savvy. Buy and use dietary supplements with the same consumer wisdom you use when you buy a car or make any major investment.

Be aware: For the same supplement in the same dosage, people may react differently. When taken without food or drinks, concentrated nutrient levels in some supplements may pose greater risks for toxicity, drug or supplement interactions, or adverse reactions.

Guidelines for Supplement Use

Keeping up with the explosion of supplements and supplement claims can be overwhelming! If you take supplements, strive to use them with good health sense, and ask for expert guidance.

Supplements: Questions to Ask an Expert

With so many supplement products and so many unknowns about them, explore these questions with qualified nutrition experts—before you take a supplement:

- What are the claims? Who's making them? Why? Are the claims valid?
- Where did the product information come from? Is the manufacturer a trusted, nonbiased source?
- Is the supplement generally safe? Can it cause harm in *any* dosage?
- Does the product come from a company that's known, or highly likely, to follow safe, appropriate manufacturing practices?
- What's known about the supplement's effectiveness for its proposed benefit?
- How do the active ingredients work in the body?
- What plant or plants and part of the plant or plants do the main active ingredients come from?
- How much of the active ingredients does the supplement have? What else does it contain?
- What are the risks and benefits of using the supplement: for anyone, for you?
- What scientific evidence supports this product formula or brand?
- What side effects might result from taking it?
- How much (dose), how often, and how long is it safe for you to take it?

Adapted from American Dietetic Association/American Pharmaceutical Association, *A Healthcare Professional's Guide to Evaluating Dietary Supplements* (2002).

For more about these supplements, see:

- Amino acid supplements—chapter 19.
- Androstenedione, or "andro"—chapter 19.
- Carnitine—chapter 19.
- Chromium picolinate—chapter 19.
- Creatine—chapter 19.
- Dehydroepiandrosterone (DHEA)—chapter 19.
- Ergogenic aids—chapter 19.
- Fiber pills and powders—chapter 6.
- Fish oil supplements—chapter 22.
- Garlic supplements—chapter 22.
- Glucosamine—chapter 22.
- Laetrile—chapter 22.
- Lecithin—chapter 22.
- Pangamic acid—chapter 19.
- SAM-e—chapter 22.
- Shark cartilage—chapter 22.
- Spirulina—chapter 19.
- Wheat germ and wheat germ oil—chapter 19.

For All Supplements . . .

Before you decide to take a dietary supplement, go with the tried-and-true as your best approach for fitness. There's plenty of scientific evidence supporting the benefits of physical activity, healthful eating, and a healthful lifestyle. If you take a supplement— any supplement—keep these general tips in mind:

- Give up the notion that dietary supplements are simple, immediate solutions to your health problems. Even supplements that offer benefits take time and ongoing use to make a difference.

- Skip the lure of this myth: "Even if a supplement won't help me, at least it won't hurt me." High dosages, taken long enough or combined with other supplements, can be harmful.

- *Best practice:* Talk to your doctor *before* you take any supplement! That's especially important if you're under age eighteen, pregnant or breast-feeding, chronically ill, elderly, or taking prescription or over-the-counter medicines. *See "Warning: Supplement Interactions!" in this chapter.*

● If you're already taking a dietary supplement, tell your doctor to make sure it's safe and appropriate for you and your health status. Be prepared to discuss:

  ● Supplement name, type, and daily or weekly dose (Bring the container if you can.)

  ● How long you have taken it and plan to take it, and why—and if you really need it!

  ● How long you've had the symptoms you're treating with supplements; if your symptoms improved

  ● Your typical day's food choices

  ● Other medications and supplements (over-the-counter and prescription) you're taking

  ● Any health problems or illnesses
    ● Whether you're pregnant or breast-feeding
    ● Whether you drink alcohol or smoke; if so, how often and how much

● If you have allergies

● If you're on a special eating plan (self-prescribed or medically prescribed)

● Known side effects (appetite loss, headaches, nausea)

● Cautions or warnings, including amount and upper limit

● If you're pregnant, planning for pregnancy, or breast-feeding, talk to your healthcare provider about supplements! Some are safe, even recommended. Others, such as some herbal and other botanicals, aren't.

● Unless your pediatrician prescribes them, avoid giving supplements to your child or teen. That includes herbals! *For more about supplements and kids see "What about Nutrient Supplements?" in chapter 16 and "Caution: Herbals Not for Kids!" in this chapter.*

● Look out for supplements with fraudulent claims. Besides being ineffective, they may be costly or harmful.

Warning: Supplement Interactions!

● *Dealing with cancer, diabetes, heart disease, immune problems, kidney problems, thyroid problems, ulcers, or other health problems?* Talk with your doctor before using dietary supplements, and about the potential for harmful interactions.

● *Taking prescription or over-the-counter medication?* Supplements—when combined with medications or other treatments—may interfere with or boost their action, even be harmful or life-threatening. *See "Food and Medicine" in chapter 22.* For example:

  ● Folic acid can interact with anticonvulsant medications.
  ● Vitamin E, garlic, and gingko biloba may thin blood—dangerous when taken with blood-thinning medication such as Coumadin and aspirin.
  ● Ginkgo can interact with some psychiatric drugs and some drugs that affect blood sugar levels.
  ● Garlic supplements may interact with drugs used in HIV therapy such as saquinavir, which is a protease inhibitor.
  ● The combination of foxglove (the source of digitalis, or digoxin) and cardiac medication is dangerous for those with heart disease.

● St. John's wort may reduce the effect of heart drugs, antidepressants, antiseizure drugs, anticancer drugs, birth control drugs, certain HIV drugs, and anti-transplant-rejection drugs.
● Ginseng can lower blood sugar levels, perhaps interfering with diabetes medication. It can also increase caffeine's effects as a stimulant.
● Calcium can interact with heart medication (such as Digoxin), thiazide diuretics (Thiazide), and antiacids with aluminum and magnesium.
● Magnesium can interact with thiazide, some cancer drugs, and antiacids with magnesium.

● *Planning for any surgery?* Avoid *all* supplements two to three weeks ahead, according to guidelines from the American Society of Anesthesiologists. Although herbal supplements may seem "innocent," their use can cause complications such as bleeding, heart instability, low blood sugar, blood pressure changes, and other drug interactions. Among those linked to surgical complications: ephedra, garlic, ginkgo, ginseng, kava, St. John's wort, and valerian.

Supplements: If You Have an Adverse Reaction . . .

● Immediately inform your healthcare provider if you think you have suffered a serious harmful effect or illness from a dietary supplement.

● Report any serious problems to the FDA's MedWatch hotline: (1-800-FDA-1088), fax (1-800-FDA-0178), or (www.fda.gov/medwatch/) online. Either you or your healthcare provider can do this. Be prepared to identify the probable product.

● For a general concern or complaint about any supplement, contact your nearest FDA District Office. Find the phone number on the www.cfsan.fda.gov/~dms/district.html Web site.

● Look for products labeled with the voluntary USP (U.S. Pharmacopeia) or NF letters, which indicates that the manufacturer self-reports voluntary standards of quality. Some reputable companies choose to pay for independent certification; often national brands from larger companies have stricter quality controls. Certification marks represent differing criteria; most important, they indicate whether a label matches the supplement contents, not its safety or effectiveness.

● Remember, "natural" doesn't mean safe or milder. For example, peppermint leaf tea is thought safe; concentrated peppermint oil from leaves can be toxic.

● Stick with the label dosage; heed warnings. The dosage is set by the manufacturer—not by FDA regulations. Boosting the dosage without medical supervision can be dangerous. An insignificant substance can be harmful when a supplement is consumed beyond the label dosage.

● Follow the label directions. Some supplements are more effective taken with food; others, on an empty stomach. Ask your healthcare provider or pharmacist for a list of foods and drinks to avoid consuming with the supplement. Usually water is the best drink.

● Keep dietary supplements in a safe place—away from places where children may reach them! Adult iron supplements are the most common cause of poisoning deaths among children in the United States!

● Keep supplements in a cool, dry place—preferably away from the stove and not in the bathroom. Heat and moisture affect their quality and effectiveness. Keep them in their original containers (label still on).

● Check the expiration date. Supplements lose some potency as they get closer to their expiration date.

● On the same note, skip the urge to "prescribe" a supplement for someone else. Even if it works for you, it may not be safe or effective for someone else.

● Want to know about a supplement's contents? Contact the manufacturer. The FDA doesn't have the resources to analyze supplements. Companies that provide scientific information about their products are more likely to be reliable resources; still, be wary and careful.

● Ask a registered dietitian, pharmacist, or your healthcare provider about the effectiveness of specific supplements—and the research behind claims. Show the supplement container; share information you gather.

● Stay skeptical of supplement marketing—even with label or advertising claims. *See "Play 'Ten Questions'" and "Spotting a Fraud" in chapter 24 to help you evaluate their claims.*

Have You Ever Wondered

. . . if supplements are safe to take if you have allergies? Remember that herbal and other botanical supplements are made from the bark, flowers, leaves, and seeds of plants. And chitosan, promoted for weight loss (with limited effectiveness), is a fiber from the shells of shellfish—a problem if you have shellfish allergies. If you're prone to allergic reactions, check with your healthcare professional before taking them. *See chapter 21 for more about allergies.*

. . . if a supplement without cautionary information on the label is safe? Warnings about potential adverse effects of a supplement's use do not need to be printed on the label. To find out, you need to contact the manufacturer directly for substantiated evidence.

Caution: Herbals Not for Kids!

Even though supplement companies aggressively target kids and parents, herbal and other botanical supplements may not be as safe or effective for your child or teen as you may think! Some supplements are useless; others, potentially harmful. Consider this: In the big picture of scientific research, little evidence exists on the safety and effectiveness of botanical supplements for adults. Their use among children and teens is virtually untested. In other words, we don't know the short- or long-term benefits, or more importantly, the risks.

Warning: Despite the FDA ban against ephedra for anyone—including those under age eighteen—medications with a form of ephedra may be available to teens. See "Herbal Ingredients: Hazardous to Health!" in this chapter.

For Vitamin/Mineral Supplements . . .

If your doctor or a registered dietitian recommends a supplement—either a vitamin-mineral combination or a single nutrient such as calcium—follow his or her professional guidance. *That includes the general guidelines in "For All Supplements . . ." on page 608.* Choose the product recommended for you.

If you're healthy and self-prescribe a dietary supplement, first ask yourself if you really need it. Think about the foods you typically eat and what they contain. If you're eating a healthful diet—following guidelines from MyPyramid—you're likely getting all the nutrients you need already. *See "MyPyramid: Your Healthful Eating Guide" in chapter 10.*

● Remember, for most healthy people: food before pills. Use supplements as supplements—not replacements—for nutrients in healthful meals and snacks. Choose food with variety, balance, and moderation in mind: plenty of fruits, vegetables and grains, especially whole grains, for their vitamins and fiber; lean meat, fish, and poultry, for their minerals; and dairy foods, for their calcium (and other nutrients).

● Choose a vitamin-mineral combination. Limit the potency to 100 percent or less of the Daily Values (DV) for your age and gender; use the label's Supplement Facts to judge the product. A supplement with 100 percent DV is likely more than enough, especially if your diet is healthful. Avoid large doses!

● Choose a supplement for your unique needs. Consider your age, gender, and medical status. *Note:* If you're under stress, don't count on a stress vitamin pill to help. Stress doesn't increase nutrient needs.

● For economy, consider the generic brand. Paying more for the same product generally offers no additional benefits. You also may save by buying synthetic rather than natural vitamins. For the most part, their chemical makeup is the same. One exception is "natural" vitamin E (d-alpha-tocopherol on the ingredient list), which is more potent than the synthetic form (dl-tocopherol). In most cases, however, your body won't know the difference between synthetic and natural. "Natural" products likely cost more.

Don't be lured by extra ingredients: inositol, lecithin, PABA, herbs, and enzymes. They add to the cost but offer no proven nutritional benefits.

● Check the expiration date on the label. Over time, nutrient supplements lose some potency.

● Take the supplement in the recommended dosage. There's no need to double dose on days when you've missed a meal. Rather than popping a pill, make up for foods you missed with your food choices on the next day. Because supplements can have druglike effects, too much taken at one time can be dangerous.

● Remember, no nutrient supplement provides the full complement of vitamins, minerals, and other important nutrients found in food that you need for health. A supplement has only what's listed on its label. If you rely on supplements, you miss out on the full variety of nutrients, as well as fiber, phytonutrients, and other substances supplied by food.

● Be cautious about doubling up on certain nutrients. If you're already taking multivitamin/mineral supplements, taking a single vitamin or mineral supplement as well may be too much! Read the label.

For Herbal and Other Botanical Supplements . . .

Helpful or harmful? Even though herbal and other botanicals are sold over the counter, use them with caution and discretion. Some offer varying degrees of health benefit—perhaps backed up by tradition or by emerging scientific evidence. Yet many may not deliver on the myriad benefits they claim. Others may have harmful, even life-threatening effects.

Besides the guidelines in "For All Supplements . . ." earlier in this chapter, follow these guidelines:

● Seek unbiased, science-based sources of information about herbals. Relying on product claims may not be a good idea. The poorly defined term "natural" doesn't mean safe or healthful. Ask a registered dietitian or other qualified nutrition expert.

● Find out about the risks and potential side effects. Then decide with your doctor if it's safe and

Have You Ever Wondered

. . . if the same supplement can be sold by several names? Yes; that adds to consumer confusion. However, the ingredient list must list the common name.

Botanical supplements may have a common name and a botanical name—for example, St. John's wort, often promoted to treat mild to moderate depression, also is known as *Hypericum perforatum.*

The common name also may refer to a category. Ginseng may refer to *Panax ginseng* or *Panax japonicus* (Asian ginsengs) or to *Panax quinquefolius L.* (American ginseng), each with different effects. Siberian ginseng *(E. senticosus)* isn't botanically related to either!

. . . what the term "high potency" on a dietary supplement label means? According to recent government regulations, "high potency" means that a nutrient in a food product, including a dietary supplement, provides 100 percent or more of the Daily Value (DV) for that vitamin or mineral. The term also can refer to a product with several ingredients if two-thirds of its nutrients contribute more than 100 percent of the DVs. *See chapter 10 for more about DVs.*

. . . if chelated mineral supplements are any better? Chelation binds minerals to other substances, supposedly making minerals easier for the body to absorb. While that may be true, many minerals found naturally in food aren't very bioavailable; that's considered when their Dietary Reference Intakes are established. In the overall picture, chelation isn't important—if you're meeting your day's mineral recommendation.

. . . if dietary supplements contain saturated and trans fats? Some may. Energy and nutrition bars are often classified as supplements. If they have 0.5 grams or more of *trans* or saturated fats, they must be listed on the Supplement Facts.

appropriate for you—or if other known health strategies would yield safe, effective results.

● Always consult a qualified health professional. Be cautious of those who call themselves a "herbalist," "herb doctor," "health counselor," or "master herbalist." These job titles aren't regulated.

● For serious illness, avoid self-medicating with herbal or other botanical supplements. That may delay known treatment that can help you.

● Tell your doctor if you take herbal supplements. Some supplements interact with medications.

● Skip herbal remedies if you take medication—either prescription or over-the-counter medications. The combination could make your medication ineffective, or create a harmful side effect.

● If you're pregnant, trying to get pregnant, or breast-feeding, avoid herbal remedies unless your doctor gives them an okay. Substances in these remedies may pass to your baby. These products aren't meant for children, either.

● If you get a doctor's okay, use herbal products only as directed. Take single-herb products, not herbal mixtures, unless recommended by a qualified practitioner with expertise in herbal therapies. If you have an adverse effect, you can identify the source more easily if you're taking single-herb products.

● If a herbal product seems to cause any negative side effects, stop taking it, and contact your doctor right away. Your doctor should contact the FDA's MedWatch hotline, which monitors adverse reactions to food and dietary supplements. *See "Supplements: If You Have an Adverse Reaction . . ." in this chapter.*

See "Herbal Teas: Health Benefits?" in chapter 8.

The Supplement Label

A supplement label looks somewhat like a food label. Required by the Dietary Supplement Health and Education Act, the label must provide specific information you can use to make an informed decision:

● *Statement of identity.* Look for the product name, perhaps "ginseng." The term "dietary supplement" or a descriptive phrase, such as "vitamin and mineral supplement," also must appear. If the product is a botanical, the plant part must be identified.

● *Net quantity of the ingredients.* That might be the number of capsules, perhaps "sixty capsules," in the package or container, or the weight.

● *Disclaimer with any structure/function claim. See "Claim Check!" in this chapter.*

● *Supplement Facts.* This gives the serving (dosage), the amount, the percent Daily Values (DVs) per serving if appropriate, and the active ingredient.

● *Directions for use.* This might indicate how often to take the supplement, perhaps "Take one capsule daily"; whether the supplement is best taken with or without food; safety tips; or storage guidelines. Suggested dosage is meaningless when little is known about the benefits and risks of many supplements.

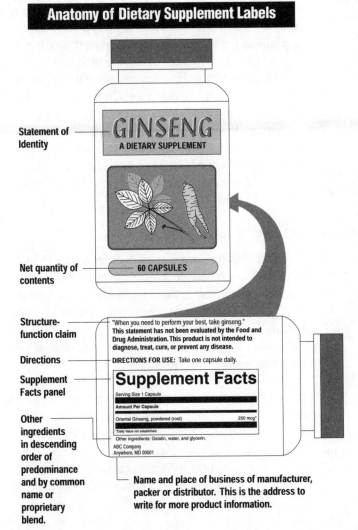

Anatomy of Dietary Supplement Labels

Statement of Identity

GINSENG
A DIETARY SUPPLEMENT

Net quantity of contents — 60 CAPSULES

Structure-function claim — "When you need to perform your best, take ginseng." This statement has not been evaluated by the Food and Drug Administration. This product is not intended to diagnose, treat, cure, or prevent any disease.

Directions — DIRECTIONS FOR USE: Take one capsule daily.

Supplement Facts panel —

Supplement Facts
Serving Size 1 Capsule
Amount Per Capsule
Oriental Ginseng, powdered (root)   250 mcg*
*Daily Value not established.
Other ingredients: Gelatin, water, and glycerin.
ABC Company
Anywhere, MD 00001

Other ingredients in descending order of predominance and by common name or proprietary blend.

Name and place of business of manufacturer, packer or distributor. This is the address to write for more product information.

● *Ingredients.* The list must be in descending order by common name or proprietary blend. *See "Ingredients Labeling, Too" in this chapter.*

● *Name and address of the manufacturer, packager, or distributor.* Use this contact information to get more product information.

As an option, supplement labels also may carry product claims: nutrient content claims, health claims, or structure/function claims.

Check the Supplement Facts

How do you know about the nutrition in a dietary supplement? Check the Supplement Facts panel, which must appear on *all* supplements. Its format is similar to the familiar Nutrition Facts you see on food products. To use the Supplement Facts panel:

● Check the serving size, or an appropriate unit, such as a capsule, packet, or teaspoonful. That's what the facts are based on. Unlike Nutrition Facts for foods, serving size isn't standardized for supplements; neither is the potency, or nutrient amount, per serving. Manufacturers make that decision.

● Check the quantity and the percent Daily Values (DVs) for any of fourteen nutrients, including sodium, vitamin A, vitamin C, calcium, and iron, if the levels are significant. Other vitamins or minerals must be listed, too, if they are added or referred to with a nutrient content claim on the label.

On the Supplement Facts, you probably won't find a nutrient if it isn't present. For example, cod liver oil lists fat on the panel, but a calcium supplement won't because it doesn't contain fat.

If the supplement has a substance with no Daily Value, the quantity per serving must be listed—for example, "15 mg omega-3 fatty acids."

Claim Check!

Confused about marketing claims for supplements? Not surprising! Some nutrient content claims and health claims are backed by scientific consensus, yet many (structure/function claims) aren't, at least not yet. One exception:

"Calcium helps build strong bones." Loose supplement regulations, including many product claims that push "over the edge" of credibility, leave many consumers misguided, bewildered, or both.

Some product claims are clearly illegal—for example, "cures cancer," "treats arthritis," " prevents impotence." According to FDA regulation, no dietary supplement can legally state or imply that it can help diagnose, treat, cure, or prevent disease.

Here's what marketers can claim about supplements—and how the claims are regulated—on package labels. *Since claims for food and for dietary supplements are similar, see chapter 11 for more information.*

Nutrient Content Claims. "High in calcium." "Excellent source of folate." "Iron-free." Like food labels, dietary supplement labels can carry nutrient content claims if they contain a specific level of a nutrient in a serving. The claims, regulated by the U.S. Food and Drug Administration (FDA), are similar to nutrient content claims for food. For example, any product with at least 20 percent of the Daily Value per serving can be labeled as "high" or "excellent source" of that nutrient.

What does a nutrient content claim tell you? It's just a clue. You need to read the Supplement Facts to know the specific nutrient content of one dose, or "serving."

Why would a supplement be "iron-free"? It's for the age fifty-plus market, when women's iron needs drop.

Health Claims. "Calcium may reduce the risk of osteoporosis." "Folic acid may reduce the risk of some neural tube defects." Health claims that describe the link between nutrients or food substances and health can be used on supplements. These FDA-regulated statements are based on scientific consensus—you can trust these claims. *For approved health claims for food and supplement labeling, see the Appendices.* Some qualified health claims have been approved for supplements but not for food products: for example, B vitamins (folic acid, vitamin B_6 and vitamin B_{12}) and reduced risk for vascular disease.

Structure/Function Claims. Echinacea: "boosts the immune system." Zinc: "helps maintain good immunity." Garlic: "helps maintain cardiovascular health." Lutein: "helps maintain healthy eyes."

Need more strategies for appropriate supplement use? Check here for "how-tos":

● Find out about *safe* supplement use for children—see chapter 16.

● Get savvy about ergogenic supplements for athletic performance—see chapter 19.

● Sort through misleading information about supplements—see chapter 24.

● Talk to a qualified nutrition expert about safe and appropriate supplements for you and your family—see chapter 24.

Structure/function claims may appear on dietary supplements as well as on food labels. They describe what the ingredient is intended to do to in the body or to promote health. Research to support these claims may be limited, with little or no scientific consensus.

By regulation, the manufacturer, not the FDA, must substantiate that the structure-function statements are truthful and not misleading. Because the FDA does not approve them, supplement labels with these claims must carry an FDA disclaimer: "This statement has not been evaluated by the Food and Drug Administration. This product is not intended to diagnose, treat, cure, or prevent any disease."

Ingredients Labeling, Too

The label shows ingredients, with their common name or proprietary blend, in descending order by weight. If an ingredient isn't in the Supplement Facts, it must be in the ingredients statement—for example, rose hips as the vitamin C source. Besides active ingredients, other substances—fillers, colorings or flavors, sweeteners—must be listed.

For herbal and other botanical supplements, potency often differs when different parts of a plant are used. If the supplement contains these ingredients, the label must identify what part of the plant it comes from—for example, ginseng may come from a root. The ingredient source may appear on an ingredients statement or near the statement of identity.

PART VI

Resources
More about
Healthful Eating

CHAPTER 24

Well Informed?

Are you well informed . . . or often confused about conflicting nutrition information? Can you easily find reliable nutrition information . . . or do you feel frustrated sorting through a maze of scientific news about healthy eating? For that matter, how do you stay up-to-date?

Probably, popular media—television, magazines, newspapers, and the Internet—are part of your health education "mix," alerting you to up-to-date food and nutrition issues, concerns, and advice. In fact, many people rely on media more than health professionals. For your own good health, you're wise to find credible sources and learn to judge the value of nutrition advice before using it to make your eating, lifestyle, and health decisions.

Where do teens and children learn about healthful eating? First and foremost, from you. So being well informed yourself ultimately teaches them. As kids get older, they learn from school, friends, and media, too. For computer-savvy kids, Web sites are an easy and private health information resource. Your challenge as a parent, caregiver, or teacher? Knowing enough to provide accurate information . . . and to direct those in your care to sources of sound eating and lifestyle guidance!

Need Nutrition Advice?

When do you need smart eating advice? Every day! Sometimes you may need to know a little more . . .

- If you're pregnant—or trying to get pregnant
- If you need guidance *and confidence* for breast-feeding
- If you're trying to deal with the "ups and downs" of infant or child feeding
- If you're trying to steer your teen toward healthier eating
- If you want to put in your peak performance for sports
- If you're struggling with your weight—or just trying to gain or lose a few pounds
- If you need to change your eating habits to prevent or manage a health problem—yours, or a family member's
- If you're caring for an aging parent or friend
- If you simply want to eat smarter to stay fit

When you need nutrition advice, ask a qualified expert. Your health—and that of your family—depend on it!

The Real Expert . . . Please Stand Up

Just who is a qualified nutrition expert? Sometimes it's hard to tell. Qualified nutrition experts, with specific academic and training credentials, know the science of nutrition. Their degrees in nutrition, dietetics, public health, or related fields (such as biochemistry, medicine, or a nutrition specialty in family and consumer sciences) come from well-respected colleges and

Who Is a Registered Dietitian?

The initials RD after someone's name mean "registered dietitian." A registered dietitian is a food and nutrition authority who has met academic and training requirements to earn the RD credential—and so provide credible nutrition guidance to the public.

As an important member of the healthcare team, an RD may have specialized expertise, perhaps in pediatric, maternal, or sports nutrition; oncology, cardiovascular, or renal nutrition; weight counseling; or diabetes education. Besides being in healthcare, education, and research, registered dietitians also provide nutrition and food expertise in business (corporate wellness, consumer affairs, product development, marketing, sales), government (public policy, government programs), food service (restaurant, institutions) management, fitness (education, training), communications (media, public relations, writing), culinary jobs (test kitchen), and in private practice counseling and consulting.

To earn the RD credential, an individual must complete a minimum of a bachelor's degree in nutrition or a related field from a U.S. regionally accredited college or university program and coursework approved by the Commission on Accreditation for Dietetics Education (CADE) of the American Dietetic Association. He or she must complete a CADE-accredited supervised practice program at a healthcare facility, community agency, or a food-service corporation, which may be combined with undergraduate or graduate studies. Typically, a practice program runs six to twelve months. Many dietetics professionals earn graduate degrees, as well.

To become registered, candidates must pass an extensive examination, administered by the Commission on Dietetic Registration, the credentialing agency of the American Dietetic Association. All RDs are required to stay current with ongoing continuing education. Only dietitians who have passed the exam and maintain their continuing education are considered "registered."

Some registered dietitians also have specialized credentials, such as Board Certified Specialists in Pediatric Nutrition (CSP) or in Renal Nutrition (CSR), or as Certified Diabetes Educators (CDE).

universities. The title "dietitian" or "nutritionist" often describes what they do.

Letters after a name don't necessarily qualify someone to provide nutrition services. Even when that person holds other academic degrees, nutrition may not be his or her specialty. Probe further.

The initials RD for "registered dietitian" or DTR for "dietetic technician, registered" mean the person has met specific educational requirements in nutrition and health. See "Who Is a Registered Dietitian?" and "Who Is a Dietetic Technician, Registered?" In states with licensing, dietitians may have more credentials, such as LD (licensed dietitian); terms differ among states. Many qualified nutrition experts also have advanced degrees, such as M.S., M.Ed., Sc.D., M.D., or Ph.D.

In many states the titles "nutritionist" and "diet counselor" aren't regulated, so terms like these may be used by those not properly qualified to give accurate nutrition information or sound advice. For example, salespeople for dietary supplements, so-called health advisers, and some authors may call themselves "nutritionists." In reality, they instead may be self-proclaimed experts, perhaps with just a little nutrition training or with only mail-order credentials.

Mail-order, diploma-mill credentials may appear impressive—but don't be fooled. The U.S. Department of Education defines a "diploma mill" as an organization awarding degrees without requiring its students to meet the established educational standards followed by reputable institutions. To see if an institution is accredited, not a diploma mill, check in your library for a list of accredited educational institutions.

Licensing qualified nutrition experts in many states helps ensure credible nutrition guidance and quality healthcare. Although qualifications for licensing differ from state to state, they often reflect the same education and training required to become an RD.

How to Find Nutrition Help . . .

Need personal nutrition counseling? Food assistance for a friend or a family member? Answers to nutrition questions? Check with health, education, and social service organizations in your community, as well as dietitians in private practice for direct services.

Who Is a Dietetic Technician, Registered?

The initials DTR after a person's name stand for "dietetic technician, registered." DTRs are trained for support roles in food and nutrition and are an integral part of the healthcare or food service management teams. DTRs often are considered partners in practice with registered dietitians. Job responsibilities may include teaching nutrition classes, offering diet counseling, performing diet histories, assessing a person's nutritional status, or managing aspects of a food-service operation. DTRs typically work in hospitals, day care, or extended care facilities; many also work in food companies, government agencies, education, retail sales and marketing, academic institutions, or fitness centers.

Currently there are two ways to attain the DTR credential. First is by completing requirements for an associate degree from a U.S. regionally accredited college or university and a CADE-accredited dietetic technician program. Second is by completing a baccalaureate degree, a didactic program in dietetics at a CADE-accredited/approved college or university, and 450 hours of supervised field experience in healthcare facilities, food-service operations, or community nutrition programs through a CADE-accredited DT program. Many DTRs earn additional degrees that complement their food and nutrition background. DTRs also must successfully complete a comprehensive registration exam administered by the Commission on Dietetic Registration, the credentialing agency of the American Dietetic Association.

Once they earn their credential, dietetic technicians, registered must stay current with ongoing continuing education. Only individuals who pass the exam and maintain their status through continuing education are considered *registered*. In addition, individuals with dietetics education and experience who are not DTRs may have job titles that include "dietetic technician," "diet tech," or "diet clerk."

To Find a Qualified Nutrition Expert

Start with these sources:

- Your doctor, health maintenance organization (HMO), or local hospital for a referral
- Your local dietetic association, public health department, Cooperative Extension Service, or the nutrition department of an area college or university

- The American Dietetic Association at *www.eatright.org* (go to "Find a Nutrition Professional"). Or call 800/366-1655 for a referral to a registered dietitian in your area.

See "The Real Expert . . . Please Stand Up" in this chapter to help you choose a qualified nutrition expert.

To Find Food and Nutrition Services

Agencies, institutions, and businesses—often staffed with qualified nutrition experts—provide direct food or nutrition services. Whether for you and for someone else who might benefit, consider:

Child Nutrition Programs. Schools, as well as early childhood centers, after-school programs, and summer camps, may provide nutritious breakfasts, lunches, milk, and snacks for children. Often local programs get support partly through the USDA's Food and Nutrition Service. By regulation, school meals and snacks must meet strict nutrition guidelines. The program also provides nutrition education. *See "For Kids Only—Today's School Meals" in chapter 16.*

Extension Service. Each state's Extension program provides consumer information on various topics, including food, nutrition, and food safety. State land-grant universities employ nutrition experts as part of the Extension staff. Look for food and nutrition information online or perhaps in your local newspaper from Extension nutrition staff.

Food Stamp Program. The food stamp program, administered by state agencies and funded by the U.S. Department of Agriculture (USDA), provides food assistance to needy families and individuals. Food stamps are used like cash in food stores and some farmers' markets. For the nearest food stamp office, check your county public health department or government pages of your phone book.

Health Organizations. For help with specific health issues, check health organizations such as the American Heart Association, the American Diabetes Association, and the Food Allergy and Anaphylaxis Network—as well as the American Dietetic Association. *Also check "Resources You Can Use," at the end of this book.* Their Web sites offer a wealth of information, and perhaps a gateway to other credible food, nutrition, and health Web sites.

Home-Delivered Meals. People who can't leave their homes or who can't prepare food independently may seek services for home-delivered meals. For those who qualify, government or community agencies provide meals at low cost. Check with a social worker, religious group, or state or area Agency on Aging.

Senior Citizens' Meal Programs. Community agencies may offer low-cost meals and social contact for senior citizens. To find services, check with a social worker, health department, religious group, or area Agency on Aging. USDA's Senior Farmers' Market Nutrition Program offers assistance with fruits and vegetables.

Soup Kitchens and Food Pantries. For those who are homeless or have limited resources for food, private and faith-based groups may provide food at no cost. Social workers, social agencies, and religious groups offer referrals.

Women, Infants, and Children (WIC) Program. This federal government program, which also has a Farmers' Market Nutrition Program, offers food assistance and nutrition education to pregnant women, infants, and preschoolers. Again, the county or other local public health department can help, or check the government pages in your phone book.

Child and Adult Care Feeding. For many low-income families, this government program provides nutritious, affordable meals and snacks daily, as part of day care for children and elderly adults.

For other government and nonprofit food assistance programs, as well as food assistance for disaster relief, talk with your healthcare provider, Extension office, or local public health department.

For More about Food Products

Food Industry Groups. Food companies and food industry groups provide information about the nutrients and ingredients in their products. Many also offer healthful eating and lifestyle information on their Web sites, package labels, and print materials or through their toll-free phone numbers (often printed on food packages). Through their consumer response services—staffed by dietitians or other qualified food and nutrition professionals—you also may find answers to your questions, perhaps through their online chat room.

When You Consult an Expert . . .

Whether you seek nutrition counseling on your own or followup from a doctor's referral, here's how you can make the most of your time with a qualified nutrition professional. For an office visit . . .

● *Have a medical checkup first.* A qualified nutrition professional needs to know your health status before providing dietary guidance. Your healthcare provider can share your blood pressure and information from blood tests, such as blood cholesterol, triglycerides, blood glucose (sugar), hemoglobin, and hematocrit levels, among others.

Some health problems are managed in part or completely by diet and perhaps physical activity. If so, your doctor may refer you to a registered dietitian for appropriate diet therapy. In many states, private health insurance and managed care plans cover nutrition counseling (also known as medical nutrition therapy) with a registered dietitian for some health conditions, such as diabetes. Ask for a referral if you qualify.

● *Share your goals.* If you seek nutrition advice on your own, know what you want to accomplish. Do you want to lose weight? Gain weight? Have more stamina for sports? Improve your blood cholesterol levels? Live a healthier lifestyle? Think about your goals ahead . . . and make them realistic.

● *Forget miracles and magic bullets.* A qualified nutrition professional will focus on changes in your lifestyle and food choices, not on quick results, miracle cures, or costly dietary supplements.

● *Tell about dietary supplements you're taking.* That includes herbal remedies and botanicals. Some supplements interact with medications (even over-the-counter types), rendering them ineffective or causing harmful side effects. *See "Food and Medicine" in chapter 22.* Dietary supplements taken in very large doses also may cause adverse health reactions. *See chapter 23, "Supplements: Use and Abuse."*

● Keep an ongoing personal health record to share and aid decisions about your nutrition and healthcare.

● *Be prepared to answer questions.* Expect to talk about your eating habits, adverse reactions to food, dietary supplements, your weight history, food preferences, general medical history, family history of health problems, medications, special diets, any nutrition instruction you've had, and your lifestyle habits. With those insights, a dietitian can help you customize food and nutrition advice for your lifestyle and health.

● *For weight counseling or sports nutrition, expect to have your weight and body composition checked*—usually height, weight, and a skinfold measurement in several spots on your body (or other techniques to measure body composition).

● *Ask for clarification.* If you don't understand the terms used in the counseling session, ask! Terms such as "blood glucose level," "HDLs," "triglycerides," "anaphylactic reaction," and "*trans* fatty acids" are nutrition-related lingo. Know what they mean.

● *Be specific with your questions.* You're the most important person on your healthcare team. You can only comply with dietary recommendations if you have a clear understanding of the advice offered.

● *Be open to professional health advice.* For example, if your healthcare provider talks about your weight, it's for your own health benefit.

● *Keep careful eating records*—if you're asked. Record everything you eat and drink, including snacks, perhaps for several days. Record the amounts (in cups, ounces, tablespoons, or the like) and how the foods were prepared, such as "fried" or "baked." *For other tips, see "Dear Diary . . ." in chapter 2.*

● *Involve your family.* If you take a nutrition class or meet with a nutrition professional, bring your family and friends along. Support helps ensure success.

● *Follow up, as advised,* so your progress can be monitored and your questions answered. Follow-up visits are great moral support, too!

● *Stick with it!* A change in body weight, blood cholesterol levels, and other physical conditions may take time. With your healthcare provider and support team, plan for gradual results.

Be Your Own Judge!

Do you rely on popular media—magazines, newspapers, TV, the Internet—for nutrition updates? Fortunately, there's plenty of reliable, consumer-friendly nutrition information available. Yet, the airwaves,

print, and the Web are also full of nutrition hype, misleading reports, and quackery. How can you be a nutrition-savvy media consumer—and sort fact from fiction?

You Can't Judge a Book by Its Cover

Although magazine racks, bookstore shelves, newspaper columns, and the Internet bombard you with healthful eating advice, being a best-seller or highly visible doesn't make the advice reliable. Despite threads of truth, the messages may be laced with misinformation or offer advice in a context that doesn't apply to you. Give what you read or hear a reliability check.

Who Wrote It?

Check the author's qualifications. A reputable nutrition author usually is educated in the field of nutrition, medicine, or a related specialty, with a degree or degrees from an accredited college or university. He or she usually is a credentialed member of a credible nutrition organization—for example, an RD or a DTR. Today you can find many books, magazine articles, newspaper columns, and online information written by qualified nutrition experts. *See "The Real Expert . . . Please Stand Up" in this chapter.*

Many credible writers are affiliated with an accredited university or medical center that offers nutrition or related health research, programs, or courses. An "accredited" institution generally is certified by an agency recognized by the U.S. Department of Education. Check the reference department of your local library for an institution's accreditation.

Why Was It Published?

For healthful eating advice, find resources with a balanced nutrition message meant to inform, not advertise. Try to analyze what's being said or implied. If it's not clear, ask a qualified nutrition expert.

Is the Nutrition Advice Credible?

Check the sources cited. Reliable advice is backed up with credible sources such as:

● *Government entities.* For example, the National Academy of Sciences/Institute of Medicine, the U.S.

Department of Health and Human Services (DHHS), the U.S. Department of Agriculture (USDA), and Centers for Disease Control and Prevention (CDC) base healthful eating and lifestyle guidelines on the most current research and consensus from scientific experts. Among the guidelines often cited: Dietary Reference Intakes, Dietary Guidelines for Americans, MyPyramid, and the CDC's body mass index and physical activity guides.

● *Credible professional nutrition and health organizations.* They base their advice on sound scientific evidence and government guidelines.

● *Peer-reviewed scientific journals.* Research reported in peer-reviewed journals goes through the scrutiny of experts before it can be printed, so in medical news stories, look for the journal citing. If you choose, you can read the original research. Among the many journals: *New England Journal of Medicine, Lancet, Journal of the American Medical Association,* and *Journal of the American Dietetic Association.*

Credible nutrition experts don't claim to have all the answers. If scientific evidence isn't conclusive or if the issues are controversial, they say so.

Have You Ever Wondered ?

. . . how to access credible scientific journals? University, medical school, and large urban libraries have them. With Internet access you can check online through MEDLINE, a database managed by the National Library of Medicine, a division of the U.S. National Institutes of Health. MEDLINE*plus* (www.nlm.nih.gov/medline plus/) is especially designed for consumer ease; the site can link you to the National Library of Medicine's PubMed Web site (www.ncbi.nlm.nih.gov/pubmed/) with access to scientific journal abstracts and articles. Some journals have their own online presence, perhaps available at no charge.

. . . how to judge today's alternative-nutrition approaches? New stories about dietary supplements, herbal remedies, and holistic therapies need to stand up to the same scrutiny as any scientific research report— and the study itself needs the same rigor and precision. Testimonials and anecdotes aren't enough.

Check "Resources You Can Use" at the back of this book for many—but not all—government and health agencies, professional organizations, and food industry groups that provide credible information.

What Do Credible Experts Say?

Look for reviews by credible experts. For a book, start inside or on the cover itself, where you may find

Words to the Wise

"May," "can"	Does not mean "will"
"Contributes to," "is linked to," or "is associated with"	Does not mean "causes"
"Proves"	Scientific studies gather evidence in a systematic way, but one study, taken alone, seldom proves anything.
"Breakthrough"	This happens only now and then—for example, the discovery of penicillin or polio vaccine. But today this word is so overworked as to be meaningless.
"Doubles the risk," "triples the risk," "risky"	May or may not be meaningful.
	Do you know what the risk was in the first place? If the risk was one in a million, and you double it, that's still only 1 in 500,000. If the risk was 1 in 100 and doubles, that's a big increase.
"Significant"	A result is "statistically significant" when the association between two factors has been found to be greater than what might occur at random (this is worked out by a mathematical formula). But people often take "significant" to mean "major" or "important."

Adapted from: © Health Letter Associates, 1996, www.WellnessLetter.com.

a list of reviewers. Like those of the author, reviewers' credentials or affiliations help you judge the reliability of nutrition information.

For an expert judgment, contact a registered dietitian or other qualified nutritionist connected with a local college, university, hospital, Extension program, public health department, or in private practice.

Read between the Headlines

Every day, nutrition and health news make headlines. In this age of instant communication, research often hits the media before nutrition experts can review and interpret the findings. Today's report may appear to contradict what you heard last week. Adding to the challenge, reporters assigned to medical stories usually need to report complex medical news quickly, in a short, simple way. The result? Confusion.

Legitimate scientists aren't out to mislead you. Responsible journalists aren't, either. Uncovering the mysteries of nutrition and the human body is a complex process. As new findings emerge, research may seem to contradict itself. But differences in two or more reports reflect how scientists continue to learn—sharing research results and questioning each step along the way. Scientific debate leads to more studies. Eventually—perhaps after years of study—recommendations based on sound science (repeated, conclusive evidence) can be shared with the public. In today's popular media, you can listen to the debate.

As science unravels more about the links among nutrition, health, and chronic disease, today's reports will eventually prove to be both true and false. You can't dissect every research report. But you can use caution and common sense before jumping to conclusions and changing your food and lifestyle choices:

● *Go beyond headlines.* An attention-grabbing headline may leave a different impression than the full newspaper article or news brief itself. Read or listen to the whole story. Often response from other experts or "bottom line" advice appears at the story's end.

● *Remember—once isn't enough!* The results of one study aren't enough to change your food choices. They're just one piece of a bigger scientific puzzle. True nutrition breakthroughs take years of study and the support of repeated findings from many scientific studies. That's why health organizations, government agencies, and health experts may appear conservative; their guidance reflects consistent, well-researched findings.

● *Check the report.* Do other studies support the evidence? And does it build on what scientists know already? Responsible scientists and careful journalists report research within the context of other studies. And one study rarely changes their nutrition advice.

● *Recognize preliminary findings for what they are—preliminary!* Read them with interest. But wait for more evidence before you make major changes.

● *Look for the human dimension.* Animal studies may be among the first steps in researching a hypothesis. But the results don't always apply to humans.

● *Learn to be research savvy.* Read more about the study itself before applying its conclusions to you. Ask yourself: Are the people studied like you—perhaps in age, gender, health, ethnicity, geographic location, and lifestyle? Did the study include a large group of people? Was the study long-range? Longer studies, with more people, more likely produce valid results. Even by asking these questions, it's hard for consumers to assess research methods. *See "Scientific Studies: Coming to Terms" in this chapter.*

● *Consider its context in the real world of healthful eating.* Does the study tell how the findings relate to overall food choices, lifestyle, and other research? A responsible report tells how research fits within the broader context of what is already known.

● *Know what the words mean.* Credible nutrition reports are careful with what they say so they won't mislead you. Research results may "suggest," but that isn't the same as "prove." And "linked to" doesn't mean "causes." *Don't jump to conclusions—get to know "Words to the Wise" on page 622.*

● *Check the source.* Ask a qualified nutrition expert. Credible research comes from credible institutions and scientists, and it's reported in credible, peer-reviewed scientific and professional journals. Before nutrition research is published in reputable journals, it must meet well-established standards of nutrition research. If research is attributed simply to "they" or to some elusive source, be wary of its results.

● *Watch for follow-up reports.* Breaking scientific

news is often followed by review and advice from nutrition experts. For example, registered dietitians often appear in media, helping to interpret news reports on nutrition issues.

Even when research has been well conducted, scientists may view the results differently. It may take time for nutrition experts to study the research methods and findings. So don't always expect an immediate response. For the best health news, look for a full perspective, not reports of one study.

● *Keep a healthy skepticism.* That's very true when evaluating news about nutrition "discoveries," "ground-breaking procedures," and "revolutionary therapy." *See "Case against Health Fraud" in this chapter.*

● *Watch out for absolutes!* Responsible scientists don't claim "proof" or "cause" until repeated studies show that the findings are conclusive.

● *Seek a qualified opinion.* Take the article with you! Before you change your eating style, consult a registered dietitian, other qualified nutrition expert, or doctor. Even promising research may not apply to you. For example, a report may suggest that red wine is heart healthy, but if you take an MAO inhibitor (an antidepressant), the combination may raise your blood pressure. Emerging science about wine may not benefit you—and drinking wine may be harmful in your case!

● *Put reports into your own reality.* For any advice, weigh the benefits and risks, as they apply to you, as an individual. And recognize that there's no such thing as "zero risk" for practically anything!

Nutrition in Cyberspace

Browsing the Web, you know that food and nutrition information is proliferating in cyberspace, with thousands of health-related sites debuting each year. Search engines can quickly direct you to Web sites and blogs with breaking nutrition news, sound eating advice, healthful recipes, government agencies, other credible nutrition resources, food product information, and even the chance to "chat" with a registered dietitian. Chat rooms, electronic bulletin boards, Listservs, and e-mail communicate nutrition information quickly and widely.

Like other media, online information is littered with nutrition misinformation. Science-based content can coexist with questionable, inaccurate, or alarming information, perhaps promoted by those holding unscientific views.

Clearing Up the Web of Confusion

How do you determine if a Web site provides information you can trust, or instead, if credible sources are quoted to "spin" a sense of legitimacy into unreliable sources? Use the same healthy skepticism with online information that you use to evaluate other nutrition information. Also ask yourself: Does it . . .

● Identify the sponsor or the owner of the site? That's your clue to the site's perspective and potential bias. The three-letter suffix on a Web site address is your first clue. Those that end in *.edu* (educational institution), *.gov* (government agencies), and perhaps *.org* (organizations, often nonprofit) tend to be the most credible. Those ending in *.com* are commercial sites and in *.net* are networks, Internet service providers, or organizations. Many *.com* sites have responsible consumer information; just be a savvy consumer.

Several new suffixes, approved for use, might be used for Web sites with nutrition and health information: *.biz* (businesses), *.coop* (business cooperatives), *.info* (general use), *.museum* (museums), *.name* (individuals), and *.pro* (professionals).

● Name contributors or perhaps an editorial board, with their credentials and perhaps an affiliation? No matter what the media, credible information comes from qualified nutrition experts. Look for a contact address or phone number.

Today many registered dietitians who work in consulting or private practice have personal Web sites. You can verify their RD credential by contacting the Commission on Dietetic Registration of the American Dietetic Association. *See "Resources You Can Use" at the back of this book for contact information.*

● Provide facts with cited sources, not just opinions? Look for information supported by established scientific findings.

● Link to credible online sites? Be aware that an unreputable site may hyperlink to a credible site— perhaps a government nutrition site—for a trustworthy perception.

Scientific Studies: Coming to Terms

You've read news reports of nutrition studies. But what do all the terms mean?

Bias. Problems in the study design that affect the reliability of the results; perhaps the subjects weren't chosen right.

Blind (single or double) study. Study (*single blind*) where the subjects don't know if they're in the experimental or placebo group until after the study's over; study (*double blind*) where the researchers don't know either, so they can't influence the outcome.

Clinical trial. Studies done to directly show the effectiveness and the safety of a supplement, medication, or treatment with a selected group of people.

Confounding variable. A "hidden" and related variable (perhaps an unknown phytonutrient) that the researcher attributes to something different.

Control group. The study group that doesn't have the treatment. A control group is used to know if a treatment has an effect.

Correlation. An association between two research variables, such as eating lycopene and reduced risk for prostate cancer. A correlation does not prove cause and effect, but may suggest further study.

Epidemiological study. Study of the incidence and prevalence of a health condition among a specific group of people, such as neural tube defects among newborns.

Generalizability. Describes how much research results apply to the general population of people who are like the studies' subjects.

Incidence. How many new cases of a disease or health condition as of a specific date, for a defined population.

In vitro study. Laboratory study with cells or tissue samples, usually done before an *in vivo* study.

In vivo study. Study with living subjects, either animal or human research.

Meta-analysis. A way to pool quantitative data from many studies to see what overall conclusions can be drawn, such as the pooling of more than forty studies on oats and more than twenty-five studies on soy protein to show their links to cholesterol-lowering.

Morbidity. Number of deaths in relation to a population.

Mortality. Number of people with an illness in relation to a population.

Observational study. Study that identifies a link between a health condition and behavior, such as overweight and TV-watching, but doesn't prove cause and effect.

Placebo. A "fake" treatment, perhaps a sugar pill, that appears to be the same as the treatment under study. It's used to remove bias when study subjects don't know which treatment they have.

Placebo effect. Positive results among subjects who think they're getting the real treatment.

Prevalence. How many *existing cases* of a disease or a health condition as of a specific date, for a defined population.

Prospective study. Study that poses the research questions, then follows groups of people, often for decades.

Random sample. A way to choose study subjects whereby anyone from a target population has an equal chance to be picked. In that way the results can be more easily generalized to a larger group.

Reliability. Describes research that is carefully controlled so the data can be reproduced. In other words, the researcher would get the same result with the same study subject several times.

Retrospective study. Study that uses recorded data or recall of the past. Because the study relies on memory or some variables that can't be easily controlled, this type of research has limitations.

Risk. The probability that something (perhaps a heart attack, stroke, cancer, diabetes, osteoporosis) will happen. "Risk" doesn't necessarily mean something will happen.

Risk factor. A factor that's statistically linked to the incidence of disease, such as a high BMI as a risk factor for heart disease. Again, it doesn't necessarily mean cause and effect.

Validity. The accuracy or truthfulness of the study's conclusion, and if the study measured what it meant to study.

Variable. A factor such as age, gender, or food choices in a study that differs among the people being studied. An *independent variable* is the one being studied; a *dependent variable*, perhaps lower blood sugar level or LDL cholesterol level, happens as a result of the treatment.

Adapted from source: Reprinted with permission of the International Food Information Council Foundation, Washington, D.C.

● Have an educational purpose, or only a hidden guise of sound nutrition advice? If it's promotional, the information is likely biased or reframed for marketing and sales. Assess information within the context of total nutrition. *Be aware:* Online charlatans sell products and "cures" with unfounded benefits or harmful side effects!

● Indicate regular updates and postings? Credible Web sites are updated often to offer the most current advice. **Caution:** Being current doesn't necessarily make it accurate. If the links don't work, it's likely old.

● Provide sound information, not just "bells and whistles"? Is it free of advertising, including pop-up ads?

● Pass other credibility tests? *See "Read between the Headlines" in this chapter.* Anyone can launch a site. Like any media report, being on the Internet doesn't ensure reliability.

● Have a nutrition expert as a host for forums and chatrooms? Many unsponsored bulletin boards bring interested people together, with chat from undisclosed sources who often aren't experts. Be wary!

"Well" Connected Links

Search engines list legitimate and less reliable Web sites side-by-side; you need skills to sort them out. That's why it's wise to tap health-related resources that indicate high standards:

● To speed your search use gateway sites that link to responsible organizations—for example, the U.S. government's site (www.nutrition.gov). The U.S. Department of Health and Human Services' Healthfinder (www.healthfinder.gov) hyperlinks to hundreds of responsible sites, as does the gateway in the American Dietetic Association's site (www.eatright.org).

● Review more than one Web site on the same nutrition topic; use several search engines. With information "sound bites," usually one site isn't complete enough.

● Look for sites with the HON-code symbol, showing they adhere to the HONcode (Health On the Net Foundation) principles. An example: the WebMD Web site, which

Have You Ever Wondered

. . . how to judge food scares that circulate through e-mail? Being 100 percent sure about these food scares takes research. What appears in your e-mail is likely a hoax (1) if it wasn't written by the e-mail sender, (2) if you're asked to forward the e-mail, (3) if it claims not to be a hoax or an urban legend, (4) if it appeals to your emotions, and (5) if it doesn't cite a legitimate source or a credible Web site. Read critically for obvious false claims, poor logic, and lack of common sense. If you're still not sure, you might want to check Web sites such as www.quackwatch.com or www.urbanlegends.com that debunk food myths.

provides online, consumer-focused health information (www.webmd.com). These sites voluntarily comply with a code of conduct for health and medical Web sites. HON is an honor symbol and system, so still be a careful online consumer.

● Ask a nutrition expert, such as an RD or a DTR, who has a quick ability to see nuances of Web site bias and inaccuracy. If you find news of interest on the Internet, such as about a phytonutrient link to health, or a dietary supplement, print the information with the name and address of the Web site; take it to your healthcare provider or a nutrition expert for a perspective.

To find reliable nutrition and health Web sites, see "Resources You Can Use" at the back of this book.

E-Nutrition Advice: Just for You

With a few mouse clicks, you can calculate your BMI, assess your food choices, even tie in to online weight control counseling. But consider this:

● If you wish, use quick, online assessments and counseling on your food choices, physical activity, and health issues, but don't replace your healthcare provider. For a reliable diagnosis and prescribed eating plan, work with a qualified healthcare provider in person, who can review your medical history. Today many registered dietitians do online counseling.

● For the same reasons, get advice or a prescription for a dietary supplement from your doctor. As an aside, buying supplements online may, or may not, cost less, and the quality is uneven.

● Even on trustworthy healthcare sites that do online nutrition assessments and counseling, there's a wrinkle: *privacy.* To protect the privacy of your records and avoid a Pandora's box of e-marketing, provide personal data on encrypted, or secured, sites only. If a "closed padlock" appears on the Web page, the data you provide are encrypted and secure. And pay attention to "alarms" on the site that warn that you're moving from secure to insecure parts of the Web site.

As you surf the Internet, keep track of your path. You may be unaware when you pass from a reliable to an unreliable source of information.

Case against Health Fraud

Can you "lose weight while you sleep"? Can a dietary supplement assure "no more arthritic pain" or "cure for AIDS"? Can a device guarantee "a bigger bustline" or "spot reduction"?

Americans spend billions of dollars annually on products and services that make such claims. Health quackery is the most common type of fraud aimed at the elderly and others. Easy remedies are hard to resist! Yet many are simply useless; others, potentially harmful. Either way, it's health fraud.

Nutrition quackery thrives among people who are uninformed or already misinformed, desperate for help, overconfident about possible risks, or alienated from traditional healthcare. And quacks can more easily manipulate those people who are already leaning in their direction, perhaps with ploys that seem reasonable: "We really care about you," "What have you got to lose?," "Science doesn't have all the answers," or "We treat medicine's failures."

Health fraud means promoting, for financial gain, a health remedy that doesn't work—or hasn't yet been proven to work. The remedy may be a device, treatment, service, plan, special foods, or other product. Although fraud is rampant in many areas of health, often it's linked to nutrition—perhaps to a dietary supplement, a herbal product, a weight-loss device, or a new diet program.

So what is quackery? The term comes from the term "quacksalver," referring to medieval peddlers of salves who sounded like quacking ducks when they used their voices to promote their wares. That's why they were called "quacks."

Quacks promote health fraud. Their motivation may be strictly financial gain. But often, quacks sincerely believe in the value of their product, treatment, or service. They don't mean to deceive you. Instead, they lack scientific understanding.

Health fraud and quackery have grown dramatically in the past several decades. Why such growth? Among the reasons, there's an unprecedented interest in personal healthcare. In general, people today take more personal responsibility for staying healthy. That interest has created a huge demand for products and services that promote health. Legitimate business uses this opportunity to provide products, treatments, and services that do have scientifically proven benefits. But this same wave of interest also has spawned a fanfare of health fraud and quackery, leaving people more vulnerable than ever.

With looser government regulation, the misuse of dietary supplements—and quackery surrounding them—have grown dramatically. Today supplement manufacturers need to prove harm, not safety. That allows claims for supplements to appear more credible than they really are. *For more about the use and abuse of supplements, see chapter 23.*

Spotting a Fraud

Does it sound too good to be true? Then it probably is! Be wary. Over the years, promoters of fraudulent weight-loss schemes have laced their claims with words and phrases like these:

all natural	exotic
ancient remedy	fast
balances hormones	guaranteed
banish fat	magical
breakthrough	miraculous
definitely no side effects	mysterious
discovered in Europe	no risk, money-
cure, cure-all	back guarantee
easy	new discovery
effortless	quick
enzymatic process	secret ingredient
exclusive product	totally safe

There's another common reason for growing health fraud: hope for a quick or easy "health fix." Some people may count on today's "medicine" to undo the results of an unhealthful lifestyle. It's not that simple—even if quacks lead you to believe otherwise.

What Are the Consequences?

Nutrition quackery exploits consumers, and it carries significant health and economic risks along the way:

● *False hopes.* Dream on! Quacks may promise—but unsound nutrition advice, products, or services won't prevent or cure disease.

● *A substitute for reliable healthcare.* False hopes, created through quackery, may delay or replace proper health promotion, medical care, or follow-up treatment. If you follow quackery, you may lose something you can't retrieve: time for effective treatment!

● *Interference with sound eating and lifestyle habits.* That happens when quackery replaces proven guidance.

● *Unneeded expense.* In the best-case scenario, some products and services touted by quacks simply don't work—and cause no harm, either. Why waste your hard-earned money on devices, products, and services that have no effect?

● *Potential harm.* Nutrition quackery also can put your health at risk. Taking very large doses of some vitamins and minerals, in the form of dietary supplements, can have toxic side effects. For example, excessive amounts of vitamin A during pregnancy increase the chances of birth defects. Inappropriate supplement use can lead to harmful drug-nutrient interactions. For example, taking vitamin K can be risky if you take blood-thinning drugs. *For more about specific vitamins and minerals, see chapter 4.*

Over-the-counter herbal products, marketed as dietary supplements, are sources of potent drugs. Yet, unlike medications, herbal products aren't well regulated. *See "Herbals and Other Botanicals: Help or Harm?" in chapter 23.*

Quackery: What You Can Do

No one has to be the victim of nutrition fraud. To protect yourself, know how to identify fraud and quackery, and where to find sound nutrition information.

● Retain a healthy skepticism as your best defense against a "quack attack." And take time to be well informed before you invest in a nutrition product, treatment, or service. *Give it the "Ten Questions" test on page 629 before you buy.*

● Seek advice from reliable sources. If you're suspicious about a statement, product, or service, contact a credible nutrition source—for example, a registered dietitian, your public health department, the medical or nutrition department of a nearby college or university, or your county Extension office. *See "Need Nutrition Advice?" in this chapter.*

● Report nutrition fraud. If you suspect that a statement, product, or service is fraudulent or false, inquire

---

Have You Ever Wondered

. . . how to check out diet scams? Besides talking with a nutrition expert, check the Federal Trade Commission (www.ftc.gov), which may list diet scams it's prosecuted.

Ten Red Flags of Junk Science

A new health or nutrition report? Before you jump to conclusions, check it out. Any combination of these signs should send up a red flag of suspicion.

1. Recommendations that promise a quick fix.
2. Dire warnings of danger from a single product or regimen.
3. Claims that sound too good to be true.
4. Simplistic conclusions drawn from a complex study.
5. Recommendations based on a single study.
6. Dramatic statements that are refuted by reputable scientific organizations.
7. Lists of "good" and "bad" foods.
8. Recommendations made to help sell a product.
9. Recommendations based on studies published without peer review.
10. Recommendations from studies that ignore differences among individuals or groups.

Source: Developed by the Food and Nutrition Science Alliance (FANSA).

with the appropriate government agency or file a complaint.

To the Postal Service. Contact your postmaster or someone else in the Postal Service if you've been the victim—or target—of nutrition fraud through the mail. It's illegal to use the Postal Service to make false claims about or to sell fraudulent products or services.

To the FDA. Make inquiries or file complaints about false claims for dietary supplements with the U.S. Food and Drug Administration (FDA). That includes concerns about inadequate information on package labels.

To the FTC. For questions or concerns about false or misleading claims in advertising, contact the Federal Trade Commission (FTC).

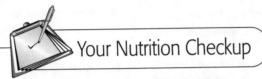 Your Nutrition Checkup

Play "Ten Questions"

Suspicious when something sounds too good to be true? To avoid the lure, arm yourself with these questions—even when you aren't suspicious!

Ask: Does the promotion of a nutrition product, regimen, service, treatment, or device . . .

Yes	No	
☐	☐	**1.** Try to lure you with scare tactics, emotional appeals, or perhaps with a "money-back guarantee" rather than proven results?
☐	☐	**2.** Promise to "revitalize," "detoxify," or "balance your body with nature"? Or does it claim to increase your stamina, stimulate your body's healing power, or boost your energy level?
☐	☐	**3.** Offer "proof" based on personal anecdotes or testimonials rather than sound science?
☐	☐	**4.** Advise supplements as "insurance" for everyone? Or recommend very large doses of nutrients? "Very large" means significantly more than 100 percent of the Daily Values (DVs). *See the Appendices for DV levels.*
☐	☐	**5.** Claim it can "treat," "cure," or "prevent" diverse health problems . . . from arthritis to cancer to sexual impotence?
☐	☐	**6.** Make unrealistic claims such as "reverse the aging process" or "cure disease" or "quick, easy approach"?
☐	☐	**7.** Blame the food supply as the source of health or behavior problems? Belittle government regulations? Or discredit the advice of recognized medical authorities?
☐	☐	**8.** Claim that its "natural" benefits surpass those of "synthetic" products?
☐	☐	**9.** Mention a "secret formula"? Or fail to list ingredients on its product label or to state any possible side effects?
☐	☐	**10.** Come from a "nutrition expert" without accepted credentials? Does that person also sell the product?

Now score yourself:

In this game of "Ten Questions," you might spot quackery with just one "yes" answer! Here's why.

1. *Fact:* Playing on emotion, misinformation, or even fear is common among nonscientific pseudo-experts. Emotional words used to promote a product can be an instant tip-off to quackery: "guar-anteed," "breakthrough," and "miraculous" are used for emotional appeal. So are false claims that most Americans are poorly nourished or that foods or additives are "deadly poisons."

2. *Fact:* Pseudo-medical jargon such as "detoxify" or "balance your body chemistry" suggests misinformation. These terms have no meaning in physiology. To sort valid medical terms from hype, ask a credible expert to decipher any confusing terms or phrases. A supplement can't increase your strength, immunity, stamina, or energy level, either. *For more about supplements promoted to athletes, see "Ergogenic Aids—No Substitute for Training" in chapter 19.* "Ergogenic" means the potential to increase work output; a supplement can't do that!

3. *Fact:* Nutrition is a science, based on fact not emotion or belief. Be skeptical of case histories and testimonials from satisfied users—if that's the only proof that a product works. Instead look for medical evidence from a reputable institution or a qualified health expert. Without scientific evidence, a reported "cure" may have other causes. Sometimes the ailment disappears on its own. The "cure" actually may be a placebo effect; its benefit may be psychological, not physical. The person may have been misdiagnosed in the first place. Even chronic ailments don't always have symptoms all the time.

4. *Fact:* Everyone does *not* need a vitamin supplement! Most healthy people can get enough nutrients with a varied, balanced eating plan from MyPyramid. Quacks rarely say who does *not* need a supplement. *See "MyPyramid: Your Healthful Eating Guide" in chapter 10.*

    For most people, there's no added benefit from taking more than 100 percent of the DVs for most vitamins and minerals. Except for a nutrition deficiency, there's no proof that nutrients alone prevent or cure anything. So ignore the hype! On the contrary, taking too much may be harmful. *See chapter 23, "Supplements: Use and Abuse."*

5. *Fact:* No nutrition regimen, device, or product can treat all that ails you. And they can't cure many health conditions, including arthritis, cancer, and sexual impotence. Even when they're part of credible treatment or prevention strategies, nutrition factors are typically just one part of overall healthcare.

6. *Fact:* Most health-promoting approaches take some effort. Claims that sound too good to be true probably are. Quacks know that's what people want to hear. Quackery thrives because people want simple cures and magic ways to change what's imperfect.

7. *Fact:* Quacks often belittle the regular food supply, government regulation, and the established medical community. They even claim that the traditional

health community is suppressing their work. Instead they call for "freedom of choice". . . and describe unproved methods as alternatives to current, proven methods. However, alternatives promoted through quackery are typically untested and may be ineffective or even unsafe. Among well-researched methods, you'll find choices.

By discrediting traditional approaches, quacks are attempting to funnel your healthcare dollars toward their own financial gain.

8. *Fact:* There's nothing magical about supplements promoted as "natural." From the standpoint of science, the chemical structure of natural and synthetic dietary supplements is essentially the same. And the body uses them in the same manner. (There's one exception: "natural" vitamin E is more potent than its synthetic form.) Herbal products aren't necessarily safe just because they're "natural." Even substances found in nature can have natural toxins, with potent, druglike effects.

9. *Fact:* By law, a medication must carry product information on its packaging. That includes the product's ingredients, use, dosage, warnings, precautions, and what to do if adverse reactions occur. However, products or regimens sold through quackery may not report all this information, including potential side effects or dangers.

10. *Fact:* Quacks are typically salespeople. Rather than offering accurate advice, their bottom line is to sell you something. Be wary when someone tries to diagnose your health status, then offers to sell you a remedy, such as a routine dietary supplement.

    Be wary of the methods used to assess your health or need for supplements. Many invalid tests may be hard to distinguish from legitimate clinical assessments. Those often used by quacks include hair analysis, iridology, and herbal crystallization analysis, among others. Computerized questionnaires can't supply enough information either to determine your need for a supplement. Get an opinion from a qualified health professional before getting these assessments or making changes based on the results.

    Quackery underlies many regimens focused on weight loss or gain, too. *To judge programs for their effectiveness and safety, see "Questions to Ask . . . About Diet Programs" in chapter 2.*

Resources You Can Use

Looking for sound nutrition information? You have many reliable resources: professional associations, health agencies, government agencies, and credible nutrition newsletters. Besides brochures, booklets, and consumer hotlines, many provide reliable on-line nutrition information. Your local hospital, public health, extension service, and many food industry groups are other reliable resources you might tap.

General Nutrition

American Dietetic Association
120 South Riverside Plaza, Suite 2000
Chicago, IL 60606-6995
www.eatright.org
Information Nutrition Line:
800/366-1655 for recorded messages, or
    to obtain a referral to a registered die-
    titian in your area

**Center for Nutrition Policy and
    Promotion**
U.S. Department of Agriculture
3101 Park Center Drive, Room 1034
Alexandria, VA 22302-1594
703/305-7600
www.usda.gov/cnpp

Cooperative Extension Service
(Contact your state's land-grant
    university.)

**Food and Nutrition Information
    Center**
National Agricultural Library
U.S. Department of Agriculture, Room
    105
10301 Baltimore Avenue
Beltsville, MD 20705-2351
301/504-5719
www.nal.usda.gov/fnic

Food and Nutrition Service
U.S. Department of Agriculture
3101 Park Center Drive
Alexandria, VA 22302
www.fns.usda.gov/fns

**International Food Information
    Council (IFIC)**
1100 Connecticut Avenue, NW, Suite 430
Washington, DC 20036
202/296-6540
www.ific.org

**National Academy of Sciences/Health
    and Medicine**
2101 Constitution Avenue, NW
Washington, DC 20418
202/334-1732
www.nationalacademies.org/health

Society for Nutrition Education
7150 Winton Drive, Suite 300
Indianapolis, IN 46268
800/235-6690
www.sne.org

U.S. Department of Agriculture
1400 Independence Avenue, SW
Washington, DC 20250
www.usda.gov

**U.S. Government (gateway to
    nutrition sites)**
www.nutrition.gov
www.healthfinder.gov
www.kids.gov

Dietary Supplements

**National Center for Alternative and
    Complementary Medicine**
9000 Rockville Pike
Bethesda, MD 20892
888/644-6226
www.nccam.nih.gov

NIH/Office of Dietary Supplements
6100 Executive Blvd.
Bethesda, MD 20892
301/435-2920
www.ods.od.nih.gov

U.S. Food and Drug Administration
www.cfsan.fda.gov/~dms/supplmnt.html

U.S. Pharmacopeia
12601 Twinbrook Parkway
Rockville, MD 20852-1790
800/227-8772
www.usp.org

Food Safety, Labeling, and Advertising

**American Association of Poision
    Control Centers**
National hotline to local centers:
    800/222-1222
www.aapcc.org

**CDC's National Prevention
    Information Network**
Clearinghouse for HIV/AIDs, STDs,
    and TB Material
P.O. Box 6003
Rockville, MD 20849-6003
800/458-5231
www.cdcnpin.org

**Center for Food Safety and Applied
    Nutrition**
Outreach and Information Center
5100 Paint Branch Parkway
    HFS-555
College Park, MD 20740-3835
888/723-3366 or 888/SAFE-FOOD
www.foodsafety/list/html

**FDA's Food Information and
    Seafood Hotline**
888/723-3366

FDA's MEDWatch Program
800/FDA-1088

Federal Trade Commission (FTC)
600 Pennsylvania Avenue, NW,
    Room 130
Washington, DC 20580
www.ftc.gov
Consumer number:
    877/FTC-HELP
(Or contact your regional FTC
    office.)

U.S. Food and Drug Administration (FDA)
Consumer Information Office
5600 Fishers Lane
Rockville, MD 20857-0001
888/INFO-FDA (888/463-6332)
(Or contact your regional FDA office.)
www.fda.gov

Food Safety and Inspection Service
U.S. Department of Agriculture
14th Street and Independence Avenue, SW
Washington, D.C. 20250
202/720-2791
www.fsis.usda.gov

USDA Meat and Poultry Hotline
888/674-6854
www.fsis.usda.gov/mph

National Lead Information Center
1200 Pennsylvania Avenue, NW
Mail Code 7404T
Washington, DC 20460
800/424-LEAD
www.epa.gov/lead

U.S. Environmental Protection Agency
Areil Rios Building
1200 Pennsylvania Avenue, NW
Washington, DC 20490
www.epa.gov
Safe Drinking Water Hotline
800/426-4791

U.S. Government (gateway to food safety sites)
www.foodsafety.gov

Water Quality Association
International Headquarters & Laboratory
4151 Naperville Road
Lisle, IL 60532-1088
630/505-0160
www.wqa.org

Food Sensitivities

American Academy of Allergy, Asthma, and Immunology
555 East Wells Street, Suite 1100
Milwaukee, WI 53202
800/822-2762
www.aaaai.org

Celiac Disease Foundation
13251 Ventura Blvd., Suite 1
Studio City, CA 91604
818/990-2354
www.celiac.org

Celiac Sprue Association/USA
P.O. Box 31700
Omaha, NE 68131-0700
402/558-0600 or 877/CSA-4-CSA
www.csaceliacs.org

Children's P.K.U. Network
3970 Via de la Valle, Suite 120
Del Mar, CA 92014
800/377-6677
www.pkunetwork.org

Food Allergy and Anaphylaxis Network
11781 Lee Jackson Hwy., Suite 160
Fairfax, VA 22033-3309
800/929-4040
www.foodallergy.org

Gluten Intolerance Group of North America
15110 10th Avenue, Suite A
Seattle, WA 98166-1820
206/246-6652
www.gluten.net

P.K.U. Parents of California
8 Myrtle Lane
San Anselmo, CA 94960
415/457-4632
www.pkuparents.org

Maternal, Infant, Child, and Adolescent Nutrition

American Academy of Pediatrics
141 Northwest Point Boulevard
Elk Grove Village, IL 60007-1098
847/434-4000
www.aap.org

La Leche League International
1400 N. Meacham Road
Schaumburg, IL 60173-4808
800/LALECHE (800/525-3243) or 847/519-7730
www.lalecheleague.org

School Nutrition Association
700 South Washington Street, Suite 300
Alexandria, VA 22314
703/739-3900
www.schoolnutrition.org

Nutrition and Aging

American Association of Retired Persons
601 E Street, NW
Washington, DC 20049
888/OUR-AARP (888/687-2277)
www.aarp.org

Elder Care Locator
800/677-1116
www.eldercare.gov

National Association of Area Agencies on Aging
1730 Rhode Island Avenue NW, Suite 1200
Washington, DC 20036
202/872-0888
www.n4a.org

National Institute on Aging
Building 31, Room 5C-27
31 Center Drive, MSC 2292
Bethesda, MD 20892
301/496-1752
www.nia.nih.gov

General Health and Disease Prevention/Treatment

General
American Academy of Family Physicians
11400 Tomahawk Creek Parkway
Leawood, KS 66211-2672
800/274-2237 or 913/906-6000
www.aafp.org

American Medical Association
515 North State Street
Chicago, IL 60610-4377
800/621-8335
www.ama-assn.org

American Public Health Association
800 I Street, NW
Washington, DC 20001
202/777-2742
www.apha.org

Centers for Disease Control and Prevention
1600 Clifton Road Northeast
Atlanta, GA 30333
404/639-3311 or 800/311-3435
www.cdc.gov

National Wellness Institute, Inc.
P.O. Box 827
Stevens Point, WI 54481-0827
800/243-8694
www.nationalwellness.org

Office of Minority Health Resource
Center
U.S. Department of Health and Human
Services
P.O. Box 37337
Washington, DC 20013-7337
800/444-6472
www.omhrc.gov

National Center for Health Statistics
U.S. Department of Health and Human
Services
3311 Toledo Road
Hyattsville, MD 20782
866/441-NCHS
www.cdc.gov/nchs

National Health Council
1730 M. Street, NW, Suite 500
Washington, DC 20036
202/785-3910
www.nhcouncil.org

National Health Information Center
P.O. Box 1133
Washington, DC 20013-1133
301/565-4167 or 800/336-4797
www.health.gov/nhic
Toll-free health information:
www.health.gov/NHIC/Pubs/
tollfree.htm
Federal health information and
clearinghouses: *www.health*
.gov/NHIC/Pubs/clearinghouses.htm

National Institutes of Health
9000 Rockville Pike
Bethesda, MD 20892
301/496-4000
www.nih.gov

U.S. Department of Health and
Human Services
200 Independence Avenue, SW
Washington, DC 20201
202/619-0257
www.hhs.gov
www.healthfinder.gov

Alcoholism

National Clearinghouse for Alcohol
and Drug Information
11420 Rockville Pike, Suite 200

Rockville, MD 20852
301/468-2600 or 800/729-6686
www.ncadi.samhsa.gov

National Council on Alcoholism and
Drug Dependence, Inc.
22 Cortlandt Street, Suite 801
New York, NY 10007-3128
212/269-7797 or 800/NCA-CALL
www.ncadd.org

Cancer

American Cancer Society
1599 Clifton Road, NE
Atlanta, GA 30329-4251
800/227-2345
www.cancer.org

American Institute for Cancer
Research
1759 R Street, NW
Washington, DC 20009
202/328-7744
www.aicr.org

National Cancer Institute
U.S. NIH
Building 31, Room 10A0331, Center
Drive, MSC 2580
Bethesda, MD 20892-2580
800/4-CANCER (800/422-6237) or
301/435-3848
www.cancer.gov

Cardiovascular (Heart) Disease

American Heart Association
7272 Greenville Avenue
Dallas, TX 75231-4596
800/AHA-USA1
(800/242-8721)
www.americanheart.org

National Cholesterol Education
Program, National Heart, Lung,
and Blood Institute
P.O. Box 30105
Bethesda, MD 20824-0105
301/592-8573
www.nhlbi.nih.gov

Diabetes

American Diabetes Association
Attn.: National Call Center
1701 North Beauregard Street
Alexandria, VA 22311
800/342-2383
www.diabetes.org

Joslin Diabetes Center
1 Joslin Place
Boston, MA 02215
617/732-2400
www.joslin.org

Juvenile Diabetes Foundation
International
120 Wall Street
New York, NY 10005-4001
212/785-9500
800/JDF-CURE (800/533-2873)
www.jdf.org

National Diabetes Information
Clearinghouse
1 Information Way
Bethesda, MD 20892-3560
800/860-8747
www. diabetes.niddk.nih.gov

Digestive Disease

Digestive Disease National Coalition
507 Capitol Court NE, Suite 200
Washington, DC 20002
202/544-7497
www.ddnc.org

National Digestive Diseases Informa-
tion Clearinghouse
2 Information Way
Bethesda, MD 20892-3570
301/654-3810 or 800/891-5389
www. digestive.niddk.nih.gov

Eating Disorders

National Association of Anorexia
Nervosa and Associated
Disorders
P.O. Box 7
Highland Park, IL 60035
847/831-3438
www.anad.org

National Eating Disorders
Organization
603 Stewart Street, Suite 803
Seattle, WA 98101
800/931-2237
www.edap.org

Oral Health

American Dental Association
211 East Chicago Avenue
Chicago, IL 60611-2678
312/440-2500
www.ada.org

Osteoporosis

National Osteoporosis Foundation
1232 22nd Street, NW
Washington, DC 20037-1292
202/223-2226 or 800/223-9994
www.nof.org

Weight

Healthy Weight Network
402 South 14th Street
Hettinger, ND 58639
701/567-2646 (fax)
www.healthyweightnetwork.com

Overeaters Anonymous
P.O. Box 44020
Rio Rancho, NM 87174
505/891-2664
www.oa.org

Shape Up America
4500 Connecticut Avenue, NW, Suite 414
Washington, DC 20008
www.shapeup.org

Sports Nutrition and Physical Activity

American Alliance for Health, Physical Education, Recreation, & Dance
1900 Association Drive
Reston, VA 20191-1598
800/213-7193
www.aahperd.org

American College of Sports Medicine
401 West Michigan Street
Indianapolis, IN 46202-3233
317/637-9200
www.acsm.org

American Council for Fitness and Nutrition
P.O. Box 33396
Washington, DC 20033
800/953-1700
www.acfn.org

American Council on Exercise
4851 Paramount Drive
San Diego, CA 92123
800/825-3626
www.acefitness.org

America on the Move Foundation
44 School Street, Suite 125
Boston, MA 02108
www.americaonthemove.org

American Running Association
4405 East-West Highway, Suite 405
Bethesda, MD 20814
301/913-9517 or 800/776-ARFA (-2732)
www.americanrunning.org

Fifty-Plus Lifelong Fitness
2483 E. Bayshore Road, Suite 202
Palo Alto, CA 94303
650/843-1750
www.50plus.org

International Center for Sports Nutrition
502 South 44th Street, Suite 3012
Omaha, NE 68105-1065
402/559-5505

National Fitness and Wellness Coalition
1800 Silas Deane Highway
Rocky Hill, CT 06067
203/721-1055

President's Council on Physical Fitness and Sports
Department W
200 Independence Avenue, SW, Room 738-H
Washington, DC 20201-0004
202/690-9000
www.fitness.gov

Women's Sports Foundation
Eisenhower Park
East Meadow, NY 11554
800/227-3988
www.womenssportsfoundation.org

YMCA of the USA
101 North Wacker Drive
Chicago, IL 60606
800/USA-YMCA (800/872-9622) or 312/977-0031

Vegetarian Eating

North American Vegetarian Society
P.O. Box 72
Dolgeville, NY 13329
518/568-7970
www.navs-online.org

The Vegetarian Resource Group
P.O. Box 1463, Dept. IN
Baltimore, MD 21203
410/366-VEGE (8343)
www.vrg.org

Food Technology/Biotechnology

Biotechnology Industry Organization
1225 Eye Street NW, Suite 400
Washington, DC 20005
202/962-9200
www.bio.org

Institute of Food Technologists
525 W. Van Buren, Suite 1000
Chicago, IL 60607
312/782-8424
www.ift.org

International Food Additives Council
5775 Peachtree-Dunwoody Road, Suite 500-G
Atlanta, GA 30342
404/252-3663

Health Fraud

National Council against Health Fraud
119 Foster Street
Peabody, MA 01960
978/532-9383
www.ncahf.org

Quackwatch, Inc.
www.quackwatch.org

Food Industry Associations

Alaska Seafood Marketing Institute
www.alaskaseafood.org

Almond Board of California
www.almondsarein.com

American Dry Bean Board
www.americanbean.org

American Egg Board
www.aeb.org

Beans for Health Alliance
www.beansforhealth.org

California Avocado Commission
www.avocado.org

California Dried Plum Board
www.californiadriedplums.org

California Fig Advisory Board
www.californiafigs.com

California Olive Industry
www.calolive.org

California Olive Oil Council
www.cooc.com

California Pistachio Commission
www.pistachios.org

California Strawberry Commission
www.calstrawberry.com

Calorie Control Council
www.caloriecontrol.org

Canned Food Alliance
www.mealtime.org

Canola Council of Canada
www.canola-council.org

Corn Refiners Association
www.corn.org

Cranberry Institute
www.cranberryinstitute.org

Distilled Spirits Council of the United States
www.discus.org

Egg Nutrition Center
www.enc-online.org

Flax Council of Canada
www.flaxcouncil.ca

Food Marketing Institute
www.fmi.org

The Glutamate Association
www.msgfacts.com

Infant Formula Council
www.infantformula.org

International Bottled Water Association
www.bottledwater.org

International Tree Nut Council
www.nuthealth.org

Mushroom Council
www.mushroomcouncil.org

National Cattlemen's Beef Association
www.beef.org

National Chicken Council
www.eatchicken.com
www.nationalchickencouncil.com

National Coffee Association
www.ncausa.org

National Dairy Council (Dairy Management, Inc.)
www.dairyinfo.com

National Fisheries Institute
www.aboutseafood.com

National Pasta Association
www.ilovepasta.org

National Pork Board
www.pork.org

National Restaurant Association
www.restaurant.org

National Turkey Federation
www.eatturkey.com

National Watermelon Promotion Board
www.watermelon.org

North Carolina Sweet Potato Commission
www.ncsweetpotatoes.com

The Peanut Institute
www.peanut-institute.org

Produce for Better Health Foundation
5-A-Day Program
www.5aday.com

Produce Marketing Association
www.pma.com

Salt Institute
www.saltinstitute.org

Snack Food Association
www.sfa.org

Salmon of the Americas
www.salmonoftheamericas.com

The Soyfoods Council
www.thesoyfoodscouncil.com

The Sugar Association
www.sugar.org

The Tea Council of the U.S.A.
www.teausa.com

United Fresh Fruit & Vegetable Association
www.uffva.org

United Soybean Board
www.soybean.org

United States Potato Board
www.healthypotato.com

USA Rice Federation
www.usarice.com

US Tuna Foundation
www.tunafacts.org

Walnut Marketing Board
www.walnuts.org

Wheat Foods Council
www.wheatfoods.org

Whole Grains Council
www.wholegrainscouncil.org

Nutrition Newsletters

Consumer Reports on Health
www.consumerreports.org

Environmental Nutrition
www.environmentalnutrition.com

FDA Consumer
www.fda.gov/fdac

Food & Fitness Advisor
The Center for Women's Health
Weill Medical College of Cornell University
www.foodandfitnessadvisor.com

Mayo Clinic Health Letter
www.mayoclinic.org

Tufts University Health and Nutrition Letter
www.healthletter.tufts.edu

University of California, Berkeley Wellness Letter
www.wellnessletter.com

Appendices

2005 Dietary Guidelines for Americans: Key Recommendations for the General Population*

Adequate Nutrients within Calorie Needs

● Consume a variety of nutrient-dense foods and beverages within and among the basic food groups while choosing foods that limit the intake of saturated and *trans* fats, cholesterol, added sugars, salt, and alcohol.

● Meet recommended intakes within energy needs by adopting a balanced eating pattern, such as the U.S. Department of Agriculture (USDA) Food Guide† or the Dietary Approaches to Stop Hypertension (DASH) Eating Plan.

Weight Management

● To maintain body weight in a healthy range, balance calories from foods and beverages with calories expended.

● To prevent gradual weight gain over time, make small decreases in food and beverage calories and increase physical activity.

Physical Activity

● Engage in regular physical activity and reduce sedentary activities to promote health, psychological well-being, and a healthy body weight.

● To reduce the risk of chronic disease in adulthood: Engage in at least 30 minutes of moderate-intensity physical activity, above usual activity, at work or home on most days of the week.

● For most people, greater health benefits can be obtained by engaging in physical activity of more vigorous intensity or longer duration.

● To help manage body weight and prevent gradual, unhealthy body weight gain in adulthood: Engage in approximately 60 minutes of moderate-to vigorous-intensity activity on most days of the week while not exceeding caloric intake requirements.

● To sustain weight loss in adulthood: Participate in at least 60 to 90 minutes of daily moderate-intensity physical activity while not exceeding caloric intake requirements. Some people may need to consult with a healthcare provider before participating in this level of activity.

● Achieve physical fitness by including cardiovascular conditioning, stretching exercises for flexibility, and resistance exercises or calisthenics for muscle strength and endurance.

---

* Recommendations for Specific Populations are presented in appropriate chapters and are listed on www.health.gov/dietaryguidelines/dga2005/document/html/executivesummary.html. *Source:* U.S. Department of Agriculture and U.S. Department of Health and Human Services.

† MyPyramid. *See chapter 10.*

Food Groups to Encourage

● Consume a sufficient amount of fruits and vegetables while staying within energy needs. Two cups of fruit and 2½ cups of vegetables per day are recommended for a reference 2,000-calorie intake, with higher or lower amounts depending on the calorie level.

● Choose a variety of fruits and vegetables each day. In particular, select from all five vegetable subgroups (dark-green, orange, legumes, starchy vegetables, and other vegetables) several times a week.

● Consume 3 or more ounce-equivalents of whole-grain products per day, with the rest of the recommended grains coming from enriched or whole-grain products. In general, at least half the grains should come from whole grains.

● Consume 3 cups per day of fat-free or low-fat milk or equivalent milk products.

Fats

● Consume less than 10 percent of calories from saturated fatty acids and less than 300 mg/day of cholesterol, and keep *trans* fatty acid consumption as low as possible.

● Keep total fat intake between 20 to 35 percent of calories, with most fats coming from sources of polyunsaturated and monounsaturated fatty acids, such as fish, nuts, and vegetable oils.

● When selecting and preparing meat, poultry, dry beans, and milk or milk products, make choices that are lean, low-fat, or fat-free.

● Limit intake of fats and oils high in saturated and/or *trans* fatty acids, and choose products low in such fats and oils.

Carbohydrates

● Choose fiber-rich fruits, vegetables, and whole grains often.

● Choose and prepare foods and beverages with little added sugars or caloric sweeteners, such as amounts suggested by the USDA Food Guide[†] and the DASH Eating Plan.

● Reduce the incidence of dental caries by practicing good oral hygiene and consuming sugar- and starch-containing foods and beverages less frequently.

Sodium and Potassium

● Consume less than 2,300 mg (approximately 1 teaspoon of salt) of sodium per day.

● Choose and prepare foods with little salt. At the same time, consume potassium-rich foods, such as fruits and vegetables.

Alcoholic Beverages

● Those who choose to drink alcoholic beverages should do so sensibly and in moderation—defined as the consumption of up to one drink per day for women and up to two drinks per day for men.

● Alcoholic beverages should not be consumed by some individuals, including those who cannot restrict their alcohol intake, women of childbearing age who may become pregnant, pregnant and lactating women, children and adolescents, individuals taking medications that can interact with alcohol, and those with specific medical conditions.

● Alcoholic beverages should be avoided by individuals engaging in activities that require attention, skill, or coordination, such as driving or operating machinery.

Food Safety

● To avoid microbial foodborne illness:

● Clean hands, food contact surfaces, and fruits and vegetables. Meat and poultry should not be washed or rinsed.

● Separate raw, cooked, and ready-to-eat foods while shopping, preparing, or storing foods.

● Cook foods to a safe temperature to kill microorganisms.

● Chill (refrigerate) perishable food promptly and defrost foods properly.

● Avoid raw (unpasteurized) milk or any products made from unpasteurized milk, raw or partially cooked eggs or foods containing raw eggs, raw or undercooked meat and poultry, unpasteurized juices, and raw sprouts.

† MyPyramid. *See chapter 10.*

Dietary Reference Intakes (DRIs): Acceptable Macronutrient Distribution Ranges
Food and Nutrition Board, Institute of Medicine, National Academies

Macronutrient	Range (percent of energy)		
	Children, 1–3 y	Children, 4–18 y	Adults
Fat	30–40	25–35	20–35
n-6 polyunsaturated fatty acids[a] (linoleic acid)	5–10	5–10	5–10
n-3 polyunsaturated fatty acids[a] (α-linolenic acid)	0.6–1.2	0.6–1.2	0.6–1.2
Carbohydrate	45–65	45–65	45–65
Protein	5–20	10–30	10–35

[a] Approximately 10% of the total can come from longer-chain n-3 or n-6 fatty acids.

SOURCE: *Dietary Reference Intakes for Energy, Carbohydrate, Fiber, Fat, Fatty Acids, Cholesterol, Protein, and Amino Acids* (2002).

Dietary Reference Intakes (DRIs): Recommended Intakes for Individuals, Macronutrients
Food and Nutrition Board, Institute of Medicine, National Academies

Life Stage Group	Total Water[a] (L/d)	Carbohydrate (g/d)	Total Fiber (g/d)	Fat (g/d)	Linoleic Acid (g/d)	α-Linolenic Acid (g/d)	Protein[b] (g/d)
Infants							
0–6 mo	0.7*	60*	ND	31*	4.4*	0.5*	9.1*
7–12 mo	0.8*	95*	ND	30*	4.6*	0.5*	**11.0**[c]
Children							
1–3 y	1.3*	**130**	19*	ND	7*	0.7*	**13**
4–8 y	1.7*	**130**	25*	ND	10*	0.9*	**19**
Males							
9–13 y	2.4*	**130**	31*	ND	12*	1.2*	**34**
14–18 y	3.3*	**130**	38*	ND	16*	1.6*	**52**
19–30 y	3.7*	**130**	38*	ND	17*	1.6*	**56**
31–50 y	3.7*	**130**	38*	ND	17*	1.6*	**56**
51–70 y	3.7*	**130**	30*	ND	14*	1.6*	**56**
> 70 y	3.7*	**130**	30*	ND	14*	1.6*	**56**
Females							
9–13 y	2.1*	**130**	26*	ND	10*	1.0*	**34**
14–18 y	2.3*	**130**	26*	ND	11*	1.1*	**46**
19–30 y	2.7*	**130**	25*	ND	12*	1.1*	**46**
31–50 y	2.7*	**130**	25*	ND	12*	1.1*	**46**
51–70 y	2.7*	**130**	21*	ND	11*	1.1*	**46**
> 70 y	2.7*	**130**	21*	ND	11*	1.1*	**46**
Pregnancy							
14–18 y	3.0*	**175**	28*	ND	13*	1.4*	**71**
19–30 y	3.0*	**175**	28*	ND	13*	1.4*	**71**
31–50 y	3.0*	**175**	28*	ND	13*	1.4*	**71**
Lactation							
14–18 y	3.8*	**210**	29*	ND	13*	1.3*	**71**
19–30 y	3.8*	**210**	29*	ND	13*	1.3*	**71**
31–50 y	3.8*	**210**	29*	ND	13*	1.3*	**71**

NOTE: This table presents Recommended Dietary Allowances (RDAs) in **bold** type and Adequate Intakes (AIs) in ordinary type followed by an asterisk (*). RDAs and AIs may both be used as goals for individual intake. RDAs are set to meet the needs of almost all (97 to 98 percent) individuals in a group. For healthy infants fed human milk, the AI is the mean intake. The AI for other life stage and gender groups is believed to cover the needs of all individuals in the group, but lack of data or uncertainty in the data prevent being able to specify with confidence the percentage of individuals covered by this intake.

[a] *Total* water includes all water contained in food, beverages, and drinking water.

[b] Based on 0.8 g/kg body weight for the reference body weight.

[c] Change from 13.5 in prepublication copy due to calculation error.

Dietary Reference Intakes (DRIs): Additional Macronutrient Recommendations
Food and Nutrition Board, Institute of Medicine, National Academies

Macronutrient	Recommendation
Dietary cholesterol	As low as possible while consuming a nutritionally adequate diet
Trans fatty acids	As low as possible while consuming a nutritionally adequate diet
Saturated fatty acids	As low as possible while consuming a nutritionally adequate diet
Added sugars	Limit to no more than 25% of total energy

SOURCE: *Dietary Reference Intakes for Energy, Carbohydrate, Fiber, Fat, Fatty Acids, Cholesterol, Protein, and Amino Acids* (2002).

Dietary Reference Intakes (DRIs): Estimated Energy Requirements (EER) for Men and Women 30 Years of Age[a]
Food and Nutrition Board, Institute of Medicine, National Academies

Height (m [in])	PAL[b]	Weight for BMI[c] of 18.5 kg/m^2 (kg [lb])	Weight for BMI of 24.99 kg/m^2 (kg [lb])	EER, Men[d] (kcal/day) BMI of 18.5 kg/m^2	BMI of 24.99 kg/m^2	EER, Women[d] (kcal/day) BMI of 18.5 kg/m^2	BMI of 24.99 kg/m^2
1.50 (59)	Sedentary	41.6 (92)	56.2 (124)	1,848	2,080	1,625	1,762
	Low active			2,009	2,267	1,803	1,956
	Active			2,215	2,506	2,025	2,198
	Very active			2,554	2,898	2,291	2,489
1.65 (65)	Sedentary	50.4 (111)	68.0 (150)	2,068	2,349	1,816	1,982
	Low active			2,254	2,566	2,016	2,202
	Active			2,490	2,842	2,267	2,477
	Very active			2,880	3,296	2,567	2,807
1.80 (71)	Sedentary	59.9 (132)	81.0 (178)	2,301	2,635	2,015	2,211
	Low active			2,513	2,884	2,239	2,459
	Active			2,782	3,200	2,519	2,769
	Very active			3,225	3,720	2,855	3,141

[a] For each year below 30, add 7 kcal/day for women and 10 kcal /day for men. For each year above 30, subtract 7 kcal/day for women and 10 kcal/day for men.

[b] PAL = physical activity level.

[c] BMI = body mass index.

[d] Derived from the following regression equations based on doubly labeled water data:

Adult man: EER = 662 – 9.53 × age (y) + PA × (15.91 × wt [kg] + 539.6 × ht [m])

Adult woman: EER = 354 – 6.91 × age (y) + PA × (9.36 × wt [kg] + 726 × ht [m])

Where PA refers to coefficient for PAL

PAL = total energy expenditure ÷ basal energy expenditure

PA = 1.0 if PAL ≥ 1.0 < 1.4 (sedentary)

PA = 1.12 if PAL ≥ 1.4 < 1.6 (low active)

PA = 1.27 if PAL ≥ 1.6 < 1.9 (active)

PA = 1.45 if PAL ≥ 1.9 < 2.5 (very active)

Dietary Reference Intakes (DRIs): Recommended Intakes for Individuals, Vitamins

Food and Nutrition Board, Institute of Medicine, National Academies

Life Stage Group	Vit A (µg/d)[a]	Vit C (mg/d)	Vit D (µg/d)[b,c]	Vit E (mg/d)[d]	Vit K (µg/d)	Thiamin (mg/d)	Riboflavin (mg/d)	Niacin (mg/d)[e]	Vit B_6 (mg/d)	Folate (µg/d)[f]	Vit B_{12} (µg/d)	Pantothenic Acid (mg/d)	Biotin (µg/d)	Choline[g] (mg/d)
Infants														
0–6 mo	400*	40*	5*	4*	2.0*	0.2*	0.3*	2*	0.1*	65*	0.4*	1.7*	5*	125*
7–12 mo	500*	50*	5*	5*	2.5*	0.3*	0.4*	4*	0.3*	80*	0.5*	1.8*	6*	150*
Children														
1–3 y	300	15	5*	6	30*	0.5	0.5	6	0.5	150	0.9	2*	8*	200*
4–8 y	400	25	5*	7	55*	0.6	0.6	8	0.6	200	1.2	3*	12*	250*
Males														
9–13 y	600	45	5*	11	60*	0.9	0.9	12	1.0	300	1.8	4*	20*	375*
14–18 y	900	75	5*	15	75*	1.2	1.3	16	1.3	400	2.4	5*	25*	550*
19–30 y	900	90	5*	15	120*	1.2	1.3	16	1.3	400	2.4	5*	30*	550*
31–50 y	900	90	5*	15	120*	1.2	1.3	16	1.3	400	2.4	5*	30*	550*
51–70 y	900	90	10*	15	120*	1.2	1.3	16	1.7	400	2.4[h]	5*	30*	550*
>70 y	900	90	15*	15	120*	1.2	1.3	16	1.7	400	2.4[h]	5*	30*	550*
Females														
9–13 y	600	45	5*	11	60*	0.9	0.9	12	1.0	300	1.8	4*	20*	375*
14–18 y	700	65	5*	15	75*	1.0	1.0	14	1.2	400[i]	2.4	5*	25*	400*
19–30 y	700	75	5*	15	90*	1.1	1.1	14	1.3	400[i]	2.4	5*	30*	425*
31–50 y	700	75	5*	15	90*	1.1	1.1	14	1.3	400[i]	2.4	5*	30*	425*
51–70 y	700	75	10*	15	90*	1.1	1.1	14	1.5	400	2.4[h]	5*	30*	425*
>70 y	700	75	15*	15	90*	1.1	1.1	14	1.5	400	2.4[h]	5*	30*	425*
Pregnancy														
14–18 y	750	80	5*	15	75*	1.4	1.4	18	1.9	600[j]	2.6	6*	30*	450*
19–30 y	770	85	5*	15	90*	1.4	1.4	18	1.9	600[j]	2.6	6*	30*	450*
31–50 y	770	85	5*	15	90*	1.4	1.4	18	1.9	600[j]	2.6	6*	30*	450*
Lactation														
14–18 y	1,200	115	5*	19	75*	1.4	1.6	17	2.0	500	2.8	7*	35*	550*
19–30 y	1,300	120	5*	19	90*	1.4	1.6	17	2.0	500	2.8	7*	35*	550*
31–50 y	1,300	120	5*	19	90*	1.4	1.6	17	2.0	500	2.8	7*	35*	550*

NOTE: This table (taken from the DRI reports, see www.nap.edu) presents Recommended Dietary Allowances (RDAs) in **bold type** and Adequate Intakes (AIs) in ordinary type followed by an asterisk (*). RDAs and AIs may both be used as goals for individual intake. RDAs are set to meet the needs of almost all (97 to 98 percent) individuals in a group. For healthy breastfed infants, the AI is the mean intake. The AI for other life stage and gender groups is believed to cover needs of all individuals in the group, but lack of data or uncertainty in the data prevent being able to specify with confidence the percentage of individuals covered by this intake.

[a] As retinol activity equivalents (RAEs). 1 RAE = 1 µg retinol, 12 µg β-carotene, 24 µg α-carotene, or 24 µg β-cryptoxanthin. The RAE for dietary provitamin A carotenoids is twofold greater than retinol equivalents (RE), whereas the RAE for preformed vitamin A is the same as RE.

[b] As cholecalciferol. 1 µg cholecalciferol = 40 IU vitamin D.

[c] In the absence of adequate exposure to sunlight.

[d] As α-tocopherol. α-Tocopherol includes *RRR*-α-tocopherol, the only form of α-tocopherol that occurs naturally in foods, and the *2R*-stereoisomeric forms of α-tocopherol (*RRR*-, *RSR*-, *RRS*-, and *RSS*-α-tocopherol) that occur in fortified foods and supplements. It does not include the *2S*-stereoisomeric forms of α-tocopherol (*SRR*-, *SSR*-, *SRS*-, and *SSS*-α-tocopherol), also found in fortified foods and supplements.

[e] As niacin equivalents (NE). 1 mg of niacin = 60 mg of tryptophan; 0–6 months = preformed niacin (not NE).

[f] As dietary folate equivalents (DFE). 1 DFE = 1 µg food folate = 0.6 µg of folic acid from fortified food or as a supplement consumed with food = 0.5 µg of a supplement taken on an empty stomach.

[g] Although AIs have been set for choline, there are few data to assess whether a dietary supply of choline is needed at all stages of the life cycle, and it may be that the choline requirement can be met by endogenous synthesis at some of these stages.

[h] Because 10 to 30 percent of older people may malabsorb food-bound B_{12}, it is advisable for those older than 50 years to meet their RDA mainly by consuming foods fortified with B_{12} or a supplement containing B_{12}.

[i] In view of evidence linking folate intake with neural tube defects in the fetus, it is recommended that all women capable of becoming pregnant consume 400 µg from supplements or fortified foods in addition to intake of food folate from a varied diet.

[j] It is assumed that women will continue consuming 400 µg from supplements or fortified food until their pregnancy is confirmed and they enter prenatal care, which ordinarily occurs after the end of the periconceptional period—the critical time for formation of the neural tube.

Dietary Reference Intakes (DRIs): Recommended Intakes for Individuals, Elements
Food and Nutrition Board, Institute of Medicine, National Academies

Life Stage Group	Calcium (mg/d)	Chromium (µg/d)	Copper (µg/d)	Fluoride (mg/d)	Iodine (µg/d)	Iron (mg/d)	Magnesium (mg/d)	Manganese (mg/d)	Molybdenum (µg/d)	Phosphorus (mg/d)	Selenium (µg/d)	Zinc (mg/d)	Potassium (g/d)	Sodium (g/d)	Chloride (g/d)
Infants															
0–6 mo	210*	0.2*	200*	0.01*	110*	0.27*	30*	0.003*	2*	100*	15*	2*	0.4*	0.12*	0.18*
7–12 mo	270*	5.5*	220*	0.5*	130*	11	75*	0.6*	3*	275*	20*	3	0.7*	0.37*	0.57*
Children															
1–3 y	500*	11*	340	0.7*	90	7	80	1.2*	17	460	20	3	3.0*	1.0*	1.5*
4–8 y	800*	15*	440	1*	90	10	130	1.5*	22	500	30	5	3.8*	1.2*	1.9*
Males															
9–13 y	1,300*	25*	700	2*	120	8	240	1.9*	34	1,250	40	8	4.5*	1.5*	2.3*
14–18 y	1,300*	35*	890	3*	150	11	410	2.2*	43	1,250	55	11	4.7*	1.5*	2.3*
19–30 y	1,000*	35*	900	4*	150	8	400	2.3*	45	700	55	11	4.7*	1.5*	2.3*
31–50 y	1,000*	35*	900	4*	150	8	420	2.3*	45	700	55	11	4.7*	1.5*	2.3*
51–70 y	1,200*	30*	900	4*	150	8	420	2.3*	45	700	55	11	4.7*	1.3*	2.0*
>70 y	1,200*	30*	900	4*	150	8	420	2.3*	45	700	55	11	4.7*	1.2*	1.8*
Females															
9–13 y	1,300*	21*	700	2*	120	8	240	1.6*	34	1,250	40	8	4.5*	1.5*	2.3*
14–18 y	1,300*	24*	890	3*	150	15	360	1.6*	43	1,250	55	9	4.7*	1.5*	2.3*
19–30 y	1,000*	25*	900	3*	150	18	310	1.8*	45	700	55	8	4.7*	1.5*	2.3*
31–50 y	1,000*	25*	900	3*	150	18	320	1.8*	45	700	55	8	4.7*	1.5*	2.3*
51–70 y	1,200*	20*	900	3*	150	8	320	1.8*	45	700	55	8	4.7*	1.3*	2.0*
>70 y	1,200*	20*	900	3*	150	8	320	1.8*	45	700	55	8	4.7*	1.2*	1.8*
Pregnancy															
14–18 y	1,300*	29*	1,000	3*	220	27	400	2.0*	50	1,250	60	12	4.7*	1.5*	2.3*
19–30 y	1,000*	30*	1,000	3*	220	27	350	2.0*	50	700	60	11	4.7*	1.5*	2.3*
31–50 y	1,000*	30*	1,000	3*	220	27	360	2.0*	50	700	60	11	4.7*	1.5*	2.3*
Lactation															
14–18 y	1,300*	44*	1,300	3*	290	10	360	2.6*	50	1,250	70	13	5.1*	1.5*	2.3*
19–30 y	1,000*	45*	1,300	3*	290	9	310	2.6*	50	700	70	12	5.1*	1.5*	2.3*
31–50 y	1,000*	45*	1,300	3*	290	9	320	2.6*	50	700	70	12	5.1*	1.5*	2.3*

NOTE: This table presents Recommended Dietary Allowances (RDAs) in **bold type** and Adequate Intakes (AIs) in ordinary type followed by an asterisk (*). RDAs and AIs may both be used as goals for individual intake. RDAs are set to meet the needs of almost all (97 to 98 percent) individuals in a group. For healthy breastfed infants, the AI is the mean intake. The AI for other life stage and gender groups is believed to cover needs of all individuals in the group, but lack of data or uncertainty in the data prevent being able to specify with confidence the percentage of individuals covered by this intake.

SOURCES: *Dietary Reference Intakes for Calcium, Phosphorous, Magnesium, Vitamin D, and Fluoride* (1997); *Dietary Reference Intakes for Thiamin, Riboflavin, Niacin, Vitamin B₆, Folate, Vitamin B₁₂, Pantothenic Acid, Biotin, and Choline* (1998); *Dietary Reference Intakes for Vitamin C, Vitamin E, Selenium, and Carotenoids* (2000); *Dietary Reference Intakes for Vitamin A, Vitamin K, Arsenic, Boron, Chromium, Copper, Iodine, Iron, Manganese, Molybdenum, Nickel, Silicon, Vanadium, and Zinc* (2001); and *Dietary Reference Intakes for Water, Potassium, Sodium, Chloride, and Sulfate* (2004). These reports may be accessed via http://www.nap.edu.

Dietary Reference Intakes (DRIs): Tolerable Upper Intake Levels (UL[a]), Vitamins
Food and Nutrition Board, Institute of Medicine, National Academies

Life Stage Group	Vitamin A (µg/d)[b]	Vitamin C (mg/d)	Vitamin D (µg/d)	Vitamin E (mg/d)[c,d]	Vitamin K	Thiamin	Riboflavin	Niacin (mg/d)[d]	Vitamin B6 (mg/d)	Folate (µg/d)[d]	Vitamin B12	Pantothenic Acid	Biotin	Choline (g/d)	Carotenoids[e]
Infants															
0–6 mo	600	ND[f]	25	ND	ND	ND	ND	ND	ND	ND	ND	ND	ND	ND	ND
7–12 mo	600	ND	25	ND	ND	ND	ND	ND	ND	ND	ND	ND	ND	ND	ND
Children															
1–3 y	600	400	50	200	ND	ND	ND	10	30	300	ND	ND	ND	1.0	ND
4–8 y	900	650	50	300	ND	ND	ND	15	40	400	ND	ND	ND	1.0	ND
Males, Females															
9–13 y	1,700	1,200	50	600	ND	ND	ND	20	60	600	ND	ND	ND	2.0	ND
14–18 y	2,800	1,800	50	800	ND	ND	ND	30	80	800	ND	ND	ND	3.0	ND
19–70 y	3,000	2,000	50	1,000	ND	ND	ND	35	100	1,000	ND	ND	ND	3.5	ND
>70 y	3,000	2,000	50	1,000	ND	ND	ND	35	100	1,000	ND	ND	ND	3.5	ND
Pregnancy															
14–18 y	2,800	1,800	50	800	ND	ND	ND	30	80	800	ND	ND	ND	3.0	ND
19–50 y	3,000	2,000	50	1,000	ND	ND	ND	35	100	1,000	ND	ND	ND	3.5	ND
Lactation															
14–18 y	2,800	1,800	50	800	ND	ND	ND	30	80	800	ND	ND	ND	3.0	ND
19–50 y	3,000	2,000	50	1,000	ND	ND	ND	35	100	1,000	ND	ND	ND	3.5	ND

[a] UL = The maximum level of daily nutrient intake that is likely to pose no risk of adverse effects. Unless otherwise specified, the UL represents total intake from food, water, and supplements. Due to lack of suitable data, ULs could not be established for vitamin K, thiamin, riboflavin, vitamin B12, pantothenic acid, biotin, carotenoids. In the absence of ULs, extra caution may be warranted in consuming levels above recommended intakes.

[b] As preformed vitamin A only.

[c] As α-tocopherol; applies to any form of supplemental α-tocopherol.

[d] The ULs for vitamin E, niacin, and folate apply to synthetic forms obtained from supplements, fortified foods, or a combination of the two.

[e] β-Carotene supplements are advised only to serve as a provitamin A source for individuals at risk of vitamin A deficiency.

[f] ND = Not determinable due to lack of data of adverse effects in this age group and concern with regard to lack of ability to handle excess amounts. Source of intake should be from food only to prevent high levels of intake.

SOURCES: *Dietary Reference Intakes for Calcium, Phosphorous, Magnesium, Vitamin D, and Fluoride* (1997); *Dietary Reference Intakes for Thiamin, Riboflavin, Niacin, Vitamin B6, Folate, Vitamin B12, Pantothenic Acid, Biotin, and Choline* (1998); *Dietary Reference Intakes for Vitamin C, Vitamin E, Selenium, and Carotenoids* (2000); and *Dietary Reference Intakes for Vitamin A, Vitamin K, Arsenic, Boron, Chromium, Copper, Iodine, Iron, Manganese, Molybdenum, Nickel, Silicon, Vanadium, and Zinc* (2001). These reports may be accessed via http://www.nap.edu.

Dietary Reference Intakes (DRIs): Tolerable Upper Intake Levels (UL^a), Elements
Food and Nutrition Board, Institute of Medicine, National Academies

Life Stage Group	Arsenic^b (mg/d)	Boron (mg/d)	Calcium (g/d)	Chromium	Copper (µg/d)	Fluoride (mg/d)	Iodine (µg/d)	Iron (mg/d)	Magnesium (mg/d)^c	Manganese (mg/d)	Molybdenum (µg/d)	Nickel (mg/d)	Phosphorus (g/d)	Potassium	Selenium (µg/d)	Silicon^d	Sulfate	Vanadium (mg/d)^e	Zinc (mg/d)	Sodium (g/d)	Chloride (g/d)
Infants																					
0–6 mo	ND^f	ND	ND	ND	ND	0.7	ND	40	ND	ND	ND	ND	ND	ND	45	ND	ND	ND	4	ND	ND
7–12 mo	ND	ND	ND	ND	ND	0.9	ND	40	ND	ND	ND	ND	ND	ND	60	ND	ND	ND	5	ND	ND
Children																					
1–3 y	ND	3	2.5	ND	1,000	1.3	200	40	65	2	300	0.2	3	ND	90	ND	ND	ND	7	1.5	2.3
4–8 y	ND	6	2.5	ND	3,000	2.2	300	40	110	3	600	0.3	3	ND	150	ND	ND	ND	12	1.9	2.9
Males,																					
Females																					
9–13 y	ND	11	2.5	ND	5,000	10	600	40	350	6	1,100	0.6	4	ND	280	ND	ND	ND	23	2.2	3.4
14–18 y	ND	17	2.5	ND	8,000	10	900	45	350	9	1,700	1.0	4	ND	400	ND	ND	ND	34	2.3	3.6
19–70 y	ND	20	2.5	ND	10,000	10	1,100	45	350	11	2,000	1.0	4	ND	400	ND	ND	1.8	40	2.3	3.6
>70 y	ND	20	2.5	ND	10,000	10	1,100	45	350	11	2,000	1.0	3	ND	400	ND	ND	1.8	40	2.3	3.6
Pregnancy																					
14–18 y	ND	17	2.5	ND	8,000	10	900	45	350	9	1,700	1.0	3.5	ND	400	ND	ND	ND	34	2.3	3.6
19–50 y	ND	20	2.5	ND	10,000	10	1,100	45	350	11	2,000	1.0	3.5	ND	400	ND	ND	ND	40	2.3	3.6
Lactation																					
14–18 y	ND	17	2.5	ND	8,000	10	900	45	350	9	1,700	1.0	4	ND	400	ND	ND	ND	34	2.3	3.6
19–50 y	ND	20	2.5	ND	10,000	10	1,100	45	350	11	2,000	1.0	4	ND	400	ND	ND	ND	40	2.3	3.6

^{a} UL = The maximum level of daily nutrient intake that is likely to pose no risk of adverse effects. Unless otherwise specified, the UL represents total intake from food, water, and supplements. Due to lack of suitable data, ULs could not be established for arsenic, chromium, silicon, potassium, and sulfate. In the absence of ULs, extra caution may be warranted in consuming levels above recommended intakes.

^{b} Although the UL was not determined for arsenic, there is no justification for adding arsenic to food or supplements.

^{c} The ULs for magnesium represent intake from a pharmacological agent only and do not include intake from food and water.

^{d} Although silicon has not been shown to cause adverse effects in humans, there is no justification for adding silicon to supplements.

^{e} Although vanadium in food has not been shown to cause adverse effects in humans, there is no justification for adding vanadium to food and vanadium supplements should be used with caution. The UL is based on adverse effects in laboratory animals and this data could be used to set a UL for adults but not children and adolescents.

^{f} ND = Not determinable due to lack of data of adverse effects in this age group and concern with regard to lack of ability to handle excess amounts. Source of intake should be from food only to prevent high levels of intake.

SOURCES: *Dietary Reference Intakes for Calcium, Phosphorous, Magnesium, Vitamin D, and Fluoride* (1997); *Dietary Reference Intakes for Thiamin, Riboflavin, Niacin, Vitamin B$_6$, Folate, Vitamin B$_{12}$, Pantothenic Acid, Biotin, and Choline* (1998); *Dietary Reference Intakes for Vitamin C, Vitamin E, Selenium, and Carotenoids* (2000); *Dietary Reference Intakes for Vitamin A, Vitamin K, Arsenic, Boron, Chromium, Copper, Iodine, Iron, Manganese, Molybdenum, Nickel, Silicon, Vanadium, and Zinc* (2001); and *Dietary Reference Intakes for Water, Potassium, Sodium, Chloride, and Sulfate* (2004). These reports may be accessed via http://www.nap.edu.

Source for pages 638–643: Reprinted with permission from Dietary Reference Intakes for Energy, Carbohydrate, Fat, Fatty Acids, Cholesterol, Protein, and Amino Acids (Macronutrients) © 2005 by the National Academy of Sciences, courtesy of the National Academies Press, Washington, D.C.

Growth Charts: Body Mass Index for Children and Teens

Body mass index (BMI) charts for adults are *not* meant for children and teens. For that reason, separate charts, using BMIs *and* percentiles, were developed by the Centers for Disease Control and Prevention for girls and boys ages two to twenty, to track their growth based on BMI (see page 645).

BMI/growth charts *are not* meant to diagnose a child's or a teen's weight status but may suggest whether a child or a teen is at risk for being overweight or underweight. A child or a teen whose BMI is at the 5 percent or less percentile *may* be underweight; at the 85 to 95 percent percentile *may* be at risk of overweight; or at the 95 percent or more percentile *may* be overweight. Healthcare professionals use these charts to track a child's or a teen's growth over time; your healthcare professional should determine if your child has a weight problem and what action to take, if any.

Body Mass Index for Adults

The table below allows you to determine your body mass index without having to perform calculations. Locate your height in the left-hand column. Scanning across that row, find the number closest to your weight. At the top of that column is your BMI. If your height or weight isn't listed in the table, here's a shortcut method for calculating BMI: multiply your weight (in pounds) by 703 and then divide this number by your height (in inches) squared (i.e., height × height). *For more information on what your BMI number means, refer to chapter 2.*

Body Mass Index

Height	19	20	21	22	23	24	25	26	27	28	29	30	35	40
4'10"	91	96	100	105	110	115	119	124	129	134	138	143	167	191
4'11"	94	99	104	109	114	119	124	128	133	138	143	148	173	198
5'0"	97	102	107	112	118	123	128	133	138	143	148	153	179	204
5'1"	100	106	111	116	122	127	132	137	143	148	153	158	185	211
5'2"	104	109	115	120	126	131	136	142	147	153	158	164	191	218
5'3"	107	113	118	124	130	135	141	146	152	158	163	169	197	225
5'4"	110	116	122	128	134	140	145	151	157	163	169	174	204	232
5'5"	114	120	126	132	138	144	150	156	162	168	174	180	210	240
5'6"	118	124	130	136	142	148	155	161	167	173	179	186	216	247
5'7"	121	127	134	140	146	153	159	166	172	178	185	191	223	255
5'8"	125	131	138	144	151	158	164	171	177	184	190	197	230	262
5'9"	128	135	142	149	155	162	169	176	182	189	196	203	236	270
5'10"	132	139	146	153	160	167	174	181	188	195	202	207	243	278
5'11"	136	143	150	157	165	172	179	186	193	200	208	215	250	286
6'0"	140	147	154	162	169	177	184	191	199	206	213	221	258	294
6'1"	144	151	159	166	174	182	189	197	204	212	219	227	265	302
6'2"	148	155	163	171	179	186	194	202	210	218	225	233	272	311
6'3"	152	160	168	176	184	192	200	208	216	224	232	240	279	319
6'4"	156	164	172	180	189	197	205	213	221	230	238	246	287	328

Weight (lbs)

OVERWEIGHT — OBESE

Source: World Health Organization.

Body mass index-for-age percentiles:
Girls, 2 to 20 years

Age (years)

Body mass index-for-age percentiles:
Boys, 2 to 20 years

Age (years)

Source: Centers for Disease Control and Prevention, National Center for Health Statistics, CDC Growth Charts: United States.
http://www.cdc.gov/nchs/about/major/nhanes/growthcharts/charts.htm. May 30, 2000.

Carbohydrates in Common Foods

"CARBO" FOODS

	SERVING	ENERGY (CALORIES)	TOTAL CARBOHYDRATES (GRAMS)*
BREAD, CEREAL, RICE, AND PASTA These foods provide a higher percentage of complex carbohydrates.			
Bagel (3½" diameter)	½	90	20
Biscuit (2½" diameter)	1	130	15
Blueberry muffin (small)	1	185	30
Bread (white, whole wheat)	1 slice	65	15
Bread sticks	2 sticks	85	15
Bun (hot dog, hamburger)	½	60	10
Cereal	1 oz. (1 cup)	110	25
Cereal (cooked Cream of Wheat)	½ cup	75	15
Corn bread (2" square)	1 piece	190	30
English muffin	½	65	15
Graham crackers	2 squares	60	10
Noodles (spaghetti)	½ cup cooked	110	20
Oatmeal (cooked)	½ cup	75	15
Oatmeal (flav. instant)	1 packet	140	30
Pancakes (4" across)	1	75	15
Popcorn (plain)	1 cup popped	30	5
Pretzels	1 oz.	110	25
Rice (brown)	½ cup cooked	110	25
Rice (white)	½ cup cooked	120	25
Saltines	5 crackers	65	10
Tortilla (flour) (6" diameter)	1	95	15
Waffles (3½" across) (4" diameter)	1	105	15
OTHER BAKED GOODS These foods provide both complex and simple carbohydrates.			
Angel food cake	1 piece	140	30
Animal crackers	5	55	10
Chocolate cake, frosted	1 piece	235	35
Fig bar	1	55	10
Granola bar, hard	1	120	15
Oatmeal raisin cookie	1	65	10
COMBINATION FOODS These foods provide a higher percentage of complex carbohydrates.			
Bean burrito	1	225	35
Pizza (cheese)	1 slice	290	35

For the carbohydrate content of specific foods, check the Nutrition Facts panel on food labels.

*Includes starches (complex carbohydrates), sugars, and fiber.

"CARBO" FOODS *(continued)*

	SERVING	ENERGY (CALORIES)	TOTAL CARBOHYDRATES (GRAMS)*
FRUITS			
These foods provide a higher percentage of simple carbohydrates.			
Apple	1 medium	70	20
Apple juice	¾ cup	85	20
Applesauce	½ cup	95	25
Banana	1 medium	105	25
Cantaloupe	½ cup	30	5
Cherries (raw)	10	45	10
Dates (dried)	5	115	30
Fruit cocktail (packed in own juice)	½ cup	55	15
Grape juice	¾ cup	115	30
Grapes	½ cup	55	15
Orange	1 medium	60	15
Orange juice	¾ cup	80	20
Pear	1 medium	95	20
Pineapple	½ cup	35	10
Dried plums (prunes)	5	100	25
Raisins (seedless)	¼ cup	125	35
Raspberries	½ cup	30	5
Strawberries	½ cup	25	5
Watermelon	½ cup	25	5
VEGETABLES			
These foods provide a higher percentage of complex carbohydrates.			
Carrot	1 med.	25	5
Corn	½ cup	90	20
Lima beans	½ cup cooked	110	20
Peas (green)	½ cup	65	15
Potato (baked, plain)	1 medium	160	35
Sweet potato	1 medium	105	25
MILK, YOGURT, AND CHEESE			
These foods provide a higher percentage of simple carbohydrates.			
Frozen yogurt (low-fat)	½ cup	110	20
Fruit flavored yogurt	1 cup	240	45
Milk (1%)	1 cup	100	10
Milk (fat-free)	1 cup	85	10
Pudding	½ cup	155	25

*Includes starches (complex carbohydrates), sugars, and fiber

Source: U.S. Department of Agriculture, Agricultural Research Service, 2005. *USDA National Nutrient Database for Standard Reference,* Release 18.

% Daily Values: What Are They Based On?

The % Daily Values (% DV) on food and supplement labels are considered average nutrient levels, not necessarily your specific nutrient needs. You may need more or less.

For daily nutrient recommendations specific to your age and gender, see the Dietary Reference Intakes (DRIs)—*shown elsewhere in the Appendices and explained in chapter 1.*

The following values are for adults and children ages four and older. Protein levels are different for infants under a year (14 grams); children one to four years (16 grams); pregnant women (60 grams); and nursing mothers (65 grams).

NUTRIENT/FOOD COMPONENT	100% DV IS EQUAL TO THIS AMOUNT
Total fat	65 g*
Saturated fat	20 g*
Cholesterol	300 mg
Sodium	2,400 mg
Potassium	3,500 mg
Total carbohydrate	300 g*
Dietary fiber	25 g†
Protein	50 g*
Vitamin A	5,000 IU
Vitamin C	60 mg
Calcium	1,000 mg
Iron	18 mg
Thiamin	1.5 mg
Riboflavin	1.7 mg
Niacin	20 mg
Vitamin D	400 IU
Vitamin E	30 IU
Vitamin B_6	2 mg
Folate	400 mcg
Vitamin B_{12}	6 mcg
Biotin	300 mcg
Pantothenic acid	10 mg
Phosphorus	1,000 mg
Iodine	150 mcg
Magnesium	400 mg
Zinc	15 mg
Copper	2 mg

*Based on a 2,000-calorie reference diet.
†Based on 11.5 grams per 1,100 calories.

Health Claims on Food Labels

WHAT DO HEALTH CLAIMS ON FOOD LABELS TELL YOU?

HEALTH CLAIMS ON FOOD LABELS	HOW IT MIGHT APPEAR ON THE LABEL
Calcium and osteoporosis	Regular exercise and a healthy diet with enough calcium help teens and young adult white and Asian women maintain good bone health and may reduce their high risk of osteoporosis later in life.
Sodium and hypertension	Diets low in sodium may reduce the risk of high blood pressure, a disease associated with many factors.
Dietary fat and cancer	Development of cancer depends on many factors. A diet low in total fat may reduce the risk of some cancers.
Saturated fat and cholesterol and the risk of coronary heart disease	While many factors affect heart disease, diets low in saturated fat and cholesterol may reduce the risk of this disease.
Fiber-containing grain products, fruits, and vegetables, and cancer	Low-fat diets rich in fiber-containing grain products, fruits, and vegetables may reduce the risk of some types of cancer, a disease associated with many factors.
Fruits, vegetables, and grain products that contain fiber, particularly soluble fiber, and their risk of coronary heart disease	Diets low in saturated fat and cholesterol and rich in fruits, vegetables, and grain products that contain some types of dietary fiber, particularly soluble fiber, may reduce the risk of heart disease, a disease associated with many factors.

WHAT DO HEALTH CLAIMS ON FOOD LABELS TELL YOU? *(continued)*

HEALTH CLAIMS ON FOOD LABELS	HOW IT MIGHT APPEAR ON THE LABEL
Fruits and vegetables and cancer	Low-fat diets rich in fruits and vegetables (foods that are low in fat and may contain dietary fiber, vitamin A, or vitamin C) may reduce the risk of some types of cancer, a disease associated with many factors. Broccoli is high in vitamins A and C, and it is a good source of dietary fiber.
Folate and neural tube defects	Healthful diets with adequate folate may reduce a woman's risk of having a child with a brain or spinal cord defect.
Sugar alcohol and dental caries	*Full claim:* Frequent between-meal consumption of foods high in sugars and starches promotes tooth decay. The sugar alcohols in [name of food] do not promote tooth decay. *Shortened claim* (on small packages): Does not promote tooth decay.
Soluble fiber from certain foods and the risk of coronary heart disease	Soluble fiber from foods such as [name of soluble fiber source], as part of a diet low in saturated fat and cholesterol, may reduce the risk of heart disease. A serving of [food name] supplies _____ grams of the [necessary daily dietary intake for the benefit] soluble fiber from [name of soluble-fiber source] necessary per day to have this effect.
Soy protein and risk of coronary heart disease	25 grams of soy protein a day, as part of a diet low in saturated fat and cholesterol, may reduce the risk of heart disease. A serving of [food name] supplies _____ grams of soy protein.
Plant sterol/stanol esters and risk of coronary heart disease (interim health claim)	1. Foods containing at least 0.65 gram per serving of vegetable oil sterol esters, eaten twice a day with meals for a daily total intake of at least 1.3 grams as part of a diet low in saturated fat and cholesterol, may reduce the risk of heart disease. A serving of [food name] supplies ___ grams of vegetable oil sterol esters. 2. Foods containing at least 1.7 gram per serving of vegetable oil stanol esters, eaten twice a day with meals for a daily total intake of at least 3.4 grams as part of a diet low in saturated fat and cholesterol, may reduce the risk of heart disease. A serving of [food name] supplies _____ grams of plant stanol esters.
Whole-grain foods and risk of heart disease and certain cancers	*Required wording:* Diets rich in whole grain foods and other plant foods and low in total fat, saturated fat, and cholesterol may reduce the risk of heart disease and some cancers.
Potassium and the risk of high blood pressure and stroke	*Required wording:* Diets containing foods that are a good source of potassium and that are low in sodium may reduce the risk of high blood pressure and stroke.

For definitions of terms such as "low," "rich," and "high," see "Label Lingo" in chapters 2, 3, 4, 5, 6, 7, and 11.

Sources: *Code of Federal Regulations,* Title 21, Parts 101.72-101.83 (Washington, D.C.: U.S. Food and Drug Administration, April 2001); *A Food Labeling Guide.* (Washington, D.C.: U.S. Food and Drug Administration, November 2000).

For a list of FDA-approved qualified health claims: www.cfsan.fda.gov/~dms/ahc-sum.html

MyPyramid

FOOD INTAKE PATTERNS *(continued)*

[5]**Meat & Beans Group** in general, 1 ounce of lean meat, poultry, or fish, 1 egg, 1 Tbsp. peanut butter, ¼ cup cooked dry beans, or ½ ounce of nuts or seeds can be considered as 1 ounce equivalent from the meat and beans group.

[6]**Milk Group** includes all fluid milk products and foods made from milk that retain their calcium content, such as yogurt and cheese. Foods made from milk that have little to no calcium, such as cream cheese, cream, and butter, are not part of the group. Most milk group choices should be fat-free or low-fat. In general, 1 cup of milk or yogurt, 1½ ounces of natural cheese, or 2 ounces of processed cheese can be considered as 1 cup from the milk group.

[7]**Oils** include fats from many different plants and from fish that are liquid at room temperature, such as canola, corn, olive, soybean, and sunflower oil. Some foods are naturally high in oils, like nuts, olives, some fish, and avocados. Foods that are mainly oil include mayonnaise, certain salad dressings, and soft margarine.

[8]**Discretionary Calorie Allowance** is the remaining amount of calories in a food intake pattern after accounting for the calories needed for all food groups—using forms of foods that are fat-free or low-fat and with no added sugars.

ESTIMATED DAILY CALORIE NEEDS

To determine which food intake pattern to use for an individual, the following chart gives an estimate of individual calorie needs. The calorie range for each age/sex group is based on physical activity level, from sedentary to active.

	Calorie Range	
CHILDREN	**SEDENTARY**	**ACTIVE**
2–3 years	1,000 →	1,400
FEMALES		
4–8 years	1,200 →	1,800
9–13	1,600 →	2,200
14–18	1,800 →	2,400
19–30	2,000 →	2,200
31–50	1,800 →	2,200
51+	1,600 →	2,200
MALES		
4–8 years	1,400 →	2,000
9–13	1,800 →	2,600
14–18	2,200 →	3,200
19–30	2,400 →	3,000
31–50	2,200 →	3,000
51+	2,000 →	2,800

Sedentary means a lifestyle that includes only the light physical activity associated with typical day-to-day life.

Active means a lifestyle that includes physical activity equivalent to walking more than 3 miles per day at 3 to 4 miles per hour, in addition to the light physical activity associated with typical day-to-day life.

MyPyramid Food Intake Pattern Calorie Levels

MyPyramid assigns Individuals to a calorie level based on their sex, age, and activity level.
The chart below identifies the calorie levels for males and females by age and activity level. Calorie levels are provided for each year of childhood, from 2-18 years, and for adults in 5-year increments.

MALES				FEMALES			
ACTIVITY LEVEL AGE	Sedentary*	Mod. active*	Active*	ACTIVITY LEVEL AGE	Sedentary*	Mod. active*	Active*
2	1000	1000	1000	2	1000	1000	1000
3	1000	1400	1400	3	1000	1200	1400
4	1200	1400	1600	4	1200	1400	1400
5	1200	1400	1600	5	1200	1400	1600
6	1400	1600	1800	6	1200	1400	1600
7	1400	1600	1800	7	1200	1600	1800
8	1400	1600	2000	8	1400	1600	1800
9	1600	1800	2000	9	1400	1600	1800
10	1600	1800	2200	10	1400	1800	2000
11	1800	2000	2200	11	1600	1800	2000
12	1800	2200	2400	12	1600	2000	2200
13	2000	2200	2600	13	1600	2000	2200
14	2000	2400	2800	14	1800	2000	2400
15	2200	2600	3000	15	1800	2000	2400
16	2400	2800	3200	16	1800	2000	2400
17	2400	2800	3200	17	1800	2000	2400
18	2400	2800	3200	18	1800	2000	2400
19-20	2600	2800	3000	19-20	2000	2200	2400
21-25	2400	2800	3000	21-25	2000	2200	2400
26-30	2400	2600	3000	26-30	1800	2000	2400
31-35	2400	2600	3000	31-35	1800	2000	2200
36-40	2400	2600	2800	36-40	1800	2000	2200
41-45	2200	2600	2800	41-45	1800	2000	2200
46-50	2200	2400	2800	46-50	1800	2000	2200
51-55	2200	2400	2800	51-55	1600	1800	2200
56-60	2200	2400	2600	56-60	1600	1800	2200
61-65	2000	2400	2600	61-65	1600	1800	2000
66-70	2000	2200	2600	66-70	1600	1800	2000
71-75	2000	2200	2600	71-75	1600	1800	2000
76 and up	2000	2200	2400	76 and up	1600	1800	2000

*Calorie levels are based on the Estimated Energy Requirements (EER) and activity levels from the Institute of Medicine Dietary Reference Intakes Macronutrients Report, 2002.
SEDENTARY = less than 30 minutes a day of moderate physical activity in addition to daily activities.
MOD. ACTIVE = at least 30 minutes up to 60 minutes a day of moderate physical activity in addition to daily activities.
ACTIVE = 60 or more minutes a day of moderate physical activity in addition to daily activities.

How Many Discretionary Calories Can You Have?

The discretionary calories allowance is based on estimated calorie needs by age/sex group. Physical activity increases calorie needs, so those who are more physically active need more total calories and have a larger discretionary calorie allowance. The discretionary calorie allowance is part of total estimated calorie needs, not in addition to total calorie needs. The chart gives a general guide.

Age and Gender	Not Physically Active*		Physically Active**	
	Estimated total calorie need	Estimated discretionary calorie allowance	Estimated total calorie need	Estimated discretionary calorie allowance
Children 2–3 years	1000	165***	1000 to 1400	165 to 170
Children 4–8 years	1200 to 1400	170***	1400 to 1800	170 to 195
Females 9–13 years	1600	130	1600 to 2200	130 to 290
Males 9–13 years	1800	195	1800 to 2600	195 to 410
Females 14–18 years	1800	195	2000 to 2400	265 to 360
Males 14–18 years	2200	290	2400 to 3200	360 ro 650
Females 16–30 years	2000	265	2000 to 2400	265 to 360
Males 16–30 years	2400	360	2600 to 3000	410 to 510
Females 31–50 years	1800	195	2000 to 2200	265 to 290
Males 31–50 years	2200	290	2400 to 3000	360 to 510
Females 51+ years	1600	130	1800 to 2200	195 to 290
Males 51+ years	2000	265	2200 to 2800	290 to 425

*These amounts are appropriate for individuals who get less than 30 minutes of moderate physical activity most days. Click here for more information about physical activity.

**These amounts are appropriate for individuals who get at least 30 minutes (lower calorie level) to at least 60 minutes (higher calorie level) of moderate physical activity most days. Click here for more information about physical activity.

***The number of discretionary calories is higher for children 8 and younger than it is for older children or adults consuming the same number of calories, because younger children's nutrient needs are lower. Therefore, less food from the basic food groups and fewer "essential calories" are needed.

Source: www.MyPyramid.com.

Produce "Package"

Vegetables and fruits, each with a somewhat different combination of "good for you" components, are chock full of nutrients and phytonutrients. Here is a brief look at vegetables and fruits that are good* sources of several key nutrients and dietary fiber.

	Carotenoids (Vitamin A)	Vitamin C	Folate	Potassium	Dietary Fiber
Vegetables					
Artichoke (1 medium)		X	X	X	X
Asparagus (½ cup)	X	X	X		
Beans, kidney (½ cup)	X		X	X	X
Beans, lima (½ cup)			X	X	X
Beets (½ cup)			X		
Black-eyed peas (½ cup)			X		X
Bok choy (½ cup)	X	X			
Broccoli (½ cup)	X	X	X		X
Brussels sprouts (½ cup)	X	X	X		X
Cabbage (½ cup)		X			
Carrots (½ cup)	X				X
Cauliflower (½ cup)		X			
Celery (½ cup)					
Chickpeas (garbanzos) (½ cup)			X		X
Collards (½ cup)	X	X	X		X
Corn (½ cup)					X
Cucumbers (½ cup)					
Eggplant (½ cup)					
Green beans (½ cup)		X			X
Green pepper (½ cup)		X			
Kale (½ cup)	X	X			
Lentils (½ cup)			X	X	X
Lettuce, iceberg (1 cup)					
loose-leaf (l cup)	X	X			
Mushrooms, raw (½ cup)					
Okra (½ cup)		X			X
Onion (½ cup)					
Parsnips (½ cup)		X	X		X
Peas, green (½ cup)	X	X	X		X
Peas, split (½ cup)			X	X	X
Pepper, red (½ cup)	X	X			
Potato without peel (1 medium)		X		X	X
Potato, with peel (1 medium)		X	X	X	X
Radishes (½ cup)		X			
Spinach, cooked (½ cup)	X	X	X	X	X

Produce "Package" (continued)

	Carotenoids (Vitamin A)	Vitamin C	Folate	Potassium	Dietary Fiber
Vegetables (continued)					
Squash, winter (½ cup)	X	X		X	X
Sweet potato (1 medium)	X	X		X	X
Tomato (1 medium)	X	X			
Turnip greens (½ cup)	X	X	X		X
Turnips (½ cup)		X			
Zucchini (½ cup)		X			
Fruits					
Apple, with skin (1 medium)		X			X
Apricot, dried (¼ cup)	X			X	X
Avocado (½ cup)		X	X	X	X
Banana (1 medium)		X		X	X
Blueberries (½ cup)		X			
Cantaloupe (½ cup)	X	X			
Figs (2 medium)					X
Grapes (½ cup)		X			
Grapefruit (½)		X			X
Grapefruit juice (¾ cup)		X			
Honeydew melon (½ cup)		X			
Kiwifruit (1 medium)		X			X
Mango (1 medium)	X	X			X
Orange (1)		X	X		X
Orange juice (¾ cup)		X		X	
Papaya (½ cup)		X			
Peach (1 medium)		X			
Pear with skin (1 medium)		X			X
Pineapple (½ cup)		X			
Plantain, cooked (½ cup)	X	X		X	
Plum (1 medium)		X			
Prunes (dried plums) (5)					X
Prune juice (¾ cup)		X		X	
Raisins (¼ cup)					
Raspberries		X			X
Strawberries (½ cup)		X			
Tangerine (1 medium)	X	X			
Watermelon (½ cup)		X			

Note: A good source of a vitamin or mineral contributes at least 10 percent of its Daily Value (DV) in a standard label serving. A source of dietary fiber contributes at least 2 grams of dietary fiber in a standardized serving.

Functional Food: What Does Research Say?

STRENGTH OF EVIDENCE FOR FUNCTIONAL FOODS CURRENTLY ON THE US MARKET [a,b]

FUNCTIONAL FOOD	BIOACTIVE COMPONENT	HEALTH BENEFIT	TYPE OF EVIDENCE	STRENGTH OF EVIDENCE	RECOMMENDED AMOUNT OR FREQUENCY OF INTAKE	REGULATORY STATUS
Fortified margarines	Plant sterol and stanol esters	Reduce total and LDL[c] cholesterol (43)	Clinical trials	Very strong	1.3 g/d for sterols 1.7 g/d for stanols	Health claim
Psyllium	Soluble fiber	Reduce total and LDL cholesterol (38)	Clinical trials	Very strong	1 g/d	Health claim
Soy	Protein	Reduce total and LDL cholesterol (22,42)	Clinical trials	Very strong	25 g/d	Health claim
Whole oat products	beta-glucan	Reduce total and LDL cholesterol (38)	Clinical trials	Very strong	3 g/d	Health claim
Cranberry juice	Proanthocyanidins	Reduce urinary tract infections (64,65)	Small number of clinical trials	Moderate	300 mL/d	Conventional food
Fatty fish	n-3 fatty acids	Reduce TG,[d] reduce heart disease cardiac deaths and fatal and nonfatal myocardial infarction (47,48,50,51)	Clinical trials; epidemiologic studies	Strong to very strong	Two fatty fish meals per week; 0.5–1.8 g EPA[e] + DHA[f]	Qualified health claim for dietary supplement
Eggs with omega-3 fatty acids	n-3 fatty acids	Reduce cholesterol (55,56)	Clinical trials	Weak to moderate	Unknown	Conventional food
Garlic	Organosulfur compounds	Reduce total and LDL cholesterol (49)	Clinical trials	Weak to moderate	600-900 mg/d (dietary supplement) or approximately 1 fresh clove/d	Conventional food and dietary supplement
Jerusalem artichoke, onion powder, ripe banana	Prebiotics/ fructooligo- saccharides	Blood pressure control; serum cholesterol reduction (59,60)	Animal studies; clinical trials	Weak	3–10 g/d	Conventional food
Green tea	Catechins	Reduce risk of certain types of cancer (57)	Epidemiologic randomized crossover study design	Moderate	4–6 cups/d	Conventional food
Black tea	Polyphenols	Reduced risk of coronary heart disease (58)				
Spinach, kale, collard greens	Lutein/zeaxanthin	Reduce risk of age-related macular degeneration (67)	Epidemiologic	Weak to moderate	6 mg/d as lutein	Conventional food, dietary supplement
Tomatoes and processed tomato products	Lycopene	Reduce prostate cancer risk (52-54)	Epidemiologic	Moderate	½ cup/d (30 mg or 10 servings/week)	Conventional food
Lamb, turkey, beef, dairy	CLA[g]	Reduce breast cancer (62,63)	In vivo and in vitro studies	Weak	Unknown	Conventional food
Cruciferous vegetables	Glucosinolates, indoles	Reduce risk of certain types of cancer (39,40,66)	Epidemiologic and in vitro	Weak to moderate	>½ cup/d	Conventional food
Fermented dairy products	Probiotics	Support GI[h] health (61)	In vivo, in vitro, and clinical data	Moderate	1 to 2 billion colony-forming units per day	Conventional food, dietary supplement
Tree nuts	Monounsaturated fatty acids, vitamin E	Reduced risk of coronary heart disease (45,46)	Clinical trial	Moderate	1–2 oz/d of nuts	Qualified health claim
Grape juice or red wine	Resveratrol	Platelet aggregation reduction (83-85)	Epidemiologic, in vivo and in vitro	Moderate to strong	8–16 oz/d	Conventional food

[a]Foods that have a Food and Drug Administration-approved health claim (sterol/stanol esters, oats, psyllium, soy) generally are supported by two dozen or more well-designed published clinical trials. For example, the soy health claim petition contained more than 40 clinical trials, whereas there are only a few clinical trials on cranberry juice and urinary tract infections.
[b]Reprinted with permission and adapted from the American Council on Science and Health: From: Hasler CM. *J Nutr.* 2002;132:3772-3781. From "Functional Food—Position of the ADA," *Journal of the American Dietetic Association*, 2004, 104:814–826.
[c]LDL=low-density lipoprotein.
[d]TG=triglyceride.
[e]EPA=eicosapentaenoic acid.
[f]DHA=docosahexaenoic acid.
[g]CLA=conjugated linoleic acid.
[h]GI=gastrointestinal.

Functions of Selected Additives

A CLOSE-UP LOOK AT ADDITIVES

Additive	Improves or Maintains Nutritional Value	Prevents Spoilage	Prevents Rancidity and Discoloration	Distributes Particles Evenly	Prevents Lumping	Retains Moisture	Makes Food Rise	Controls pH	Gives Smooth, Thick, or Uniform Texture	Improves Baking Quality	Gives Color	Gives or Enhances Flavor	Sweetens
Acetic acid								X					
Acidulants or acidifiers			X					X				X	
Agar									X				
Alginate									X				
Annatto											X		
Aspartame													X
Baking powder (sodium bicarbonate and acid salts)							X						
Baking soda (sodium bicarbonate)							X						
BHA/BHT			X										
B vitamins	X												
Caffeine												X	
Calcium	X												
Calcium bromate	X									X			
Calcium proprionate	X	X											
Calcium silicate	X				X								
Calcium sulfate	X								X				
Caramel color											X		
Carob gum				X					X				
Carotene	X										X		
Carrageenan				X					X				
Cellulose						X			X				
Citric acid			X					X				X	
Corn syrup												X	X
Dextrin						X			X				
Disodium gyanylate or inosinate												X	
EDTA			X										
Gelatin									X				
Glycerine						X							
Glycerol monostearate						X							
Guar gum									X				
Herbs												X	
Hydrolyzed vegetable protein												X	
Iodine	X												

657

A Close-Up Look at Additives *(continued)*

	Improves or Maintains Nutritional Value	Prevents Spoilage	Prevents Rancidity and Discoloration	Distributes Particles Evenly	Prevents Lumping	Retains Moisture	Makes Food Rise	Controls pH	Gives Smooth, Thick, or Uniform Texture	Improves Baking Quality	Gives Color	Gives or Enhances Flavor	Sweetens
Iron	X												
Iron ammonium					X								
Lactic acid		X						X					
Lecithin			X	X									
Modified food starch				X	X				X				
Mono- and diglycerides				X									
Monosodium glutamate (MSG)												X	
Paprika											X		
Pectin				X					X				
Phosphoric acid								X					
Polysorbate				X									
Potassium sorbate		X											
Proprionic acid		X											
Propyl gallate			X										
Saffron											X	X	
Salt												X	
Silicon dioxide					X								
Sodium benzoate		X											
Sodium citrate				X									
Sodium nitrate/nitrite		X											
Sorbitan monostearate				X									
Sorbitol						X							X
Spices												X	
Sugar		X										X	X
Turmeric											X	X	
Vanilla												X	
Vitamin A	X												
Vitamin C	X		X										
Vitamin D	X												
Vitamin E (tocopherols)	X		X										
Xanthan gum									X				
Yeast							X						

Index

kale, 190
kamut, 193
kava, 599, 600
kelp, 190–191
ketoacidosis, 568
ketosis, 48
kidneys, 152, 578. *See also* sodium
kitchen safety, 280–306
  for children, 424–426
  cleanliness, 288–290
  ecological conservation and, 306
  foodborne illness and, 280–288
  food preparation and service, 295–305
  food storage and, 290–295
  injury prevention, 305
  for people with special needs, 477–478
  See also food preparation; safety
kitchen scales, 332
kitchen scissors, 332
kohlrabi, 190
kosher foods, 252, 539
kosher salt, 150
kumquat, 191

labels. *See* food labels
lactase, 461, 525
lactation consultants, 379. *See also* breast-feeding
lactitol, 110, 126, 129
lactobacilli, 111, 603
lacto-ovo-vegetarian diet, 505. *See also* vegetarian diet
lactose, 112, 113, 122
lactose intolerance, 104, 113, 266, 408, 524–526
lacto-vegetarian diet. *See* vegetarian diet
laetrile, 564
La Leche League, 379
lard, 57
L-arginine, 507
latching on, in breast-feeding, 377
latte, 167–169
lauric acid, 65
LDL ("bad") blood cholesterol (low-density lipoproteins), 55, 58, 64, 136, 173, 545, 546
lead, 164–165, 291, 449
learning, breakfast and, 235–236
leavening agents, 198, 199
lecithin, 585, 605
leeks, 190
leftover foods, 292, 293, 303
legumes, 222
  adding to recipes, 329
  fiber in, 143–144
  vegetarian diet, 516–518
  See also beans; peanuts
lentils, 329
leucine, 507
lifestyle
  aging and, 467–472
  goals for, 16–18
  meal planning and, 233

modifications to manage blood pressure, 554
  overweight risks and, 29
  vegetarian diet and, 505
lignan, 110, 134, 139, 454
lignin, 132, 133, 139
lime, 91
linoleic acid, 16, 53, 56
lipids, 55, 57. *See also* blood (serum) cholesterol
lipoproteins, 55, 550–551
liposuction, 51
liquid diets, very-low-calorie, 48–49
liquid smoke, 300
Listeria monocytogenes, 282, 284, 286, 449
"lite" salt, 150
liver, 173
lobelia, 600
longan, 191
loquat, 191
lotus root, 190
low-"cal" foods, 39, 53, 120. *See also* calories
low-"carb" diet, 42, 47, 120. *See also* carbohydrates
low-fat diet, 12, 39, 53, 70, 505. *See also* dietary fat
L-tryptophan, 601
lunch menu ideas, 234
lung cancer, 88
lutein, 109, 317, 606
lychee, 191–192
lycopene, 109, 317, 606

macrobiotic diet, 505
macronutrients, 452
mad cow disease, 285
magnesium, 93–94, 609
magnolia-stephania preparation, 600
ma huang, 599
mainnitol, 110
major minerals, 91–95, 99–107
malt beverages, 178
maltitol, 126
maltose, 112
malt syrup, 123
malt vinegar, 528
manganese, 90, 92, 98
mango, 192
mangosteen, 192
mannitol, 126, 129, 570
manufacturer information, for foods, 252
MAO (monoamine oxidase inhibitors), 601
maple syrup, 123
margarine, 28, 57–59
marinades, 297, 299, 335, 528
mature adults, 458–478
  alcohol and, 172
  biomarkers of aging, 459
  caffeine and, 169
  fiber and, 140
  fitness and, 5–6
  fluids needed by, 155

foodborne illness in, 466
health challenges of, 472–478
heart disease and, 544
lifestyle change and, 467–472
meal preparation alternatives for, 620
menu suggestions for, 464, 469
metabolism of, 43
"miracle" anti-aging products for, 463
nutrients for, 458–465
osteoporosis and, 577
physical activity for, 11, 465–467
poor nutrition signs, 469
"sandwich generation" responsibilities and, 471
sodium intake for, 148, 151
tooth loss in, 118
vegetarian diet for, 512–513
women and weight, 440
maturing agents, 198, 199
mayonnaise, 281
meal planning
  for athletes, 500
  blood cholesterol levels and, 545–547
  breakfast, 233–237
  diabetes and, 568–574
  doctor-prescribed eating plans, 584
  eating habits, 38–40, 40–41, 44, 402, 403
  feeding plan for infants, 394
  frequency of meals, 43, 402
  frozen meals, 268
  "grazing," 240
  location of meals, 44
  for mature adults, 464, 467–468
  medication interactions and, 587–589
  preparation alternatives, 620
  for preschoolers, 403, 404
  for school-age children, 415
  school meals, 416–418, 429–431
  skipping meals, 27, 572–573
  snacking, 237–240
  time for, 233
  timing of, 28
  vegetarian diet and, 513–520
  workplace and, 240–242
  See also food choices; food preparation; recipes; supermarket shopping
meal replacement products
  "complete nutrition products," 499
  effectiveness of, 49
  as snacks, 239
  very-low-calorie liquid diets, 48–49
  for weight gain, 43
meat
  biotechnology and, 209
  dry heat cooking methods, 321
  in ethnic dishes, 189
  fast food meals, 349–350
  food labels, 260
  garnishes for, 311
  hormones in, 206
  for infants, 393
  lean cuts, low-fat cooking methods, 319
  less common types, 228
  mad cow disease, 285